FOCUS ON EVIDENCE

PROCEDURE

Infusion Nurses Society

INFUSION NURSING

AN EVIDENCE-BASED APPROACH

Third Edition

Infusion Nurses Society

INFUSION NURSING

AN EVIDENCE-BASED APPROACH

Mary Alexander, MA, RN, CRNI®, CAE, FAAN
Chief Executive Officer, Infusion Nurses Society
Editor-in-Chief, Infusion Nursing: An Evidence-Based Approach
Norwood, Massachusetts

Ann Corrigan, MS, RN, CRNI®
Nurse Manager
Wellstar Kennestone Hospital
Marietta, Georgia

Lisa Gorski, MS, HHCNS-BC, CRNI®, FAAN
Clinical Nurse Specialist
Wheaton Franciscan Home Health & Hospice
Milwaukee, Wisconsin

Judy Hankins, BSN, CRNI®
Infusion Specialist/Training Coordinator (Retired)
Moses Cone Health System
IV Admixture/Pharmacy Department
Greensboro, North Carolina

Roxanne Perucca, MS, CRNI®
Director of Magnet/Nursing Excellence
Department of Nursing
University of Louisville Hospital
Louisville, Kentucky

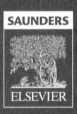

SAUNDERS

ELSEVIER

BP45

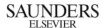

11830 Westline Industrial Drive
St. Louis, Missouri 63146

Infusion Nursing: An Evidence-Based Approach   ISBN: 978-1-4160-6410-7
Copyright © 2010, 2001, 1995 by Saunders, an imprint of Elsevier Inc.

Notice

Library of Congress Cataloging-in-Publication Data
Infusion nursing: an evidence-based approach / Mary Alexander, editor-in-chief;
  Ann Corrigan ... [et al.]. -- 3rd ed.
     p. ; cm.
  Rev. ed. of: Infusion therapy in clinical practice / Judy Hankins ... [et al.]. 2nd ed. c2001.
  Includes bibliographical references and index.
  ISBN 978-1-4160-6410-7 (alk. paper)
1. Intravenous therapy. 2. Nursing. I. Alexander, Mary, 1955- II. Corrigan, Ann, 1948- III. Infusion Nurses
  Society. IV. Infusion therapy in clinical practice.
  [DNLM: 1. Infusions, Parenteral--nursing. 2. Evidence-Based Medicine. 3. Fluid Therapy--nursing.
     4. Parenteral Nutrition--nursing.   WB 354 I425 2010]
  RM170. I515 2010
  615' .6--dc22   2009009134

ISBN: 978-1-4160-6410-7

Editor: Tamara Myers
Senior Developmental Editor: Laura M. Selkirk
Publishing Services Manager: Jeff Patterson
Project Manager: Jeanne Genz
Designer: Mark Oberkrom

Working together to grow
libraries in developing countries

www.elsevier.com | www.bookaid.org | www.sabre.org

ELSEVIER   BOOK AID International   Sabre Foundation

Printed in the United States of America

Last digit is the print number: 9 8 7 6 5 4 3 2

3/29/11

CONTRIBUTORS

Mary Alexander, MA, RN, CRNI®, CAE, FAAN
Chief Executive Officer, Infusion Nurses Society
Editor-in-Chief, *Infusion Nursing: An Evidence-Based
   Approach*
Norwood, Massachusetts
Chapter 4: Legal Issues of Infusion Nursing

Sherri Barnhill, MA, RN
Director, Education Services
Connecticut Hospital Association
Wallingford, Connecticut
Chapter 7: Clinician and Patient Safety

Jeannine M. Brant, PhD, APRN, AOCN®
Oncology Clinical Nurse Specialist/Nurse Scientist
Billings Clinic
Billings, Montana
Chapter 27: Intraspinal Access and Medication Administration

Melody Bullock-Corkhill, BSN, BS, MS, CRNI®
Interim Director, VAS Team/DICC Services
Moses Cone Health System
Greensboro, North Carolina
Chapter 24: Central Venous Access Devices: Access and Insertion

Ann Corrigan, MS, RN, CRNI®
Nurse Manager
Wellstar Kennestone Hospital
Marietta, Georgia
Chapter 1: Infusion Nursing as a Specialty
Chapter 9: Financial Considerations

Lynn Czaplewski, MS, ACNS-BC, CRNI®, AOCNS®
Clinical Nurse Specialist
Oncology Alliance
Wauwatosa, Wisconsin
Chapter 6: Clinician and Patient Education

Brenda Dugger, MSHA, RN, CRNI®, CNA-BC
Senior Vice President, Patient Care Services
St. Mary's Health Care System
Athens, Georgia
Chapter 28: Documentation

Beth Fabian, BA, RN, CRNI®
Branch Manager
Coram—Specialty Infusion Services
An Apria Healthcare Company
Lansing, Michigan
Chapter 30: Infusion Therapy in the Older Adult

Anne Marie Frey, BSN, RN, CRNI®
Clinical Nurse Level Four
Vascular Access Service
The Children's Hospital of Philadelphia
Philadelphia, Pennsylvania
Chapter 29: Infusion Therapy in Children

Lisa Gorski, MS, HHCNS-BC, CRNI®, FAAN
Clinical Nurse Specialist
Wheaton Franciscan Home Health & Hospice
Milwaukee, Wisconsin
Chapter 8: Infusion Therapy Across the Continuum
Chapter 9: Financial Considerations
*Chapter 25: Central Venous Access Devices: Care, Maintenance,
   and Potential Complications*

Lynn C. Hadaway, MEd, RN, BC, CRNI®
President
Lynn Hadaway Associates, Inc.
Milner, Georgia
Chapter 10: Anatomy and Physiology Related to Infusion Therapy
Chapter 20: Infusion Therapy Equipment

Mary E. Hagle, PhD, RN, AOCN®
Manager/Research Scientist
Center for Nursing Research and Practice, Aurora Health
   Care
Adjunct Clinical Assistant Professor, University of
   Wisconsin-Milwaukee
Milwaukee, Wisconsin
Chapter 2: Evidence-Based Practice

Judy Hankins, BSN, CRNI®
Infusion Specialist/Training Coordinator (Retired)
Moses Cone Health System
IV Admixture/Pharmacy Department
Greensboro, North Carolina
Chapter 9: Financial Considerations
Chapter 11: Fluids and Electrolytes
Chapter 15: Pharmacology

Karin Henderson, MSN, RN, CCRN, CS-GNP
Director of Nursing Services
Moses Cone Health System
Greensboro, North Carolina
Chapter 26: Alternative Infusion Access Devices

Mark R. Hunter, RN, CRNI®
Senior Manager, Clinical Development
Baxter Healthcare Corporation
Global Infusion Systems
Round Lake, Illinois
Chapter 25: Central Venous Access Devices: Care, Maintenance,
*   and Potential Complications*

Elizabeth A. Krzywda, MSN, ANP
Nurse Practitioner
Medical College of Wisconsin
Department of Surgery
Milwaukee, Wisconsin
Chapter 17: Parenteral Nutrition

Rose Anne Lonsway, BSN, MA, RN, CRNI®
Chief Executive Officer
R.A. Lonsway Consulting, LLC
Worthington, Ohio
Chapter 22: Patient Assessment as Related to Fluid &
*   Electrolyte Balance*

Mary McGoldrick, MS, RN, CRNI®
Home Care and Hospice Consultant
Home Health Systems, Inc.
St. Simons Island, Georgia
Chapter 12: Infection Prevention and Control

Doug Meyer, RPh, MBA
Assistant Director of Clinical Practice
Froedtert Hospital Pharmacy Department
Milwaukee, Wisconsin
Chapter 17: Parenteral Nutrition

Crystal Miller, BSN, MA, RN, CRNI®
IV Therapy Nurse
IV Therapy Department
St. Francis Hospital Medical Center
Hartford, Connecticut
Chapter 8: Infusion Therapy Across the Continuum
Chapter 21: Product Selection and Evaluation

Nancy Mortlock, BSN, CRNI®, OCN®
Infusion Consultant/Clinical Research Consultant
Spokane, Washington
Chapter 8: Infusion Therapy Across the Continuum

Marilyn Parker, MSN, ACHPN, ACNS, BC
Clinical Nurse Specialist, Palliative Care
Nursing Clinical Excellence
University of Kansas Hospital
Kansas City, Kansas
Chapter 26: Alternative Infusion Access Devices

Roxanne Perucca, MS, CRNI®
Director of Magnet/Nursing Excellence
Department of Nursing
University of Louisville Hospital
Louisville, Kentucky
Chapter 9: Financial Considerations
Chapter 23: Peripheral Venous Access Devices
Chapter 25: Central Venous Access Devices: Care, Maintenance,
*   and Potential Complications*

Janet Petit, MSN, NNP-BC, CNS
Neonatal Nurse Practitioner/Clinical Nurse Specialist
Doctors Medical Center
Assistant Nurse Manager, Perinatal Region
Kaiser Foundation Hospital
Modesto, California
Chapter 29: Infusion Therapy in Children

Lynn Phillips, MSN, RN, CRNI®
Professor Emeritus, Butte College
Nursing Education Consultant
Chico, California
Chapter 13: Parenteral Fluids

Kathryn Schroeter, PhD, RN, CNOR
Assistant Adjunct Professor of Bioethics
Medical College of Wisconsin
Milwaukee, Wisconsin
Chapter 5: Ethics

Lisa Schulmeister, MN, RN, APRN-BC, OCN®, FAAN
Oncology Nursing Consultant
New Orleans, Louisiana
Chapter 18: Antineoplastic Therapy

Patricia Senk, BSN, RN
Research Associate
Center for Nursing Research and Practice, Aurora Health
   Care
Doctoral Student, University of Wisconsin-Milwaukee
Milwaukee, Wisconsin
Chapter 2: Evidence-Based Practice

Grace P. Sierchio, RN, MSN, CRNI®, CPHQ
Director of Quality Assurance and Regulatory Compliance
Vital Care, Inc.
Meridian, Mississippi
Chapter 3: Quality Management

Melanie H. Simpson, PhD, RN-BC, OCN®, CHPN
Pain Management Team Coordinator
The University of Kansas Hospital
Kansas City, Kansas
Chapter 19: Pain Management

Candace K. Stearns, MN, FNP-BC, ONP-C
Hospitalist
St. Vincent Healthcare
Billings, Montana
Chapter 27: Intraspinal Access and Medication Administration

Nancy L. Trick, RN, CRNI®
Manager, Clinical Education
Teleflex Medical
Research Triangle Park, North Carolina
Chapter 14: Blood Component Therapy

Michelle S. Turner, PharmD, BCPS
Clinical Pharmacist
Department of Pharmacy
Moses H. Cone Memorial Hospital
Greensboro, North Carolina
Chapter 15: Pharmacology

Cora Vizcarra, MBA, RN, CRNI®
Infusion Nurse Consultant/CEO
MCV & Associates Healthcare, Inc.
Indianapolis, Indiana
Chapter 16: Biologic Therapy

Hugh K. Webster, Esq.
Attorney
Webster, Chamberlain & Bean
Washington, DC
Chapter 4: Legal Issues of Infusion Nursing

REVIEWERS

Patricia T. Alpert, DrPH, MSN
Assistant Professor
University of Nevada, Las Vegas
Las Vegas, Nevada

Jan Belden, MSN, FNP-C
Nurse Practitioner, Pain Management
Advanced Practice Nursing
Loma Linda University Medical Center
Loma Linda, California

Susan Dempsey, RN-BC, MN, CNS
Clinical Nurse Specialist
Pain Management
Scripps Memorial Hospital, La Jolla
La Jolla, California

Dora Hallock, RN, MSN
Oncology Clinical Nurse Specialist
UMass Memorial Health Care
Worcester, Massachusetts

Barbara Harvey, RN, BSN, MSHSA, OCN®, CRNI®
Chemotherapy/Biotherapy Instructor
Independent Contractor
Phoenix, Arizona

Joan Ralph Webber, RN, MSN, CNS, OCN®, CRNI®
Oncology Clinical Nurse Specialist
Banner Desert Medical Center
Mesa, Arizona

Nancy L. Whitehill, MSN, RN, AOCNS®, CRNI®
CNS Oncology
Outpatient Infusion Center
Mercy Hospital
Fairfield, Ohio

PREFACE

Infusion nursing is a dynamic and constantly evolving specialty practice, and infusion therapy has become ubiquitous in the patient care experience. The invasive nature of infusion therapy and its risk for developing complications require that all health care professionals who are involved in infusion therapy have access to the most up-to-date relevant information. Whether the clinician is actually performing the procedure or monitoring a patient with a venous access device, knowledge of the principles of infusion therapy is imperative for the delivery of safe patient care.

Today's health care environment demands that data and research support our clinical practice. Health care professionals must question the health care myths and traditional practices that are not based on best evidence or current research. What is needed is a better understanding for reviewing and critiquing research, coupled with the necessary tools for applying the principles to clinical practice.

To reflect the primary focus of the text, this edition has a new title, *Infusion Nursing: An Evidence-Based Approach*. Acknowledging the significance of research and its direct correlation to best practice, the content of the book is heavily referenced with the most current scientific literature. To underscore this point, most chapters feature a "Focus on Evidence" box that highlights published research and its impact on infusion therapy practice.

This authoritative text is a comprehensive reference for all health care professionals involved in the delivery of infusion therapy. Providing safe infusion care requires a vast body of knowledge; topics in this volume range from the fundamentals to advanced concepts that reflect the increased responsibility and accountability expected of health care professionals. The text begins with an overview of infusion nursing, including quality management and legal and ethical concerns. The foundations of practice require knowledge of anatomy and physiology, basic information on the effects of fluid and electrolytes, and the core principles of infection prevention and control.

To achieve desired patient outcomes, specific therapies are used to treat various patient conditions and diseases. Infusion-related treatments include the administration of parenteral fluids, blood and blood components, parenteral nutrition, pain medications, and pharmacological medications, including antineoplastic drugs and biologic agents, all of which are addressed herein.

With rapid technological advances and increasingly sophisticated equipment, the need for education continues. The section on infusion delivery systems includes details about infusion-related products and equipment as well as information that contributes to prudent product selections and evaluations. The section on infusion nursing practice begins with patient assessment, followed by information on peripheral and central venous access devices, including procedures for device placement, as well as material on care and maintenance procedures and identification and treatment of infusion-related complications. As the field has expanded, the infusion nurse's responsibilities have increased; therefore alternative choices of administration, such as continuous subcutaneous infusions, intraosseous access, and intraspinal access, are discussed.

This edition has responded to growth and change in the specialty practice of infusion therapy by adding several new chapters. "Evidence-Based Practice" sets the stage and provides a basis from which to begin incorporating research and evidence into best practice. The cost of health care is directly related to the cost of the therapies that treat specific diseases as well as the costs associated with treating preventable infusion-related complications. "Financial Considerations" discusses the concepts of revenue generation and reimbursement activities that impact infusion care. The chapter on "Patient and Clinician Safety" presents critical elements of safety as they relate to infusion care. "Biologic Therapy" sheds light on the new agents that are being developed and how they affect patient care.

Delivery of infusion therapy takes place across the continuum of health care settings, from acute care hospitals to ambulatory infusion centers, skilled nursing facilities and physicians' offices, and the home. Information on the unique approaches needed within a particular patient care setting is included in the text. In addition, providers of infusion therapy care for all patient populations with varying degrees of acuity, from the neonate to the elderly patient. These health care professionals represent varied levels of education, skill, and competence in infusion practices; besides infusion nurse specialists, there are physicians, pharmacists, nurse generalists, and nurses in other specialties, such as oncology or intensive care, who contribute to infusion therapy delivery. Information has been provided to address the special needs of their patients.

A great deal of knowledge is needed before a nurse can provide safe, competent care. Readers are encouraged to use this text to expand their knowledge and enhance their practice. In the current context of health care reform, rising patient acuity, and new technology, the infusion nursing specialty calls for resources that promote and guide the delivery of safe, cost-effective patient care while increasing the confidence and satisfaction of both the patient and the clinician. The intent of this book is to provide sound evidence that supports our clinical practice while preparing infusion nurse professionals for opportunities and challenges that may arise as health care systems adjust to shifting realities.

Mary Alexander, MA, RN, CRNI®, CAE, FAAN
Editor-in-Chief

ACKNOWLEDGMENTS

The specialty practice of infusion nursing is changing at a rapid pace. Key components that guide our practice are advanced technology, accompanied by evidence-based practice and data-driven research. Incorporating these factors into a book with a format that will benefit the reader is an enormous challenge. Only through the efforts of many dedicated individuals was this project completed.

First, I want to acknowledge the editors, Ann Corrigan, Lisa Gorski, Judy Hankins, and Roxanne Perucca, a group of highly respected infusion nurse experts, for their commitment and willingness to be part of this revision project. The countless hours they spent reviewing and revising drafts, working with authors, and also contributing chapters is greatly appreciated. Without their dedication and perseverance, our ambitious deadlines would not have been met.

Without the contributing authors who shared their knowledge, expertise, and time, there would be no textbook. I would like to express my gratitude for their participation in this considerable undertaking.

I would like to thank the Infusion Nurses Society Board of Directors for supporting the efforts of the editors on this entire project. Their recommendations and encouragement were more than welcome. I am also grateful for assistance from the INS staff throughout the revision process.

I am indebted to the Elsevier staff, whose professionalism and skill greatly improved this work. I want to thank Tamara Myers, Acquisitions Editor; Laura Selkirk, Senior Developmental Editor; Jeanne Genz, Project Manager; and Angela Perdue, Editorial Assistant, for their assistance and guidance during each phase of the revision process.

Finally, sincere appreciation is expressed by the editors to their departmental administrations, staffs, and families for their patience and support. We hope you will share our pride in the publication of this edition.

Mary Alexander, MA, RN, CRNI®, CAE, FAAN
Editor-in-Chief

CONTENTS

SECTION VI—SPECIALTY POPULATIONS

1

INFUSION NURSING AS A SPECIALTY

Ann Corrigan, MS, RN, CRNI®*

Infusion therapy is a highly specialized form of treatment that has evolved from an extreme measure used only on the most critically ill to a therapy used for 90% or more of all hospitalized patients. No longer confined to the hospital setting, infusion therapies are now delivered in alternative care sites such as the home, skilled nursing facilities, and physician offices. Infusion therapy refers to the administration of solutions, medications, nutritional products, and blood and blood components via the parenteral route.

EARLY HISTORY

The practice of using veins to inject substances essentially began in the 17th century. The first documented use of infusion therapy was administering blood as a treatment in 1492, when blood from three young boys was administered to Pope Innocent VIII (Greenwalt, 1997). It was not until 1615, however, that the concept of infusing blood from one person to another was again considered by Libavious. It would be several centuries before person-to-person transfusion became possible, and even longer before it became a safe practice.

In 1628 William Harvey's experimental work resulted in the development of the theory of circulation, which led to an understanding of blood flow and of the presence and importance of valves. This new information about the circulatory system led others to experiment with injecting substances into the vascular system to observe the effect on the recipient. One of the earliest to document this type of experiment was Sir Christopher Wren, famed architect of St. Paul's Cathedral in London. In 1656 he experimented with injecting opium and wine into the veins of dogs using a quill and animal bladder (Weinstein, 2007). The first successful injection into humans was accomplished in 1662 by J. D. Major. About

this time, Richard Lower presented a paper before the Royal Society in England on intravenous (IV) feeding and blood transfusion in dogs. He was able to demonstrate his transfusion theory with a successful animal-to-animal transfusion (Greenwalt, 1997).

The first documented animal-to-human transfusion is credited to Jean Baptiste Denis. In 1667 Denis, a physician to the French royalty, successfully transfused 9 ounces of lamb's blood into a 15-year-old boy suffering from madness (Cosnett, 1989; Greenwalt, 1997). Subsequent transfusions to the boy were not successful and resulted in the first transfusion reaction. This initial success of Denis led to the promiscuous use of transfusions, with fatal results. As a result of the many fatalities, the Church and the French parliament banned the transfusion of blood from animals to humans in 1687.

Following the 1687 edict banning blood transfusions, little growth in the field of infusion therapy was noted for the next 150 years. The one significant event in the 18th century occurred in 1795, when Philip Syng Physick, from the University of Edinburgh, noted that the use of blood transfusions in obstetric hemorrhage had some success in decreasing mortality from this complication.

19th CENTURY

Infusion therapy, as practiced today, had its real beginnings in the 19th century, which was a time of rapid advancement in medicine. In 1818 James Blundell performed the first man-to-man transfusion in London (Greenwalt, 1997). In 1834 Blundell again used human blood to transfuse women who were threatened by hemorrhage during childbirth. Blundell is further credited with the correlation between blood loss and hypoxemia during hemorrhage.

One complication of early transfusions was coagulation of the blood during the transfusion. In 1821 Jean Louis Prevost, a French physician, experimented with preventing this coagulation. Prevost and Jean B. Dumas were the first to use defibrinated blood in animal transfusions (Weinstein, 2007). By 1875

---

*The author and editors wish to acknowledge the contributions made by Nancy M. Delisio as author of this chapter in the second edition of *Infusion Nursing in Clinical Practice.*

Landois had discovered lysing between the serums of different animals, which later resulted in an understanding of antigen-antibody reactions.

The cholera epidemic of 1831 was an important event in the advancement of infusion therapy. Dr. William O'Shaughnessy, an Edinburgh physician, identified the significance of water and salt loss from the blood of cholera victims. In 1832 Dr. Thomas Latta of Leith, Scotland, is credited with taking this information and experimenting with administration of a saline solution to a patient. He described the patient as one who "apparently had reached the last moments of her earthly existence and now nothing could injure her. Indeed, so entirely was she reduced that I feared that I shall be unable to get my apparatus ready, ere she expire" (Cosnett, 1989). Latta was successful in resuscitating the patient initially, but the patient relapsed and eventually died. Dr. Latta wrote in *Lancet* of June 12, 1832, "I have no doubt the case would have issued in complete reaction, had the remedy, which had already produced such effect, been repeated" (Cosnett, 1989). The initial success of the saline injection led to further use of this therapy during the epidemic, but these efforts met with only limited success. Of the first 25 reported cases so treated, 8 recovered and there was much criticism, most often from outside the medical journals.

Further work continued and in 1853 Claude Bernard, a French physiologist, experimented with injecting sugar solutions into dogs. For the next two decades, he continued to experiment and infused not only sugar solutions but also egg whites and milk into animals, with some success.

In 1852 the importance of protein in relation to nitrogen balance, weight gain, and general well-being was observed by Bidder and Schmidt and confirmed by Voit in 1866. This correlation between protein and health led to the concept of nutritional support, although the effect of this relationship would not be fully known for another 75 to 100 years.

Major advances were made during the 1860s that would have an impact on infusion nursing and on all of medicine. Louis Pasteur developed the germ theory of disease, and demonstrated that fermentation and putrefaction result from the growth of germs. Building on this theory, Joseph Lister, Professor of Surgery at the University of Glasgow, hypothesized that microbes might be responsible for wound suppuration. He further postulated that infection could be prevented by destroying organisms and preventing contaminated air from coming into contact with the wound (Lyons and Petrucelli, 1987). Lister's studies describing the use of carbolic acid spray as an antiseptic were published in 1867.

Many physicians began observing strict rules of cleanliness without understanding the implications. In France, surgeons continued to focus on the use of antisepsis during procedures instead of asepsis. Not until the early 1900s were the principles of asepsis fully understood. By then, it was common practice that only sterile items could contact the patient.

The use of gloves for procedures was introduced in 1889, when William Halsted of Johns Hopkins Hospital had the Goodyear Rubber Co. make a pair of rubber gloves for his operating room nurse (Weinstein, 2007). The use of gloves became popular, and by 1899 rubber gloves were being used on all clean cases. Today, gloves provide protection not only for the patient but also for the practitioner.

The last half of the 19th century also saw advances in the field of nutritional support. In 1869 Menzel and Perco of Vienna wrote a paper on the use of fat, milk, and camphor injected subcutaneously. The successful administration of a glucose solution is credited to Biedl and Krause in 1896 (Millam, 1996).

20th CENTURY

For almost 250 years, experiments in which different substances were injected into the body had yielded limited results. As with most of medicine, major advances occurred during the 20th century. By this time, the use of saline and glucose solutions was a more widely accepted practice, although they were still used only on the critically ill patient. Equipment was cleaned and sterilized between uses as a routine measure with the advent of heat sterilization in 1910, and with the medical profession's acceptance that everything coming into contact with the patient needed to be sterile. The discovery of pyrogens in 1923 led to measures that helped eliminate them from fluids and drugs. Dr. Florence Seibert of the Phipps Institute in Philadelphia solved the serious problem of pyrogenic reactions to IV infusions in 1925, thus paving the way for safer practice (Greenwalt, 1997).

ADVANCES IN THERAPIES

Early in the 20th century, Karl Landsteiner discovered naturally occurring antibodies in the blood that led to a reaction when mixed with blood from another subject. This discovery eventually led to the identification of the ABO blood groups in 1901. By 1907 Reuben Ottenberg began using blood type differences as a basis for donor selection. By 1908 Epstein had set forth the hypothesis that ABO blood groups are inherited. Even with this information, transfusion therapy was still potentially fatal. Matching donor and recipient blood types helped reduce the incidence of transfusion reactions, but coagulation during the procedure continued to be a problem. During World War I, Oswald Robertson introduced the use of preserved anticoagulant blood, and by 1915 sodium citrate was being used successfully as an anticoagulant in blood transfusions (Greenwalt, 1997).

Levine and Stetson discovered the anti-Rh antigen in 1939, and in 1941 Levine and Burnham recognized that the anti-Rh antigen is responsible for alloimmunization during pregnancy and causes hemolytic disease of the newborn. These developments were important steps in the safe transfusion of blood.

World War II is important in the history of transfusion therapy because transfusions were used more widely during this time than ever before. Out of necessity, blood was being administered to the wounded troops in an effort to save more lives. Plasma was the first component to be used, and new techniques for the separation of plasma were developed in 1941. It was soon recognized, however, that plasma transfusions could not meet all the needs of the wounded, and by 1943 red blood cells were being salvaged and transfused. In 1962 the first filter to reduce white cell contamination and help reduce fibrin clots was designed. This helped solve an undesirable effect of transfusion therapy that had been recognized for more than four decades.

Today, blood can be separated into many different components, and each component is administered to correct a specific deficiency. Improved techniques make it possible to obtain, test, store, and administer these components. The risk of transfusion therapy has diminished as a result of the discovery and understanding of antigen-antibody reactions and of the development of improved methods for detecting bloodborne diseases. Administration sets, filters, infusion and warming devices, and other types of equipment are constantly being modified and improved. Agents were developed in the late 20th century that help the body to stimulate its own production of certain blood components, thereby reducing the need for transfusions and further reducing risks. In addition, there continues to be research to look at alternatives to the use of blood.

During the 20th century, advances were also being made in the area of nutritional support. Between 1904 and 1906, research on maintaining nitrogen balance for general well-being was conducted, and the rectal administration of protein for nutrition was documented. By 1918 Murlin and Riche were experimenting with the administration of fats to animals as a source of nutrition. The 1930s became a time of intense experimentation in nutritional support. In 1935 Emmett Holt of Baltimore administered an infusion of cottonseed oil, and has since been credited with the first infusion of a fat emulsion. By 1939 Dr. Robert Elman, along with Weiner, infused a solution of 2% casein hydrolysate and 8% dextrose without adverse effects. Following this success, various protein hydrolysates were studied, and in 1940 Schohl and Blackfan infused synthetic crystalline amino acids into infants. By 1944 Helfich and Abelson were able to provide nutritional support to a 5-day-old infant with a solution of 50% glucose and 10% casein hydrolysate, alternated with a 10% olive oil-lecithin emulsion.

With the assistance of Dr. Harry Vars at the Harrison Department of Surgical Research at the University of Pennsylvania, Stanley Dudrick conducted a series of experiments on beagle puppies in an attempt to support them totally by the parenteral route. By the early 1970s Dudrick had proven the effectiveness of protein and dextrose solutions for nutritional support. Today, primarily because of Dudrick's work, patients can receive parenteral nutrition through the intravenous route and survive diseases and conditions that had formerly resulted in death.

The use of fat emulsions as a caloric source was also investigated, but the severe adverse reactions encountered with the IV administration of these substances led the U.S. Food and Drug Administration (FDA) to ban their use in the United States in 1964. Fats were still being administered in Europe, however, and an emulsion derived from soybean oil was developed. This refined product, which produced no significant side effects, led the FDA to reverse its ban on the IV administration of fat emulsions in 1980, and soybean and safflower oil emulsions were approved for IV administration.

ADVANCES IN EQUIPMENT

Advances in fluids and medications used for IV administration continued to evolve. Medical science provided the information necessary to replace and maintain the body's fluid and electrolyte balance, to maintain or improve nutritional status, and to treat many disease states intravenously. The technology for administering IV solutions and medications has also advanced since Sir Christopher Wren used the quill, vein, and bladder of an animal for his treatments (Weinstein, 2007).

During the early trials with transfusion therapy, scientists and physicians used feather quills (sometimes with metal tips), animal veins, and animal bladders. This equipment was described in a 1670 Amsterdam publication called *Clysmatic Nova*. The crude apparatus of Wren was later replaced by metal needles, rubber tubing, and glass containers. Originally, the

equipment was designed to be reused and required cleaning and eventually sterilization between uses. The first fluid containers consisted of an open glass flask that was covered with a piece of gauze to keep debris out. By the 1930s the container had evolved into a closed, vacuum glass bottle. The technology for refining plastics has done much for the improvement of infusion therapy equipment. Rubber was the precursor for the use of the plastic (polyvinyl chloride) that was applied to administration sets first and then fluid containers. Today, plastic containers and administration sets are state of the art for infusion therapy equipment.

Devices for accessing the vein have also progressed rapidly in the last 60 years. Metal cannulas and crude metal needles that required cleaning and resharpening between uses were first used in the 19th century. Problems with infiltration, however, led to the development of the plastic cannula in 1945. These first catheters were made of flexible plastic tubing that required either a cutdown (incision to access the vein) or a needle for introduction into the vein. In 1950 the Rochester needle was introduced by Gautier and Maasa, and revolutionized the IV catheter (Weinstein, 2007). The over-the-needle type of catheter is state of the art and used to deliver almost all peripheral infusions. The metal needle is still available, but it is now a disposable device modified for short-term use.

Another catheter available is the through-the-needle device, which allows the plastic catheter to be threaded into the vein through the needle after venipuncture has been completed. This device was first introduced in 1958 by the Deseret Pharmaceutical Co., and its successors are still used today for the placement of percutaneous central catheters and peripherally inserted central catheters (PICCs).

Peripheral IV catheters, both metal and plastic, are available in a variety of gauge sizes to allow for the delivery of different therapies to all age groups. Gauges range from a large lumen (12 gauge) to a neonatal size (27 gauge). Central catheters also come in a variety of sizes from 1.8 French to 13 French. Catheters are available in varying lengths, from 0.75 to 30 inches or longer. The length is generally determined by the route of administration, peripheral or central, and the size and age of the patient. The *Infusion Nursing Standards of Practice* recommends that the shortest length, smallest gauge catheter be used to accommodate the prescribed therapy (INS, 2006).

Before 1949 IV therapy could be administered only through a peripheral vein. At that time, Meng and colleagues documented the use of a catheter placed in the central venous system of a dog for administering a hypertonic dextrose and protein solution. The subclavian puncture for accessing the central veins was more frequently used after its description by Aubaniac from Vietnam in 1952. In 1967 Dudrick adapted the subclavian approach for the administration of high concentrations of dextrose and proteins, which produced minimal side effects caused by the tonicity of the solution.

Further expansion on this concept led to the development of a catheter that is placed in the subclavian vein and then tunneled under the subcutaneous tissue to exit on the chest wall. Originally designed for use with children, this catheter became known as the *Broviac catheter*. A size appropriate for adults, the Hickman catheter, was developed soon after. The evolution of the Hickman-Broviac catheter has allowed for the administration of therapies over long periods, with minimal technical complications. It has also revolutionized infusion therapy by allowing safer administration of solutions in the home setting.

The 1980s saw further evolution of the use of central venous access with the introduction of the totally implanted system. This system consists of the central catheter and a device referred to as a *port*. The catheter is placed by percutaneous puncture into the subclavian vein, and the port is placed in a subcutaneous pocket generally on the chest wall. Access to this port is by puncture through the skin with a specially designed needle for the portal septum. By the end of the 20th century, venous ports were being placed in the arm with the catheter threaded into the superior vena cava via the basilic or cephalic vein, and ports were being placed for other therapies such as epidural pain management.

The PICC was introduced in the last quarter of the 20th century. The advantages of using this catheter are that there is less risk involved; fewer injuries are caused during insertion and also there is reduced risk of infection. It can be inserted by the registered nurse (RN) who is trained in its placement.

Peripheral catheters primarily consist of a single lumen, although experiments have been carried out with dual lumen catheters. Central catheters—percutaneous, PICC, tunneled, and ports—are available in both single lumen and multilumen design. The multilumen design makes it possible for multiple therapies to be delivered through one device, thus sparing the patient from numerous venipunctures.

To make the delivery of infusion therapy safer, various administration devices have been developed. Filters were first used in 1943 to remove fibrin clots during blood transfusions. Filters are now of two types—screen and depth—and are available in a number of micron sizes. Filters remove particulate matter from the solution and, depending on the micron size, can also eliminate air and remove endotoxins.

In addition to filters, administration devices that provide the close regulation of flow rate were developed. Before the use of this technology, infusions were administered by gravity and the flow rate was regulated primarily by a screw or roller clamp on the administration set. This mode of delivery allowed for a variation in flow rate being dependent on gravity, and as a result could lead to complications of the therapy being delivered. The development of electronic infusion devices has improved the accuracy of administration. Factors that affect flow rate, such as head height and internal pressure, are overcome by the use of these devices. This made the delivery of the various therapies safer for the patient.

The first electronic infusion device developed was the syringe pump, and the quantity of solution it delivered depended on the syringe size used. It was used primarily to administer fluids at a slow rate, especially to infants and children. The syringe device is still available, and is often used to control medication administration. The concept of the syringe pump was modified further to allow large volumes of fluid to be administered. The controller, first developed by IVAC in 1972, allowed for gravity infusion but controlled it through a drop-counting system that triggered an alarm when the number of drops deviated from the preset number. Subsequently, infusion pumps were designed to deliver a solution at a prescribed rate under positive pressure. These devices have multiple alarms that can alert the practitioner to potential problems and thereby promote patient safety. Infusion devices can also deliver simultaneous or multiple infusions at prescribed intervals.

Ambulatory infusion devices allow for continuous or intermittent infusions outside the hospital setting. These devices allow patients to receive necessary therapy while maintaining, as much as possible, a normal lifestyle. The quality of life for many patients has been dramatically improved by the use of these ambulatory devices.

Another technological advance that has improved the quality of patient care is the patient-controlled analgesia (PCA) pump. This device enables patients to control their pain by allowing them to administer their pain medication as they need it. This method of medication administration has proven especially effective in the management of postoperative pain.

During the 1970s the administration of pain medication was expanded to alternative routes. As early as 1976 Yaks and Rudy had demonstrated the successful administration of morphine directly into the subarachnoid space of animals. In 1977 Wang proved that an intrathecal injection of morphine provided profound relief in humans. Today, the intrathecal and epidural routes have proven effective for the administration of specific therapies, especially the control of postoperative and cancer pain. The intrathecal route has also been used for administering some antineoplastic agents.

Using the bone marrow as a route for transfusion was first advocated by Drinker in 1922. In the 1940s Tocantins established the basis for the widespread use of this technique for fluid administration, but it was used only briefly. By the late 1950s intraosseous administration had fallen into obscurity. The 1980s saw resurgence in the use of this mode of fluid administration. The resurgence of this method of administration occurred as a result of advances in pediatric resuscitation and emergency medicine. The successful use of this mode of administration has proven it to be an important advancement in infusion therapy.

21st CENTURY

As infusion nursing moved into the 21st century, advances in technology continued. In radiology, certain diagnostic tests yielded better results when contrast agents were administered under pressure. Most central venous access devices (CVADs), however, could not withstand the amount of pressure being used, and the potential for rupturing the catheter was high. Patients with CVADs were requiring peripheral IV access to undergo the test, and frequently these patients did not have suitable peripheral venous access. Catheter manufacturers responded by developing power-injectable CVADs including PICCs and implanted ports. These catheters were designed to withstand the pressure exerted by the power injector.

Electronic infusion devices now assist with patient safety by allowing the health care organization to develop a predetermined drug library that includes upper and lower dose limits in an effort to reduce harmful medication errors. Many devices can also be connected to the organization's information systems that allow for computerized documentation, report generation, and nurse alerts when a problem is detected.

The scope of practice of the infusion nurse has expanded. Infusion nurses have been inserting PICCs since the 1980s. However, they were limited by being able to access only those veins that they could visualize or palpate. Bedside ultrasound technology evolved and as a result has significantly increased the number and the success rate of PICCs inserted by infusion nurses.

A relatively new role emerging is that of the infusion nurse being allowed to view chest radiographs to confirm distal tip placement of PICCs. After infusion nurses are trained in the reading of x-ray films and have undergone competency validation, radiologists are allowing infusion nurses to determine the initial location of the catheter tip, with confirmation by the radiologist within a specified period of time. This has allowed for more timely administration of therapies to the patient, thereby improving care.

Even though infusion nursing is a specialty practice, infusion nurses and infusion teams have had a tenuous history. In 2002 the Centers for Disease Control and Prevention (CDC) published a *Morbidity and Mortality Weekly Report* entitled *Guidelines for the Prevention of Intravascular Catheter-Related Infections*. These guidelines rate having "trained personnel for the insertion and maintenance of intravascular catheters" as a category 1A, which means it strongly recommends implementation, and this recommendation is strongly supported by well-designed experimental, clinical, or epidemiological studies (CDC, 2002).

INFUSION NURSING

In 1966 Barbara Levenstein's article *Intravenous Therapy: A Nursing Specialty* was published in the *Nursing Clinics of North America*. In this article she stated, "Modern medicine is making bold new demands upon the professional nurse. She is required to extend her scope of knowledge and skills to areas once considered the physician's realm .... One of the functions inherited by nursing service is the administration of intravenous therapy. Hospitals adopting this policy are finding it favorable to delegate this activity to a group of specially trained nurses. This is done to maintain a control for patient safety against indiscriminate practices. The patient also benefits by receiving a specialized efficient service. Thus has been created a new specialty in professional nursing" (Levenstein, 1966).

Nursing involvement in the practice of infusion therapy was new in the 20th century. It is only since the 1940s that nurses have been allowed to perform IV procedures. Before this, nurses only assisted the physician with the venipuncture and the administration of solutions. Their role was primarily that of monitoring the patient.

It was after World War II that there was debate as to whether nurses should perform intravenous therapy. Before this intravenous therapy was strictly a physicians' responsibility as it was considered highly dangerous because of the risk of introducing infectious agents in the course of penetrating the vein. In 1943 the attorney general of New York declared venipuncture by anyone other than a physician to be an illegal practice of medicine. The controversy surrounding the practice of venipuncture as a medical or nursing act continued into the 1960s. In 1961 New York's ruling was finally reversed. Maryland, however, had a ruling requiring physicians to administer IV medications until as late as 1962.

In 1940 the Massachusetts General Hospital of Boston was the first to allow a nurse, Ada Plumer, to be responsible for the administration of IV therapies, and eventually she developed the first IV team (Box 1-1). The nurse at that time was expected to be technically competent and able to perform successful venipuncture.

During the last 60 years, the role of the nurse in infusion therapy has evolved to more than that of a "therapist." The

---

Box 1-1   GENERAL RESPONSIBILITIES OF THE IV NURSE IN THE 1940s

- Administering IV solutions and blood transfusions
- Cleaning and sharpening needles for reuse
- Cleaning the infusion set
- Maintaining patency of the needle
- Ensuring unobstructed infusion flow

---

infusion nurse of the 21st century is expected to be more than a technician; the nurse is expected to be capable of integrating the holistic principles of medicine and nursing, management, marketing, education, and performance improvement into the patient's plan of care. Clinical expertise is as important as technical expertise in the practice of infusion nursing in the 21st century.

The concerns of the mid-20th century that infusion therapy was highly dangerous to administer were not and are not unfounded. The complications of the therapies administered today have the same life-threatening or life-altering potentials that early therapies had. In the early stages of infusion therapy the risk of life-threatening infections was the major concern. Although infection continues to be a risk, there is also the risk today posed by the many different agents delivered intravenously alone or in combination. Once these agents are administered, there is no recall, and therefore it is essential the infusion nurse know and understand the impact of what is being administered.

Since the 1980s there has been rapid growth in the specialty practice of infusion nursing as evidenced by the following developments:

- Development of the 1980 *Infusion Nursing Standards of Practice* (revised 1990, 1998, 2000, 2006)
- Declaration by the U.S. House of Representatives on October 1, 1980, that January 25th of each year will be recognized as Infusion Nurse Day
- Development and administration of the first national certification examination for infusion nurses (1985)
- Development by the Centers for Disease Control and Prevention of "standard precautions" (1987)
- Publication of the CDC *Guidelines for the Prevention of Intravascular Catheter-Related Infections* supporting the use of trained personnel (2002)
- Initiation of central line bundling recommendations from the Institute for Healthcare Improvement (2006)

Infusion therapy continues to grow. It is no longer used only for the most critically ill patients. A majority of all hospitalized patients will experience some form of infusion therapy during their hospitalization, and many will be discharged with therapy to continue in an alternative setting. The ability to deliver these therapies in alternative settings has kept pace with the rapidly expanding specialty. No longer must patients be confined to the hospital to receive their care. Therapies can be delivered in the home setting, skilled nursing facilities, physician offices, and clinics. The infusion nurse working in these settings has the same responsibility to be knowledgeable about the therapies in order to provide safe, quality care to the patient. The pharmacological and technological advances demand that the nurse be more specialized and knowledgeable in order to offset any risk involved and maximize value for the patient and the health care organization.

INFUSION NURSES SOCIETY

Considered to be the premier specialty nursing organization for infusion nursing, the Infusion Nurses Society (INS), as known today, was established in 1973. Other organizations existed that were multidisciplinary or focused on a given geographical location.

In November 1972 two IV nurses, Ada Plumer from Massachusetts General Hospital in Boston and Marguerite Knight from the Johns Hopkins Hospital in Baltimore, wrote an organizational letter asking individuals to unite to form the American Association of IV Nurses. By the time 16 charter members assembled in Baltimore on January 25, 1973, there was some concern that the term "nurse" would restrict membership to nurses exclusively, whereas the proposed bylaws were more expansive. The name was then changed to the National Intravenous Therapy Association (NITA), and the stated purpose of the organization was to standardize the specialty practice of IV nursing and to ensure the provision of quality, cost-efficient patient care.

By the 1980s growth continued in both the organization and the specialty practice. There was some confusion, however, among other health care professionals, consumers, and legislators about what NITA represented even though the organization was comprised of 99% nurses. As a result, the membership voted in 1987 to officially rename the organization Intravenous Nurses Society. In 2001, on approval of the membership, the name of the organization was changed again to Infusion Nurses Society. The rationale for this change was that infusion nurses were involved in more than just intravenous administration. The practice had expanded to include obtaining access to and/or administering solutions and medications through routes such as arterial, epidural, intraosseous, and intracavity. Therefore the term "intravenous" was no longer a true description of the practice.

Growth of the organization was seen in the establishment of local chapters across the country. Membership continues to grow to the point where INS is an international nursing organization with members around the world. Nurses are involved in infusion nursing in many different settings that include the hospital, home, skilled nursing facilities, physician offices, private enterprises, and industry.

The vision of INS is to exceed the public's expectations of excellence by setting the standard for infusion care, and its mission statement describes how this is to be achieved (Box 1-2). The INS value statement defines the commitments of the organization (Box 1-3).

INS recognized the need for standards and published the first *Intravenous Nursing Standards of Practice* in 1980. The document has since undergone four revisions to address the changing aspects of the practice. The changing dynamics of infusion nursing lead to frequent review of these *Standards,* and documented evidence is required before consideration is given to a change in any of the *Standards.* The *Standards* are often referred to in litigation cases involving infusion nursing.

The flagship publication of the INS is its peer-review journal entitled *Journal of Infusion Nursing (JIN)*. The journal, published bimonthly, highlights clinical, technical, ethical, and managerial issues relevant to the infusion nurse practice. Besides the *Standards of Practice* and the *Journal of Infusion Nursing,* INS has an additional number of publications and learning tools to assist the infusion nurse and those interested in infusion nursing (Box 1-4).

Box 1-2 INFUSION NURSES SOCIETY VISION AND MISSION STATEMENTS

VISION

Recognized as the global authority in infusion therapy, INS is dedicated to exceeding the public's expectation of excellence by setting the standard for infusion care.

MISSION

INS sets the standard for excellence in infusion nursing by:
- Developing and disseminating standards of practice
- Providing professional development opportunities and quality education
- Advancing best practice through evidence-based research
- Supporting professional certification
- Advocating for the public

Box 1-3 INS VALUE STATEMENT

INS is committed to:
- **Excellence**—We are dedicated to continually improving ourselves, our programs, and services.
- **Integrity**—We are committed to honesty, trust, and respect in all we do.
- **Inclusiveness**—We encourage and respect diversity of thought and of individuals.
- **Innovation**—We promote creativity and inventiveness of ideas and processes.

Box 1-4 INS TOOLS AND PUBLICATIONS

- *Journal of Infusion Nursing*
- *Infusion Nursing Standards of Practice*
- *Core Curriculum for Infusion Nursing*
- *Policies and Procedures for Infusion Nursing*
- *Policies and Procedures for Infusion Nursing of the Older Adult*
- Clinical Competency Validation Program
- Patient Education Workbook and Work Mat
- Infusion Therapy Team Implementation Module
- PICC Education Module
- Fundamentals of Infusion Therapy
- Flushing Protocols

 CERTIFICATION

The National Organization for Competency Assurance (NOCA, 2008) states that certification of specialized skill sets affirms a knowledge and experience base for practitioners in a particular field, their employers, and the public at large. The American Board of Nursing Specialties (ABNS) recently defined certification as the formal recognition of specialized knowledge, skills, and experience demonstrated by achievement of standards identified by a nursing specialty to promote optimal health outcomes (Niebuhr and Biel, 2007). It is further stated that while basic nursing licensure indicates a minimal professional practice standard, certification denotes a high level of knowledge and practice, with the intent to protect the public (Niebuhr and Biel, 2007).

Through the certification process, the specialty organization recognizes individuals who have met the qualifying requirements and successfully completed the examination. Certification is recognition for knowledge and experience over and above that required for general licensure. Certification also provides control to the professional organization by forcing it to establish a clear identity, define the area of practice, and set performance standards (Crudi, 1987).

Certification is believed to have started as early as 1912, when it was used as a credentialing measure for public health nurses out of concern for the inadequacy of hospital-based training for diversified roles. This first program required the nurse to complete a postgraduate program to earn the certificate. The American Nurses Association began investigating the process of providing a certification program in the 1950s. The American Association of Critical Care Nurses was one of the first to offer a credentialing program to its members. In 1983 the Infusion Nurses Certification Corporation (INCC) began the process to develop a certification examination for infusion nursing, and offered its first examination in March 1985.

Consumers during this first decade of the 21st century have become more aware and demanding of quality care. They have become more knowledgeable of the type of care they want to receive and expect the caregiver to have this knowledge. Certification programs help instill a system of accountability that directly affects the quality of care that the consumer can expect to receive.

Certification programs continue to grow in many specialty nursing organizations. All offer an examination, with some specialties offering two levels of certification: basic and advanced. The number of certified nurses has also grown. One of the major influences on certification comes from health care organizations applying for Magnet status from the American Nurses Credentialing Corporation (ANCC). Magnet is a program developed by ANCC to recognize health care organizations that provide excellence in nursing (Weinstein, 2007). The number of credentialed nurses within a health care organization is considered in the application process. This has helped to foster an increased awareness of credentialing by both the public and the professional.

INFUSION NURSES CERTIFICATION CORPORATION

The Infusion Nurses Certification Corporation (INCC) oversees the CRNI® examination. The mission of INCC is for the benefit and protection of the public, thus the separation of INS and INCC. INS is a member organization working to meet its members' needs, while INCC exists for public protection, meeting the public's needs and not those of a particular membership. INCC's vision statement addresses the public's expectations of certification, while the organization's core values consist of integrity, public protection, and excellence (Box 1-5). INCC recognizes the certified infusion nurse with the certified registered nurse infusion (CRNI®) designation.

In order for an individual to become certified, the RN must pass a written examination. However, before being able to sit

---

Box 1-5 INFUSION NURSES CERTIFICATION CORPORATION

VISION

Certification, by INCC, is the standard of excellence that nurses will seek in order to provide optimal infusion care that the public expects, demands, and deserves.

MISSION

INCC promotes excellence in infusion nursing certification by:
- Developing and administering a comprehensive, evidence-based program
- Advocating the importance of the CRNI® credential
- Supporting continuing infusion nursing education and research

VALUES
- **Integrity—**We are committed to providing a psychometrically sound, legally-defensible certification program.
- **Public Protection—**We support the role certified nurses play in promoting optimal health outcomes and ensuring that our program is driven by the needs of the public.
- **Excellence—**We are committed to providing a program of high quality and are dedicated to a process of continuous improvement.

---

for the examination the RN must meet certain requirements. These requirements are the following:
- The RN must hold a current, active, unrestricted RN license in the United States or Canada. If not licensed in the United States or Canada, the application must include an educational evaluation and license equivalency report from an approved organization.
- The RN must have a minimum of 1600 hours of experience in infusion therapy as an RN within 2 years prior to the exam.

CRNI® EXAMINATION

There are nine major content areas on the certification examination. The content areas reflect those recommended for the basic curriculum of infusion nursing. The core content areas are as follows: technology and clinical application, fluid and electrolyte therapy, pharmacology, infection control, transfusion therapy, antineoplastic and biologic therapy, parenteral nutrition, performance improvement, and pediatrics.

Successful completion of the examination results in the nurse being awarded the CRNI® designation.

RECERTIFICATION

The CRNI® credential is valid for a 3-year period following successful completion of the examination. Recertification is required to be eligible to continue using the credential. To become recertified one must be an active CRNI®; possess a current, active, unrestricted RN license or equivalent as previously described; and be able to document 1000 hours of clinical practice in infusion nursing within the previous 3 years. In addition, the nurse must either document 40 recertification units earned during the previous 3 years or recertify by examination.

INFUSION NURSE SPECIALIST

Patient safety is a major focus in today's health care environment. It is necessary in any setting where infusion therapy is delivered to have highly trained and knowledgeable infusion nurses to insert and monitor IVs and to assess infusion products for use. The infusion nurse specialist works autonomously and is held accountable for knowing what to do and how to do it. The nurse must also be able to collaborate with other health care professionals to ensure that the patient is receiving the best quality of care in a safe environment.

The infusion nurse specialist has the responsibilities of collaborating with others to coordinate patient care and of communicating patient care information to other health care professionals. The infusion nurse specialist is a resource to others by virtue of having a specialized body of knowledge and through collaboration helps ensure that the patient will receive high-quality care. The infusion nurse specialist also functions as an educator, mentor, and preceptor. In her 8th edition of *Plumer's Principles and Practice of Intravenous Therapy*, Sharon Weinstein refers to this role of the infusion nurse specialist as that of knowledge-sharer.

The infusion nurse specialist also participates in performance improvement initiatives as a function of this role. Performance improvement should be an ongoing initiative as health care strives to provide safe, quality patient care.

Research is another role that many infusion nurses are participating in today. The emphasis on evidence-based practice requires that research be done to support best practice. Research provides the clinician the opportunity to trial new ideas to advance the practice and/or improve patient care.

INS recognizes the licensed practical nurse/licensed vocational nurse (LPN/LVN) as being the minimum-level clinician qualified to assist in tasks delegated by the RN for the administration of infusion therapy (INS, 2006). The role of the LPN/LVN in infusion therapy is defined by a state's Nurse Practice Act, the Board of Nursing, organizational policies and procedures, and practice guidelines. The LPN/LVN works under the auspices of the RN.

ROLE DELINEATION

According to the *Infusion Nursing Standards of Practice* the practice of infusion therapy encompasses various levels of knowledge and expertise. The continuum of expertise extends from the nurse who is practicing infusion therapy to the nurse who is qualified to practice in an extended role. The CRNI® credential identifies the nurse who is educated in infusion therapy and is capable of practicing in an expanded role. With the increasing attention to patient safety and quality care, the certified infusion nurse specialist is prepared to participate in the benchmarking of quality indicators for infusion nursing.

SCOPE OF PRACTICE

A specialist is a generalist, but a generalist has not acquired the knowledge and skill in a defined area to be designated a specialist (INS, 2006). Basic nursing education prepares the candidate to become a generalist with a global approach to nursing practice. Specialty practice takes that global approach and focuses on a defined area that requires advanced knowledge and skill. Some specialization can be achieved by formal education at the graduate level and beyond as evidenced by becoming a nurse practitioner or nurse anesthetist. Specialization can also be achieved as a result of concentrated study, continuing education, and skill development in a specific area of interest. Infusion nursing is such a specialization.

The infusion patient represents a diversity of cultures and ethnic backgrounds, diagnoses, and degrees of illness and is found in a variety of different settings. These patients also represent a spectrum of ages from the neonate to the geriatric population. Each age on that spectrum can present opportunities and challenges that the infusion nurse needs to be prepared to meet.

The infusion nurse is accountable for practicing within the defined scope of practice for either the RN or the LPN/LVN and is committed to providing safe, quality care (INS, 2006). The infusion nurse's practice is based on the following:

- Knowledge of anatomy and physiology
- Specific knowledge and understanding of the vascular system and its relationship with other body systems and infusion therapy modalities
- Participation in the establishment of the patient's ongoing plan of care
- Possession of skills necessary for the administration of infusion therapies
- Knowledge of state-of-the-art technologies associated with infusion therapies
- Knowledge of psychosocial aspects, including sensitivity to the patient's wholeness, uniqueness, and significant social relationships, and knowledge of community and economic resources
- Interaction and collaboration with members of the health care team and participation in the clinical decision-making process (INS, 2006)

In caring for the patient, the infusion nurse uses the nursing process of assessment, problem identification, intervention, and evaluation. The infusion nurse strives for safe, high-quality patient outcomes. By constantly monitoring patient and process outcomes, the infusion nurse is able to identify areas that will benefit from performance improvement, thereby improving the quality of care.

COMPETENCY

Infusion nurses, regardless of the age and condition of the patient population they serve and the setting in which they practice, require the same basic clinical competencies to perform their role. Clinical competencies describe practice and educational requirements and provide validation for professional infusion nursing practice (INS, 2006). These competencies serve as guidelines as to what knowledge the infusion nurse should have and are used in developing orientation and continuing educational programs.

Clinical competencies include the many tasks that infusion nurses perform on a daily basis—from initiating, monitoring, and terminating infusion therapy to educating the patient or caregiver to collecting and analyzing data. Each health care organization must define in policy and procedure the competencies that are the responsibility of the infusion nurse in that organization.

More than clinical competency is required of the infusion nurse. In the *Infusion Nursing Standards of Practice* there are 10 additional areas of competency identified in which the infusion nurse may be expected to participate. These are communication, patient education, technology, continuing education, legal issues, performance improvement, research, consultation, clinical management, and the budgetary process. The first six areas are competencies in which proficiency should be demonstrated by every infusion nurse, while the last two are needed by those involved in management.

EDUCATION

The infusion nurse must demonstrate accountability, reliability, initiative, and effective communication and technical skills as well as complete certain education requirements before practicing infusion nursing. The education includes both theoretical and clinical components. Entry level into infusion nursing requires that the individual have a current RN or LPN/LVN license to practice and 2 years of acute care nursing experience.

CURRICULUM DESCRIPTION

The curriculum of study recommended to become an infusion nurse is described in the *Infusion Nursing Standards of Practice*. Any program of study for infusion nursing should be based on outcome criteria established by behavioral objectives. Both theoretical knowledge and clinical experience should be represented in the curriculum.

Box 1-6 NINE CORE AREAS TO BE INCLUDED IN A THEORETICAL CURRICULUM

1. Technology and clinical application
2. Pharmacology
3. Neonate and pediatric patients
4. Antineoplastic and biologic therapy
5. Performance improvement
6. Fluid and electrolytes
7. Infection control
8. Transfusion therapy
9. Parenteral nutrition

THEORY

The theoretical portion of the curriculum for infusion nursing should encompass the nine core areas of the practice (Box 1-6).

CLINICAL EXPERIENCE

The nurse should be supervised in all clinical aspects of infusion nursing until proficiency is determined to be acceptable and competency has been validated through a competency assessment program.

SUMMARY

Many factors influence health care today and as a result provide expanding possibilities for the infusion nurse. Advances in pharmacology and technology, the changing demographics of the patient population, resource shortage, and the economic issues surrounding reimbursement for health care are opportunities and challenges that face the specialty practice and the infusion nurse specialist in the 21st century.

REFERENCES

Centers for Disease Control and Prevention: Guidelines for the prevention of intravascular catheter-related infections. *MMWR* 52(RR10):1-37, 2002.

Cosnett, JE: Before our time: the origins of intravenous fluid therapy, *Lancet* 4(8641):768-771, 1989.

Crudi C: Certification: is the payoff worth the price? *RN* 50(7):36-44, 1987.

Greenwalt TJ: A short history of transfusion medicine, *Transfusion* 37(5):550-563, 1997.

Infusion Nurses Society: Infusion nursing standards of practice, *JIN* 29(suppl 1S), 2006.

Levenstein B: Intravenous therapy: a nursing specialty, *Nurs Clin North Am* 1(2):259-267, 1966.

Lyons AS, Petrucelli RJ: *Medicine: an illustrated history*, New York, 1987, Harry N Abrams.

Millam D: The history of intravenous therapy, *J Intravenous Nurs* 19(1):5-14, 1996.

National Organization for Competency Assurance: *What is certification?* Accessed 3/17/08 from www.noca.org/GeneralInformation/WhatisCertification/tabid/63/Default.aspx.

Niebuhr B, Biel M: The value of specialty nursing certification, *Nurs Outlook* 55(4):176-181, 2007.

Weinstein SM: *Plumer's principles and practice of intravenous therapy.* ed 8, Philadelphia, 2007, Lippincott Williams & Wilkins.

2 EVIDENCE-BASED PRACTICE

Mary E. Hagle, PhD, RN, AOCN® and Patricia Senk, BSN, RN

Nursing practice requires current best evidence to provide care that meets our standards, partners with patients, and is effective and efficient. Nurses must question their personal beliefs, health care myths, and traditional practices that are not based on research and current best evidence. How many nurses continue to lock a peripheral IV with heparin because this is the way "it has always been done" or the order is written for this? It has been more than 17 years since two meta-analyses were published with the practice recommendation that 0.9% sodium chloride is an effective locking solution for peripheral IVs (Goode et al, 1991; Peterson and Kirchhoff, 1991). Seventeen years is the time it takes to translate research findings into practice; based on this fact, all peripheral IVs in adults in acute care settings with nonthrombogenic catheters should be locked with 0.9% sodium chloride. Is your practice research based? An interesting survey would be to validate this research-based practice in the United States and in other developed countries. Unfortunately, most nursing practice assessments or interventions do not have a meta-analysis, let alone two, as their current best evidence. Thus obtaining current best evidence is a process composed of key steps for the individual nurse, the health care organization, professional nursing organizations, and nursing as a profession.

The use of best evidence in practice is now a measurable goal, as identified by the Institute of Medicine (IOM). They set a goal that by 2020, "90% of clinical decisions will be supported by accurate, timely, and up-to-date clinical information, and will reflect the best available evidence" (IOM, 2007, p. ix). This goal is the result of a 2001 recommendation that care needs to be effective and based on the best available scientific knowledge (IOM, 2001). There is also acknowledgment that evidence is more than expert consensus-based guidelines yet not necessarily only randomized controlled trials. Current best evidence is just that—the synthesized knowledge a nurse has at the time to provide effective care. As the body of evidence is synthesized and gaps are identified, research is justified to provide support for our care. The knowledge loop is closed when new evidence is integrated into current systems in a way that is timely and efficient.

Evidence needs to be transparent for both nurses and patients. Nursing practice is the care of patients or clients; patients are one half of the partnership. Every nursing theory involves a nurse and a patient. Current best evidence is implemented with the patient's decision and is tempered by the patient's personal knowledge and skills, beliefs, preferences, and values in the context of the situation. It is the nurse's knowledge, skill, experience, and expertise that integrate these components for a quality health care outcome.

STANDARDS OF PRACTICE

The standards of both the American Nurses Association (ANA) and the Infusion Nurses Society (INS) recognize the importance of incorporating best current evidence into nursing. Standard 13 of the ANA's *Scope and Standards of Practice* (ANA, 2004) requires that "the registered nurse integrate research findings into practice" (p. 40). Nurses practice according to this standard by using the best evidence available to guide their decisions and actively participate in research activities. A continuum of research activities can include the following: identifying a clinical problem; participating in data collection; using research in policies, procedures, and standards of practice; and *critically appraising and interpreting research* for use in the practice setting (ANA, 2004). *Nursing's Social Policy Statement* (ANA, 2003) identifies the nurse's relationship with, and obligation to, the patient. It calls upon the nurse to (1) use research to expand the science of nursing; (2) use evidence-based knowledge when assessing, planning, implementing, and evaluating care; and (3) use evidence to improve care (ANA, 2003). The *Infusion Nursing Standards of Practice* (INS, 2006) promote evidence-based practice and research. Standard 18 specifically addresses the utilization of research "to expand the base of nursing knowledge in infusion therapy, to validate and improve practice, to advance professional accountability, and to enhance evidence-based decision making" (INS, 2006, p. S24). This is accomplished by participating in research activities, *critically appraising research outcomes*, and implementing research findings into clinical practice.

DEFINITION OF EVIDENCE-BASED PRACTICE

The components of current best evidence with the patient's decision-making and personal knowledge carried out by nurses with expertise have been espoused by medical and nurse authors as comprising evidence-based practice (EBP). The Institute of Medicine (2001, p. 147) legitimized EBP for all health care practitioners with their definition:

> *Evidence-based practice is the integration of best research evidence with clinical expertise and patient values.* Best research evidence *refers to clinically relevant research, often from the basic health and medical sciences, but especially from patient-centered clinical research into the accuracy and precision of diagnostic tests (including the clinical examination); the power of prognostic markers; and the efficacy and safety of therapeutic, rehabilitative, and preventive regimens.* Clinical expertise *means the ability to use clinical skills and past experience to rapidly identify each patient's unique health state and diagnosis, individual risks and benefits of potential interventions, and personal values and expectations.* Patient values *refer to the unique preferences, concerns, and expectations that each patient brings to a clinical encounter and that must be integrated into clinical decisions if they are to serve the patient.*

EBP provides a framework and culture for quality health care. Each component needs to be supported in the full sense of the word by the organization and by a culture of daily practice by the individual nurse. The micro level of EBP is at the nurse-patient relationship. In daily practice, the current best evidence needs to be integrated through computerized clinical decision support information for access by nurses and into care plans that are patient-centered and based on appropriate assessments and risk factors (Hook, Devine, Lang, 2008; IOM, 2007; O'Neill, Dluhy, Hansen et al, 2006). Unnecessary traditional practices need to be eliminated based on current best evidence. Imagine a nurse at 2 AM faced with an unusual and unique patient situation. In an EBP environment, the nurse is able to rapidly access research-based resources and has the skills and knowledge to evaluate the evidence at hand to effectively care for his/her patient. In addition, the current best evidence is provided for the patient in language the patient understands with content to aid his or her decisions (Figure 2-1).

At the system or organizational level, EBP is supported and expected. Financial and human resources are available to obtain and appraise evidence, translate it into practice, and evaluate effectiveness. Current best evidence is incorporated into policies, procedures, professional standards, protocols, care plans, and computerized clinical decision support. Education is widespread and easily available for all health care personnel and patients/families to understand EBP and the processes that support it. System level outcomes are transparent for nurses and patients.

There are two additional levels, meso and macro, for EBP that are gaining attention. The meso level involves negotiations between health care organizations and payers. "In the future, the implementation of evidence-based procedures will become an important criterion for the financial reimbursement of nursing provision by health-insurance funding" plans, which may lead to high-quality nursing care that is effective and cost-efficient (Hasseler, 2006, p. 222). The political machinations or strategies are at the macro level, that is, the level where health policy, health

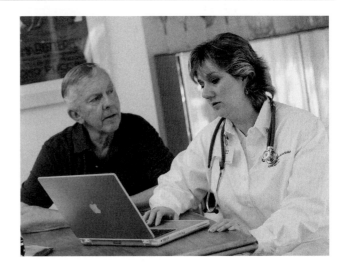

FIGURE 2-1 EBP in action. (From Aurora Health Care, Milwaukee, Wis.)

care funding, and other measures are decided (Hasseler, 2006, p. 223): "If the nursing profession fails to become involved in the debate on drawing up and developing evidence-based nursing procedures and standards in the new programs, other professional groups will step in and take over the fields of activity...."

Using current best evidence can be an automatic and an active process. By accessing EBP policies, procedures, professional standards, protocols, and care plans that are already in place, nurses are incorporating best evidence into practice through an automatic mechanism. For example, because fluoride is added to drinking water, tooth decay in children and adults is prevented without active participation at the time. Nurses also may be actively involved in EBP through any of the steps, such as identification of the key clinical question, the initial evidence review, appraisal, or integration into organizational processes. EBP also engages nurses through the triggers, alerts, decisions, or tasks within a computerized clinical decision support mechanism. Regardless of the practice setting (long-term care, acute care, home health, primary care, or elsewhere), it is critical that EBP is the culture of daily practice for nurses.

COMPONENTS OF EVIDENCE-BASED PRACTICE

Having a culture of EBP involves, at a minimum, understanding each component of EBP. Expertise develops as nurses and teams become more familiar with EBP. The following sections address the components of EBP: best evidence; clinician experience and expertise; and patient beliefs, preferences, and values in the context of the practice setting and current patient situation.

BEST EVIDENCE

Evidence is defined as "a thing or things helpful in forming a conclusion or judgment"; it is the proof. As such, evidence may come from a variety of sources including published and unpublished reports, internal quality improvement project summaries, and expert opinion.

The best evidence is not necessarily a research report, because research may not have been done or reported in your area

TABLE 2-1 PICO Method to Format a Clinical Question

PICO method	Explanation	Example
Patient population	Individual or groups of individuals you are interested in studying	Adults in acute care setting with short-term central venous access device
Intervention	The intervention in which you are interested	Saline solution for locking
Comparison	The intervention that you want to use for comparison	Heparin for locking
Outcome	The effect of the intervention	The length of time the catheter is patent with both locking solutions

Data from Nollan R, Fineout-Overholt E, Stephenson P: Asking compelling clinical questions. In Melnyk BM, Fineout-Overholt E: *Evidence-based practice in nursing and healthcare: a guide to best practice,* Philadelphia, 2005, Lippincott Williams & Wilkins.

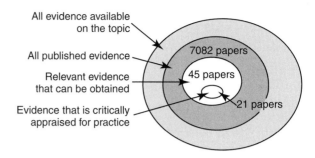

FIGURE 2-2 Finding the evidence.

of interest. Best evidence can be evaluated against objective criteria and categorized into a hierarchy of usefulness. The body of evidence is synthesized for the practice recommendation. The steps to identify, obtain, evaluate, and synthesize the evidence are important to ensure reaching the best evidence for the topic.

Asking the clinical question

The search for evidence begins with asking a clinical question. Nurses' clinical questions come from a variety of sources, which may include a newly published study or clinical guideline, a novel clinical experience, an unexpected outcome, a questioning of tradition, or unclear benchmarking data. A structured format during question formation assists nurses, novice to expert, in including the key elements in their question. These elements are the study population, which is similar to your patients, the intervention of interest and the comparison intervention, and the outcome of interest. One method to aid in forming the question is the "PICO" (**P**atient population; **I**ntervention; **C**omparison; **O**utcome) method (Nollan, Fineout-Overholt, Stephenson, 2005), as outlined in Table 2-1. This format for the clinical question also assists in identifying the key terms that might be used during the literature search.

The patient population identifies the group of individuals who are the focus of the question and about whom information is needed. The population may be individuals with a specific disease or condition, or of a certain age, gender, or ethnicity. For example, your clinical interest is the adult population in the acute care setting with a short-term central venous access device (CVAD). If the pediatric population were included in the search, the evidence obtained would not be useful to answer the clinical question. Knowing the population helps to narrow down the potentially large amount of literature to be reviewed and will allow the focus to be on what is important to the clinical practice area. For example, if the interest is in the effect of an intervention on adult males and the study included only adult females, the results may not pertain to the question. Including additional words commonly used to describe a disease, treatment, or device is also helpful when searching for

evidence. A CVAD is sometimes called a subclavian catheter in clinical practice; both of these terms could be used when performing a literature search. Of course, using the accepted subject heading is recommended as well, and each nurse and librarian has their own method for doing searches. As a result, directions on doing literature searches are beyond the scope of this chapter.

The specific intervention or interventions of interest should be identified, and may include a treatment, a screening assessment, risk factor, or prevention strategy. In the preceding example, the interest was in the locking solution for a CVAD. Your institution uses saline solution, but several articles have been reviewed related to the use of heparin when locking a CVAD. Identifying this intervention will help exclude literature that examines the recommended replacement time for a CVAD. While this may be a clinically important question, the desired clinical question is focused on the recommended locking solution. Use only literature that addresses the desired clinical question; if it is not related, exclude it from the list of evidence to consider.

A comparison group can be a group that receives no treatment or several groups in which each receives a different treatment or intervention. The comparison group in the example is the patient group receiving the heparin solution for locking.

The outcome of interest is the effect of the treatment. In the preceding example, the outcome or effect is patency of the CVAD; the treatment option is either saline solution or heparin. In the example, identifying this specific outcome will exclude literature that examines the infection rate of the CVAD. After identifying the appropriate content for each element of PICO, the clinical question is developed: Should saline solution or heparin be used when locking a CVAD in adult patients in the acute care setting?

Searching for evidence

Once the key clinical question is identified, it is used to guide the evidence search. Working with a librarian is advised, especially if there is a lack of previous experience in completing a literature search. An overwhelming amount of evidence is often available; many times there are thousands of papers. The reality of how difficult it can be to find relevant evidence that answers a clinical question is demonstrated in Figure 2-2. The outer ring identifies all the evidence that is available on a topic or problem of interest. This includes both published and unpublished evidence, ranging from rigorous studies, to expert opinion, to internal quality improvement reports. Only a portion of the evidence that exists is published. Published sources include journals, conference proceedings, a dissertation or thesis, and textbooks. When a literature search is completed, only a portion of all available published evidence is obtained; this may be due,

Box 2-1 SAMPLE DATABASES FOR A LITERATURE SEARCH

Database	Subject matter
National Guideline Clearinghouse www.guideline.gov/	Provides guidelines on health care topics; initiative of U.S. Agency for Healthcare Research and Quality (AHRQ)
Cochrane Database of Systematic Reviews www.cochrane.org/reviews	Provides systematic reviews on health care topics; independently supported; based in U.K.
National Institute for Health and Clinical Excellence www.nice.org.uk/	Provides national guidelines (guidance) on health promotion and treatment; an independent organization based in U.K.
PubMed www.pubmed.gov	Includes citations from MEDLINE and other journals; service of U.S. National Library of Medicine
Cumulative Index of Nursing and Allied Health Literature (CINAHL)	Includes journals from nursing and allied health; by subscription
MEDLINE	Includes journals from medicine, nursing, and dentistry; by subscription
PsycINFO	Includes literature from psychology and related disciplines; by subscription

Box 2-2 ORGANIZATIONS PROVIDING EVIDENCE SUMMARIES, STANDARDS, AND OTHER EVIDENCE

National organizations	Website address
Agency for Healthcare Research and Quality (AHRQ)	www.ahrq.gov
Centers for Disease Control and Prevention	www.cdc.gov
Institute for Healthcare Improvement (IHI)	www.ihi.org
National Quality Forum (NQF)	www.qualityforum.org
TRIP Database: Turning Research into Practice	www.tripdatabase.com

Sample professional nursing organizations	Website address
American Association of Critical-Care Nurses	www.aacn.org
American Nurses Association	www.nursingworld.org
Infusion Nurses Society	www.ins1.org
Oncology Nursing Society	www.ons.org

in part, to the specific search words that were used. Additionally, only some of the available evidence may be obtained; costs of retrieving dissertations or requesting articles may be a deterrent, along with the time lag to obtain such evidence.

Once the available evidence is obtained, an initial review is done. Although an article may be identified when using specific search terms, it does not mean that the sample, tool, or disease state is the same as the patient population or area of interest. Each article needs to be examined for its relevance to answering the clinical question. If interested in the rate of phlebitis for peripheral intravenous infusions (PIVs) with routine catheter replacement every 96 hours in adults in the acute care setting, one search would yield 7082 papers. When limiting this search to the last 10 years, papers only in English, with adults, and human populations, then the evidence that can be obtained and reviewed would include 45 papers. These papers would be reviewed for pertinence to the topic, population, and setting; for example, several papers are eliminated since the catheters in the study were peripherally inserted central catheters (PICCs) and not PIVs. The 21 remaining papers are then critically appraised, content is abstracted onto an evidence table, and the quality of the evidence is rated. High-quality applicable evidence would be synthesized and used in a practice recommendation.

A database of guidelines or systematic reviews is a good place to start searching for evidence (Box 2-1). Many of the databases have tutorials to assist clinicians in searching for information on their topic. These databases are easily accessible via the Internet and the guidelines are free and downloadable. Other databases contain citations and abstracts for journals specific to a discipline, such as CINAHL (Cumulative Index to Nursing and Allied Health Literature) for nurses and allied health professionals. The published papers can be purchased by individuals or through a library subscription. The school, hospital, or local

library can help locate articles and may have subscriptions to journals that are unfamiliar to the nurse or researcher. Often, university alumni have access to the school's library and search services, as another means to obtain resources.

National organizations interested in health care quality and patient safety are another source for evidence. Several national organizations, as well as professional clinical organizations, have websites with additional sources of evidence and may provide practice guidelines they have endorsed (Box 2-2). These lists are not all-inclusive and other summaries sometimes are published (Dee, 2005). More organizations are taking responsibility to support practice with best evidence. As quality and safety become major outcomes, bodies of evidence and synthesis are needed to identify best practice and stop ineffective or possibly harmful practices.

Critical appraisal and rating the evidence

Each paper, report, or quality improvement project can be a type of evidence. The evidence that is used depends on the body of evidence available and the quality of each piece of evidence. A health care organization may have results from a quality improvement project or benchmarking data that also can be used to support the use of a specific intervention. Initially, evaluate the available evidence by considering the following questions. Some papers will be put aside after this review.

- What are the setting, sample, and interventions used in the article? Are the setting and sample the same, or similar, to the subject of interest? There would be no need to review articles from the home care setting if the population of interest is in the acute care setting. The interventions of interest or technology need to be similar to the clinical question.
- Is the article from a peer-reviewed journal? Articles in a peer-reviewed journal have gone through a rigorous content review for scientific and statistical accuracy, which usually involves individuals who are experts in the field.

- Who are the authors, and what are their credentials? Are the author's experts in the field? While not every author has to be an expert, what are the individuals' credentials? If it is a research study, is one author an individual with the education to perform research?
- Are there any conflicts of interest? Did a group or corporation that may have an interest in the results sponsor the study?

When the evidence is pared after this initial review, it is sometimes helpful to sort the evidence chronologically and determine what is the most recent information on the topic. Another way of becoming familiar with the evidence is to sort by a hierarchy of research design, which is the plan for conducting the study. It is the manner of selecting the sample and administering the intervention. Generally, evidence such as a meta-analysis and systematic review of randomized controlled trials (RCTs) are considered the highest rank of research design; however, these are also the fewest types of evidence available. Evidence such as a case study has a low ranking in the hierarchy of research design. Because research used to support nursing practice encompasses a variety of research designs, it is important to include qualitative design in a hierarchy (Melnyk and Fineout-Overholt, 2005). A common hierarchy of research designs and their definitions are outlined in Box 2-3.

Research studies are only one type of evidence. Other evidence high in the rating hierarchy, but not a research design, is a clinical practice guideline based on a systematic review or a systematic review of one phenomenon using studies and other evidence on the topic. A systematic review is a rigorous methodical search, review, and critical appraisal of research evidence, by two or more researchers to answer a specific clinical question (Collins et al, 2005; Guyatt et al, 2008). Other review types are available too, such as an integrative review or a narrative review, all having varying levels of evidence and rigor in their development. These types of evidence may be available on a topic when a meta-analysis or systematic review of RCTs is not. The benefit of these types of evidence is that they merge findings from several studies and other sources on the same clinical topic. A variety of practice guidelines are available, and it is important to determine how the recommendations were developed. A guideline may be based on a rigorous systematic review or it may be based on consensus of experts. If none of these evidence types are available, then look for a single RCT. If an RCT is not available, then look for correlational, case control, descriptive, qualitative, or other studies. Last, examine expert opinions, reports, or quality improvement projects.

Once the main pieces of evidence are identified and sorted, a critical appraisal is done of each piece. A critical appraisal, or a quality analysis, of the evidence examines the study or paper for three domains: design, methodology, and how it was analyzed, all to minimize bias (Agency for Healthcare Research and Quality [AHRQ], 2002). Criteria in each of these domains may include, for example, blinding, adequate sample size, and preciseness of the results (AHRQ, 2002; Ebell et al, 2004; Schünemann et al, 2008). Often a checklist is used to rate each criterion, such as whether the subjects were randomized or if appropriate statistical analysis was used. As part of the critical appraisal system, a value may be assigned to each piece of evidence, or a hierarchy of quality is established, so that some evidence is more valuable as compared to the remaining evidence. This is helpful when looking at the final body of evidence. There are many systems for the critical appraisal and rating of individual evidence, especially quantitative studies, as well as available systems for guidelines and qualitative

Box 2-3   HIERARCHY OF RESEARCH DESIGNS AND THEIR DEFINITIONS

Research design	Broad definition
Meta-analysis	A specific statistical analysis to combine findings of several studies examining the same phenomenon to determine the overall effect of an intervention
Systematic review of randomized controlled trials (RCTs)	A methodology to identify, appraise, and synthesize RCTs on the same phenomenon
Randomized controlled trial (RCT)	A study where subjects are randomly assigned to groups; one group receives a treatment and the other group does not; the groups are blinded to the treatment, or in other words, they do not know which treatment they are receiving
Correlational design	A study that focuses on the relationship between two variables in the same population
Case control design	A study of two matched samples at the same time; one sample has the characteristic or variable of interest and one does not
Cohort design	A study of one sample that is followed over time to describe and identify a relationship between a variable and an outcome
Descriptive design	An examination of a phenomenon as it naturally occurs; there is no manipulation of variables. Data collected may include: Quantitative, such as a survey: descriptive analysis of numerical data Qualitative: analysis of verbal or written data, such as interviews, textbooks, or observational notes
Case study	An exploration and description of a single unit, such as a person, organization, community, or group at one point in time or over time

Data from Collins S et al: Finding the evidence. In DiCenso A, Guyatt G, Ciliska D, editors: *Evidence-based nursing: a guide to clinical practice*, St Louis, 2005, Mosby; and Burns N, Grove S: *The practice of nursing research: conduct, critique, and utilization*, ed 5, St Louis, 2005, Saunders.

evidence (Box 2-4). When selecting a system, consider one that is clear, concise, reproducible among various research teams, and understandable to clinicians as well as researchers. This is an opportunity for professional nursing organizations to adopt or develop a common system that crosses specialties.

Summarizing the evidence

The next step in evaluating evidence for implementation into practice is to summarize the evidence that will be used. Depending on the topic or clinical question that has been asked, there may be only a few articles or many to summarize and synthesize into a recommendation for practice. One method to help with this process is to create an evidence table. Each piece of evidence is abstracted, or key points summarized, using a structured approach through a table. An example of an evidence table with commonly used column headings and explanations for abstracting evidence is provided in Table 2-2. A sample of how one study was abstracted is provided in Table 2-3.

An evidence table helps to organize the information and can be arranged alphabetically by author, chronologically by publication year, assembling similar evidence or study results together, or arranging content by steps in the nursing process (assessment, diagnosis/problem, intervention, outcomes) (Lang et al, 2006). Another consideration is separate evidence tables for each aspect of practice, such as peripheral IV dressings, peripheral IV routine replacement, or phlebitis assessment. Additional column headings can be inserted, depending on the focus of the clinical question. For example, if evaluating which tool to use for phlebitis assessment, there may be a need to add a column in the evidence table to describe the tool that was used in each study, including reliability and validity. If evaluating an intervention, there may be a need to note any cost considerations, special personnel, equipment needed, or other factors to consider in specific settings. The critical appraisal or quality system for evidence evaluation may determine some of the columns for abstracting as well. Some authors restrict their evidence searches to English-only journals, or research only from developed countries, which may maintain a similarity of technology or health care for comparison. As identified in Table 2-2, it is helpful to include the country where the study was done. Lastly, topics of emerging importance to include when evaluating individual evidence include costs of the intervention to the patient and other patient-centered factors or outcomes, such as pain, inconvenience, or possible adverse

effects from the intervention (Ebell et al, 2004; Schünemann et al, 2008). Only high-quality evidence that contributes to answering the clinical question is used. Sometimes all that is available is evidence based on anatomy, physiology, or common practice; then it is included with the appropriate evidence rating. The evidence that comprises "current best evidence" may consist of as few as 2 to 3 studies or as many as 21 studies, or more.

The goal of an evidence table is to provide enough information from the study, article, or other evidence so that there is no need to keep returning to the original study to answer questions. On the other hand, including every detail for each article is not needed. Keep in mind the overall purpose, and the clinical question. Add any general notes or personal observations about the study as comments.

Synthesis

Once all the evidence is retrieved, appraised, and entered into an evidence table, the evidence is synthesized. Synthesis of evidence is a process that pulls together the abstracted content to make a practice recommendation. This process begins with examining each piece of evidence again. Critically evaluate the evidence; determine if the population meets the population of interest, if the intervention studied is safe and is useful to practice, or whether the benefits outweigh the risks (DiCenso and Guyatt, 2005; Pearson, Field, and Jordan, 2007). If study findings are quantitative (for example, the rate of phlebitis), then results for each intervention can be compared for preciseness and significance. Many times the samples are not comparable and statistical comparison is not possible. However, consistent findings toward one intervention across many studies provide support for one intervention over another.

For a variety of study or evidence types, examine all of the results together as a whole; note if there is a theme, or intervention, that emerges. Determine the quality, quantity, and consistency of the evidence and how well it answers the clinical question (AHRQ, 2002). The most rigorous synthesis is based on evidence in a systematic review. Eventually, most nursing practices from assessment to intervention will be based on a synthesis from a systematic review of the body of evidence available at the time. New knowledge comes from individual studies as well as the synthesis of a body of evidence. Nurses from all areas of practice, including direct care, leadership, education, and research, need to conduct systematic reviews as part of their program of research in order to advance our science and identify the gaps in knowledge.

Practice recommendations

Based on the cumulative information in the evidence table and individual synthesis, practice recommendations can be developed. They take the form of a clinical statement, such as that from O'Grady et al (2002, p. 22): "Do not routinely replace CVCs, PICCs, hemodialysis catheters, or pulmonary artery catheters to prevent catheter-related infections. Category IB." (This statement then has a rating with it, such as Category IB, as in the previous example.) It is helpful if the rating titles are self-evident, such as those adopted by the GRADE Working Group (DiCenso and Guyatt, 2005), which include "Do it," "Don't do it," "Probably do it," and "Probably don't do it." These are extremely clear! Other self-evident recommendation rating titles include "Effective, Possibly effective, Not effective, and Possibly harmful" (Ackley et al, 2008) or "Level 1-Good,

TABLE 2-2 Evidence Table with Typical Column Headings for Study or Evidence Content

Citation/Country/ Quality of individual evidence	Type of evidence/ Study design	Research question/Purpose	Sample/Setting	Intervention	Results/Findings
Author (year) Country *Where study was conducted* Quality *Rating system for each study or individual article/evidence COMMENTS by the abstractor can be noted in any section. Use different print or color to note that comments are not from author of evidence*	Type of evidence *Meta-analysis, systematic review of randomized controlled trials (RCTs), single RCT, other type of study, practice guideline, expert opinion, internal data* Study design *if other type of study*	Research question *Or* Purpose of guideline/ expert opinion article	Who was studied or what group of individuals was included? Include age, gender, and ethnicity if applicable. Inclusion/exclusion criteria Sample size *Note if a power analysis was used to determine sample size; that is, size of sample that was statistically determined, thus allowing for strongest statistical analysis to be conducted with accuracy and reliability*	What intervention was done and with what was it compared? *Or* What intervention is recommended in the guideline or article? *Or* What was current practice that resulted in findings? *Or* What was focus for abstracting, such as risk assessment tool?	What are the results of the study? *Or* What are the expected results using the guideline? *Or* What is the result of current practice? *Or* Is an outcome measure recommended?

TABLE 2-3 Sample Evidence Table with Content from One Study Abstracted

Citation/Country/ Quality of individual evidence	Type of evidence/ study	Research question/ purpose	Sample/Setting	Intervention	Results/Findings
Lai (1998) United States Fair	Descriptive, correlational	Is the phlebitis rate lower for peripheral IVs left in place for 72 hours vs. those left in place for 96 hours?	2503 evalulatable peripheral IV lines; 80 IVs remained for 96 hours or more Adult Gender not provided Med-surg patients admitted to hospital Acute care teaching hospital; urban	Phlebitis tool described in paper; no other description or citation Peripheral IV lines were left in place beyond 72 hours if IV access needed for only 24 more hours or if patient had access problem *COMMENT Only 1 month studied. Not randomized. Tool not thoroughly described with reliability and validity. Small sample at 96 hours.*	Phlebitis rates for IVs left in for 72 hours vs. 96 hours were not significantly different: 3.3% vs. 2.6%, respectively, p = 1.000 by Fisher's exact test 215 IVs were removed at 72 hours per policy without signs of phlebitis *COMMENT Large sample overall, but small sample for 96-hour evaluation. Could change practice with proper QI monitoring. Benefit outweighs risk. Feasible to do: good for patient, lower cost.*

Level 2-Fair, and Level 3-Poor" (Pearson, Field, and Jordan, 2007).

In many published guidelines, the rating schema is in the beginning of the publication. For example, the CDC (O'Grady et al, 2002, p. 13) provides this statement immediately before its full set of recommendations:

... Each recommendation is categorized on the basis of existing scientific data, theoretical rationale, applicability, and economic impact. The...system for categorizing recommendations is as follows:

Category IA. *Strongly recommended for implementation and strongly supported by well-designed experimental, clinical, or epidemiologic studies.*

Category IB. *Strongly recommended for implementation and supported by some experimental, clinical, or epidemiologic studies, and a strong theoretical rationale.*

In the preceding example, at the end of the recommendation statement, there is the term Category IB. It is clearer to the reader now that the recommendation has a rating of "Category IB" and is supported by *some* studies and rationale. It can be surmised from this second level recommendation that further research is warranted.

Recommendations need to be effective, safe, ethical, efficient, and practical. Recommendations need to weigh the benefits against any possible harm. And benefits need to be evaluated against resources and costs for the patient, the population, and possibly the organization. A recommendation would be simple to make when there is a body of high-quality evidence; however, this is rarely the case. Because a synthesis is composed of evidence with varying quality and consistency, a recommendation may have varying levels of strength or force supporting it. The GRADE system contains a method to rate recommendations based on several factors, including evidence quality and patient considerations; its format helps with understanding what is recommended and what is its basis (Schünemann et al, 2008).

Just as with research design and evidence types, there is a system of evaluation for recommendations. One evaluation system is composed of three domains: quality, quantity, and consistency (AHRQ, 2002). It is this ongoing process of checks and balances to rate and then evaluate evidence and recommendations that provides for quality and safety in EBP. The rating system and evaluation mechanism that may be proposed for implementation in a practice setting need to be discussed with clinicians, researchers, administrators, and possibly patients, and may need to take into consideration the population and setting. Despite having a schema and a systematic method for evidence evaluation and synthesis, a practice recommendation is difficult because no one person or patient is the same as another. Thus the nurse and patient relationship is at the crux of EBP.

Integration into practice

It is important to have EBP recommendations readily available to the nurse when they are needed, in a manner that is easy to use. One of the most common ways to integrate evidence into practice is through the development of policies and procedures. Nursing policies and procedures help develop nursing practice. When built on evidence, nursing practice moves away from tradition to one that is research based. EBP is also built into standards of care that are created by specialty practice organizations, such as INS. Professional standards provide criteria for professional competence, thus protecting the patient in addition to the nurse (INS, 2006). The practice criteria established by INS are based on the best available evidence.

The integration of policies and procedures or professional standards into a computerized informatics system (CIS) can provide a nurse with quick access to clinical information when needed. As clinical decision support is built into a CIS, the nurse is provided with the current best evidence at the point of care. Clinical decision support can be as simple as calculating the dose of a needed medication. The nurse can also be provided with a link to information on a medication, such as how the medication is titrated and the recommended dose range. The clinical decision support can be integrated with decision reminders presented to the nurse based on a documented patient assessment. In this instance, the nurse may be presented with a reminder to start a care plan based on the patient's identified risk for a medication-related side effect (Lang et al, 2006). Finally, data from the practice recommendations need to be retrieved from the electronic health record and analyzed for the effectiveness of nursing actions based on the recommendation. This provides a feedback loop for evaluation and research of the recommendation.

CLINICIAN EXPERIENCE AND EXPERTISE

When research evidence is not readily available, or is nonexistent, clinical experience and expertise are used to answer a clinical question or solve a problem. Clinical experience builds knowledge and expertise through repeated observation and nursing practice with similar situations over time. It is through experience that a nurse is able to make the connection from one clinical condition to another. If a clinical experience has not previously been encountered, then support from other nurses and additional information are necessary to care for and support the patient (Benner and Leonard, 2005).

A nurse's knowledge needs to be based on more than tradition. Relying on tradition may produce more harm than good for the patient and the system. As a nurse acquires knowledge, based on experience, she or he develops a competence or expertise in a specific clinical area. Clinical expertise combines current patient data, past clinical experience, and personal knowledge (DiCenso, Guyatt, and Ciliska, 2005). Clinical expertise allows for self-reflection on practice along with personally analyzing a clinical situation. This includes evaluating the clinical situation that occurred, the part played in the clinical situation, the observed outcomes, and experiences reported by the patient. Self-reflection must also include an examination of one's personal beliefs, health care myths, and traditional practices that are not based on research. It is essential to the development of EBP that the health care environment supports this type of personal reflection, life-long learning, and questioning of tradition.

PATIENT BELIEFS, PREFERENCES, AND VALUES

Patient values and preferences play an important role in EBP. The patient must be included as part of the health care team to ensure that a treatment aligns with his or her values and preferences. The patient understands his or her body, social life, and response to previous experiences that are unfamiliar to health care members. A treatment option that works for one individual may not work for another because of personal beliefs. If the treatment does not match the patient preference or style, there is a greater possibility that the patient will not adhere to the treatment plan. A partnership approach between the nurse and patient allows the patient to determine if a structured treatment plan is preferred over a plan that allows for flexibility. The patient may prefer to have a treatment regimen closer to home rather than closer to work. A patient's ability to participate in health care decisions is based on many factors, which include willingness to participate, current health status, and personal support system. Based on these factors, the patient's ability to participate fluctuates, and as a result, the health care team must continually evaluate the treatment plan and adapt.

When health care providers develop a partnership relationship with the patient, an improvement in health outcomes is realized. The Joint Commission, the Agency for Healthcare Research and Quality, and the Institute of Medicine support involvement of the patient in the development of the health care plan and decision-making. For a long time, nursing has practiced patient and nurse partnerships within a caring and therapeutic relationship (McQueen, 2000). A partnership promotes sharing the responsibility and accountability for the planning, implementation, and evaluation of the intervention plan of care. As the patient builds knowledge about his or her health status, positive effects on health care costs are realized with increased prevention action and health promotion.

Additionally, individuals are becoming more educated about health conditions and treatment options from a variety of sources, such as books, magazines, newspapers, the Internet, friends, and relatives (Tu and Cohen, 2008). This has provided individuals with increased knowledge about health conditions, specific information to discuss with their health care team, and information on how to manage and maintain their overall health (Tu and Cohen, 2008). However, this information needs to be treated with caution since sources are not always credible. The health care team has a responsibility to evaluate the source of information and assist the patient to evaluate the source and content of all information.

An ethical conflict can develop for the health care team when a patient selects a treatment option, including no treatment, that does not correlate with the current best evidence for treatment, or the preference of the health care provider. To facilitate a fully informed decision, the patient must be provided with information on all the available treatment options with recommendations. The health care provider must present the information without bias so as not to persuade the patient to follow one treatment path over another (Sidani et al, 2006). Providing information only on known effective treatment options is one option to reduce the ethical conflict.

SITUATIONAL CONTEXT

Context is another factor to consider in relation to EBP. Context has been referred to as the setting in which evidence is implemented; this refers specifically to culture, leadership, and measurement (McCormack et al, 2002) as well as leadership roles, actions of the organization, institutional support, monitoring and feedback processes, and internal and external facilitation for change (Ellis et al, 2005). Context has been recognized as one of the core elements in implementing EBP.

Context should be considered not only in relation to implementation of EBP but also, more importantly, in relation to patient care. Aspects of each individual patient's situation may impact the care provided, such as access to family or community support, logistics of the home environment, ability to afford medications, literacy and comprehension, or other factors. The care environment is another contextual consideration as practice may change based on whether the patient is in a long-term care facility, urban teaching hospital, or small rural community hospital. In addition, this may affect any practice recommendation being considered, from the viewpoint of the patient, nurse, and setting.

 ## EBP AT THE POINT OF CARE: NURSE AND PATIENT

What begins as a nurse questioning usual practice, or reading a recent journal article, or wanting to find out more about a new intervention, can lead to the development of a practice recommendation that is based on the best evidence. Organizationally, it is crucial that the practice recommendation, based on evidence, be brought to the nurse at the point of care. As previously stated, this can be done in a number of ways, through the use of policies, procedures, professional standards, protocols, care plans, and computerized clinical decision support. The patient benefits from quality outcomes when the best evidence is brought to the nurse. It is not enough that the nurse carries

out the practice recommendation; the nurse must determine with the patient if the practice recommendation is appropriate for the patient at that point in time. For example, when considering the type of dressing to use on a tunneled CVAD when the patient is discharged home, the nurse must consider many factors. This might include the cost of the dressing, how often the dressing must be changed, the location of the catheter, and whether the patient needs assistance. If assistance is needed, who is available and how often that person is available are all questions that must be discussed. Practicing in partnership with the patient and using best evidence at the point of care provide an optimal experience to promote recovery and meet the outcomes for patient preference, safety, professional accountability, and organizational quality.

 ## MODELS OF EBP

A variety of models have been developed to promote EBP or integrate research findings into practice. These models range in detail from specific algorithmic decision steps to conceptual components. Since EBP may involve a variety of nurses and disciplines in an organization, including staff nurses, clinical leaders, administrators, librarians, and researchers, it may be most productive to review, discuss, and agree as a group to adopt or adapt a published model or even develop a new model. Criteria on which to evaluate a model are helpful during discussions; sample criteria used by one nursing-shared governance group to make a decision are listed below:

- *Principles of EBP:* Integrate best research evidence with clinical expertise and patient preferences and values
- *Principles of ANA nursing research standard:* Integrate research findings into practice (ANA, 2004)
- Clarity
- Simplicity
- Nursing philosophy/nursing framework compatibility

A model serves many purposes. It is helpful in planning the steps for promoting EBP and in securing resources to achieve a change in infrastructure and culture, which is a priority for leaders (Melnyk et al, 2005). It guides the integration of best evidence into the systems of practice. A model will focus the educational efforts for nurses and other disciplines on the need to use the best evidence, how to evaluate evidence, and methods of integration of best evidence into practice. Additionally, the environment must be inclusive of patients' and families' beliefs, preferences, and values. A detailed model is an aid to a nurse who may be a novice in some parts of EBP, such as finding the evidence, or evaluating a guideline, or even in knowing where to start. Equally important, a model aids the process of evaluation: a nurse to evaluate the outcome of his or her care, the organization to evaluate the culture of EBP, and researchers to evaluate the implementation and effectiveness of best evidence. Several models of EBP are listed in Box 2-5 with their sources.

 ## EBP SUPPORT AND OPPORTUNITIES

Organizational support is identified as one area that is needed and frequently lacking, which in turn can prevent the incorporation of evidence-based findings into practice. Two nurse

Box 2-5 **MODELS OF EVIDENCE-BASED PRACTICE AND THEIR SOURCE**	
Model	**Sources**
ACE Star Model of Knowledge Transformation	Stevens (2004)
ARCC Model (Advancing Research & Clinical Practice Through Close Collaboration)	Fineout-Overholt et al (2005)
ASPAN EBP Model	Mamaril (2005)
Built on Kitson Model	Kitson et al (1998)
Evidence Based Multidisciplinary Practice Model	Goode and Piedalue (1999)
Framework for adopting evidence-based innovation in an organization	Dobbins et al (2005)
HHS Model for EBN Practice	Mohide and Coker (2005)
Iowa Model of EBP	Titler et al (2001)
JBI Model of Evidence-Based Health Care	Pearson et al (2007)
Johns Hopkins EBP Model	Newhouse et al (2005)
Knowledge-Based Nursing Initiative of ACW	Lang et al (2006)
Model for Change to EBP	Rosswurm and Larrabee (1999)
PARIHS Framework	Rycroft-Malone (2004)
PRISM (Practical, Robust Implementation, and Sustainability Model)	Feldstein and Glasgow (2008)
Stetler Model	Stetler (2001)
Trinity Model of EBP	Vratny and Shriver (2007)

all disciplines may need to be used, and team members from business, finance, and accounting to help with the cost-benefit analysis are useful. Infusion therapy practitioners work closely with infection preventionists, and certainly with product manufacturers. Consider expanding the EBP team to include staff nurses, administrators, a librarian, a financial analyst, and a patient. Many efforts are now including patients, such as Planetree (a program enabling patients to be active in their health care), and action research (a focused inquiry to improve quality or processes and frequently involving patients or consumers) among others (Eastwood, O'Connell, and Gardner, 2008).

SUMMARY

EBP extends beyond the clinical setting between nurse and patient. The disciplines of education, informatics, leadership, and management benefit from the principles of EBP and these in turn inform nursing practice (Fawcett and Garity, 2009; Finkelman and Kenner, 2007; Geibert, 2006; Levin and Feldman, 2006; Pipe and Caruso, 2008; Scott, 2006). In the broader definition, EBP means that, "to the greatest extent possible, the decisions that shape the health and health care of Americans—by patients, providers, payers, and policy makers alike—will be grounded on a reliable evidence base, will account appropriately for individual variation in patient needs, and will support the generation of new insights on clinical effectiveness" (IOM, 2007, p. 2).

REFERENCES

Ackley BJ, Ladwig GB, Swan BA et al: *Evidence-based nursing care guidelines: medical-surgical interventions*, St Louis, 2008, Mosby.

Agency for Healthcare Research and Quality (AHRQ): *Systems to rate the strength of scientific evidence* (AHRQ Pub No. 02-E016), Washington, DC, 2002, U.S. Department of Health and Human Services.

American Nurses Association (ANA): *Nursing's social policy statement*, ed 2, Silver Spring, Md, 2003, Author.

American Nurses Association (ANA): *Nursing: scope and standards of practice*, Washington, DC, 2004, Author.

Benner P, Leonard V: Patient concerns, choices, and clinical judgment in evidence-based practice, In Melnyk BM, Fineout-Overholt E, editors: *Evidence-based practice in nursing & healthcare: a guide to best practice*, (pp 163-182), Philadelphia, 2005, Lippincott Williams & Wilkins.

Boutron I, Moher D, Altman DG, CONSORT Group: Extending the CONSORT statement to randomized trials of nonpharmacologic treatment: explanation and elaboration, *Ann Int Med* 48:295-309, 2008.

Burns N, Grove S: *The practice of nursing research: conduct, critique, and utilization*, ed 5, St Louis, 2005, Saunders.

Collins S, Voth T, DiCenso A et al: Finding the evidence. In DiCenso A, Guyatt G, Ciliska D, editors: *Evidence-based nursing: a guide to clinical practice*, (pp 20-43), St Louis, 2005, Mosby.

Cummings G, Estabrooks C, Midodzi W et al: Influence of organizational characteristics and context on research utilization, *Nurs Res* 56(4S), S24-S39, 2007.

Dee C: Making the most of nursing's electronic resources, *Am J Nurs* 105(9):79-85, 2005.

DeWalt DA, Berkman ND, Sheridan S et al: Literacy and health outcomes: a systematic review of the literature, *J Gen Int Med* 19:1228-39, 2004.

DiCenso A, Guyatt G: Interpreting levels of evidence and grades of health care recommendations. In DiCenso A, Guyatt G, Ciliska D, editors: *Evidence-based nursing: a guide to clinical practice* (pp 508-525), St Louis, 2005, Mosby.

surveys and a national summit found that lack of support at the organizational and managerial levels is an identified barrier to the implementation of EBP in clinical practice (Estabrooks et al, 2007; Fink, Thompson, and Bonnes, 2005; Melnyk et al, 2005). However, transformational and passionate leaders with knowledgeable and enthusiastic nurses can transform a culture into one of EBP. Facilitators of EBP include champions, clinical and academic partnerships, and clearly written research reports (Melnyk et al, 2005).

A culture and leadership that supports EBP comes from a learning organization and will increase research utilization and staff development, and decrease rates of adverse events for nurses and patients (Cummings et al, 2007; Rycroft-Malone, 2004). A variety of resources are needed for an EBP environment. However, with more cost analysis of EBP outcomes (including cost-benefit and cost avoidance) and more validated downstream effects (such as recruitment, retention, and staff satisfaction), organizational support may be more enthusiastic and forthcoming. Some studies have documented reduced cost through integration of EBP (Goode and Piedalue, 1999; Goode et al, 2000); therefore obtaining additional resources to support EBP may be cost neutral. The current health care environment requires creativity, both in the innovation of process and intervention and also in staffing and resources.

EBP should be an interdisciplinary effort in many clinical situations. All disciplines can be part of the team, literature from

DiCenso A, Guyatt G, Ciliska D: *Evidence-based nursing: a guide to clinical practice*, St Louis, 2005, Mosby.

Dobbins M, Ciliska D, Estabrooks C et al, Changing nursing practice in an organization, In DiCenso A, Guyatt G, Ciliska D, editors: *Evidence-based nursing: a guide to clinical practice*, (pp 172-200), St Louis, 2005, Mosby.

Eastwood GM, O'Connell B, Gardner A: Selecting the right integration of research into practice strategy, *J Nurs Care Quality* 23(3):258-264, 2008.

Ebell M, Siwek J, Weiss B et al: Strength of recommendation taxonomy (SORT): a patient-centered approach to grading evidence in the medical literature, *J Am Board Family Pract* 17:59-67, 2004.

Ellis I, Howard P, Larson A et al: From workshop to work practice: an exploration of context and facilitation in the development of evidence-based practice, *Worldviews Evidence-Based Nurs* 2(2):84-93, 2005.

Estabrooks C, Midodzi W, Cummings G et al: Predicting research use in nursing organizations, *Nursing Research, 56*(4S), S7-S23, 2007.

Evans D: Hierarchy of evidence: a framework for ranking evidence evaluating healthcare interventions, *J Clin Nurs* 12:77-84, 2003.

Fawcett J, Garity J: *Evaluating research for evidence-based nursing practice*, Philadelphia, Pa, 2009, FA Davis.

Feldstein AC, Glasgow RE: A practical, robust implementation and sustainability model (PRISM) for integrating research findings into practice, *Joint Commission J Qual Patient Safety* 34:228-43, 2008.

Fineout-Overholt E, Melnyk BM, Schultz A: Transforming health care from the inside out: advancing evidence-based practice in the 21st century, *J Profess Nurs* 21(6):335-344, 2005.

Fink R, Thompson C, Bonnes D: Overcoming barriers and promoting the use of research in practice, *JONA, 35*(3), 121-129, 2005.

Finkelman A, Kenner C: *Teaching IOM: implications of the IOM reports for nursing education*, Silver Spring, Md, 2007, American Nurses Association.

Geibert RC: The journey to evidence: managing the information infrastructure. In Malloch K, Porter-O'Grady T, editors: *Introduction to evidence-based practice in nursing and health care* (pp 125-148), Boston, 2006, Jones and Bartlett.

Giacomini M, Cook D: Qualitative research. In Guyatt G, Rennie D, Meade M et al, editors: *Users' guides to the medical literature: a manual for evidence-based clinical practice*, ed 2 (pp 341-360), New York, 2008, McGraw Hill Medical.

Goode CJ, Piedalue F: Evidence-based clinical practice, *J Nurs Admin* 29(6):15-21, 1999.

Goode CJ, Tanaka DJ, Krugman M et al: Outcomes from use of an evidence-based practice guideline, *Nurs Economics* 18(4):202-207, 2000.

Goode C, Titler M, Rakel B et al: A meta-analysis of effects of heparin flush and saline flush: quality and cost implications, *Nurs Res* 40:324-330, 1991.

Guyatt G, Jaeschke R, Prasad K et al: Summarizing the evidence. In Guyatt G, Rennie D, Meade M et al, editors: *Users' guides to the medical literature: a manual for evidence-based clinical practice*, ed 2, (pp 523-542), New York, 2008, McGraw Hill Medical.

Hasseler M: Evidence-based nursing for practice and science. In Kim HS, Kollak I, editors: *Nursing theories: conceptual and philosophical foundations*, ed 2, (pp 215-235), New York, 2006, Springer.

Hook M, Devine E, Lang N: Using a computerized fall risk assessment process to tailor interventions in acute care. In Henriksen K, Battles JB, Keyes MA et al editors: *Advances in patient safety: new directions and alternative approaches, Vol 1. Assessment* (AHRQ Pub No. 08-0034-1), Rockville, Md, 2008, Agency for Healthcare Research and Quality.

Infusion Nurses Society: Infusion nursing standards of practice, *J Infus Nurs* 29(1 suppl):S1-S92, 2006.

Institute of Medicine (IOM): *Crossing the quality chasm: a new health system for the 21st century*, Washington, DC, 2001, The National Academies Press.

Institute of Medicine (IOM): *The learning healthcare system: workshop summary*, Washington, DC, 2007, The National Academies Press.

Kitson A, Harvey G, McCormack B: Enabling the implementation of evidenced-based practice: a conceptual framework, *Qual Health Care* 7(3):149-158, 1998.

Lai KK: Safety of prolonging peripheral cannula and IV tubing use from 72 hours to 96 hours, *Am J Infect Control* 26:66-70, 1998.

Lang NM, Hook ML, Akre ME et al: Translating knowledge-based nursing into referential and executable applications in an intelligent clinical information system. In Weaver CA, Delaney CW, Weber P et al, editors: *Nursing and informatics for the 21st century: an international look at practice, trends and the future* (pp 291-303), Chicago, 2006, HIMSS.

Levin RF, Feldman HR, editors: *Teaching evidence-based practice in nursing: a guide for academic and clinical settings*, New York, 2006, Springer.

Mamaril ME: ASPAN's evidence-based practice model—introduction of ASPAN's evidence-based practice model, *J PeriAnesthes Nurs* 20: 236-238, 2005.

McCormack B, Kitson A, Harvey G et al: Getting evidence into practice: the meaning of 'context,' *J Adv Nurs* 38(1):94-104, 2002.

McQueen A: Nurse-patient relationships and partnership in hospital care, *J Clin Nurs* 9:723-731, 2000.

Melnyk BM, Fineout-Overholt E: Making the case for evidence-based practice. In Melnyk BM, Fineout-Overholt E, editors: *Evidence-based practice in nursing & healthcare: a guide to best practice* (pp 3-24), Philadelphia, 2005, Lippincott Williams & Wilkins.

Melnyk BM, Fineout-Overholt E, Stetler C et al: Outcomes and implementation strategies from the first US Evidence-Based Practice Leadership Summit, *Worldviews Evidence-Based Nurs* 2:113-121, 2005.

Mohide EA, Coker E: Toward clinical scholarship: promoting evidence-based practice in the clinical setting, *J Profess Nurs* 21(6):372-379, 2005.

Newhouse R et al: Evidence-based practice: a practical approach to implementation, *J Nurs Admin* 35(1):35-40, 2005.

Nollan R, Fineout-Overholt E, Stephenson P: Asking compelling clinical questions. In Melnyk BM, Fineout-Overholt E, editors: *Evidence-based practice in nursing & healthcare: a guide to best practice* (pp 25-37), Philadelphia, 2005, Lippincott Williams & Wilkins.

O'Grady NP, Alexander M, Dellinger EP et al: Guidelines for the prevention of intravascular catheter-related infections, *Morbid Mortal Weekly Rep* 51(RR-10):1-26, 2002. Erratum for Appendix B, *MMWR* 51(32), 711.

O'Neill ES, Dluhy NM, Hansen AS et al: Coupling the N-CODES system with actual nurse decision-making, *CIN: Comput Informatics Nurs* 24(1):28-36, 2006.

Pearson A, Field J, Jordan Z: *Evidence-based clinical practice in nursing and health care: assimilating research, experience and expertise*, Malden, Mass, 2007, Blackwell.

Peterson F, Kirchhoff K: Analysis of the research about heparinized versus nonheparinized intravascular lines, *Heart Lung* 20:631-642, 1991.

Pipe TB, Caruso E: Leadership strategies: inspiring evidence-based practice at the individual, unit, and organizational levels, *J Nurs Care Quality* 23(3):265-271, 2008.

Rosswurm MA, Larrabee JH: A model for change to evidence-based practice, *Image* 31(4):317-322, 1999.

Rycroft-Malone J: The PARIHS framework—a framework for guiding the implementation of evidence-based practice, *J Nurs Care Qual* 19:297-304, 2004.

Schünemann HJ, Vist GE, Jaeschke R et al: Grading recommendations. In Guyatt G, Rennie D, Meade M et al, editors: *Users' guides to the medical literature: a manual for evidence-based clinical practice*, ed 2 (pp 679-701), New York, 2008, McGraw Hill Medical.

Scott KA: Managing variance through an evidence-based framework for safe and reliable health care. In Malloch K, Porter-O'Grady T, editors: *Introduction to evidence-based practice in nursing and health care* (pp 149-181), Boston, 2006, Jones and Bartlett.

Sidani S, Epstein D, Miranda J: Eliciting patient treatment preferences: a strategy to integrate evidence-based and patient-centered care, *Worldviews Evidence-Based Nurs* 3(3):116-123, 2006.

Stetler CB: Updating the Stetler Model of research utilization to facilitate evidence-based practice, *Nurs Outlook* 49(6):272-279, 2001.

Stevens KR: *ACE model of evidence-based practice: knowledge transformation*, 2004, Academic Center for Evidence-Based Practice. Accessed at www.acestar.uthscsa.edu.

Titler MG, Kleiber C, Steelman VJ et al: The Iowa model of evidence-based practice to promote quality care, *Crit Care Nurs Clin North Am* 13(4):497-509, 2001.

Tu HT, Cohen GR: *Striking jump in consumers seeking health care information—tracking report no. 20*, Washington, DC, 2008, Center for Studying Health System Change. Accessed at www.hschange.com.

Vratny A, Shriver D: A conceptual model for growing evidence-based practice, *Nurs Admin Quart* 31:162-170, 2007.

QUALITY MANAGEMENT

Grace P. Sierchio, RN, MSN, CRNI®, CPHQ

Quality management is an organizational culture committed to achieving excellence. It is not a singular activity or a singular department or project team. Instead, it is an ongoing set of processes that are the very "fabric" of an organization. The National Association of Healthcare Quality defines "total quality" as "an attitude, an orientation that permeates an entire organization, and the way that an organization performs internal and external business" (Claflin, 1998).

In health care, quality management seeks to improve customer outcomes by improving the processes of patient care. Many "models" or approaches to quality management exist. New conceptual models are developed and new tools and methodologies wax and wane in popularity. In the end, they all strive to achieve the same goal: they seek to improve customer satisfaction and outcomes by producing products or services that are consistent, reliable, free of defects, safe, and effective. They also seek to improve the operational and financial health of the organization by improving internal processes and minimizing cost while maximizing potential profitability.

When studying quality management, the reader must consider that the provision of a health care *service* to a patient is distinctly different from the manufacture of a health care *product*. The number of variables is greatly increased. As a result of patient condition, co-morbidities, and the complexity of health care programs, the process of producing a service for a patient is much less consistent and predictable than the production of a product for a patient. The ordering, planning, insertion, and monitoring of a peripherally inserted central catheter (PICC) are markedly different than the manufacture of the PICC.

With that said, the ultimate goal in the management of service quality is to reduce inconsistency, and to strive for achieving a "perfect" service, free of defects (errors) and resulting in the desired patient outcome without causing complication or harm.

Infusion nursing is a service. It is a service grounded in evidence-based professional nursing practice that seeks to contribute to the overall desired patient outcome. That outcome might be the consistent maintenance of a continuous subcutaneous infusion site so that pain is successfully treated, or the successful completion of chemotherapy resulting in health status improvement. It might be the successful initiation of home parenteral nutrition resulting in a return to an ideal body weight, or the successful completion of intravenous antibiotics resulting in the elimination of cellulitis. Whatever the ultimate patient goal might be, the infusion nurse's contribution is to provide services coordinated with other disciplines towards that goal. The infusion nurse's goal is to provide quality care (services) so that the patient can meet *his or her* goal.

An organization with a true quality management culture involves every discipline, organizational level, and department in the process of improvement. The infusion nurse must act as the advocate for patient outcomes and safety related to infusion equipment and therapies by actively participating in the process. The infusion nurse is the "SME" or "subject matter expert" when an improvement study or project involves infusion therapy. No one is better equipped and experienced to provide expertise in the improvement of infusion services.

This chapter seeks to educate the infusion nurse about common models and methods for quality management. It provides an overview of basic quality improvement techniques. Practitioners who are interested in learning more are encouraged to contact quality and health care related organizations, such as the National Association of Healthcare Quality (NAHQ), for additional information and resources.

Throughout this chapter, there are numerous references to The Joint Commission (TJC). Quality management requirements have always been part of TJC's accreditation process and TJC standards are one of several national and international benchmarks for quality in health care. There are a growing number of organizations that can accredit hospitals and alternative site organizations. All have standards related to the improvement of services. TJC standards are only one method of achieving improvement. However, since many hospitals and home care organizations maintain TJC accreditation, their quality improvement standards still serve as an industry standard, and their published guidelines for quality improvement will be described frequently in this chapter.

THE IMPETUS FOR CHANGE

It has been acknowledged that for decades the quality of health care in the United States has been greatly mismanaged. Patient morbidity and mortality continued to rise through the 1980s and 1990s, while at the same time the national expenditures for health care skyrocketed (Institute of Medicine, 2000). Health care industry leaders, reacting to adverse events occurring to patients in hospitals and in other health care settings, called for immediate research to determine the degree of our nation's health care quality crisis. In 2000 the Institute of Medicine (IOM) published the first of a set of groundbreaking papers entitled *To Err Is Human: Building a Safer Health System.* The study results provided a sober look at the overusage, underusage, and misusage of health care services in the United States. In 2001 the IOM published *Crossing the Quality Chasm: A New Health System for the 21st Century.* It described strategies that might be used to effectively "fix" what was perceived as a "broken" health care delivery system (Institute of Medicine, 2001). The Joint Commission's publication of its *Agenda for Change* drastically shifted the focus in accredited organizations from structural issues (e.g., written policies) to process and outcome consistency and included the development of accreditation standards mandating effective quality management programs (TJC, 1990). These papers created a ripple effect through the health care industry, resulting in increased attention being given to quality assurance and quality improvement. The publication of these documents proved to be a turning point in the history of health care quality in the United States.

DEFINING AND PERCEIVING QUALITY

While health care leaders agreed that quality needed to be improved, the concept of quality as it pertains to health care services remained difficult to define. *Quality* has been broadly described by many as the comprehensive positive outcome to a product. In health care, however, the service is multifaceted and multidimensional, which contributes to different perceptions of quality. Five patients and five clinicians might all be asked, "What is a high-quality venipuncture?" and you might receive seven different responses. Our perception of quality is frequently influenced by our own expectations of outcome, needs, prior experiences, and emotional and cognitive status at the time the question was asked. A precise definition of quality health care attempts to acknowledge these differences and includes the services delivered *and* their perceived value to the consumer (Figure 3-1).

PATIENT CARE

Quality of care has been described as the effective technical application of medical science to prevent, diagnose, treat, and cure disease. This is the simplest description of quality because it concentrates on the technical aspects of patient care. Theoretically, "care" is a product or process that can be observed, measured, tested, and controlled through statistical methodologies.

Any discussion of quality principles can become confusing since different organizations, authors, and quality improvement methods define and describe terms differently. This chapter

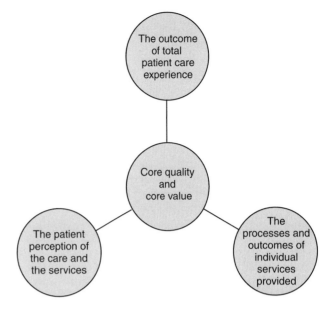

FIGURE 3-1 Elements of health care quality.

defines the term "patient care" as the total sum experience provided to a patient by the health care system. The system might be one facility (e.g., a hospital), or it might be coordinated home care organizations (e.g., a home care agency coordinating with a home infusion pharmacy). Patient care can include both services and products. It can include both products that are "consumed," such as dressing kits, and products that are durable medical equipment, such as an infusion pump. It can include educational, technical, and support processes. An example would be a patient that receives patient education about self-administering IV antibiotics, instructions concerning IV equipment and supplies; and financial counseling regarding the funding for the home infusion services.

Many departments, disciplines, and organizational "layers" contribute to the patient care provided. In the example in the previous paragraph, nurses, equipment managers, pharmacists, and delivery staff *each* contributed services and/or products that were part of the total patient care experience. Taking the example one step further, different layers of organizational structure contributed to the patient care. From the CEO that approved the purchase of new infusion pumps, to the project team that designed new patient education materials, to the first-line providers of care that packed and delivered the supplies, every layer of the organization contributed their "service" to the total patient care experience.

To measure the "quality" of patient care, the optimal method would somehow measure how the coordinated services of everyone involved resulted in the intended patient outcome and did not result in any complications or adverse event. Likewise, it would measure not only the clinical outcome but also the patient's perception of the total patient care experience.

It is significant to note that, since services provided by different departments or disciplines make up the total patient care experience, the failure by one service to deliver "quality" can influence the patient's perception of the whole experience. A classic example is the patient that is provided the most technologically advanced medical care by the most caring and professional staff, but that has a negative perception of the entire hospitalization experience because his or her food plate always arrives cold. It is the classic "weak link in the chain" concept.

PERCEIVED QUALITY OF SERVICES

As stated, multiple services make up "patient care." Each service provided by an individual clinician or department, in turn, has its own desired procedure outcome based on established practice standards and protocols or pathways developed by consensus.

When the infusion nurse provides a peripheral IV catheter insertion (service) to a patient, the intended outcome is to insert the catheter aseptically, on the first attempt, with minimal discomfort, in an appropriate catheter site. These procedure outcomes are based on researched and published performance standards for the specific procedure (service) provided.

Quality patient care is the major product delivered in health care, but *service* is the subjective aspect that influences the consumer's perception of quality. Each service provided must meet two basic goals to be successful. The service must be provided correctly in terms of the technical aspect, and the service must be provided in a way that leaves the patient with the sense that it was performed correctly, with professionalism and care. The nursing procedure may be technically correct, but the patient judges the care according to how the service was delivered. In the previous example, the nurse can insert the catheter, meeting all of the listed criteria (such as aseptic placement and first attempt, for example), but if done so in an unfriendly or brusque manner the patient's perception of the quality of that service will be influenced.

TJC refers to this as *patient perception of care*. Measuring patients' perceptions of the care they receive is an important component in the performance improvement program of any health care organization.

PERCEIVED VALUE OF SERVICES

Perception of "quality" and perception of "value" are intertwined but are different. "Value" is a function of the quality of the service *in relation to its cost*. Historically, patients might have been insulated from the cost of their health care because their health insurance provider paid the cost and the patient's portion was minimal or waived. In today's health care arena, patients are responsible for an increasingly larger portion of their health care costs. Because of larger deductibles, heftier co-payments, and a growing list of noncovered services and medications, consumers are becoming increasingly analytical about their health care options, the perceived value, and their out-of-pocket costs. Therefore consumers are now more conscious of the value of the care they receive, and they expect the highest caliber care in relation to the cost. Taking this concept a step further, the "customer" in today's health care is frequently not just the patient, but also the insurance company or payment source. Third-party payers that are accredited by the National Committee on Quality Assurance (NCQA) must maintain quality control and quality management standards. They, in turn, expect the same of the providers of care that bill for the services. This is the basis of managed care, which attempts to create a balance of acceptable value and a controlled cost of health care.

Governmental payers have spoken loudly in the past several years by establishing long awaited quality standards. The Centers for Medicare & Medicaid Services (CMS) published quality standards for Part B Suppliers in 2006. The document clearly demonstrates the government's dedication to controlling the cost of health care while, at the same time, assuring the quality of the care provided to Medicare beneficiaries. Specific standards within that document mandate the establishment of formal quality management programs that include mandatory third-party accreditation and patient outcome monitoring (Centers for Medicare & Medicaid Services, 2006).

"Pay for Performance" or (P-4-P in quality management terms) is another quality/value concept that is currently being studied by governmental payers and may some day be used by public and private sector payers of health care services in both hospitals and alternative settings. The concept of P-4-P is simply that providers of health care are reimbursed in accordance to how well they provide the care. Financial incentives are provided to organizations that achieve clinical and other benchmarks of performance (DeBoer, Iyenger, Dudhela, 2008). It is, basically, a patient outcome–based sliding scale for payments. Although at first this might seem bizarre, remember that health care in the United States is one of the few industries where a provider can bill and be entitled to payment even if the service was provided in an incorrect manner and resulted in poor outcomes and adverse events. Instinctively, we as an industry know this has to change. As part of the P-4-P concept the health care industry has taken on the mission of developing performance measures that can be used to compare the performance of one organization to that of another. To accurately and validly compare performance and establish the benchmarks, all organizations must collect the same performance measures in the same way. These measures are known as "core performance measures" (TJC, 2008d). Further discussion of core measures and performance measures follows later in this chapter.

LEADERS IN QUALITY MANAGEMENT

Three names often mentioned in discussions of quality are Juran, Crosby, and Deming. These leaders defined, refined, and popularized the concept of quality in the manufacturing world, but their teachings serve as the groundwork for the quality initiative in health care. These "thought" leaders were historically the founders of the quality movement in the United States as well as in other countries. Many new "thought" leaders have expanded upon their work in recent years, creating industrial and service models. Some of these new "thought" approaches to quality will be reviewed as well as the "foundation" theories.

J. M. JURAN

Dr. Juran was among the first to recognize that product quality requires careful planning, control, and improvement. These basic managerial processes are known as the *Juran trilogy*. Although his teachings were initially applied to Japanese business, Juran's principles of quality planning, quality control, and quality improvement have since been used in American industry (Juran, 1989).

Quality planning

Quality does not occur by accident; it is the result of meticulous preparation. The major aspects of planning are determining customer needs and developing products that meet those needs. The primary emphasis is on external customers, who are the end users of the product, but consideration must also be given to the internal customers, who assist in product development.

Quality control

The process of quality control requires that product performance be evaluated and compared with product goals, and that the differences between performance and goals be resolved. To achieve quality control, all employees must be accountable and make use of a feedback loop.

Quality improvement

Quality improvement requires organized change to attain unprecedented levels of performance. It represents a transition from little *q* (a narrow scope of quality limited to clients and products) to big Q (a broad concept of quality that defines *customers* as those who are affected and *products* as all goods and services). In addition, it exchanges the reactionary practices of "putting out fires" and "ready, fire, aim" for a proactive, systematic process that concentrates on improving all aspects of business. One of the best known methods for achieving quality improvement is by means of quality councils, also known as *quality circles*.

Juran's teachings regarding the involvement of every level of worker in the improvement process are carried forward today in many new models of quality management. It is a foundation of every successful quality system.

PHILIP B. CROSBY

Crosby is a management consultant who worked his way up through the ranks of business. He introduced the philosophy of "do it right the first time," which conveys his belief that quality is free; it is the nonquality products that cost money because they require rework. To explain the concept, Crosby used the phrase *zero defects*. This expression emphasizes that compliance with defined standards and specifications is necessary to achieve quality; poor quality is the result of lack of compliance and nonconformance. However, it was also Crosby's contention that conformance requirements must be based on input from the workers who produce the product (Crosby, 1979).

Most quality experts in health care agree that the concept of zero defect is not easily applicable to health care services. As stated earlier, providing health care services is, by its nature, very different from manufacturing a product. Although the latter can be controlled by specifications and procedures to the degree that a 100% perfection rate can be attained, the unpredictability of human physiology, psychology, and circumstances make this a challenge in health care, including infusion nursing.

However, "thought" leaders in health care have been reexamining some of Crosby's teachings and adapting them for use in health care. Six Sigma, a growing model for quality improvement in health care, is based on Crosby's foundational teachings and will be described later.

To place Crosby's teachings in the context of infusion nursing, we can use the example of a PICC insertion program. When planning the program, the team manager faced the decision of purchasing task lighting for the procedure rooms. She selected lighting (Lamp B) that was significantly less expensive than the recommended lamp (Lamp A). She perceived that Lamp B was a better value because it was 40% less expensive. When purchasing six lamps, the "savings" were significant. However, 4 months into the program the lamps began to fail, producing flickering during the procedures. The infusion nurses or their technical assistants frequently needed to interrupt the insertion to replace the lamp or reposition it to provide adequate light. In eight situations, the interruption required restarting the procedure with a new insertion kit. The team manager quickly realized that the "value" of the lamps was poor, and the rework needed to correct the problem cost more than the reduced lamp prices.

W. EDWARDS DEMING

Dr. Deming, the "guru" of quality, is best known for helping the Japanese achieve world-class quality in product manufacturing, but many American industries have since adopted his teachings. Like Crosby, Deming's philosophy of quality is based on the premise that problems with quality reside predominantly in an organization's systems and processes, not in its employees (Deming, 1989). Deming's strategy stresses continuous quality improvement and is based on the 14-point system for managing quality (Box 3-1).

Using our PICC program example to illustrate some of Deming's philosophy, the team manager, through quality control, detects that the incidence of unsuccessful first attempts is increasing. She evaluates the problem and sees that it is not limited to one particular nurse but to several. By meeting with the staff and using quality improvement methods (e.g., root cause analysis, brainstorming, and process mapping, to be described later), the team manager realizes that the increase is not due to nursing error, but is due to a combination of a recent change in PICC insertion kits (*materials*), poor task lighting (*materials*), and a change in how patients are positioned in the procedure chairs (*methods or procedures*).

BILL SMITH

Bill Smith is frequently referenced in quality management literature as a new thought leader in quality management. Bill Smith is considered to be the "Father of Six Sigma." Six Sigma is loosely based on the work of Crosby and the concept of "zero defect." Smith, who was the quality assurance director for the Land Mobile Products Sector of Motorola, developed this method of quality management. Its premise is that, through the proper control of variables and the consistent application of internal processes, you can limit the number of defects in the products you produce to less than 3.4 per 1 million opportunities. For example, you could manufacture 1 million IV catheters and less than 3.4 in the million would be defective. Six Sigma uses statistical models to measure and analyze defects. It is rapidly becoming one of the most commonly used quality management models in industries internationally (George et al, 2005; Gygi et al, 2005; Pande, Neuman, Cavanagh, 2000). Jack Welch (then the well-known and respected industry leader and CEO of General Electric) and others quickly recognized the potential value and profitability of using Six Sigma techniques and helped make them mainstream in industry. There are many authors and quality leaders who have examined how to adapt Six Sigma for health care, and many feel its use will grow in health care over the next decades.

Box 3-1   DEMING'S 14-POINT SYSTEM FOR MANAGING QUALITY

1. *Create consistency of purpose for product improvement.* The vision of the organization must be directed at continual refinement of the product. For an organization to become and remain competitive, there must be a strategy for achieving continuous improvement.
2. *Adopt the new philosophy.* Mistakes and negativism cannot be tolerated. Instead, the philosophy of the organization must be dedicated to improving quality.
3. *Cease dependence on inspection.* Quality is the result of improved production processes, not the identification of defective products. Prevention reduces the need for inspection to produce a quality product.
4. *Avoid awarding business on price alone.* If the concentration is on quarterly dividends alone, quality and productivity suffer.
5. *Constantly improve.* Quality improvement is a continual process, not a one-time activity. Improvement is the result of a never-ending pursuit to reduce waste and improve systems.
6. *Institute training.* Workers must be properly trained to perform effectively and efficiently. The organization must invest in training; failure to do so may be detrimental to survival of the organization.
7. *Institute leadership.* Management and leadership are different. Managers tell the worker what to do; leaders create a vision and guide the workers in achieving progressively improved outcomes.
8. *Drive out fear.* Fear inhibits innovation. If workers are fearful of expressing their ideas or asking questions, the job may continue to be done ineffectively or incorrectly.

9. *Break down barriers between staff areas.* Competition and rivalry between departments stem from conflicting goals. A unity in mission and promotion of teamwork within and among departments help identify opportunities for improvement.
10. *Eliminate slogans, extortions, and targets for workforce.* Quality is not a management-defined slogan and is not achieved by coercing workers to achieve optimal results. Workers must be involved in identifying methods to improve quality and determining how these expectations are communicated to others.
11. *Eliminate numerical quotas.* Quotas are counterproductive because they concentrate on numbers instead of processes that can be improved.
12. *Remove barriers to pride of workmanship.* Workers need to be empowered to have pride in the quality of their work. To accomplish this, the organization must eliminate barriers, such as defective materials, that hinder the quality of the product.
13. *Institute vigorous program of education.* Quality improvement activities require that both managers and workers be educated about statistical techniques and team-building exercises.
14. *Take action to achieve transformation.* All workers must be involved in the change from quality control to quality improvement. The change must be led by a dedicated team of those in top management who have established a precise plan of action to improve quality.

"14-Point System," from *Deming Management at Work* by Mary Walton, ©1990 by Mary Walton. Used by permission G.P Putnam's Sons, a division of Penguin Putnam, Inc.

FREDERICK WINSLOW TAYLOR

F. W. Taylor was a mechanical engineer. His contribution to quality management thought was the principle of increased efficiency and reduced waste through the use of standardized procedures. This concept of increasing both quality and profitability by using standards and by reducing waste was coined the "Efficiency Movement" (Carreira, 2005). It was adopted by industry leaders such as John D. Rockefeller and Henry Ford. Ultimately it served as a foundation for a current quality management philosophy known internally as "lean manufacturing."

Lean manufacturing has recently been popularized by the Toyota Motor Corporation through its use of the Toyota Product System (TPS). It emphasizes the improvement of the quality of a product through the most efficient manufacturing processes that emphasize standardization, minimal waste, and constant measurement and monitoring. Lean manufacturing principles are often connected to Six Sigma principles, creating a hybrid that is called "Lean Six Sigma."

INTERNATIONAL ORGANIZATION FOR STANDARDIZATION (ISO)

Lastly, a discussion of quality management history and theories would be incomplete without discussion of ISO standards. The International Organization for Standardization (ISO) is an international organization that publishes standards for a large scope of manufacturing and service industries. To become ISO registered, a company must apply the principles of ISO

standardization in the workplace, and use the standards to continually improve the products and services provided to its customers (Anton and Anton, 2006).

ISO 9000 and ISO 9001 registration are internationally accepted symbols of good quality management practices within a company. Throughout the world, ISO has been commonly used in manufacturing. Although a small number of health care organizations in the United States are ISO certified, the U.S. health care sector still has not fully embraced the use of ISO 9001 to improve patient care. However, its impact has been seen in improving products and equipment manufactured for patients.

NATIONAL ORGANIZATIONS AND ACCREDITING BODIES

The interest in improving health care in the United States and in controlling the escalating costs of health care has lead to a tremendous growth in the number, size, and activity of organizations and public and private institutions that aim to improve health care outcomes and efficiencies. Some aim to educate practitioners and consumers, while others aim to develop theories, strategies, and tools for quality management.

The Institute for Healthcare Improvement (IHI) is an example. IHI is an independent not-for-profit organization whose mission is to improve health care globally through research and education. This organization holds conferences that bring together some of the most progressive thought leaders in health care quality, and strives to teach organizations how to use quality improvement tools to improve outcomes while controlling costs. Additional information is available at www.ihi.org.

The National Quality Forum (NQF) is another highly active and visible organization in health care improvement. The NQF is a not-for-profit membership that seeks to improve outcomes, stabilize or reduce costs, and improve efficiencies in our health care industry. The NQF has also been very involved in the review and evaluation of core performance measures for various health care sectors, including home care. This organization was established as a public-private partnership organization. Its membership includes representatives from consumers, practitioners, employers/purchasers, labor unions, health care associated industries, and national, regional, and local health care organizations. Additional information is available at www.qualityforum.org.

The value of third-party accreditation was underscored in 2006 when the Centers for Medicare & Medicaid Services (CMS) established a mandatory requirement for accreditation in order to participate in the CMS Part B Supplier program (Centers for Medicare & Medicaid Services, 2006). This program provides payment for durable medical equipment for enrolled Medicare beneficiaries with Part B coverage. Included in Part B is reimbursement for infusion therapy pumps and other infusion-related devices. Organizations providing these products now must be accredited by a third-party accreditor that has been granted deemed status by CMS. Accreditors include The Joint Commission (TJC), Accreditation Commission for Health Care (ACHC), Community Healthcare Accreditation Program (CHAP), and others. The accrediting agencies work to develop meaningful patient care standards for health care organizations, as well as to educate practitioners and consumers regarding health care quality and effectiveness.

APPROACHES TO QUALITY MANAGEMENT

With the increasing emphasis on quality in health care, organizations have initiated programs to control, ensure, assess, improve, and manage quality. The leadership team will select a quality management model based on a variety of factors including cost, the availability of local expertise, and possibly the quality "trend" at the time. Regardless of which model of quality management is selected, the end result should be that the organization embraces methods that continually improve patient care. Defining some of the terms used is a challenge because of the different models. The same term might be used differently by two different quality management (QM) models. This section will offer typical definitions and descriptions of the various terms. The terms *quality control, quality assurance, quality assessment, continuous quality improvement,* and *total quality management* are not synonymous but may appear to "overlap," much like circles in a Venn diagram.

QUALITY CONTROL

Quality control (QC) is the evaluation of the production of a product or a service, by means of statistical methodologies. This approach consists of "on-line" inspection that compares a random sample of products with a predetermined, acceptable level of defects. Primary components of QC include data collection and statistical analysis of data. It was originally used for

the inspection of manufacturing equipment and manufactured products, and has been referred to as *statistical quality control.* Six Sigma, described earlier in this chapter, is based on the principles of quality control.

Using the PICC program example to illustrate quality control, two elements of the program can be reviewed. The first is the PICCs used, and the second is the average wait time for insertion (one product and one service). Quality control principles would take a random sampling of catheters from the assembly line and would test the internal diameter French size. The aggregate, or averaging of the French sizes for the sample of catheters, would be calculated and would yield statistics used by the factory's quality manager. Using quality control for the service component is similar. The PICC program for this large facility places 60 PICCs per day, and an average (statistical mean) of 280 per week. The acceptable standard set by the PICC team for an insertion wait time was 5.5 hours. The program's quality committee meets weekly and randomly audits 30 insertion records per week. The results show that the statistical average for the week was 4.3 hours. The quality circle discusses the results, evaluates that there is no need for further action, and documents the result on an ongoing trend chart.

The major disadvantages of QC are its emphasis on statistical methods and the "pass/fail" nature of the process. Data analysis should serve as the basis for decision making, but in quality control, there is a tendency for the statistical tools to become an end in themselves. Results are monitored and reported after goods or services have been produced, without emphasis on improving outcomes. In this case, the PICC team is happy with a wait time of 4.3 hours and no discussion ensues on how to, over time, gradually reduce the wait time to improve patient care.

Hence, this tool-oriented approach is being replaced by problem-oriented and results-oriented techniques (Juran, 1989).

QUALITY ASSURANCE

It was once assumed that most health care was of high quality, so the primary objective of "traditional" quality assurance was to ensure that the acceptable level of care was maintained. *Quality assurance* (QA) may be defined as the determination of the degree of excellence through monitoring and evaluation. Before the publication of the IOM reports, quality assurance typically meant retrospective chart reviews by a dedicated quality assurance staff member. The reviews focused on the documentation of certain specific aspects of care. "Thresholds" of compliance were arbitrarily set, and typically no activity was taken to move the threshold to improve quality. A PICC program at that time might have audited 10% of 3 months of charts to see if the catheter length was documented. A threshold of 95% would have been set, and the program would "pass" or "fail." In reality, what was being assessed was not the patient care, or even the specific PICC service, but instead the *documentation* of a particular element of a PICC insertion.

When the IOM reports were published, health care industry thought leaders accepted that a major change in how we manage quality must occur. The industry began to adopt components of the industrial models of quality management. During the transition, quality programs in health care progressed from quality assurance to quality improvement, and have now progressed towards total quality management in progressive organizations.

In 1990 TJC developed the *Agenda for Change,* which initiated the transition from QA to continuous quality improvement. The goal was to create outcome monitoring and evaluation processes to help organizations improve the quality of care provided (JCAHO, 1990). Consistent with this change, TJC began the paradigm shift by renaming their chapter on quality *Quality Assessment and Improvement.* TJC explained that the underlying rationale for the shift to assessing and improving quality was to overcome several weaknesses inherent in QA practices. First, QA is often focused solely on one specific aspect of a service provided by one particular department or discipline. It does not tend to focus on the total patient care experience. It does not reflect the interdisciplinary or cross-service nature of patient care, and the interrelated managerial, governance, support, and clinical processes that affect patient care outcomes. Each of these tendencies inhibits the organization's ability to improve processes and thus improve patient care outcomes. Table 3-1 highlights the differences between QA and quality improvement (QI).

The term *quality assurance* might still be used by individuals as a "trailing remnant of earlier days," but it does not accurately convey the intent of the current quality management paradigm. Quality cannot be ensured; it can only be assessed, managed, or improved.

QUALITY ASSESSMENT AND IMPROVEMENT

Changing from quality "assurance" to quality "improvement" was much more than a renaming of a hospital or home care department. It was a major paradigm shift in health care culture. Through the continued work of the Institute of Medicine and the creation of private and governmental work groups focused on changing quality management processes, the health care system has survived the paradigm shift. Although much more work needs to be done, it is commonly accepted among providers that organizations must always strive to improve quality in order for health care facilities to survive and thrive. The antiquated cliché of "If it ain't broke don't fix it" is rarely heard in health care today. Instead, what is heard is, "If it ain't broke, let's see how we can make sure it *never* breaks." To do so, the two steps of quality assessment and improvement methods must be used.

Quality assessment

Quality assessment is the first component of the two-step concept. It consists of data collection and data analysis. Quality assessment can be a highly complex process. It requires extensive planning and expertise to develop a successful quality assessment process. Many facilities hire professionals certified in health care quality as internal staff or as consultants to help design an assessment program. As discussed earlier in the chapter, because patient care is multifaceted, and because "quality" can be a very subjective term, quality assessment is challenging.

As nurses, there is an understanding of assessment; it is a basic component of the nursing process. Assessment requires observation and measurement of a problem or condition, and in quality assessment, the quality of care is observed and measured.

Imagine that the PICC program quality committee meets to discuss quality assessment. The question of whether or not absence of postinsertion phlebitis is a sign of a "quality" procedure is debated. Some felt it reflects more than just the performance of the team. It could be impacted by actions taken by the home care nurse or the medical unit staff. Patients with certain co-morbidities might be predisposed to phlebitis. After extensive debate, the group agreed to collect data on phlebitis. Discussion then ensued on which definition of phlebitis to use, and what severity or phlebitis rating would be considered a "defect" and counted. Further discussion (argument) ensued on what the appropriate time frame was for monitoring the site for phlebitis, and what to do if the patient had already been discharged to home. Ultimately, the team, with the help of the hospital's QI director, develops the phlebitis data collection including the procedure, sample size, rating scale, paper logs, and desired graphics display.

Quality improvement

Quality improvement is the process necessary to initiate corrective actions or seize opportunities to improve the effectiveness and efficacy of services through the ongoing monitoring and assessment of a performance measure. It is the second step of the QA/QI model. It is the step (or phase) during which action steps are planned and performed. A critical point is that improvement *cannot* occur without valid and reliable assessment. "One cannot manage what one cannot measure" is a common phrase used by quality managers. It is not appropriate for a quality committee or team to embark on an improvement study based on anecdotal stories or situations. In order for true improvement and quality management to occur, the level of quality must be assessed first. Once assessment has been completed, improvement can take place.

Imagine that the PICC program studies postinsertion mechanical phlebitis rates. Based on a 100% sample size monitored 48 hours postinsertion, the phlebitis rate was 24 PICCs out of 280 PICCs inserted, or 8.6%. The industry benchmark

TABLE 3-1 Quality Assurance versus Quality Improvement

Quality assurance	Quality improvement
Problem oriented	Results oriented
Focuses on inspection	Focuses on identification and correction
Uses "snapshot" data to evaluate performance	Uses "trend" data to identify appropriate areas for action
Focuses on negative aspects of care	Focuses on positive aspects of care
Monitors nursing tasks	Monitors patient processes and outcomes
Retrospective	Concurrent
Evaluates documentation	Evaluates care, services, and outcomes
Random monitoring	Planned, systematic monitoring
May be unrelated to standards	Based on standards and benchmarks
Fixed process	Dynamic process
Reactionary	Proactive
Responsibility of QA coordinator/ designee	Organization-wide commitment and involvement

found in the literature was 8.3%. (This is not an evidence-based statistic. Rather, it is a hypothetical statistic used for the purposes of this example.) The PICC team asks the QI director if a problem exists based on the data. By using statistical techniques, the QI director informs them that their slightly higher percentage is not statistically significant. In other words, they are within acceptable limits if only comparing to the benchmark.

However, the PICC team asks itself what it could do to lower the phlebitis rate the following month. Ideas are shared, strategies are planned and implemented, and over the course of the next 14 days changes are made in the postinsertion procedures. The only step remaining is to *assess* whether the steps taken lowered the phlebitis rate (improvement). To do so, the team used the same data collection study, and found the phlebitis rate decreased to 7.8%.

CONTINUOUS QUALITY IMPROVEMENT

We have described quality assessment and quality improvement (QA/QI), but what is *"continuous quality improvement"* (CQI)? CQI builds on the foundation of QA/QI. CQI broadens the focus from only the clinical aspects of care to all the facets of the organization that affect patient outcomes. It sometimes requires a change in management philosophy and organizational culture, because there must be a visible commitment to CQI for the process to be effective. Current Joint Commission standards emphasize that managers and leaders in the organization contribute to the process by establishing expectations, providing necessary resources, and fostering communication and coordination of activities (TJC, 2008a).

The scope of CQI is more extensive than the activities of quality assessment and improvement. CQI considers processes by determining how well they are performed, coordinated, and integrated and by developing strategies for further improvement; it recognizes both internal customers (all employees) and external customers (patients, physicians, third-party payers) and values their perceptions of the care and services delivered; and it promotes the pursuit of objective data to evaluate and improve patient outcomes. In other words, CQI includes a broad organizational assessment of the total patient care experience.

An essential characteristic of CQI is that it is a continuous process. Quality is not achieved and then discarded; quality is the result of long-term commitment to the ongoing evaluation and improvement of patient outcomes. CQI is based on the assumption that outcomes are never optimized but may be constantly improved.

Another distinctive feature of CQI is that it emphasizes improvement in the interdisciplinary processes involved in patient care delivery, not just individual activities. Applying this concept to infusion nursing requires that all factors contributing to the quality of care be examined. An example is the administration of IV medication. Steps involved in this process in the hospital setting include receipt of a prescription for the medication by the physician, transcription of the order on the nursing unit, preparation and delivery of the medication by the pharmacy, and administration of the scheduled dose(s) by the nurse. Coordination of these various steps affects the quality of the desired outcome, which is efficient and effective administration of IV medication. Therefore with CQI, monitoring IV medication administration entails all functions contributing to the actual nursing procedure.

PERFORMANCE IMPROVEMENT

TJC continues to influence how organizations design and implement quality management programs. As a result, terminology and theoretical models recommended by TJC have significant impact, much like the ripples on a pond's surface.

With the publication of their hospital and home care standards for 1999 and 2000, TJC introduced the term *performance improvement*. Its standards on quality referred to the "assessment and improvement of organizational *performance*" rather than on the assessment and improvement of *quality.*

Once again, the shift from "quality improvement" to "performance improvement" was not just *another* retitling of a hospital or home care company department. It was another shift in quality management philosophy. Although not as revolutionary as the shift from QA to QI, this shift focused on the difference between improving "quality" and improving "performance." One must first differentiate between the two. Earlier in the chapter "quality" was defined, including a description of how "quality" is difficult to assess because it is highly subjective. On the other hand, "performance" is much more discreet. It is a specific aspect of the patient's experience that can more clearly be defined, described, and measured.

Using the PICC team as an example, the overall "quality" of the program might be difficult to define and measure in a way that takes into consideration technical aspects as well as customer perceptions. However, the "performance" of the PICC team can be more easily measured. The number of PICCs inserted per day is measurable. The average wait time until insertion is measurable, and the incidence of infection per 1000 catheter days is measurable. One can see that performance, compared to quality, lends itself more easily to data collection and analysis.

The challenge facing hospitals and other providers of care is determining which discreet aspects of performance are most important. That is, which measurements of performance have the greatest ability to describe the overall patient care experience and which measurements have the ability to create the most positive improvements in patient care (Harrington and White, 2008)? Consensus groups continue to work diligently to determine what "core performance measures" should be collected and analyzed in every organization so that performance improvement can have the greatest impact.

Other than shifting the conceptual framework toward evaluating *performance* versus *quality,* the elements of assessment, analysis, improvement, and reassessment remain relatively unchanged from CQI. In addition, like CQI, performance improvement is leadership driven; crosses all key functional areas of an organization, including clinical, managerial, and support; and recognizes both internal and external customers.

TOTAL QUALITY MANAGEMENT

With the shift from QA to CQI and now performance improvement (PI), health care organizations have recognized that quality is not a fixed commodity defined by health care professionals but is a strategic mission that must be shared by the entire organization. As a result, several health care organizations have adopted a management system that fosters continuous improvement at all levels and for all functions by focusing on maximizing customer satisfaction. This system is aptly named *total quality management* (TQM).

Because TQM and CQI are based on the teachings of the quality gurus Deming, Crosby, and Juran, the two approaches to quality management share several characteristics. First, both programs are customer focused. The goal is to meet the expectations of internal and external customers. Second, continuous process improvement is stressed. A culture conducive to ongoing quality improvement is the critical link between customer requirements and outcomes. Last, and most important, there must be total organizational involvement. Those in top management must be committed to the program and provide a clear vision for the organization; employees must be empowered to participate actively in the quality improvement process.

Unlike CQI, TQM is not unique to health care. It has been successfully implemented as a strategic resource management system in various sectors of the service industry. Application of the system to health care has been prompted by the current regulated, cost-competitive environment of the health care industry. No longer can health care providers deliver merely *acceptable* care and services. Health care affects patients' lives, so any outcome that is less than optimal may have serious ramifications. Box 3-2 illustrates the effects of reducing quality by just one tenth of 1%.

There are several distinctive characteristics of TQM. First, TQM contributes to a positive work environment by emphasizing horizontal cross-functional coordination and vertical integration. The clinical, managerial, and support staffs within the organization function as an interconnected network linked laterally, over time, in a collaborative culture. This is in contrast to the typical functional hierarchy in which the organization is a loose collection of separate individuals or departments. Second, TQM fosters collaboration by recognizing the underlying psychosocial principles affecting individuals and groups within the organization. There is a natural tendency for individuals to make judgments based on biases, but through careful and continual training, TQM overcomes these biases and creates an environment of trust. Third, TQM promotes teamwork as a means to break down barriers to communication and enhance interdepartmental collaboration. Active involvement and cooperation within the organization create a common bond among team members by encouraging them to reach consensus on goals and collaborate on solutions.

To realize total quality as a strategic management vision, the costs of quality versus the costs of not supporting quality must be acknowledged. The costs of not supporting quality have been depicted as an iceberg. Above the surface are the visible costs

---

Box 3-2 EXAMPLES OF LESS THAN 99.9% QUALITY

- 2 million documents will be lost by the IRS this year.
- 22,000 checks will be deducted from the wrong bank accounts in the next hour.
- 12 babies will be given to the wrong parents each day.
- 2 plane landings daily at O'Hare International Airport in Chicago will be unsafe.
- 292 pacemaker operations will be performed incorrectly this year.
- 268,500 defective tires will be shipped this year.
- 20,000 incorrect drug prescriptions will be written in the next 12 months.
- 5,517,200 cases of soft drinks produced in the next 12 months will be flatter than a bad tire.
- 107 incorrect medical procedures will be performed by the end of the day today.

(e.g., patient complaints, repeat work, loss of revenue because of customer dissatisfaction); the less obvious but larger costs (e.g., excessive employee turnover, lack of teamwork) are hidden below the surface. Applying the principles of TQM helps uncover and eliminate these hidden costs. The visible costs of quality (e.g., quality management team expenses) may then be deemed as either necessary or avoidable so that unnecessary expenditures are reduced.

TQM is also effective because it strengthens the customer-supplier chain. All employees are customers *and* suppliers, linked in a chain that runs through the organization to the ultimate, external customer. Alignment and execution determine the strength of the chain. *Alignment* is defined as "doing the right thing," whereas *execution* is "doing the thing right." When both alignment and execution are achieved throughout the chain, "right things are done right."

As an integrated internal management system, TQM focuses on organizational improvement. The system is broader than the clinical aspects of infusion nursing, but an organizational culture fostered by TQM facilitates improvements necessary to deliver quality infusion nursing care.

Six Sigma and lean manufacturing are examples of TQM models. Both work by integrating the organization down the chain of command as well as across department lines. Six Sigma is focused on eliminating variations completely so that defects cannot occur (Gygi, DeCarlo, Williams, 2005). An example would be the use of a written standard procedure for setting up a PICC insertion tray 100% of the time, leading to a decreased chance of accidental contamination of the sterile field. Lean manufacturing is focused on the reduction of waste and rework by using standardized procedures (Sayer and Williams, 2007). An example would be the design of a customized PICC insertion tray containing only the supplies used for that team's insertion procedure, resulting in a lower priced insertion tray and no waste of unused supplies. In both examples, one sees that a critical element is the use of standardized procedures. This leads into the following section on standards of practice.

 ## STANDARDS: STATEMENTS OF EXPECTED QUALITY

Effective quality management is based on well-defined statements of quality. The statements are the criteria by which the levels of excellence are established and are a basis for quality assessment, evaluation, and improvement. However, establishing statements of quality in health care is a complex process. The delivery of patient care services does not result in a tangible product; the service is consumed as it is delivered. Traditional technical quality-of-conformance measures are therefore ineffective unless they are combined with behavioral norms that describe how the service is to be provided and criteria that outline the intended results of care.

Statements of quality that integrate the technical features, behavioral aspects, and desired outcomes of health care are known as *standards*. Standards represent the levels of excellence agreed upon by a consensus expert group. They do not necessarily depict the optimal level of achievement (known as "best practice standards") but refer to the levels of achievement that are acceptable based on the realistic availability of resources and the current state of knowledge. Discrepancies between best practice and acceptable levels of performance provide incentive for continual improvement. As a result, standards are dynamic and reflect progressively higher levels of acceptable achievement in the continual refinement of quality patient care.

TYPES OF STANDARDS BY DOMAINS OF CARE

Standards determine whether the delivery of health care services is properly established, implemented, and evaluated. *Properly established* implies that the organization has put in place infrastructure to support the acceptable levels of achievement. This could include equipment, physical environment design, written procedures, and adequate staffing. *Properly implemented* implies that the staff of the organization uses the infrastructure to provide the services in a way that is described in standard procedures. This could include the insertion of a peripheral catheter by a properly educated nurse according to an established procedure using appropriate equipment. *Properly evaluated* implies that the organization measures the outcome of the care provided. Hence, standards can be divided according to patient care structures, processes, or outcomes.

Structure standards

Structure standards refer to the conditions and mechanisms that provide support for the actual provision of care. They are the framework that facilitates patient care by defining the rules of the organization and its governance. Examples of structure standards are the mission, philosophy, and goals of the organization, which serve as a foundation for the commitment to quality.

Policies are a critical component of structure. They are the established rules that guide the organization in the delivery of patient care. A unique characteristic of policies is that they are not negotiable. This means that under no circumstances may a policy be modified unless it undergoes an official review and revision procedure. If an organization's policy specifies that only registered nurses are permitted to administer IV medications, a licensed practical nurse may not perform the procedure. Very rarely are staff members permitted to deviate from written policy; deviation is typically limited to situations where the written policy could cause harm because of a unique patient situation.

Process standards

Process standards have been described as "working" standards because they describe the functions performed by health care providers in the delivery of patient care. Structure standards specify what must be done, but process standards describe how it is done. As such, process standards focus on the practitioner and include job descriptions, performance standards, procedures, practice guidelines, protocols, and critical pathways.

A *job description* or *job summary* is a written record of the job qualifications, scope of responsibilities, and principal duties. It is a generic instrument that describes the basic functions of the position. *Performance standards* evolve from the job description and define the level of performance required for the job. For example, the job description for an infusion nurse may state that a basic function is the performance of venipuncture, but the performance criteria specify that the infusion nurse must adhere to aseptic technique, follow established policies and procedures, and demonstrate proficiency in the insertion of peripheral IV catheters. Some organizations carry the concept of performance standards further by specifying the expected performance standard data. For example, the performance standard might state that the nurse successfully inserts peripheral catheters on the first attempt a minimum of 92% of the time.

Procedures involve psychomotor skills performed by health care providers in the delivery of patient care. Written procedures contain a series of precise steps that outline the recommended manner in which the skills should be performed.

Practice guidelines are used by organizations to help make clinical care decisions based on the current state of knowledge about a specific disease state or therapy. For example, a hospital may use practice guidelines for the use of narcotic analgesics in oncology pain treatment. Nursing practice guidelines are based on the nursing process and can assist with decision making in the delivery of nursing services.

Protocols complement procedures and practice guidelines because they provide a basis for clinical decision making in specific patient care issues. For example, the infusion nurse follows the written procedure and practice guidelines for the performance of venipuncture. The practice guidelines might suggest that based on the patient's age and condition an intradermal injection of lidocaine as a local anesthetic is recommended. The infusion nurse might then follow a protocol for the combination of sodium bicarbonate with lidocaine, the drug concentration and dosing, and the administration of the anesthetic.

Critical pathways are a hybrid of a practice guideline, a protocol, and a data collection tool to measure process compliance and outcome. Critical pathways are used by many industries to "map" the critical steps along a process that *must* occur in order for the expected or desired outcome to occur. Critical pathways, when used in health care and nursing practice, are known as "clinical pathways." Clinical pathways typically list interventions required by different health team members in a day by day timeline. The value of pathways is their ability to coordinate the interventions of more than one discipline, and their ability to detect when one particular patient's process veers "off course" from the pathway. This "variance" can be studied and evaluated to determine what must be done for that patient to meet the desired outcome of care. Variance data are collected and evaluated by quality management professionals to improve the process within the organization (TJC, 2008b).

Although structure standards are not negotiable, process standards may be modified based on the decision of the practitioner and as the situation demands. For example, a written process standard specifies that insertion sites are to be prepared with chlorhexidine solution before venipuncture. However, one patient is allergic to the agent. In that situation, alcohol or povidone-iodine may be substituted to prepare the intended venipuncture site.

Outcome standards

Outcome standards are statements of the intended end results of patient care. They are patient focused and reflect the desired goals of the care provided. Historically, outcome standards have been expressed in negative terms such as *mortality rates, infection rates, phlebitis rates,* and *medication errors.* Although it is important to monitor the incidence of these potential adverse events, other more positive patient outcomes can be expressed as standards. Statements such as *patient satisfaction, resolution of infection, control of pain, prevention of rehospitalization, and maintenance of desired nutritional status* better communicate the ultimate goal of patient care.

Because the outcome of care is typically a consequence of how the care was delivered, outcome standards are linked to at least one process standard. For every process standard, there is at least one associated outcome; the process influences or determines the results to be achieved. For example, the process of "proper skin antisepsis prior to venipuncture" is linked to the outcome of "absence of infection."

TYPES OF STANDARDS BY DOMAINS OF ORGANIZATIONAL STRUCTURE

Another way to look at the division of standards is by domain. Patient care services can encompass three domains: the organization leadership, the practitioner (health care professional), and the patient/consumer. In the previous section, there was a discussion of how each of these domains was linked to a type of standard. Leadership was linked to structural standards, practitioners were linked to process standards, and the patient was linked to outcome standards.

In this section, another set of terminology is used that more appropriately describes the statements of quality in health care in these three domains. They are (respectively) *standards of governance, standards of practice,* and *standards of care.*

Standards of governance

TJC is placing greater emphasis on the role of the health care organization's leaders in providing the necessary support and resources to improve patient care. Such expectations and responsibilities of managers and other key leaders can be established by means of standards of governance. Likewise, ISO standards mandate that the organization's processes be "transparent" from the very top of the leadership hierarchy through every level of the organization so that deficiencies or variances from the standard operating procedure can be detected rapidly and acted upon immediately. Standards of governance define the administrative domain and establish parameters to measure the levels of excellence in leadership. An example of a standard of governance is the statement, "Organizational leaders will provide an environment that fosters the highest quality of patient care and employee satisfaction." All models of TQM and CQI mandate that standards of governance be clearly defined and written, and that those standards support the continual improvement of internal processes.

Standards of practice

Standards of practice focus on the provider of care and clearly state the acceptable levels of practice in patient care delivery. Practice standards address the clinical aspects of patient care services that are linked to patient outcomes. However, standards of nursing practice define nursing accountability and provide a framework for evaluating professional competency in the delivery of patient care services. They are consistent with valid research findings, national norms, and legal guidelines, and they complement expectations of regulatory agencies. In Table 3-2, fundamental aspects of infusion therapy are written as both standards of care and standards of practice.

Based on the premise that nurses, individually and collectively, are responsible and accountable for their practice, professional nursing associations have researched, developed, and published standards of nursing practice. These standardized statements reflect commitment to quality patient care and

include generic *and* specialty standards of practice. Generic standards, such as the *Standards of Nursing Practice* from the American Nurses Association, are universal for all types of nursing; specialty standards are applicable to a specific area of practice, such as the *Infusion Nursing Standards of Practice* (Infusion Nurses Society, 2006).

Because published standards of nursing practice define criteria relative to nursing accountability and professional competency, they may be adopted by health care organizations. This differs from standards of care, which must be developed and individualized by the organization in which the care is delivered. For example, the *Infusion Nursing Standards of Practice* defines the autonomy, accountability, and requirements of the specialty practice of infusion nursing and are applicable to all practice settings where infusion therapy is delivered (Infusion Nurses Society, 2006). Box 3-3 is an example of the standard of practice for hand hygiene as presented in the 2006 revision of *Infusion Nursing Standards of Practice* (Infusion Nurses Society, 2006).

Standards of care

The consumer of care, the patient, is the focus of the standards of care. Standards of care are statements of the expected patient care experience or outcome. To measure quality based on expectations, TJC has indicated that standards of care must be developed within the organization. The standards either may be generic, addressing patient care throughout the organization, or may be specific to the care delivered in or by a specialty area (TJC, 2008a). For example, a generic standard of care might state, "the patient will remain free of hospital acquired infection"; a specific standard of care, relative to infusion nursing, further stipulates that "patients will remain free of hospital acquired blood stream infection associated with the PICC."

 ## METHODS OF MEASURING PERFORMANCE

In the past, literature written about the QA model described the use of *indicators* as statements of performance that are measured and monitored to see whether the organization met predetermined goals. The term *indicator* is used less often today, and instead performance improvement teams refer to *performance measures.* Measures are numerical (statistical) representations of one aspect of care or an outcome of care that has been evaluated.

Performance improvement cannot occur without the ability to measure current performance. How can a hospital's leadership know improvement is necessary if they cannot measure performance? In addition, most areas of performance should be monitored over time, looking at the trends and patterns in the performance rather than basing improvement on a single "snapshot." A mistake frequently made in the past, particularly by inexperienced leadership teams, was to create improvement studies and projects based on specific isolated adverse events. Tremendous resources have been spent studying and improving services without careful evaluation of the scale and magnitude of the problem. The result is frequently a short-term, nonsustainable improvement aimed at fixing a specific situation and not an organizational process (Harrington and White, 2008).

Today's accreditation standards demand the use of more complex statistical methods than in the past. Likewise, TQM models are based on the use of statistical techniques to properly

TABLE 3-2 **Examples of Standards of Care and Standards of Practice Regarding Fundamental Aspects of Infusion Therapy**

Aspect of care	Standard of care	Standard of practice
Care plan or clinical pathway	Patient has health care needs identified.	Care plan is established within 24 hours of completion of initial patient assessment.
Initiation of infusion	Patient has infusion initiated for therapeutic or diagnostic purpose.	Therapy is initiated on physician's order using the nursing process.
Catheter site preparation	Patient is free of infection related to infusion therapy.	Peripheral insertion site is aseptically cleansed with antimicrobial solution before catheter insertion.
Monitoring infusions	Patient receives infusions at prescribed flow rate.	Patient assessments are performed at routine intervals and as required during the infusion.
Disposal of sharps	Patient is safe from preventable hazards in the environment.	Needles and stylets are disposed in nonpermeable, puncture-resistant, tamper-proof containers.
Patient education	Patient has the right to receive information on all aspects of care.	Patient is informed of each treatment in clear, concise terminology.

Box 3-3   STANDARD OF PRACTICE FOR HAND HYGIENE

STANDARD

- Hand hygiene shall be performed before and immediately after all clinical procedures and before donning and after removal of gloves.
- The nurse shall not wear artificial nails or nail products when performing infusion therapy procedures.
- In cases where the nurse's hands are visibly contaminated with blood or body fluids, hand hygiene with either nonantiseptic or antiseptic (preferably antiseptic-containing) liquid soap and water shall be performed.

PRACTICE CRITERIA

- Hand hygiene should be a routine practice established in organizational policies and procedures, and in practice guidelines.
- Chosen hand hygiene products should provide high efficiency with low potential for skin irritation. Towelettes and non–alcohol-based hand rubs should not be used for hand hygiene. Hand hygiene products should be used according to the manufacturer's labeled use(s) and directions.

- Use of alcohol-based hand rub products or handwashing with soap and water is appropriate for hand decontamination when hands are not visibly soiled, before performing aseptic infusion procedures, after contact with objects or equipment in the patient's immediate vicinity, and after removing gloves.
- Bar soap should not be used as it is a potential source of bacteria; however, liquid soap and water are adequate for hand hygiene.
- Dispensers of liquid soap/antiseptic solutions are recommended. Containers should be filled or refilled, discarded, and replaced according to organizational policies and procedures and practice guidelines.
- Single-use soap scrub packets or waterless antibacterial products should be used when running water is compromised or unavailable.
- The infusion nurse should be involved with product evaluation to assess for product feel, fragrance, and skin irritation. Other products for skin care such as gloves, lotions, and moisturizers should be assessed for compatibility with hand antisepsis products.

From Infusion Nurses Society: Infusion nursing standards of practice, *JIN* 29(suppl 1S), 2006.

---

monitor performance and detect and evaluate improvements. Leaders and performance improvement teams in hospitals and home care need to become familiar with the terminology and methods of performance measurement and statistical process control that have been used for decades in other industries. Staff and infusion team nurses should help monitor performance trends and patterns as part of their unit's or team's PI activities (TJC, 2008b). To this end, the remaining chapter sections provide an overview of some of the important principles of using performance measures and the statistical methods used to display and analyze those measures.

TYPES OF PERFORMANCE MEASURES

There are two different ways of looking at how measures are categorized. One is by placing measures into categories based on what aspect (domain) of patient service is being evaluated, and the other is to look at what *statistical* type of measure it is.

Performance measures by domains of care

There are at least three types of "aspect of care" or "domain" categories: structure measures, process measures, and outcome measures. The previous section in this chapter provided detailed definitions of the terms *structure, process,* and *outcome,* which will not be repeated here. These same domains of care are considered when planning performance measurement. Just as each of these domains has "statements of excellence" (standards), they also have "measures of excellence," or performance measures.

A *structure measure* is a quantitative tool to measure an aspect of the organization's infrastructure that can impact patient care. An example is the percentage of infusion pumps audited that met rate reliability criteria when tested by technicians between patient uses. Assuming that equipment is considered as part of the organization's structures, this would be a structure measurement.

A *process measure* is a quantitative tool to measure an aspect of actual patient services that can impact patient outcome. An example is the percentage of PICCs inserted within 12 hours of the physician's request for the insertion.

An *outcome measure* is a quantitative tool to measure the outcome of the patient's treatment. An example is the incidence of extravasation in patients receiving chemotherapy per 1000 chemotherapy treatment days.

Of the three measures, quality thought leaders recommend the use of outcome measures as the most accurate measurement of the organization's *overall* performance because they tend to cross departmental lines. Patients who have positive outcomes generally do so because all departments worked effectively and in unison for the welfare of the patient. Patients with poor outcomes may have had complications as a result of the actions of one or of several departments. Because of this "global" or "universal" nature of outcome measures, they can more clearly reflect *organizational* performance versus performance of an *individual or department*.

There are four other measures that are sometimes used to evaluate an organization's performance but are not strictly clinical in nature. These are patient perception and operational, utilization, and financial measures.

The appropriateness of using patient perception measures has been debated by health care experts for some time. Nursing literature has endorsed the use of a satisfaction measure if it is composed of four different functional perspectives. These include health status, knowledge function, skill function, and psychosocial function. When a satisfaction survey includes each of these elements, it offers a comprehensive evaluation of how the care was delivered (processes) and the patient's perceptions of the results (outcomes). TJC recommends that the organization use either clinical performance measures or patient perception measures to meet accreditation requirements.

Organizations may also choose to measure and monitor utilization and operational and financial performance. Every well-run organization should be able to report its financial performance and act on negative or positive trends to increase financial efficiency and profitability. However, measures of this kind are not related to the quality of care provided to patients and are therefore not customarily accepted by licensing agencies, accrediting bodies, or payers as part of a *clinical* QA program. A common example of a financial measure is *"days sales outstanding"* (DSO), which is the number of days between the billing of services and the receipt of payment from a third-party payer. An example of an operational measure is the percentage of staff turnover. An example of a utilization measure is the percentage of patients using formulary versus nonformulary medications.

PERFORMANCE MEASURES BY STATISTICAL TYPE

Another way to categorize performance measures is by how they are expressed numerically.

Continuous variable measures

A continuous variable measure (sometimes called a *measure of central tendency*) is a measure that is expressed as a number along a continuous scale. The value is a single discrete number that rises and falls at each measurement (Murray, 2007).

A hospital-based example of a measure of central tendency, or continuous variable, would be the average wait time between the ordering of a PICC placement by a physician and the time of PICC placement. For example, for one month an evaluation of all patients who had PICCs ordered and placed may indicate an average wait time of 6.3 hours. This value might rise and fall each month as staffing, volume, or other variables affect the system. An example for home care might be the average (mean) time elapsed between an initial referral and the delivery of home medical equipment.

Rate-based proportion measures

Rate-based measures are measures that compare the total number of times something occurred to the total number of times that it could have occurred. This type of measure has a numerator and denominator and is often expressed as a percentage. Note that the numerator is a subset of the denominator.

A home care–based example of a rate-based proportion measure is the percentage of patients receiving home pain management infusion therapy who expressed satisfaction with their pain relief. In this outcome/patient-perception measurement, the PI team assesses the total number of high satisfaction ratings for pain management returned on surveys, compared with the total number of patients who received pain management. If all questionnaires are returned, this would give an accurate measurement of the success of the pain management program (from the patient's perspective).

Rate-based ratio measures

A *rate-based ratio measure* compares the number of times something occurred with an unrelated phenomenon. This type of measure also has a numerator and a denominator, but the numerator is not a subset of the denominator as in the previous type. (Therefore this measure is never expressed as a percentage.) Rather, the denominator is usually a common denominator used for comparison purposes and benchmarking.

An example of a rate-based ratio measure often used by hospitals and home care organizations is the incidence of cases of catheter infections (numerator) per 1000 catheter care days (denominator). Another common example is the number of adverse drug reactions per 1000 drug therapy days, or the number of adverse drug reactions per 1000 drug doses administered.

SELECTING APPROPRIATE MEASURES

One of the most difficult decisions for an organization is which measures to use as indications of quality and performance. Writers have described a health care "dashboard," or the development of a concise set of performance measures that can be reviewed regularly to give the "driver" (or leadership) of the organization a clear view of its performance (Enrado, 2007). This area of quality management in health care is still evolving. Much needs to be learned about the development and use of measures that not only can assess an organization's performance but also can be used by similar organizations to compare themselves with each other. These are sometimes referred to as *core measures*.

The best recommendations available from experts are to use measures that do the following:
- Reflect areas of service that are high risk, problem prone, high cost, or high volume, and that directly reflect the outcome or potential outcome of the patient's care.
- Address (crossover to) all key functions of an organization: managerial, clinical, and support services, and that cross departmental lines.

- By consensus, are meaningful and useful for the improvement of the organization.
- Can be used to benchmark (compare) performance against the performance of another organization.

CHARACTERISTICS OF GOOD MEASURES

Because the criteria for acceptable measures can be demanding, performance improvement teams often elicit the help of statisticians or research designers when developing measures.

For a measure to be statistically appropriate and useful, it must possess the following characteristics (TJC, 2008b):

- *Reliability* denotes the ability to measure the variable regardless of who is gathering the data, when the data are collected, or from which source the data are obtained.
- *Validity* requires that the indicator measures what it is intended to measure. A valid indicator identifies situations in which quality is lacking or confirms circumstances in which quality is present.
- *Measurability* is the ability to translate the important aspects of care into measurable, quantifiable terms to detect the level of quality.
- *Specificity* implies that indicators characterize a specific event. Each indicator must be precise and unique to the event to be measured.
- *Relevancy* requires that the indicator relates to and only to the critical aspect of care being measured.

SENTINEL EVENTS

Another type of performance measure that should always be monitored is the sentinel event measure. A *sentinel event* is "an unexpected occurrence involving death or serious physical or psychologic injury, or the risk thereof." Serious injury specifically includes loss of life or function. The phrase *risk thereof* includes any process variation for which a recurrence would carry a significant chance of a serious adverse outcome (TJC, 2008c).

Examples of sentinel events used by hospitals include the death of a patient from a hemolytic blood transfusion reaction, surgery on the wrong body part, retention of an unintended foreign body postoperatively, patient suicide in an inpatient setting, rape, and abduction of a patient.

Sentinel events used by home care agencies and home care pharmacies include the death of a patient related to administration or dispensing of an incorrect drug or incorrect dosage, emotional or physical abuse perpetrated on a patient by a home care worker, or permanent organ dysfunction as a result of insufficient or incorrect drug monitoring.

Because of the very serious nature of a sentinel event, any occurrence must instigate a performance improvement review by the PI team. After a sentinel event, the organization's leaders generally assemble a task force comprised of PI, leadership, and risk management staff to investigate and act on the issue. A root cause analysis must be performed and corrective measures taken (TJC, 2008c). The threshold, or acceptable level, for sentinel events in any organization should always be 0%.

Reporting of a sentinel event is a controversial issue. Experts in risk management have voiced concern over any policy or standard that mandates the reporting of a sentinel event to an outside organization, whether it is a governmental or consulting agency. TJC has encouraged but not mandated the voluntary reporting of these occurrences as part of the accredited organization's performance improvement efforts. The benefit of reporting events is that other organizations can learn to prevent sentinel events by reviewing the aggregated information gathered by organizations such as the MedWatch program and TJC. However, each organization must develop its own internal policies and procedure on this issue.

ESTABLISHING THRESHOLDS

Once performance measures are selected and approved, the accepted minimum or maximum value for that measure must be determined. In some cases, the answer is self-evident. As described earlier, the acceptable threshold for sentinel events should always be 0%. In this way, even a single occurrence would raise a quality improvement "flag" and initiate investigation and action.

However, most events are not sentinel in nature. They are "rate-based" events that can and will occur from time to time. The PI team must determine the extent to which rate-based events can occur and still be deemed acceptable. In those cases, the value is set based on comparison to national benchmark data. Regardless of how the acceptable value is set, it will serve as a "trigger point," prompting an improvement project if the value is not met.

In addition to comparing a performance measurement with a predetermined threshold, there are other recommended statistical methods to detect positive or negative changes in the organization's processes. These are discussed further in the section Methods of Displaying and Analyzing Data.

DETERMINING SAMPLE SIZE

Standard research methodologies should be used when designing performance measures for performance improvement. One of the most important considerations is the sampling technique, sampling frequency, and sample size to be used. The technique selected should ensure the accuracy and reliability of the data. The sample size should be sufficient so that conclusions can be drawn from the data.

Possible sampling techniques include probability and nonprobability methods. Probability methods are the most scientific because they involve random selection of the sample. By using numerical tables, each case has an equal chance of selection for the review process. Nonprobability sampling reflects qualitative judgment and does not ensure selection based on chance. Convenience and quota sampling are examples of nonprobability methods.

Sample size is a controversial issue. Because the sample size must be representative of the total population under examination, application of the research process is the most accurate means to determine an appropriate sample size. However, some authors have offered general guidelines for sampling. They have suggested a sample size of 5%, or 20 cases (whichever is greater), for routine review; 10%, or 40 cases (whichever is greater), if the threshold for monitoring has been triggered; and 15%, or 60 cases (whichever is greater), for intensive review. Because of the seriousness of sentinel events, a 100% review is always required.

COLLECTING DATA

Data collection may involve either retrospective or concurrent review. Retrospective review entails collecting data after the care has been provided. In the past, such data collections were known as *chart audits* because they focused on the documentation of care after the patient was discharged. Retrospective reviews are the easiest to perform but are the least effective in changing practice. In contrast, concurrent reviews are done while patients are still hospitalized or on service. Interviews and observations are examples of concurrent review, and the timeliness of such activities is instrumental in improving the quality of the care delivered.

METHODS OF DISPLAYING AND ANALYZING DATA

To get the most benefit from the data collected, the QI/PI team should monitor data over time. Monitoring data over time allows the team to detect trends and patterns that can lead to problem identification and resolution.

The methods of displaying and analyzing data reviewed in this section have been used extensively in other industries for decades. The health care industry is now evolving to a level of sophistication where statistical techniques are used to detect variations in the system, prioritize problems and possible solutions, and evaluate the effects of changes. The infusion nurse, whether direct caregiver or manager, is now expected to be familiar with basic statistical models so that he or she can participate in performance improvement cycles. Nurses and other quality team members should no longer rely on "gut feelings" or informal observations of problems to design improvement projects. Projects and improvements should be based on sound statistical design, collection, and analysis. TJC has several standards specifically related to the appropriateness of the data aggregation, display, and analysis used by an organization.

RUN CHART

A run chart displays a numerical value over a period of time. The number on the chart might represent anything from the incidence of PICC infections, to the wait time for special meal orders from the hospital food service, or to the adverse drug reaction rate on a pediatric unit.

Most persons are familiar with run charts in either their workplace or an outside setting because they offer an easy, at-a-glance view of a trend. Many people use run charts to monitor stock prices, average daily temperatures, and so on. Figure 3-2 depicts a run chart of peripheral IV infiltrates.

Run charts are useful in that the viewer can easily see if the trend is upward, downward, or static. Unfortunately, run charts have limited value outside of this. Some experts believe that run charts can be analyzed for statistically significant patterns. However, most PI practitioners use them only to demonstrate the most basic and obvious of trends.

Most experts in statistical process control agree that to best detect variations in a system (and to determine whether the variation is statistically significant), the run chart's more complex relative, the control chart, should be used.

CONTROL CHART

The control chart is one of the most valuable, versatile, and informative tools that health care providers can use to detect variations in the system. These variations might be positive or negative (improvements or problem areas). Figure 3-3 shows an example of a control chart.

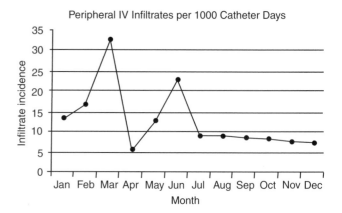

FIGURE 3-2 Run chart of peripheral infiltrations for 2007.

At first glance, a control chart appears similar to a run chart. A numerical value is plotted on the chart over time, and the movement of this value can be easily observed for upward or downward movement. Upon closer inspection, however, the user will note two *thresholds (or "limits")*, usually indicated as colored lines or dotted lines. One of these limits, referred to as the *upper control limit* (UCL), is found somewhere above the average value on the chart. The other, the *lower control limit* (LCL), is found below the average value on the chart.

Researchers and performance improvement experts use the UCL, LCL, and average (mean) to tell them when the organization's process has gone "out of control," referring here to statistical control. The UCL and LCL values are *not* arbitrarily set by the PI team. Unlike thresholds of QA indicators discussed earlier, these values are not determined by literature review or benchmarking. They are set statistically by the values on the chart. The values of the UCL and LCL are determined by using the mathematical formula for standard deviation (sometimes referred to as *sigma*). Most PI teams set the UCL and LCL values for a total of two or three standard deviations (or two or three sigma) from the mean or average.

An important lesson that control charts teach as they are used is that there is always movement upward and downward in a system. Upward movement is not always positive, and downward movement is not always negative. This constant fluctuation is a result of the normal variations in a system, such as hospital staffing, changes in equipment, and so forth. It is referred to as *common cause variation* and should not concern the PI team. However, control charts can show us when significant fluctuations are out of the ordinary. These changes, referred to as *special cause variations,* may be cause for concern if they negatively affect patient welfare.

There are many ways that a control chart can tell if the process is statistically out of control (if special cause variation exists). The most obvious is if one of the observed values falls outside of the upper or lower control limit. There are many other trends and patterns that PI teams look for on control charts that are beyond the scope of this text.

PARETO CHART

The Pareto chart is considered by many experts in performance improvement to be the most useful type of bar graph. It is named for its creator, Vilfred Pareto, who is also credited with development of the Pareto principle, commonly known as the

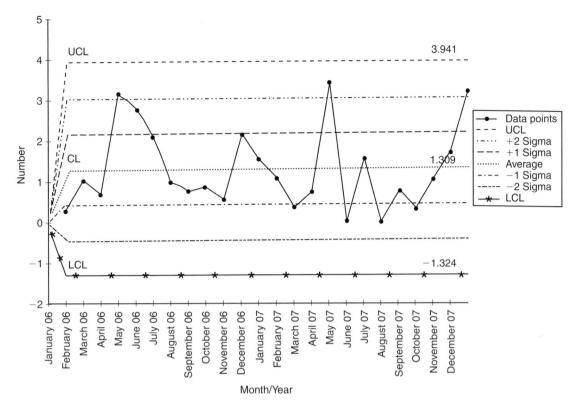

FIGURE 3-3 Control chart of unscheduled hospitalizations of home care patients.

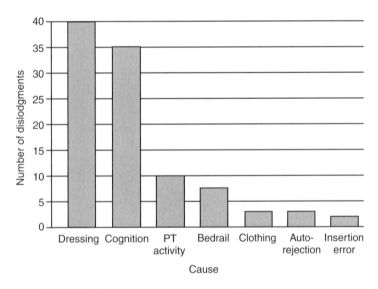

FIGURE 3-4 Pareto chart ranking causes of midline catheter dislodgment.

80/20 rule. Supporters of the Pareto principle believe that, in most cases, 80% of the root causes of a problem are attributed to 20% of the factors.

When data are displayed on a Pareto chart, they are always ranked in sequence from the most common result or cause to the least common. Therefore the bar on the extreme left will always be the largest, and each bar will gradually decrease in size. Users of Pareto charts will focus their attention on the one or two bars immediately to the left of the y axis. Figure 3-4 is an example of a Pareto chart.

The Pareto chart is used to help the PI team prioritize. The chart helps distinguish between the one or few possible causes

of a problem that have the most impact and cost, from the many other possible causes that have little significance.

For example, the PI committee of an area hospital needed to reduce their midline catheter dislodgment rate. A control chart created from an outcome measure on catheter dislodgment showed that for the last 2 months the rate of dislodgment of midline catheters had been above the upper control limit, signaling that the process was "out of control" and required correction. To determine the most common causes of dislodgment, the team brainstormed, listed eight possible causes, and collected data through survey to determine the distribution of the causes. The Pareto chart in Figure 3-4 shows the results. The team determined that 75% of the dislodgment occurred for one of two reasons: the dressing technique used did not hold the catheter in place securely, or cognitive impairment of patients caused them to remove the catheter. By using the Pareto principle, the team was able to concentrate its efforts to these two causes, rather than spending valuable time and resources correcting other causes that had little bearing on the overall picture.

HISTOGRAM

The histogram is also a bar graph. Instead of showing prioritization of causes, the histogram shows the distribution of data, or patterns in variation (Murray, 2007).

The histogram in Figure 3-5 shows the distribution of the following data: time elapsed between delivery of specimen to the laboratory and return phone report of results for stat chemistry values.

On viewing the histogram, it shows the majority of laboratory results were returned between 30 and 40 minutes from the time of specimen delivery, with a normal distribution both above and below this time frame.

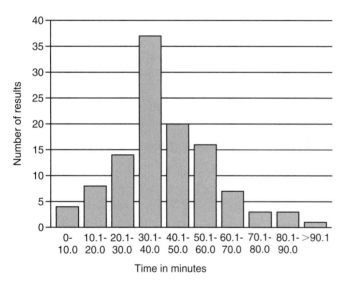

FIGURE 3-5 Histogram displaying time elapsed for phoned stat lab results.

If the laboratory director wished to improve this elapsed time and implement corrective (improvement) actions, he or she could repeat the same survey 2 months later and look at the distribution of the results. Has the distribution changed by moving toward the lower values of the time interval?

SCATTER DIAGRAM

The scatter diagram is a useful tool that illustrates the relationship (or lack thereof) of two variables. On a scatter diagram, each of the two variables is assigned an axis. The point where the two intersect is marked with a dot or other symbol.

By looking at the clustering of these symbols, one can hypothesize whether there is a relationship between the variables. Points clustered in an area going from lower left to upper right indicate a positive correlation. Points clustered in an area going from upper left to lower right indicate a negative correlation. If the points do not cluster at all but are randomly located throughout the grid, it is presumed that there is no correlation at all.

For example, the scatter diagram in Figure 3-6 shows the possible relationship between the number of infusion nurses staffing the hospital at any given time and the time elapsed between a request for an IV start and the actual insertion. Observe that as the number of nurses increased, the wait time decreased. There is a negative correlation between these two variables, showing the organization leadership that staffing most probably does affect the efficiency of services.

Note that a relationship cannot be absolutely proven by the use of a scatter diagram. However, the probable relationship or lack thereof between two variables can be supported.

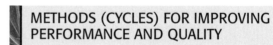

METHODS (CYCLES) FOR IMPROVING PERFORMANCE AND QUALITY

THE SHEWHART CYCLE (PDSA OR PDCA)

The PDSA cycle (also called the *Plan-Do-Study-Act cycle*) is attributed to Walter Shewhart, a quality improvement specialist with Bell Laboratories in the 1920s and 1930s. This cycle model was introduced to Mr. Shewhart's student, W. Edwards Deming,

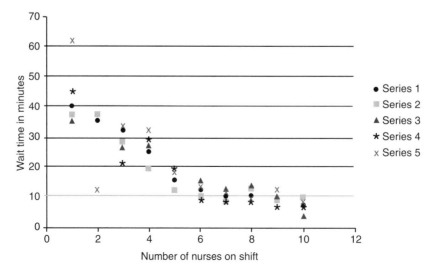

FIGURE 3-6 Scatter diagram of the correlation between staffing and wait time for IV starts.

who then described the PDSA cycle in many of his writings and teachings. This cycle, which has also been referred to as the *PDCA cycle* (Plan-Do-Check-Act cycle), is depicted in Figure 3-7.

The PDSA cycle has been adopted by many organizations in health care and other industries because of its flexibility, logic, and simplicity. It is adaptable to many different situations, making it a powerful and convenient tool. The following description provides an overview of the process.

Plan

The Plan phase of the PDSA cycle is the starting point of a project. It is triggered by data collected and evaluated that signal the improvement team about an area of deficiency or an area that could be improved. Examples would be a rise in infection rate, a decrease in overall patient satisfaction, or an increase in the average wait time for catheter insertion. The Plan phase calls for the development of the overall plan for the improvement. It is recommended that the number of improvement strategies agreed on during this phase be no more than than four. In addition to deciding what changes will be made, the PI team must decide how to test the changes. In other words, how will the team know that the change they made in fact led to an improvement? In almost all cases, the team will collect the same data that led them to decide that an improvement needed to be made in the first place. What type of data or observations will need to be collected and recorded to show the team the effect of the changes?

Other questions answered during the planning phase of the cycle include the following:
- What is the team trying to accomplish?
- What staff members will be involved in these changes?
- What resources are available to make the changes?
- What obstacles may prevent the changes?
- What time frames will be in effect for making the changes and collecting the data?

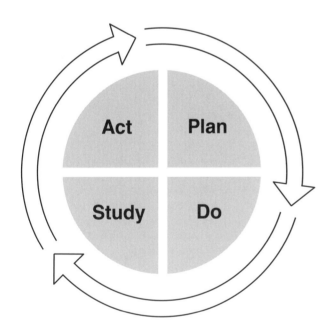

FIGURE 3-7 The PDCA (Plan, Do, Check [or "Study" as shown here], Act) cycle.

Do

During the Do phase of the cycle, the changes are actually made. This is the "working" phase of the cycle. Most improvement teams use task lists, checklists, computer software for project management, or other tools to make sure that the tasks assigned are completed correctly and on time. Some improvement teams use a "critical pathway" approach during this phase, similar to those used to guide patient care. In most large organizations, the changes made during this phase are limited to only one area, such as one department or one hospital unit. As a result, many references refer to this phase as the *pilot test* phase because changes are made on a limited scale. For example, a hospital may institute a change in patient admission assessment procedures on a medical unit and test the results. If successful, the changes would then be phased into all medical units. Likewise, a home infusion company might make changes to the type of equipment dispensed by one branch, evaluate the results, and then expand the changes to all branches of the company.

Study or check

During the Study or Check phase of the cycle, the team must objectively review data collected during the previous phase and ask itself, "Did the changes improve our process or our outcomes?" The team must assess whether it met its objectives.

It is important that the improvement team collect data using the same methods and tools during this phase as it did during the Plan phase. As described earlier, an improvement cycle (project) should never begin until a valid data collection is performed. Without reliable and valid data, the improvement team cannot possibly know if the change made during the improvement cycle truly resulted in an improvement.

As an example, to properly conduct an improvement cycle on PICC wait time, the team would not begin improvement planning simply because a physician complained about an excessive wait time. If several complaints are received, it would be appropriate to perform a valid data collection to calculate the *statistially accurate* mean wait time. If a problem is detected and improvement strategies are implemented, the team must then *check* or *study* its result by collecting wait time data in exactly the same way as during the Plan phase.

A question often asked is, "How do we know how much of a change to expect?" The degree of success is assessed by comparing the baseline data to the data collected after the changes were made. Did the degree of change meet the team's target? The target must be mutually agreed upon and described in the Plan phase of the cycle. It may be based on group consensus, a patient care standard, a practice standard, a clinical pathway, or national benchmarking data.

Act

During the Act phase of the cycle, the team must decide whether to move forward with the changes that were made, incorporating them fully into the organization's structure, policies, procedures, and educational processes. If the Do phase was a "pilot" test, the changes made are tested during the Check phase. If they were found to be successful, the changes made would then be incorporated systemwide throughout the hospital or home care company. Changes that brought about improvements should be phased into all applicable areas of the organization as part of its standard operating procedures.

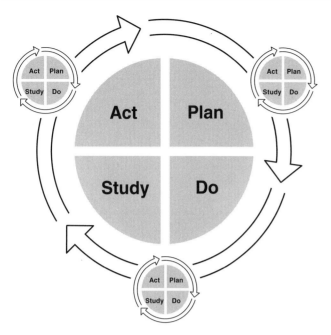

FIGURE 3-8 Rapid cycle improvement.

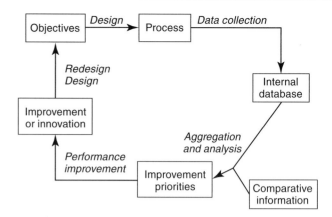

FIGURE 3-9 The JCAHO cycle for performance improvement. (From JCAHO: *1999-2000 comprehensive accreditation manual for home care,* Oakbrook Terrace, Ill, 2000, Joint Commission Resources.)

Those that did not should be either abandoned or redesigned and tested again.

RAPID CYCLE IMPROVEMENT

As the use of PDSA became increasingly popular, an off-shoot of the process evolved known as "rapid cycle PDSA" or "rapid cycle improvement." Frustrated by the seemingly long time it can take to complete a PDSA project, organizations looked for ways to see improvements quickly (Picker Institute, 2000). In health care this is especially important since improvements can positively affect patient health, and improvement teams are appropriately eager to implement changes that they clearly see are of benefit.

The principle of rapid cycle improvement is simply that the improvement team takes a larger PDSA project and divides it into smaller PDSA cycles, each of which can be accomplished in a short period of time. A larger project that may take 6 months to complete would be divided into four to six cycles. Each cycle could be completed in 3 to 4 weeks, so that the successful improvement noted in that cycle would then be incorporated systemwide and not need to wait the full 6 months in order to be implemented. A rapid cycle improvement model is depicted in Figure 3-8.

THE JOINT COMMISSION CYCLE FOR IMPROVING PERFORMANCE

Publications by TJC introduced a new cycle methodology for improving performance. Replacing the traditional Ten Step Model was a cyclical model that integrates several theories of performance improvement. This model, depicted in Figure 3-9, differs from its predecessor in that the model is cyclical in nature, can be entered at any point in the cycle, and is flexible enough to meet the needs of many types of organizations, from large projects to small. The reader will note that there are many similarities between The Joint Commission

model and the traditional industrial model of PDSA. In many aspects they are congruent, but the terminology used is different.

The four basic components of The Joint Commission's cycle are as follows:

1. Design
2. Measure
3. Assess
4. Improve

For the sake of consistency with TJC publications, the discussion of this improvement cycle begins with the design phase. Remember, however, that the improvement process can begin at any point in this cycle.

Design

The design phase of the cycle refers to the design of a new process within the organization to meet the needs of the consumer. Infusion-related examples are the creation of an assessment procedure and documentation form for epidural analgesia patients, the creation of a 24-hour help line for post-discharge surgical patients with central catheters, and development of patient education materials for patients going home with parenteral nutrition.

There are many issues that the leadership and staff of an organization should take into account when designing a process, including the following:

- The organization's mission, vision, and goals
- Expectations and needs of the consumers
- Preexisting knowledge about the same type of process at other organizations (which can be obtained from the literature or through peer networking)
- The necessary data, resources, and time to make the process successful
- The cost versus the benefit of creating the process
- The benefit to the consumer resulting from function, process, product, or service

Measure

To determine whether a process is meeting its intended goal of benefiting the consumer, data must be collected and analyzed. Without data it is impossible to objectively determine whether a process, product, or service is "good enough" as it exists or whether it requires redesign for improvement. In addition, data should be collected after changes are made to assess the degree to which improvement occurred as a result of the changes.

TJC recommends that an organization continually collect performance measurement data related to services that have significant impact on the patient or consumer. The guideline of measuring processes that are high risk, high volume, and problem prone applies to this segment of the cycle. Variations or unacceptable levels of performance would then initiate an improvement process.

The results of this phase of the improvement cycle are statistical data. There are many methods of collecting and displaying data for performance improvement. These were discussed earlier in the section titled Methods of Displaying and Analyzing Data.

Assess

The assessment phase of this cycle involves using the collected data to make judgments to determine whether an opportunity for improvement exists. The data are translated into usable information. The analysis of data can answer the following questions:

- Where can the organization improve? What are its strengths versus weaknesses?
- How can the organization prioritize improvement activities? Certain statistical graphs, such as a Pareto chart, can point out areas that require more immediate attention.
- How can the organization improve? If an opportunity for improvement is found, planning methods (discussed later) such as root cause analysis and brainstorming will find reasons for the organization's weaknesses and strategies for improvement.
- Did the organization improve? Once changes are made, assessment can determine whether the change resulted in improvement.

The result of this phase of the cycle is a list of improvement priorities.

Improve

This is the action phase of the improvement cycle, during which the team actually institutes the changes proposed during the assessment phase. During this phase, the team determines what must be done, who should do it, how it should be done, and how to decide whether the action was successful. TJC recommends instituting changes on a limited test basis and measuring their effect before instituting them throughout the entire organization. The result of this phase of the cycle is actual change to the process being improved.

 ## TOOLS FOR PLANNING IMPROVEMENTS

Regardless of the conceptual model used to guide the improvement process, the organization can use any one of several tools available for planning improvements. In other words, whether the organization uses The Joint Commission cycle for improvement, the PDSA cycle, or rapid cycle PDSA, there will be a certain phase of the cycle where the team must decide what improvements need to be made and how they should be made.

When that time comes, the PI team can select from many available tools to guide the planning process. Some of the most well-known and commonly used tools are described next.

THE ISHIKAWA DIAGRAM (CAUSE-AND-EFFECT DIAGRAM)

The Ishikawa diagram, named for its originator Kaoru Ishikawa, is often referred to as the *cause-and-effect diagram,* or the fishbone diagram. The cause-and-effect diagram is an excellent tool for documenting why things happen. For example, if a hospital notes an increase in its central venous catheter infection rate, the PI team might draw a cause-and-effect diagram to document the possible reasons why the infection rate has risen. Being able to view the list of reasons on a cause-and-effect diagram can help the PI team decide which reasons merit the most attention and require corrective action.

The Ishikawa diagram is used extensively in what is termed *root cause analysis,* meaning the development of hypotheses of why an event occurred. The importance of root cause analysis has increased since TJC has required every organization to have a method for root cause analysis for any sentinel event (TJC, 2008c).

An example of a cause-and-effect diagram is found in Figure 3-10. In the original, popularized by W. Edwards Deming, the segments of the "fishbone" were materials, methods, manpower, management, and machines. Users of the diagram assigned and listed potential root causes into one of these five sections. As this diagram became adapted to health care situations, the segments were listed in TJC literature as materials, people, equipment, and methods. Some versions of the diagram included a fifth segment titled *environment.* Users can create or delete segments to the fishbone as warranted by the specific setting and information.

When all the potential causes have been listed on the diagram, the team should study the diagram to determine any obvious root causes and causes that can be readily solved. A plan for correcting each cause is then developed.

BRAINSTORMING

Brainstorming is a group process used to develop a list of ideas for improvement in a minimal amount of time. It is often a starting point for teams faced with a problem that needs resolution. Many teams brainstorm regularly but do not recognize it as an accepted tool for improvement and therefore do not document the activity in performance improvement records. However, brainstorming is an effective tool, especially at the beginning of the planning phase of the improvement cycle.

Brainstorming should be directed, not haphazard. Usually, the PI team leader directs the group. The leader should define the subject and keep the brainstorming session on track by steering members back to the subject as needed. Team members should be given time to think about the subject at hand, but the time should be limited. The goal of this creative process is to have members contribute ideas without overanalyzing them. Too much analysis of an idea can hamper the creative flow.

The leader should set a short time limit (10 to 20 minutes is adequate) during which the team members contribute ideas to the list. An unstructured approach has members voicing ideas as they come to mind, in no apparent order. The leader must carefully guide this group to encourage participation from everyone while staying on track. In a structured approach,

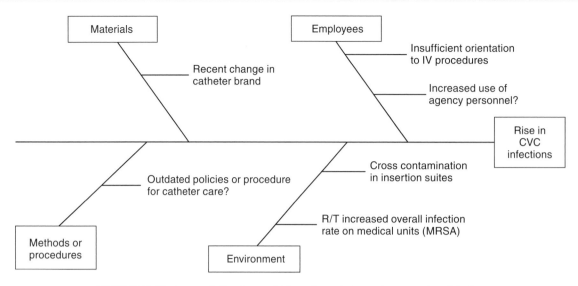

FIGURE 3-10 Cause-and-effect diagram (Ishikawa diagram) of central venous catheter infections. *CVC,* central venous catheter; *MRSA,* methicillin-resistant *Staphylococcus aureus; R/T,* related to.

members voice ideas by going around a circle or in some order until all ideas are exhausted.

Many groups write the ideas down as they are contributed onto a wipe board, easel and pad, or overhead projector, or they use computer technology to project the typed ideas onto a screen. No matter which method is used, members can benefit from seeing the submitted ideas (Box 3-4). No effort should be made to discuss the ideas, rank them, or analyze them in any way.

AFFINITY DIAGRAMS

Many teams use affinity diagrams after a brainstorming session. Affinity diagrams are used to organize large volumes of ideas or issues into logical groups. Once a brainstorming session generates a list of ideas, an affinity diagram can help the team organize those ideas into manageable projects or subgroups, as shown in Figure 3-11.

Most often, affinity diagrams are created by listing each brainstorm idea onto an index card or sticky note. The ideas are displayed on an easel or on a table top. Team members then sort the ideas into groups silently. The ideas should not be discussed. Team members can move a card into another grouping. Once all the cards are sorted and a consensus is reached, the sorting ends. The team then creates headers for each group and draws the diagram using the groups created.

MULTIVOTING

Multivoting is a strategy used to narrow down a large list of ideas to a list that is more manageable, uses resources more wisely, and will lead to better improvement. By using this technique, the team can rank ideas in an order that will guide the improvement planning process toward ideas with greatest impact.

The principle of multivoting is that each member of the team is given a certain number of points to distribute to the ideas on the list. A general guideline is to take the total number of ideas on the list and divide by 4. For example, if there are 20 ideas on the list, each member is given 5 points to distribute.

The team members independently assign number values to items on the list, up to five (in this example) in any way they choose. They can give one item all five points or distribute

Box 3-4 BRAINSTORMING SESSION: HOW TO IMPROVE PATIENT SATISFACTION WITH IV TEACHING

The performance improvement team and the home care agency's IV team were asked to brainstorm for possible improvements to be made in order to increase patient satisfaction ratings with the education provided. The following list was generated:
- Spend more time on initial visit.
- Have an inservice for staff on teaching skills.
- Provide a fourth teaching visit instead of the usual three.
- Develop new patient education literature for IV teaching.
- Use videos, podcasts, and mp3 technologies.
- Use practice models (to practice procedures).
- Call the patient before the first independent dosing to review steps.
- Hire an education specialist for teaching only.
- Ask the patient to have a caregiver or family member attend teaching visits.
- Make the pamphlets easier to understand.
- Find out what the patients do not like if they give a bad rating (e.g., What are the causes of dissatisfaction?).
- Prepare patient before hospital discharge (e.g., minimize fear, frustration) for the fact that he or she will need to learn skills.

points as they wish to any or all of the items. The points for each idea are tallied, and the ideas are ranked in order of total points assigned, as shown in Table 3-3.

FLOWCHARTING

Another tool used extensively for root cause analysis and process improvement is the flowchart. A flowchart is a graphic representation of a process. It is "a simple form of process mapping that uses symbols to represent points of decisions and events that collectively form a 'picture' of an organizational process." Flowcharts help team members understand steps in a process, identify costly redundancies and omissions, and plan for changes (Anderson, 2008).

How can we improve our patient satisfaction rating for teaching IV therapy skills to patients?

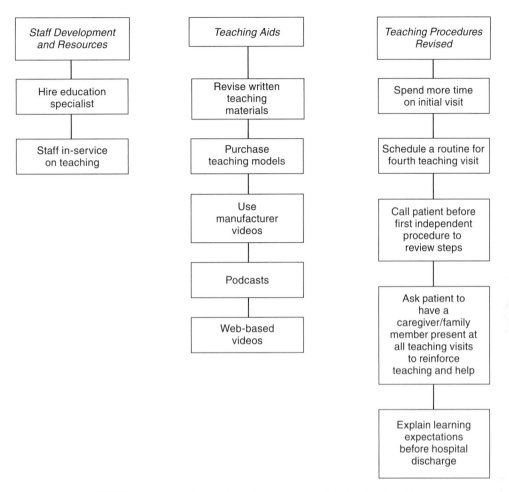

FIGURE 3-11 Affinity diagram: how to improve patient satisfaction with IV teaching.

Flowcharts are often drawn or reviewed during the planning phase of the improvement cycle to detect weak links in the process that may cause problems and therefore warrant improvement. Flowcharts can also be used during the planning phase when designing new processes or solutions.

An interesting observation has been that many important and valuable issues are raised for discussion during the creation of a flowchart because team members may have different concepts of how a process is intended to run. Flowcharting and brainstorming often occur simultaneously. Flowcharting can take some time, especially when there is a problem in the process and resulting confusion about how it should be charted. However, because this is a very effective PI tool, the time is well spent.

To create an effective flowchart, the team must determine the start and end points of the process, list all of the steps or events and decision points in the process, arrange them in sequence, and then use universal symbols to create a flowchart that can be analyzed. A sample flowchart is depicted in Figure 3-12.

OTHER TOOLS FOR PLANNING IMPROVEMENTS

Some of the more common tools used by performance improvement teams to plan what must be improved and how improvements can be prioritized and implemented have been

described. This is only a partial listing, however, and library sources on quality management can provide detailed descriptions of additional tools and methodologies.

TOOLS FOR DOCUMENTING IMPROVEMENT ACTIONS

All improvement cycles, whether PDSA or The Joint Commission cycle, include a phase for implementing the planned improvements or changes. This occurs after the team delegates responsibility for tasks to specific team or staff members.

To expedite the activities and document that they are completed according to the team's desired time frame, many teams use a documentation tool. The two most common tools are task lists and action plans; however, project management software and story boards are also used for documentation.

TASK LISTS

A task list is simply a list of things to be done or obtained. They are used to keep track of what needs to be completed. In some situations, a task list can be expanded into an action plan.

TABLE 3-3 Multivoting: How to Improve Patient Satisfaction with IV Teaching

Points	Item
The IV team and PI team were given the list created during the brainstorming session. They were asked to consider which ideas were most feasible and would improve the satisfaction ratings most significantly. Each member (total of 10 members) was allowed 3 points to allot to 1 or more items on the list. The result of the multivoting was as follows:	
5	Spend more time on the initial visit.
0	Provide a fourth teaching visit instead of the usual three.
10	Develop new patient education literature for IV teaching.
0	Use videos.
3	Develop mp3 podcasts.
3	Develop and post web-based videos.
6	Use practice models.
2	Call the patient before first independent dose to review the steps of the procedure(s).
1	Hire an education specialist for teaching only.
2	Ask the patient to have a caregiver or family member attend teaching visits.
0	Make the pamphlets easier to understand.
0	Find out what the patients do not like if they give a bad rating (determine the causes of dissatisfaction).
4	Have a staff inservice on teaching skills.
0	Review teaching plan in the hospital before discharge.

ACTION PLANS

Action plans contain more detail than simple task lists. Most action plans include a detailed description of the task, the name of the person to whom the task has been delegated, and the target completion date. Some action plans also have a column for the initials of the person who has completed the task and the date of completion. One suggested format for an action plan is shown in Figure 3-13. Since most users today complete forms onscreen with a computer, this type of "rolling form" is easily expanded and updated by adding additional rows in any word processing software. The continual "movement" of the PDSA project as it progresses through its phases and even through several smaller PDSA cycles (rapid cycles of improvement) can easily be documented on the same form. Figure 3-14 depicts a more traditional "paper and pencil" style form that can be completed.

Action plans and task lists are important quality improvement documents that should be kept with the organization's performance improvement records.

PROJECT MANAGEMENT SOFTWARE

Professionals in today's health care organizations are increasingly dependent on computerization to plan activities, communicate with each other, monitor patient status, measure performance, and evaluate quality of care. As such, the use of software to expedite quality and performance improvement is greatly encouraged.

If the organization has an information technology (IT) department, it might be beneficial to involve that department

in the selection of quality management software and project management software. Many software packages are available that combine these two functions. The organization leadership should optimally provide infrastructure resources (e.g., software and hardware) so that the organization can rapidly measure, assess, and improve performance.

STORY BOARDS

A story board is a posterlike display of the steps of an improvement project. It is intended for public display. Some story boards are laid out using the specific improvement cycle method used such as PDSA. Other boards simply use a timeline sequence to tell the viewer the story of how an improvement was planned, implemented, and evaluated.

Story boards provide an easy, visual way of explaining the PI team's accomplishments to other members of the organization and keep the PI team members focused on the project.

 INTEGRATING QUALITY MANAGEMENT

As discussed earlier, quality management continues to evolve from a "silo" scenario, where each discipline or department collects its own data and acts on it, to an integrated approach, where data are collected that reflect systemwide performance. Improvement teams today are generally composed of representatives from multiple departments and services. The trend is to integrate monitoring and evaluation activities within the health care organization.

TJC standards specify that infection control, utilization review, and risk management be included in the organization-wide performance assessment and improvement activities (TJC, 2008a). Although each activity has a distinct purpose, they all indicate trends that are useful in identifying opportunities for improvement. Infection control is directed at the surveillance and control of the transmission of disease; utilization review relates to the appropriate use of the patient care services; and risk management focuses on identifying and preventing potential risks to the patient, health care worker, and organization. Merging these various functions under the umbrella of "total quality management" offers a comprehensive approach to systemwide improvement.

Quality management activities are not new to infusion nursing. Monitoring and evaluation of infusion nursing care have always included trending of infusion-related infections, determination of appropriateness of infusion therapy, and prevention of infusion-associated risks and complications. Cheryl Gardner, one of the pioneers of infusion quality management, endorsed comprehensive monitoring as early as 1981. In fact, the role of quality improvement in nursing is historically based. Florence Nightingale championed the concepts of infection surveillance, evaluation, root cause analysis, and improvement in her classic text *Notes on Nursing*, originally published in 1860 (Nightingale, 1969).

Quality management integration can pose a challenge for infusion nursing. In the hospital setting, "integration" implies that the infusion therapy PI program can no longer be limited to care provided by the infusion team. Patients receive infusion nursing care on units and in departments other than those serviced by the infusion team, such as the critical care unit and emergency, surgery, and radiology departments.

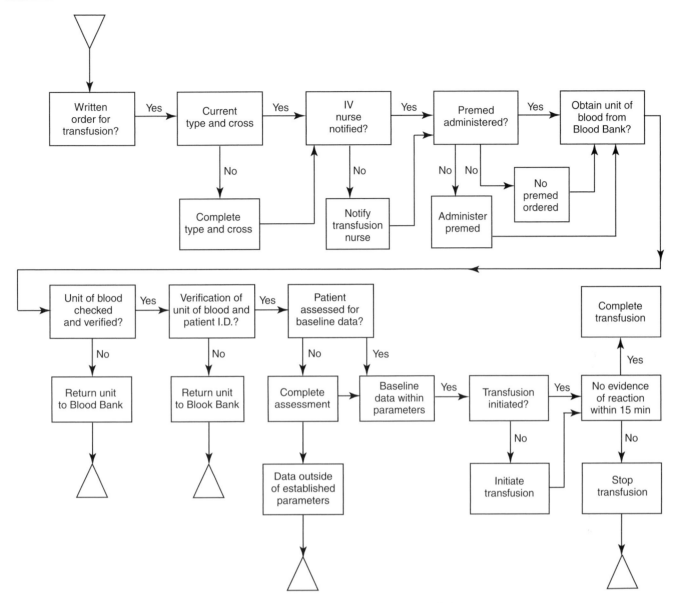

FIGURE 3-12 Flowchart of administration of a transfusion.

In the home care setting and other alternative sites, this means that the infusion quality management program must integrate the organization's pharmacy staff, nursing staff, associated professionals (e.g., physical therapists, occupational therapists, dietitians), nonprofessional staff (e.g., nurse aides and delivery personnel), and administrative personnel. Each member of the team provides important and valuable services to the patients and should contribute to the infusion team's PI process.

Integrating quality assessment and improvement activities requires that the infusion team work with others to identify opportunities for improvements in infusion nursing care throughout the organization.

FUTURE OPPORTUNITIES AND CHALLENGES

The health care system has begun a major cultural and paradigm shift. As an industry, it continues to grapple with the need to improve performance and patient care quality, while at the

same time surviving within difficult financial constraints. A perfect example of this dichotomy is the recent CMS "value-based purchasing policy," which was enacted on October 1, 2008. The premise and intent of this policy are the withholding of CMS reimbursement for expenses associated with certain hospital-acquired conditions (sometimes referred to as "never events"), including pressure ulcers and catheter infection (Collier, 2008). To balance both patient care quality and expenses, the organization must put its performance improvement resources to best use. The PI program must select improvement priorities that carry the greatest benefit to the greatest number of patients.

Another challenge facing our national health care system is the development of a national strategy for data measurement. Simply stated, there is a need to move from the internal collection of performance data that differ from one organization to another, to a unified approach where data are collected across health care organizations in a manner that allows data warehousing, analysis, and reporting. The creation of a framework for national performance measurement system will be a massive undertaking, but one that would most certainly result

Patient Name:_____

Start Date: 2/13/08

New Action Items Based On:

	Desk review:
✓	Phone conference attended by: (IV Team) Nancy P., John S. (QA) Grace Q., (Media Relations/Graphics) Lisa V.; (Purchasing) Eric P.
	On site meeting attended by:

Complete	Item	Person	Updates/comments
	PDSA Section: Development of New Patient Teaching Materials		
	Review current booklets for readability, grade level, graphics content; outsource to patient education consultant (Target 3/13)	John S	3/13: John met with PatientConnect; they are currently reviewing current pamphlets and will submit feedback within 30 days.
✓	Establish list of newer therapies/ procedures not already in the booklet library (Target 3/13)	Nancy P	Three booklets deleted; seven booklets added to the list (completed 3/13)
	Booklet design: produce 2-3 versions of prototype booklet using four-color printing with itemization of cost to produce (Target 3/13)	Lisa V	3/13: Two designs presented to group on 3/13. Team preferred design #1 using larger font (Antigoni font). We still need pricing estimate for production before project can be approved
	PDSA Section: Practice Models		
✓	Review of available companies and pricing (Target 3/13)	Eric P; John S	Eric and John presented catalogs from three companies. Group felt that Acme Models had best value and widest selection (completed 3/13)
	RFP to Acme Models; Send request for proposal to Acme for the twelve training models selected. See attached list of models. Obtain price commitment (Target 4/18)	Eric P	
	Section:		

FIGURE 3-13 Format of action plan.

in the ability to improve patient outcomes on a large scale (TJC, 2008d).

As an industry, health care must adopt quality principles to the same degree as automobile manufacturing and the aviation industry. To accomplish change, there is a need to encourage our professionals and clinicians to become educated and proficient in quality techniques. The National Association for Healthcare Quality publishes excellent study resources to this end. The field of quality management can be an excellent career path for infusion nurses interested in quality improvement theories and methods. Mark Chassin, MD, MPP, MPH, and the President

of TJC, was interviewed for an article in the *Journal for Health-care Quality*. When asked if he had any final "words of wisdom" to share, his reply was the following:

"In the coming years, healthcare quality professionals will be among the most valued resources that hospitals and other healthcare organizations have. The most effective organizations will invest in the development of these professionals, place them in central roles in the organizations, and equip them with appropriate resources for achieving their most critical strategic goals in safety

Issue	Desired Outcome	Target Date	Actions	Completion Date		Person Responsible	Actual Outcome
				Projected	Actual		

FIGURE 3-14 Traditional action plan format.

and quality. As the tide of demand for improved safety and quality continues to rise on all sides—government, private sector, consumers—healthcare quality professionals will be lifted by that tide. So my word of advice would be "Get ready for that tsunami" (Harrington and White, 2008).

 SUMMARY

As the infusion patient population continues to increase in number and acuity, and the cost of providing care continues to escalate, it has become critically important for health care organizations to provide quality-driven care, achieve acceptable patient outcomes, and implement efficiencies to contain costs.

The role of the infusion nurse in accomplishing these goals is an important one. The infusion nurse today should be familiar with current methods to measure, assess, and improve quality of care. As a valuable member of quality improvement committees, the infusion nurse can positively impact processes and outcomes related to infusion therapy.

This chapter has provided a historical perspective to quality measurement and improvement, and has described tools and techniques used in health care and other industries to continually improve outcomes and services. Nurses in clinical and administrative roles can adopt these techniques to provide cost-effective quality infusion services.

 REFERENCES

Anderson B: *Mapping work processes,* American Society for Quality, Milwaukee, Wis, 2008, Quality Press.

Anton D, Anton C: *ISO 9001 survival guide,* ed 3, Ashland, Ore, 2006, AEM Publishing.

Carreira B: *Lean manufacturing that works: powerful tools for drastically reducing waste and maximizing profits,* New York, 2005, AMACOM, a division of American Management Association.

Centers for Medicare & Medicaid Services: *Quality standards: suppliers of durable medical equipment, prosthetics, orthotics and supplies,* August 14, 2006. www.cms.hhs.gov/DMEPOSCompetitiveBid/downloads/CMS_DMEPOS_Quality_Standards_081406.pdf.

Claflin N, editor: *NAHQ guide to quality management,* ed 8, Glenview, Ill, 1998, National Association of Healthcare Quality.

Collier S: The executive's guide to value-based purchasing, *HealthLeaders Media,* March 7, 2008.

Crosby PB: *Quality is free: the art of making quality certain,* New York, 1979, New American Library.

DeBoer A, Iyenger A, Dudhela T: Tools for competing successfully in a pay-for-performance environment, *HealthLeaders Media,* February 4, 2008.

Deming WE: *Out of crisis,* Cambridge, Mass, 1989, MIT Center for Advanced Engineering Study.

Enrado P: California heart center sees dashboard benefits, *Healthcare Finance News,* May 1, 2007.

George ML, Maxey J, Rowlands DT et al: *The lean six sigma pocket toolbook: a quick reference guide to 100 tools for improving quality and speed,* New York, 2005, McGraw-Hill.

Gygi C, DeCarlo N, Williams B et al (foreword): *Six sigma for dummies,* Indianapolis, 2005, Wiley.

Harrington L, White SV: Interview with a quality leader: Mark Chassin, new president of The Joint Commission, *J Healthcare Quality* 30(1): Jan/Feb 2008.

Infusion Nurses Society: Infusion nursing standards of practice, *JIN* 29(suppl 1S), 2006.

Institute of Medicine, Committee on Quality of Health Care in America: *Crossing the quality chasm: a new health system for the 21st century* (Corrigan JM, Donaldson MS, Kohn LT et al, editors), Washington, DC, 2001, National Academies Press.

Institute of Medicine, Committee on Quality of Health Care in America: *To err is human: building a safer health system* (Kohn LT, Corrigan JM, Donaldson MS, editors), Washington, DC, 2000, National Academies Press.

Joint Commission on the Accreditation of Healthcare Organizations: *Agenda for change,* Chicago, 1990, Author.

Joint Commission on the Accreditation of Healthcare Organizations: *1999-2000 comprehensive accreditation manual for home care,* Oakbrook Terrace, Ill, 2000, Joint Commission Resources.

Juran JM: *Juran on leadership for quality,* New York, 1989, Free Press.

Murray S: *Using data for improvement: the toolkit (DVD and workbook),* Glenview, IL, 2007, NAHQ.

Nightingale F: *Notes on nursing: what it is, and what it is not,* New York, 1969, (original publication 1860), Dover Publishing.

Pande PS, Neuman RP, Cavanagh RR: *The six sigma way: how G.E., Motorola, and other companies are honing their performance,* New York, 2000, McGraw-Hill.

Picker Institute: Service quality update: rapid cycle improvement, *New visions for health care,* Issue 17, Boston, 2000, Author.

Sayer NJ, Williams B: *Lean for dummies,* Indianapolis, 2007, Wiley.

The Joint Commission: *Comprehensive accreditation manual for home care,* Oakbrook Terrace, Ill, 2008a, Joint Commission Resources.

The Joint Commission: *Tools for performance improvement in healthcare: a quick reference guide,* ed 2, Oakbrook Terrace, Ill 2008b, Joint Commission Resources.

The Joint Commission: *Understanding and preventing sentinel events in your healthcare organization,* Oakbrook Terrace, Ill, 2008c, Joint Commission Resources.

The Joint Commission: *Healthcare at the crossroads: development of a national performance measurement data set,* Oakbrook Terrace, Ill, 2008d, Joint Commission Resources.

4 LEGAL ISSUES OF INFUSION NURSING

Mary C. Alexander, MA, RN, CRNI®, CAE, FAAN and Hugh K. Webster, Esq.

Nowhere in professional nursing has the role of the nurse grown as fast, as effectively, and as favorably as in infusion nursing. The development of infusion nursing reflects a general trend in the nursing profession. Nurses today monitor complex physiologic data, operate sophisticated life-saving equipment, and coordinate the delivery of health care services. More importantly, nurses now have responsibility for exercising discriminatory judgment. No longer do nurses blindly follow physicians' orders; they collaborate with physicians to ensure that their patients receive the highest quality of care.

The expanding responsibility of infusion nurses has advantages and disadvantages. The nurse's emerging role offers rewards such as intellectual stimulation and professional satisfaction. However, the heightened status also means increased legal risks for the nurse and the added potential for liability. It is therefore the intent of this chapter to broaden awareness of the legal issues of infusion nursing. Four major topics are discussed: the legal standard of care, legal terminology, legal principles, and risk management strategies.

 ## LEGAL STANDARD OF CARE

Nurses have a duty to provide reasonable, prudent patient care as required by the situation. The care delivered by the nurse must comply with what is expected, given the circumstances in which the care is provided. This is known as the *legal standard of care.*

The legal standard of care is used to evaluate the quality of nursing conduct and has several important characteristics (Beare and Myers, 1998). First, the standard of care is a reasonable expectation of the nursing care. This means that the care represents the typical performance of a professional nurse who has special knowledge and skill beyond that of an ordinary person. For example, an infusion nurse is expected to be able to perform a successful venipuncture on the first attempt. Second, the standard of care is measurable. The care can be evaluated based on what a similarly prepared nurse would do in the same situation. For example, a nurse who has been educated to insert a peripherally inserted central catheter (PICC) would know the appropriate site preparation procedure to prevent a catheter-related bloodstream infection (CRBSI). Third, the standard of care is valid based on where the care was delivered. There is

variability based on the state where the care is delivered, thus influencing the established standard by which the care may be evaluated. An example of such variability is whether a registered nurse is allowed to determine PICC tip placement on a chest radiograph. There are some states that allow this practice, while a few others specifically limit it within the scope of nursing practice. Fourth, the standard of care must be applicable based on the current state of knowledge. Standards evolve with increasing knowledge and experience, so the care must be evaluated within the historical context of when the care was delivered. For example, the 2006 revision of the *Infusion Nursing Standards of Practice* is applicable only to infusion nursing care delivered since that document was published.

Standards can be voluntary, such as those promulgated by professional groups, or they may be mandated legislatively. Nursing, like most other professions, is regulated by these dual controls, both of which are aimed at providing quality patient care. Professional standards are the forerunners of legal standards. What has become the customary, usual nursing practice, as defined by the profession, later translates into the legal duty the nurse owes to the patient.

To clarify, the difference between standard of care and standard of practice is that the focus with a standard of care is on the recipient of care, the patient, while the focus with a standard of practice is on the provider of care, in this case the nurse. The legal standards of care for infusion nursing are derived from four sources: federal statutes and regulations, state statutes, professional standards, and institutional standards.

FEDERAL STATUTES AND REGULATIONS

Federal statutes are laws that have been enacted by Congress and are published in the *United States Code.* Regulations interpreting and implementing these laws are promulgated by numerous federal agencies, including the Occupational Safety and Health Administration (OSHA), the Food and Drug Administration (FDA), and the U.S. Department of Health and Human Services (USDHHS). Agency regulations are published in the *Code of Federal Regulations.* The most applicable federal statutes and regulations relative to infusion nursing concern occupational safety and health, infection prevention and control, medical device safety, federally funded insurance programs, and patient self-determination.

Occupational Safety and Health Administration

By law, the Occupational Safety and Health Administration (OSHA) has the authority to both establish and enforce regulations to promote job safety and protect the health of workers. One of OSHA's regulations is the Hazard Communication Standard, or "right-to-know" law, which requires that employees be informed of the hazardous potential of chemicals encountered in the workplace (Federal Register, 2001). Hence, infusion nurses must be knowledgeable of warning labels on hazardous chemical containers used within the health care organization, and in completing material safety data sheets (MSDSs).

In 2001 OSHA revised the 1991 Final Rule of the Occupational Exposure to Bloodborne Pathogens; Needlesticks and Other Sharps Injuries which expands on standard precautions and addresses the risk of occupational exposure to bloodborne pathogens. The standard specifies that all body secretions can be potentially infectious, and that personnel having contact with patients must adhere to strict guidelines. The revision includes examples of engineering controls, and requires exposure control plans, solicitation of employee input, and recordkeeping. Compliance with the guidelines is subject to comprehensive enforcement procedures (Federal Register, 2001).

Centers for Disease Control and Prevention

The Centers for Disease Control and Prevention (CDC) is a federal agency under the USDHHS, whose mission is to promote health and quality of life by preventing and controlling disease, injury, and disability by means of surveillance, research, and demonstration projects. Although this agency does not regulate health, the CDC is responsible for providing guidance in the form of recommendations, which are considered voluntary standards. An example related to infusion nursing is the *Guidelines for the Prevention of Intravascular Catheter-Related Infections* (CDC, 2002; Bennett and Brachman, 2007). Sometimes, the voluntary guidelines issued by the CDC may be adopted by a federal agency and, in effect, become regulations. Such was the case when OSHA adopted the standard precautions developed by the CDC for compliance interpretation.

Food and Drug Administration

Since 1938 the Food and Drug Administration (FDA) has been responsible for regulating products such as food, cosmetics, prescription and over-the-counter medications, and biological agents to ensure that they are safe and effective for their intended purposes. In 1976 this authority was extended to medical devices. With enactment of the Safe Medical Device Act of 1990 (SMDA), device-user facilities, such as hospitals, ambulatory surgical centers, nursing homes, and outpatient treatment facilities, are legally required to report to the FDA and the manufacturer, if known, incidents in which a medical device may have contributed to the serious injury, serious illness, or death of a patient. The term device is broadly defined and may include infusion-related equipment such as venous access devices, solution containers, and electronic infusion devices (FDA, 2002). It is the infusion nurse's professional responsibility, regardless of the practice setting, to inspect product integrity before use and to report any suggested or potential medical device problems (INS, 2006). To report significant adverse events, product problems, or product use errors, the health care professional is

---

Box 4-1 PRODUCT PROBLEM REPORTING PROGRAM

WHEN TO REPORT

Problems with medical devices should be reported if the event observed involves, or has the potential to cause, a death, serious injury, or life-threatening malfunction. This includes problems such as the following:

- User error is the cause (the design of the device or unclear/incomplete labeling may have contributed to the problem).
- A decision is made to no longer use the device because of a malfunction that has occurred.
- Repeated repairs fail to solve the problem.
- Design or repair changes by the manufacturer have adversely affected the performance, safety, or efficacy of the device.
- The problem was the result of incompatibility between devices of different manufacturers and labeling failed to warn the user of this potential for problems.
- The malfunction results in prolonged hospitalization, readmission, or repeated surgical procedures.

WHAT TO REPORT

A complete description of the problem and information regarding the device needs to be submitted, including the following:

- Product name
- Manufacturer's name and address
- Identification numbers of the device (lot number, model number, serial number, expiration date)
- Problem noted (including any actual or potential adverse effects)
- Name, title, and practice specialty of the user of the device

HOW TO REPORT

Problems are reported to MedWatch, the Food and Drug Administration (FDA) safety information and adverse event reporting program. Reports can be made by telephone: 1-800-FDA-1088; by facsimile: 1-800-FDA-0178; by mail: MedWatch, Food and Drug Administration, 5600 Fishers Lane, Rockville, MD 20852-9787; or on-line: www.fda.gov/medwatch/report.htm.

---

to use the FDA's MedWatch program. Guidelines for voluntary reporting to the FDA are listed in Box 4-1.

Centers for Medicare & Medicaid Services

The Centers for Medicare & Medicaid Services (CMS), formerly known as the Health Care Financing Administration (HCFA), is a federal agency created in 1977 to administer the Medicare program and the federal portion of the Medicaid program. Because CMS is responsible for ensuring the quality of health care for beneficiaries participating in these federally funded health insurance programs, the agency sets standards for health care providers receiving Medicare/Medicaid reimbursement. Nurses employed by such providers must comply with the applicable standards, which are commonly referred to as *CMS regulations*.

Patient self-determination

The Patient Self-Determination Act of 1990 requires that all health care providers accepting Medicare and Medicaid payments provide written information regarding advance directives. An advance directive is a document by which an adult patient may legally decide about future medical treatment. The information is provided at the time of admission to the facility, and it recognizes the patient's rights as a competent adult to decide about the use of do-not-resuscitate orders and the withdrawal of life-sustaining equipment (Monarch, 2002). Although this requirement is federally mandated, each state is responsible for overseeing this program; thus there may be implementation variations from state to state.

STATE STATUTES

A *jurisdiction* is a legally established geographic area, such as a state. Variations exist among state statutes because each state government may enact laws specific for that geographic area. A state cannot enact a law that conflicts with federal laws, but it may pass additional regulations (Monarch, 2002). The primary types of state statutes that affect the delivery of infusion nursing care are the Nurse Practice Acts, requirements for nurse licensure, joint policy statements, and licensing of health care facilities.

Nurse Practice Acts

The practice of nursing is regulated by a legislatively enacted Nurse Practice Act (NPA). Although each NPA is unique, most contain similar provisions such as a scope of practice, definitions, description of the composition of the boards of nursing (BON), and requirements for initial licensure and licensure renewal. NPAs, along with administrative rules, and the Administrative Procedures Act (APA) determine what nurses regulated by the BON can and cannot do within the jurisdiction (Monarch, 2002).

NPAs may be general or specific in their guidance for a particular procedure or action. Those states that publish only general standards in the NPA announce specific criteria for nursing behavior in bulletins or newsletters. Some states may have specific position statements allowing or limiting the inclusion of activities within the state's scope of practice. In other states, a decision tree may be used to assist in determining whether an act is within the scope of practice. Each nurse is responsible for familiarizing himself or herself with the NPA of the state in which the nurse practices (Monarch, 2002; Markovich, 2008).

Requirements for nurse licensure

Each NPA specifies that the nurse must be licensed to practice nursing within the state. The minimum requirements for licensure are established by the state board of nursing (BON). The state BON is also empowered to suspend or revoke the license of any nurse for violation of the specified norms of conduct for that state.

The mutual recognition model of nurse licensure allows a nurse to have one license (in his or her state of residency) and to practice in other states (both physically and electronically), subject to each state's practice law and regulation. Under mutual recognition, a nurse may practice across state lines unless otherwise restricted. To achieve mutual recognition, each state must enact legislation or regulation authorizing the nurse licensure compact (NLC). The nurse must legally reside in an NLC state to be eligible to have a multistate license (National Council of State Boards of Nursing [NCSBN], 2008).

Joint policy statements

When questions regarding the professional responsibility of nurses to perform specific therapeutic procedures cannot be answered by existing state statutes, a joint policy statement may be issued. Sponsors of joint policy statements include the state's nursing association, medical society, and hospital association (Weinstein, 2007).

Licensing of health care facilities

Each state has a department of health that sets standards for the licensing of health care facilities. Although these standards are generally directed toward the physical facilities, qualifications of employees, and maintenance of records, they are interrelated with nursing practice. For example, the state health department may mandate how and where medications are to be stored, and the nurse's conduct must not violate these standards.

PROFESSIONAL STANDARDS

Professional standards are not merely the minimum criteria enacted by the legislature, but represent an attempt by a peer group to establish a level of competency that is expected by the profession and has been recognized as such by courts (*Koeniguer v. Eckrich*, 1988).

In health care, professional standards may apply to the entire industry or may pertain only to a specific profession or specialty. The American Nurses Association (ANA) has developed generic standards that address nursing practice, while The Joint Commission has accreditation standards that health care organizations use to measure their delivery of patient care. In contrast, the Infusion Nurses Society (INS) has developed the *Infusion Nursing Standards of Practice* that specifically address infusion nursing practice. In addition, standards, guidelines, criteria, and recommendations from other professional organizations—such as the AABB (formerly known as the American Association of Blood Banks), the American Society of Health-System Pharmacists (ASHP), the American Society for Parenteral and Enteral Nutrition (A.S.P.E.N), the Association for Professionals in Infection Control and Epidemiology (APIC), and the Oncology Nursing Society (ONS)—also influence the professional standards for infusion nursing.

American Nurses Association

The ANA has published *Nursing: Scope and Standards of Practice* that describe a competent level of nursing care as demonstrated by the critical thinking model known as the nursing process. The nursing process includes the components of assessment, diagnosis, outcomes identification, planning, implementation, and evaluation (ANA, 2004). As such, they are considered the foundation for nursing practice.

The Joint Commission

The Joint Commission (TJC), formerly known as the Joint Commission on Accreditation of Healthcare Organizations (JCAHO), is a private, nongovernmental accrediting body that defines optimal, achievable standards for health care organizations such as hospitals, home care services, nursing homes, and ambulatory care centers. The intent of the standards is to improve the quality of health care provided to the public by stimulating health care organizations to meet or exceed the standards through accreditation.

Infusion Nurses Society

INS introduced the first standards for the specialty practice of infusion nursing in 1980. The standards are reviewed routinely, and subsequent revisions reflect changes in clinical practice and technological advances based on evidence-based practice and research. The *Infusion Nursing Standards of Practice* are specific to the specialty practice of infusion nursing and are applicable in all practice settings in which infusion care is delivered (INS, 2006).

INSTITUTIONAL STANDARDS

In addition to governmental and professional standards, each institution or agency specifies its own practice through policies, procedures, protocols, and guidelines. *Policies* are general statements as to when a particular procedure, method, or action is to be used. In contrast, *procedures* are step-by-step outlines of how actions or methods are to be performed. A *protocol* is a formal plan for a course of medical treatment, patient care activity, or research project. *Guidelines* describe a process of patient care management that has the potential for improving the quality of clinical and patient decision-making (ANA, 2004). As systemically developed statements based on available scientific evidence and expert opinion, practice guidelines address the specific care of specific patient populations or phenomena, whereas standards provide a broad framework of practice. Standards should remain stable over time, as they reflect the philosophical values of the profession (ANA, 2004).

 LEGAL TERMINOLOGY

In an age that greatly emphasizes the legal rights of people, nurses have a responsibility to understand the basic precepts of law. Our society is founded on a system of legal principles and processes by which people can resolve problems and disputes without resorting to physical force. The term *law* has been broadly defined as those standards of human conduct that are established and enforced by the authority of an organized society through its government. To comprehend this legal system and apply the principles to the practice of infusion nursing, the nurse must be cognizant of the terminology commonly used to discuss legal matters.

CATEGORIES OF LAW

There are numerous types of laws and various methods by which they are categorized. Often, laws are categorized in relation to the four sources from which they originate and may be identified as follows: (1) *constitutional law,* originating from the federal and state constitutions; (2) *statutory law,* enacted by the legislative branch of government; (3) *administrative law,* issued by administrative agencies that have been established by the legislature or appointed by the executive branch; and (4) *common law,* which results from interpretation of the laws by the judicial system. Some texts also classify laws as public and private law. Constitutional, statutory, and administrative laws are considered *public law* because they deal with public

welfare. In contrast, *private law* is concerned with the rights, duties, and legal relations involving private individuals. Contractual law and laws regarding negligence and malpractice are components of private law (Holmes, 2004).

Laws may also be categorized as to their intent. Such a classification emphasizes how the law affects nurses, and which laws are applicable to practice. Therefore the categories of law relative to infusion nursing include administrative, criminal, contractual, and civil law.

Administrative law

Statutes are laws that are enacted by the legislature and are known as *statutory law*. When the legislature enacts statutes to regulate business or confer benefits on its citizens, it may be difficult to foresee variations necessary for proper execution of the law. To provide for this eventuality, the legislature may establish an administrative agency empowered to make rules and regulations that have the force of laws. Examples of federal administrative agencies include the FDA, OSHA, and CMS. Regulations from these agencies affect the practice of infusion nursing. FDA regulations emphasize product safety, rules issued by OSHA focus on protection of the health care worker, and CMS guidelines affect providers participating in the Medicare/Medicaid programs.

States may also have administrative agencies that are created by the legislature. The primary example is the state board of nursing, also referred to as the board of nurse examiners, nurse licensing board, or nursing board. These boards set requirements for and grant approval to nursing schools, conduct licensing examinations, and issue and renew licenses for nurses. In addition, they are empowered to revoke or annul a nurse's license if there is evidence of incompetence, fraud, or deceit in securing the license; unprofessional conduct; practicing while impaired; criminal acts; or gross negligence.

Criminal law

Laws relating to an offense against the general public that results in a harmful effect against society as a whole are classified as *criminal law*. The primary emphasis of criminal law is defining behaviors that are prohibited or controlled by society. Criminal offenses are prosecuted by a governmental authority and punishment may result in fines and/or imprisonment. Performing infusion nursing procedures in a manner that violates the Nurse Practice Act or the Medical Practice Act is an example of a criminal offense.

Contractual law

A *contract* is an agreement between two or more persons that creates, changes, or eliminates a legal right or obligation. Most nurses do not have employment contracts, but rather enter into general, flexible arrangements with their employers. However, even if the employing agency has no written contract, there is still a binding legal commitment based on a mutual understanding. The nurse has a duty to perform the nursing assignment in accordance with the standards of professional nursing practice; the employer's duty is to provide a safe workplace and properly trained and qualified workers.

As infusion nurses become entrepreneurs, there is an increasing need for nurses to understand how to negotiate written contracts for their services. Consideration must also be given as to how the contract may be terminated. If the nurse fails to perform the obligations required by the contract, a breach of contract may be committed and the nurse may be required to pay damages. The term *damages* usually refers to a sum of money awarded to a person or organization whose rights have been violated by another.

Civil law

The legal rights and obligations of private citizens are the focus of civil law. This category is commonly referred to as *case law* because it is decided by a judge and/or jury. By law, individuals and groups are protected from harm and, if injured by the actions of another, may file a civil action seeking damages. If the civil offense is a private wrong against another's person or property, it is referred to as a *tort.* Torts are the result of a private act or omission and may be further classified as intentional, unintentional, or quasi-intentional.

Intentional torts

An intentional tort involves the purposeful invasion of a person's legal rights. The two best known intentional torts are assault and battery. Although the two terms are often linked, they have separate and distinct meanings. *Assault* is the unjustifiable attempt to touch another person or the threat to do so, communicated in such a way as to cause the person to believe it will be done. For example, if a competent adult patient refuses to have a venipuncture performed but the nurse proceeds to assemble the venipuncture equipment and to prepare to perform the procedure, the patient has been assaulted. *Battery* is defined as the unlawful carrying out of threatened physical harm. If, in the previous example, the nurse proceeds to apply the tourniquet and actually perform the venipuncture, the action would be considered battery.

The term *coercion* is often used to explain assault and battery. Coercion is the forcing of another person to act in a certain manner by means of threat or intimidation. Hence, coercing a rational adult patient to accept a venipuncture constitutes assault and battery.

Another example of an intentional tort is *false imprisonment,* which involves placing individuals in a confined area against their will. In the practice of infusion nursing, it is sometimes necessary to restrain a patient's extremity to stabilize and secure the catheter. In such situations, the nurse must follow policies and procedures governing the use of restraints and resort to restraints only when the patient's safety is in jeopardy. Failure to follow these guidelines may result in allegations of false imprisonment.

Unintentional torts

An inadvertent act, or failure to act, that results in injury or harm to a person is an *unintentional tort.* An unintentional tort may involve an action that is unreasonable and inappropriate, or the lack of an action that is reasonable and appropriate. Two types of unintentional torts are negligence and professional malpractice.

Negligence is not doing something that a reasonable layperson would do given the situation. For example, if a store owner knows that the store parking lot is icy, yet takes no corrective action and a customer slips and falls, the owner may be deemed to have been negligent. However, the opposite also constitutes negligence, because a person who does something that a reasonable person would not do in similar circumstances is also negligent.

When negligent conduct occurs on the part of a member of a profession, it is considered *malpractice.* Medical malpractice has been further defined as deviation from the professional standard of practice that a qualified health care provider of the same specialty would follow given similar circumstances. In this context, malpractice may be considered synonymous with *professional negligence* because the failure to act in a reasonable and prudent manner, as defined by the profession, may result in harm to the patient (Monarch, 2002). For example, the death of a patient as a result of the administration of 1000 mL of 3% sodium chloride infusion, instead of the prescribed 1000 mL of 5% dextrose in 0.33% sodium chloride, may be ruled as malpractice.

Although malpractice implies the failure to act in a reasonable and prudent manner, it also denotes stepping beyond one's authority. Each state has a Nurse Practice Act that defines the scope of nursing practice. If the nurse performs a procedure outside the boundaries of nursing practice, it may be ruled an illegal "practice of medicine" in violation of the Medical Practice Act for that state. For example, removing a tunneled or implanted vascular access device is a medical act; if a nurse performs this procedure, it could be malpractice.

Quasi-intentional torts

The categories of civil wrongs that involve a person's reputation or peace of mind are considered quasi-intentional torts. *Defamation* damages a person's reputation through false and malicious statements. If the statements are written, they are known as *libel,* and if spoken as *slander.* A person's peace of mind may be violated through *invasion of privacy* or by a *breach of confidentiality.* Patients are vulnerable to unauthorized release of private and confidential information concerning their diagnosis, prognosis, treatment, and plan of care. Hence, nurses have a legal duty and professional responsibility to ensure that these civil rights of patients are not violated.

LEGAL PROCESSES

In our legal system, there are three forums in which legal disputes are settled, and each has unique rules of procedure and rules of evidence. Disciplinary disputes and violations of regulations set by an administrative agency are settled within the administrative law forum. For example, state board of nursing decisions are governed by the state administrative laws. Criminal charges are heard in a criminal law forum. An example is the use of criminal laws to try a nurse charged with a criminal offense. Tort disputes, such as negligence or malpractice, are referred to as civil law forum, which is typically a court. In a civil action, the person who has been wronged seeks compensation for the harm or injury suffered. This differs from criminal or administrative law, which seeks to punish the wrongdoer.

Two basic rights are paramount in the legal process—the right to use courts to settle disputes and the right to due process. There are two sides to a dispute—the plaintiff and the defendant—and both have the right to use the legal system to settle the conflict. In a case questioning the nurse's care, the *plaintiff* may be the injured patient who initiated a civil suit, or the state agency or prosecutor if the offense involves an administrative or criminal action. The *defendant* is the person accused of violating the standard of care (civil law), acting unprofessionally (administrative law), or committing a criminal offense (criminal law).

The second basic legal right is the right to due process. This means that certain principles must be followed within a fair and just forum, including proper notice, arrangement of an opportunity to be heard, presentation of evidence, and cross-examination of witnesses.

 ## LEGAL PRINCIPLES

As a result of the growth and increasing complexity of infusion nursing, the greatest legal risk for nurses practicing this specialty is negligence, also known as *negligent conduct* or *malpractice*. The plaintiff may believe the nurse was negligent, but legal action cannot be initiated unless several rules are followed.

ELEMENTS OF NEGLIGENCE

If a patient (plaintiff) believes that an act performed by a nurse or the nurse's failure to act has resulted in injury or harm, the legal process begins once he or she selects a lawyer to represent his or her interests. The counsel for the plaintiff (the allegedly injured patient or heirs) must then determine whether there is a basis for the lawsuit. This involves reviewing the medical record, collecting data, interviewing witnesses, and arranging for the case to be reviewed by an expert. Because the plaintiff has the burden of proof, counsel must determine whether there is evidence of the elements of negligence.

In a lawsuit, the plaintiff (patient) must present evidence that the defendant (nurse) failed to use the degree of skill and judgment commensurate with the nurse's education, experience, and position. In other words, there must be evidence of failure to conform to what a reasonably prudent nurse would have done, or would not have done, if placed in the same situation. As stated by one court, "A nurse who undertakes to render professional services is under a duty to exercise reasonable care and diligence in the application of her knowledge and skill to the patient's case and to use her best judgment in the treatment and care of patients" (Miller-Slades, 1995). The four elements necessary to prove negligence are duty of care, breach of duty, causation, and legally compensable injury.

Duty of care

The first element that must be proven by the plaintiff is that the defendant owed a duty of care. This means that the nurse was in some way responsible for the patient. For example, if the nurse performs a venipuncture on a patient to initiate an infusion, there is a duty of care to the patient. However, if the mother of the patient becomes faint during the venipuncture procedure and falls, injuring her wrist, the duty of care to the patient's mother is questionable. The nurse owed a duty of care to the patient but not to the patient's mother, unless there was a prior realistic agreement to do so. Hence, the mother (as a plaintiff) will probably not be successful in proving duty of care.

Breach of duty

The second critical element that must be proven is that the defendant violated, or breached, the duty of care owed to the patient. A breach in the standard of care must have occurred according to standards dictated by the state NPA and reasonable, prudent clinical practice. The breach of duty may be the result of an act (commission) or of a failure to act (omission). For example, necrosis and tissue sloughing resulting from infiltration of a peripheral infusion of 10% dextrose in water may be the result of failure to monitor a peripheral venipuncture site, an act of omission. On the other hand, injury caused by initiating an infusion without a physician's order is an act of commission. Both may be considered breaches of duty. Other examples of breach of duty relative to infusion nursing are as follows:

- *Delay in drug administration:* A lidocaine infusion has been prescribed for a patient experiencing ventricular tachycardia. Although the infusion is to be initiated immediately, the order is not communicated to the nurse and there is a 3-hour delay until the infusion is initiated.
- *Failure to administer an infusion at the prescribed rate:* A dehydrated patient is to receive an IV infusion at 150 mL/hr, but the rate is incorrectly calculated and the solution infuses at 50 mL/hr.
- *Inappropriate administration of a drug:* Phenytoin is administered at a rate of 100 mg/min and the patient experiences a severe adverse reaction.
- *Failure to provide patient education:* A patient is discharged home with a long-term central venous access device (CVAD). No arrangements are made for home health care, and the patient is not instructed on care of the CVAD or protocols to address an emergency situation.

Breach of duty may also result from barriers to the delivery of patient care. In home care, for example, a patient who refuses to follow the treatment regimen may affect the agency's ability to manage the patient's care. However, termination of care without reasonable notice and adequate time for the patient to secure additional care may be interpreted as patient abandonment. When an agency contracts to provide services, a duty is owed to the patient. Regardless of the reasons, termination of care without adequate notice or provision for continued care represents a breach of duty.

In the case of a private citizen, such as a landlord, the jury can generally comprehend what a reasonably prudent landlord would have done based on the circumstances, and the law allows jurors to use their common sense in reaching a verdict. A nursing negligence case, however, is far more complex because the allegation is that the nurse breached the standard of reasonable nursing care. Because the law recognizes that the average juror does not understand medical terminology, the nursing process, or the legal standard of nursing care, it is often mandated that qualified witnesses educate the jury as to the circumstances of the case (*Gibson v. Bossier City General Hospital,* 1991). This is the role of the expert witness.

An *expert witness* in a medical or nursing malpractice case is a health care provider who is called on to educate the judge and jury regarding the appropriate standard of care and to identify any deviation from the established standard. The law requires the use of expert witness testimony when assessments and conclusions of fact depend on scientific and technical information that is more than common knowledge. Qualifications of the nurse expert include current professional licensure and clinical expertise in the area of nursing. Typically, the expert witness is of the same profession, has similar experience as the defendant, and has demonstrated expertise in the specialty practice (Diehl-Svrjcek et al, 2007). For example, an infusion nurse holding the CRNI® credential with extensive experience in home infusion therapy would be qualified to offer expert testimony in a case involving the actions of a home care infusion nurse.

In offering expert testimony, the witness may rely on personal knowledge and experience, professional articles, published standards of practice, and nursing documentation contained in the patient's medical record to educate the jury. Once the jury understands the applicable standard of care, the expert may offer an opinion as to whether the defendant deviated from that standard. Because nursing negligence is a complex issue, expert witnesses may be used to testify both for and against the defendant. The plaintiff's expert witness will attempt to convince the jury that the defendant (nurse) deviated from the accepted nursing standards; the expert witness for the defense will testify that the defendant's actions represented reasonable nursing care. The jury, however, is not governed by the opinions of the experts and can reject either or both testimonies.

Causation

The third element that must be proven is causation or proximate cause. By law, the injury to the plaintiff must be the result of negligent conduct on the part of the defendant. Patients may be injured because of the conduct of the nurse, but if the nurse was performing in a reasonable, safe manner, the nurse is not responsible for the harm. For example, if a nurse administers penicillin intravenously to a patient and an allergic reaction ensues, the nurse is responsible only if he or she failed to check for possible allergies before administration of the drug. However, if the patient had no known allergies, there is no liability on the part of the nurse.

Legally compensable injury

The final element of negligence is that the patient suffered injury, and that the injury is a type for which the law allows compensation. Because the plaintiff must prove that negligent conduct was actually responsible for harm or injury, it is possible to have severe negligence but no lawsuit. For example, the nurse performs a venipuncture and initiates an infusion of 5% dextrose in 0.9% sodium chloride, but 5% dextrose in 0.45% sodium chloride was prescribed. If the nurse discovers the error before initiating the infusion and no harm has come to the patient, then there can be no lawsuit. Often, potential clients contact malpractice attorneys and relate how they were "almost" injured by a nurse or physician. However, the common reply is that by law, "almost" does not count. If there is no injury, there can be no lawsuit.

COMMON AREAS OF NURSING NEGLIGENCE

To avoid the risks of negligence, the nurse needs to be aware of those areas most commonly associated with negligent conduct and act in such a way as to prevent liability. Areas of negligence specific to infusion nursing include medication administration, equipment use, failure to act, failure to monitor and assess clinical status, failure to prevent infection, lack of communication, and negligent conduct of another.

Medication administration

The actions of nurses related to the administration of medications have been the subject of more lawsuits than any other area of nursing. Examples include giving the wrong medication (*Habuda v. Trustees of Rex Hospital, Inc.,* 1968), not being familiar with the possible harmful effects of a medication (*Polonsky v.*

Union Hospital, 1981), failure to administer medication at proper intervals (*Harrington v. Rush Presbyterian-St. Lukes Hospital,* 1990), administering medication in an improper manner (*Belmon v. St. Francis Cabrini Hosp.,* 1983; *Hill v. Ohio University,* 1988); and failure to obey a physician's instructions (*Georgetti v. United Hospital Medical Ctr.,* 1992). However, there also can be a duty to correct the erroneous orders of a physician (*Jensen v. Archbishop Bergen Mercy Hosp.,* 1991). If the nurse fails to meet the professional expectations relative to medication administration and the failure results in injury to the patient, the nurse is liable. Many cases involving medication errors are settled before reaching a jury because the health care organization's records furnish ample proof of the error.

Equipment use

Protecting the patient from equipment hazards is a responsibility the nurse assumes when using items such as venous access devices, solution containers, administration sets, and electronic infusion devices. The nurse has the duty to reasonably inspect, maintain, use, and supervise equipment to prevent obvious harm to the patient. Nurses have been held responsible for improper use and disposal of equipment, for not supervising the use of equipment, and for leaving equipment in an inappropriate area. If the patient cannot prove when, where, or by whom he or she was injured, courts have found nurses responsible by applying a doctrine called *res ipsa loquitur* (*Guilbeaux v. Lafayette General Hospital,* 1991; *Dixon v. Taylor,* 1993; *Maciag v. Strato Medical Corp.,* 1994). This doctrine means that the injury is so obvious that it "speaks for itself." For example, when an unconscious patient sustains injury from a hematoma caused by an unsuccessful venipuncture attempt, he or she certainly is unable to testify as to how or by whom the injury occurred. In this situation, the law allows the patient to prove, by virtue of the obviousness of the situation, that it was the negligence of the nurse performing the venipuncture that caused the injury.

If, however, the nurse can prove that ordinary precautions were taken to protect the patient from danger, the nurse is not liable, even though the patient was subsequently injured. Such may be the case when a peripheral IV catheter breaks off and harms the patient during an IV infusion. If the nurse inspected the catheter before insertion and detected no visible defect, the nurse is not responsible for the manufacturer's defective product.

Failure to act

Affirmative actions are the subject of most lawsuits against nurses, but the nurse's failure to act may also injure the patient. An example of negligent failure to act is a nurse who receives an order to administer a potassium infusion to a patient experiencing cardiac arrhythmia, but who fails to respond to the order. If the arrhythmia becomes life-threatening because of the failure to act and subsequently results in death, the nurse is liable for the patient's demise.

Failure to monitor and assess clinical status

For any patient with a venous access device (VAD), monitoring and continuous assessment are critical components of the patient's care. Ongoing assessment would include observing the patient's current clinical status and response to therapy, the skin-catheter junction and surrounding tissues, the flow rate and appropriateness of the solution, and potential side effects and complications (Benvenuto, 2004). Failure to monitor and assess may include not checking the infusion site according to the clinically appropriate frequency and not addressing patient complaints in an expeditious manner. Patient complaints of pain and tenderness may indicate a phlebitis or infiltration, which could be the precursor to permanent tissue damage or necrosis (Diehl-Svrjcek et al, 2007).

Failure to prevent infection

Because of the invasive nature of VAD placement, patients are at risk to develop a CRBSI. It is vital that nurses are knowledgeable of infection prevention measures that reduce the risk of infection. Examples of failure to prevent infection would include nonadherence to organizational policy for changing administration sets or dressings, performing site care, or replacing VADs, and failure to report suspected signs of infection (Diehl-Svrjcek, et al, 2007).

Lack of communication

Although failure to communicate is closely related to the failure to act, it may be the sole specific cause of injury. Examples of nursing negligence resulting from lack of communication are the failure to inform the physician of abnormal findings noted during the nursing assessment (*Roach v. Springfield Clinic,* 1991) or the failure to notify the physician of a patient's deteriorating condition (*Vogler v. Dominguez,* 1993). Clearly, nurses have an obligation to exercise sound clinical judgment as to what is significant regarding the patient's status and to communicate that information (*Berdyck v. Shinde,* 1993).

Negligent conduct of another

Along with the person who is primarily responsible, a nurse may be liable for allowing or aiding the negligence of another person. For example, if a physician fails to specify the route of administration for a drug and the nurse administers the drug without checking the route with the prescribing physician, the nurse and physician are jointly responsible if an injury occurs. Merely attempting to contact the physician is not enough to release the nurse from liability. If there is a lack of action by the physician, the nurse is required to advise authorities within the organization to ensure intervention on behalf of the patient.

TOOLS OF DISCOVERY

Once the complaint is filed in court and served on the defendant, the discovery phase of litigation begins. Two tools of discovery often used are interrogatories and depositions. The first step in discovery is for both sides of a lawsuit to develop lists of questions called *interrogatories.* Interrogatories can be presented to the plaintiff, defendants, and witnesses for either side and the questions must be answered in writing. Although the questions can encompass more than the issues of the specific case, the goal of interrogatories is to uncover relevant facts regarding the dispute.

In contrast, a *deposition* is a statement taken from the witness under oath but outside the courtroom. This is a formal procedure in which the opposing party's attorney asks questions of the witness and the entire exchange is recorded by a court reporter. Depositions can be used as testimony in court.

A key component of the discovery phase is the use of written standards of care. Interrogatories and depositions of the

defendant concentrate on the extent of the nurse's familiarity with professional standards of practice. A lack of familiarity with applicable standards seriously detracts from the defendant's credibility as a witness. Conversely, a well-prepared defendant can take advantage of the opposing attorney's questions. By effectively communicating familiarity with the standards cited, the nurse may retaliate against any inference of negligence, and point out how the nursing actions met or exceeded the written guidelines.

PERSONAL LIABILITY

Liability denotes that a person has a legal responsibility to fulfill an obligation. Because nurses are responsible for delivering reasonable, prudent nursing care, they are liable for deviations from the established standard and any resultant harm. This is known as the *rule of personal liability,* where each person is responsible for his or her actions. For example, the nurse administers a prescribed medication, but rapid injection of the drug results in harm to the patient. In this situation, the physician who prescribed the medication is not responsible for the nurse's negligence in administering the drug; the harm was the result of the nurse's actions, not the physician's.

Although the nurse is responsible for nursing actions, in select circumstances the physician may be held jointly accountable for the negligence of a nurse. This primarily concerns the operating room, where the nurse is considered the "borrowed servant" of the physician. This legal principle is derived from agency law, and it places responsibility on the person who is clearly in charge of the situation and who has the greatest control over all present. It is often referred to as the *captain-of-the-ship* doctrine because it analogizes the surgeon to a captain who is the master of the operating room "crew." Outside the operating room, physicians have rarely been found to be responsible for nurses' negligent acts.

Another concept that must be considered in determining responsibility is the doctrine of *respondeat superior,* or "let the master answer." According to this legal principle, an employer is liable for damages caused by a servant's wrongful act performed within the scope of his or her employment. As a result, even when the nurse is held liable for negligence, the employer may also be held responsible for the nurse's actions. The doctrine does not absolve the nurse from responsibility, but it allows both the nurse and the employer to be named in the lawsuit. Application of this legal principle is common in cases in which a nurse does not have liability insurance and the plaintiff must rely on the employer's insurance to cover the injury.

Nursing assistive personnel (NAP) may be part of a health care team. The registered nurses must know who has the appropriate skills and competencies to meet a patient's needs when assigning a portion of care to someone else. Appropriate delegation and supervision of the person carrying out the assignment are imperative as the nurse is still responsible for the patient's care. Knowledge of what the state BON allows when delegating to others is imperative as some states do not specify which duties may be delegated, while others give clear guidance on which tasks can be assigned to others (Potter and Grant, 2004; Austin, 2008).

Statute of limitations

There is a time frame within which a plaintiff may file a lawsuit or lose the chance to have a day in court. If the plaintiff does not contact an attorney until shortly before the statute of limitations expires, there may not be enough time to investigate the facts of the case fully. To protect the client's interests, the attorney may name every person who could possibly be responsible for the injury. For example, if a patient dies as a result of an overdose of heparin and four different nurses administered the medication to the patient during the last 2 days of the patient's life, the attorney may name all four nurses as defendants. Those nurses determined to be fault free are then removed from the lawsuit before the trial.

 RISK MANAGEMENT STRATEGIES

Risk management is a system used by health care organizations to identify, analyze, and implement strategies for eliminating, minimizing, and coping with liabilities. In practice, risk management strategies combine the elements of loss reduction *and* loss prevention. Through a series of reactive and proactive activities, the potential for risk exposure is managed. The following are examples of risk management strategies that may decrease the risk of potential liability.

PATIENT RIGHTS

A critical responsibility of nurses is the duty not to violate patient rights. State and federal regulations governing health care mandate that every patient receiving health care be afforded certain rights. Hence, nursing care should be delivered in a manner that honors the rights of the patient. The five major topics pertaining to these rights are informed consent, refusal of treatment, discharge planning, freedom from restraints, and confidentiality. These issues, which are based on a professional obligation to the patient, carry legal consequences.

Informed consent is one of the most effective proactive risk management strategies. In general, consent is not required for procedures that are considered simple and common, and for which the risks are commonly understood. If a contemplated procedure inherently involves a known risk of death or serious harm, this risk must be disclosed to the patient, along with the complications that might possibly occur (Cady, 2005). Patients must be provided with sufficient information to enable them to rationally decide whether to undergo treatment. For the consent to be valid, the patient must be capable of granting consent, receive sufficient information to make an informed decision, and freely grant consent without coercion.

Although consent may be obtained verbally, a written agreement may also be required. Such may be the case with specialized procedures such as a PICC insertion. Documentation of the consent generally consists of evidence that the patient has received the necessary information, and that the patient has agreed to the proposed procedure. Because such documentation may protect both the patient and the nurse, consent forms are used as a risk management tool. However, the patient's signature on the form does not necessarily imply understanding of the informed consent. Informed consent is not simply the patient signing a consent form, but is a process of a detailed discussion between the health care provider and the patient (Tay, 2005).

Refusal of treatment refers to the right of every competent adult patient to decline therapy. Because the patient's wishes are paramount to any decision regarding health care, health care professionals are legally required to honor the patient's

decisions and any advance directives. For example, a patient has the right to refuse a transfusion. The patient must be informed of the consequences of such a decision, and should be required to sign forms documenting receipt of the information and confirming the decision. If a risk-free test or treatment is recommended, and the patient refuses to consent, the provider must advise the patient of all material risks of which a "reasonable person" would want to be informed before deciding not to undergo the procedure (Cady, 2005).

Refusing care may also take the form of leaving the health care facility against medical advice. Unless patients pose a danger—to themselves or others—that necessitates emergency detention for observation or psychiatric care, patients cannot be held against their will. Patients must be informed of the consequences of leaving, provided with adequate discharge instructions, and requested to sign forms confirming that they are leaving the facility against medical advice.

Discharge planning concentrates on preparing the patient for eventual discharge from the health care facility. Because patients are discharged when care is no longer medically necessary, governmental regulations mandate that patients be informed of and prepared for their date of discharge. Preparing the patient for discharge begins at the time of admission to the facility and continues throughout the patient's stay. For example, if a patient is admitted for insertion of an implanted port, instructions regarding care of the port should be initiated at the time of admission and continued until discharge. By doing so, the patient should be adequately prepared to care for the port, and discharge does not need to be postponed until patient teaching has been completed.

Freedom from restraints is a basic right of every patient. The only exceptions are in behavioral management situations, or if the patient's safety is in jeopardy. All restraints must be ordered by a physician in accordance with state and federal rules and regulations, with face-to-face evaluation of the patient within 1 hour if the purpose is behavioral management. An armboard used for the purpose of catheter stabilization at an area of flexion is not considered a restraint (INS, 2006).

Confidentiality means that information about the patient must be kept private, and should not be released without the patient's permission. This includes information contained in the patient's medical record, and details regarding the patient's diagnosis, treatment, and expected length of stay. The Health Insurance Portability and Accountability Act of 1996 (HIPAA) is meant to protect the privacy of patients' health information (Federal Register, 2003). All health care providers need to be educated related to HIPAA policies so that violations do not occur (Levine, 2006; Brous, 2007; Knox and Smith, 2007). Unauthorized disclosure carries fines, and if the disclosure results in economic, bodily, or psychological harm, the person who disclosed the information may be liable for damages.

UNUSUAL OCCURRENCE REPORTS

Documenting an unusual occurrence is a reactive risk management strategy that provides the facts concerning an event that may result in risk exposure. It is an internal reporting mechanism that notifies the organization that an event has occurred, and provides an opportunity to investigate the situation while the circumstances are still clear. Such documents were once referred to as *incident reports,* but because of the negative connotation, the terminology has been replaced with *reports of an unusual occurrence* or *variance reports.*

Unusual occurrence reports are confidential internal reporting mechanisms. If the patient's medical record contains evidence of a report and the patient later files a lawsuit, the report must be presented in court.

DOCUMENTATION

Accurate documentation in the medical record objectively describes the care rendered and the patient's response. Because a lawsuit may be filed years after the event occurred, the documentation in the medical record is often the only factual information available to determine whether there was a deviation from the standard of care. However, the reliability of the medical record may be discredited if there are inconsistencies, contradictory entries, unexplained time gaps, alterations, obliterations, omissions, or illegible entries (Ferrell, 2007; Monarch, 2007).

Nurses know that documentation in the medical record must be objective, legible, timely, complete, and accurate. The problem with documentation is often the result of a lack of compliance, not a lack of education. Substandard or absent documentation, in conjunction with significant patient injury, may lead to legal action against the nurse. Common legal claims for departure from standards of care include failure to make prompt, accurate entries in a patient's medical record and altering a medical record without noting it as a correction with signature, date, and time of change (Diehl-Svrjcek et al, 2007). Documentation is the only evidence to demonstrate that nursing actions met the legal standard of care.

PROFESSIONAL LIABILITY INSURANCE

Insurance is a risk management strategy whereby the nurse may transfer financial risk to an insurer. Because of the doctrine of *respondeat superior,* health care facilities and agencies usually carry insurance for negligent acts of their employees performed within the scope of their job responsibilities. However, many nurses also carry their own individual professional liability insurance.

The decision to purchase liability insurance is a personal one, and many factors must be considered. First, without insurance, the nurse may be required to use personal assets to compensate for a patient's injuries. However, if the actions were within the scope of employment, the damages may be covered by the employer's insurance policy. Second, potential risks must be evaluated. If there is high risk of personal liability because of the practice setting and nursing interventions employed, purchasing individual insurance may be warranted. Third, purchasing insurance requires that the nurse enter a contract with the insurer. As part of the contract, the nurse agrees to pay premiums and the insurer agrees to compensate the patient if the nurse is found guilty of malpractice. The nurse must evaluate the price of the premiums and understand that compensation is limited to the terms set in the insurance policy. Because insurance can be complex, the nurse must consider all benefits and risks before purchasing professional liability insurance.

PATIENT RELATIONS

It has been said that it is easier to sue an enemy than a friend. A patient who perceives the nurse as an impersonal, aloof person who is unconcerned with the patient's welfare is more apt to initiate legal action if an injury occurs. However, if the lines of communication are open between the nurse and patient, and expressions of anger, fear, and complaints by the patient are promptly investigated and resolved, claims of negligence may be avoided.

PERFORMANCE IMPROVEMENT

Performance improvement is the continuous effort to improve patient care by focusing on elements of an organization's performance. It serves as a risk management strategy because of its proactive approach to identify opportunities for improvement. Problems not only are identified and resolved, but outcomes also are improved by enhancing the processes involved in patient care. The focus is taken away from managing negative outcomes, but rather achieving positive results (Benvenuto, 2004).

CONTINUING COMPETENCY

Recognizing that passing a licensure examination does not ensure public health and safety throughout the career of a nurse, the National Council of State Boards of Nursing (NCSBN) has focused on continuing competency. They have defined *continued competence* as the ongoing ability to render safe direct nursing care, or the ongoing ability to make sound judgments upon which nursing care is based. Mechanisms identified that evaluate continuing competency include the following: professional certification and recertification, peer review, testing and retesting, continuing education, self-assessment, chart audits, electronic and clinical simulation, and a combination of activities that are reflected in professional portfolios (Monarch, 2002; NCSBN, 2008).

 SUMMARY

In today's increasingly cost-conscious and litigious health care environment, infusion nurses must provide safe, quality infusion nursing care. It is the nurse's responsibility to be knowledgeable of the legal risks and potential liabilities associated with this specialty practice. If care is rendered appropriately, the patient adequately monitored, actions accurately documented, and the physician informed of changes in the patient's condition, patient injury and litigation may be avoided.

 REFERENCES

American Nurses Association: *Nursing: scope and standards of nursing practice,* Washington, DC, 2004, Author.

Austin S: Seven legal tips for safe nursing practice, *Nursing2008* 38(3):34-39, 2008.

Beare PG, Myers JL: *Principles and practice of adult health nursing,* ed 3, St Louis, 1998, Mosby.

Belmon v. St. Francis Cabrini Hosp., 427 So.2d 541 (La. App. 1983) (failure to notice hemorrhage at needle puncture sites, a "major known-complication" and "well-known" risk of certain anticoagulant).

Bennett J, Brachman P: *Hospital infections,* ed 5, Philadelphia, 2007, Lippincott Williams & Wilkins.

Benvenuto DB: Performance improvement. In Alexander M, Corrigan A, editors: *Core curriculum for infusion nursing,* ed 3, Philadelphia, 2004, Lippincott Williams & Wilkins.

Berdyck v. Shinde, 613 N.E. 2d 1014 (Ohio 1993) (nurse who did not report nausea, headaches, and stomach pain of patient was negligent).

Brous EA: HIPAA vs. law enforcement, *AJN* 107(8):60-63, 2007.

Cady RF: Nurse executive's legal primer, *JONA Healthcare Law, Ethics, Regul* 7(1):10-20, 2005.

Centers for Disease Control and Prevention: Guidelines for the prevention of intravascular catheter-related infections, *MMWR* 51(RR-10):1-29, 2002.

Diehl-Svrjcek BC, Dawson B, Duncan LL: Infusion nursing: aspects of practice liability, *JIN* 30(5):274-279, 2007.

Dixon v. Taylor, 431 S.E. 2d 778 (N.C. Ct. App. 1993) (failure to keep code cart restocked).

Federal Register: Health insurance reform: security standards; final rule, *Fed Regist* 68(34):8334-8381, 2003 (to be codified at 45 CFR §§160, 162,164).

Federal Register: Occupational exposure to bloodborne pathogens; needlestick and other sharps injuries; final rule, *Fed Regist* 66:5317-5325, 2001 (to be codified at 29 CFR §1910).

Ferrell KG: Documentation, part 2: the best evidence of care, *AJN* 107(7):61-64, 2007.

Georgetti v. United Hospital Medical Ctr., 611 NYS2d 579 (1992) ("It is clear that when an attending physician gives direct and explicit orders to hospital staff, nurses are not authorized to unilaterally depart from them.").

Gibson v. Bossier City General Hospital, 594 So. 2d 1332 (La. Ct. App. 1991) ("[T]he events and circumstances [of the case] were beyond the knowledge of the average person" and therefore an expert witness was needed regarding alleged improper injection of medication).

Guilbeaux v. Lafayette General Hospital, 589 So. 2d 629 (La. Ct. 1991) (nurse committed malpractice by improperly removing Jackson-Pratt drain, leaving a strip of tube in the patient's back).

Habuda v. Trustees of Rex Hospital, Inc., 164 SE2d 17 (N.C. Ct. App. 1968) (nurse administered pHisoHex antibacterial scrub, instead of Milk of Magnesia, which was similar in appearance and location).

Harrington v. Rush Presbyterian-St. Lukes Hospital, 569 NE2d 15 (Ill. App. 1990).

Hill v. Ohio University, 610 NE2d 634 (Ohio Ct. Cl. 1988) (alleged failure to give "deep intramuscular injection" of Kenalog, as required).

Holmes HN, *Nurses legal handbook,* ed 5, Philadelphia, 2004, Lippincott Williams & Wilkins.

Infusion Nurses Society: Infusion nursing standards of practice, *JIN* 29(suppl 1S), 2006.

Jensen v. Archbishop Bergen Mercy Hosp., 459 NW2d 178 (Neb. 1991).

Knox C, Smith A: Handhelds and HIPAA, *Nursing Management* 38(6):38-40, 2007.

Koeniguer v. Eckrich, 422 NW2d 600 (S.D. 1988) ("standards published by the ANA and various general practices treatises" relevant in nurse malpractice cases).

Levine C: HIPAA and talking with family caregivers, *AJN* 106(8):51-53, 2006.

Maciag v. Strato Medical Corp., 644 A.2d 647 (N.J. Super. Ct. 1994) (*res ipsa* applied when subclavian venous catheter fractured inside unconscious patient).

Markovich MB: The expanding role of the infusion nurse in radiographic interpretation for peripherally inserted central catheter tip placement, *JIN* 31(2):96-103, 2008.

Miller-Slades D: Liability theories in nursing negligence cases, 33 *Trial Liability* 43 Clev. St. L. Rev. 57 (1995).

Monarch K: Documentation, part 1: principles for self protection, *AJN* 107(7):58-60, 2007.

Monarch K: *Nursing and the law: trends and issues,* Washington, DC, 2002, American Nurses Publishing.

National Council of State Boards of Nursing. Meeting the ongoing challenge of continued competence [concept paper]. Accessed 5/19/08 at https://www.ncsbn.org/Continued_Comp_Paper_TestingServices.pdf.

National Council of State Boards of Nursing: *Nurse licensure compact administrators.* Accessed 5/19/08 at www.ncsbn.org/nlc.htm.

Polonsky v. Union Hospital, 418 NE2d 620 (Mass. Ct. App. 1981) (nurse found negligent for not knowing of dangers of giving sleeping drug Dalmane to elderly patient recovering from a heart attack).

Potter P, Grant E: Understanding RN and unlicensed assistive personnel working relationships in designing care delivery strategies, *JONA* 34(1):19-25, 2004.

Roach v. Springfield Clinic, 585 NE2d 1070 (Ill. App. 1991) (failure to notify physician of abnormal fetal heart tones detected by monitoring system).

Tay CSK: Recent developments in informed consent: the basis of modern medical ethics, *APLAR J Rheumatol* 8:165-170, 2005.

U.S. Food and Drug Administration: *Medical device reporting (MDR): general information.* Accessed 5/30/08 at www.fda.gov/cdrh/mdr/mdr-general.html (updated 9/22/02).

Vogler v. Dominguez, 624 NE2d 56 (Ind. Ct. App. 1993) (failure to report "abnormalities" or changes in a patient's condition can be negligent).

Weinstein SM: *Plumer's principles and practices of intravenous therapy,* ed 8, Philadelphia, 2007, Lippincott Williams & Wilkins.

5 ETHICS

Kathryn Schroeter, PhD, RN, CNOR*

In the current climate of health care reform, nurses may have difficulty with such ethical issues as patient rights, societal needs, and allocation of resources. Every day, nurses are asked to assist patients and families in dealing with ethical concerns. Since nurses work in an environment where patients are vulnerable, it becomes imperative that nurses be able to understand and articulate the ethical issues that surround their practice.

Bioethics is a branch of applied ethics that studies the philosophical, social, and legal issues that arise in medicine and the life sciences. It is no longer a topic that is discussed only from a philosophical perspective. The principles are being applied to everyday health care decisions and the importance is growing as the current practice changes. There may also be physiological responses that occur as a result of the stress incurred from the attempts by individuals to cope with their situations. Some ethical situations may evolve into legal battles as the perceptions of the patients, families, health care providers, and organization administrators may not always be in agreement. Nurses benefit from understanding and using ethical frameworks to better manage health care dilemmas.

In a report on the nursing shortage, the U.S. General Accounting Office (U.S. GAO) reported that nurses' sources of dissatisfaction included poor working conditions such as inadequate staffing, heavy workloads, increased use of overtime, and lack of sufficient support staff (U.S. GAO, 2001). Perhaps, while not directly stated as such, these factors may be influenced by nurses' experiences of moral distress, and this could further compound the current nursing shortage as nurses continue to leave the workforce.

Moral distress is a serious problem in nursing (Nathaniel, 2002). It may be a significant contributing factor to loss of nurses' integrity and dissatisfaction with their work. It may also contribute to problems with nurse-patient relationships, and thus affect the quality, quantity, and cost of nursing care. Loss of nurses from the workforce is a compelling threat to patient care.

While nurses are often the first to become aware of patients' ethical quandaries, they often feel unprepared or unqualified to deal with ethical decision-making. Nurses need useful, proactive, and relevant strategies in order to more effectively deal with ethical issues, and ultimately lead to improved clinical practice.

Nurses are responsible for nursing decisions that are not only clinically and technically sound but also morally appropriate and suitable for the specific problems of the particular patient being treated. The medical (technical) aspects of the decision answer the question, "What *can* be done for this patient?" The moral component involves patient wishes and answers the question, "What *ought* to be done for this patient?" (Schroeter et al, 2002).

This chapter is designed to educate infusion nurses about principles and applications for the effective management of ethical concerns and issues. By offering an overview of bioethics along with implications for the profession of nursing, this information both enlightens and enhances the professionalism of nurses by guiding decision-making and communication and promoting an understanding of current trends and practices.

ETHICS

As nurses are all too aware, there are ethical conflicts inherent to health care. An ethical conflict can be described as a presenting event that requires commitment to a single obligation when two or more genuine duties exist; the resultant outcomes have option-specific variability; and moral regret is a residual, demonstrative manifestation of the selection process (Beauchamp and Childress, 2001). It is also helpful to have a working definition of the terms "ethics" and "moral" even though they are often used interchangeably:

- Ethics: a mode of inquiry that helps one understand the moral dimensions of human conduct (Fry, 1989)
- Moral: overlaps with "ethical" but is more aligned with personal belief and cultural values (American Nurses Association [ANA], 2001)

Ethical behavior is an extremely complex phenomenon. It reflects society and how the actions of people living in groups

*The author and editors wish to acknowledge the contributions made by Lorys Oddi as author of this chapter in the second edition of *Infusion Therapy in Clinical Practice*.

affect each other. Discussions of ethics commonly divide the content area into thoughts, behaviors, and emotions. There are subsequent variables within the disciplines that impact ethical behavior. However, the relationships among these elements seem uncertain. The discipline of nursing, with its own history and evolution, has elements that both describe and impact nurses' ethical reasoning and behavior.

ETHICS CODES

Fortunately, the profession of nursing has standards, practices, and an ethical code to provide some guidance for the discipline (ANA, 2001). According to the American Nurses Association (ANA), nurses have a duty to provide ethical care for patients, but also an ethical duty to care for self and family. The duty to care as an ethical component of the nurse-patient relationship can be inferred from the second provision of the ANA's *Code of Ethics for Nursing*, which notes that the nurse's primary commitment is to the patient (ANA, 2001).

At times, nurses must decide how, when, or if they should take action on behalf of a patient; whether to intervene if a professional colleague (nurse, physician, or other health care worker) is violating the rights of other individuals or is endangering patients; and how they can balance legitimate self-interest against the demands of the institution, patients, and physicians. A nurse must recognize that there is a duty to the patient, but also a duty to self. Professional nurses practice autonomously and also as members of the health care team. Nurses may find themselves in practice situations in which they are expected to conform to institutional routines and practices regardless of their views of appropriate courses of action for patient care.

While issues such as patient/human rights as evidenced in topics like end-of-life decision-making, do-not-resuscitate orders, informed consent, and the right to refuse treatment may be woven throughout, it may be true that some issues are more prevalent in certain nursing specialties than others. For example, end-of-life issues may be encountered more often in the intensive care, hospice, and oncology practice settings than in other outpatient environments. The issues may not only vary in intensity from practice setting to practice setting, but also there may be other factors that affect the nurse's ability to address ethical issues.

According to Biton and Tabak (2003), work satisfaction is known to be one of the major factors related to nurses' quality of care. They argued that professionalism, as manifested by the ethical code of practice, needs to be applied on a daily basis in the workplace. These researchers examined nurses' perceptions of the everyday strains on their work to assess how they experienced the amount of energy invested in following an ethical code of practice. It has become vital that nurses know how to manage ethical decisions appropriately, so that patients' rights can be honored without compromising the nurse's own moral conscience.

In today's climate of cost containment, nurses may feel pressure to "cut corners" in delivering care, to accept understaffing that they feel may jeopardize patient care, and to sacrifice their personal welfare and that of their families to work double shifts or forego earned days off when staffing problems arise. Whether the nurse is employed in a hospital, the community, a clinic, or a home, the employing institution exerts a significant effect on professional practice.

Over the years, the nursing profession has been increasingly articulate in declaring the need for nurses to have autonomy in their professional practice. Improved education and the broadening of nursing responsibilities have certainly contributed to increasing this autonomy. Professional organizations also stress that nurses' primary responsibility is to their patients. Although they overtly promote the ideal of patients' needs as their primary concern, institutions may actually expect nurses to be primarily concerned with the agency's welfare. Incorporating the code of ethics into daily practice and understanding the issues are the beginning of comprehensive and competent nursing practice.

EXPLICATIONS FOR PRACTICE

Each specialty area of nursing practice takes the ANA's *Code of Ethics* and derives explications for practice. Nurses who practice infusion therapy must develop knowledge and skill to analyze the ethical aspects of their specific care if they are to effectively fulfill their professional responsibilities. The code can serve as a starting point but there needs to be more understanding and knowledge to provide ethical nursing practice.

How, then, can the moral dimensions of infusion nursing be explained? The nursing literature consistently suggests that patient advocacy provides a model of professional nursing that is highly desirable. Patient advocacy is viewed as an essential component of the role of the professional nurse, but how does the nurse view the component of advocacy? Assuming the stance of a patient advocate involves acting on ethical principles and values.

Nurses in a variety of patient care settings, such as infusion nurses, are available to patients to hear their concerns and wishes. Nurses have always been on the front line and, in that position, are often the first to advocate for their patients. As patient advocates, nurses are in a position where they must act to secure patients' safety, and this includes acting to prevent an impaired coworker from providing patient care while under the influence of substances such as alcohol or drugs.

However, some nurses who raise questions about ethical aspects of patient care with a physician or other health care provider may risk personal reprimand, verbal abuse, or disciplinary action within the institution or by the licensing board. Although physicians and other health care providers legitimately need nurses to carry out some medical aspects of patient care, they are not entitled to interfere with aspects of nursing practice that lie outside of their medical expertise, or to expect nurses to abandon their responsibility to patients and the institution because of a physician's demands. This is a difficult position for nurses to be in and that is why most organizations have a confidential number or contact that employees can use to report unethical practice. Each nurse needs to be aware of the steps within an organization that are available to help deal with ethical issues in practice.

The traditional view that nurses must sacrifice personal and family interests and concerns to meet the demands of patients and the employing institution may occasionally place nurses in ethical dilemmas. A nurse could feel obliged to work extra shifts and holidays to such an extent that primary commitments to family members (e.g., spouse, children, aged parents) would suffer. In these situations, the nurse's physical and psychological health and well-being could be impaired.

To the extent that nurses feel they cannot fulfill the expectations of society, they may also experience confusion and conflict about such activities as providing artificial feeding, resuscitating terminal patients, and engaging in other life-prolonging efforts when such efforts appear futile. Each nurse must personally reflect on the ethical issues that are evident in his or her own practice, and make a decision about how he or she can continue to practice without compromising individual moral and professional integrity. Whatever the cause, repeated violations of one's integrity are harmful to oneself and, ultimately, to patient care. The whole reason for the existence of nursing is to contribute to the health of patients.

Furthermore, if nurses fail to comply with demands or cannot meet the expectations of others, they may suffer consequences in their personal and professional lives. Failure to act in accordance with one's beliefs violates one's conscience and places one in moral jeopardy. Unfortunately, the correct course of action is not always obvious. In addition, numerous other factors come into play, such as the seriousness of the violation of another's rights and well-being; the harshness of the consequences for all concerned; and the scope of the nurse's authority, control, and responsibility.

For example, if a nurse risks negative repercussions from the institution or the physician by fulfilling perceived obligations to the patient, he or she may be tempted to avoid the risk and act in self-interest and for self-protection. Failure to act in accordance with one's conscience can cause acute discomfort and, as discussed later, can be very detrimental if it develops into an ongoing pattern of behavior. Conflicting demands and potentially serious consequences mitigate nurses' moral responsibility for actions taken or avoided in a situation.

Nurses should not be required to be heroic in their disagreements with an institution, but rather need to develop a realistic view of others' duties in ethical dilemmas and to recognize the limits of their own responsibility. The consequences to all parties involved should be considered before the nurse takes any action, and the nurse must make every effort to make sound ethical decisions before choosing a course of action. Incurring a reprimand or the displeasure of a colleague is a small price to pay for taking appropriate action.

However, extreme personal sacrifices, such as losing one's job or facing legal or professional disciplinary action, should not ordinarily be required to maintain one's moral integrity, unless the ethical violation involved is sufficiently grave to warrant such sacrifice. In other words, an important question to ask in nurses' ethical decision-making may be, "How far must I go to resolve this situation?" In some cases the demands of other parties may be so unreasonable and the consequences of failure to comply with those demands so drastic that nurses may have to make a conscious choice about whether or not to continue to work in a given situation.

Fortunately, heroic sacrifice is not routinely required. Even if nurses cannot always successfully and openly confront issues, engaging in ethical analysis may clarify the issue and open the door for realistic efforts at resolution. In any situation, nurses can and must critically examine questionable health care decisions, analyze the constraints and contingencies involved, and ask for reasons or justification for actions taken. The nurse is not justified in standing by passively when ethical dilemmas arise.

In summary, the conflicting expectations of multiple roles (professional, employee, family member, and individual) place nurses in ethical dilemmas. Nurses may feel they are obliged to be "all things to all people" and are adversely affected when they are unable to please everyone in a given situation. Feeling caught between opposing duties is stressful and demoralizing for the nurse, who may retreat into inaction in an effort to escape psychological conflict.

VALUES AND VALUING

To function as competent, caring, and professional health care providers, today's nurses must use strategies that develop values into motivational and collaborative visions and goals. Values influence the relational and behavioral aspects of patient care and the functioning of organizations.

Nurses who understand how values impact on recruitment and retention can provide staff enrichment and enhance multidisciplinary partnerships. Aiken, Havens, and Sloane (2000) reported that the organizational context in which nurses practice is important. The values and ethics inherent to nursing are also inherent to creating a Magnet culture of nursing practice. The Magnet program designated by the American Nurses Credentialing Center (ANCC) recognizes those hospital facilities that foster an environment that attracts and retains competent nurses through respect for the values, art, and science of nursing. Magnet hospitals allow nurses to focus on patients, resulting in positive outcomes that can be directly attributed to nursing care.

Values are integral to creating a Magnet culture and can enhance the practice environment. The strength in understanding culture lies in the relationships that can be made between beliefs and values that are inherent to various cultures. Value and valuing are notions intrinsic to ethics, culture, and social behavior.

Within the nursing process, the nurse uses values that have been acquired through education and experience; these values are involved, perhaps unconsciously, in the day-to-day decisions the nurse makes about nursing practice. The values involved in the ethical decision-making process may not be obvious to the nurse. Many of these values have their origins in the nurse's religious, cultural, and ethnic childhood experiences. They are an integral part of the nurse's personality, and play a major role in the nurse's intuitive response to ethical dilemmas encountered in practice. Furthermore, each nurse has a different value system. Many of the beliefs, assumptions, and attitudes that contribute to the value system may need to be examined systematically before they are put into action in ethical decision-making.

 ## NURSES AS ADVOCATES

It is important to examine advocacy as a concept in its relation to the discipline of nursing since it presents as a common theme throughout the current literature. Primarily, it has been argued that the ethical constraint facing nurses is that they are not free to be ethical because they are dispossessed of the free action of moral agency, the ability to act independently for one's patient(s).

In the discipline of nursing, advocacy is viewed as a duty or obligation. This relates to the ANA code statement (2001, p. 14) that "as an advocate for the patient, the nurse must be alert to and take appropriate action regarding any instances of incompetent, unethical, illegal, or impaired practice...." This duty arises from the nurse's role as continual observer of the patient's condition. Deontology, or duty-based ethics, prescribes actions to be done solely out of obligation. It is questionable whether such action(s) can be, or is (are), demonstrated consistently, and nurses may have differing perceptions of this concept.

ADVOCACY

The concept of advocacy reflects the confusion, and potential conflict, between the responsibility of nurses to support the patient as well as the institution, and also the need of nurses to support themselves. Empirical evidence is sparse and philosophical arguments prevail in the field of patient advocacy (Hewitt, 2002). There are other health care providers, such as physicians, social workers, and therapists, who fill the role of patient advocate.

Nurses follow their code of ethics and that directs them to be patient advocates; however, they may not always be working in partnership with other health care providers who are also advocates for the patient. As nurses collaborate with these other health care providers, they can involve them in the process of facilitating ethical decision-making and may promote improved patient care. Nurses may invite other health care providers to participate in family care conferences related to ethical concerns, or even in ethics consultation meetings that may occur within the sphere of patient care.

How can advocacy, as it relates to the role of the nurse, be described? Kohnke (1980) suggests that the nurse's role as a patient advocate has three basic components: (1) to inform patients of their rights in a particular situation, (2) to ensure that patients are given all the information necessary to make an informed decision, and (3) to support patients in decisions they make. This research is reflective of what can be found in many hospital or health care organizational policies that address nursing care and responsibilities.

The third point in Kohnke's definition may be perceived as relativistic in that it tells the nurse to support whatever the patient decides. This implies an "anything goes" philosophy of ethics, but the definition does not, however, reflect the concept of choice. The nurse still has the ability to choose whether or not to support the patient's decisions. Some nurses can support patients' decisions while other nurses cannot if there is too great a disparity between the decision and the nurse's moral conscience.

Since patients and nurses are individuals, they may not have the same beliefs or values, but this does not necessarily mean that they must cross a line within their personal moral code that they do not wish to cross. If nurses are to value individuality and treat patients objectively and without judgment, then nurses may need to opt out of providing care in those situations where they feel ethically compromised.

An example of patient advocacy as identified in the role of the infusion nurse is described by Gorski (2008):

"I made a visit to a long term home infusion therapy patient whom I had never seen before. This patient was independent with fluid administration in management of her conditions including short bowel syndrome and malabsorption. The purpose of my home visit was to perform a routine monthly assessment to address any changes in condition and infusion needs. She immediately shared with me that she had a small crack in her Hickman catheter near the hub. This occurred when she accidentally forgot to open the catheter clamp during line flushing. She did not call the home infusion pharmacy but had sought help through her physician. The physician gave her a prescription to have the catheter repaired. She took the prescription to the outpatient department and was referred to the nurse who was known as the clinic's infusion 'expert.' This nurse told her that her catheter was not repairable and that she would need to have it replaced...in terms of additional background to this case, the patient's Hickman catheter was over one year old and the exit site looked good—other than the small crack near the hub—and that this patient had several catheters over quite a few years...and a previous physician was unable to place a catheter due to thrombotic changes in her vasculature... The patient voiced frustration because she still believed her line could be repaired. During the visit, I called and spoke to the clinic infusion nurse who was insistent that the catheter could not be repaired. The end result was that I ordered the appropriate repair kit through the home infusion pharmacy and successfully performed the procedure. Six months later, all continues to go well with this patient and her catheter and she was pleased to avoid another procedure."

In this example the author discusses two infusion nursing standards—Standard 57: Access Device Repair; and Standard 7: Ethics (INS, 2006). The *Infusion Nursing Code of Ethics* related to standards of practice (INS, 2001) provides clarification and guidance for the nurse practicing in this specialty area. Key to note in the standard is the focus on advocacy for nursing practice. The standards stress that ethical principles shall be the foundation for decision-making and patient advocacy and that the principles of beneficence, nonmaleficence, fidelity, protection of patient autonomy, justice, and veracity shall dictate nursing action (INS, 2006). The nurse shall act as a patient advocate; maintain patient confidentiality, safety, and security; and respect, promote, and preserve human autonomy, dignity, rights, and diversity.

According to Gorski (2008), when the possibility of access device repair is considered, the RN must be competent in performing the procedure, and if the device is not repairable, it must be removed. Gorski suggests, however, that nurses may lack the knowledge that some catheters are repairable and that catheter damage is a relatively uncommon occurrence. Because much infusion therapy is provided by nurses and other health care providers who are not specialists in infusion therapy and who are not familiar with the *Infusion Nursing Standards of Practice*, we as infusion nurses must continually address this lack of knowledge (Gorski, 2008). While the infusion nurse has an ethical obligation to act as a patient advocate, his or her lack of knowledge may interfere with taking the necessary action. In the previous example, the clinic nurse might not have known that the catheter was repairable and, though she may have wanted to provide the best care possible for her patients, she was unable to consider the risks and benefits of catheter replacement. The potential benefits of catheter repair included avoiding a potentially difficult catheter replacement, the risks associated with another surgical procedure, disruption in the patient's life, and the out-of-pocket costs to the patient as well as insurance costs. When objectively weighing the risks versus the benefits, the benefits of catheter repair outweighed the risks of catheter replacement (Gorski, 2008). Repairing the catheter was following the principle of beneficence, doing "good" for the patient, and, as such, being able to act as a patient advocate.

To clarify advocacy, it is important to note that nurses may be able to identify ethical obligations, or duties, but each nurse may bring a different knowledge base and describe a different motivation behind his or her actions. Speculation might offer that the frustration that nurses experience when attempting to function in the role of patient advocate reflects the confusion between advocacy and empowerment. In other words, nurses must feel a level of empowerment that will allow them to take action(s) as appropriate to provide safe, competent, and ethical patient care.

NURSING CARE PROVIDED IN THE HOME HEALTH ENVIRONMENT

Nurses who care for patients in their homes often develop relationships with their patients as they provide care over multiple home visits and often over a relatively long time. This aspect of time can influence the infusion nurse's perception of the patient's ethical issues and needs.

A qualitative study by Oberle and Tenove (2000) focused on 22 public health nurses, 11 in rural settings and 11 in urban settings, who described ethical problems that they had experienced in practice. The nurses in this study most often described a relational response rather than a choice between options when they described their ethical concerns. Their goal was to maintain the "good" while simultaneously maintaining a supportive relationship with their patients. The themes that emerged from these data included relationships, respect for persons, systems' issues, and putting self at risk. The infusion home health nurse may have opportunities to talk in depth about such factors as family and issues of feelings, for example, which puts the nurse in a position to advocate for his or her patients.

In addition, the relationships in home health nursing tend to emphasize more than the nurse/patient link by stressing the nurse/patient/family relationship (Ladd et al, 2000). By virtue of caring for patients in their homes, it is easy to see that home health nurses would function in more of a triad relationship, as it would be difficult to remove the family or significant others with whom the patient lives. Therefore it becomes imperative for the infusion nurse to consider his or her relationship to the patient when providing care in the patient's home.

CULTURAL COMPETENCE

Cultural competence is an integral part of nursing practice and a component of ethically competent care. In essence, to disallow the cultural differences of individual patients would be tantamount to unethical patient care by nurses or any other type of health care providers. It is thus necessary to explore the issue of cultural competence and the perception of nurses as related to this aspect of ethical practice. Nurses providing infusion therapy care for patients across the social and cultural spectrum. They identify cultural differences of individuals, and they assess these factors in order to provide care that will meet the cultural needs of their patients.

Nurses who provide infusion therapy need to be able to differentiate between culturally sensitive care and culturally competent care. They need to be able to note if the care they provide is adequate (i.e., they need to be sensitive to or aware of an individual's cultural needs when providing care). They need to be able to note if they or other nurses are competent to address cultural needs in practice. For example, if the infusion nurse notes that another member of the health care team is unable or unwilling to incorporate specific cultural aspects to patient care, then this action or lack of action can become either a benefit or a burden to any related ethical decision-making.

▍ APPROACHES TO ETHICAL DECISION-MAKING

Nurses are most likely familiar with ethical decision-making. There are many different methods that can be used to facilitate ethical decision-making in the health care environment. The nurse should be able to apply his or her already acquired skills to the ethical decision-making process and then build on them as needed.

Ethical decision-making requires a systematic approach; the nurse must collect facts from many sources, analyze those facts, and arrive at a conclusion. How do nurses attempt to resolve ethical conflict situations? Spielman (1993) asserts that there are five basic approaches to ethical conflict resolution: (1) avoidance, characterized by evasion and unwillingness to engage in problem solving; (2) accommodation, a one-sided approach characterized by behavior that conforms to the other party's values and sacrifices one's own values; (3) coercion, a one-sided approach characterized by conforming to one's own values and sacrificing the other party's values; (4) compromise, a joint approach characterized by give and take and some sacrifice of each participant's values; and (5) collaboration, a joint approach that produces a solution requiring little or no sacrifice of either party's values. Spielman argues that the resolution of conflict need not depend only on abstract theory, intuition, communication skills, and time constraints. It is important to understand why a nurse may or may not report unethical practice as it may have a direct impact on patient care and safety.

An overview of ethical theory and practice models can help nurses understand how to use ethics in practice. The models can be classified as action-based, agent-based, and situation-based.

ACTION-BASED

Principles of bioethics recognize and define the moral obligation on the part of nurses to further the welfare, health, and well-being of their patients. Acting on principle is necessary if nurses are to exhibit integrity, which requires that one's actions be consistent with one's beliefs. People who lack integrity, who vacillate from one value system to another, quickly become known as unreliable, capricious, or untrustworthy among professional colleagues. They are dangerous because their actions, based on personal values, may violate the rights of those with whom they come in contact.

The principle of beneficence, in particular, is understood and generally accepted by health care professionals and the public to be a foundational principle of the patient-provider relationship (Ruderman et al, 2006).

The principlist approach applies the principle of respect for autonomy, the principle of beneficence, the principle of non-maleficence, and the principle of justice to contemporary ethical dilemmas. Although this approach is sometimes criticized for its lack of foundational theory and its Western-dominated methodology, principlism is widely used as a starting point for practical ethical decision-making in the clinical, technological, and epidemiological professions.

This approach to ethics is one designed specifically to facilitate identification, analysis, and resolution of dilemmas relevant to concerns within the health care sciences (Beauchamp and Childress, 2001). The values of autonomy, beneficence, nonmaleficence, and justice are fundamental elements of principlism, because of their common acceptance. It is important to recognize while reviewing these values that they contain no hierarchical order. No one value will trump another value. These values are complementary and, in some instances, one value will conflict with another.

These principles frequently conflict with the values of those involved in ethical decision-making. It is often difficult to prioritize between principles as the context of each situation may vary. The primary principles are autonomy, beneficence, non-maleficence, justice, veracity, and fidelity.

Autonomy is the self-determination of an individual. It encompasses respect for persons as it allows individuals to make voluntary, uncoerced decisions about all life situations. Beneficence is the principle of doing good. It is what health care providers strive to do for their patients (i.e., to do good, to benefit, or to act in the best interests of the patient). Non-maleficence is the principle that directs health care providers to do no harm. Justice is the principle that treats individuals according to what is fair or owed to them. Patients in the hospital expect to be treated fairly and to receive equal care. Veracity is the principle of truth telling. In American society, it is expected that health care providers will be truthful about all aspects of the patient's care. It is also an expectation of health care providers to keep the promises of the patient. This principle is fidelity and is demonstrated in the health care providers' responsibility to maintain the confidentiality of patient information.

The principlist approach uses the aforementioned principles to represent and codify certain values and understandings of ethics. Depending on the situation, one or more principles may take precedence over the others. The interaction between the principles will generate a resolution to the conflict, and the interaction will vary depending on the dynamics of the ethical situation encountered. One principle usually will carry more weight and, thus, result in a particular decision or choice of action being made. This theory argues that the principles in a given ethical situation are weighted and prioritized according to the individual's or group's perspective.

Consequentialism refers to a group of normative ethical theories that maintain that the moral status of an action is determined by the goodness or badness of its consequences. One common type of consequentialism is utilitarianism, where a decision is made regarding the best course of action by simply applying a cost-benefit analysis to the situation. A commonly accepted utilitarian calculus for determining an action's moral acceptability is "the greatest happiness for the greatest number." Thus a consequentialist would typically attempt to calculate the consequences or outcome of a decision, and if the benefits of the outcome are outweighed by the risks of either not performing the action or performing some other action, then the action is considered as morally desirable.

Critics of consequentialism often cite situations in which the application of a consequentialist theory runs into trouble. For instance, consequentialism would allow actions of slavery or torture if the benefits to the majority outweighed the harms to those who were enslaved or tortured. More specific versions of consequentialism have attempted to address this problem with some success.

Nonconsequentialism is given to a group of ethical theories that do not determine the moral status of an action solely by the goodness or badness of its consequences. Rather than calculating the consequences of an action and then deciding whether the benefits of performing that action are outweighed by its risks, a nonconsequentialist will tend to take other considerations into account when deciding the morally right course of action.

The most cited nonconsequentialist ethical theory is deontology. A deontologist simply judges the moral acceptability of an action using a rights-based or duty-based system of analysis. In other words, a person who adopts a deontological system of ethical decision-making will typically think in terms of "a person's right to act in some way" or "a right to possess something." Decisions are also made using duty-based justifications such as "a duty to act on a certain principle" or a "duty not to hinder some course of action." Deontologists are sometimes confronted with the problem of conflicting duties or rights. Thus a morally right course of action may reveal that there are in fact two opposing rights applicable in any one situation.

AGENT-BASED

The agent-based model of ethical decision-making focuses on the moral nature of the agent(s) or the one(s) making the ethical decisions. The primary agent-based model or theoretical approach involves virtue as the means to the end. Such virtue-based approaches to ethics place importance on the character of the person performing the action rather than on the action itself. Virtue ethics has its roots in Greek philosophy in the work of Aristotle. Hierarchies of virtues, like vices, have changed over time but generally include justice, temperance, charity, mercy and wisdom to name a few.

Generally, virtue ethicists believe that traditional moral theories fail to acknowledge the importance of the role of inner character traits in ethical decision-making. Thus if a nurse makes a decision to take ethical action in the care of a patient and the patient inadvertently becomes injured or has a negative outcome from the care provided, the nurse is still said to have acted in an ethical manner since it was the intent of the nurse to do good. The negative consequences of the action(s) do not negate the good that was originally intended by the nurse.

SITUATION-BASED

Casuistry is the name given to a newly revived school of ethical thought originating in sixteenth century Spain. Casuists argue that specific cases inform moral principles, not vice versa. Thus the best starting point for ethical decision-making is examining particular cases and the respective decisions made about those cases. Casuistry is most easily applied to dilemmas in medical ethics where case study provides for effective teaching practices.

Casuistry is a case-based method that supports the premise that sometimes it makes more sense to start with cases rather than principles. This approach uses analogical reasoning, which allows valid comparisons among cases, much like precedent in case law. The guidelines in casuistry reflect both insights from specific examples and larger ideas embodied in principles. The process of casuistry begins with a paradigm case and then discerns which aspects of the paradigm, when examined together, make the case morally unambiguous. The approach known as casuistry works on the premise that routine daily living and social institutions exemplify moral principles. Nurses can then reflect upon the practices and situations that are done well and in which the right actions are clear or paradigmatic. Concepts or principles are the by-product of the case analysis.

Casuistry emphasizes practical problem solving by means of subtle interpretations of individual cases based on paradigm cases. The cases used are real, and it is important to make them long, richly detailed, and comprehensive in order to promote the best understanding. Additionally, the cases should reflect the perspectives of all the involved participants. Ethical principles are applied in casuistry, but are discovered in the cases themselves and emerge gradually from reflection upon our responses to particular cases.

Relativism is the view that moral appraisals are essentially dependent upon a moral code that is specific to a time, place, and culture. There are no absolute criteria with which moral actions may be appraised. A relativist may cite geographical, historical, or anthropological data in support of his or her case. In short, moral relativism accepts what all human beings do as appropriate in their contexts. There is no basis for ethical argument or discussion. Relativism, when used as an excuse for action, may not always be appropriate, nor may it avoid violating the rights of any, or all, involved in the ethical situation.

Each situation we encounter is unique because each patient and relevant circumstances are unique. A set of rules rigidly and automatically applied can lead to highly unethical decisions. This inability to apply rules rigidly leads some nurses to draw the erroneous conclusion that all ethical decisions are arbitrary and subject to personal whim. Nothing could be further from the truth: exercise of arbitrary and unpredictable decisions in the ethical aspects of care can create much harm and injustice. A consistent, thoughtful approach is mandatory for those responsible for the care of patients.

Feminist approaches to ethical analysis purport that contemporary fundamental moral principles generally fail to consider the importance of moral relationships and the role of emotion in moral reasoning. This alternative approach to ethical analysis turns attention from moral judgments to focus on the importance of the moral impulse or moral attitude. Sometimes called an ethic of care, this approach to ethics concentrates on the "being" of ethics rather than on the "doing," much like a virtue ethics position. The central focus of an ethic of care is on loving, caring, empathy, and sensitivity.

The strength of the ethical perspective is its prescriptive nature. It promotes an action guide for nurses to follow in the realm of patient care. As ethics is a branch of philosophy, there are multiple approaches to take when it comes to applying actions to real life situations. Thus each nurse may not only experience a situation differently but also address the situation; identify and analyze the ethical conflict issues, feelings, behaviors, and actions; and resolve the situation differently.

ETHICAL THEORIES

The process skills that nurses bring to ethical decision-making are not sufficient to enable sound ethical decisions. When nurses and other health care providers are involved in ethical decision-making, it is often evident that not everyone analyzes the issues from a similar view. There are many theories that are used to help us deal with ethical issues. Ethical theories consider the motive or intent of the practitioner/agent, the means used by the agent to accomplish the act, and the consequences of the act. A few of the more commonly used theories are as follows:

- *Utilitarianism:* This theory is often interpreted as purporting that the way to decide is based on the numbers (i.e., the greatest good for the greatest number). An action or means of practice is right if it focuses on maximizing the good consequences and minimizing the bad consequences as a whole.
- *Deontology:* This theory is based on the concept of duty or binding obligation. The means of an action are intrinsically or inherently right or wrong. Nurses are bound by their professional duty to always do right by their patients. In essence, what we do for our patients is good because it is our duty to care for them properly.

- *Virtue:* Virtue theory might also be known as Aristotelian ethics as it has evolved from the philosophy of Aristotle. In this theory, the intent of the agent (person taking the ethical stand or action) is what determines whether or not the act was good or moral. If the intent was to do good, then even if the outcome was bad, the act would still be considered ethical.
- *Egoist:* Objectivism, a philosophy developed in the latter half of the twentieth century, puts forth an ethical theory or system of rational self-interest. It does not, however, treat ethics as an isolated field; rather, it builds on two prerequisite branches of philosophy: metaphysics (our world around us) and epistemology (how we know what we know). It uses objectivism, metaphysics, and epistemology as a foundation for its theories on politics. While this growing philosophical movement carries with it some controversy, such as selfishness as a virtue, it deserves investigation.

Individuals must always remember that they may have inadequate or incorrect information about a situation. They may have engaged in faulty reasoning or may lack the insight or experience necessary to make the sound decision. Furthermore, health care situations are dynamic, and new developments may change the ethical aspects of any situation. These limitations mean that nurses must remain flexible and consider new information. Respect for others is absolutely critical. If nurses enter ethical conflicts with a rigid and judgmental attitude, satisfactory resolution of conflicts will be delayed, inhibited, or prevented. In addition, interpersonal conflicts will develop if others feel devalued by the nurse's negative attitudes.

 ## APPLICATIONS TO INFUSION NURSING PRACTICE

An examination of the nursing literature reveals that many rules, principles, and philosophies are available to help nurses in their ethical decision-making endeavors. Sometimes, this variety of information can be more a hindrance than help because the resulting detail and complexity can overwhelm the reader and lead to a sense of paralysis and despair. Each nurse should study and adopt a coherent approach that makes sense to him or her.

The principles involved with the framework presented in this chapter are not discussed comprehensively in the following paragraphs. Rather, discussion is limited to the essential elements of each principle, an overview of their importance, and examples of situations in which the infusion nurse may encounter conflicts relating to the principles.

 ## ETHICAL PRACTICE FOR INFUSION NURSING

Infusion nurses may encounter potential violations of patients' rights of autonomy with every patient contact. Some obvious practices that may be questionable include the initiation, continuation, or discontinuance of parenteral nutrition or experimental drugs; unusual dosages or combinations of drugs; and artificial hydration and similar procedures. To make autonomous decisions about undergoing any treatment, patients must be informed (using language and concepts that are appropriate to their educational level) about the associated risks, anticipated benefits, available alternative treatments, and consequences of accepting or rejecting the treatment.

The patient's perception of his or her quality of life is also important to assess in order to promote ethical decision-making. The term *quality of life* is used in many ways. Factors that might be considered include the following: the symptoms of the illness and side effects of treatment; the patient's functional ability to perform basic activities of living; the patient's experiences of happiness, pleasure, pain, and suffering; and, finally, the patient's independence, privacy, and dignity (Lo, 2005).

Patients must be given adequate information with which to make their decisions; in addition, they must have adequate time to consider their choices without being pressured to comply, even if the staff believes that a certain treatment is the only choice a patient has. Remember, only the patient can choose what is best for him or her. The health care worker can only create the appropriate climate within which the decision can be made.

If patients lack decision-making capability (e.g., because of changes in level of consciousness, emotional distress, effects of age, inability to understand and judge alternatives), an attempt should be made to ascertain what the patient would choose if he or she were able. Advance directives, documentation of patient wishes before mental impairment, and information provided by significant others all make it easier for the system to respect patients' autonomy. These resources are available to infusion nurses in any practice setting. Nurses must recognize that patients do not lose their rights of autonomy merely because their capacity to make decisions is impaired; therefore every effort must be made to discover the patient's preferences. In cases in which the patient's wishes cannot be determined, health care workers must rely on other ethical principles to guide care.

Infusion nurses have brief encounters with patients over varying lengths of time. In some respects, the nature of this contact is a disadvantage because the infusion nurse may lack vital insight and opportunity to determine whether autonomy has been respected. Alternatively, these brief encounters over time enable the infusion nurse to view the situation from a fresh perspective, free from activities on the unit that may have a desensitizing effect on the unit staff. In the community or home situation, the infusion nurse may be the only health care professional available to note changes in patients' conditions or attitudes. The infusion nurse in any setting may be viewed by the physician as a collaborator whose expert opinion is valued because of his or her extensive knowledge and experience.

Thus infusion nurses are often in a position to enhance the autonomy of patients within their care. The nature of their contact with patients and their unique perspective require that they be sensitive to situations in which patients' rights of autonomy are in jeopardy. Sometimes, the conversation of a patient will suggest to the infusion nurse that the patient does not fully understand the implications of a particular procedure. A patient's chance remark ("I don't want to go through all of this") may trigger a question about the patient's desire to begin or continue a course of therapy (Oddi, 2001). A patient who lacks the mental capacity to understand what is being explained may appear to be suffering without hope of benefiting from a procedure. In all such instances, the infusion nurse should explore the situation more fully—with the patient if possible. Collecting relevant data and raising questions based on personal observations can help clarify the existence of an ethical problem and provide additional facts with which the situation can be analyzed. Ethical analysis can then be used to resolve conflicts associated with the violation of a patient's autonomy.

Infusion nurses can avoid causing physical harm to their patients by exercising care when performing procedures, administering proper dosages of infusion medications and nutrients, keeping current with developments in the field, remaining alert to signs of untoward effects of treatments, and intervening early to prevent further damage when complications arise. Educating the patient, caregivers, and other staff about the specific care required for treatments provided by the infusion nurse is another way of preventing harm.

Physical harm may also be prevented when the infusion nurse raises questions about poor care that he or she observes and takes action to promote safe care for patients. One group of infusion nurses in a community setting was instrumental in changing policy regarding home administration of a chemotherapeutic agent that had a greater than 50% risk of systemic anaphylaxis (Oddi, 2001). Their concerns about patient safety and their own ability to handle such a complication were expressed to their management and the physician. The expression of concern led to a resolution that was satisfactory for all.

If disclosure is regarded as essential to the patient's care, the nurse should obtain the patient's permission to reveal the information to the appropriate individuals on the health care team, or should encourage the patient to make the disclosure. When disclosure of confidential information is mandated, such as the legal requirement to report suspected child abuse, the patient needs to know that the nurse will report information to the appropriate individuals.

Infusion nurses can contribute to the well-being of their patients by carrying out the patient's care in a safe, compassionate manner. Questioning management's decision to control expenses by using less expensive peripheral catheters instead of central venous access devices for patients on public aid is a beneficent action. Listening to patients' concerns and providing follow-up for problems also promote beneficence. Intervening to ensure that the patient receiving nursing care at home or in the hospital obtains the services of physicians, chaplains, or other resource personnel is also a means of actively promoting the welfare of patients.

If infusion nurses are aware of dishonesty in billing patients or governmental agencies for services, they may be required to take action to have such practices investigated. Ultimately, such practices may result in a loss of essential services to all because of the legal and professional sanctions that may result.

ACTIONS TO PROMOTE ETHICAL PRACTICE

Infusion nurses can take many actions to improve their ability to practice ethically and ensure ethical care of their patients. First, infusion nurses should actively improve their knowledge of and sensitivity to the ethical aspects of patient care. Attendance at workshops and conferences dealing with ethics is a good way to learn more about ethics. Continued independent learning is essential to understanding the theoretical basis for ethics. Professional nursing journals are increasing their publication of articles that deal with specific ethical conflicts through the presentation of case studies.

Infusion nurses need to develop insight and sensitivity to questionable practices that they encounter. Such insight requires a willingness to investigate further when one feels a sense of discomfort or questions some aspect of care. The nurse must embark on a systematic process of ethical analysis to determine whether an ethical conflict truly exists and to define the nature of the conflict.

However, reliance on a sense of discomfort is only one aspect of assessment. Serious violations of ethics may go unrecognized by the nurse whose value system is not attuned to the area of the violation. Thus the nurse is obliged to go beyond relying on an intuitive sense that ethical concerns exist, and must make a conscious effort to learn more about the ethical implications of nursing practice. Such efforts include conducting a thorough review of the literature dealing with nursing ethics, attending meetings, discussing ethical issues with colleagues, investigating ambiguous areas, and consulting journal articles.

Infusion nurses must show respect and faith in all members of the team as ethical practitioners who share concern for the ethical care of patients. In addition, the infusion nurse must raise questions where doubt or insufficient information exists. Silence may result in the violation of another's rights. On the other hand, the nurse must appreciate the complexity of any health care situation and must not leap to conclusions without being certain that unethical practice is being used.

The infusion nurse's efforts to explore further any situation in which a patient's rights may be threatened or violated are an invaluable asset for ensuring ethical practice. Simple actions such as asking questions to see whether patients understand and accept their therapy, reminding physicians and other personnel to explain options fully to patients and families, and asking whether advance directives are available and encouraging their use are all means of anticipating and preventing ethical dilemmas throughout the course of an illness.

Infusion nurses should be especially alert to patients' comments that indicate their states of mind in relation to such issues as prolonging life with technology; these comments are invaluable should a patient lapse into coma and be unable to make necessary choices at a later time. Verbatim documentation of such comments in the chart is essential in case evidence of the patient's state of mind is required at a future date.

A useful approach that will increase sensitivity to ethical aspects of care is to copy information dealing with ethics for distribution and discussion among peers on the infusion team. Group discussion can help sensitize everyone to the range of ethical issues involved in an area of practice. Open discussion may encourage a cohesive approach to resolving problems and helps develop consensus among the staff.

Resources available in the agency should be used to help define and address ethical concerns. Hospitals and nursing homes may have access to ethicists, legal counsel, or pastoral staffs that can help clarify and facilitate resolution of ethical dilemmas. Nurses practicing in the community, who may not have ready access to such personnel, nonetheless can consult community religious leaders or the staff of the local hospital to obtain a referral for discussing such problems.

Volunteering to serve on the agency's ethics committee is an excellent way to gain knowledge and experience in the ethical aspects of care. Networking, which can widen the nurse's awareness of available resources, is an added bonus to such service. The creation of unit-based ethics committees, either for the infusion team itself or for members of the unit staff with the infusion nurse in attendance, may also be helpful. Such local ethics committees may improve problem solving, communication, and support for all individuals involved in patient care.

A critical mechanism for helping the individual nurse address ethical concerns in a systematic and constructive way is to create a reflective journal. Any perceived problems or concerns should be fully and objectively described by the nurse. The situation, dates and times, and the people involved should be included. Journal entries can provide evidence of the prevalence and seriousness of problems. The continuing occurrence of some types of problems will become obvious through content analysis of the entries, and can serve as an impetus for corrective action.

Nurses who practice infusion therapy should become familiar with the ethics-related policies and procedures of each organization in which he or she practices. There are many policies related to ethics, including but not limited to, do-not-resuscitate orders, end-of-life care, advance directives, withholding or withdrawing life-sustaining treatment, informed consent, patient rights and responsibilities, and staff accommodation.

A policy on staff accommodation is important because it outlines the steps that a nurse must take if he or she is unable to provide patient care based on his or her personal values or religious beliefs.

DISASTER ETHICS

The expertise of nurses, physicians, and other health care providers is an integral component of the response to a pandemic or disaster. How many other segments of society can realistically and legitimately be expected to fulfill this role and to assume this level of risk? Each health care professional should make a personal and professional decision about his or her "duty to care" when working conditions become unsafe. Unsafe working conditions will cause severe conflicts for health care workers, knowing that they have an obligation to care for their patients and also an obligation to care for themselves. An example of such a situation occurs when supplies of personal protective equipment are no longer available to health care providers. Nurses have the training that puts them in the thick of such things. That is why, in light of this level of responsibility, nurses must determine what level of risk they are willing to assume.

One action that can be taken by infusion nurses is to decide what aspects of your role and duties will or will not be able to be fulfilled in times of disaster. In essence, if the organization is preparing a list of staff members who are going to commit to being able to work in a disaster situation, the nurse should not volunteer if she or he has dependents that will become helpless in a disaster. In planning a facility's disaster response, potential emergency responders should think carefully about committing to what could be a 1-day disaster—or a 2-week cataclysmic response. Nurses and others must ask themselves if they can secure their dependents and make the commitment to staying if needed.

Each nurse has a responsibility to consider his or her "duty to care" commitments and how they will be carried out in a disaster *before* any incident. A nurse makes a commitment to his or her professional responsibilities. At the same time, the nurse has commitments to family and other personal interests. The nurse cannot make these decisions in isolation but, professionally, should involve his or her colleagues and, personally, should involve his or her family in discussions about these "duty to care" decisions (Schroeter, 2008).

Nurses should be encouraged to participate in preparedness committees and councils at all levels. Involvement in legislation can also assist nurses in defining their own ethical limitation and improve their overall knowledge base.

Education, both for the professional health care provider and for the public, is needed to clarify realistic expectations of all involved. Most importantly, however, nurses, as individual members of society, need to reflect on their own personal values and integrity to determine what actions they will consider to be morally appropriate for themselves during times of disaster.

ETHICS COMMITTEES AND CONSULTATION

The purpose of an ethics consultation is to bring the expertise and experience of others to bear on a situation that requires clarification of issues and values related to patient care (Schroeter, 2004). It is imperative that nurses be represented on organizational ethics committees. Ethics committees work through initial analysis of case problems by one of several ethics consultants who are members of the ethics committee. As appropriate, the consultant may act as sole consultant, may assemble and lead an ethics team from available members of the ethics committee, or may ask the chair of the committee to convene the entire ethics committee. The request for the consultation may be made by the attending physician, by the patient (surrogate for the nondecisional patients), by immediate family members, by involved nursing staff or house staff, by involved social workers, or by a chaplain.

The ethics consultant will determine the nature of the ethical problem and whether an ethics consultation is appropriate. The attending physician and the director of nursing will be notified of an ethics consult. Once a determination is made that an ethics consultation is appropriate, the ethics consultant may attempt to resolve the problem through a telephone consultation. If the problem cannot or, in the consultant's judgment, should not be resolved in this manner, the consultant should proceed as follows:

Under most circumstances, the consultant will see the patient. If the patient is decisional, the consultant will notify him or her of the nature of the visit. If the patient objects to the consultation, it should be discontinued. If the patient is not decisional or decision-making capacity is uncertain, the agent or proper surrogate must be notified of the ethics consultation at the earliest reasonable opportunity. If the surrogate or agent objects, the consultation should be discontinued.

Following the patient's or the surrogate's consent to consultation, the ethics consultant will, as appropriate:

a. Discuss the case with the attending physician, house staff, and involved nursing staff.
b. Interview family members and other involved persons and caregivers.
c. Review the chart.

If the problem is uncomplicated, common or previously encountered by the committee and the assessment of the ethics committee can be anticipated, the consultant may resolve it without the full ethics committee meeting. If, in the judgment of the ethics consultant, the full ethics committee should review the case, the chair of the committee should convene a meeting. All present will be reminded of the need for confidentiality and cautioned not to discuss the case in any context in which the patient can be identified. Discussion will then proceed along the general guidelines that follow:

Assessment of the Ethical Problem (by consultant or full ethics committee)
1. Medical facts
2. Patient preference, if known
3. Other relevant factors

Problem Assessment and Recommendation(s)
1. The ethical problem should be delineated.
2. Ethically appropriate recommendation(s) should be made.

A note of a full committee or in-person consultation will be placed in the patient's medical record by a member of the ethics committee, unless the attending physician requests otherwise.

 ## SUMMARY

The willingness and ability of infusion nurses to participate in ethical decision-making in clinical practice is influenced by numerous historical and organizational factors. The types of ethical dilemmas encountered and nurses' ability to intervene as autonomous practitioners are both affected by the values and the power of colleagues in the work situation. Nurses must be alert to the influence of these factors on their willingness to intervene. At all times, the nurse's primary obligation is to act to safeguard the patient's welfare, although other aspects of the situation must be investigated and balanced so that an ethically acceptable resolution is reached.

Although a concern for ethics is evident throughout the history of nursing, nurses may lack the knowledge and skills in ethical decision-making that would give them the confidence and credibility to be full participants in this process. Nonetheless, nurses can and must always raise questions about the ethics of clinical practice. They should embark on a conscious effort to improve their knowledge of ethical theory and their ability to engage in ethical analysis. This chapter provides an overview of introductory material and suggestions for further study to improve the knowledge base of infusion nurses in this area.

Nurses have a duty to uphold the standards of their profession. As such, they have a commitment to help regulate nursing to protect this public right to quality nursing services while also protecting their own right to self-preservation and self-care. The pivotal position of infusion nurses gives them an opportunity to recognize ethical problems in care that may not be evident to others of the health care team. Especially in the community, the infusion nurse may be the only professional contact who has insights relating to ethical concerns. Hence infusion nurses must assess possible ethical problems, act as a role model for ethical care, and adopt a problem-solving approach in situations that give rise to ethical concerns. Infusion nurses, like other nurses, have a critical role to play in ensuring ethical practice in today's health care environment.

Ethical issues will become more complex as technology becomes more sophisticated and medical care resources become more limited. For example, infusion nurses have been made aware of cost-containment issues such as resource allocation in both the hospital and home care environments.

Ethical actions, such as ensuring patients' rights or speaking for patients for which the infusion nurse may be responsible, are often difficult but necessary during the care of the patient. Some of these behaviors can be difficult to predict, but disrespectful, unprofessional, or incompetent care is hard to dismiss. Nurses must acknowledge patients' right to self-determination and the corresponding duty to protect it. The ability of the nurse and other members of the health care team to recognize ethical conflicts within the team and to constructively deal with them is important to the future of patient care.

The ANA's *Code of Ethics* (2001) asserts that the nurse does not necessarily have to agree with or condone certain individual choices, but that the nurse respects the patient as a person.

As health care increases in complexity, nurses will continue to encounter ethical issues in their practice. Education must be available for these nurses so that they may be better able to meet the expectations required of them by patients, families, employers, and colleagues. Nurses can also use data from ethics research to develop curricula with ethics content designed to meet the needs of students as they begin to move into their professional role. Ethics education must be a part of continuing education throughout any nurse's professional career.

REFERENCES

Aiken LH, Havens DS, Sloane DM: The Magnet nursing services recognition program—a comparison of two groups of magnet hospitals, *Am J Nurs* 100(3):26-35, 2000.

American Nurses Association: *The code for nurses with interpretive statements*, Kansas City, Mo, 2001, Author.

Beauchamp TL, Childress JF: *Principles of biomedical ethics*, ed 5, New York, 2001, Oxford University Press.

Biton V, Tabak N: The relationship between the application of the nursing ethical code and nurses' work satisfaction, *Int J Nurs Pract* 9(3):140-157, 2003.

Fry ST: Toward a theory of nursing ethics, *Adv Nurs Sci* 11(4):9-22, 1989.

Gorski LA: Speaking of standards: standard 7: ethics. Ethical decision making and repair of a patient's catheter: a case example, *J Infus Nurs* 30(4):203-204, 2008.

Hewitt J: A critical review of the arguments debating the role of the nurse advocate, *J Adv Nurs* 37:439-445, 2002.

Infusion Nurses Society: Infusion nursing code of ethics, *J Infus Nurs* 24(4):242-243, 2001.

Infusion Nurses Society: Infusion nursing standards of practice, *J Infus Nurs* 29(1S):S1-92, 2006.

Kohnke A: The nurse as advocate,, *Am J Nurs* 80:2038-2039, 1980.

Ladd RE, Pasquerella L, Smith S: What to do when the end is near: ethical issues in home health care nursing,, *Public Health Nurs* 17:103-110, 2000.

Lo B: *Resolving ethical dilemmas: a guide for clinicians*, ed 3, Baltimore, Md, 2005, Williams and Wilkins.

Nathaniel A: Moral distress among nurses, *Ethics and human rights update* 1(3), Washington DC, 2002.

Oberle K, Tenove S: Ethical issues in public health nursing, *Nurs Ethics* 7:425-439, 2000.

Ruderman C, Tracy CS, Ethics LOddi: In Hankins J, Lonsway RA, Hedrick C, editors: *Infusion therapy in clinical practice*, ed 2, Philadelphia, 2001, Saunders (pp 637-646).

Ruderman C, Tracy CS, Bensimon CM, et al: On pandemics and the duty to care: whose duty? who cares?, *BMC Med Ethics* 7(1):E5), 2006.

Schroeter K: *Doing the right thing: nurses' experiences of ethics in perioperativepractice*, PhD Dissertation, Milwaukee, 2004, University of Wisconsin.

Schroeter K: Duty to self versus duty to care, *J Trauma Nurs* 15(1), 2008.

Schroeter K, Derse A, Junkerman C et al: *Practical ethics for nurses and nursing students*, Frederick, Md, 2002, University Publishing Group.

Spielman BJ: Conflict in medical ethics cases; seeking patterns of resolution, *J Clin Ethics* 4:212-217, 1993.

U.S. General Accounting Office: Nursing workforce—emerging nurse shortages due to multiple factors, July 2001. Accessed 5/25/08 at www.gao.gov/new.items/d01944.pdf.

6 CLINICIAN AND PATIENT EDUCATION

Lynn Czaplewski, MS, ACNS-BC, CRNI®, AOCNS®*

 ## CLINICIAN EDUCATION

INTRODUCTION

Currently and historically, many schools of nursing do not include infusion therapy in basic nursing curriculums. Curriculums filled to capacity, faculty shortage, and lack of faculty knowledge in infusion therapy often prohibit its inclusion in the program (Smith, 2006). Infusion therapy skills or tasks may be taught in a skills' laboratory but the theoretical knowledge necessary for safe practice may not be included. Theory, including peripheral and central catheter site selection, infusate properties, and infusion-related infection prevention and complications, is often not addressed or is imbedded in basic nursing information. A graduate nurse can leave school with little or no skill in infusion therapy or knowledge of the theory applicable to infusion practice. Some health care facilities offer a review of infusion therapy during orientation while others expect that the nurse is already equipped with those skills and knowledge. This results in fear and anxiety for the nurse, and patient dissatisfaction as a result of lack of nurses' competency. In addition, litigation may result from a nurse's lack of knowledge and poor skills. Integration of infusion therapy principles and standards into nursing curriculums is essential in a time when the majority of hospitalized patients receive some type of infusion therapy, and when infusion therapy is delivered in outpatient facilities, infusion clinics, and physicians' offices, and in the home, schools, and workplace. It is likely that practicing nurses in most clinical settings require knowledge of infusion therapy. The *Infusion Nursing Standards of Practice* (Infusion Nurses Society [INS], 2006) recommend a curriculum for intravenous (IV) education to ensure the competency of nurses practicing infusion therapy (Box 6-1). These recommendations are intended for all nurses who care for patients requiring infusion therapy.

Infusion nurses who have earned the CRNI® (Certified Registered Nurse Infusion) designation by successfully completing the CRNI® certification examination have become consultants and educators in all practice settings. The CRNI® may have the responsibility for staff development related to infusion therapy and competency assessment.

INFUSION-RELATED COMPETENCIES

Staff development is the process of assessing nursing competency and developing competencies, quality, and excellence in patient care (Kelly-Thomas, 1998). During orientation it is imperative to assess the competencies of the nurse. Typically nurses learn aspects of infusion therapy "on-the-job," picking up information and skills that may or may not be accurate. "We've always done it this way" is a frequent mantra among nurses; misinformation and substandard care can result. Many nurses are unfamiliar with the *Infusion Nursing Standards of Practice* (INS, 2006), the Centers for Disease Control and Prevention (CDC) *Guidelines for the Prevention of Intravascular Catheter-Related Infections* (O'Grady et al, 2002), or even the Occupatioal Safety and Health Administration (OSHA) regulations. Nursing practice can become "tradition" in that the information is passed from nurse to nurse. It becomes the responsibility of the education department or staff development educator to correct misconceptions and teach evidence-based practice. It may be difficult to change those who are "set in their ways." Evidence-based practice may be more readily accepted when nurses recognize and identify actual infusion-related complications and the cost to the patient in terms of pain, loss of income, and dissatisfaction if appropriate care is not provided.

Competencies are defined as the knowledge and skills required to safely practice an aspect or aspects of nursing. Competency assessment is an evaluation measuring a set of skills and knowledge required to provide care. It takes into consideration technical skills and critical thinking, and the ability to apply these competencies at the right time (Kelly-Thomas, 1998). Minimum nursing competency is demonstrated by a novice nurse who passed the National Council Licensure Examination (NCLEX®). Certification in infusion therapy by the Infusion Nurses Certification Corporation (INCC) validates through examination entry-level competencies in infusion therapy. Standards of practice, professional guidelines, and facility policies and procedures are the framework from which competencies are developed. Competency assessment is not

*The author and editors wish to acknowledge the contributions made by Rebecca Kochheiser Berry and Mary A. Banks as authors of this chapter in the second edition of *Infusion Therapy in Clinical Practice*.

Box 6-1 INFUSION NURSES SOCIETY RECOMMENDATIONS FOR AN INFUSION CURRICULUM

1. Technology and clinical applications
   a. Use, function, care, maintenance of supplies and equipment (Examples: catheters, administration sets, infusion control devices, needleless valves, dressings)
   b. Potential risks and complications of supplies and equipment
   c. Anatomy and physiology of vascular system
2. Fluid and electrolyte balance
   a. Pathophysiology
   b. Laboratory values
   c. Types of fluids and electrolyte imbalances
   d. Recognition of fluid overload, dehydration, abnormal acid-base balance
3. Pharmacology
   a. Classifications of parenteral drugs including actions, pharmacokinetics, chemical properties, dosing, monitoring, side effects, toxicities, compatibilities, and stabilities
4. Infection control
   a. Microbiology
   b. Mode of transmission
   c. Laboratory values
   d. Surveillance
   e. Prevention
   f. Aseptic technique
5. Neonate and pediatric patients
   a. Growth and development
   b. Fluids and electrolytes
   c. Dose calculations
   d. Infusion delivery systems
   e. Site and device selection
   f. Psychological implications
6. Transfusion therapy
   a. Immunohematology
   b. Blood typing
   c. Blood products
   d. Equipment
   e. Reactions
7. Antineoplastic and biologic therapy
   a. Cell cycle
   b. Goal of therapy
   c. Laboratory values
   d. Chemotherapeutic and biotherapeutic agents
   e. Side effects and toxicities
   f. Dosing
   g. Administration and safe handling
8. Parenteral nutrition
   a. Indications
   b. Available solutions and additives
   c. Metabolic processes
   d. Monitoring
   e. Potential complications
   f. Monitoring
9. Performance improvement
   a. Legal and ethical aspects
   b. Outcome measurement
   c. Standards of practice
   d. Principles of continuous performance improvement

From Infusion Nurses Society: Infusion nursing standards of practice, *J Infus Nurs* 29(1 suppl), 2006.

---

a one-time-only process. It requires ongoing appraisal of skills and knowledge associated with high-risk procedures. Continuing evaluation of competency in health care organizations is necessary to meet the standards of accrediting bodies, such as The Joint Commission, and to ensure safe patient care. Methods of collecting evidence of staff competency may include performance evaluations, performance checklists, and written examinations. A list of examples of infusion-related competencies can be found in Figure 6-1.

ADULT LEARNING

Whether teaching nursing staff or adult patients, consideration must be given to research-based learning theories to be effective. Cognitive learning pertains to perception, judgment, memory, and reasoning. Cognitive learning theories are based on Gestalt (German meaning to shape and form) psychology (Merriam-Webster, 2008). Gestalt laws are organizing principles that are part of perception. One law, the law of Pragnanz, states that we are innately driven to experience things as regular, orderly, and simply as possible. The law of closure says that a person will complete a thought, picture, or figure if something is missing, in other words "close the gap." The tendency of a person to group similar items together forms the basis of the law of similarity. Insight learning is a well-known concept of Gestalt theory, which means solving a problem by means of recognizing an organizing principle. In essence, when a learner recognizes

meaning in the experience, learning occurs (Merriam, Caffarella, and Baumgartner, 2006). This theory can be readily adapted to the process of infusion therapy competency development. A teaching plan that is organized and logical facilitates learning. For example, when preparing to teach peripheral IV insertion, including basic, preparatory information at the beginning of the lesson, such as recognizing types of peripheral IV catheters and selecting an appropriate gauge and length of catheter, is logical. This allows the learner to start to build upon basic concepts to the more difficult aspect of the lesson, which would be the venipuncture. Organizing information so that it follows the progression of steps to the venipuncture, dressing, and securement assists the learner in remembering the steps to be successful in that procedure. If the lesson skips important steps, such as allowing the antiseptic to dry, the learner may "close the gap" by assuming the venipuncture can be made through wet antiseptic. Presenting complications of peripheral venipuncture as part of the peripheral venipuncture lesson helps the learner to understand the meaning and implications of each step of the procedure.

Bruner (1966) identified three processes, occurring at the same time, that result in learning. The first process is acquiring new information; the second is taking the new knowledge and synthesizing it to see if it applies to a new task. During the third and last process—evaluation—the learner assesses whether the way the information was manipulated is adequate to the task. Learning through discovery is also emphasized. This approach

INFUSION COMPETENCY ASSESSMENT

Name : _____   Date of Hire : _____

COMPETENCY	PROFICIENT	NEEDS REVIEW	NEEDS INSTRUCTION	MEETS EXPECTED CRITERIA
1. Blood Draw—Peripheral				
Peripheral access device				
Syringe method				
Vacutainer method				
2. Blood Draw—Central Venous Access Device				
Implanted port				
Tunneled catheter (Groshong, Neostar, Hickman, etc.)				
PICC				
Nontunneled catheter (Arrow, triple-lumen, etc.)				
Syringe method				
Vacutainer method				
3. Blood Draw Processing				
Select appropriate tube for test ordered				
Proper order of tubes drawn				
Labeling tubes				
Completing lab order form with ICD-9 codes				
Safety needles/winged steel needle set				
Blood transfer device				
4. Peripheral Venous Access: Insertion and Maintenance				
Anatomy and physiology of veins				
Site selection based on vein assessment and therapy prescribed				
Vein distension				
Skin antisepsis with chlorhexidine				
Aseptic technique				
Standard precautions				
Use of gloves				
Atraumatic insertion of IV catheter				
Identification of vein patency				
Sterile dressing application and labeling				
Catheter stabilization				
Use of extension tubing				
Identification of infiltration, phlebitis, extravasation				
Initiates appropriate action for infiltration, phlebitis, extravasation				

FIGURE 6-1 Infusion-related competencies.

(Continued)

5. Central Venous Access Devices: Accessing and Maintenance				
Aseptic technique				
Assessing patency				
Appropriate use of clamps				
Troubleshoot for withdrawal occlusions				
Use of antithrombolytic for thrombotic occlusions: total occlusion (stopcock method) and withdrawal occlusions				
Push, pause, positive pressure locking 0.9% sodium chloride flushing and heparin				
Use of positive pressure valves				
6. Implanted Ports				
Accessing implanted port using aseptic technique				
Skin antisepsis with chlorhexidine				
Use of safety noncoring needle				
Sterile dressing application and labeling				
Device stabilization				
Initiating an infusion				
Deaccessing port				
Identification of complications: infiltration, occlusion, local infection, port pocket infection, sepsis, skin reactions, port dislodgement, pinch-off syndrome				
Initiate appropriate action for each complication				
7. Tunneled Catheters (Groshong, Neostar, Hickman)				
Aseptic site care and labeling				
Catheter stabilization				
Initiating an infusion				
Discontinuing an infusion				
Identification of complications: occlusion, local site/tunnel infection, skin reactions, pinch-off syndrome, catheter damage				
Initiate appropriate action for each complication				
8. Peripherally Inserted Central Catheter (PICC)				
Aseptic site care and labeling				
Catheter stabilization with securement device, sterile tape, or surgical strips				
Initiating an infusion				
Discontinuing an infusion				
Identification of complications: occlusion, local infection, phlebitis, sepsis, skin reactions, catheter damage				
Initiate appropriate action for each complication				

FIGURE 6-1, cont'd Infusion-related competencies.

is valuable because it helps the learner associate new information with something that is familiar. For example, a patient must learn how to use an ambulatory pump for home infusion. The patient has a microwave with a touch keypad. Using the knowledge about how to program the microwave may assist the patient in adapting that knowledge to the working of the pump. Programming the total time for the infusion, pressing a "start" key, and identifying alarms can be used as an example of knowledge familiar to the patient so that information can be applied to learning about the pump. Learning about the pump involves the acquisition of new information—why it is used, how it works, how to start and stop the pump, and how to identify troubleshooting alarms. New information can be "cubbyholed" into previous knowledge; therefore the information is more organized, easier to understand, and applicable to the use of a pump.

Three subconcepts to increase learning competence are recognizing the needs of the learner, taking into account the learner's style of learning, and involving the learner in an organized activity (Smith, 1982). These concepts also align with the theories of the father of adult education, Malcolm Knowles. Learning is more likely to occur if there is some immediacy in the need to learn, that is, if the information can be immediately applied (Merriam et al, 2006). A nurse needs to learn how to change a peripherally inserted central catheter (PICC) dressing and cleanse the site. The nurse has a patient that needs a PICC dressing change. There is immediacy in the nurse's need to learn this procedure. The nurse is more likely to assimilate that procedure because it will be applied immediately. If any problems occur during the dressing change, such as assessment of erythema at the insertion site, the nurse will be able to identify this complication and will learn to manage it based on the new information presented with the lesson on PICC site care. Smith (1982) also identifies that learning is very individualized, since each person learns best through different means. Some people learn new material most effectively visually, such as by watching a video or learning via the Internet. Others prefer to listen, using the sense of hearing, to learn. Listening to CDs while driving in a car is an illustration of that concept. "Learning while doing" or a hands-on approach is best for others. A combination of techniques for teaching and learning often strengthens the learning process and contributes to recall of the lesson. The learner may be shown a DVD regarding choices for venous access to illustrate the types of devices and how they are used. The nurse can reinforce that learning by discussing with the patient pros and cons of each device based on the patient's lifestyle. By handling demonstration models of devices and manipulating a mannequin that has the devices, the patient is most likely to choose an appropriate device. In essence, the cognitive approach to learning is valuable because it helps the learner associate new information with something that is familiar.

The adult learning theory of Malcolm Knowles focuses on involving adult learners in the learning process. The theory is based on the following five assumptions about the adult learner:

1. Adults are autonomous and self-directed. They must be actively involved in the learning process and their perspectives about their learning needs must be sought.
2. Adults have a variety of life experiences and knowledge, prior education, work-related activities, and family responsibilities. Identifying what the learner already knows and building and relating educational experiences on prior knowledge engage the learner.
3. Adults are more problem-centered in learning and goal-oriented. If the learning can be immediately applied, it is more likely to occur.
4. Adults expect an organized program with defined objectives. Learners must clearly understand how the learning will help them achieve their goals.
5. Adults are relevancy-oriented and practical. Educational programs must be applicable to their work; they must see the value and be interested (Lieb, 1991).

In addition, adults need to feel respected. "Talking down" to an adult learner and not recognizing the learner's current knowledge and expertise hamper learning. The following is an example of application of Knowles' theory: Nurses in orientation in an outpatient oncology clinic need to learn how to assess and manage catheter occlusions. Central venous access device occlusions occur frequently in the oncology setting. As self-directed adults, the nurses can choose to learn the information or, if previously exposed to the information, can "tune out." Whether or not the procedure is learned is up to the learner. Comparing catheter occlusion to clogged plumbing can be easily related to a commonplace household problem. Knowing that the assessment and skill of relieving occlusions will be used frequently in daily practice motivates the nurse to carefully learn the techniques.

ASSESSMENT OF LEARNING NEEDS

The first step in a successful program is determining the need for a program. Performing an educational needs assessment identifies what the learners believe is important information needed to safely and competently perform their job. It also helps the educator prioritize the requirements and interests of the learners. A needs assessment can be accomplished through a variety of methods. Methods may include using a questionnaire or survey, reviewing incident reports, observing nurses' performance, or collecting data from exit interviews or from quality improvement activities. This might include results of chart audits, individual nurse feedback, nursing satisfaction surveys, written test results, new product evaluation, or implementation of new or revised policies and procedures, or feedback from orientation. An example of a nursing needs assessment survey can be found in Figure 6-2.

TEACHING STRATEGIES

Once learning needs have been established and prioritized, methods for teaching and learning are determined. Selecting an appropriate format to use should be based on a number of factors such as urgency, availability of time, number of learners, and type of information to be learned. Urgency is a highly motivating factor creating a readiness to learn. If a patient is to have an implanted pump placed for pain management and the staff has never seen or worked with this device, the need to learn is urgent. Under these circumstances, education of staff involved in the care of the patient may need to occur within hours of caring for the patient. Time availability also impacts strategies for learning. If nurses can only attend educational programs when "off-duty" because of short staffing during work hours, creative methods need to be implemented. Motivating the learners to attend after-hours programs may be difficult. Personal and family responsibilities may deter the nurse from attending.

The number of learners also affects how learning is to occur. While a "just-in-time" inservice may be easily facilitated for

EDUCATIONAL NEEDS SURVEY FOR INFUSION THERAPY

The goals of this survey are:

1. To prioritize what type of information and training you need to effectively care for the patient requiring infusion therapy

2. To present the information at times, at locations, and in formats that would be most beneficial to you

Desired outcomes:

- A report will be distributed to each nurse and administrator.
- A priority list of education topics will be compiled.
- A continuing education calendar will be established.
- A plan for future needs will be developed.

INFUSION THERAPY

_____	Difficult peripheral IV insertions	_____	Catheter-related infections
_____	Vascular access device selection	_____	Catheter occlusion prevention & management
_____	Catheter migration	_____	Infusion equipment choices
_____	PICCs	_____	Catheter malposition
_____	Tunneled catheters	_____	Catheter leaks/fractures
_____	Implanted ports	_____	Catheter removal
_____	Nontunneled catheters	_____	Extravasation prevention & management
_____	Pinch-off syndrome	_____	Port dislodgement
_____	Dialysis/plasmapheresis catheters	_____	Port erosion
_____	Dressing materials	_____	Flushing protocols

Other: _____

CONTINUING EDUCATION FORMAT SUGGESTIONS

Please indicate your learning style:

- Visual learner (learn through seeing)
- Auditory learner (learn through hearing)
- Tactile/kinesthetic learner (learn through touching, doing)

List in order of preference your preferred methods of receiving information (1 = most preferred, 5 = least preferred):

_____ Paper handouts

_____ Poster presentations

_____ Email newsletters

_____ PowerPoint® presentation with no auditory component

_____ PowerPoint® presentation with voice-over

_____ Classroom in a group

_____ Self-study package

_____ Video

_____ One-on-one hands-on discussion

_____ Computer program

_____ Vendor presentations

_____ Other: _____

FIGURE 6-2 Educational needs survey.

What day(s) of the week is (are) best for you to participate in an educational program/inservice/self-study? List in order of preference (1 = best, 5 = worst):

_____ Monday

_____ Tuesday

_____ Wednesday

_____ Thursday

_____ Friday

_____ Saturday

What time(s) of the day might work out best for you? List in order of preference (1 = best, 5 = worst):

_____ Before work (7 AM to 8 AM)

_____ During work, mornings

_____ During work, afternoons

_____ After work (5 PM)

_____ Evenings (6 PM to 7 PM)

Where would you consider meeting? (1 = first choice, 5 = last choice)

_____ One central location

_____ Rotating office sites

_____ At an office nearest to my location

_____ Only at the office location where I work

_____ Other: _____

Your ideas and suggestions are very valuable. Please list any other ideas, suggestions, concerns, or issues (use additional sheet of paper or other side of this paper if you need more space).

FIGURE 6-2, cont'd Educational needs survey.

a small group of nurses, a facility-wide program requires intense planning and creative interventions. The type of information that is to be learned affects program planning as well. The standard framework used for developing programs has long been *Bloom's Taxonomy of Educational Objectives*. This framework identifies levels of learning within the cognitive, psychomotor, and affective domains (Harton, 2007). In each domain learning occurs by building on previous knowledge from the simple to the complex. The *Revised Bloom's Taxonomy* (Anderson et al, 2001) identifies four types of knowledge: factual, conceptual, procedural, and meta-cognitive. Factual knowledge is basic, "must know" information such as knowing the types of central venous access devices and distinguishing characteristics. Conceptual knowledge is more complex, involving relationships and theories. Learning why a subclavian catheter tip position is not considered central placement based on the anatomy of the veins and the physiology of blood flow uses conceptual knowledge. When skills must be learned, procedural knowledge is used. Changing a PICC dressing using aseptic technique is using procedural knowledge, that is, task-oriented learning. Meta-cognitive knowledge involves the use of critical thinking to solve problems. The learner's self-awareness and self-regulation come into play. When a nurse identifies a possible catheter-related sepsis and appropriately intervenes, meta-cognitive knowledge is applied. Box 6-2 lists examples of types of educational interventions. Not all types of programs are appropriate for all types of learning (Table 6-1).

Box 6-2 TEACHING STRATEGIES: EXAMPLES OF LEARNING ACTIVITIES

- Traditional lectures
- Discussions
- Self-learning modules
- CD-ROMs
- Games
- Simulations
- Train-the-trainer programs
- Computer-based programs
- Demonstrations
- Hands-on experiences
- Poster presentations
- Journal clubs
- Microsoft PowerPoint® presentations
- Case studies

PROGRAM PLANNING

The program curriculum can be planned after educational needs of the nursing staff are assessed, data are collected and analyzed, a list of priorities is developed, and the teaching topics are identified. In order for the right information to be taught in the right way, the target audience must be identified. Is the

TABLE 6-1 Suggested Teaching Strategies Based on Content to be Learned

Type of information and examples	Strategies	Considerations
Facts • New policy • Definitions • Anatomy/physiology • Fluids and electrolytes • Drugs	• Lecture • Self-study package • Webinar • Games • Handouts • Posters • CD-ROM	• Consider learner's previous knowledge and build on it • Use pictures, drawings, algorithms • Include rationale
Concepts • Advantages of one antiseptic over another • How catheter occlusions occur • Transfusion reactions	• Lecture • Slides • Self-study package • Webinar • Group discussion • Posters • Journal club • CD-ROM	• Involve learners • Use pictures, drawings, algorithms, concept maps • Use *Infusion Nursing Standards of Practice* • List resources/research
Procedures • Insertion of a peripheral catheter • Site care • Handling a chemotherapy spill • Implanted port access	• Hands-on workshop • Demonstration • Practicum • Simulation • DVD/video • "Just-in-time" inservice • Posters	• Allow for practice time and return demonstrations • Use *Policies and Procedures for Infusion Nursing* • Identify best practice • Include rationale
Meta-cognition • Troubleshooting a catheter occlusion • Evaluating lab values in a patient receiving parenteral nutrition • Choosing an appropriate vascular access device	• Case studies • Role playing • Simulation • Group discussion • Use of preceptors • Nursing rounds • Journal club	• Requires higher levels of thinking • Previous clinical experiences help to develop this domain

intended program meant for nurses new to the standards, policies, and procedures of the organization? Is it meant for nurses unfamiliar with the *Infusion Nursing Standards of Practice* and current research related to infusion nursing? Is the purpose of the program to teach experienced infusion nurses to perform an advanced procedure such as PICC insertion? Is the program for generalist nurses needing the basics of infusion therapy? Nurses working in a long-term care facility may rarely care for a patient requiring an IV antibiotic. Program goals of an IV program will differ greatly for that audience than for a group of interventional radiology nurses. Providing education for medical assistants or nursing assistants will not be at the same level as education for an experienced registered nurse (RN) nor will the goals be the same. A "one-size-fits-all" type of program cannot possibly meet the objectives for different types of learners. The

program must be geared to the specific needs and objectives of the intended learners. An example of an intended audience statement is the following: "This program is intended for the graduate nurse with minimal or no experience in peripheral IV insertion."

An essential part of every educational program is fun. Imbedding the program with appropriate cartoons, games, prizes, or treats helps keep the learner involved. A serious lecture program not only may be boring but also may allow the learner to mentally retreat from the task at hand.

To stimulate the learner, consideration of the generation of the learner is needed. Most programs will be comprised of learners from a variety of generations. The greatest number of nurses in today's workforce were born from 1943 to 1960, the "Baby Boomers." This generation values life-long learning and likes mentoring others. They enjoy taking a leadership role. "Generation X" consists of those born from 1961 to 1980. They comprise the second largest percent of the nursing workforce. Descriptions of this generation include intensely independent, self-directed, and resourceful. Work-life balance is important to them and they are very savvy with technology. Those nurses born from 1980 to 2000 are called "Millenials." Social connections and networking are vital to them and they are interested in continuous learning. They value structure and need coaching (Sherman, 2008). To be successful in facilitating an educational program for a multigenerational audience, as an example, involve the Baby Boomers in the development of the program and in mentoring the younger staff. Schedule the program during the workday because Generation X'ers are not as likely to attend an off-hours program. Allow time for interaction and socialization to draw in the Millenials. Awareness of these generational differences will help to create a program that will be valued by all participants.

The next step is determining the objectives for the educational offering. *A Taxonomy of Cognitive Objectives* was developed by Benjamin Bloom in the 1950s and serves as a planning tool for learning objectives. In the 1990s, one of Bloom's students, Lorin Anderson, revisited the taxonomy. The taxonomy provides a method of organizing thinking skills into six levels, from the most basic to the higher order of thinking (Table 6-2) (Anderson et al, 2001).

It is often challenging to determine the best time and date for the program, and the optimal time needed to present the program. After determining the objectives, an anticipated 1-hour program may be greatly insufficient to achieve the outcomes. The program may need to be broken down into concise, short offerings, or a variety of methods may need to be used over an extended time. For instance, a program on peripheral IV insertions may require 4 to 6 hours but most nurses are not able to attend a lengthy program because of clinical requirements or home responsibilities. The realistic attention span of the learners is considered when determining the length of the program and the methodology used in planning the program. If a program is planned after working hours, attention spans may be very short due to fatigue and other factors. Finding a convenient time for all staff may be impossible. One way to cover the necessary information and the hands-on portion would be to break it down into five 1-hour classes. An alternative method would be to cover the factual and conceptual aspects of the program in a self-study module or an on-line PowerPoint® presentation, followed by two 1-hour hands-on sessions and then a "take-home" post-test and evaluation. The hands-on practicum is an integral part of any infusion-related program. A gap exists

TABLE 6-2 Using Bloom's Revised Taxonomy to Develop Program Objectives

Taxonomy	Sample verbs used in objectives	Examples of objectives
1. Remembering—retrieving, identifying, and recalling relevant knowledge from long-term memory	Acquire Define Label Match Recognize List Describe Retrieve Name Locate Distinguish Repeat Know Choose Review Record Select Sort	• The nurse will be able to *recognize* the signs of a catheter-related sepsis. • The nurse will be able to *distinguish* a tunneled catheter from a nontunneled catheter. • The nurse will *choose* the correct blood collection tube when drawing a PT/INR. • The nurse will be able to *define* hypo- and hypertonic solutions.
2. Understanding—comprehending meaning from oral, written, and graphic messages through interpreting, exemplifying, classifying, summarizing, inferring, comparing, and explaining; understand uses and implications of terms, facts, methods, procedures, concepts	Interpret Compare Demonstrate Differentiate Exemplify Infer Group Outline Predict Represent Trace Summarize Classify Explain	• The nurse will be able to *interpret* the signs and symptoms of hypoglycemia in the patient receiving PN. • The nurse will be able to *classify* the types of pain. • The nurse will be able to *differentiate* a febrile nonhemolytic reaction from anaphylaxis.
3. Applying—executing or implementing a procedure; formulating interventions	Implement Convert Demonstrate Discuss Examine Prepare Carry out Use Execute	• The nurse will be able to *demonstrate* methods to distend peripheral veins. • The nurse will be able to *implement* a patient teaching plan for hand hygiene.
4. Analyzing—breaking information into parts to explore understandings and relationships; evaluate relevancy	Compare Organize Find Classify Categorize Select Determine	• The nurse will be able to *select* a peripheral catheter insertion site based on the type of therapy and condition of the veins. • The nurse will be able to *determine* hypervolemia based on the patient's signs and symptoms.
5. Evaluating—justifying a decision or course of action	Check Interpret Verify Hypothesize Critique Experiment Judge	• The nurse will be able to *verify* a patient's identification using two methods. • The nurse will be able to *critique* four infusion control devices based on selected criteria. • The nurse will be able to *interpret* a culture and sensitivity lab report.
6. Creating—putting elements together to form a coherent or functional whole	Design Devise Organize Construct Plan Produce Invent	• The nurse will be able to *design* a method for evaluating safety products. • The nurse will be able to *plan* a quality improvement project related to phlebitis rates.

Retrieved from http://social.chass.ncsu.edu/slatta/hi216/learning/bloom.htm

between learning and understanding theory and principles and the technical skills required to be successful. It is challenging to identify preceptors with expert skills along with the knowledge of the *Infusion Nursing Standards of Practice* to work one-on-one with the learner. Not every nurse is a preceptor. In addition to expertise in infusion therapy, the preceptor must be interested in teaching, understand the principles of adult education, know how to give constructive feedback, and validate clinical performance (Lockhart, 2004). The preceptor must be a suitable role model for teaching specific techniques.

The use of current technology has expanded the options for learning the skills necessary for infusion therapy. Professional-looking presentations can be created using a scanner and digital camera to download pictures and illustrations in the Microsoft PowerPoint® program (Hendrickson, 2007). Virtual simulation software programs allow the learner to simulate procedures, such as peripheral venipuncture, on the computer. Text, anatomy, video, and a virtual reality simulator are provided with the software. Simulation models—such as rubber skin flaps with veins in mannequin arm models, chests in sophisticated human-sized mannequins, and studios that provide realistic scenarios and opportunities for venipuncture, PICC insertion, and central venous access device placements—assist the educator in providing hands-on experiences that spare the patient a learner's practice. There is no substitution for the practice needed to master a skill at the clinical level, but simulation can help the learner gain confidence with a procedure before performing it on a patient. See Table 6-3 for simulation models and mannequins.

Another consideration in program planning is cost. Budgetary considerations involve the educator's and preceptors' time in planning and implementing the program, marketing, cost of supplies and duplicating handouts, speaker fees, room rental, audio-visual equipment, and food and beverages. Computer-based programs described earlier tend to be costly. Limited resources compel the educator to use creative program planning. The use of email to advertise a program and post the handouts is one way to decrease costs. In-house staff with expertise in the subject matter and the desire to teach eliminate the cost of an outside speaker. Allowing participants to bring in their own beverages or lunch eliminates the need for purchased food.

Offsetting the cost of a program can be achieved by charging a small fee for employees. One theory about motivating a learner to attend a voluntary educational program is to charge a fee rather than to provide a free program. The prepaid fee is a motivating factor for the learner to attend. Mandatory programs are free to the employee and require the facility to pay the employee's hourly salary, which increases the cost of the program. A strategy that is useful is allowing employees to attend without any fee but creating revenue by opening the program to the general nursing community and charging those attendees a fee (Figure 6-3).

Creating handouts or self-study modules can be an expensive and time-consuming undertaking. However, handouts help to reinforce instruction and demonstration and can be a resource to the learner in the future. Handouts can be as simple as printing the slides from a PowerPoint® presentation or as sophisticated as a textbook or a printed document. Incorporating

TABLE 6-3 Examples of Infusion Teaching Models

Simulation models for infusion therapy	Capabilities	Manufacturer/Distributor
Laerdal IV torso	External jugular insertion	Laerdal
Life/form® Venatech IV trainer	Peripheral IV placement and arterial blood gas	Life/form®
Life/form® infant crisis mannequin	Arm and leg IV insertion, intraosseous placement, and umbilical cannulation Advanced life support	Life/form®
CentraLine Man	External jugular cannulation	Simulab Corp.
Geriatric IV training arm	Peripheral IV placement with rolling veins	Nasco Health Care
Infant IV arm	IV placement in superficial veins of arm	Nasco Health Care
Life/form® advanced venipuncture and injection arm, white or black	Peripheral IV placement, phlebotomy, intramuscular and intradermal injections	Life/form®
Nita Newborn™ infant venous access simulator	Venous access for newborns and infants	Nasco Health Care
Life/form® IV leg	Infant leg for greater and lesser saphenous veins and dorsal venous arch IV placement	Life/form®
Life/form® pediatric head	IV access of temporal and jugular veins of infant head	Life/form®
Life/form® hemodialysis practice arm	Accessing fistulas	Life/form®
Deluxe IV training arm	Peripheral IV placement and intramuscular injections	Simulaids
Chester Chest™	PICC, implanted port, peripheral IV, and peripheral port care and maintenance	VATA
Port—"Body in a Box"™	Port palpation and accessing	VATA
Dermalike™ Advanced four-vein venipuncture training aid, latex-free	Easy to difficult peripheral IV placement	VATA
Peter PICC Line™	For PICC placement	VATA

pictures, diagrams, concept maps, or algorithms can create interest in the handout and strengthen a lecture or computer-based program. Whatever method is used to develop handouts, the copy must be well-organized and easy-to-read, using a font and type size that are conducive to reading. As an example, using a Times New Roman or Arial font creates a more readable copy. Also, the reader may struggle to read a small font size. When creating handouts from PowerPoint® slides, if there is too much print on a slide the handouts will be unreadable because of the tiny print.

PROGRAM CONTENT

Program content based on one or all of the nine core areas of infusion therapy assists the educator in planning a program. Identification of what the learner needs to know to achieve the objectives is the first step in developing the content. The next step is to identify how to best involve the learner in achieving the objectives (Kelly-Thomas, 1998). Content on any topic should include the following questions:
- What are the goals and objectives (i.e., what is the crucial information to learn)?
- Who needs to learn the information (i.e., what is the target audience)?
- How will the necessary information and skills be taught (i.e., how will the content be developed; what resources will be used)?

In the development of the content, appropriate resources must be used in order to ensure the content is accurate and evidence-based (Krugman, 2003). A good place to start is to review this textbook and other infusion therapy publications, such as the *Infusion Nursing Standards of Practice* (INS, 2006) and *Policies and Procedures for Infusion Nursing* (INS, 2006). Scientific books on anatomy, physiology, and physics may also be helpful in collecting information. To target the most up-to-date information, a literature search on the specific topic should be done using a database such as CINAHL or MEDLINE. These online databases are typically available in most hospital and academic libraries, and are generally available to the public. A librarian can assist the educator in using the databases to locate specific information needed. These databases allow the searcher to locate evidence-based articles. The online database of evidence-based literature is the Cochrane Library and is accessible to the public as well.

EVALUATION

Evaluating the achievement of program objectives is an integral part of any educational encounter. The evaluation determines if the objectives have been met. In addition, the evaluation should include opinions related to the effectiveness and knowledge of the speaker and the learning environment. The evaluation is a valuable tool that is used to determine the effectiveness of the program and is also used in future program planning.

EXPENSES			
ITEM	**SET COST**	**VARIABLE COST**	**ACTUAL COST**
Planner's time		# hr × hourly salary:	
Educator's time: preparation time and presentation time	Can be a standard fee	# hr × hourly salary:	
Room rental			
AV rental			
Refreshments			
Copy cost of handouts			
IV or other supplies used for demonstrations or practice			
Advertisement/marketing			
Certificates and other office supplies			
Other			
Total			

INCOME		
ITEM	**EXPECTED**	**ACTUAL**
Attendees fee		
Vendor support		
Total		

FIGURE 6-3 Budget worksheet.

See Figure 6-4 for a sample of an evaluation form. A post-test can also help the educator evaluate if the goals of the program have been met by assessing the knowledge of the learner on key points.

The execution of clinical staff education requires careful planning; understanding principles of adult education, teaching, and learning; and using creative methods to educate. This awareness is helpful whether facilitating a "just-in-time" bedside teaching session or a day-long seminar. See Figure 6-5 for a sample education planning record.

 PATIENT EDUCATION

PATIENTS' RIGHTS

Patients have the right to know about their illnesses, medications, treatment, and expected outcomes. With this knowledge the patient is better equipped to make health care decisions, to give informed consent, and to be an active participant in care. In the *Infusion Nursing Standards of Practice,* Standard 11.1

EVALUATION OF VASCULAR ACCESS WORKSHOP

Please rate how well each objective was met on a scale of 1 to 5, with 1 = strongly agree and 5 = strongly disagree

The participant will be able to select appropriate veins for peripheral IV access.	1	2	3	4	5
The participant will be able to implement troubleshooting strategies for patients with difficult veins.	1	2	3	4	5
The participant will be able to demonstrate the steps to achieving successful peripheral IV access.	1	2	3	4	5
The participant will be able to identify implanted ports, PICCs, and tunneled catheters and describe how they are used.	1	2	3	4	5
The participant will be able to demonstrate safe access of an implanted port, PICC, and tunneled catheter.	1	2	3	4	5
The participant will be able to demonstrate aseptic care of central catheters.	1	2	3	4	5
The participant will be able to demonstrate catheter flushing strategies to prevent catheter occlusion.	1	2	3	4	5

(Continued)

FIGURE 6-4 Sample program evaluation form.

The participant will be able to describe troubleshooting strategies for catheter occlusions.	**1**	**2**	**3**	**4**	**5**
The participant will be able to identify complications related to peripheral and central catheter access.	**1**	**2**	**3**	**4**	**5**
The presentation was effective.	**1**	**2**	**3**	**4**	**5**
The content reflected the objectives.	**1**	**2**	**3**	**4**	**5**
The presenter was knowledgeable.	**1**	**2**	**3**	**4**	**5**
The teaching methods were effective.	**1**	**2**	**3**	**4**	**5**
The seminar met your expectations.	**1**	**2**	**3**	**4**	**5**
Physical facilities were appropriate for program.	**1**	**2**	**3**	**4**	**5**
What aspects of this program pleased you?					
Did any aspects of the program disappoint you?					

FIGURE 6-4, cont'd Sample program evaluation form.

states that nurses will educate the patient and/or caregiver. Patient education is a basic part of nursing care and an essential independent nursing function (Kozier et al, 2004). The Institute of Medicine's landmark report in 2001, *Crossing the Quality Chasm. A New Health System for the 21st Century,* identified the need for health care organizations to provide the education and information that patients need and want (IOM, 2001). As an example, a patient receiving peripheral IV hydration in an acute care setting needs to know why the hydration is being provided, what a peripheral IV is, how it is inserted, what the patient may experience, and how to recognize signs of local and systemic complications. After that information is provided, the patient has the right to consent or refuse that treatment. In a life-threatening emergency, consent may be implied based on the general consent for treatment on admission to a facility. Patients are encouraged to take an active role in their care, and the nurse facilitates that process by empowering the patient through education. The amount of teaching that is required is based on the practice setting and the anticipated amount of patient involvement. Patients requiring infusion therapy or living with long-term venous access devices can be found in almost every health care and non–health care environment—acute care (emergency department, inpatient, surgery center), home care, ambulatory care/outpatient services, subacute or

intermediate care, long-term care, the patient's workplace, elementary and secondary schools, and physicians' offices (e.g., oncology, infectious diseases, rheumatology). Focusing the teaching on the most important aspects of what is to be learned is crucial. Too many unnecessary details can confuse the patient.

GOALS OF PATIENT EDUCATION

The following are some goals of patient education:
- To ensure that the patient and/or caregivers understand the purpose of the therapy, reasonable alternatives, desired outcomes, and potential adverse reactions
- To improve the health of the patient
- To improve the management of symptoms
- To allow the patient and/or caregivers the opportunity to ask specific questions and receive information
- To prevent hospital readmissions
- To decrease the cost of care
- To improve quality of life
- To ensure patient satisfaction
- To provide the information necessary for the patient and/or caregivers to make a decision about the plan of care (American Hospital Association, 1991)

EDUCATIONAL OFFERING PLANNING RECORD

ITEM	INTERVENTION	COMPLETION
Needs assessment		
Brochure/announcement		
Reserve room		
Reserve audiovisual supplies		
Other supplies needed		
Notify staff (e.g., email)		
Order supplies/books		
Confirmation letters to attendees		
Select food		
Handouts copied		
Collate folders		
Certificates		
Evaluations		
Participant list		
Name tags		
Evaluation summary		
Lists of attendees to directors		

FIGURE 6-5 Sample program planning list.

PREPARE FOR PATIENT EDUCATION

To plan an educational intervention that will be effective and patient-centered, the following objectives should be considered:

- Determine the goals of patient teaching.
- Develop a clear understanding of what the patient needs to learn; information that will help the patient learn how to identify problems and learn self-care skills should be included. This information is gleaned from the patient's medical record, from collaboration with other members of the health care team, and from an assessment of the patient's learning needs (Table 6-4).
- Thoroughly review the patient's medical record, the diagnosis, pertinent laboratory values, the treatment plan, and desired outcomes.
- Determine barriers to learning by conducting an assessment of the patient's physical and psychosocial status. Examples of such barriers include psychomotor limitations, pain, fatigue, and any medications that may cause drowsiness, clouding of consciousness, or decreased mental alertness. Other barriers include memory deficits (dementia, forgetfulness), visual impairments, or hearing loss; any social issues or lifestyle factors, such as support system, caregiver availability, homelessness, lack of refrigeration, lack of plumbing, or poor personal hygiene; cultural or religious issues, such as values, language, or restrictions to treatment; and literacy (ability to read and comprehend).
- Perform an assessment of the patient's psychological status, such as personal and social adjustment to illness, anxiety, fear, suspicion, defensiveness, or feelings of alienation or hopelessness. Any of these factors may prevent the patient from wanting to learn or may preclude the patient's ability to learn.

- Determine how the patient learns best (that is, through listening, by performing return demonstrations, or by reading).

Other common barriers to effective patient education are a shortage of nursing time to teach and lack of reimbursement for teaching if a patient will be receiving infusion therapy at home. A patient's stay in an acute care facility is frequently very short. Discharge planning is started on the day of admission or shortly afterward. At times there is little warning that a patient may be discharged. This limits the amount of time available for patient education. Reimbursement for patient education in the home care setting is often very limited. Using efficient and creative teaching methods is often required to achieve the desired level of patient self-care. Based on a thorough assessment of the patient's needs, a plan is devised based on what needs to be taught, how the patient will be taught, overcoming barriers to effective teaching, and when and in what time frame the patient will be taught.

TEACHING METHODS

Consideration of the patient's learning style helps the patient learn more effectively and increases recall of the material taught (Black, 2004). Most people learn through a combination of styles. The visual learner will be interested in pictures, diagrams, CD-ROMs, and the written word. Teaching about devices such as venous access devices or procedures such as flushing a PICC is facilitated by having the actual supplies available and demonstrating the procedure or device. Pictures of anatomy help the patient understand the placement of a PICC from the basilic vein in the upper arm to the superior vena cava. Using a mannequin such as Chester Chest™ helps the visual learner understand how an implanted port will look under the skin and what a port looks like.

TABLE 6-4 Teaching Guidelines for Staff and Patient Education

Therapy	Patient education	Staff education content
Peripheral catheter placement Central venous access device placement Arterial catheter placement Implanted pump access Intraperitoneal catheter access	• Describe the device • Reason for placement • Alternatives • How it will be placed • Aseptic technique • Level of discomfort patient may experience • Methods of decreasing discomfort • Potential complications • Prevention of complications • Management of complications • Catheter/device flushing • Site care and frequency	• Anatomy/physiology of vasculature • Types of devices and features • Placement procedure • Patient selection • Dwell time • Peripheral site selection • Peripheral sites to avoid • Peripheral vein dilation • Skin antisepsis • Catheter securement • Catheter flushing solutions, frequency • Site care and dressings • Infection prevention measures • Complications: occlusion, infection, thrombosis, etc. • Prevention of complications • Complication management • Desired outcomes

Ambulatory pumps
Pole-mounted pumps
Specialized pumps
	• Rationale
	• Desired outcome
	• On/off and start/stop
	• Programming
	• Checking for proper functioning
	• Alarms/troubleshooting
	• Initiating an infusion
		• Pump features
		  • On/off
		  • Start/stop
		  • PSI
		  • Maximum/minimum infusion rates
		  • Volume to be infused
		  • Infusion rates
		  • Alarms: air-in-line, occlusion, low battery, needs maintenance, infusion not started
		  • Battery life
		• Setting alarm volume
		• Changing batteries or recharging pump
		• Programming primary and secondary infusions
		• Taper mode
		• Delayed start
		• Troubleshooting

Hydration	• Rationale
	• Desired outcome
	• Anticipated duration of treatment
	• Type of fluids
	• Potential complications
		• Assessment for hydration status
		• Types of IV solutions and properties (isotonic, hypertonic, hypotonic)
		• Electrolytes
		• Vitamins
		• Complications
		  • Fluid overload
		  • Dehydration
		  • Electrolyte imbalances
		• Prevention of complications
		• Management of complications
		• Monitoring parameters
		  • Vital signs
		  • Weight
		  • Lung sounds
		• Desired outcomes

Anti-infective therapy	• Rationale
	• Desired outcome
	• Frequency of administration
	• Method of delivery
	• Potential complications
	• Management of complications
		• Assessing culture and sensitivity reports
		• Drugs
		  • Type of antimicrobial
		  • Dose
		  • Administration frequency
		  • Duration of therapy
		• Method of administration (peripheral catheter, central venous catheter, intracavitary, intraosseous)
		• Side effects
		• Management of side effects
		• Pharmacokinetics monitoring
		• Laboratory monitoring

(Continued)

TABLE 6-4 Teaching Guidelines for Staff and Patient Education—cont'd

Therapy	Patient education	Staff education content
Parenteral nutrition	<ul><li>Rationale</li><li>Alternatives</li><li>Desired outcome</li><li>Anticipated length of therapy</li><li>Composition of formula</li><li>Method of delivery</li><li>Potential complications</li><li>Monitoring laboratory studies</li><li>Monitoring weight</li><li>Monitoring of blood glucose level</li><li>Possible changes in formula based on labs</li><li>Strict aseptic technique</li><li>Potential complications</li><li>Prevention of complications</li><li>Management of complications</li><li>Reimbursement</li></ul>	<ul><li>Patient selection</li><li>Desired outcomes</li><li>Nutritional needs</li><li>Calorie calculation</li><li>Solutions and additives</li><li>Carbohydrates<ul><li>Amino acids</li><li>Lipid emulsions</li><li>Vitamins</li><li>Electrolytes</li><li>Trace elements</li></ul></li><li>Central venous access placement</li><li>Filters</li><li>Rate of administration</li><li>Continuous versus intermittent</li><li>Tapering requirements</li><li>Monitoring<ul><li>Vital signs</li><li>Temperature</li><li>Weight</li><li>Lung sounds</li><li>Fluid overload</li><li>Dehydration</li><li>Laboratory values</li></ul></li><li>Complications</li><li>Management of complications</li></ul>
Blood and blood products	<ul><li>Rationale</li><li>Alternatives</li><li>Desired outcome</li><li>Infusion times</li><li>Type and crossmatching process</li><li>Risks and safety issues</li><li>Potential adverse reactions</li><li>Management of adverse reactions</li></ul>	<ul><li>CBC assessment</li><li>Assessment of patients requiring blood/blood products</li><li>Types of blood products and compositions</li><li>Securing blood products from a blood bank</li><li>Criteria for transfusions</li><li>Compatibilities</li><li>Blood types</li><li>Antigens</li><li>Filtering</li><li>Verification of blood product and patient identification</li><li>Initiating a transfusion</li><li>Monitoring parameters</li><li>Transfusion reactions</li><li>Prevention of reactions</li><li>Managing reactions</li></ul>
Blood withdrawal	<ul><li>Rationale</li><li>Tests required</li><li>Method of withdrawal: peripheral or central venous access, fingerstick, heelstick</li><li>Level of patient discomfort</li><li>Potential complications: vasovagal response, hematoma, infection, phlebitis</li></ul>	<ul><li>Selecting a peripheral venipuncture site</li><li>Vein dilation</li><li>Accessing a central venous catheter for blood withdrawal/blood discard volume</li><li>Devices used for venipuncture</li><li>Order of draw of required tubes</li><li>Use of Vacutainer versus syringe method</li><li>Tube labeling</li><li>ICD-9 codes for tests prescribed</li><li>Tube processing</li></ul>
Therapeutic phlebotomy	<ul><li>Rationale</li><li>Alternatives</li><li>Desired outcomes</li><li>Method of venous access</li><li>Potential patient discomfort</li><li>Length of procedure</li><li>Pre- and post-hydration requirements</li><li>Potential complications</li><li>Management of complications</li></ul>	<ul><li>Criteria for patient selection</li><li>CBC assessment</li><li>Assessing patient symptoms</li><li>Skin antisepsis</li><li>Antecubital venipuncture</li><li>Use of phlebotomy collection bag</li><li>Determining amount of blood to be withdrawn</li><li>Weighing the blood bag</li><li>Monitoring the patient</li><li>Hydration requirements</li><li>Potential complications</li><li>Management of complications</li></ul>

TABLE 6-4   **Teaching Guidelines for Staff and Patient Education—cont'd**

Therapy	Patient education	Staff education content
Intravenous immunoglobulins (IVIG)	• Rationale • Alternative • Goal of treatment • IVIG name, dosage, infusion rate • Length of treatment • Monitoring required • Possible adverse reactions • Prevention of adverse reactions • Management of adverse reactions • Reimbursement	• Types of immunoglobulins • Assessment of immunoglobulin assays • Assessment of immune-deficient patient • Criteria for administration • Specific products and their uses • IV versus subcutaneous routes of administration • Dosages • Infusion rates • Handling, storage, and disposal of IVIG/supplies • Patient monitoring • Potential adverse reactions • Management of adverse reactions
Antineoplastic and biologic therapies	• Rationale • Alternative • Goal of treatment • Antineoplastic drugs • Biotherapeutic drugs • Drugs given to prevent side effects • Length of treatment • Number of cycles • Side effects of each drug • Symptom management • Reimbursement • Method of administration of each drug • Monitoring of labs, scans • Use of ambulatory infusion pump	• Criteria for patient selection for various treatments • Classification of agents • Method of action • Principles of biotherapy • Dose-limiting toxicities • Doses • Diluents • Methods of administration: continuous, intermittent, IV push • Dose calculations • Incompatibilities • Storage and disposal • Safe handling of biohazard drugs • Immediate complications: extravasation, infusion reactions, flare, spills • Side effects • Side effect prevention • Side effect management • Monitoring
Pain management	• Rationale • Alternative • Goal of treatment • Name and method of action of each drug • Time of onset and duration • Dosage • Possible side effects • Side effect management • Evaluation of effectiveness • Method of delivery • Use of PCA infusion pump	• Parenteral analgesics and uses • Pain assessment • Categories of analgesics • Dosage • Methods of administration: IV, subcutaneous, intrathecal, epidural • Monitoring • Side effects • Side effect management
Anticoagulation therapy	• Rationale • Alternative • Goal of treatment • Name and action of drug • Time of onset and duration • Dosage and adjustment • Monitoring laboratory studies • Method of administration • Side effects • Potential complications • Self-administration of subcutaneous drugs	• Assessment of coagulation studies • Drug categories • Dose parameters and adjustments based on labs • Incompatibilities • Methods of administration: IV or subcutaneous • Potential side effects • Management of side effects
Inotropic therapy	• Rationale • Alternative • Goal of treatment • Name(s) and action of drug(s) • Dosage • Monitoring of labs • Method of administration • Side effects • Potential complications	• Criteria for therapy • Assessment of patient with cardiac disease • Drug categories • Dose parameters • Potential side effects • Toxicities • Management of side effects • Monitoring parameters

Tactile learners need to touch and feel objects. Learners are more likely to retain information if allowed to do a procedure rather than just observing. Auditory learners learn best through the spoken word. When teaching patients, attention must be paid to the words the nurse is using. Medical jargon or complex words are distracting to the patient and deter the learning process. For instance, discussion and one-on-one teaching are useful when giving the rationale for therapy and information about drugs and side effects. The use of stories and acronyms will assist the learning. Asking questions to validate what was learned can enhance recall (Suter and Suter, 2008).

OVERCOMING BARRIERS

Before learning can occur, physical barriers, learning barriers, and psychosocial issues must be resolved or minimized.

Physical barriers

A patient in acute pain or discomfort from nausea will not be able to absorb concepts or procedures provided in a teaching session. The challenge is helping the patient achieve an acceptable pain level while preventing somnolence. The comfort of any patient must be a serious consideration in any teaching setting. The patient may be easily fatigued because of an illness, lack of rest, difficulty coping, or medications. Short teaching sessions are more likely to hold the patient's attention and help the patient retain what was taught. Sessions scheduled when the patient is well-rested improve attention and retention. A patient with decreased vision may learn best with one-on-one instruction and tactile experiences. Providing the teaching in a well-lit area aids patients with visual impairments. If the patient wears glasses, make sure the patient is wearing them and they are clean. Holding the teaching session in a quiet, private area will assist the patient with hearing deficits.

Psychosocial barriers

Anxiety interferes with the patient's ability to learn and concentrate. A psychosocial assessment includes the determination of the patient's level of anxiety. Some of the patient's anxiety may be due to fear of the unknown and the teaching session alone may answer some of the patient's concerns (Stephenson, 2006). Addressing other patient concerns and worries such as insurance coverage of the therapy, family concerns, and other issues helps to clear the patient's mind of pressing and anxiety-filled issues. Assessing for the level of anxiety includes observing verbal and nonverbal cues; inquiring about patient concerns such as physical, financial, and social issues; and determining prior coping skills and prior experiences in the health care system. Professional counseling for the patient may be warranted. The use of psychoeducational methods involves health education, support groups, venting of emotions, and behavioral techniques to deal with illness (Bush, 1998). In some cases pharmacological treatments may be needed (Barsevick, Sweeney, Haney et al, 2002). Establishing rapport with the patient is essential for the development of trust and a therapeutic relationship.

Health literacy

Literacy is "using printed and written information to function in society, to achieve one's goals, and to develop one's knowledge and potential" (National Assessment of Adult Literacy [NAAL], 2003). About 93 million American adults have very poor or marginal literacy skills (NAAL, 2003). It is estimated that 75% of low literate adults have not told their health care providers about their inability to read, write, or comprehend the written word. The strongest predictor of a patient's health status is the patient's literacy skills and not the patient's educational level. Literacy also includes the ability to understand the predominant language. Health literacy is: "The degree to which individuals have the capacity to obtain, process, and understand basic health information and services needed to make appropriate health decisions" (U.S. Department of Health and Human Services, 2000). The patient must be able to navigate the health care system and make decisions regarding care and treatment. These tasks are difficult for even the most schooled individuals. A patient with limited literacy skills has a greater amount of difficulty with adhering to medication schedules, filling out registration and insurance forms, following physician's orders, and understanding how to use the health care system efficiently (Edmunds, 2005). Awareness of the problems of literacy and health literacy is essential to providing teaching that the patient will understand. Studies have shown that patients with a low level of literacy tend to be less compliant with treatment and less likely to refer back to printed materials given to them as teaching aids. They are more likely to not adhere to a plan of care and are more likely to be hospitalized. Their fear level may be quite high because of a lack of understanding and feeling overwhelmed by what health care professionals feel they need to learn.

It is very difficult for health care professionals to determine the patient's literacy level. Patients with low health literacy are not likely to acknowledge it and often use excuses to hide it. A patient unable to read can pretend to read and understand printed materials to prevent embarrassment (Mayer and Villaire, 2004). Even a patient with a strong educational background feels vulnerable when faced with an illness and may have a difficult time understanding medical terms and navigating the system. Using simple language, avoiding medical jargon, explaining terminology, and talking in short sentences assist the patient in understanding what is being taught. Using terminology that anyone can understand is not "talking down" to a patient. For instance, using x-ray instead of imaging and using tube versus catheter are words most people will understand. Brochures or any printed material needs to be tested to ensure a fifth-grade reading level. Most health-related materials are written at a level too high for the average patient's understanding. About 40% of seniors read at or below the fifth-grade level (Doak, Doak, and Root, 1996). Typically, the readability goal is a fifth- or sixth-grade level. Microsoft Word 2003® and Word 2007® have the capability of computing readability statistics.

The *Ask Me 3™* patient education program developed by the Partnership for Clear Health Communication (National Patient Safety Foundation, 2008) promotes effective communication between health care providers and patients in order to improve health outcomes. These three questions are used to ensure the patient leaves the health care setting with essential information that will bring about positive health outcomes. Consider the following three questions when teaching patients:

1. What is my main problem (cognitive)?
2. What do I need to do?
3. Why is it important for me to do this?

Example: An IV antibiotic has been prescribed for a patient with a catheter-related infection. It will be administered through a newly-placed PICC. The patient will be receiving short-term home care to learn how to self-administer the antibiotic and flush the catheter.

- *What is my main problem?* You have an infection from the tube you had in your chest. You will be receiving a medicine through the tube in your arm that will get rid of the infection.
- *What do I need to do?* You need to learn to give the medicine into the tube. A nurse will show you how to do this when you get home and how to take care of the tube.
- *Why is it important for me to do this?* So that you will get well and then have the tube removed from your arm.

Cultural issues

Cultural issues may present as barriers to learning. Currently minorities comprise one third of the U.S. population. By 2050 minorities will become the majority of the population. One third of the population will be Hispanic. The black population is projected to increase from 41.1 million, or 14% of the population in 2008, to 65.7 million, or 15% of the population, in 2050. During this same time, the Asian population is projected to climb from 15.5 million to 40.6 million. Its share of the nation's population is expected to rise from 5.1% to 9.2%. Among the remaining race groups, American Indians and Alaska Natives are projected to rise from 4.9 million to 8.6 million (or from 1.6% to 2% of the total population) in the period 2008 to 2050. The Native Hawaiian and other Pacific Islander population is expected to more than double, from 1.1 million to 2.6 million from 2008 to 2050. During this same time, the number of people who identify themselves as being of two or more races is projected to more than triple, from 5.2 million to 16.2 million (U.S. Census Bureau, 2008).

To be effective, the integration of culture into patient teaching is necessary. Nurses may have negative feelings towards patients from a different ethnic background than their own (Taylor, 2005). Interactions with the patient are likely to be shorter, involve the patient less, and be less therapeutic. Reasons that nurses may react in a less than therapeutic manner include the lack of knowledge about cultural diversity, an absence of skills to work with patients of other cultures, and a lack of confidence. Nurses may also lack experience and educational preparation in working with diverse patients. Personal prejudices also may come into play (Cutilli, 2006). To be effective as a teacher and caregiver, the nurse must first be aware of cultural differences and then take on the task of learning more about different cultures (McHenry, 2007). Methods for assessing the patient's understanding of their condition based on their cultural values are to use the L-E-A-R-N model (Berlin and Fowkes, 1983) or the Kleinman model (Hollinger, 2001) (Box 6-3).

Language is another possible barrier. Teaching may need to be done through an interpreter. An interpreter must be knowledgeable about medical language and should not be a family member. Family members are unsuitable as interpreters because the patient's confidentiality will be compromised; family, especially if it is a son or daughter, may be embarrassed by the content of the teaching; and the family member may not be totally truthful in the interpretations for fear of upsetting the patient. A qualified professional interpreter should be used. Teaching a patient through an interpreter may take twice as long as expected (Box 6-4).

Box 6-3   MODELS TO ASSESS THE PATIENT'S UNDERSTANDING OF ILLNESS AND TREATMENT

L-E-A-R-N model	**Kleinman model**
Listen to the patient's perception of the problem.	What do you call your problem?
Explain your perceptions of the problem.	What do you think caused your problem?
Acknowledge and discuss similarities and differences.	What has your sickness done to you?
Recommend treatment.	How bad is it?
Negotiate treatment.	What do you fear most?
	What do you think should be done about it?

Box 6-4   TIPS FOR WORKING WITH AN INTERPRETER

- The interpreter must understand that confidentiality must be maintained.
- Avoid the use of medical terms.
- Be aware of nonverbal communication—it should match the content of the discussion.
- Look at the patient, not the interpreter, when teaching.
- Provide written materials in the language of the patient to reinforce what was taught.
- Repeat important points.
- Ask the patient to repeat the important points.
- Learn some phrases in the patient's language.
- Be aware that if the patient nods during the teaching it may be out of politeness and may not indicate comprehension.

Age differences

Older adults

In 2050 the number of people age 65 and older will be doubled what it is today. All the baby boomers will have reached 65 and older by 2025, and the number of people 85 years old and older will have tripled. Awareness of changes in the older patient will help facilitate effective learning (Jansen et al, 2007). Changes include a shortening of the attention span and sensory memory deficits. The patient may have increased anxiety because of the awareness that memory has shortened. When an older patient receives information, the reaction time to these messages is slower. The patient may have difficulty grasping information that is fast-paced and intensive (Palmer, 2006). Changes in cognitive function and comprehension may result in the patient not able to ask questions and may lead to misunderstanding of the material taught. For more information on working with an older patient, see Box 6-5.

Pediatric patients

Teaching children involves awareness of the developmental stage of the child and involvement by the parents or primary caregiver. To elicit cooperation from the child, involve the child in his or her care as much as possible. If a child requires an infusion in the home setting, depending on age and ability, the

Box 6-5   GUIDELINES FOR TEACHING AN OLDER ADULT

- Sit with the patient and face the patient.
- Speak slowly.
- Use short teaching sessions.
- Ensure the patient is well-rested.
- Repeat the main points.
- Summarize the main points at the end of the teaching session.
- Use printed materials that have large, well-spaced lettering.
- Eliminate background noise.
- Encourage the patient to participate and provide feedback.
- Be aware that the patient may have limited finances.
- If the teaching is outside of the patient's environment, transportation may be a problem.
- Include supportive family if possible.

Polzien G: The ABCs of teaching older adults: implications for home care and hospice, *Home Healthcare Nurse* 24(8):487-489, 2006.

fun for children and can be personally focused (Rassin et al, 2004).

EVALUATION AND DOCUMENTATION

For the most common teaching scenarios, a patient teaching checklist is effective to ensure that all staff give the patient the same information and to prevent omission of important teaching concepts. See Figure 6-6 for an example of an oncology teaching checklist.

Evaluation of the effectiveness of patient education is required to determine if the most important topics of the education have been assimilated. Asking the patient to "teach" the nurse the information or procedure, or having the patient write down the steps, or devising scenarios to determine if the patient understands what to do are all effective ways to evaluate the success of the teaching. Repetition is essential to reinforce major concepts. Documentation of patient education ensures the patient was taught, identifies what was taught, and records the patient's responses.

child may be involved in gathering supplies, opening packages, skin cleansing, or applying a dressing. The parent or guardian must learn the procedures thoroughly and serve as the child's "consultant" in matters of double-checking what the child has done. Determining what the child fears most will assist in developing a teaching plan. If the child fears needles and needs an implanted port accessed, utilizing methods for anesthetizing the area will help to eliminate the fear. Children also enjoy rituals as coping strategies. Doing a procedure at the same time every day and using a step-by-step process assist with accuracy and understanding, although with children flexibility must be incorporated. Allowing the child to practice a procedure on a doll or child mannequin is less threatening than taking the steps for the child to do the procedure on himself or herself. Include rewards in teaching, such as special Band-Aids, small gifts, or a special event (Ott, 2005). Computer learning is another way to interest a child in the learning process. Computer games are

PATIENT OUTCOMES

The patient and/or caregiver will be able to:
- Learn the topic and be able to apply the knowledge
- Engage in self-care activities
- Improve/stabilize his/her health condition
- Relieve symptoms of condition
- Relieve anxiety due to lack of knowledge
- Improve in function
- Reduce costs related to a decrease in number of interactions with healthcare providers (including emergency room visits)
- Patient satisfaction related to the teaching intervention

PATIENT TEACHING DOCUMENTATION

PREPARATION FOR TEACHING:

_____ Teaching packet

_____ Record appointments on calendar (if known) and any scheduled medications

_____ Teaching sheets for chemotherapy agents, any drugs the patient needs to take *before* treatment, and side effect sheets appropriate to agents

GENERAL INFORMATION/INTRODUCTION:

1. Language patient speaks? _____Can he/she understand English? **Yes No** Can he/she read English? **Yes No** Will an interpreter be needed? **Yes No**

2. What kind of cancer do you have?
   _____

3. How and when did you find out about it?
   _____

4. Have you ever been treated for cancer before now?
   _____

5. What did you receive? _____ What kind of side effects did you have? _____
   _____

6. What has the doctor told you about your cancer and the treatment? _____
   _____

7. What do you already know about chemotherapy? _____
   _____

8. Do you have any problems with your vision, hearing, or memory? _____

9. Do you have any pain right now? _____

10. Are you experiencing any other symptoms right now like nausea, vomiting, or loss of appetite? _____

11. Do you have advance directives? _____ Would you like information about it? **Yes No** Copy in patient's medical record? **Yes No**

12. Do you smoke? **Yes No** Would you like any information about stopping smoking? **Yes No**

13. Do you have any cultural or religious beliefs/practices that will affect treatment? _____

14. What do *you* want to know? _____

   _____ Review "What is cancer?"

   _____ How chemotherapy works

   _____ Review treatment plan & calendar

   _____ Overview of specific agents and *major* side effects (list agents)

   _____

(Continued)

From Mueller PS, Glennon CA: A self-developed prechemotherapy education checklist, *Clin J Oncol Nurs* 11(5):715-719, 2007.

FIGURE 6-6 Oncology teaching checklist.

CHECK SIDE EFFECTS RELATED TO AGENTS PRESCRIBED:

GI

_____Nausea/vomiting

Emetogenic rating of agents (Check all that apply)

_____ Age 50 or less

_____ History of motion or morning sickness

_____ Female

_____ Nausea/vomiting with previous treatment

If 2 or more are checked:

Increase emetogenic level by 1 level

_____ Final emetogenic rating

_____ Diarrhea

_____ Constipation

_____ Mucositis

_____ Anorexia

_____ Taste changes

Hematologic

_____ What is CBC?

_____ Neutropenia

_____ Thrombocytopenia

_____ Anemia

_____ Overview of growth factors

Skin

_____ Hair thinning

_____ Alopecia

_____ Hand/foot syndrome

_____ Skin & nail changes

_____ Phototoxicity

_____ Rash

_____ Radiation recall

GU

_____ Hemorrhagic cystitis

_____ Nephrotoxicity

_____ Contraception

_____ Infertility

_____ Intimacy

_____ Menopause (premature)

_____ Alteration in urine color

Infusion Reactions

_____ Signs/symptoms

_____ Prevention

_____ Hepatotoxicity

_____ Secondary malignancies

Neuro/Psych

_____ Neuropathies

_____ Ototoxicity

_____ Depression

_____ Fatigue

Cardiac

_____ MUGA scan

Date: _____

Results: _____

Respiratory

_____ Pulmonary fibrosis

_____ Pulmonary edema

_____ PFTs done

FIGURE 6-6, cont'd Oncology teaching checklist.

_____ Chemotherapy precautions

_____ Chemotherapy day tips

_____ Help yourself booklets given:

    _____ *Keeping Your Exercise Program on Track*   _____ *Thermometer*

    _____ *Benefits of Good Nutrition*   _____ *Cancer Counseling*

    _____*Will I Be Able to Work during Treatment?*   _____ *ACS TLC*

    _____ *Chemotherapy & Your Emotions*   _____ *Look Good/Feel Better*

    _____ *Eating Hints*   _____ *Disease/treatment-related info*

Other: _____

_____ IV access:

    _____ Discuss options—chest port, arm port, PICC; use Venous Access Assessment

    _____ CVAD already placed: copy of card, PICC or port booklet; and review complications

    (infections, occlusion, PICC migration)

_____ Coping: refer to Help at Home and Resources

Who lives with you? _____

Who will be the person most supportive for you? _____

Who will help you take care of tasks at home should you need help (e.g., meal preparation,

shopping, laundry, cleaning, errands)? _____

How will you get to your appointments and treatments? _____

_____ When to call the doctor: phone number magnet

_____ General information

Office hours

Tour of infusion clinic

_____ Patient and/or caregiver verbalized understanding of teaching information

FIGURE 6-6, cont'd Oncology teaching checklist.

SUMMARY

Addressing the needs of the patient is crucial for successful patient education. Using the principles of adult education, learning theories and methods for teaching apply to any educational intervention whether it be for staff or patients.

REFERENCES

American Hospital Association: *A patient's bill of rights,* revised 1991. Retrieved 10/20/08 from http://www.patienttalk.info/AHA-Patient_Bill_of_Rights.htm.

Anderson LW, Krathwohl DR, Airasian PW et al, editors: *A taxonomy for learning, teaching, and assessing: a revision of Bloom's taxonomy of educational objectives* (abridged ed.), Sudbury, Mass, 2001, Jones and Bartlett.

Barsevick AM, Sweeney C, Haney E et al: A systematic qualitative analysis of psychoeducational interventions for depression in patients with cancer, *Oncol Nurs Forum* 29:73-87, 2002.

Berlin EA, Fowkes WC, Jr: A teaching framework for cross-cultural health care—application in family practice. In Cross-cultural medicine, *West J Med* 12:(139):93-98, 1983.

Black JM: Assessing learning preferences, *Plast Surg Nurs* 24(2):68-69, 2004.

Bruner J: *Toward a theory of instruction,* Cambridge, Mass, 1966, Harvard University Press.

Bush NJ: Anxiety and the cancer experience, In Carroll-Johnson RM, Gorman LM, Bush NJ, editors: *Psychosocial nursing care: along the cancer continuum* (pp 125-138), Pittsburgh, 1998, Oncology Nursing Society.

Cutilli CC: Do your patients understand? Providing culturally congruent patient education, *Orthopedic Nurs* 25:(3)218-224, 2006.

Doak CC, Doak LG, Root JH: *Teaching patients with low literacy skills,* ed 2, Philadelphia, 1996, J.B. Lippincott.

Edmunds M: Advocacy in practice. Health literacy, a barrier to patient education, *Nurse Pract: Am J Primary Healthcare* 30(3):54, 2005.

Harton BB: Clinical staff development. Planning and teaching for desired outcomes, *J Nurs Staff Develop* 23(6):260-268, 2007.

Hendrickson T: Electronic staff education, *J Nurs Staff Develop* 23(6), 2007.

Hollinger B: Integration of cultural systems and beliefs. In Rankin SH, Stallings KD, editors: *Patient education: principles & practice*, ed 4, Philadelphia, 2001, Lippincott Williams & Wilkins.

Infusion Nurses Society: Infusion nursing standards of practice, *J Infus Nurs* 29(1 suppl), 2006.

Infusion Nurses Society: *Policies and procedures for infusion nursing*, ed 3, Norwood, MA: author.

Institute of Medicine: *Crossing the quality chasm. A new health system for the 21st century*, Washington, DC, 2001, National Academy Press.

Jansen J, van Weert J, van Dulmen S et al: Patient education about treatment in cancer care: an overview of the literature on older patients' needs, *Cancer Nurs* 30:(4)251-260, 2007.

Kelly-Thomas KJ: *Clinical and nursing staff development. Current competence, future focus*, ed 2, Philadelphia, 1998, Lippincott.

Kozier B, Erb G, Berman A et al: *Fundamentals of nursing. Concepts, process, and practice*, ed 7, Upper Saddle River, NJ, 2004, Pearson Prentice Hall.

Krugman M: Evidence-based practice: the role of staff development, *J Nurs Staff Develop* 19(6):279-285, 2003.

Lieb S: *Principles of adult learning*, 1991. Retrieved 4/16/08 from http://honolulu.hawaii.edu/intranet/committees/FacDevCom/guidebk/teachip/adult.

Lockhart JS: *Unit-based staff development for clinical nurses*, Pittsburgh, 2004, Oncology Nursing Society.

Mayer GG, Villaire M: Low health literacy and its effects on patient care, *JONA* 34:(10)440-442, 2004.

McHenry DM: A growing challenge: patient education in a diverse America, *J Nurs Staff Develop* 23(2):83-88, 2007.

Merriam SB, Caffarella RS, Baumgartner LM: *Learning in adulthood*, ed 3, San Francisco, 2006, Jossey-Bass.

Merriam-Webster Online. Retrieved 6/20/08 from www.merriam-webster.com/.

Mueller PS, Glennon CA: A nurse-developed prechemotherapy education checklist, *Clin J Oncol Nurs* 11(5):715-719, 2006.

National Assessment of Adult Literacy: (2003). *A first look at the literacy of American adults in the 21st century*, U.S. Department of Education, 2003. Retrieved 5/27/08 from http://nces.ed.gov/NAAL/PDF/2006470.pdf.

National Patient Safety Foundation, Partnership for Clear Health Communication: *Ask Me 3*™. Retrieved 7/7/08 from http://www.npsf.org/askme3/PCHC/what_is_ask. php.

Oermann MH: How effective is your patient teaching? *JWOCN* 30:122-125, 2003.

O'Grady NP et al: Guidelines for the prevention of intravascular catheter-related infections, *MMWR Recommend Rep* 51(RR10):1-26, 2002.

Ott MJ: "I want to do it myself!" Interferon self-injection for children with chronic viral hepatitis, *Gastroenterol Nurs* 28:(5)406-409, 2005.

Palmer JA: Nursing implications for older adult patient education, *Plastic Surg Nurs* 26:(4)189-192, 2006.

Polzien G: The ABCs of teaching older adults: implications for home care and hospice, *Home Healthcare Nurse* 24(8):487-489, 2006.

Rassin M, Gutman Y, Silner D: Developing a computer game to prepare children for surgery, *AORN J* 80:(6)1095-1102, 2004.

Sherman RO: One size doesn't fit all: motivating a multigenerational staff, *Nurs Manag* 39(9), 2008.

Smith EL: Staff development through a patient safety lens, *J Nurs Staff Develop* 22(4):210-212, 2006.

Smith RM: *Learning how to learn: applied learning theory for adults*, Chicago, 1982, Follett.

Stephenson PL: Before the teaching begins: managing patient anxiety prior to providing education, *Clin J Oncol Nurs* 10(2):241-245, 2006.

Suter PM, Suter WN: Timeless principles of learning. A solid foundation for enhancing chronic disease self-management, *Home Healthcare Nurse* 26:(2)82-88, 2008.

Taylor R: Addressing barriers to cultural competence, *J Nurs Staff Develop* 21:(4)135-142, 2005.

U.S. Census Bureau: *An older and more diverse nation by mid-century*, U.S. Department of Commerce, 2008. Retrieved from http://www.census.gov/Press-Release/www/releases/archives/population/012496.

U.S. Department of Health and Human Services: *Healthy People 2010: understanding and improving health*, ed 2, Washington, DC, 2000, U.S. Government Printing Office.

7 Clinician and Patient Safety

Sherri Barnhill, MA, RN*

In today's complex world of health care, clinician and patient safety is paramount now more than ever. Most health care organizations have dedicated staff whose job it is to improve safety for their employees as well as their patients. There are many professional groups that have formed in recent years to support the patient safety teams in hospitals to design safer practices. In this chapter, the following information will be provided: reasons why errors occur in the health care setting, barriers to improving safety, the pathophysiology of errors, and ways to improve patient safety in an organization, with specific examples included for infusion nurses. The last section of the chapter is dedicated to regulatory, accrediting, and professional organizations that are looking at clinician and patient safety from a higher level. Their perspectives on the topic and the ways that they desire adherence or expect compliance are outlined. As each organization approaches clinician and patient safety from a different perspective, the lessons received from each will provide a broad base in which to practice safety in any health care setting.

INTRODUCTION

The purposeful study of improving the safety of both clinician and patient intensified after the Institute of Medicine (IOM) report *To Err is Human: Building a Safer Health System* was published in 2000. The IOM estimated that between 44,000 and 98,000 lives are lost each year through medical errors, of which 7000 are from medication errors (IOM, 2000). In patient safety circles, that number is routinely quoted. However, to help put these numbers in perspective, consider that many towns across the United States have far fewer residents. Medical errors are the eighth leading cause of death in the United States. More people die from medical errors than acquired immunodeficiency syndrome (AIDS), motor vehicle deaths, or breast cancer (IOM, 2000). Where does one start to tackle this huge problem in a health care environment that continues to grow in complexity

every day? First of all, there is a need to grasp why errors occur in the first place in order to identify ways to prevent them.

BARRIERS TO IMPROVEMENT

No clinician, be it a physician, nurse, or other health care provider, drives to work each morning and ponders, "How can I mess up today?" On the contrary, clinicians from all specialties arrive at their health care organizations ready to meet the complex demands of caring for their patients every day. So what are their barriers? They fall into three categories: lack of awareness, complex environment, and culture of blame.

LACK OF AWARENESS

The first barrier is a *lack of awareness*. This refers to lack of awareness of the magnitude of the problem. (This barrier is not referring to lack of clinical knowledge.) Although there are between 44,000 and 98,000 deaths annually, there are approximately 2.5 million nurses and 900,000 physicians practicing in 7500 hospitals across the United States (American Medical Association [AMA], 2006; U.S. Census Bureau, 2008). Given these figures, a clinician would, statistically speaking, rarely be involved in a serious incident. Therefore it is not uncommon for nurses and physicians to believe that provision of health care is safer than it actually is in the day-to-day world.

COMPLEX ENVIRONMENT

The second barrier to safety improvement involves the *complex environment* in which health care providers work. Until fairly recently nurses worked without the benefit of computerized axial tomography (CAT) scans, magnetic resonance imaging (MRI), and peripherally inserted central catheters (PICCs). No one knew that one day a gallbladder could be removed through a laparoscope or that a diseased heart could be repaired without using a heart bypass machine. Neonatal intensive care units several years ago could not imagine successfully caring for infants weighing 1 pound. However, along with the tremendous life-giving benefits of technology has come the stress

* We would like to acknowledge of Mary R. Heisey and Maxine B. Perdue for their contributions to Chapter 34: Management of Hazardous Substances in IV therapy used in the second edition of *Infusion Therapy in Clinical Practice*.

of harnessing that knowledge and making the right decision each and every time. The problem is that clinicians, no matter how well educated, are human and mistakes are going to happen. Vigilance will not prevent human error. Health care is so complex that no one can predict all the possible complications that can occur when providing care to a patient. Therefore because events are tightly interlinked, when an error occurs downward spiraling events develop in rapid succession.

Consider, for example, an infusion nurse who is asked to assist a nurse on a medical-surgical floor who is unable to obtain a peripheral line in one of her patients. The medical-surgical nurse provides the infusion nurse what she believes is the necessary information. The infusion nurse prioritizes care based on the information provided and arrives on the unit within 30 minutes to provide assistance. What the infusion nurse sees, however, is incongruent with the message that was received from the patient's nurse. The infusion nurse arrives to find a room full of health care personnel quickly trying to manage a patient who is hemodynamically compromised and is being closely monitored. One nurse's lack of communication dominoes into a scenario in which the patient's survival can be at risk.

In all work environments, there are two basic kinds of errors that people make. James Reason (2000), a British professor of psychology, defined them as either active errors or latent errors. Active errors, also known as "errors at the sharp end of health care," occur at the point of interaction between the person (for example, a nurse) and a larger system (for example, a medication cart). An example of an active error is the nurse pulling the wrong medication out of the drawer and administering it. Active errors are considered to occur on the frontline of the job and are in direct control of the clinician on the sharp end of health care. In this example, it would be at the bedside where the medication was given to the patient.

The second type of error is called a latent error. Latent errors are also known as "errors at the blunt end of healthcare." This is an error that contributed to or gave rise to the active error and is not necessarily apparent when it happens. In the preceding example, the latent error might have been that the incorrect medication was either a look-alike or sound-alike medication. Practicing in a hectic chaotic environment, the nurse mistakes the look-alike medication for the intended medication. Initial review of the incident often focuses on the active error and the nurse on the sharp end at the bedside often gets blamed for the mistake. When that occurs, no attention is focused on the latent error, increasing the likelihood that the error will be repeated. Only when it is recognized that the latent error is actually the root cause of the error that needs to be fixed will the medical errors be reduced or eliminated.

CULTURE OF BLAME

So what is worse than knowing that mistakes are going to happen? The third barrier to decreasing errors is working in an environment in which a *culture of blame* is the foundation. Who has not heard someone on a nursing unit say, "If the nurse had only been more careful, this would not have happened"? Using the preceding example, when the mistake occurred, did the medical-surgical nurse have all the information to give the infusion nurse? Was the medical-surgical nurse a new graduate? And once the infusion nurse arrived, were all the needed supplies available? Were policies or protocols in place to safely practice? Many organizations have infused their facilities with the belief that if something bad happens, it must be assigned to someone and that person should be blamed, disciplined, or terminated for the mistake. How likely are nurses working in punitive environments willing to come forward and acknowledge a medication error, or a near miss of any kind? Historically, hospitals have stopped the investigation at the active error level rather than researching the latent error or root error creating an unhealthy environment. Reporting near misses is vital for improving patient safety. Not until reporting these events becomes routine will an organization be able to see trends in a certain type of occurrence. When trends are identified, change in practice can occur and a near miss will not become a direct hit. For example, several nurses report choosing a certain medication and at the time of administration it is determined by each to be incorrect. As a result of each nurse reporting a near miss, an investigation occurs that determines two look-alike medications are located side-by-side in the medication drawer. The solution could be to physically separate the two medications. Working in an environment that encourages reporting near misses will improve overall patient safety immeasurably.

 ## PATHOPHYSIOLOGY OF ERROR

There is a "pathophysiology of error," coined by Lucian Leape, MD, faculty member at the Harvard School of Public Health and renowned expert on health care safety. This phrase applies to all work environments including health care. In the next section, several examples of why and how mistakes are made will be covered.

RELIANCE ON WEAK ASPECTS OF COGNITION

Humans often desire to rely on their memory in order to complete tasks. This is the way many people were taught from primary school through nursing or medical school. Memorization often starts with the ABCs, and then the multiplication tables. From there, the expectation may lead to using memory as a tool to learn much more complicated facets of training such as scientific formulas, calculations, and equations. What nursing students and medical students may not be taught is that memory is faulty and not to be fully trusted. The social science term for this is "reliance on weak aspects of cognition," and this is the first cause of error. Because something is very clear at the moment it is presented, people tend to think that it will stay that clear throughout that day and tomorrow. On a busy nursing unit, however, a nurse may be interrupted five times while walking down the hall to restart an IV. What are the chances that the nurse will remember all five of those messages accurately when charting hours later?

INTERRUPTIONS

Interruptions are the second type of cause of error. When a person stops the nurse in the hallway to deliver a message, the message deliverer does not intend to assist in causing an error but the potential is there. Some health care organizations are so aware of the danger of interruption that when a nurse is preparing medications to be administered, a vest is worn with the following inscription: "Thank you for helping me provide safe care to my patients by not disturbing me while I prepare and administer these medications."

FATIGUE

Another cause of error is simple fatigue. While historically a badge of honor in health care, fatigue is being acknowledged as a major factor in many types of errors. Lucian Leape, MD, has said many times, "Healthcare is the only profession where fatigue is not considered a factor in errors." Known as a sleep-deprived nation, American health care providers take that one step further by having nurses work double shifts or historically by the number of hours physicians in training spend on duty at one time. It has been estimated that being awake for 24 hours is the equivalent to having a blood alcohol level of 0.1% (Dawson and Reid, 1997). If it is illegal to drive a motor vehicle because of the impact on the body when exceeding the blood alcohol level, should it be permissible to care for patients? Health care is slowly realizing the concerns and implications. In 1984 an 18-year-old girl was admitted to a New York hospital complaining of flulike symptoms. Seven hours later she was dead. Out of this tragedy came the review of medical residents' level of fatigue and the role it had in her death. State legislation in New York mandated limiting the hours that medical residents may work in any given week. Known as the Bell Commission, Dr. Bertrand Bell, the chairman of the committee that investigated this case, remarked, "How is it possible for anyone to be functional working an 85 hour work week? A bus driver can not do it, a pilot can not do it, so why should a neophyte doctor do it?" (Josefson, 1998). In 2001 the Accreditation Council for American Medical Education (ACAME), the agency that oversees the accreditation of medical education (similar to the oversight of hospital accreditation by The Joint Commission), now requires a limitation on the number of work hours for physicians in training. Many hospitals have taken this lesson and expanded it to nursing by instituting a policy that does not allow nurses to work more than 12 hours at a time. However, in this time of nursing shortages, many organizations do allow nurses to work extra hours in order to meet the staffing demands. Patients come first, and when there are vacancies or illnesses in the health care organization, nurses will step up and do what it takes to provide patient care.

TIME PRESSURE

Time pressure in health care also adds to the problem of inducing errors in the workplace. In the American environment, where federal reimbursement is decreasing, health care resources are stretched thin, and shortages of nurses abound, time pressures add to the pathophysiology of error. Fewer nurses are caring for more and sicker patients, leaving greater room for error. Because patients are having more diagnostic tests and surgeries, patients are more mobile across the health care settings than ever. Also known as "performance pressure," the stress to move patients through the health care system has a domino effect on the entire health care system, leaving everyone fatigued, stressed, and accident-prone.

HAND-OFFS

Communication "hand-offs" are another very common way that patient safety is compromised. Most clinicians do not realize how many times information is passed from one person to another in the course of one patient transaction. Hand-offs are like the children's game of "rumor," where a sentence is whispered in the ear of one child and the message is whispered to another and another until the last child verbalizes the sentence. As would be expected, the final version of the sentence bears no resemblance to the original statement; so it is with passing information from one clinician to another. Infusion nurses often receive orders that are hand-written and nonstructured, where deciphering the exact order is sometimes difficult. Equally unsafe, the infusion nurse may receive instructions from a nurse who is verbally passing the instructions to another caregiver in a nonstructured format from yet another nurse.

Errors can occur anywhere along the chain of information hand-offs in a multifaceted, complex health care system. Some of these providers will have multiple patients who could be traveling anywhere along this continuum of care, with the likelihood for error increasing exponentially.

MEDICATION TERMINOLOGY

Adding to the contributing factors for error already discussed is a world of medications that have hundreds of look-alike/sound-alike names. The United States Pharmacopeia (USP) is a nonprofit organization whose mission is, among other things, to advance public health by promoting safe and proper use of medications. MEDMARX® is an anonymous Internet-based program that is used by health care organizations to report, track, and analyze medication errors. Since it was created in 1998, hospitals across the nation have voluntarily provided 1.2 million reports of medication errors. The eighth annual USP MEDMARX® report, published in 2008, indicated that more than 1400 commonly used drugs are involved in look-alike/sound-alike drug errors. The MEDMARX® report found that 1.4% of these errors resulted in patient harm. It was also estimated that seven of these errors either caused patient death or significantly contributed to death. From these 1400 drugs, the USP determined that there were 3170 pairs of drugs that are often mistaken for the other (Thompson, 2008; USP, 2008).

STANDARDIZATION

Nonstandard procedures and nonstandard environments are also a cause for clinicians to inadvertently compromise patient safety. The way to perform any procedure may differ when practices are determined by individual practitioners. Until the Institute for Healthcare Improvement (IHI) began its drive to standardize the process for the placement of central lines, each caregiver tended to perform the insertion as trained by the individual's instructor or mentor. Not until clearly defined steps were outlined and the concept of "bundling" taught, did the infection rate for bloodstream infections start to significantly decrease in health care organizations. Bundling is the concept that multiple steps in a process must be followed 100% of the time in order to decrease the likelihood of error. Environments that are standardized improve efficiency and decrease error for infusion nurses. Safety is improved for infusion nurses when the following occur:

- Carts are fully stocked with items clustered related to use.
- Shelves are labeled.
- Carts and equipment are consistently found in the same place.

Although individuality is to be commended, standardized procedures, treatments, and environments increase safety and decrease error in health care.

KNOWLEDGE BASE

An expanding knowledge base is another cause of error in health care. Information that was learned while in nursing school becomes outdated and sometimes obsolete within a couple of years of postgraduate practice. Within the field of medicine, one study indicated that an internist would need to read 20 newly published articles a day, 365 days a year (and remember all that new information) to keep abreast of the latest scientific information in that chosen specialty (Shaneyfelt, 2001). Nursing would be no different. Obviously this is an impossibility; errors will be made because of the expanding knowledge base within one's field.

PARADIGM SHIFTS

Although the term "paradigm shift" has become clichéd in many ways, the concept is quite relevant in health care. A paradigm is the way one thinks based on his/her beliefs and environment. Thomas Kuhn (1970), a professor and writer on the history of science, coined the phrase "paradigm shift" in 1960 to indicate the ways humans shift or transition one way of thinking to another. Clinicians in health care often feel comfortable practicing the way they were trained during school, even though science may indicate that new ways of practice are better. This line of thought reflects back to the expanded knowledge base where a nurse cannot practice according to the idea that information learned 5 or 10 years ago is the current method of practice.

Lacking the ability to address a paradigm shift is another way patient safety can suffer. The key components of the central line bundle are hand hygiene, maximal barrier precautions upon insertion, chlorhexidine skin antisepsis, optimal catheter site selection (with the subclavian vein as the preferred site for nontunneled catheters), and daily review of line necessity with prompt removal when unnecessary. One of the biggest drawbacks by many clinicians who have been inserting PICCs for years was the need to wear maximal barrier precautions. It was considered highly unnecessary and would slow down patient care (remember the "time pressure" contribution to error). Infusion nurses had not been trained to wear maximal barrier precautions; so why would one start now (expanding knowledge base)? Only when clinicians could see that changing a traditional process could actually decrease infection did the thought of changing one's practice—shifting one's paradigm—demonstrate reductions in infection rates.

 PATIENT SAFETY

Most nurses were trained that education was all that was needed to make improvements and then, if needed, to re-educate. While no one would disagree that education is crucial in the delivery of safe health care, the idea that education alone will improve safety is faulty. The role of human factors' research is a concept that nurses most likely were not taught in school. However, the impact it makes on safety in the workplace is enormous. The science of studying humans and the environments in which they work is termed human factors. For example, under what conditions is the work completed? What kinds of tools are used in order to complete the work? What constraints occur in the workplace? By taking these variables into account,

work environments can be made safer and more efficient. In infusion nursing, one of the best examples is how human factors influenced the design of the "smart pump." Before the new design, a nurse would stand at an IV container/administration set and count drops to calculate flow rates. Medications would be added and tape would be placed on the container indicating such factors as dosing and flow rate. This was dangerous in many ways, but at the time there was no safe alternative. Historically, one of the most common causes of medication errors is that resulting from reliance on these weak aspects of cognition. Often, medications being infused are "high-hazard" medications and, as discussed previously, once an error reaches a patient, the chain of events is so tightly coupled that it is difficult to mitigate its effects. The smart pump has made a positive impact in this area. A smart pump utilizes special software targeted at eliminating the reliance on weak aspects of cognition. This design has incorporated the human factors associated with the infusion and the staff nurses performing this task but has eliminated much of the human variability of administering fluid and medication. Infusion pumps are now fitted with safeguards that have the ability to identify and correct many nurse programming errors before the error reaches the patient. The infusion pump can trigger an alarm that notifies a nurse when drug parameters are either too high or too low. Infusion pumps also have the ability to stop the administration of medication doses identified to be extremely unsafe. Calculating the rate into the pump allows for more consistent administration of the prescribed amount of the solution or medication. However, errors are still possible when an infusion pump allows clinicians to override limits or warnings.

WAYS TO IMPROVE SAFETY AND EFFICIENCY

This section will address several ways that using human factors' research improves the safety and efficiency of the nurse. In 2006 The Joint Commission (TJC) identified communication breakdowns, estimated at roughly 65%, as the number one root cause of sentinel events in hospitals. A sentinel event is an unexpected occurrence that involves serious physical or psychological injury to a patient or one that causes death (TJC, 2008a). By root cause, The Joint Commission means that while the actual sentinel event may have been "wrong site surgery," the real root cause of that sentinel event was the result of a communication breakdown between the surgeon and the nurse, which led to the sentinel event.

Reduce and improve hand-offs

Improving communication hand-offs is the first example of how human factors' research will improve patient safety. Historically, the way in which patient information is communicated, whether it is transferred from one unit to another or at change of shifts, has been determined by the nurse. The report might be communicated by phone, in person, or on a tape recorder. Also, in the past the order in which the information was given and the comprehensiveness of the content were often determined by the individual. Recalling the concept of weak aspects of cognition (where the nurse relied on memory to convey a comprehensive report), there was no assurance that the correct information was reported every time. There was often the illusion that communication had occurred on the part of the nurse giving a report. Communication hand-off tools have become widely used to ensure that vital information is passed

COMMUNICATION HAND-OFF INFORMATION

Name of patient:_____ Age:_____ Time of request: _____

Patient location: _____Diagnosis:_____ Priority: _____

Emergent ☐   1 hour ☐   4 hours ☐

Code Status: Full ☐   Limited ☐   No code ☐

Current lines in place: PICC ☐   Peripheral ☐   Central ☐

Line needed placed: PICC ☐   Peripheral ☐   Central ☐

Diabetic: No ☐   Yes ☐   Anticoagulant therapy: No ☐   Yes ☐

Infection: No ☐   Yes ☐   Do not stick: Right ☐   Left ☐   Arm ☐   Leg ☐

Isolation: No ☐   Airborne ☐   Contact ☐   Droplet ☐

LOC: oriented   x1 ☐   x2 ☐   x3 ☐   Responsive to verbal stimulus ☐
                                                                      Responsive to pain ☐
                                                                             Comatose ☐

Communication barriers: No ☐   Yes ☐   Hearing ☐   Vision ☐   Language ☐

FIGURE 7-1 Communication hand-off information.

on to the next caregiver. A communication form template encourages the nurse giving report to systematically proceed through vital information by having a tool on hand. The nurse is no longer relying on memory to communicate everything that needs to be conveyed.

Hand-off tools

Hand-off tools can be used in a variety of settings whether it is a change of shift report or whether a patient is being temporarily transferred into another department's care for a specific procedure. For infusion nurses, a hand-off tool can be used when a call is made requesting infusion nursing services. One of the most common error types in infusion nursing is the lack of consistent information obtained from the requesting unit before arrival. The tool will assist in the prioritization of care and arriving at the new site better prepared to immediately begin providing care. There is no one standard hand-off tool and organizations can modify current tools to fit their individual needs (Figure 7-1).The bottom line is to improve patient safety in any way that can be accomplished.

SBAR

It comes as no surprise to say that nurses and physicians are educated differently, not only in content but also in style. Nurses are encouraged to be collaborators and to seek consensus, and they are taught that although they can describe patient conditions, they cannot diagnose them. So in discussing patient care with colleagues, narrative, descriptive explanations are used. Physicians, on the other hand, are taught to be decision-makers, to problem-solve, and then to diagnose. So in crucial situations when vital information needs to be conveyed between these two clinicians, many times each is left frustrated with the other. Communication styles just do not necessarily mesh. A bridge to that communication conflict is a communication

tool that actually had its origins in the nuclear submarine field. After the IOM study was published in 2000 and the gravity of up to 98,000 lost lives annually was realized in the health care community, a group of health care providers at Kaiser Permanente met to discuss how medical errors could be decreased. Out of one of these discussions came the communication tool SBAR (pronounced S-BAR). A team member, a former safety officer on a nuclear submarine, explained how vital information was communicated quickly, succinctly, and in the same manner each time. During this strategy session, the concept of SBAR was born (Monroe, 2006), which indicates the following:

- **S**ituation—State the problem (the reason for the call) in 5 to 10 seconds.
- **B**ackground—Put the situation in context. Provide objective information.
- **A**ssessment—State the problem.
- **R**ecommendation—Recommend what needs to be done. What does the physician need to do?

By standardizing communication through developing a template, efficiency is increased and patient safety improved (Figure 7-2). Health care organizations across the nation have adopted this communication strategy for use in a variety of situations. Although SBAR is most commonly used when nurses and physicians communicate with each other about a patient issue, it is being used successfully with pharmacists and others. The most important point is this communication strategy works both ways. In health care organizations that have fully integrated this method, physicians call and convey information using SBAR and nurses call and communicate patient information via SBAR to the physicians as well. The following is an example of how this communication technique is used:

- S (Situation)—Dr. Smith, this is Susan Carter. I am the nurse taking care of Daniel Mason in room 1069. He has developed pain and burning at his left forearm IV site.

S	**Situation:** I am calling about (patient's name_____). The problem is_____. Vital signs are BP:_____ Pulse:_____ Resp:_____ Temp:_____. I am concerned about _____ because _____.
B	**Background:** The patient's mental status is_____, skin is _____, patient is/is not on O$_2$. Pulse oximetry is_____.
A	**Assessment:** I think the problem is_____. **OR** The problem seems to be _____. **OR** I am concerned that the patient is unstable.
R	**Recommend:** I would like to recommend that you _____. (See the patient? Transfer? Obtain tests? Other?)

FIGURE 7-2 SBAR communication tool. *(Adapted from* Dingley C, Daugherty K, Derieg MK, and Persing R: *Improving patient safety through provider communication strategy enhancements,* Accessed 1/5/09 from www.ahrq.gov/downloads/pub/advances2/vol3/advances-dingley_14.pdf).

- B (Background)—Mr. Mason is a 63-year-old male with a history of hypertension, renal insufficiency, and congestive heart failure (CHF), admitted with exacerbation of his CHF. He was started yesterday on intravenous dopamine in an attempt to enhance his urine output. The dopamine is infusing into the site where he has developed symptoms.
- A (Assessment)—His venipuncture site is reddened and edematous. It appears that he has a dopamine extravasation.
- R (Recommendation)—I have discontinued the IV catheter and elevated the arm. I feel he may benefit from phentolamine and would like you to evaluate the patient.

This method of communication will only occur with acceptance from all disciplines. Training on how to use the tool is vital. After training, many hospitals place a laminated SBAR form near telephones and in dictation areas to use as a visual trigger in utilizing this strategy.

Medication "tall man lettering"

Eliminating look-alike and sound-alike medications through human factors' research is in process. The Center for Drug Evaluation and Research (CDER), a part of the U.S. Food and Drug Administration, conducted a study in 2001 that, "requested manufacturers of sixteen look-alike name pairs to voluntarily revise the appearance of their established names in order to minimize medication errors resulting from look-alike confusion" (USP, 2008). The revision of the names is what is known in the process improvement world as "tall man lettering." By emphasizing the differences in closely similar words, those differences will trigger the clinician's eye to see the drug in a new and distinct way. Tall man lettering is using the capital alphabet as a visual trigger to decrease the chance for medication mix-up. Box 7-1, from the CDER, provides recommended names for drug pairs using the tall man lettering technique.

As in life, too much of any one thing is not good. While the FDA has proposed this list for specified drugs, manufacturers have extended that list to other drugs (Lesar, 2008). While at first this might make sense, standardization is actually impacted as a result of companies independently choosing their own way of lettering drugs. If every drug is lettered this way, it will cause "alert fatigue" and in doing so clinicians will not see any differentiation (Lesar, 2008). It simply defeats the purpose.

Cues

Affordance is a quality improvement term meaning that which "affords" the nurse the opportunity to do the right thing. Working in a hectic and complex environment such as health care, developing cues to trigger nurses to remember to complete certain tasks is an affordance. For the nurse who

Box 7-1   FDA CDER LOOK-ALIKE/SOUND-ALIKE MEDICATIONS

Established Name	Recommended Name
acetohexamide	acetoHEXAMIDE
acetazolamide	acetaZOLAMIDE
bupropion	buPROPion
buspirone	busPIRone
chlorpromazine	chlorproMAZINE
chlorpropamide	chlorproPAMIDE
clomiphene	clomiPHENE
clomipramine	clomiPRAMINE
cyclosporine	cycloSPORINE
cycloserine	cycloSERINE
daunorubicin	DAUNOrubicin
doxorubicin	DOXOrubicin
dimenhydrinate	dimenhyDRINATE
diphenhydramine	diphenhydrAMINE
dobutamine	DOBUTamine
dopamine	DOPamine
ephedrine	epHEDrine
epinephrine	epINEPHrine
glipizide	glipiZIDE
glyburide	glyBURIDE
hydralazine	hydrALAZINE
hydroxyzine	hydrOXYzine
medroxyprogesterone	medroxyPROGESTERone
methylprednisolone	methylPREDNISolone
methyltestosterone	methylTESTOSTERone
nicardipine	niCARdipine
nifedipine	NIFEdipine
prednisone	predniSONE
prednisolone	prednisoLONE
sulfadiazine	sulfADIAZINE
sulfisoxazole	sulfiSOXAZOLE
tolazamide	TOLAZamide
tolbutamide	TOLBUTamide
vinblastine	vinBLAStine
vincristine	vinCRIStine

From the FDA/Center for Drug and Evaluation Research: *Name differentiation project.* Accessed November 25, 2008 from http://www.fda.gov/cder/drug/mederrors/nameDiff.htm.

is mentally processing a specific task and not thinking about performing hand hygiene, a cue could prove to be helpful. A colorful, attention-grabbing sign placed outside a patient's door reminding health care workers to perform hand hygiene before entering the patient's room offers a visual cue triggering the nurse to do the right thing. When developing cues, providers take advantage of a nurse's various senses. Depending upon the type of task involved, triggers can be visual, auditory, or tactile. Even when a cue is not purposefully placed in a caregiver's path, making things visible to a nurse is another way to increase patient safety. In the previous example of using tall man lettering to decrease medication errors, the USP (2008) recommended that the indication of the drug also be added to prescriptions so that it would cue a clinician to think about why it is being ordered as another way to catch a medication

error. By combining two triggers, tall man lettering and a visual cue, it improves the chance that a medication error will not occur (USP, 2008).

Workspace standardization

Standardizing the layout or design of nursing work areas such as medication rooms, infusion carts, or storerooms may not at first appear to be a clinician or patient safety tool. However, human factors research is linked with the environment in which a person works and the tools that assist a person to perform his or her job. Standardizing the workspace can improve efficiency and safety. The term "parking lot" has been used in process improvement parlance for a while. It is a phrase meaning that every piece of equipment, big or small, should have its own "parking space" on a unit, enabling a staff member to know the exact location. These parking spaces are often outlined with colored tape that demarcates where a piece of equipment should be housed. Sometimes the space will also be marked with the name of the equipment. Once a team understands and accepts this concept, precious time can be saved, efficiency improved, and safety increased. The less time a nurse spends hunting for a piece of equipment, the more time is available at the bedside to provide patient care. The same concept is true of standardizing a storeroom or an infusion cart. Members of the infusion team should be involved in the process. For example, brainstorming about which supplies are needed on a daily basis, the amount of those supplies needed to provide safe patient care, and the layout of those supplies in order of importance or use will increase safety as a nurse will always know where every item (work tools) is at any given time. Standardization decreases errors.

Product standardization

To take the concept of standardization one step further, when hospitals understand that product standardization is a significant factor in patient safety, product acquisition takes on a different tone. Each physician has tools and equipment that are preferred because of previous training with a certain type of equipment or learning to perform a task using a certain kind of tool. However, as variability of equipment or supplies increases, safety decreases. If a nurse must learn a different process for each physician who uses a different tool, mistakes may occur as a result of the variability, and the weak aspects of cognition will ensure errors at some point. In hospitals that have standardized equipment and decreased tool variation, safety and efficiency have improved, and errors have decreased.

Care standardization

Errors are also decreased with standardization of care. The standardization of central line placement is a good example of how determination of the logical sequence and correct way to place a central line is now a standardization of care. Safety is reinforced when practitioners standardize order sheets to accompany the process. Instead of each physician writing different orders manually, some evidence-based and some not, the order sheet can be standardized. Therefore handwriting illegibility is not an issue and there are no surprises in the orders, leading to optimal care. The orders are routine, known, and accepted. The more ways care can be standardized, the safer it is for all.

Checklists

Checklists also play a role in health care as they provide a mechanism to ensure nurses do not forget steps in processes. Many departments in hospitals are now using checklists as part of their treatment regimen. Preoperatively, both nurse anesthetists and operating room (OR) nurses use them so as not to miss important information before surgery. Intensive care units (ICUs) use checklists to ensure all steps are being performed to prevent ventilator-associated pneumonia in patients. Like communication hand-offs, these written cues trigger the nurse to verify the same thing every time, thus improving patient safety.

Process improvement techniques

As was mentioned in an earlier section, while education is an obvious part of preparing a nurse for practice, there are many other ways to improve delivery of safe patient care. There are three levels of process improvement techniques that include forcing functions, constraints, and affordances.

Forcing functions

Forcing functions are processes that "force" a person to do the right thing. Several years ago, patients were being inadvertently harmed by anesthesia personnel when the gas lines were connected incorrectly, connecting what was thought to be oxygen to the nitrous oxide line and vice versa. When this pattern of error was discovered, the gas lines were redesigned so oxygen would only connect with oxygen and nitrous oxide would only connect with nitrous oxide. Hence the redesign "forced" the nurse to do the right thing. The redesign prevented a misconnection from occurring.

A second example can be seen as more and more hospitals adopt electronic medical record (EMR) charting. Nurses, physicians, and pharmacists, in collaboration with informational systems staff, have worked together in some organizations to determine what parts of the chart are absolutes, thus requiring the clinician to chart in the way the record is configured. For example, if a clinician does not chart a patient's allergies, a window pops up (visual cue) and, until the practitioner acknowledges the cue and charts appropriately, the computer will not allow charting to proceed to the next step. It forces the clinician to do the right thing and chart the missing information.

Constraints

Constraints, another process improvement tool, are one step down from forcing functions. An example of a constraint is a patient bed that defaults to 30 degrees automatically after a nurse provides patient care, such as initiating infusion therapy. Thirty degrees is the optimal angle at which patients are typically placed as one of the steps in decreasing ventilator-associated pneumonia. The difference in a forcing function versus a constraint is that if for some reason the 30 degrees is contraindicated, the nurse can override that setting. If it were a forcing function, the nurse would not be able to make the change.

Natural mapping (which is a type of constraint) is another way that improves both clinician and patient safety. Natural mapping is the concept that, if the order or placement of something is logical or natural, a person will have to depend upon his or her memory less to know how something works. Remember, reducing the reliance on weak aspects of cognition is essential in safety. This was a concept coined by the cognitive scientist Donald Norman (Norman, 1988), who has devoted his life to the wonders and pitfalls of human design. In this world there are good natural mappings and poor natural mappings. A classic example of both a good and a poor natural mapping is the illustration that Dr. Norman uses when comparing the design of knobs on stoves. When each knob corresponds with its burner, it is a good mapping. There are many manufacturers who chose aesthetics over design, and the placement of the knobs has nothing to do with how the stove operates. The new infusion pumps are an example of good mapping for infusion nurses. The pumps are designed logically or well mapped such that an infusion nurse is able to stand at an infusion pump and determine fairly readily which knob controls which function.

Affordances

The third technique is affordance. As mentioned earlier, affordance is a visual cue, like a hand hygiene poster. Another example is a picture of a clock posted at the head of the bed that indicates a 2-hour turning schedule for the patient at high risk for pressure ulcers. While affordances can improve patient safety, nothing will stop a nurse from walking by a sign encouraging hand hygiene and not performing hand hygiene, nor from seeing the clock and inconsistently turning patients every 2 hours. It is simply a reminder and does not have the ability to change behavior in and of itself.

RECOVERY PLAN

Even with all of the tools that health care providers can use to improve safety, it should be assumed that errors will occur along the way. Donald Berwick (Berwick, 2001), President and CEO of the Institute of Healthcare Improvement, said it eloquently when he was speaking about health care and human limitations: "So long as it involves humans, and thank God it does, healthcare can never be free of errors. But it can be free of injury." To that end, a plan of recovery is often wise. Though a plan cannot be provided for every potential error, those situations where there might be a higher than normal risk should have a plan of recovery. These plans might involve a visual cue (affordance) in which drug calculations are posted in order to provide quick help in a crisis situation. In some ICUs, a vial of Narcan (naloxone hydrochloride injection, USP) is placed near a patient who is at risk of an overdose. The vial is placed in the same place (standardization) each time it is used for this patient situation. Another example is the plan of recovery for malignant hyperthermia, which can occur in a surgical setting. In response to a dangerous and often fatal response in some patients to certain anesthetic drugs, operating rooms will maintain a malignant hyperthermia cart stocked and ready for use at a moment's notice. This cart is kept in the same location in the OR (parking lot) for quick access. And because this is such a rare phenomenon, the company that produces the drug used to counteract malignant hyperthermia, Dantrium intravenous (dantrolene sodium), has published a poster that is placed on the cart for the clinician to use during the stressful situation.

Finally, health care organizations that have put "defaults" into place in certain areas of clinical practice have seen great improvements. Some organizations have received approval to have certain protocols in place that will always occur, unless a physician specifically writes an order against the protocol. For example, in the emergency department (ED), defaults have been written and adopted in some hospitals that if a patient enters the ED complaining of chest pain, the patient will be given an aspirin before any diagnosis. This default will allow the benefits of the aspirin to begin, so precious time is not wasted. Another common default in hospitals is the pneumococcal vaccination. When a patient is admitted, and meets predetermined criteria, that patient will receive a pneumococcal vaccination without a specific order. This practice, when it can be done, improves safety, efficiency, and compliance with important standards of care.

 ORGANIZATIONS

There are a variety of organizations devoted to improving clinician and patient safety through improving the quality of care that a patient receives. Each organization's perspective on how that is accomplished, however, can be quite different (Box 7-2).

CENTERS FOR MEDICARE & MEDICAID SERVICES (CMS)

President Lyndon B. Johnson signed the Social Security Act on July 30, 1965, establishing both Medicare and Medicaid. The Centers for Medicare & Medicaid Services (CMS), as it is now called, is responsible for the coordination of Medicare and Medicaid across the United States (CMS, 2008a). This Social Security Act includes a provision where hospitals accredited by The Joint Commission are deemed to be in compliance with most CMS regulations, known as "Medicare Conditions of Participation for Hospitals," and therefore are permitted to participate in Medicare and Medicaid. In recent years, CMS has become increasingly interested in moving from being a passive payer to an active purchaser of health care services. In doing so, CMS has become more active in attempting to measure and lead hospitals in the improvement of quality of health care (CMS, 2008b). (Refer to Chapter 9, Financial Considerations, to review additional information on the link between reimbursement and documented quality improvement. Also, refer to Chapter 3, Quality Management.)

OCCUPATIONAL SAFETY AND HEALTH ADMINISTRATION (OSHA)

In 1970 Congress established the Occupational Safety and Health Administration (OSHA) "to assure so far as possible every working man and woman in the nation safe and healthful working conditions" (OSHA, 1999b). Under the Department of Labor, OSHA compiled a comprehensive set of rules and regulations that set standards for workplace safety through the establishment of the Occupational Safety and Health (OSH) Act. OSHA regulates numerous safety and health aspects, including material labeling and information communication, personal protective equipment, workplace monitoring, medical surveillance, and training requirements. In addition, numerous chemicals are regulated individually. Because of the nature of an infusion nurse's work, this section on employee safety will be more comprehensive than other organizational information.

Hazardous Communication Standard

A key OSHA rule that has affected facilities managing hazardous materials and hazardous wastes is the Hazardous Communication Standard (HCS), which was passed by the U.S. Congress in 1988. It requires every employer to develop, implement, and maintain a written, comprehensive communication program for the workplace. The standard identifies three areas that must be covered within each employer's comprehensive program (ASHP, 1998) (Box 7-3).

Box 7-2   ORGANIZATIONS DEVOTED TO IMPROVING CLINICIAN AND PATIENT SAFETY

Organization	Type of Agency
Centers for Medicare & Medicaid Services (CMS)	Regulatory
Occupational Safety and Health Administration (OSHA)	Regulatory
The Joint Commission (TJC)	Accreditation
Hospital Quality Alliance (HQA)	Patient safety and quality improvement
Agency for Healthcare Research and Quality (AHRQ)	Patient safety and quality improvement
National Quality Forum (NQF)	Patient safety and quality improvement
Institute for Healthcare Improvement (IHI)	Patient safety and quality improvement
The Leapfrog Group	Patient safety and quality improvement
United States Pharmacopeia (USP)	Patient safety and quality improvement

---

Box 7-3   COMPREHENSIVE PROGRAM FOR MANAGEMENT OF HAZARDOUS WASTE AREAS REQUIRING COVERAGE

- *A means to identify and warn employees of hazardous chemicals:* Employers must post a notice (prepared by the Department of Labor) of employee rights under the OSH Act, and labels must be maintained on all chemical containers, including stationary containers.
- *MSDSs:* Material safety data sheets are comprehensive data sheets that must be maintained on each hazardous chemical or medication. All medications must be classified to indicate a potential for significant health hazard. Each safety data sheet should provide information regarding proper handling and storage procedures, accident and fire prevention, special hazards, and emergency procedures for each chemical used in the work area. MSDSs must be available and accessible to employees at all times.
- *An employee information and training program:* The training program must be established in writing and kept at the facility. The program must provide education regarding the potential hazards, preparation, transportation, administration, management of accidental exposure, and disposal of all chemical agents used by the employee.

General duty clause—Occupational Safety and Health Act

The OSH Act of 1970 and its amendments pertain mainly to workplace safety. It established a set of regulations that set standards for both employers and employees. The clause stipulates that the employer must furnish each employee a place of employment that is free from recognized hazards that could cause death or serious physical harm and that the employer must comply with occupational safety and health standards given under this act. It further stipulates that each employee must comply with occupational safety and health standards and all rules, regulations, and orders issued by the Act that apply to the individual's own action and conduct.

Noncompliance with the stipulations of the OSH Act can result in a fine being placed on the organization for the actions of both the employer and the employee. Therefore it is essential that organizations have well-developed policies and procedures for their employees to follow. In many organizations and agencies, compliance standards have been written into performance appraisals as safety standards.

Work-practice guidelines for personnel dealing with cytotoxic (antineoplastic) drugs

In 1986 the Office of Occupational Medicine, a division of OSHA, developed a set of guidelines for health professionals to use during the course of handling hazardous substances to prevent exposure to cytotoxic drug therapy. They were not issued as mandatory standards, but rather as guidelines designed to assist all health care personnel who may be exposed to cytotoxic drugs through inhalation, skin absorption, or trauma, including physicians, nurses, pharmacists, aides, and the numerous and diverse health care support staff. The guidelines were developed because of the concerns of health care personnel regarding the potential harm that may result from exposure to cytotoxic drugs.

Two elements were recommended as being essential to ensure proper workplace practices: (1) the education and training of all staff involved in any aspect of cytotoxic drug handling and (2) the use of a biologic safety cabinet (BSC). The costs of implementing education and training and the installation of the BSC are relatively minor. The potential benefits are major.

In 2004 the National Institute for Occupational Safety and Health (NIOSH) issued an alert to increase awareness to employees and employers of the hazards of working with hazardous drugs. NIOSH listed detailed steps that employees and employers must take to protect themselves from harm. The list can be viewed on the World Wide Web at www.cdc.gov/niosh/docs/2004-165/#sum (NIOSH, 2004).

Bloodborne pathogen standards

In 1991 OSHA published regulations for occupational exposure to bloodborne pathogens (OSHA, 1991). In 1992 OSHA issued a directive mandating that employers implement certain rules and regulations when there is a potential for exposure to blood or other potentially infectious materials. The mandate was comprehensive and included rules and regulations mandating everything from an exposure control plan to the use of a ducted exhaust-air ventilation system. This mandate required nurses to use personal protective equipment and engineering controls (e.g., sharps disposal containers and self-sheathing needles) when performing venipunctures and when there was a potential for contact with bloodborne pathogens. The mandate further stipulated that these controls be evaluated and replaced on an ongoing basis.

In 1999 OSHA issued a new compliance directive to the bloodborne pathogens standard that covered all U.S. employees at risk for occupational exposure to blood or other potentially infectious materials (OSHA, 1999a). The directive updated the regulations enacted in 1992 and contained a number of provisions that forced health care facilities to take a more proactive approach to the prevention of sharps injuries. Although the directive did not place requirements

---

Box 7-4   OSHA'S 2001 REVISED BLOODBORNE PATHOGENS STANDARD: *Recommendations for Prevention of Occupational Exposures to Bloodborne Pathogens*

1. Comprehensive Exposure Control Plan
   - A written plan to eliminate employee exposures to bloodborne pathogens
   - Reviewed and updated annually
   - Reflects changes in technology
   - Emphasizes engineering controls
   - Includes annual documentation of consideration and implementation of safer medical devices
   - Solicits input from nonmanagerial employees in the identification and selection of safer medical devices
2. Engineering Controls
   - Used to reduce (remove, eliminate, or isolate) employee exposure
   - Evaluated to reduce exposure before, during, and after use of products
3. Staff Education
   - Ongoing
   - Annual program to address what employees can do to eliminate potential exposures
4. Tracking and Follow-up of Injuries
   - Documentation of injuries (incident report log) with follow-up treatment
      - Includes employee job category, department, and body part affected
      - Includes type and brand of device, circumstances, and procedure
   - Documentation of procedure for evaluation of circumstances surrounding exposure incidents

---

on the employees, it did recognize and emphasize the advances made in medical technology and reminded employers that they must use readily available technology in their safety and health programs. As health care has become more complex and in many ways more dangerous, OSHA revised the regulations again in 2001 in response to the Needlestick Safety and Prevention Act (see details in the next section) (OSHA, 2001) (Box 7-4).

Needlestick Safety and Prevention Act

Federal action to protect health care workers from the risks of sharps injuries passed the House of Representatives and Congress in 2000. The Needlestick Safety and Prevention Act called for revisions to the bloodborne pathogens standard as stated in the preceding section. The changes affect four key areas, imposing requirements on employers of individuals who have the potential for exposure to bloodborne pathogens. The following four key areas incorporate the OSHA revised bloodborne pathogen standards (OSHA, 2001; Needlestick Safety and Prevention Act, 2000a, 2000b):

1. *Redefine engineering controls.* The Act redefined engineering controls to include safer medical devices such as sharps with engineered protections and needleless systems. The phrase "sharps with engineered sharps injury protections" (SESIP) is defined as "a non-needle

sharp or a needle device with a built-in safety feature or mechanism that effectively reduces the risk of an exposure incident." "Needleless systems" are defined as systems "that do not use needles for (a) the collection of bodily fluids or withdrawal of body fluids, (b) the administration of medication or fluids, or (c) any other procedure with percutaneous exposure to a contaminated sharp."

2. *Update bloodborne pathogens exposure control plans to reflect changes in technology*. The Act requires employers to update exposure control plans to reflect changes in technology that reduce or eliminate exposure to bloodborne pathogens. Employers will have to "document annually consideration and implementation of safer medical devices and solicitation of input from nonmanagerial employees."

3. *Maintain a sharps injury log*. The employer is required to establish and maintain a sharps injury log for the recording of percutaneous injuries from contaminated sharps. Information should be maintained in a manner to protect the confidentiality of the injured employee. The sharps injury log must minimally contain "(a) the type and brand of device involved in the incident, (b) the department or work area where the exposure incident occurred, and (c) an explanation of how the incident occurred."

4. *Solicit input from nonmanagerial employees*. Employers must involve nonmanagerial employees, that is direct caregivers, in the identification, evaluation, and selection of safety devices. In addition, these employees must represent a cross-section of the employees within the facility to ensure that a representative sample is making the final decision on these engineering controls.

THE JOINT COMMISSION (TJC)

In 1952 the American College of Surgeons along with the American College of Physicians, the American Hospital Association, the American Medical Association, and the Canadian Medical Association formed the Joint Commission on Accreditation of Hospitals (JCAH). As discussed previously, in 1965 Congress passed the Medicare Act, which included a provision that hospitals accredited by the JCAH were deemed to be in compliance with most of the Medicare Conditions of Participation, permitting accredited hospitals to participate in Medicare and Medicaid. In 1986 Dennis O'Leary was chosen to head JCAH as an agent of change. In 1987, in an attempt to emphasize this change along with the changing scope of the organization, the name was changed to the Joint Commission on Accreditation of Healthcare Organizations (JCAHO), eventually changing in 2007 to The Joint Commission (TJC). Dr. O'Leary began the process of shifting the focus of the accreditation process to actual organizational performance. As part of this shift, focus was placed on creating an indicator measurement system to support performance improvement. This began in 1988 as the Indicator Measurement System (IMSystem), eventually evolving into the current Core Measure System (TJC, 2008b).

In an attempt to increase the focus on critical patient safety concerns and promote improvement in patient safety, The Joint Commission created the first list of National Patient Safety Goals (NPSGs). The first list included the following six goals and was released on January 1, 2003:

Goal 1: Improve the accuracy of patient identification

Goal 2: Improve the effectiveness of communication among caregivers

Goal 3: Improve the safety of using high-alert medications

Goal 4: Eliminate wrong-site, wrong-patient, and wrong-procedure surgery

Goal 5: Improve the safety of using infusion pumps

Goal 6: Improve the effectiveness of clinical alarm systems

Each year, TJC reevaluates the list, adding new goals based on sentinel event reports and national trends. They also retire other goals that have been universally implemented. Organizations accredited by The Joint Commission are expected to demonstrate compliance with all past and current NPSGs, and The Joint Commission evaluates compliance with these goals during each hospital accreditation survey. Of the current list of NPSGs, the ones that most affect infusion nurses include, but are not limited to the following:

- Improving the accuracy of patient identification
- Improving the effectiveness of communication among caregivers
- Improving the safety of using medications
- Reducing the risk of health care–associated infections
- Accurately and completely reconciling medications across the continuum of care
- Encouraging patients' active involvement in their own care as a patient safety strategy
- Improving recognition and response to changes in a patient's condition

For more information on The Joint Commission's National Patient Safety Goals, visit http://www.jointcommission.org/PatientSafety/NationalPatientSafetyGoals/.

FOCUS ON EVIDENCE

Needlestick Prevention

- A prospective observational study was conducted for 2 years after the introduction of safety-engineered devices (SEDs) and compared with prospectively collected pre-intervention needlestick injury (NSI) data from the 2 year prior period. The study concluded that introduction of SEDs resulted in a fall of 49% in hollow-bore NSI, contributed to by the virtual elimination of NSI related to accessing IV lines with minimal cost outlay (Whitby, McLaws, and Slater 2008).

- A multicenter observational prospective survey with a 1-year follow-up period was conducted to evaluate SEDs with respect to their effectiveness in preventing NSIs in healthcare settings and their importance among other preventive measures. Data were prospectively collected for a 12-month period. The procedures for which the risk of NSI was high were also reported 1 week per quarter to estimate procedure-specific NSI rates. Device types were documented. The study found that the use of SEDs during phlebotomy procedures was associated with a 74% lower risk of NSI and was probably the most important preventive factor (Lamontagne et.al 2007).

- A prospective observational study was conducted over a 7-year period in a 3600-bed tertiary care university hospital in France to determine the effectiveness of 2 protective devices in preventing needlestick injuries to health care workers. Needlestick-related injury incidence rates decreased significantly after the implementation of the 2 safety devices, representing a 48% decline in the incidence rate overall (Rogues et al. 2004).

HOSPITAL QUALITY ALLIANCE (HQA)

In 2002 CMS joined forces with The Joint Commission (TJC), the American Hospital Association, the American Medical Association, the American Nurses Association, and other professional organizations along with insurance companies and consumer and employer groups to form the Hospital Quality Alliance (HQA). The HQA is dedicated to identifying a set of standardized hospital quality measures that would be used to improve the quality of care across the nation (CMS, 2008c). To that end, HQA created the website "Hospital Compare" to function as a consumer-focused site that posts participating hospital results of these quality indicators. CMS, TJC, and HQA continue to work to expand these quality indicators. CMS plans to begin to associate hospital reimbursement to performance on these quality indicators (CMS, 2008c).

AGENCY FOR HEALTHCARE RESEARCH AND QUALITY (AHRQ)

The Agency for Healthcare Research and Quality (AHRQ) is an agency within the U.S. Department of Health and Human Services. It is the nation's federal agency for research as it relates to health care quality and patient safety. Its complement is the National Institutes of Health (NIH), which primarily focuses on biomedical research. The goal of AHRQ is to provide patients with objective data with which to make enlightened decisions regarding health care (AHRQ website). In addition, AHRQ assists clinicians by providing a web-based mechanism in which to obtain information on evidence-based clinical practice guidelines. This web-based program is the National Quality Measures Clearinghouse and can be accessed through the Internet at www.qualitymeasures.ahrq.gov.

NATIONAL QUALITY FORUM (NQF)

One challenge that all health care providers face in improving the quality and safety of the health care environment is the lack of standardization of performance measurement indicators. Hospital clinicians and administrators across the nation struggle with a multitude of regulatory organizations, payer and private organizations, all creating their own performance standards and all expecting compliance. In an attempt to address this issue, the creation of the National Quality Forum (NQF) was proposed through a report issued in 1998 by the President's Advisory Commission on Consumer Protection and Quality in the Health Care Industry. As a result, the NQF was launched in May of 1999. NQF's mission "is to improve the quality of American health care by setting national priorities and goals for performance improvement, endorsing national consensus standards for measuring and publicly reporting on performance, and promoting the attainment of national goals through education and outreach programs" (NQF, 2008). CMS has agreed not to propagate new standards until they have been endorsed by NQF through this process. With increasing focus on errors in medicine and the push for reporting of these errors, NQF began to look at creating a standardized list of reportable serious events in health care. In 2002 the National Quality Forum published *Serious Reportable Events in Healthcare: A Consensus Report* (NQF, 2006). The list currently contains 28 serious reportable events. Many states and health care organizations have adopted this list as the core of their reporting system. Examples of serious reportable events that would most likely involve infusion nurses include, but are not limited to the following:

- Patient death or serious disability associated with the use of contaminated drugs, devices, or biologics provided by the health care facility
- Patient death or serious disability associated with the use of or the function of a device in patient care in which the device is used for functions other than is intended
- Patient death or serious disability associated with intravascular air embolism that occurs while receiving care in a health care facility
- Patient death or serious disability associated with a medication error (e.g., errors involving the wrong drug, wrong dose, wrong patient, wrong time, wrong rate, wrong preparation, or wrong route of administration)
- Patient death or serious disability resulting from a hemolytic reaction caused by the administration of ABO/HLA-incompatible blood or blood products (NQF, 2006)

INSTITUTE FOR HEALTHCARE IMPROVEMENT (IHI)

The Institute for Healthcare Improvement (IHI) was founded in 1991 by a group of individuals who desired to improve the level of health care worldwide. IHI believes that by joining forces with individuals who are committed to patient safety and quality outcomes, there can be profound changes made in health care (IHI, 2008a). The overarching aim of IHI is that there be:

- No needless deaths
- No needless pain or suffering
- No helplessness in those served or serving
- No unwanted waiting
- No waste (IHI, 2008a)

IHI enables change in a couple of ways. First, IHI coordinates collaboratives, which are teams in hospitals from across the nation that are committed to making positive change on a given health care topic. They work at their home hospitals with facilitation and support from IHI and then, during "learning sessions" as they are called, these teams meet and share their successes and failures, providing a rich learning experience for all. Examples of collaboratives include reducing surgical site infection, transforming care at the bedside, and improving patient flow in hospitals. By providing these teams with experts in process improvement strategies and by supporting teams as they make changes at their hospitals, dramatic improvements have been seen across the country. IHI is committed to bringing people and organizations together so that sharing of ideas and strategies can be used to make improvements. Another way IHI encourages improvements is by its annual conference attended by nurses, physicians, and senior hospital leadership from across the country. In December of 2004 at IHI's 16th Annual National Forum on Quality Improvement in Healthcare, President and CEO Donald Berwick launched the 100,000 Lives Campaign. At one of the plenary sessions, Dr. Berwick challenged the conference attendees that the way in which health care providers often "quantify" lives improved or lives saved needed to be changed. To drive that point home, Dr. Berwick coined the phrase, "Some is not a number. Soon is not a time." He then challenged those in the session to save 100,000 lives (the number) by June 14, 2006, at 9:00 AM EST (the time) (IHI, 2008b). He stated that the following six improvement strategies save lives:

1. Development of rapid response teams
2. Development of reliable care for acute myocardial infarctions

3. Prevention of ventilator-associated pneumonia bundles
4. Prevention of central line infections
5. Prevention of surgical site infections
6. Prevention of adverse drug events with medication reconciliation

At that conference, members could enroll their hospital to participate in the campaign. Not to be left to their own devices, IHI provided free resources in which to assist hospitals to begin addressing one or all of the preceding initiatives. Ongoing support throughout the 18 months was available through IHI as hospital teams worked on these improvements. Hospitals collected mortality data and sent it to IHI for compilation as a way of tracking overall improvement. In the end, a total of 3000 hospitals signed up, which equaled 75% of the total hospital beds in the United States, and an estimated 122,000 lives have been estimated to be saved from needless death by the June 16, 2006, deadline (IHI, 2008b).

After the 100,000 Lives Campaign, improvement experts began to discuss those patients who do not die from substandard care but are otherwise harmed by it. And from those discussions, a second campaign at IHI was launched—the 5 Million Lives Campaign—which was designed to protect patients from 5 million incidents of medical harm. The time period for this campaign was from December 2006 to December 2008. IHI defined harm as, "unintended physical injury resulting from or contributed to by medical care (including the absence of indicated medical treatment), that requires additional monitoring, treatment, or hospitalization, or that results in death." IHI expanded upon the six interventions from the 100,000 Lives Campaign and added six more:

1. Prevent harm from high-alert medications
2. Reduce surgical site complications
3. Prevent pressure ulcers
4. Reduce methicillin-resistant *Staphylococcus aureus* (MRSA)
5. Deliver reliable evidence-based care for congestive heart failure
6. Get boards on board

The same supportive tools were available. For hospitals that had not joined the 100,000 Lives Campaign, many joined in December 2006 and worked on interventions from both lists (McCannon, Hackbarth, and Griffin, 2007).

THE LEAPFROG GROUP

From regulatory agencies and quality improvement agencies comes a group with a completely different perspective on quality. More than 150 purchasers of health care insurance—employers such as Boeing, 3M, FedEx, and Microsoft—founded The Leapfrog Group in 2000. These purchasers recognized that they were spending billions of dollars on health care and wanted to influence improvement in not only quality and safety but also affordability. This group wanted to know they were getting their money's worth. The Leapfrog Group made its mission to trigger giant "leaps" forward in these areas (The Leapfrog Group). As business leaders, they also took a business approach by offering incentives for those hospitals that showed they had made these "leaps." The Leapfrog Group believes that the nation's health care is lacking in safety and quality and that it is often not of good value. In addition, improvements would occur if purchasers rewarded superior patient care. Therefore the group established the following four leaps, which they believe hospitals should adopt as a step in improving quality:

1. Computer physician order entry
2. Evidence-based hospital referral
3. Intensive care units staffed by intensivists
4. The National Quality Forum endorsed safe practices (see the preceding section on the NQF)

UNITED STATES PHARMACOPEIA (USP)

Finally, the United States Pharmacopeia (USP) is a public health organization that sets the safety and quality standards for prescriptions and over-the-counter medications. USP provides two services to the health care industry, one of which is the USP Medication Error Reporting Program that allows health care clinicians to self-report errors. From that information, USP provides a mechanism through their MEDMARX® Internet-based reporting system that allows health care organizations to track medication error trends. This was outlined in more detail earlier in this chapter.

 SUMMARY

While the IOM report was difficult for many to believe at first, it has been the catalyst for improvements worldwide since its publication (IOM, 2000). As a result of the impact of realizing that 44,000 up to 98,000 lives are needlessly lost each year, clinicians from all specialty backgrounds have been working to make their specific areas safer. Understanding why errors occur and then applying techniques to each clinical area can and does improve patient safety.

 REFERENCES

Agency for Healthcare Research and Quality: *What is AHRQ?* Accessed 3/3/08 from http://www.ahrq.gov/about/whatis.htm.

American Medical Association: *Total physicians by race/ethnicity—2006.* Accessed 2/25/08 from http://www.ama-assn.org/ama/pub/category/12930.html.

American Society of Health System Pharmacists, Tools for Health-System Pharmacists, Bethesda, Md, 1998:HM-1.

Berwick D: Not again! preventing errors lies in redesign—not exhortation, *Br Med J* 322(7281):247-248, 2001.

Centers for Medicare & Medicaid Services: *History,* 2008a. Accessed 3/3/08 from http://www.cms.hhs.gov/History/.

Centers for Medicare & Medicaid Services: *Certification and compliance,* 2008b. Accessed 3/3/08 from http://www.cms.hhs.gov/CertificationandComplianc/08_Hospitals.asp.

Centers for Medicare & Medicaid Services: *Hospital quality initiatives: hospital quality alliance,* 2008c. Accessed 3/3/08 from http://www.cms.hhs.gov/HospitalQualityInits/15_HospitalQualityAlliance.asp.

Dawson D, Reid K: Fatigue, alcohol and performance impairment, *Nature* 388:235, 1997.

Dingley C, Daugherty K, Derieg MK, and Persing R: *Improving Patient Safety Through Provider Communication Strategy Enhancements.* Accessed 1/05/09 from http://www.ahrg.gov/downloads/pub/advances2/vol3/advances-dingley_14.pdf.

Institute for Healthcare Improvement: *About us,* 2008a. Accessed 3/3/08 from http://www.ihi.org/ihi/about.

Institute for Healthcare Improvement: *Overview of the 100,000 lives campaign,* 2008b. Accessed 3/3/08 from http://www.ihi.org/IHI/Programs/Campaign/100kCampaignOverviewArchive.htm.

Institute of Medicine, Committee on Quality Health Care in America: *To err is human: building a safer health system,* Washington, DC, 2000, National Academy Press.

Josefson D: New York's junior doctors work illegally long hours, *Br J Med* 316:1630, 1998.

Kuhn T: *The structure of scientific revolutions,* Chicago, 1970, University Press.

Lamontagne F, Abiteboul D, Lolom I, Pellissier G, Tarantola A, Descamps JM, Bouvet E. Role of safety-engineered devices in preventing needlestick injuries in 32 French hospitals. *Infect Control Hosp Epidemiol* 28(1):18-23, 2007.

Lesar T: IV product labeling: practices to improve patient safety, *Pharm Purch Prod* 5(1):2-4, 2008.

McCannon J, Hackbarth A, Griffin F: Miles to go: an introduction to the 5 million lives campaign, *Jt Commis J Qual Patient Safety* 33(8):447-484, 2007.

Monroe M: SBAR: a structured human factors communication technique, *Am Soc Safety Eng Healthcare Specialty* 5(3):1-3, 2006.

National Quality Forum (press report): *Serious reportable events,* Oct 2006. Accessed at http://www.qualityforum.org/pdf/news/prSeriousReportableEvents10-15-06.pdf.

National Quality Forum: *Mission,* 2008. Accessed 3/3/08 from http://www.qualityforum.org/about/mission.asp.

Needlestick Safety and Prevention Act (H.R. 5178), 106th Congress, 2nd session, Washington, DC, 2000a.

Needlestick Safety and Prevention Act (introduced in the Senate), S. 3067 IS, 106th Congress, 2nd session, Washington, DC, 2000b.

NIOSH: *Preventing occupational exposure to antineoplastic and other hazardous drugs in healthcare settings,* 2004. Accessed 10/4/08 from http://www.cdc.gov/niosh/2004-165#sum.

Norman D: *The design of everyday things,* New York, 1988, Basic Books.

OSHA: *Enforcement procedures for the occupational exposure to bloodborne pathogens,* Directive CPL2-2.44D, November 4, 1999a.

OSHA: Occupational exposure to bloodborne pathogens: final rule, *Fed Regist* 56(235):29 CFR Part 1910.1030, 1991.

OSHA: *Safety topics: bloodborne pathogens and needlestick prevention,* 2001. Accessed 10/4/08 from http://www.osha.gov/SLTC/bloodbornepathogens/index.html.

OSHA: Strategic plan, Occupational Safety & Health Administration, 1999b.

Reason J: Human error: model and management, *Br J Med* 320:768-770, 2000.

Rogues AM, Verdun-Esquer C, Buisson-Valles I, Laville MF, Lasheras A, Sarrat A, Beaudelle H, Brochard P, Gachie JP: Impact of safety devices for preventing percutaneous injuries related to phlebotomy procedures in healthcare workers, *Am J Infect Control* 32(8):441-444, 2004.

Shaneyfelt T: Building bridges to quality, *JAMA* 286(20):2600-2601, 2001.

The Joint Commission: *Sentinel event statistics,* 2008a. Accessed 2/20/08 from http://www.jointcommission.org/SentinelEvents/Statistics/.

The Joint Commission: *A journey through the history of The Joint Commission,* 2008b. Accessed 3/3/08 from http://www.jointcommission.org/AboutUs/joint_commission_history.htm.

The Leapfrog Group: How and why leapfrog group started. Accessed 3/3/08 from http://www.leapfroggroup.org/about_us/how_and_why.

Thompson C: USP says thousands of drug names look or sound alike, *Am J Health-Systems Pharm* 65:386-388, 2008.

U.S. Census Bureau: *Facts for features.* Accessed 2/25/08 from http://www.census.gov/Press-Release/www/releases/archives/facts_for_features_special_editions/004491.html.

U.S. Pharmacopeia 8th annual MEDMARX® report indicated look-alike/sound-alike drugs lead to thousands of medication errors nationwide, (press release), Rockville, Md, Jan 29, 2008.

Whitby M, McLaws M-L, Slater K: Needlestick injures in a major teaching hospital: the worthwhile effect of hospital-wide replacement of conventional hollow-bore needles, *Am J Infect Control* 36(3):180-186, 2008.

8 INFUSION THERAPY ACROSS THE CONTINUUM

Lisa Gorski, MS, HHCNS-BC, CRNI®, FAAN,
Crystal Miller, BSN, MA, RN, CRNI®, Nancy Mortlock, BSN, CRNI®, OCN®*

Infusion therapy is administered in every patient care setting. This chapter is divided into three sections with an overview presenting issues related to acute care and non–acute care settings such as outpatient and long-term care. In the acute care section, the focus is on the implementation of the infusion therapy team. The history of alternative sites for infusion delivery is explored in the alternative site and home care sections. Options for, and advantages of, alternative site infusion administration as well as criteria for safe infusion delivery are addressed.

ACUTE CARE

The challenge in the health care industry in the United States is to deliver the highest quality of care to the greatest number of people, using all available resources in the most cost-effective manner. With each advance in technology and each breakthrough in health care intervention, the challenge becomes greater and the solution more complex. In the past, budget management of a facility was often a matter of determining where and how to use the available funds. Payment was based on charges and fees for services, so attention to volume and operational costs was primary. Higher operational costs and decreased payment have changed the focus of management. As in the past, it is mandatory to the success of an organization for managers to be astute in all aspects of health industry standards. The emphasis for nurse managers has expanded from managing not only care delivery but also the fiscal aspects of health care delivery.

A health care worker from 50 years ago would likely find the current health care system barely recognizable. We have seen a gradual decrease in the number of hospitals in this country. With projected closures, increased expenditures, and dwindling resources, reform was inevitable. The delivery of nursing care has been affected dramatically. One aspect that has felt the greatest impact is the delivery of infusion therapy. Maintaining quality and cost-effectiveness in delivering this aspect of care alone is of great concern. Criteria for the justification of hospital admission often include the clinical necessity for a venous access device (VAD) or an infusion medication. Although it is not a criterion for remaining in the hospital after the acute phase of illness as it once was, it is rare to find a patient who has not had infusion therapy by the end of a hospital stay.

Because registered nurses (RNs) manage most aspects of infusion therapy administration and infusion access, shortages in the RN workforce have led to changes in the way nursing care is delivered. Primary nursing and patient-focused care have placed more demands on the generalist nurse. Many services that were once delivered by specialists, such as infusion therapy, are now the responsibility of generalist staff nurses. The use of nursing assistive personnel (NAP) to assist in tasks has also expanded. In addition to assessing and providing direct patient care needs in the hospital, RNs serve also in the role of case managers, planning for safe and appropriate care beyond the hospital environment. High costs and decreasing reimbursement make earlier discharge to alternative settings a necessity. The demand for providing complicated infusion therapies outside the zones of acute care has expanded the role of the infusion therapy nurse. A high quality of care requires infusion nursing expertise. Clearly in the acute care environment, the specialized skills of an infusion team enhance the process for managing patient care.

Formerly, acute care facilities were reimbursed for the ancillary (versus routine) services provided by an infusion team. This reimbursement provided an incentive for implementing hospital infusion teams. Another impetus to establish such teams was the cost savings realized when infusion care was managed by specialists; there were fewer clinical complications, fewer supplies were used, and procedures were performed more quickly. With the institution of the prospective payment system, direct reimbursement for infusion therapy teams could no longer be assumed and teams were at risk with justification for their services under the close scrutiny of cost-benefit analyses. Maintaining existing infusion teams has often been a challenge for institutions, and establishing new teams even more so, despite evidence of the potential benefits infusion teams provide to patients and facilities.

FOCUS ON EVIDENCE

Impact of Infusion Teams in the Acute Care Setting

- Specialized "IV teams" have shown unequivocal effectiveness in reducing the incidence of catheter–related infections and associated complications and costs (O'Grady et al, 2002).
- A randomized controlled trial examined the incidence of infection when an intravenous team provided infusion services. There were significantly less local and infectious-related complications in peripheral catheters started and maintained by an IV team. The occurrence rate of local complications was 21.7% in catheters inserted by medical housestaff and maintained by floor nurses and 7.9% in catheters inserted by the IV team. There was a 35% overall decrease in infection (Soifer et al, 1998).
- A 12-month descriptive study was conducted to assess the value of services provided by an infusion resource team. Data were analyzed from the 789 consults received for infusion services from a randomized sample of 250 patients. Requests for venipuncture services were received from the noncritical medicine and surgical wards, with 31% requested from the general and vascular surgery wards. Vascular access was fair to good for 50% of the consults, but 39% of consults had poor access. Most consults (81%) resulted in the optimal initiation of peripheral catheters in areas of nonflexion and a 96% overall successful insertion of peripheral catheters (Bosma and Jewesson, 2002).
- A prevalence study was undertaken to assess the impact of a dedicated infusion therapy team on the reduction of catheter-related nosocomial infections. Before establishing an IV team, the total number of bloodstream infections annually was 47; the number of infections decreased to 18 per year after formation of the IV team (Brunelle, 2003).
- A 2-year study conducted at a 300-bed acute care facility supported previous data that personnel specially trained to maintain intravascular devices provide a service that effectively reduces catheter-related infections and overall costs. The implementation of an IV team on medical-surgical units resulted in a decrease in infusion-related bacteremias from 4.6% to 1.5% per 1000 patient discharges, decreased morbidity, and an estimated cost savings of $124,906 (Miller et al, 1996).
- This prospective study explored the impact of a dedicated infusion team on nosocomial bloodstream infection rates in an acute care setting. Before the introduction of an infusion team, the bloodstream infection rate was 1.1 infections per 1000 patient days (p < .01). After the introduction of the infusion team, there was a 35% reduction in nosocomial infections (1.1 to 0.7 infections per 1000 patient days, p < .01), which included a 51% decrease in infections caused by *Staphylococcus aureus* (Meier et al, 1998).

Acute care organizations are again facing significant changes in reimbursement as a "pay for performance" strategy is being implemented for hospitalized patients whose care is reimbursed under Medicare (i.e., Centers for Medicare & Medicaid Services [CMS]). Effective in October 2008, CMS implemented a plan that limits reimbursement for certain preventable complications. This includes vascular catheter–associated infections. This major change in reimbursement will compel organizations to reconsider the infusion team. Improved outcomes of care including decreased risk of infection led to CDC support for infusion teams in their 2002 practice guidelines (O'Grady et al, 2002).

ORGANIZATIONAL STRUCTURE

To maintain their viability, hospitals have been forced to become more knowledgeable and strategic in business plan development. While some facilities have become casualties, unable to maintain financial solvency with implementation of the reforms, other institutions, recognizing the economic necessity and the potential benefit of changes, have merged to form multifacility health systems. Controlling cost expenditure has forced hospitals to implement strategies that may compromise the quality of care they deliver.

Infusion care delivery models

Advances in health care delivery and related technologies, along with the adoption of more healthful lifestyles, have led to an increase in life expectancy with a subsequent increase in the average age of the hospitalized patient. This older population has frequent acute and chronic illnesses, often requiring complicated therapies, increasing the need for complex care and nursing interventions. Models of care that offer relief for some routine, high-volume tasks that nurses perform are often implemented. Such models often incorporate the use of NAP to provide routine care under the direction of the RN. Of note, while the Infusion Nurses Society (INS) supports the assistance of NAP in routine care, INS does not support the use of NAP in the direct provision of infusion therapy (e.g., catheter insertion, site care, drug/solution administration) (INS, 2009). Computerized systems help the nurse document and communicate aspects of unit management and patient care coordination. Specialized nursing management of infusion therapy has often been delegated to teams of infusion nurse specialists. Infusion specialists offer the means for maintaining consistency and quality in infusion nursing care throughout the acute care facility. Their early assessments and interventions have an impact on the discharge planning of infusion therapy needs. Even the most complicated infusion therapy needs can be met in the outpatient and home settings by these specialists.

With decreased lengths of stay, streamlined resources, and a reduced workforce, nursing is challenged to develop a care model that maintains both cost-effectiveness and quality of care. Reengineering and decentralization continue the transition of many services to the unit level. Skill-mix staffing has moved care delivery from the primary-care model to a patient-focused model.

Today's professional practice models focus on enhanced efficiency, improved quality, and desired patient outcomes. It is important for the infusion team to function within these models to have the most positive impact on patient care outcomes. The mode of practice is setting and service dependent and contributes to the success of the infusion team and the organization. When the focus of care is quality and patient satisfaction, hospitals operate cost-effectively and safely, reducing the incidence of litigation.

Infusion therapy has moved beyond the realm of technical skills. Today's infusion nurse provides clinical knowledge and serves as the primary resource for infusion therapy education. What better way to ensure positive outcomes than with a group of specialized nurses whose expertise benefits both the patients and the organization.

Operational designs

Each organizational structural design is associated with distinct advantages and disadvantages that must be evaluated carefully. A major consideration is to enhance the ability of the infusion team to meet its own established goals, objectives, and standards of care while remaining cost-effective. The ability to positively affect the maximum number of patient outcomes must be preserved. The positive impact of an infusion team directly relates to the scope of services offered and the commitment to providing exceptional service while obtaining quality outcomes. Autonomy, accountability, and collaboration are vital for the existence of an infusion department.

For the infusion team to perform at an optimal level and to derive maximum benefit from the infusion nurse's specialty skills to the patient and the organization, the infusion nurse should be assigned exclusively to infusion-related functions, without crossover into general nursing activities. It is important to note that successful high-quality infusion teams are operating as closed staff units reporting within nursing departments. Advantages may be seen in maximizing the infusion nurse specialist's collaboration and working in partnership with peers to meet established goals and strategic initiatives. It is important that collaborative relationships be maintained with other departments, such as nursing, infection prevention, case management, and pharmacy. The infusion nurse should be an active participant in the interdisciplinary health care team, and is essential in meeting the patient care objectives of providing timely and effective infusion therapy in the most appropriate setting, without complications.

Some infusion teams are placed under the pharmacy department because of the relationship between infusion therapy and the administration aspects of IV admixtures, solutions, and medications. Delivering IV medications and solutions is an integral function of all infusion teams. An association with the pharmacy affects the organizational structure and the workload responsibilities of the infusion team in various ways. There are other benefits afforded to the team reporting to pharmacy; for example, infusion team nurses gain knowledge about the safe administration of IV medications. An infusion nurse working within the pharmacy department can be an invaluable liaison between two major health care departments.

There are many instances in IV drug and solution administration in which drug compatibilities, characteristics, interactions, and filtration needs require specific administration supplies or venous access. The pharmacy staff benefits from the infusion nurse's expertise with access devices and their use and maintenance requirements. Knowledge of proper, safe IV medication administration prevents infusion drug–related complications. Interaction with the infusion nurse gives the pharmacy staff the opportunity to participate more directly in infusion-related patient care. The pharmacy director's membership on the pharmacy and therapeutics committee is an asset to the infusion therapy team, because the committee is often the hospital's approval body for policies and procedures.

Establishing a collaborative partnership with other hospital departments is essential for an infusion team. In many hospital environments, establishing the communication necessary to ensure this close relationship may not be accomplished easily. In recent years, professional practice models based on shared or collaborative governance have provided an alternative to the hierarchical management structures of most institutions. These practice models provide staff nurses with the opportunity to share the responsibility and accountability for the nursing organization. Committees are established in which nurses from the various areas of the hospital are responsible for activities such as setting standards for their practice, developing policies and procedures, and evaluating the quality of practice and its outcomes. Collaborative governance offers potential advantages for infusion teams inside and outside the nursing department.

The infusion team that actively participates in shared governance models benefits from a strong communication system that would otherwise not be available to an ancillary department. Such involvement offers decision-making opportunities at the unit level and the ability to address hospital-wide concerns. Participation in shared governance activities strengthens the infusion nurse's ties to the nursing structure, allows increased visibility, and enhances the team's value to the organization. It provides infusion nurses with the opportunity to have a voice not just about infusion-related issues, but about all facets of nursing. The viability of an infusion team rests on the value the organization places on the department's contribution to hospital goals, and on meeting department-specific goals.

The Infusion Nurses Society (INS) encourages infusion nurses to collaborate with or participate in committees that regulate the practice of infusion nursing and interact with the members of the health care team to provide safe, quality infusion therapy and care (INS, 2006). Representatives from the infusion therapy department should be active participants in committees such as pharmacy and therapeutics, infection control and prevention, nutritional support, transfusion therapy, safety, quality assurance, and risk management.

SCOPE OF SERVICES

With the majority of acute care patients receiving infusion therapy at any given time, the infusion nurse is an integral part of the nursing process for each patient. The infusion nurse's role is no longer viewed as a technical position but is one that consolidates knowledge regarding infusion therapy and incorporates sound clinical assessment and intervention into the patient's care plan. It is essential that the infusion nurse be given time for thorough patient assessment before preparing the patient's infusion plan of care. When establishing the scope of practice of the infusion therapy department, it is important to evaluate the practice setting carefully, looking at current and potential demands for infusion services. The present scope of services for infusion therapies must be reviewed, the current demand for services and how that demand is being met must be ascertained, and the future demand for services must be carefully estimated. It is important to remember that as the infusion therapy concept gains acceptance from medical and nursing staffs, the demand for services is likely to increase. This increase will affect the demand for existing services and will include requests for more sophisticated technological procedures. Quality management data related to infusion therapy are critical, providing valuable information for determining the essential functions needed to improve infusion care. While infusion teams deliver infusion therapy with a high level of expertise and have a positive impact on the quality of care, it can be difficult to quantify the impact this has on the organization. Quality assurance data for evaluating infusion care are not consistently kept in hospitals without infusion teams and often must be estimated from random checks of individual units or obtained from other facilities of comparable size. Consideration also needs to be given to the scope of pharmacy services currently in place and changes

Box 8-1 INFUSION NURSING TEAM SERVICES

While many possible services are listed, any combination of services may be provided:

- Venipuncture (as needed)
- Routine peripheral catheter site changes
- Initiation of blood components
- Assistance to physicians in central venous access device (CVAD) insertion
- Routine and as-needed CVAD dressing care
- CVAD blood withdrawals
- Daily peripheral site checks
- Implanted port access
- Declotting of CVADs and peripherally inserted central catheters (PICCs)
- Insertion and maintenance of PICCs
- Insertion and maintenance of specialty peripheral catheters
- Consultation and teaching for long-term CVADs
- Preparation of selected large-volume parenteral solutions and IV medications
- Administration of intraspinal medications
- Care of intraspinal catheters
- Therapeutic phlebotomies
- Participation as member of code team
- Chemotherapy administration
- Care and maintenance of arterial catheters; obtaining blood gases
- Administration of parenteral nutrition
- Evaluation of infusion therapy–related equipment
- Data collection of infusion-related statistics
- In coordination with the pharmacist, consultation on pharmacokinetics scheduling and compatibility issues
- Staff education through clinical validation and inservice training
- Patient teaching for catheter care and home or outpatient infusion therapies
- Provision of outpatient infusion therapies, patient monitoring, and education

anticipated with the addition of the infusion team. Once these have been determined, the desired team functions and service hours can be better defined.

The ideal infusion therapy department should be staffed to provide the total spectrum of infusion therapy services 24 hours a day, every day of the week. The infusion nurse performs all functions connected with the administration of IV solutions, medications, chemotherapeutic agents, blood and blood components, and parenteral nutrition. Specific responsibilities performed by infusion nursing teams are listed in Box 8-1. Benchmarking statistics to quantify infusion therapy department services, productivity, and patient outcomes are an important function of the infusion team staff. There are compelling data that specialized education lowers the risk of infection and complications associated with vascular catheters (Sheretz, 1999; Catney et al, 2001).

In addition to providing a full spectrum of infusion therapy services, the ideal team provides these services to all areas of the hospital. If this is not possible, a realistic alternative is for critical care, emergency department, and other high-volume areas of the facility to provide their own infusion-related care. However, it remains important for the infusion team to be as involved as possible with these areas to provide whatever support is necessary and feasible.

An infusion team's functions include some type of routine patient service rounds to designated areas of the institution. Rounds by the infusion team may be made routinely, at specific intervals, or a set number of times per shift or day, depending on such factors as the size of the facility, the workload type and volume, and staffing resources.

If the infusion team's staffing is limited, it may be necessary to designate some of the more routine technical aspects of initiating and maintaining infusion care to the staff nurse. The nursing staff must be educated regarding the functions of the infusion therapy department and be clear as to their own responsibilities regarding their patients' infusion therapy needs. Regardless of functions performed by the infusion team, every nurse is responsible for routine monitoring of a patient's IV site and infusions, and for ongoing patient assessment of the response to the therapies delivered. This monitoring, as described in the *Infusion Nursing Standards of Practice,* should be related to the patient's condition, age, and practice setting and should follow established infusion therapy policy and procedure. An infusion team's functions may include routine site checks performed on each shift or selected shifts, but the staff nurse must perform site checks in the interim, and initiate appropriate nursing interventions as necessary.

MANAGEMENT CONSIDERATIONS

The organizational structure and the roles of the various managers and staff members who constitute the infusion team vary depending on the size of the department and hospital, functions and services provided by the team, hours of service, and budgetary constraints. It is critical to ensure that an infusion team has precisely the right staff and is the right size to perform its services. Typically, infusion teams consist of a management or supervisory position, nursing staff, and an educational coordinator. However the team is organized, concise position descriptions for all members of the team are essential and should be reviewed annually and revised when necessary.

Staff qualifications

Entry-level requirements for the RN entering the infusion nursing specialty include current licensure and successful completion of an organized program of study on infusion therapy, including the opportunity to apply principles and practices of infusion therapy (INS, 2006). INS also recommends, but does not require, the bachelor of science degree in nursing. For nurses to be called an "Infusion Nurse Specialist," according to the *Infusion Nursing Standards of Practice* (2006), the nurse must be certified in infusion nursing. It is important for all infusion team members to obtain national certification in the specialty of infusion nursing through the Infusion Nurses Certification Corporation (INCC). Although most professional nursing certification programs are voluntary, certified team members validate the competency and advanced skill level of the staff; they are often used as a marketing tool by institutions. Certification enhances the professional credibility of the nurses and demonstrates their high level of commitment to their specialty practice. In a consumer-driven marketplace, credentialed professionals demonstrate an organization's dedication to professional development through continuing nursing education.

Because of the types of invasive procedures performed by infusion nurses, infusion teams are primarily staffed with registered nurses. Infusion-related procedures and activities require the level of theoretical and clinical knowledge and expert technical skill provided by RNs. The use of RNs on infusion teams has been an especially important component of the patient care delivery models implemented by many institutions in response to changes in the health care reimbursement structure. With much of direct patient bedside care often being delivered by unlicensed personnel, the extra support of an infusion RN can be very valuable to the generalist RN who now has to manage many more patients than in the past. The knowledge and expert skills of the infusion RN are needed more than ever to ensure quality of care in the delivery of infusion therapies.

Although the use of RNs may be optimal, to provide cost-effective services many infusion teams have also found it beneficial and necessary to use licensed vocational nurses (LVNs) or licensed practical nurses (LPNs). Consideration must be given to limitations in job functions of LVNs/LPNs when using them in the role of the infusion nurse. Infusion therapy–related practice guidelines for the LVN/LPN vary by state and may be further restricted by institutional policy. When an LVN/LPN is a member of the infusion team, all functions must, as defined in their licensure, be under the supervision of an RN. The supervising RN may be on the infusion team or on the patient care unit where the LVN/LPN is performing infusion care. LVNs/LPNs are limited in their role regarding infusion therapy and may not perform advanced technical procedures such as peripherally inserted central catheter (PICC) insertions. After completing education and training requirements and depending on the scope of practice as defined by the state's Nurse Practice Act, the LVN/LPN may be permitted to perform venipunctures, monitor solution administration and VAD sites, and administer certain solutions and blood products.

An infusion therapy team should be managed by a licensed RN. Five years of recent experience in an acute care hospital setting is preferred, with a minimum of 2 years of experience in nursing management. Experience preparing and managing budgets is desirable. Certification in infusion therapy (CRNI®) should be required, or a candidate should at least meet the eligibility criteria for certification in the specialty of infusion therapy. The individual must demonstrate good organizational and communication skills. To establish and maintain a successful infusion team, the manager must have a high degree of interest and experience in the delivery of infusion therapy. Maintaining skills and expertise in all aspects of the specialty is necessary for recognizing needs and implementing appropriate adjustments in services. The infusion manager is held accountable for his or her own practice and work performed under his or her supervision. The infusion nurse manager should be well respected in the organization and be capable of dealing effectively with all hospital departments. The title for this position (e.g., manager, director, supervisor) may vary, depending on the department to which the team reports and the responsibilities of the position.

The infusion therapy department manager's responsibilities are typically diverse and require good organizational and delegation skills. The manager's responsibilities may include writing and reviewing policies and procedures based on evidence-based practice recommendations and current standards, keeping abreast of the latest developments in technology, budgeting, and conducting performance evaluations. The infusion therapy nurse manager provides infusion therapy–related orientation and continuing education programs within and often outside the organization, keeps the staff motivated, and develops and maintains a quality management program. It is also crucial for the infusion manager to serve on committees within the hospital related to infusion therapy, such as pharmacy and therapeutics, infection prevention, product evaluation, nutritional support, safety, tumor board, and transfusion. Along with the clinical specialty rationales for membership on these committees, it is important that the infusion therapy team participate in product evaluation, selection, and standardization and conduct inservice training.

An infusion therapy department manager must carefully design and implement an effective quality management program to ensure that acceptable care parameters are met. The program should address the delivery of necessary and appropriate care, while minimizing complications and ensuring that all complications are investigated. The program should evaluate negative outcomes to determine whether they are attributable to such factors as nurse practice, procedural or systems' issues, equipment failure, or supply defects. The infusion team staff can provide the data from infusion therapy monitoring. The manager reports findings, assesses impact, and develops recommendations for corrective actions to improve outcomes.

An important and challenging responsibility for the infusion manager is ensuring technical and clinical expertise and maintaining staff morale in an arena in which most activities are carried out independently. It is crucial to hold regular staff meetings so that team members can openly share problems, raise questions, and identify educational needs. Staff meetings also provide an excellent opportunity for inservice training and review of procedures and equipment. Unit-based governing councils, which are part of a shared governance system, can also play an integral role in the success of the team and satisfaction of the staff. Through shared governance, nurses are empowered to make decisions that can impact their practice. The infusion therapy manager must be aware of the aspects of shared governance that enhance the philosophy and meet the objectives of the infusion team.

An important supplemental role to be considered for inclusion in the infusion therapy department is the educational coordinator. The educational coordinator's job description should include creating and maintaining an orientation program for new staff and providing continuing education and staff development programs and ongoing infusion-related inservice training. The educational coordinator should also act as liaison to the medical and nursing staff and encourage staff to attend outside educational meetings and be active in their specialty organizations.

Teams in large facilities may find it appropriate to incorporate within the team infusion nurses who are dedicated to specific subspecialty areas of the discipline. The role could be defined as that of clinical resource person. For example, a staff member may be dedicated to all aspects of managing central venous catheters, nutritional support, or transfusion therapy or may be the nurse who places PICCs or administers chemotherapy. If there is a large and diverse pediatric population, there may be an infusion team specialist for all aspects of pediatric infusion therapy. It is important to recognize the specialist as a valuable resource available throughout the organization for consultation.

Staffing

To provide cost-effective patient care and reduce the incidence of complications related to infusion therapy, ideally an infusion therapy team should provide full-service coverage 24 hours a day, every day of the week. The number of registered nurses on the team is determined by the number of hospital beds or patients served by the organization or agency, the type and volume of hands-on procedures performed, and the infusion therapies delivered. The ideal infusion team is organized so that it consists of the management, educational, and infusion nurse full-time equivalents (FTEs) needed to provide optimal service levels to all patients receiving infusion therapy.

In reality, FTEs available for the infusion therapy team are not always adequate to meet the ideal situation, and infusion therapy department resources vary depending on the organization. Most infusion teams probably do not have sufficient staffing resources to provide all specialty services and the related levels of care for their specialty. Having to work within such limitations, a choice must be made regarding how best to use the expertise of the team within the facility. A good approach is the implementation of team functions over time. Initial services should address the most pressing needs and should be based on a realistic workload to establish the team. Once the team is organized, is operating smoothly, and is successfully performing designated functions, additional services can be proposed as needs are recognized and resources become available.

When a full-service team cannot be justified, a limited-service team, although not ideal, may be able to provide quality team services for some aspects of infusion care. Budget considerations will define the limited-service hours. Limited-service teams can vary widely in the allocation of service hours. Typical options include covering day and evening hours, with no coverage during the night shift. Time studies related to workload volume help define the greatest hours of need. Some teams can flex their shift coverage into the late night and early morning hours, leaving only a 4- to 6-hour period without infusion team coverage. This is obviously preferred when there are no resources for a full-service team because it offers the least interruption of service. Other teams may offer services only during expanded day-shift hours (i.e., early morning to early evening). This provides some consistent, quality care by infusion nurses but leaves primary responsibility related to infusion care to staff nurses during the hours when there is no infusion team coverage. This may lead to inaccurate data collection and inconsistent quality of care. When a limited-service infusion team is in place, responsibility for infusion functions during off-service hours must be clearly defined and understood to minimize the interruption of therapy. It is important to the ongoing collection of clinical data and to the workload management of the infusion team that services performed by the general nursing staff are clearly communicated.

Initially, to secure the hours needed for core or basic staffing, many of the nurses and nursing hours can be transferred from the general nursing department and dedicated to infusion therapy services. This eliminates the need for massive recruiting and hiring. There is a period of orientation and inservice education required during the initial phase. Ongoing monitoring of staff and systems at this time is crucial to address any problems that might arise. To determine staffing requirements, time studies must be completed for each infusion function, keeping in mind that productivity and efficiency improve after implementation. A time study should collect data on the average number of infusion patients, the number of VADs per patient, infusion functions performed on each shift, and admixtures prepared for each nursing unit. With the average time for each activity determined from current literature or

for each facility, staffing needs can be estimated. Subsequently, the number of hours spent to perform infusion therapy can be determined, as can the number of FTEs. Using time study estimates and estimated volume data to define distribution of the workload, staffing levels for each shift can be determined. For greater accuracy, provisions for fatigue, delays, and travel time can be estimated when determining staffing levels. Orientation, vacation, holiday, and sick time relief can be estimated based on the benefits provided to team members and on historical data for even more accurate staffing estimates.

Infusion teams that are also responsible for outpatient therapy need to plan for additional staffing hours. Outpatient services may be provided in a dedicated room in the hospital setting or in an alternative setting. For smaller, hospital-based outpatient service operations, in-hospital infusion nurses may be able to cover staffing needs, especially for scheduled services. Ideally, an infusion nurse should be assigned exclusively to cover outpatient and home settings. To be cost-effective, all members of the infusion team, whether in the hospital or an outpatient setting, should be able to function when needed in either environment. Twenty-four-hour service departments can also use their evening and night shifts in a cost-effective manner to cover off-hour calls from outpatients. They can be a valuable resource for the home health staff in problem solving when they are managing the patient in the home setting, and for the staff of skilled nursing facilities. Coordinating with the home health agency to make the necessary interventions in the home when the patient cannot visit the infusion nurse is an acceptable option. The initial contact and assessment for infusion therapy-related issues should remain with the infusion nurse.

One problem encountered in staffing for the infusion team is meeting emergency needs. How to cover that last-minute sick call or the extended illness of an employee is a dilemma that needs careful consideration by the infusion team manager before it happens. It is more difficult for smaller teams that offer specialized services to maintain flexible staffing. For such teams, it is difficult to draw qualified staff from the general nursing population or even from outside agencies. Thought must be given to maintaining reliable on-call RN resources. One solution is to cross-train interested nurses from the critical care specialty or the emergency department, where venipuncture skills are most likely to be maintained. The workload distribution may need to be adjusted temporarily to integrate nonspecialist staff. For example, routine IV restarts should be assigned to the per diem staff and care of central line dressings to the infusion nurse. In areas where there are a number of infusion teams or home infusion organizations that might provide infusion nurses, those resources could be used and shared. This practice will give infusion nurses a wide experience base to meet the community's needs. The possibility for establishing community-wide adherence to standards in infusion care becomes more realistic with large numbers of specialists involved in the practice.

Of course, for organizations with 24-hour infusion team coverage, staffing problems are magnified. Without careful attention to maintaining resources, the cost in overtime and the decline in levels of quality or service could be detrimental to the objectives of the infusion team. Smaller teams should plan carefully for meeting staffing needs in many situations. Crisis staffing has a decidedly negative effect on the operations of the infusion team.

ADDITIONAL CONSIDERATIONS

Fiscal restraints and organizational redesign necessitate that hospitals consider both internal and external environmental factors. An analysis of internal factors should begin by identifying the institution's priorities and then demonstrating how the infusion team relates to those priorities. For example, if the facility has placed a high priority on improving the quality of infusion care because of current deficiencies, the justification should focus on the advantages brought to the institution by the specialized knowledge and skill of the infusion team. A complete internal analysis should also include the institution's financial status, political structure, and the attitudes and perceptions of physicians, floor nurses, and patients. The external analysis should examine the effect of regulatory and demographic changes, changes in third-party payer reimbursement, competitor activities, limited human resources (e.g., shortage of nurses in the community), changes in availability or cost of supplies, and new technology.

The justification for an infusion team centers on the benefits associated with delivering infusion therapy by a team of specially educated nurses. Benefits inherent in the use of infusion teams include standardization of equipment, improved productivity with better utilization of nursing resources, fewer patient complications, and improved risk management because an expert is monitoring care. To justify the importance of maintaining infusion teams or of creating infusion teams based on enhanced patient care and cost savings, infusion supervisors and managers should build their case on a foundation that addresses the environment, demand, costs, and benefits. Each area must be thoroughly researched and carefully analyzed, and the findings of this study must be skillfully presented to the organization's decision-makers. It is important to remember the reasons the team was established; those reasons should be assessed again when justifying the team's continued operation. Refer to Chapter 9 for additional information on validating and maintaining an infusion therapy team.

The future of infusion teams continues to depend on the issues of quality care and allocation of resources. Commitment to quality in any setting also requires careful analysis of how close adherence to standards of practice affects patient outcomes. For those committed to the philosophy of the infusion therapy specialty, the challenge remains to provide rationale and data-driven justification to support their services. It is the challenge of the infusion nurses to provide this expertise efficiently and cost-effectively within a carefully managed health care system.

ALTERNATIVE SITE: OUTPATIENT AND LONG-TERM CARE SETTINGS

The high cost of health care and decreasing reimbursement have made earlier discharge to alternative sites for infusion administration a necessity. In some cases hospitalization for uncomplicated conditions can be avoided by delivery of needed infusion therapy in an alternative site. It is now the norm for chemotherapy to be given in an alternative infusion setting, whether in an oncologist's office or a free-standing infusion clinic, or with an ambulatory infusion pump at home for those receiving continuous infusions. The durability and dependability of long-term central venous catheters and ambulatory

infusion pumps and a greater knowledge of the stability of chemotherapeutic agents have allowed tremendous freedom and flexibility for patients with cancer. Infusion centers with private examination rooms provide an ideal alternative setting for immunocompromised patients. They are safe places to be examined by the physician, visit with the pharmacist, and have dressing changes, pump refills, or assessments performed by the nurse. Like chemotherapy, the outpatient use of infusion antimicrobials has proven to be an efficacious, safe, and preferred delivery modality for infectious diseases. Common diagnoses associated with home and outpatient antimicrobial administration include skin and soft tissue infections, osteomyelitis, endocarditis, bacteremia, and wound infections (Tice et al, 2004).

Outpatient infusion therapy is successfully delivered in sites such as infusion departments or centers, physicians' offices, extended and long-term care facilities, and the home setting. Each setting has its own advantages and disadvantages. Because of the uniqueness of the home as the only non–institution-based setting, it is addressed separately in the final section of this chapter.

Patients treated outside the hospital, whether in an outpatient facility, long-term care facility, or at home, avoid problems inherent in the hospital system, including unfamiliar, sometimes frightening surroundings; isolation from friends and family; and lack of privacy. Avoiding or leaving the hospital setting also may facilitate the transition from the role of "sick patient" back to the familiar, functioning self, thus speeding adaptation and recovery (Tice et al, 2004). While patient safety is the primary consideration of clinicians administering infusion therapy in all practice settings, safety is magnified because of the intermittent nature of patient contacts and care in alternative settings.

HISTORY AND EVOLUTION OF OUTPATIENT INFUSION ADMINISTRATION

Since the first reporting of outpatient intravenous infusion therapy in the 1970s, outpatient antimicrobial therapy has grown into an industry affecting millions of Americans and generating billions of dollars annually. It has demonstrated that infusion therapies can be safely and effectively delivered in alternative settings while overall reducing health care expenditures. Bernard and colleagues (2001) showed an average cost savings of $4732 per week for treatment of osteomyelitis, while another study with varying infection diagnoses demonstrated average cost savings of $4130 per week (Dalavisio et al, 2000). Reasons for this rapid growth include the many benefits outpatient therapy provides to patients, new technologies that make it possible, and well-documented cost savings (Tice et al, 2004). Factors accounting for the shift in the delivery of infusion therapies to alternative settings are listed in Box 8-2.

In the early 1970s Rucker and Harrison (Tice et al, 2004) reported on outpatient IV medications used to manage children with cystic fibrosis. The first experience administering outpatient IV antibiotics to adults was by Antoniskis and colleagues (1978), who described 13 patients who self-administered parenteral antibiotics, primarily for osteomyelitis, resulting in positive outcomes, including safety and significant cost savings as compared to a hospital-treated control group. Subsequently, the literature supports the efficacy, safety, and cost-effectiveness of treating patients with parenteral antimicrobials on an outpatient basis. Practice guidelines for outpatient antimicrobial therapy were first published in 1977 and have been updated

Box 8-2 FACTORS CONTRIBUTING TO ALTERNATIVE SITE INFUSION THERAPY

- Fixed or declining reimbursement for inpatient care
- Decreasing length of hospital stay
- Emphasis on preventive care
- Patient choice
- Revenue potential
- Availability of long-term VADs and ambulatory infusion devices
- Scientific data supporting prolonged parenteral drug stability
- New antimicrobial agents and infusion drugs and biologicals
- Research supporting safe outpatient delivery of complex regimens

Box 8-3 EXAMPLES OF INFUSION THERAPIES ADMINISTERED IN OUTPATIENT AND HOME SETTINGS

- Antimicrobial, antifungal, and antiviral drugs
- Parenteral nutrition
- Antineoplastic therapy
- Analgesics for pain management: subcutaneous, intravenous, epidural, intrathecal
- IV hydration solutions
- Inotropic medications in end-stage heart failure (generally palliative care)
- Intravenous immunoglobulin therapy
- Biologic drugs
- Factor replacement in hemophilia
- IV diuretics
- IV methylprednisone
- Tocolytic therapy in pregnancy
- Antiemetic therapy in pregnancy/adjunctive to antineoplastic therapy

by the Infectious Diseases Society of America (Tice et al, 2004). Infusion therapies administered in alternative site settings are listed in Box 8-3.

ALTERNATIVE SITES

The infusion center

An infusion center may be developed in a variety of medical settings, including a physician's office, hospital clinic, urgent care center, emergency department, or as a free-standing infusion clinic. Infusion centers have a medical staff on site and ready availability of medications, supplies, and equipment needed to respond to venous access problems or emergencies. The nurse, physician, pharmacist, social worker, dietitian, and administrative staff work together to provide an effective and efficient communication system for designing treatment programs and following the outcomes of therapy.

Infusion centers allow for coordination of resources and efficient delivery of services. Several patients can receive infusions and be monitored at the same time, saving money by efficient use of professional staff. With staffing, equipment, and physician involvement similar to those of the hospital, the infusion center is a practical way to initiate extended outpatient

care. Because of this similarity, some patients may perceive the transition from the hospital to the infusion center as less traumatic and perhaps better supervised than transitioning directly to home care and self-administration. Specialized infusion services provided in the infusion center include venous access device care; antimicrobial, antifungal, and antiviral infusions; continuous or intermittent chemotherapy administration; various intramuscular and subcutaneous injections; infusions of IV immunoglobulin, hydration solutions, and analgesics; and parenteral nutrition administration.

One limiting factor of the infusion center model is the difficulty of treating patients who require infusion therapy and/or other nursing interventions more than once a day. For these patients, a combination of self-administration in the home and visits to the infusion clinic may be helpful. Patients may also be taught to self-infuse by the infusion center nurses. Self-administration is considered a model of outpatient antimicrobial therapy (OPAT) (Tice et al, 2004; Tice, 2006) and is differentiated from the home care model as addressed later in the chapter. In a retrospective analysis of more than 2000 outpatient antimicrobial episodes over a 13-year period, self-administration was compared to health care provider administered infusion therapy and was found to be safe with no excess complications or hospitalizations in the self-care group (Matthews, 2007). It is important that patients are carefully selected for this model of self-administration.

Teaching patients and their families to provide long-term infusion therapy has allowed the population of chronically ill patients to return to work or school and function as normally as their disease will allow. Children needing infusion therapy may benefit from self-administration when a parent or responsible person is taught to administer the therapy. Parents can be remarkably adept when properly educated in the sterile procedures of IV administration but are sometimes overlooked as caregivers.

Self-administration also offers considerable financial savings, particularly for prolonged courses of treatment, afforded by significant reductions in personnel and overhead costs associated with outpatient center visits. However, consistent support is necessary for patients and caregivers who administer medication to ensure adherence to the prescribed treatment plan and to monitor patient response. Intermittent patient visits to the infusion center are necessary for ongoing assessment of the venous access device, drug and supply distribution, and clinical assessment. A major liability concern and common criticism of the self-administration model is the perceived lack of medical supervision. Patient failure to adhere to the medication schedule or administration methods may result in medications given too quickly, too slowly, or not given at all, potentially increasing the risk for fluid overload, electrolyte imbalance, arrhythmias, harmful drug interactions, or continued infection. Delayed or immediate allergic or anaphylactic reactions may occur in any setting, but they are harder to manage when they are associated with self-administration. To reduce the risk for self-administration problems, patients and caregivers must be carefully selected, well-educated in infusion administration, and monitored for adherence by intermittent phone communications. Home health care should be considered for patients at risk. A major advantage of home health care is that it allows the nurse to evaluate the home situation. The nurse can assess physical limitations, environmental hazards, domestic issues, and any drug or alcohol abuse that would affect patient compliance. Problems in these areas are difficult to observe apart from a home visit.

Clinic designs and space considerations

Acquiring the right kind of space for a free-standing infusion center allows flexibility in designing and building a work area that will provide adequate work space and facilitate good communication for all of the members of the outpatient infusion team. An infusion center should provide a reception area, private examination and counseling rooms, a pharmacy, administrative space, treatment areas for central venous catheter insertion and sterile procedures, and isolation rooms. All rooms should be equipped with closable doors.

Experience has demonstrated that having a "group" infusion room can be therapeutic and provide an atmosphere for patients to visit and share their personal experiences. This area should be comfortable for patients who may spend 2 to 3 hours per day receiving infusions. Games, TV, DVDs, and magazines are helpful in providing the infusion patient enjoyable distractions. It is advisable to provide comfortable reclining chairs. State departments of health and the Occupational Safety and Health Administration (OSHA) provide information regarding acceptable upholstery fabrics, floor surfaces that can be easily cleaned and disinfected, and rules regarding eating and drinking in an infusion room. Natural light is important for accurate assessment of skin color. Ventilation and temperature control will add comfort and enhance a pleasing environment.

The pharmacy area should include an office for the pharmacists and pharmacy technicians, an anteroom where pharmacy personnel change into scrub clothing to prepare for mixing solutions, and a compounding or "hood room" that meets USP 797 guidelines. The compounding room should be sealed off from traffic areas and vented, either to the outside or to the filtered duct system of the building. Each state's board of pharmacy provides certification specifications and regulatory requirements. The manufacturers of laminar flow hoods are helpful in providing installation information for these products. The Joint Commission has guidelines to help develop policies and procedures for the pharmacy. State law dictates the legalities of physician involvement in dispensing medication through an office. In some states, the pharmacy cannot be owned and operated by a physician. A physician will often purchase compounding services from a free-standing pharmacy near the physician's office.

Communication and staff reporting are optimal if all members of the infusion team work in proximity. The nursing area, where nurses assemble IV solutions and administration sets and stock IV equipment and supplies for initiating venipunctures, should be near the infusion area. Nurses should locate their work area within observation range of the patient; this will enhance productivity by allowing the nurse to document the treatment while it is happening. Supplies, phones, computers, nursing assessment equipment, and emergency equipment, such as oxygen tanks, masks, nasal cannulae, emergency medications, an Ambu bag, and resuscitation supplies, should be readily accessible.

If the infusion nurses are performing phlebotomies for laboratory studies, the state department of health provides guidelines for an acceptable blood drawing area and proper specimen handling. Often, the infusion nurse analyzes blood samples in the laboratory of the infusion clinic, thus eliminating the waiting period for the sample to be taken to an outside reference laboratory and analyzed.

Nurse productivity is enhanced when easy access to the pharmacist, physician, dietitian, secretarial staff, and equipment and supplies is provided. Regular discussion about the patient's treatment, response to treatment, order changes, dietary needs, and laboratory findings can improve treatment outcomes.

Secretarial, billing and personnel offices should be positioned to enhance communication and reporting. Computer access, electronic billing and reimbursement capabilities, patient records, and a storage area for supplies and equipment should be located centrally to enable all staff access and availability. The size of the infusion clinic should be based on the number of patient visits anticipated daily.

Long-term care facilities

Long-term care facilities such as nursing homes or rehabilitation institutions provide another potential setting for outpatient infusion therapy. The long-term care facility can provide many benefits to clinicians as they strive to maintain the quality of care outside of the acute care setting. In these institutions, physicians are able to manage patient care through more aggressive supervision. Physician supervision occurs in three different ways. The prescribing physician can admit the patient to a facility for infusion and serve as the patient's attending physician throughout the patient's stay. All the duties and privileges of an attending physician, including the history and physical examination, daily progress documentation, and discharge summary, are inherent in this model. Many long-term acute care hospitals require that a patient be seen daily by the attending physician, similar to an acute care hospital, regardless of the patient's needs. In the second model of physician supervision, the prescribing physician acts as a consultant to the attending physician. The follow-up and documentation requirements are fewer and there is less clinical management. In the final model, physicians may act as administrative consultants for the long-term care facility to provide medical and technical assistance to patients, physicians, and staff.

Long-term care facilities are particularly appropriate venues for delivering infusion therapy to patients with functional or cognitive limitations or to patients insured by third-party payers who do not allow payment for home or office infusion therapy. They provide a safe environment for patients who require a substantial amount of monitoring, or those with substance abuse problems who are not sick enough to require hospitalization yet are not safely managed in the outpatient or home setting (Tice et al, 2004).

Commonly, an outpatient infusion pharmacy will provide the infusion medications, supplies, and equipment to the long-term care facility by contract. Experienced infusion nurses often provide "back-up call" to the facilities because nurses working in long-term care often lack sufficient infusion experience and expertise.

The limited availability of laboratory and radiology services in some long-term care facilities may contribute to the difficulty in managing a course of treatment with infusion therapies. It may be necessary to transport a patient to an acute care or outpatient setting for a chest radiograph to verify the location of a central venous catheter tip or for other diagnostic studies.

CHOOSING THE APPROPRIATE DELIVERY MODEL

The choice of delivery model depends on the individual patient, the provider's expertise, community resources, and geographic limitations. Third-party payers may also have preferred infusion models selected for their insured participants. Physicians experienced in managing outpatient therapies may prefer a

TABLE 8-1 Advantages and Disadvantages of Alternative Care Settings for Infusion Therapy

Setting	Advantages	Disadvantages
Infusion clinic; hospital-based infusion center	• Team of health care professionals together in one facility • Physician oversight readily available • Safe for first-dose administration and monitoring • Medications readily available for changes in treatment	• Patient must travel to facility • May not be available in rural communities • Overhead costs • Cost for storage of supplies and equipment • Costs associated with space
Hospital emergency department	• Team of health care professionals together in one facility • Physician oversight readily available • Safe for first-dose administration and monitoring • Medications readily available for changes in treatment • Available in rural communities	• Patient must travel to facility • Unpredictable census and staffing • Risk for lengthy wait for medication administration and medication changes
Home care	• Patient and family convenience • Home delivery of medications and supplies by home infusion pharmacy • Allows patient to return to normal activities, school, and work • Ability to assess home environment • Ability to treat terminal or homebound patients • Ability to teach patients self-administration • Decreased risk for health care–associated infections	• Commuting costs • Intrusion on privacy • Decreased physician oversight • Risk for nonadherence • Home laboratory services may be unavailable in areas, requiring patient to go to outpatient setting for laboratory studies • First doses of infusion medications require special considerations and availability of emergency medications in the home • Patient and family must participate in care and must report changes in condition between home visits for timely management of potential complications
Long-term care facility	• Safer environment for patients with history of substance abuse • Safer environment for patients with functional and/or cognitive limitations	• Increased risk of health care–associated infections • Lack of experienced infusion nurses • Decreased physician oversight

certain delivery model. If a patient is unstable or is having difficulty with the infusions or venous access, the physician may prefer a model that provides direct monitoring and continuity of care among personnel caring for the patient.

Given the cost constraints of managed care, models that allow multiple patients to receive infusions simultaneously may be the most cost-effective. They require the least nursing time when the entire infusion team is in the same building. Choice of an appropriate alternative setting depends on the specialized training and expertise of the programs' personnel and the resources available to them. Regardless of the model chosen, a continued and ongoing team effort among the health care professionals is crucial to the effectiveness and outcomes of treatment. Advantages and disadvantages of the various models are summarized in Table 8-1.

PATIENT SELECTION

The patient is the central member of the outpatient infusion team and must participate in his or her own care. Perhaps the most important role for the patient is reporting significant changes in vital signs and symptoms, including rash, nausea, vomiting, diarrhea, phlebitis, erythema, or purulence at the site of the access device insertion. Educating patients to be reliable team members involves encouraging them to communicate often with the nurse, physician, and sometimes the pharmacist.

The criteria for patient selection and monitoring of patients who receive outpatient infusion therapies have been gradually established by various professional groups. In terms of venous

access devices, peripheral catheters may be appropriate for short-term infusion therapies. The PICC is frequently the VAD of choice; long-term catheters such as tunneled catheters or implanted ports present another option, especially when frequent blood draws are necessary, or in very active patients, or in infants and children (Tice et al, 2004; Chary, Tice, and Martinelli, 2006). In the Infectious Diseases Society of America (IDSA) guidelines (Tice et al, 2004), considerations for outpatient antimicrobial infusion administration include the following:
- There is a documented need for outpatient antimicrobial therapy.
- The patient's medical resource needs are available at the proposed outpatient site.
- Safety of the home or other outpatient site for supporting needed care is addressed.
- Patient and/or caregiver willing to participate in care.
- Mechanisms are in place for rapid and reliable communications for patient monitoring.
- Patient and/or caregiver understand the risks, benefits, and economic considerations.

The patient's mental and physical abilities, self-confidence, anxiety, and fears should all be assessed during discharge planning. Limitations on ambulation, prolonged sitting, and access to transportation may weigh heavily against outpatient treatment. Yet, home care may not be appropriate for patients who live alone and are not able to adequately self-monitor their infusion related care.

The risk of IV narcotic or other drug abuse must always be considered in patient selection. Although drug abusers could potentially use a reliable IV line for other than prescribed IV medications, prolonged hospitalization may be difficult to justify and may not necessarily prevent the problem. Patients who are likely to use their VADs are generally poor candidates for outpatient infusion administration and the long-term care facility may be the best site for care; alternatively, daily infusions with removal of the catheter may be an option (Tice et al, 2004).

Home circumstances must be evaluated carefully. Family support is particularly important if self-administration or family administration of the infusion is planned. The presence of a family member who can be educated to recognize potential difficulties and evaluate the patient's condition is valuable for the patient and physician. The distance from a patient's residence to the nearest medical facility must also be considered. The patient should have adequate venous access if a peripheral IV catheter is to be used or there will be placement of (or plans for placement of) an appropriate central venous access device.

A patient being evaluated for admission into a self-administration program should be evaluated against the following criteria before being admitted:

- Mental or psychosocial evaluation (the patient should be alert and oriented to person, place, time, and environment)
- Demonstration of adequate memory, problem-solving skills, and abilities to manage
- Ability to demonstrate required tasks to comply with therapy
- Willingness and ability to accept responsibilities and risks involved in home infusion
- Demonstration of the manual dexterity and acuity of sight and hearing required to manage tasks and equipment and to seek help in the event of emergency

If the patient does not meet the admission criteria in terms of mental and physical capabilities, a primary caregiver must be identified who will be available to support home infusion. The home environment may be assessed via conversation with the patient in the clinic or hospital, or over the phone (Box 8-4).

COORDINATION OF CARE

The professional team

Although the three primary team members, physician, nurse, and pharmacist, have distinct roles, they also have overlapping functions. As in constructing a workable design for the facility, it is imperative that the personnel be qualified, work as a cohesive unit, and have advanced knowledge in infusion skills.

Box 8-4   ASSESSING THE HOME ENVIRONMENT

- Is there an adequate area to prepare and administer IV infusions and perform dressing changes?
- Is there adequate refrigeration and storage space for medications and supplies?
- Are electrical outlets available and intact, especially if required for equipment?
- Can equipment, infectious waste, and medications be safely stored out of the reach of children or pets?
- Is there telephone access—landline or cellular?
- Are there home/neighborhood issues affecting the safety of the staff who are making home visits and home delivery of medications/supplies?

Physician

Physician involvement in care in an alternative setting is crucial in a number of areas. First, physicians must be instrumental in the development of and promotion of adherence to clinical practice guidelines. As treatment protocols for various disease processes are developed based on the latest research, physicians must have input into such factors as patient selection criteria, appropriate safety measures for alternative site care delivery, and measurements for assessing the progress of treatment. Policy and procedure manuals should include the input of a physician.

As managed care drives costs downward, the physician must help make decisions regarding resource utilization and ensure that low resource levels remain appropriate and adequate for safety and efficacy. Physicians make an important contribution to risk management in managed care organizations. In a system with some degree of vertical integration, physicians can provide leadership in identifying, developing, and coordinating multidisciplinary disease-management programs.

Nurse

Although some aspects of the nurse's role remain the same in any setting, responsibilities vary from one alternative setting to the next. Advanced knowledge and infusion skills are essential for any nurse employed by an infusion service. The nurse must demonstrate an understanding and expertise with central venous catheters, insertion procedures, routine maintenance and standards of care associated with each device, peripheral IV starts, site selection, site management, and provision of medications and supplies. The nurse maintains the most regular contact with the patient and thus is pivotal in coordinating care and alerting the physician to problems. In all settings, the nurse provides a critical role by being involved in patient selection, education, vascular access, and central venous catheter maintenance; helping patients deal with their illness and the prescribed plan of treatment; maximizing patient's self-care potential; evaluating patient progress; and monitoring and reporting of the patient's adaptation and response to therapy. The infusion nurse can be the catalyst between the patient and the other members of the health care team. The roles and responsibilities of the RN in an outpatient setting vary somewhat depending on the model.

Assessment and planning include making initial decisions with the patient and the physician regarding appropriateness of the intended setting, method of venous access, how and when the antimicrobial or solution will be administered, and determination of the patient's other needs. The nurse continually monitors the success of the treatment plan by evaluating the patient's compliance, clinical response, and reported satisfaction. The nurse may be responsible for selecting, initiating, and maintaining the venous access device and for monitoring its status between doses, if necessary.

Administration of medications or solutions may be performed by the nurse, or the nurse may teach the patient or caregiver to infuse the drug and manage the infusion device between nurse visits. The nurse will often collect laboratory samples, evaluate clinical data reflecting the patient's response, and relay all information to the physician. Nurses share in the responsibility for distributing information to the other health care providers involved in the patient's care. Nurses in all settings provide patients with information regarding possible side effects and adverse reactions associated with the medication. Nurse availability should be provided 24 hours per day.

Pharmacist

The pharmacist plays an important and often varied role in providing medications within the alternative care setting and is the most knowledgeable about medication storage, preparation, dosing, and delivery.

Decisions and activities in which pharmacists should participate include the following:

- Researching and evaluating the direct or comparative efficacy, safety, and cost-effectiveness of specific drug delivery systems and administration devices
- Reviewing the patient's history of drug reactions and current medications; choosing and dispensing the particular drug and dosage delivery system or administration device/supplies
- Educating patients regarding side effects, drug interactions, pharmacokinetics, stability, appropriate dosage, and costs of medications
- Monitoring ongoing clinical information and laboratory data

Up-to-date policies and procedures for compounding sterile products should be written and available to all pharmacists. All pharmacy-prepared sterile products should bear an appropriate expiration date. The expiration date assigned should be based on currently available drug stability information and sterility considerations. Sterile products should be labeled with at least the following information: patient's name and other appropriate patient information; solution name; volume, strengths, and concentrations of all ingredients; expiration date and time; prescribed administration regimen; appropriate auxiliary labeling; storage requirements; name of the person performing the admixture and/or the responsible pharmacist; device-specific instructions; and any additional information in accordance with state or federal requirements.

The pharmacist must inspect the container for leaks and integrity, and the solution for cloudiness, particulates, color, and volume; this inspection should be performed when the preparation is completed and again when the product is dispensed. The pharmacist should be knowledgeable of pharmacokinetics and pharmacodynamics. Knowledge of the pharmacokinetics of antimicrobials and the pharmacodynamics predictive of antimicrobial efficacy enables the pharmacist to design reasonable outpatient IV regimens for most agents. Once-daily antimicrobial drug administration is advantageous and simplifies the regimen for alternative site infusion therapy (Tice et al, 2004). Understanding the characteristics of aminoglycosides, vancomycin, and the long half-life β-lactams, which allow once-daily dosing intervals, enables the pharmacist to help the physician develop a treatment plan to achieve positive treatment outcomes. Documentation of the pharmacy's activities should be maintained on file and be sufficient to comply with state and federal laws and regulations and the organization's policies and procedures. State and federal law also establish how long records must be kept.

ALTERNATIVE SITE: HOME CARE

During the 1980s the specialty practice of home infusion therapy emerged as patients were increasingly transitioned from the hospital to the home setting. Early categories of home infusion therapy primarily included antimicrobial drugs and parenteral nutrition. Today, infusion therapy includes not only intravenous drugs and fluids but also therapies delivered via the subcutaneous and intraspinal routes. Although antimicrobial drugs and parenteral nutrition remain two of the most commonly administered home therapies, antineoplastic drugs, opioid analgesics, cardiac medications such as inotropic drugs and diuretics, immune globulin, and other biologic drugs are also administered in the home. Essential to the success of home infusion therapy are careful planning to ensure safety of infusion administration and patient education. The high degree of patient and family involvement in their own care is what makes the specialty of home infusion therapy unique. A broad overview of home infusion therapy is presented in this section. It describes its evolution and history, reviews basic concepts related to the field, and describes the home care process and the roles and responsibilities of the service providers involved.

HISTORY AND EVOLUTION OF HOME HEALTH CARE AND HOME INFUSION THERAPY

While community-based care has been practiced for centuries, home health care was formalized by Florence Nightingale, William Rathbone, and their colleagues in England during the 1800s, while the late 1800s saw the beginning of Visiting Nurse Associations in the United States (American Nurses Association [ANA], 2008). Significant growth in the home care industry occurred when Medicare legislation enacted in 1965 introduced a home health benefit. In the 1980s the practice of home health care and home infusion therapy grew even more, becoming a well-accepted alternative to hospital-based infusion therapy. The main impetus for the rapid development of home programs at that time came in response to changes in hospital reimbursement based on diagnosis-related groups (DRGs). The DRG system changed reimbursement from a retrospective case-per-day payment system to a fixed-fee prospective payment system based on the diagnoses. Patients began to be discharged earlier and sicker, requiring assistance with care posthospitalization.

The term "high-tech" home care emerged (Haddad, 1987; Gorski, 1998), which included delivery of infusion therapies as well as respiratory support and monitoring systems, care of medically fragile children, and complex case management of patients with multiple complex needs such as those with AIDS or post–bone marrow transplant. Placement of access devices in the home, including peripherally inserted central catheters (PICCs), by highly skilled home health nurses contributed to the growth of home infusion therapy. Today, PICCs are not placed in the home as often because of the logistical difficulties in verifying tip placement as well as the difficulty implementing the latest technology in vein identification (e.g., bedside ultrasound). One must acknowledge, however, those "pioneer" home health nurses who placed these catheters in the 1980s and early 1990s contributed to the advancement of home infusion therapy. The first two IV therapies to be self-administered in the home were total parenteral nutrition (TPN) and antibiotics. Poretz (1991) studied 150 patients in the Cleveland Clinic Home Antibiotic Program; results showed that adverse reactions were mild and infrequent, and demonstrated better than a 90% treatment success rate.

The first standards of practice for home health care were published by the American Nurses Association in 1986, followed by revisions in 1992, 1999, and 2008 (ANA, 2008). While the current *Infusion Nursing Standards of Practice* addresses infusion nursing in all settings, a separate document addressing specific standards for home care was first published in 1984 (National Intravenous Therapy Association, 1984) as rapid growth in home infusion therapy was occurring.

In 1982 the Visiting Nurse Associations of America (VNAA) and the National Association of Home Care (NAHC) were formed, and continue to provide strong, national leadership for the overall home health care industry. Later, the National Home Infusion Association (NHIA) was formed and currently serves as a trade association to represent and advance the interests of organizations and individuals who provide infusion and specialized pharmacy products and services to the entire spectrum of home-based patients. The Infusion Nurses Society continues to be the nursing voice for infusion therapy across all settings.

Medical advances including new infusion therapies and drugs and also technological advances in equipment (such as long-term venous access devices and compact, ambulatory pumps with complex infusion-programming capability) contribute to the continued growth and possibilities for home infusion therapy. Research continues to document overall patient satisfaction with home infusion therapy, positive clinical outcomes, and a low rate of complications as presented in the subsequent sections of this chapter.

HOME CARE ADVANTAGES

Patients and families experience psychosocial, emotional, financial, and health benefits while receiving care in the home setting. Patients are more comfortable in the privacy and familiarity of their own homes than in the hospital. In addition, patients maintain a higher degree of control over their therapy and their lives with home care. Often, patients return to work or other activities and still maintain their infusion therapy regimen.

An important patient benefit is reduced risk for acquiring health care–associated infections. Overall, the rate of complications, including catheter–related bloodstream infections (CRBSIs), among patients receiving home infusion therapy appears to be low. Studies documenting the relatively low rate or risk of infection for patients receiving home infusion therapy are cited in the Focus on Evidence box in Chapter 12. However, there is need for more research in identifying home care–related risk factors, including replication of existing studies, and identifying the best interventions to reduce such risk. As the rate of CRBSIs in hospitals is plummeting because of implementation of the central line bundle (Institute for Healthcare Improvement) and improved adherence to infection control measures, home health care must also analyze infection risk factors and develop a "zero-tolerance" attitude toward home care–associated infections (McGoldrick, 2008).

While not widely studied, clinical outcomes are generally comparable to those seen in other settings with a tendency towards patients preferring the home as the treatment setting (see the Focus on Evidence: Home Infusion Advantages). The stress experienced by family members and caregivers when their loved ones are hospitalized is most often lessened when patients are treated at home. Home care requires family participation, allowing significant others to be active in the care of the patient to the degree they and the patient feel most comfortable. Additional assistance with care may be obtained based on the severity and acuteness of the illness. Additional home health services include home health aides for assistance with

activities of daily living; professional therapy services including physical, occupational, and speech and language; and social services. Some organizations provide respiratory and dietitian services. Reimbursement for such services varies based on the patient's sources of health insurance (see Chapter 9).

FOCUS ON EVIDENCE

Home Infusion Advantages

- In a randomized controlled trial, patients with relapses of multiple sclerosis were assigned to a 3-day regimen of IV methylprednisolone either at home (n = 51) or in an outpatient clinic (n = 54). Using a researcher-developed tool (MS Relapse Management Scale), coordination of care was significantly better in the home treatment group (p = .024). Other dimensions measured by the tool (access to care, information, interpersonal care) did not differ between the two groups. Cost of care was either approximately the same or less in the home setting (Chataway, Porter, Riazi et al, 2006).
- In a survey of adults requiring enzyme replacement therapy for Fabry's or Gaucher's disease, the majority of patients preferred home over hospital visits for infusion administration, reporting increased comfort, less stress, and less impact on family life (Milligan, Hughes, Goodwin et al, 2006).
- In a small study comparing outcomes between home and hospital treatment with IV antibiotics for patients with cystic fibrosis, the patients treated at home achieved greater improvements in quality of life measurements although forced vital capacity measurements improved more in the hospital group (Esmond, Butler, and McCormack, 2006).
- In a retrospective study comparing adults age 60 and older to younger adults who received home IV antimicrobial therapy, clinical outcomes were similar in both groups with the exception of a significant increase in nephrotoxicity occurring more often in the older patient group (p = .02) (Cox, Malani, Wiseman et al, 2007).
- In a 2-year study, patients were successfully treated with enzyme replacement therapy at home for mucopolysaccharidosis type I. Of 17 patients, 13 patients transferred to home after hospital infusions; 6 months of hospital infusions were required before doing infusions at home. Over 1000 home infusions were performed without serious complications (Cox-Brinkman, Timmermans, Wijburg et al, 2007).

Home care is less expensive than hospital therapy. While there are regional variations in health care costs, the cost of infusion therapy administered in the home care setting is much less than the cost of inpatient treatment (National Home Infusion Association, 2008). In a randomized trial comparing home to hospital-based IV antibiotic therapy, the cost of home care was approximately one half of inpatient care (Wolter, Cagney, and McCormack, 2004). Home infusion therapy has allowed an increasing number of patients to be treated without ever being admitted to the hospital, avoiding the significant costs associated with hospitalization. Other financial benefits are also experienced by the family. Because the patient is treated in the home setting with clinicians going to the patient, family members are no longer burdened with making special arrangements to transport their loved one for treatments and evaluations. Home infusion allows the family to spend time in their own home and eliminates the need for special arrangements for child care and other responsibilities often made difficult during periods of hospitalization. The home environment and activities return to as near normal as possible.

PLANNING FOR HOME CARE

Discharge planning and preparation for home care addresses factors such as the patient's ability to participate in care, the stability of the patient's clinical condition, caregiver availability, use of an appropriate infusion access device, and home environmental issues (Gorski, 2005a). Most often, infusion therapy is continued after hospitalization, or transitioned after outpatient services. Infusion therapy may also be initiated in the home without prior hospitalization or outpatient care. Diagnoses commonly associated with home infusion therapy include infections, cancer, cancer-related and chronic pain syndromes, gastrointestinal diseases affecting normal functioning of the gastrointestinal system, heart failure, and immune disorders. Infusion therapies that are administered in home care are listed in Box 8-3.

Patient participation in care

It is critical that patient motivation, ability, and willingness to participate in care are assessed as part of the planning process. Patients must be informed of their expected level of participation in care. Most often, particularly with infusion of antimicrobials and parenteral nutrition, it is expected that the patient or caregiver will learn how to independently administer the infusions. If the patient is not able to fully or partially participate in care, the potential for family members or other caregivers to assist with care must be addressed. For patients in managed health care plans, insurance case managers often authorize a limited number of home visits (see Chapter 9 for more details). It is absolutely essential that patients are informed of home care expectations and reimbursement issues. Even if the home health nurse is expected to administer all infusions, which is often the case with infusion of biologicals or some chemotherapy drugs, patients must assume responsibility for living safely with the infusion access device, and in some cases for living day to day with an IV solution and/or medication constantly infusing via an infusion pump. Patients must be able to appropriately respond to alarms, potential complications such as signs of infection, or adverse reactions to the infusion. Patients and families are often anxious or fearful about going home with a catheter in place or about the home infusion drugs. The nature of the infusion and associated diagnosis or impact of the illness (e.g., cancer, inability to eat) may evoke additional anxiety as well as coping issues (Gorski, 2005a). During the planning process, the discharging organization, usually the hospital, should communicate significant concerns and fears to the home care agency, thus preparing the home health nurse to be aware of, acknowledge, and address patient concerns.

Clinical condition and stability

Before transitioning the patient to the home setting, the patient should be clinically stable. Vital signs should be within normal limits for the patient, and the patient should demonstrate tolerance of the intended home infusion therapy without evidence of adverse reactions or unmanageable side effects.

Laboratory results, pertinent to the patient's intended infusion therapy and diagnoses, are made available to the home health provider, such as renal function tests, electrolyte levels, and blood counts.

First dosing at home

The OPAT practice guidelines from the IDSA (Tice et al, 2004) recommend that first doses of antimicrobial drugs be given in a monitored setting with access to emergency drugs. The reality is that risk of anaphylaxis is very low, and that first doses are given by many home care organizations. In a study of more than 700 home care patients receiving more than 1000 courses of IV antibiotics, there were no episodes of anaphylaxis (Dobson, Boyle, and Loewenthal, 2004). In this study, first doses were administered under direct supervision, patients had ready access to a telephone and transport, and if the patient had a history of a drug reaction, that drug was not given. The researchers did report that 90% of the antibiotics were given by continuous infusion versus a bolus or intermittent infusion, which may have influenced the low rate of reactions. Based upon a literature review focused on first and second doses of IV antibiotic administration, Trowbridge and Kralik (2006) concluded that it is safe to administer first doses in a community setting when protocols are in place. To reduce risks associated with first-dose administration, the following criteria should be in place (Gorski, 2005b; Trowbridge and Kralik, 2006):

- The home infusion pharmacy/nursing agency should have clear policies in place for first-dose administration.
- The patient should have no history of severe drug reactions and minimal medication allergies.
- All nursing staff should be knowledgeable about potential drug reactions and certified in basic life support.
- Orders for and presence of emergency medications (e.g., epinephrine and diphenhydramine) for use in the event of an anaphylactic reaction should be available in the home.
- The home care nurse should remain with the patient for the entire duration of the first-dose administration.
- Environmental factors should include telephone access (landline or mobile).

Continuation of therapy from other setting to home care

In most cases the patient's home infusion therapy will be started at home with the next dose or infusion at the scheduled time. Adjustments should be made for an appropriate home schedule. For example, the patient receiving an IV antibiotic every 12 hours may have been receiving the medication at 5 AM and 5 PM in the hospital but may need to be adjusted to a more realistic home schedule of 8 AM and 8 PM.

In some cases, infusions cannot be interrupted as the patient transitions from the hospital to home care, such as with continuous analgesic infusions, inotropic drug infusions, or continuous parenteral nutrition. The results of such interruptions might result in worsening pain, cardiac decompensation, or hypoglycemia, respectively. In these types of cases, the home infusion pharmacy delivers the infusion solutions, needed supplies, and infusion pump to the hospital for the home care nurse to convert the patient to the home infusion before leaving the hospital.

Venous access

Selecting the most appropriate venous access device (VAD), in relation to both the type of infusion therapy to be administered and the patient's needs, is another essential step in planning for home infusion therapy. While most often the patient is referred for home infusion therapy with a VAD already in place, the home health nurse must ensure that the device is appropriate for the intended therapy. In some cases, the nurse will educate patients in selecting the best VAD for their condition and infusion therapy needs.

A variety of factors guide the process. PICCs are the most common type of catheter used in home care (Moureau et al, 2002; Gorski and Czaplewski, 2004). Peripheral catheters are used less often because courses of home infusion therapy are often long in duration or characteristics of the medication or fluid require central venous access. However, peripheral IV catheters, including midline catheters, are associated with a very low risk of catheter-related bloodstream infection (Maki, Kluger, and Crnich, 2006). Peripheral IV catheters are an appropriate, cost-effective choice for infusion therapies expected to last 7 to 10 days or when therapy is being administered infrequently (for example, weekly or monthly drug infusions such as methylprednisone or alpha$_1$-proteinase inhibitor [e.g., Prolastin]). Long-term VADs such as tunneled catheters or implanted ports are also common in home care, most often with patients who require long-term or even life-long infusion therapies such as parenteral nutrition and chemotherapy.

Home environment/Safety issues

The home setting should be reasonably safe and clean for storage of medications and supplies and for infusion administration. Electricity, telephone access, and refrigeration are also critical issues. Most often, the home infusion pharmacy delivers medications and infusion-related supplies on a weekly basis. The medications must be stored in a clean area of the refrigerator and supplies must be kept in a clean area safe from children and pets. If an infusion pump is required, electricity may be needed to recharge the battery, although many pumps can run on disposable batteries. Home environment issues are summarized in Box 8-4. Safety issues in relation to home care providers must also be considered during home care planning, such as unsafe neighborhoods or substance abuse. However, once the patient is admitted, unforeseen safety issues may arise and will need to be addressed. Staff safety is addressed in the last section of this chapter.

INFUSION ADMINISTRATION

The simplest administration method is selected for IV antibiotics to promote ease of patient teaching and cost-effective care. Elastomeric pumps, IV push, and simple gravity infusion are common methods for IV antimicrobial drug administration. While elastomeric ("balloon") pumps are more expensive, cost savings are realized when fewer home visits are required to teach patients. Ambulatory programmable pumps are used for medications or solutions that need to be accurately controlled (e.g., parenteral nutrition, analgesics), when patient compliance is a concern, or if the frequency of the dose would lend itself to the use of such a device. In some situations, such as with IV antibiotics, the infusion device is connected only intermittently.

The access device is flushed after administration. In other situations, such as continuous medication infusion or high-frequency dosing of antibiotics, the infusion pump is connected continuously. For pump infusion of antibiotics, the medication infuses at preprogrammed intervals, and during the "off" cycle the infusion device maintains positive pressure and administers a minute amount of solution to keep the infusion access device patent. Some pumps are also capable of delivering multiple antibiotics according to independently timed schedules.

Some home infusion programs are successfully administering selected antibiotics, such as certain cephalosporins, IV push (Miano and Wood, 1998; Poole and Nowobilski-Vasilios, 1999). Cost efficiency and simplicity of administration combined with no increase in phlebitis rates between traditional administration methodologies and the IV push method have led to more frequent use of IV push. However, patients should be carefully selected to ensure safety with IV push administration.

PATIENT EDUCATION

Effective patient education is absolutely critical to the success of home care. Unlike outpatient or acute care settings where the nurse most often administers and directly monitors the infusion drugs, in the home setting patients and/or caregivers are expected to participate, to learn how to administer their antimicrobial medications, and to self-monitor for adverse reactions and response to the infusion therapy. Factors that impact the degree to which technical procedures are taught may include the patient's cognitive ability and willingness to learn, the complexity of the technique, the number of available home visits, the patient's distance from the organization, and the standard of practice. While patients or their caregivers are commonly expected to administer solutions and medications, change administration sets, and give injections, they are not routinely expected to place peripheral IV catheters or draw blood.

The patient's readiness to learn and any potential factors affecting readiness must be assessed. The patient's physical condition, such as weakness, fatigue, or anxiety over being at home with an IV catheter and medications, will impact ability to learn. Functional limitations may also be a concern, such as the patient's manual dexterity or poor memory. Family or other caregivers are often willing to learn if the patient exhibits limitations or is just not ready. As mentioned earlier, whenever possible, the timing of the medication dose(s) should be scheduled to best meet the patient's needs and work and sleep schedule. It must be recognized that depending on the source of reimbursement, the number of home visits authorized by the insurance company for teaching the patient may be limited. Each home visit must be used efficiently to teach, and when patients or caregivers exhibit difficulty in learning, the teaching-learning process must be evaluated and questions must be asked (Gorski, 2005b). For example, has there been consistency in teaching (especially a concern when multiple nurses see the patient)? What types of issues are affecting the patient—anxiety, functional or cognitive limitations, lack of motivation? Will additional teaching home visits help? If so, the home health nurse will need to advocate for this with the insurance case manager, as appropriate. Could procedures be simplified? Would an outpatient setting be a better setting?

When planning for patient teaching, utilization of standardized teaching handouts and a skills checklist will decrease teaching time and the number of home visits (Grimes-Holsinger,

Box 8-5 TEACHING TOPICS FOR THE HOME INFUSION THERAPY PATIENT

- Medications and supplies
  - Regular delivery day
  - Taking inventory
  - Safe storage of supplies and sharps container
  - Clean area in refrigerator for medication/solution storage
- Infection prevention
  - Handwashing before and after each IV-related procedure
  - Aseptic technique
    1. Disinfect injection cap/valve with alcohol wipe before *each* access; use friction
    2. Maintain sterility of the syringe tips and end of tubing
- Catheter care procedures
  - Site care procedure (Will nurse or patient perform procedure?)
  - Injection cap/valve changes
  - Catheter clamping
  - Flushing
    1. Preparing flush syringes
    2. Technique
    3. How often
  - Activity limitations (if imposed)
  - Safe dressing and bathing
- Infusion administration procedures
  - Medication label (correct name, medication, expiration date)
  - SASH technique: saline-administer-saline-heparin (SASH) or saline-administer-saline (SAS)
  - Administration set changes
  - Infusion administration method
    1. Gravity drip
    2. IV push
    3. Elastomeric pump
    4. Infusion pump
       a. Changing infusion container
       b. Resetting program parameters
       c. Setting pump alarms
       d. Scheduling battery changes
- Signs of potential complications and how/when/what to report
  - Venous access device related
  - Infusion therapy related

Data from Gorski LA: *Pocket guide to home infusion therapy,* Sudbury, Mass, 2005b, Jones and Bartlett.

2002). A checklist of teaching topics is found in Box 8-5. Goals for self-care should be clearly established with the patient and family. The goals may include self-administration of a twice-daily dose of IV cefepime to be administered by the patient, with weekly site care and changing of the PICC securement device and dressing to be done by the nurse. Teaching strategies should be based on how the patient best learns. Home care agencies and pharmacies will provide a folder of written teaching materials; however, some patients do not read well or prefer to learn by observing. Some additional teaching strategies are summarized in the following list (Gorski, 2005b):

- Pay attention to the teaching environment; a location with an easily cleanable surface and good lighting, such as a kitchen table, is ideal.
- Organize all needed supplies for each infusion.
- Foster an unhurried and relaxed atmosphere to reduce anxiety.
- Teach procedures in small portions and in a way that maximizes learning during each home visit. Example: focus on flushing procedures first; during the first home visit, the nurse can demonstrate the first 0.9% sodium chloride flush and administer the medication; following the medication, the nurse can attach the second 0.9% sodium chloride flush and have the patient administer the 0.9% sodium chloride; then the patient can independently complete the heparin flush; a significant amount of hands-on teaching has occurred during the first visit, giving the patient a sense of accomplishment and reducing anxiety for the next home visit.
- Be alert to patient expressions of fear, frustration, and/or anxiety to learning the procedure.

COORDINATION OF CARE

Along with the patient, the infusion nurse, pharmacist, and physician are the primary health care professionals involved in home infusion therapy. However, other members of the team may also include a case manager and other home health professionals (e.g., physical therapist, social worker, dietitian). Communication among the health care team is essential to a well-coordinated home infusion program (Oselan and Querciagrossa, 2003). For example, detailed communication among nurse, pharmacist, and patient is essential before starting care to establish supply needs based on the venous access device. The pharmacy will need to know not only the prescribed infusion but also the type of IV catheter and number of catheter lumens, type of dressing, catheter securement device, antiseptic dressings (if indicated), and flushing solution and frequency. In general, pharmacies deliver supplies to the patient once a week, perhaps less or more often based on the stability of the IV solutions or drugs. To maintain cost of care, supply needs must be carefully assessed up front and on an ongoing basis to avoid extra deliveries and delays in therapy. Most aspects of patient care such as changes in orders, reporting laboratory values, and patient assessments are communicated through telephone or facsimile. As electronic health records evolve, communication of health care information also occurs with the interfacing of computer systems between organizations.

Infusion nurse

The infusion nurse's responsibilities include performing the initial patient assessment, reviewing body systems, reviewing medical history, conducting the psychosocial assessment, evaluating available support systems, and assessing functional limitations, environment, and cognitive and technical skills. Based on the assessment, nursing diagnoses and expected outcomes of care are identified and the care plan is developed and implemented. Ongoing responsibilities include patient teaching, monitoring, and evaluation; assessment of adherence to the medication regimen; performance of technical procedures of infusion therapy; psychosocial support; and 24-hour emergency availability. The nurse communicates with the patient, pharmacist, and/or physician to address ongoing supply needs, adherence to the medication regimen, limitations related to self-care and options for simplifying the procedure (e.g., elastomeric pumps), and home environmental issues such as cleanliness or safety impacting care. Communication is essential to facilitate timely response to changes in patient status, deliver care efficiently, decrease costs, and maintain patient satisfaction.

Pharmacist

In some geographic locations, the pharmacist and the infusion nurse visit the patient when necessary for evaluation and assessment. Whether the pharmacist provides home care depends on the philosophy of the organization and the demands of the marketplace. The pharmacist's responsibilities include reviewing medical records for current and past medical, nutritional, and medication history; reviewing laboratory data; obtaining physician orders; and conducting interviews with patients. The pharmacist also prepares, dispenses, and delivers medications, solutions, supplies, and equipment; plans patient care; monitors therapeutic response; analyzes laboratory data; and is available 24 hours a day for emergencies. A therapeutic evaluation is made based on patient assessment (when possible), the physical examination and history, and information conveyed by nursing staff, patients, family members, caregivers, and other members of the health care team. Pharmacists are experts in medication therapy and can receive additional certification in home infusion therapy from the National Home Infusion Association (NHIA).

Physician

The primary care physician and other specialists involved in the care of the patient are responsible for establishing a diagnosis, assessing therapeutic response, monitoring laboratory data, and maintaining communication with team members. In addition, the physician is responsible for approving and ordering changes in the infusion regimen and updating the patient's treatment plan.

Patient

The patient and the family are active participants in home infusion therapy. The patient is involved in every aspect of the care and must learn about his or her condition requiring infusion therapy, the plan for treatment, expected outcomes of care, potential complications, and how to communicate with the health care team members.

STAFF SAFETY

While home infusion therapy is an excellent, cost-effective option for many patients, the issue of staff safety must also be addressed. Nurses and pharmacy staff, whether the pharmacist or delivery staff, may find themselves in unsafe neighborhoods. In a home care agency survey (Sylvester and Reisener, 2002), safety issues identified most often by staff included isolated locations, illegal drugs, threatening animals, gangs, vandalism, inadequate lighting, and verbal abuse. Based on the survey, a form was developed that patients are required to sign; in essence, the form states patients must assist in reducing potential safety threats (e.g., isolate threatening animal) or services may be terminated. Agency admission criteria also were revised to address safety of the home to provide safe care. Safety protocols must be established, security or escort services must be in place, and an annual plan for reviewing the home safety plan are recommendations from Anderson (2008) based upon a

Box 8-6 SECURITY SUGGESTIONS FOR HOME VISITS

- Survey the area before getting out of the car.
- Plan visit carefully using directions or global positioning systems (GPS) to improve navigation and avoid getting lost in neighborhoods.
- Do not leave visible belongings in the car (e.g., computers, purses); rather, lock them in the trunk.
- Schedule visits in the morning when going to high-risk areas.
- Ask for and use a security escort as needed.
- Dress appropriately, comfortably, and professionally.
- Walk purposefully and be attentive to surroundings.
- If home situation appears unsafe during the visit, leave immediately.
- Preprogram emergency numbers into cellular phone.
- Consider alternative site care settings such as an outpatient infusion center when safety issues cannot be adequately addressed.

Data from Sylvester BJ, Reisener L: Scared to go to work: a home care performance improvement initiative, *J Nurs Care Qual* 17(1):71-82, 2002; Anderson NR: Safe in the city, *Home Healthcare Nurse* 26(9):534-540, 2008.

literature review. Yearly training covering violence prevention, risk factors, early warning signs, methods to diffuse situations, and alarm systems are just a few things recommended by OSHA (2004). Safety suggestions are summarized in Box 8-6.

SUMMARY

Infusion therapy is administered across all health care settings. When patients are stable in the acute care setting yet still require ongoing infusion therapy, the most appropriate alternative setting should be selected. Increasingly, infusion therapies are safely initiated in a non–acute care setting without prior hospitalization. The patient's specific infusion therapy needs along with functional and cognitive status, availability of caregiver or family support, home environment, and patient and physician preference are important factors influencing the optimal alternative setting, whether it be the home, an outpatient clinic, or a long-term care setting. Most infusion therapies can be safely administered in one of the alternative sites. Regardless of the setting, the role of the specialty infusion nurse is essential in ensuring the best possible outcome for the patient.

REFERENCES

American Nurses Association: *Home health nursing scope and standards of practice*, Washington, DC, 2008, Author. Accessed at Nursebooks.org.

Anderson NR: Safe in the city, *Home Healthcare Nurse* 26(9):534-540, 2008.

Antoniskis A, Anderson BC, Van Volkinburg EJ et al: Feasibility of outpatient self-administration of parenteral antibiotics, *West J Med* 128(3):203-206, 1978.

Bernard L, El H, Pron B et al: Outpatient parenteral antimicrobial therapy (OPAT) for the treatment of osteomyelitis: evaluation of efficacy, tolerance and cost, *J Clin Pharm Ther* 26(6):445-451, 2001.

Bosma LT, Jewesson P: A infusion program resource nurse consult service: our experience in a major Canadian teaching hospital, *J Infus Nurs* 25(5):310, 2002.

Brunelle D: Impact of a dedicated infusion therapy team on the reduction of catheter-related nosocomial infections, *J Infus Nurs* 26(6):362, 2003.

Catney MR, Hillis S, Wakefield B et al: Relationship between peripheral intravenous catheter dwell time and the development of phlebitis and infiltration. *J Infus Nurs* 24(5):332-341, 2001.

Chary A, Tice AD, Martinelli LP: Experience of infectious diseases consultants with outpatient antimicrobial therapy: results of an emerging infections network survey, *Clin Infect Dis* 43:1290-1295, 2006.

Chataway J, Porter B, Riazi A et al: Home versus outpatient administration of intravenous steroids for multiple sclerosis relapses: a randomized controlled trial, *Lancet Neurol* 5(7):565-571, 2006.

Cox AM, Malani PN, Wiseman SW et al: Home intravenous antimicrobial infusion therapy: a viable option in older adults, *J Am Geriatr Soc* 55(5):645-650, 2007.

Cox-Brinkman J, Timmermans RG, Wijburg FA et al: Home treatment with enzyme replacement therapy for mucopolysaccharidosis type I is feasible and safe, *J Inherit Metab Dis* 30(6):984, 2007.

Dalovisio JR, Juneau J, Baumgarten K et al: Financial impact of a home intravenous antibiotic program on a Medicare managed care program, *Clin Infect Dis* 30(4):639-642, 2000.

Dobson PM, Boyle M, Loewenthal M: Home intravenous antibiotic therapy and allergic drug reactions: is there a case for routine supply of anaphylaxis kits? *J Infus Nurs* 27(6):425-430, 2004.

Esmond G, Butler M, McCormack AM: Comparison of hospital and home intravenous antibiotic therapy in adults with cystic fibrosis, *J Clin Nurs* 15:52-60, 2006.

Gorski L: Hospital to home care: discharge planning for the patient requiring home infusion therapy, *Top Adv Pract Nurs eJournal* 5(3), 2005a. Accessed 1/7/07 from http://www.medscape.com/viewarticle/507906.

Gorski LA: *High-tech home care manual*, Gaithersbury, Md, 1998, Aspen Publishers.

Gorski LA: *Pocket guide to home infusion therapy*, Sudbury, Mass, 2005b, Jones and Bartlett.

Gorski LA, Czaplewski LM: Peripherally inserted central & midline catheters for the home care nurse, *Home Healthcare Nurse* 22:758-771, 2004.

Grimes-Holsinger V: Comparing the effect of a skills checklist on teaching 'ime required to achieve independence in administration of infusion medication, *J Infus Nurs* 25(2):109-120, 2002.

Haddad AM: *High tech home care: a practical guide*, Gaithersburg, Md, 1987, Aspen.

Infusion Nurses Society: Infusion nursing standards of practice, *J Infus Nurs* 29(1 suppl):S1-92, 2006.

Infusion Nurses Society: The use of nursing assistive personnel in the provision of infusion therapy [position paper], *J Infus Nurs* 32(1):21-22, 2009.

Institute for Healthcare Improvement: *Implement the central line bundle*. Accessed 9/28/08 from http://www.ihi.org/IHI/Topics/CriticalCare/IntensiveCare/Changes/ImplementtheCentralLineBundle.htm.

Maki DG, Kluger DM, Crnich CJ: The risk of bloodstream infection in adults with different intravascular devices: a systematic review of 200 published prospective studies, *Mayo Clin Proc* 81(9):1159-1171, 2006.

Matthews PC, Conlon CP, Berendt AR et al: Outpatient parenteral antimicrobial therapy (OPAT): is it safe for selected patients to self-administer at home? A retrospective analysis of a large cohort over 13 years, *J Antimicrob Chemother* 60(2):356-362, 2007.

McGoldrick M: Infection prevention and control: achieving a culture of zero tolerance, *Home Healthcare Nurse* 26(1):67-68, 2008.

Meier PA, Fredrickson M, Catney M et al: Impact of a dedicated intravenous therapy team on nosocomial bloodstream infection rates, *Am J Infect Control* 26(4):388-392, 1998.

Miano B, Wood W: Implementation of the IV push method of antibiotic administration using the FOCUS/PDCA approach, *Home Healthcare Nurse* 16(12):831-837, 1998.

Miller JM, Goetz AM, Squier C et al: Reduction in nosocomial intravenous device-related bacteremias after institution of an intravenous therapy team, *J Infus Nurs* 19(2):103, 1996.

Milligan A, Hughes D, Goodwin S et al: Intravenous enzyme replacement therapy: better in home or hospital? *Br J Nurs* 15(6):330-333, 2006.

Moureau N, Poole S, Murdock MA et al: Central venous catheters in home infusion care: outcomes analysis in 50,470 patients, *J Interv Radiol* 13:1009-1016, 2002.

National Home Infusion Association: Infusion FAQs. 2008. Accessed 2/24/08 from http://www.nhianet.org/faqs.htm.

National Intravenous Therapy Association: Home I.V. therapy, *NITA X* 7(2):93, 1984.

Occupational Safety and Health Administration (OSHA): *Guidelines for preventing workplace violence for healthcare and social service workers*, 2004. Retrieved 10/26/08 from www.osha.gov/Publications/OSHA3148/osha3148.html.

O'Grady NP, Alexander M, Dellinger EP et al: Guidelines for the prevention of intravascular catheter-related infections, *MMWR Recomm Rep* 51(RR-10):1-29, 2002.

Oselan SA, Querciagrossa AJ: Collaboration of nursing and pharmacy in home infusion therapy,, *Home Healthcare Nurse* 21:818-824, 2003.

Poole SM, Nowobilski-Vasilios A: Intravenous push medications in the home, *J Infus Nurs* 22:(4)209, 1999.

Poretz DM: High tech comes home, *Am J Med* 91:453, 1991.

Sheretz R: Look before you leap: discontinuation of an infusion therapy team, *Infect Control Hosp Epidemiol* 20:99, 1999.

Soifer NE, Borzak S, Edlin BR et al: Prevention of peripheral venous catheter complications with an intravenous therapy team: a randomized controlled trial, *Arch Intern Med* 158:473, 1998.

Sylvester BJ, Reisener L: Scared to go to work: a home care performance improvement initiative, *J Nurs Care Qual* 17(1):71-82, 2002.

Tice A, Rehm S, Dalovisio J et al: Practice guidelines for outpatient parenteral antimicrobial therapy, *Clin Infect Dis* 38(12):1651-1672, 2004.

Tice AD: *Handbook of outpatient parenteral antimicrobial therapy: for infectious diseases*, Tarrytown, NY, 2006, CRG.

Trowbridge K, Kralik D: Evidence for intravenous antibiotic therapy in the community, *Austral Nurs J* 13(9):28-31, 2006.

Wolter JM, Cagney RA, McCormick JG: A randomized trial of home vs. hospital intravenous antibiotic therapy in adults with infectious diseases, *J Infect* 48:263-268, 2004.

9 FINANCIAL CONSIDERATIONS

Ann Corrigan, MS, RN, CRNI®, Lisa Gorski, MS, HHCNS-BC, CRNI®, FAAN, Judy Hankins, BSN, CRNI®, and Roxanne Perucca, MS, CRNI®*

Creating and maintaining a viable health care system requires the meshing of clinical and financial services. Health care facilities are constantly faced with escalating costs while revenue is decreasing. The higher costs are a result of increased salaries, new facilities or facility renovation, new products and technology, and education and services that address higher patient acuity. Many years ago, charges would be increased for services rendered. This is no longer a viable answer as often there is a maximum allowable reimbursement returned to the health care facility. Health care professionals often make patient care decisions that increase the cost of day-to-day care while administrators try to set financial limits in which the clinicians must operate. Therefore it is important for clinical, administrative, and financial staff to work together to provide quality services within or less than the budgeted dollars.

This chapter will provide general information related to the value of services required by third-party purchasers, reimbursement and revenue concepts, and budgeting functions. Information will also be provided about infusion team justification, including cost factors, implementation methods, and ongoing analyses of services. Specific regulations and guidelines change rapidly and will not be included in this chapter. Therefore it is important to continually seek information from financial resources within your health care facility, from regulatory organizations, and from third-party payers to ensure that relevant and accurate data are used to support financial decisions.

THIRD-PARTY PURCHASERS OF VALUE

The need for specialized clinicians is recognized as important to patient safety and quality of care. One of the specialty areas that has become an ever-increasing component of health care is infusion therapy. Infusion nurses have demonstrated "infusion care can be accomplished with more efficiency, fewer complications, and at lower costs" (INS, 2005).

Patients expect to receive quality infusion care. Clinicians strive to provide care based on national standards of practice and guidelines. Third-party payers (e.g., Centers for Medicare & Medicaid Services [CMS] and insurance companies) also expect their customers to receive quality care at a reasonable cost. Standards and guidelines are established, as well as individual contracts, to help meet this expectation. The health care industry receives payment for the services provided in a manner that is different from other industries. The reasons for the differences of the revenue function within health care include the following:

- A vast majority of payment comes from a source other than the individual receiving the services (e.g., third-party payers).
- The level of payment for identical services may vary based on the third-party payer.
- Actual payment schedules may be based on preestablished or negotiated rules of payment often related to codes entered in the patient's bill.
- The government, one of the largest payers, defines their reimbursement rules for given services (Castro and Layman, 2006).

CENTERS FOR MEDICARE & MEDICAID SERVICES (CMS)

The Centers for Medicare & Medicaid Services (CMS), a federal agency, was established in 1977 to administer the Medicare program and the federal portion of the Medicaid program. Its purpose is to ensure quality health care for beneficiaries receiving services through these federally funded health insurance programs. Any health care provider must meet the established standards to receive reimbursement for Medicare and Medicaid customers. Hospitals not reporting quality data receive a reduced percentage in their annual payments.

CMS has established quality measures that will provide a greater awareness of the quality of care provided by a facility. These data will allow patients to make more informed decisions related to their health care. CMS is continually looking at standards and guidelines developed by other quality groups and organizations, such as the National Quality Forum, to update their program for quality improvement.

*The author and editors wish to acknowledge the contributions made by Crystal Miller in the second edition of *Infusion Therapy in Clinical Practice.*

Patients receiving health care services under the Medicare/Medicaid umbrella have the opportunity to provide feedback and concerns to the agency. All concerns are followed up by CMS personnel, and the validity of the concern is determined. If a complaint is valid, the health care facility must provide documentation related to how standards will be met in the future. Failure to comply with established standards in the established time frame could result in elimination of reimbursement for care rendered to CMS beneficiaries, leading to a large financial impact to the health care facility.

INSURANCE COMPANIES

Health insurance was developed to help offset services for individuals requiring health care. In 1847 the first "sickness" clause was added to an insurance document. Health insurance became fully established in 1929 when an insurance company covered school teachers in Texas. After World War II, the health insurance industry became a widespread means of reimbursement for health care services (Castro and Layman, 2006).

The majority of health insurance plans are directly related to employment. These plans may require partial payment for the cost of the plan as well as partial reimbursement for services received. Insurance companies may establish individual contracts with a given health care facility. These contracts may require the health care facility to meet certain quality measures to receive payment.

HEALTH CARE REIMBURSEMENT METHODOLOGIES

The two major types of unit of payment include fee-for-service reimbursement and episode-of-care reimbursement.

Fee-for-service reimbursement

In fee-for-service reimbursement, providers of health care services receive payment for each service received. The provider submits a claim to the third-party payer listing the charges for each service rendered. This form of reimbursement allows the patient to make decisions about health care services, including who will provide them as well as where the services will be provided. Often this method requires a higher deductible or co-payment.

Included in this methodology may be individuals who use a self-pay plan for each service received. Often this type of payment results from the lack of health insurance or benefits under governmental health programs. With the self-pay plan, the patient assumes responsibility for the cost of his or her health care.

Fee-for-service may include the retrospective payment method where providers are reimbursed for each service rendered. It may also include managed care reimbursement where the third-party payer manages the costs of health care.

Episode-of-care reimbursement

The episode-of-care form of reimbursement is a method where health care providers receive a lump sum for all services related to a condition or disease. The following are examples of forms of this type of reimbursement:
- *Capitation*—fixed payment set for a specific period of time
- *Global payment*—one combined payment for services of multiple providers treating a single episode of care

- *Prospective payment*—payment rates for services are established in advance for a specific time period (Castro and Layman, 2006)

Episode-of-care reimbursement rewards effective and efficient delivery of health care services while penalizing ineffective and inefficient services. The case-based payment rates are based on averages of costs for all patients within the group (Casto and Layman, 2006). Facilities providing effective care make money, and lose money for ineffective services and outcomes. The bottom line is health care delivered in an efficient, effective manner reaps greater operating margins.

The concern for case-based payment relates to the potential for use of less expensive diagnostic and therapeutic procedures. At times, there may also be refusal to pay for certain procedures or treatments.

In the quest to provide quality care in a cost-effective manner, researchers and third-party payers, including governmental health agencies, continue to review and update payment methods nationally and internationally. Therefore as mentioned earlier, it is important for health care professionals to review and update health care services as well as stay abreast of the financial changes.

 REIMBURSEMENT AND REVENUE

Reimbursement and revenue generation brings an added value to an inpatient infusion team. In today's competitive health care environment, it is essential for an infusion therapy department to establish a budget that has a revenue and expense cost center. Because of the complexity of health care billing, the infusion nurse must work in partnership with billing compliance personnel to establish appropriate billing codes and charges for the services provided and supplies used. Billing rules and regulations are frequently changing and organizations are being more proactive in reviewing their charging processes. The billing process is also under heavy scrutiny by consumers, government agencies, and insurers. Price transparency is encouraged by many consumer groups and is being mandated in some states.

HOSPITAL REIMBURSEMENT

Currently, reimbursement is based on a system that reflects the work performed and the resources consumed in the delivery of the service. Resources include the supplies used and the time required to perform the procedure. Each procedure is identified by a code that is listed in a schedule that is identified by various payers. In the schedule, each procedure is assigned a charge, commonly called "relative value units (RVUs)," for the time worked, supply expense, and a mark-up percentage that incorporates overhead costs including liability and operational costs such as utilities. Table 9-1 lists infusion therapy procedures and the average nursing time to perform the procedure.

It is important for any new procedure or service to undergo the code development process. Billing compliance personnel will also conduct a valuation of the expenses involved by determining the geographic difference in labor, supply, and liability costs. Each of these elements is adjusted by a "geographic practice cost index" for each Medicare locality (Thorwarth, 2004).

The next step after a charge or relative value has been determined for a procedure is to assign a CPT (current procedure terminology) code. The CPT coding system contains more than 8000 codes and is the building block for medical care reimbursement and record-keeping (Thorwarth, 2004). Each procedure performed is assigned a CPT code or a series of HCPCS (healthcare common procedural coding system) codes within the CPT. The CPT code is used to file reimbursement claims, as well as to track procedures for research, utilization review, and other purposes. A variety of reimbursement codes are available for different payers of patients in various health care settings.

TABLE 9-1 Infusion Therapy Procedures and Average Nursing Time to Perform Procedure

Infusion procedures/ Services	Time (standard time/ minutes)
Peripheral insertion*	15
Midline insertion	32.5
PICC insertion with ultrasound	90
Fibrolytic treatment	22
Central dressing change	15
Peripheral dressing change*	5
Access implantable port	17.5
Repair tunneled catheter	20
Lab blood draws	12
Site assessment*	4.5
D/C peripheral catheter*	4.5
D/C central catheter*	10
Patient phone calls*	3
Inservice/teaching time*	
Student shadow hours*	
RN validation hours*	

* No charge for performing.

Uniform bill, or UB-92, codes are used by hospitals for inpatient and outpatient billing to major third-party payers.

Medicare uses diagnostic-related groups (DRGs) to reimburse inpatient stays. The DRG reimbursement system was instituted so that health care organizations would receive a fixed payment based on diagnosis and not on the facility's charges. The prospective payment system (PPS) produces a list of prices that Medicare pays for services delivered for each DRG. With the advent of changes in Medicare payment, the health care facility is reimbursed at a prospectively determined rate for treating a specific case, irrespective of the charges accumulated during the patient's stay. This places the burden of reducing health care costs on facilities and requires them to be more efficient in their delivery of care (Niedzwiecki, 2006). With the advent of the PPS, hospitals have implemented other measures to generate revenue, such as inserting peripherally inserted central catheters (PICCs) not only in the inpatient setting but also in an outpatient ambulatory clinic or an alternative care setting.

Revenue codes are used by payers to categorize the items used and charges incurred during a patient's stay with a health care provider. All items on a patient's bill must be assigned a revenue code for payers to process the bill. All health care charges must be accurate and follow standard guidelines. To facilitate this, health care organizations set up charges on a chargemaster. The chargemaster is a large computer file that contains all patient charges. Table 9-2 is an example of a chargemaster account for infusion therapy charges.

Because of the frequent changes in rules and regulations, procedure codes and charges are frequently reviewed by billing compliance personnel. It is important for the infusion nurse to perform an annual review with billing compliance personnel to evaluate current procedures and charges. In the annual review process, consideration should be given to adding any new infusion procedures that are being performed as well as adjusting supply costs for any changes in contractual agreements. It is important for the infusion nurse to stay informed and knowledgeable regarding the constantly changing rules and regulations that govern reimbursement.

TABLE 9-2 Sample Chargemaster

Procedure	UB-92	CPT 5	FY09 New price	Medicare fee payment	Medicare APC payment	Peer mkt avg price	MSA mkt avg price
Blood draw	300	36415	$28.00			$22.27	$20.25
PICC insertion single lumen	361	36569	$1,194.00		$666.42	$1,768	$1,525.3
PICC insertion dual lumen	361	36569	$1,283.00		$666.42	$1,768	$1,525.3
PICC insertion triple lumen	361	36569	$1,315.00		$666.42	$1,768	$1,525.3
PICC insertion power	361	36569	$1,074.00		$666.42	$1,768	$1,525.3
PICC replace single lumen	361	36584	$1,040.00		$666.42	$2,072	$1,414.9
PICC replace dual lumen	361	36584	$1,191.00		$666.42	$2,072	$1,414.9
Declotting access/catheter	361	36593	$532.00		$151.64	$1,198	$623.79
US-guided needle placement	402	76937	$573.00			$988.8	$720.62
Midline catheter kit	270		$800.00				
Noncoring needle	270		$88.00				
Transparent dressing	270		$48.00				
Micro extension set	270		$24.00				
Hickman repair kit single lumen	270		$743.00				
Hickman repair kit dual lumen	270		$989.00				
Catheter securement device	270		$50.00				

HOME CARE REIMBURSEMENT

Reimbursement for home infusion therapy is complex because of the different models of home infusion delivery as well as the varying sources of, and gaps in, insurance reimbursement. Depending on patient needs, geographic differences in the model of care, availability of resources, and reimbursement requirements, there may be differences in how home infusion services are provided. The following are two examples of home infusion services:

1. A full-service home infusion pharmacy provides all needed services including both drugs and supplies delivered to the patient's home as well as nursing services.
2. A home infusion pharmacy provides pharmaceutical needs but refers or works with a home care agency to provide nursing and other needed home care services (e.g., physical therapy).

While a detailed presentation of the intricacies of home care reimbursement is beyond the scope of this chapter, an overview of key concepts is provided.

Most private health insurance plans consider home infusion therapy as a medical service, and reimburse clinical services (e.g., nursing visits), medications, and needed supplies under the medical benefit rather than the prescription drug benefit. Payments are generally separate for the drugs and nursing visits. Many, if not most, health insurance plans require preauthorization for home care and/or co-payments; therefore patients must be informed of any charges they may incur. If home infusion services are not covered by insurance, the patient may choose to pay for the home infusion therapy, receive the therapy in the hospital or physician's office, or obtain funding through charitable organizations.

Organizations are often required to make one home visit to assess the patient's needs in the home environment and then establish a plan of treatment that includes the type and frequency of service necessary to return the patient to his or her optimal level of functioning. This information is then communicated to the insurance case manager, who authorizes a finite number of visits that must occur within a specified amount of time. For example, three daily visits are authorized to teach the patient home IV antibiotic therapy. After the third visit, if goals are not met, the agency must obtain additional authorization to continue services.

In making the decision to authorize additional visits and ongoing services, the case manager is dependent upon the nurse's assessment of patient progress and clinical documentation. The home health nurse must clearly communicate any barriers limiting the patient from achieving goals and hindering return to independence. For example, the home health nurse might find that the patient is very anxious about learning to perform his IV infusion, slowing down progress. The home health nurse asks for two more visits, anticipating that these visits will provide the opportunity for this patient to learn to safely perform his infusion independently. The home health care nurse becomes the "eyes and ears" of the insurance company, and many patient-related decisions involve collaboration with the case manager. Any unauthorized visits may not be reimbursed; therefore the home health organization must meticulously track both visits and authorizations to assure reimbursement for services rendered to the patient.

Government health plans such as Medicaid, TRICARE, and the Federal Employees Health Benefits Program reimburse for home infusion therapy (NHIA, 2008). Because Medicaid coverage is administered by the state, there are differences in the extent of coverage and there are often gaps. Coverage under Medicare is complex and limited. Medicare's fee-for-service program (Parts A, B, and D) is the only major health plan in the country that has not recognized the clear benefits of adequately covering provision of infusion therapies in a patient's home. Because most Medicare beneficiaries are enrolled in the fee-for-service program, when seniors and the disabled find they may need infusion therapy they often find it unaffordable to receive this care in the comfort of their homes (NHIA, 2008).

When home nursing visits are needed for beneficiaries receiving infusion therapy, there may be Medicare Part A coverage under Medicare's home health benefit when the following conditions are met: the patient is serviced by a Medicare-certified home health agency, the patient meets homebound criteria, and the patient requires intermittent (not 24 hour) home nursing. Agencies that are Medicare certified must complete an OASIS (Outcome and Assessment Information Set) assessment in addition to the routine home care assessment (CMS, 2007). The OASIS assessment is a data collection tool used to quantify demographic, clinical, and functional information about the patient's health status. This information is submitted to the state and to CMS and becomes part of an outcome assessment database that is used to measure and assess the quality of patient care and delivery of services. Medicare provides a payment in a lump sum to the home health agency to provide all the beneficiary's home care services required for a 60-day period, or "episode of care," under the prospective payment system (PPS). The Medicare PPS, originally implemented in 2000, was revised for the first time effective January 2008 (CMS, 2008b). Accurate coding of the patient's diagnoses along with accurate completion of certain OASIS items is essential as OASIS scores determine the PPS payment. PPS reimbursement to the agency is based on averages. With some patients, the agency may achieve a profitable episode, and with others the agency may experience a financial loss. The mechanism by which this balance of profit and loss is achieved is called case mix adjusting or case mix management.

Under Medicare Part B, there is some coverage for a few infusion therapies administered using durable medical equipment such as mechanical or electronic external infusion pumps. Infusion therapies covered under Part B include a few anti-infective drugs, certain chemotherapy infusion drugs, inotropic drugs including dobutamine and milrinone, and infusion analgesics. Parenteral and enteral nutrition infusion therapies may be covered under Medicare Part B, but only if the need for the therapy is documented to be for at least 90 days and other coverage criteria are met. Coverage for intravenous immune globulin (IVIG) for primary immune deficiency patients exists but supplies and equipment are not reimbursed. More specific information can be obtained by contacting the Medicare entities called Durable Medical Equipment Medicare Administrative Contractors through the website http://www.cms.hhs.gov/center/dme.asp (CMS, 2008a). While most infusion drugs may be covered by the Medicare Part D prescription drug benefit, the Centers for Medicare & Medicaid Services (CMS) has determined that it does not have the authority to cover the infusion-related services, equipment, and supplies under Part D. As a result, many Medicare beneficiaries are effectively denied access to home infusion therapy and are compelled to receive infusion therapy in hospitals and skilled nursing facilities at a significantly higher cost to Medicare and at great inconvenience to the patients (NHIA, 2008). Increasingly, more participants in the Medicare program are enrolling in the Medicare Advantage (Part C) program. Similar to most commercial health plans, many Medicare Advantage health plans will cover home infusion because they recognize it will reduce their overall health care costs and achieve high levels of patient satisfaction. NHIA is working on legislation to address the gaps and limitations in coverage by Medicare and is an excellent resource for seeking the most up-to-date information about reimbursement for home infusion therapy (www.nhianet.org).

As a result of the complexity of home infusion reimbursement, home infusion pharmacies and home health care agencies have the expertise and internal resources to check and verify coverage for nursing care, medications, and needed supplies. This includes evaluating the reimbursement potential for the prescribed infusion therapy, necessary supplies, and required nursing or other services as well as verifying insurance coverage. Financial service representatives can help the patient explore reimbursement possibilities and will often negotiate with insurance companies. Such services assist the patient by interpreting and clarifying policy limits, negotiating rates and services covered under the policy, and determining which services are not covered.

INFUSION TEAM VALIDATION AND IMPLEMENTATION

As stated previously, reimbursement and revenue from infusion teams bring added value to health care organizations. In addition to this added value, other important infusion-related issues should be considered:

- Nearly all hospitalized patients receive some form of infusion therapy.
- Some patients continue to receive infusion therapy after inpatient discharge.
- Patient satisfaction increases with timely, efficient infusion therapy.
- Patient dissatisfaction with the skill level of the person inserting the catheter is documented in a 2003 Press Ganey survey (INS, 2005).

With this information in mind, it is important to look at the concept of infusion teams. The use of infusion teams has been increasing; however, there is still a void in recognizing the value of infusion therapy as a specialty service. Therefore it is important to provide information related to the value of infusion therapy teams. This information along with expert input from infusion-related professional organizations and health care organization infusion teams can be a great asset in planning and implementing a quality infusion service.

Validation for infusion teams centers largely on the benefits associated with delivering infusion therapy by a group of infusion nurses. The following guidelines may be considered when establishing an infusion team or validating the continuation of an established team.

FUNDAMENTAL CONSIDERATIONS

Validation

To validate the need for an infusion team, the external environment, internal organizational environment, demands for services, cost factors, and associated benefits should be thoroughly researched and carefully analyzed.

Maintenance

An established team may have to research or analyze only specific areas as needed to validate its continuation. However, an established team should always be one step ahead and able to address all the factors used to validate a new team.

Environmental analysis

To justify an infusion team within an institution, first analyze external and internal environmental factors to assess any demands on the organization that can offset its ability to support new services, financially and professionally. The information may be obtained from administrators, financial managers, professional associations, and peer review organizations.

External environmental factors that should be considered include the following:

- Impact of regulatory and demographic changes
- Payer and competitor activities
- Worker supply changes
- Technological changes
- Licensing changes
- Other area institutions (Do other local hospitals have infusion teams? If so, how do the functions, responsibilities, and coverage of the teams differ? If not, what is different about a non–infusion team hospital that enables the hospital to not require an infusion team?)

The following internal environmental factors should be analyzed:

- Identify the priorities of hospital management and the infusion team, and then show how the infusion team's strengths and weaknesses relate to those priorities. For example, identify how an infusion team can control costs while maintaining a high quality of patient care.
- Who makes decisions for the organization, and who influences the decision-makers? Analyze the data from the perspective of the decision-makers: what are their goals; what is important to them?
- Examine the health care organization's financial status.
- Consider the organization's internal power, political structure, and the overall climate for acceptance of services offered by the infusion team, by floor nurses, and by physicians.
- What is the health care organization's mission?
- How is the health care organization performing financially? What changes are being implemented to control costs or improve reimbursement?
- In what way is the existing or proposed infusion team compatible with the goals of the organization (i.e., improved, cost-effective quality care)?
- What is the purpose of the infusion team? Is this purpose recognized by administration?
- What is the health care organization's case mix? What are the implications for the infusion team?

Demand for service analysis

If the environmental analysis suggests that the infusion team concept would receive support, the demand for services should be assessed to show the relative merits of an infusion team to the organization. The following should be considered:

- Evaluate the number and type of infusion services that are being performed (e.g., IV starts and restarts, peripherally inserted central catheter [PICC] insertions, central venous catheter [CVC] maintenance procedures, administration set changes, infusion device manipulations, blood component administration).

- Evaluate the number of patients receiving infusion therapy and the intensity of infusion therapy (e.g., days receiving therapy, procedures performed, materials and nurse time needed per patient, department performing therapy).
- Quantify the potential for infusion therapy by calculating the average infusion costs and charges per patient, and total and average patient days.
- Assess the severity of illness of the organization's patients. Infusion therapy increases with the severity of illness, as determined by secondary diagnosis, age, malnutrition, dehydration, and surgical versus medical stay.

Cost-benefit analysis reference

Once an analysis of the organization and demand for services has been performed, the next strategy is to "sell" the concept of the infusion team and its associated benefits. Major emphasis should be placed on the fact that infusion teams can reduce costs through savings in labor and materials.

Labor

Labor is the largest element of cost associated with infusion therapy. It is important to show that labor can become more efficient by using infusion nurses. Compare the workload unit requirements of infusion nurses with those of non–infusion nurses to demonstrate the efficiencies and salary differentials that provide savings. An infusion team requires fewer workload unit requirements. Labor costs vary, depending on the salaries of the individuals providing infusion therapy. Emphasize that time saved can be redirected to other patient care activities and that improved efficiency can result in decreased full time equivalent (FTE) requirements on the units.

Supplies

Show that infusion teams can reduce material costs through more efficient use of supplies and standardization of infusion-related materials and equipment. Evaluate the impact of an infusion team in terms of total materials used and material usage efficiency. Compare this information with the materials that would be required without an infusion team and then compare the total costs per procedure related to materials used with and without an infusion team. It has been shown that an infusion team may use as little as one third of the materials used by a non–infusion team.

Improved quality of care

Reports that infusion teams improve quality of care may be regarded as subjective, rather than objective. It is important to define in quantitative ways the quality improvements offered by the infusion team concept. This may be accomplished in the following manner:

- Make a list of those characteristics that define good or poor quality in infusion care.
- Obtain information from medical records, infection prevention program reports, and infusion incident reports. A controlled study, either retrospective, concurrent, or prospective, may be necessary for more accurate documentation.
- Select two similar nursing units for a quality study. Using your list of quality measurements, perform random checks of infusion patients and establish quality indices

on both units; then, on one unit implement a pilot study using the infusion team concept. After implementation, conduct a new study on both units and compare with previous results. Use statistical methods in the studies and use unbiased observers. Typically, phlebitis and infection rates are studied.

- Improved quality of care must provide clear cost savings.

For maintaining an existing team, it is important to establish a continuing quality management program. Conduct studies to demonstrate the improvements the team has accomplished, and identify problem areas. For example, all members of the team should document selected quality management data (e.g., number of patients with phlebitis, infiltrations, infections, clotted venous access devices). This should be done every shift and can be best accomplished while documenting daily workload data.

Length of stay

To determine how an infusion team affects length of stay, identify patients with abnormally long stays and determine the reasons for those extended stays (e.g., severity of disease, nosocomial infection, medical complications, lack of venous access device placement and resultant interruption of therapy, delayed laboratory results, failure to discontinue infusion therapy). After considering reasons for extended stays, examine a population for which an infusion team would have a major impact. Call attention to the infusion team's role in preventing extra patient days, and calculate the percentages of incremental preventable cost and incremental avoidable delays attributable to an infusion team.

For existing teams, all staff members should record, at the end of their shift, any interventions undertaken that would have an impact on length of stay or costs. This provides ongoing data for justification of the infusion team. A simple way to collect data is to maintain a logbook in the department for each infusion nurse to note these interventions quickly. For example, there could be columns for the date, room number, patient's name, intervention, results, time required by the infusion nurse, and signature of the person carrying out the intervention.

Risk management

Plot the frequency and costs of lawsuits, which might disclose trends that support the need for an infusion team. Identify lawsuits that involved infusion complications and then calculate the dollars spent for legal fees, court costs, employee time, court awards, and settlements for these suits against the hospital.

Marketing advantage

Market an infusion team as a potential source of referrals or admissions. The infusion team can be promoted as a time saver and more efficient resource of infusion therapy. The team can also provide outpatient services, such as education and infusion services for home care patients and outpatients. Emphasize the improved quality of care delivered by the organization with infusion nurses providing care, based on national standards. Work with the organization's marketing department to investigate strategies for marketing to the hospital administration and community.

Organization and functions of the infusion team

Once the infusion team concept has been proposed and accepted as a valuable service, several factors must be considered when establishing the organization and functions of the team.

Identify the organizational structure that best benefits and enhances the team within the institution. Each organizational structure is associated with advantages and disadvantages, depending on the institutional environment. It is important to look for a structure that allows the team to meet its objectives, goals, and philosophy of care while remaining cost-effective. Note that INS recommends that the infusion team be established as an independent department that reports directly to administration.

Analyze current responsibilities

Compare current infusion practice with the proposed practice of the infusion team, including the following responsibilities: admixture preparation; venipuncture, site care and maintenance, and follow-up; PICC insertions; central venous access device care; blood product administration; infusion-related activities performed by various classifications of employees; and current nursing policies regarding infusion techniques.

Volume of infusion therapy activities

Establish daily volumes of infusion therapy activity for each nursing area. Sources of data include patient medical records, pharmacy records, purchasing, and various documents maintained on the nursing units. Establish current volumes of infusion therapy activities to provide information for comparison of the institution with other health care organizations, and establish a baseline for comparison of growth and mix changes.

Analyze facility layout

Study the layout in the facility, including unit location and size, and types of infusion therapy services that are required.

Resources and staffing

The following factors influencing resources and staffing should be analyzed:

- What resources are available for designing an infusion team? What role is played by a group such as the nursing division or education department?
- How many employees does the team need?
- Is there a significant shortage of nurses? Is it difficult to staff and provide 24-hour coverage?
- What role will an LVN/LPN have on the team?
- What resources are available to train the staff?

Functions of the infusion team

The following functions of the infusion team should be considered:

- What services are most needed by the institution? If unable to justify all the services, it is desirable to provide an alternative and phase-in functions over time.
- Is the team to provide 24-hour coverage every day of the week? (Remember that this is preferred for optimal functioning of the team.) What are the implications if it does not? If the team is part-time, who is responsible for infusion-related functions during the other hours?
- In what areas can the team provide services (e.g., general care areas, pediatrics-nursery, intensive care areas, emergency department, labor and delivery)?
- Identify team functions.

Costs for the infusion team (use the hospital accounting division as a resource)

The following factors should be considered when determining costs for the infusion team:

- What are the projected costs of the necessary staffing (include salary, benefits, sick leave, vacation)?
- What are supply costs (projected or actual) for infusion therapy activities?
- What are the methods for charging?
- Are they part of general nursing care charges or are they special charges? What is included in the charge structure?

Analyze reimbursement and revenue

Demonstrate how the infusion team concept results in increased revenues—project potential increases. Obtain information from other hospitals that have implemented teams. Examine current reimbursement issues, such as fee for service, discounted fee for user, per diem rate, per case rates, and capitation.

Develop budgetary goals

For the development of budgetary goals the following factors should be considered:

- Evaluate organizational goals.
- Determine long-range objectives.
- For established teams, forecast levels of activity for the coming year.
- Continually analyze how the team's role can expand, and reevaluate services provided. Remember that with the continual changes in health care and technology, the primary functions of the team may be altered.

Developing units of service

Develop units of service standards for labor hours needed to provide particular services. These standards provide productivity data. Determine units of service through time estimates, historical data averages, service logs, work sampling, predetermined accepted standards, and time and motion studies.

Units of service need to be logged by the staff daily on each shift. This can be accomplished efficiently by using computer and bar coding systems. Data can also be easily recorded manually on daily tally sheets. Each nurse can log procedures performed at the end of the shift and each procedure can then be converted to units of service.

Plan of care

It is important to establish the infusion team's role in patient assessment and plans of care specific to infusion therapy. Establish a system for integrating the infusion nursing plan of care into the overall plan of care.

Additional strategies for maintaining an infusion team

- Become indispensable. For example, provide and be responsible for highly specialized services such as PICC insertions.
- Provide educational and inservice programs. For example, have members of the team be actively involved in nursing orientation, hospital-wide inservice training, and hospital and community educational programs.
- Continually evaluate the function and success of other infusion teams in the area.
- Meet regularly with other infusion team managers in the community.

BUDGET

Any organization or service in existence must have monies available to cover expenses. The expense of doing business must also be covered by incoming revenue. With these two factors in place, it is important that a budget be in place to maintain a viable business.

Understanding the concepts of budgeting is considered to be a basic skill set required of management. The discussion in this chapter will attempt to acquaint the reader with the basics of the budgeting process.

A budget is a financial plan of an organization that covers a specific period of time. It helps to provide financial guidelines for the organization to meet strategic goals.

The goal of organizations that plan to operate in the future is to obtain the cash needed to cover operating expenses and other needs, for example, capital expansion. Nonprofit organizations, such as many health care organizations, need to make a profit in order to ensure that they can continue to provide their anticipated level of service, have capital for maintenance and expansion, and maintain a cash reserve to cover unanticipated expenses. A major difference between nonprofit organizations and for-profit organizations is that nonprofit organizations reinvest their profits into the organization, whereas a for-profit organization may return part of their profits to their shareholders (and, must also pay taxes on their profits).

Budgets are a financial forecast for the organization of estimated income and expenses over a specified period of time. Budgeting therefore is planning for expected needs and ensuring that there are sufficient resources. An accurate budget can be the difference between success and failure and is essential to the solvency of an organization. *Finance for Managers,* from the Harvard Business Essentials series, defines budget as the translation of strategic plans into measurable quantities that express the expected resources required and the anticipated returns over a certain period (Harvard Business Essentials, 2002).

BASIC FUNCTIONS

There are four basic functions to creating a successful budget. The four functions are planning, coordinating and communicating, monitoring progress, and evaluating performance.

Planning

Planning is key to budget development. In planning, three steps need to be followed: choosing goals, reviewing options and predicting results, and deciding on the most desirable course of action.

1. *Goals.* When developing a budget, one of the first steps is to determine the goal that is hoped to be accomplished in the specified period of time. Frequently, the board of directors sets the overall goals for the institution, which is conveyed to all levels of management in the planning phase. Is a new program to be added, is a current service expected to grow at a higher rate secondary to increased population, or is a new technology wanted or required to improve overall patient care without growth? These questions need to be answered in the planning phase so that the organization or department knows what to expect, what

resources are required, and what the expected return is for both new and existing services.

2. *Options for attaining goal.* Once the decision is made about the goal, it is time to look at all the options for attaining the goal. If the goal is to provide ultrasound-guided placement of peripherally inserted central catheters, two of the decisions that would need to be made are who will provide the service (infusion nurses, interventional radiology, a contract agency) and what equipment will be required. When anticipating the need for equipment, should it be purchased or rented, or does the organization already have existing equipment to meet the need? The various options associated with the goal need to be reviewed and a cost-benefit analysis of each option completed.

3. *Desirable course of action.* The final step in planning is choosing the option that will best allow the organization to meet the desired goal. The cost and the benefit of each option help determine the direction the organization or department wants to pursue, and the budget should reflect these decisions.

Coordinating and communicating

Since each department submits a budget reflecting their needs, the overall impact of the sum must be taken into account as the budget is built for the entire organization. This is where the master budget, which is discussed later, is developed, taking into account the strategic goals of the organization and the goals of the individual departments. The financial department is most likely the department responsible for coordinating individual budgets into the master budget. Frequently, departmental submissions must be adjusted to make certain that the entity as a whole meets the overall objectives.

Communication is extremely important in this phase. Before the planning phase, the strategic objectives for the organization are communicated to all management levels. These objectives need to be considered in the development of the budgets for the individual departments. Individual department leaders need to also communicate with other department leaders if their goals have the potential to impact another department's budget. For example, the marketing department should be aware of the new program that needs to be promoted and include it in their budget development.

Once individual budgets have been developed and are ready to be sent to upper management for coordination, it is essential for the department leaders to communicate their needs, assumptions, expectations, and goals. Knowledge of the departmental budgets facilitates the development of the master budget to meet the strategic goals of the organization. It is typical that adjustments are processed to ensure that all affected departmental needs are addressed. These adjustments may result in some departmental requests being denied or reduced in order to meet overall budget goals.

Monitoring progress

As important as it is to develop a good budget, it is equally important to monitor progress in meeting the budget. The organization may give a department $100,000 to spend on supplies. If that department then orders supplies without regards to the budget, the department will most likely exceed their supply budget. If all departments exceed the budgeted monies, the organization's master budget would soon be meaningless, resulting in a decreased expected net income at year-end.

A variance report is a budgetary report card for management. Variance reports can be developed at all levels of the budgetary process. Review of these reports allows leaders to be more time-efficient in locating and correcting problems by highlighting the differences between actual and budgeted revenue and expenses for a particular area (Siciliano, 2003). A budgetary variance can be either favorable (above budget in revenues or below in expenses) or unfavorable (below budget in revenue or above in expenses). A variance may also be controllable or uncontrollable. The excessive supply budget discussed earlier is an example of a controllable variance. Monitoring what is bought and maintaining a par level can help bring that variance back into acceptable range. There may be unexpected price variations in supplies (such as pharmaceutical price increases higher than expected) but these must be offset by better management of other expenses. An example of an uncontrollable variance would be the need to repair a piece of equipment because of unexpected maintenance problems.

Variance reports may use the actual versus the budgeted amount or the actual versus a variable (or flexed) budget amount. The variable budget is based on changes in activity level—if more activity occurs than was planned, the department would be allocated more resources for meeting the higher activity levels (the opposite is also true: if activity levels are lower than those that were budgeted, flex budgets are reduced at the department level). The original budgeted amount may also be shown to demonstrate the difference between the variable budget and the planned budget.

Once leaders have had the opportunity to review the variance report, they can develop a plan of action to bring their department into compliance with the approved budget. An effective leader will review each line item and determine the reason for the variance and what can be done to improve the budget/expense ratio. Variances occur for a number of reasons; it may be inefficiency on part of the staff, overstocking supplies, or even poor forecasting of the original budget. The first two problems can be addressed quickly and the actual budget can be adjusted to achieve compliance with the budgeted amount. Poor forecasting, however, will impact the budget for the entire time the budget is in effect. This therefore stresses the importance of the first function of the budget cycle, and that is planning. Poor planning by a leader can result in poor long-term performance.

Evaluating performance

Budgets are also an effective performance evaluation tool by which leaders can be evaluated. Leaders are accountable for the fiscal responsibility of their departments. As a result, they are involved in the planning and implementation decisions related to budget and are held accountable for achieving results. Successful results at the departmental level help in the achievement of the organizational goals while unsuccessful results can be a hindrance to the organization meeting these goals.

TYPES OF BUDGETS

There are a number of different types of budgets designed to meet a variety of needs. Not every organization uses the same time period or the same criteria in developing their budget.

Some of the different criteria used to develop budgets will be explained in the following section.

Short-term budget versus long-term budget

Budgets are designed to cover a specific period of time. This time period depends on the organization and the purpose of the budget. A start-up company may develop short-term budgets that cover only several months at a time as the company sets the foundation for the organization. Companies may also have long-term goals that cover several years, addressing capital projects such as building new facilities. Typically, most budgets cover a span of 1 year.

Fixed budget versus rolling budget

A fixed budget covers a specific period of time—most often the period is for 1 year. This yearly time frame is referred to as the fiscal year for the organization. A new budget is prepared before the beginning of each specified time period. Although the budget may be reviewed at intervals during the specified time period, the basic budget remains unchanged.

The fixed budget is considered to be rigid as it does not allow for changes in the budget during the allotted time frame. Businesses in rapid change environments find that the fixed budget limits them too much. Therefore the mechanism of choice is one that is continually updated. This is referred to as a rolling budget. The rolling budget has a consistent time frame but the actual period covered by the budget changes. The overall time frame is a year with the budget reviewed on a monthly basis, reflecting changes within that month.

With the rolling budget, leaders are required to be consistently planning, reevaluating, and making necessary revisions to meet the established goals. Therefore a major disadvantage of rolling budgets is that the process can be very time-consuming for management.

Zero-based budget versus incremental budget

Zero-based budgeting creates a new budget from the beginning each time a budget is developed. Development of a zero-based budget requires the leader to review all assumptions and projections; it is back to the planning phase each time. Although this provides a more in-depth analysis of each line item on the budget, it is also very time-consuming. Zero-based budgets are typically used for discretionary purchases, such as travel.

In developing the incremental budget, information is extrapolated from historical data (Harvard Business Essentials, 2002). The previous budget period is reviewed taking into account what was budgeted and the actual results. In addition, expectations for the future are incorporated into the new budget. The advantage of this is that it allows for history, experience, and future expectations to be included. The disadvantage with this process is that leaders may not take the time to plan; instead the leader may just take the information from the past budget period and increase it by a percentage for the next budget year. Another disadvantage to the incremental budget is the "use it or lose it" concept. With this concept, the thought process is if the allocated resources are not used within the budget period, these resources will not be allocated for the new budget. As a result, departments sometimes purchase unnecessary items to ensure the same resources are allocated the following year.

Master budget

The master budget is the accumulation of all the pieces of the picture for the organization. It includes the operating budget and the financial budget in one comprehensive document. It is a summary of every department's financial projections for the specified time. Development of the master budget is a senior leadership responsibility. It is their role to review budgets from all the departments and to determine how they mesh with the strategic goals of the organization. Adjustments may have to be made based on the final decisions. Harvard Business Essentials (2002) states that the following three questions should be asked by senior management before preparing a master budget:

1. Do the tactical plans being considered support the larger and longer-term strategic goals of the organization?
2. Does the organization have, or have access to, the required resources (that is, the cash it needs to fund the activities throughout the immediate budget period)?
3. Will the organization create enough value to attract adequate future resources (that is, profits, loans, or investors) to achieve its longer-term goals?

Operating budget

The operating budget addresses the revenue and expenses of a department for the coming budget period. It is not a forecast of what is expected; it is a target based on the forecasting done in the planning phase by the department leader. The operating budget of each department helps comprise the master budget; therefore agreement must be reached between senior leadership and the department manager on the final operating budget. Once the final budget reaches consensus and is allocated (or spread by month) throughout the budget year, department leaders are responsible for meeting the targeted budget. A variance report discussed earlier in this chapter is developed using the initial operating budget to help leaders monitor the results.

The operating budget is a line-by-line description that includes revenue expectations, salaries, and supply costs along with other expenses. Revenue expectations are based on what the revenue statistics are for the department. In health care, statistics may vary by department; for example, pharmacy may be the number of agents dispensed, infusion therapy may be the number of procedures performed, nursing may be based on the average patient days for that particular unit, and for home health it may be the number of patient visits. Revenue statistics may vary from organization to organization or department to department; thus it is important to know how an organization determines the revenue statistics for each department.

Salary costs include both the productive and nonproductive costs related to a full-time equivalent (FTE). A FTE is generally based on 2080 hours per year. So someone who works 40 hours per week is considered 1 FTE, while someone who works 20 hours per week is considered a 0.5 FTE. Productive costs are incurred for the employee performing critical job functions and include overtime and shift differentials. Nonproductive costs are costs associated with employee expense while not performing critical job functions, such as vacation, education, and jury duty pay.

The number of FTEs can be calculated in a number of different ways. It is important to have the appropriate number of staff needed to provide the care required for the hours and days the department operates. A department that operates 8 hours per day Monday through Friday will require less staff than the department that operates 24 hours per day 7 days a week. Another consideration is the skill mix required when different skill levels are used. A hospital inpatient nursing unit needs more registered nurses than nursing assistive personnel to meet the needs of their patients while a skilled nursing facility may use more nursing assistive personnel than registered nurses. In calculating the FTE budget, it is also important to provide for time off coverage. An individual who works 40 hours per week is considered 1 FTE. However, if this individual's job requires a replacement for time off, additional hours must be allocated when planning the number of FTEs needed for this position.

Other expenses are the direct expenses associated with that particular department's activity. These are often separated into subaccounts to better identify what is required for that department to operate. The subaccounts depend on the particular organization. Some examples of subaccounts are medical-surgical supplies, drugs, office supplies, and minor equipment. Additional accounts may include purchased services, biomedical services, professional fees, and travel expenses. Some of these expenses will be fixed expenses, indicating that the cost essentially remains unchanged regardless of activity. Variable expenses are expenses that fluctuate in relation to the volume of activity. If the inpatient census is lower than normal in a hospital, there should be a reciprocal decrease in the need for certain supplies, decreasing the expenses associated with those supplies. See Box 9-1 for examples of fixed and variable expenses.

Capital budget

The capital budget refers to those items that require a large outlay of monies for either the organization itself or the department. The capital budget is incorporated into the master budget. The amount of dollars identified as being a capital expense is determined by the organization and its size. A small organization may determine that anything costing more than $1000 may be a capital expense while larger organizations may identify items costing greater than $5000 to $10,000 as capital items. It is important for the department leader to understand what constitutes a capital expense when preparing the budget.

Box 9-1   VARIABLE VERSUS FIXED EXPENSES

VARIABLE EXPENSES

These are expenses that are directly impacted by changes in volume. These items include:
- Medical-surgical charge items (items that have a charge associated with them)
- Medical-surgical noncharge items
- Drugs
- Paper/forms

FIXED EXPENSES

These are expenses that have been set and are not affected by changes in volume. These items include:
- Maintenance agreements
- Rent
- Pager services
- Professional development

The monies for capital budget requests are most often allocated differently than the monies for the operating budget, requiring leaders to submit separate requests for these funds. Major users of capital funds include surgery, pharmacy, laboratory, radiology, and critical care units. However, all departments may have needs for equipment that meet the capital budget definition at some time. An example of a capital expense for an infusion therapy department would be the purchase of a bedside ultrasound device.

Senior leadership has the responsibility of reviewing all capital budget requests, and determining how each meets the mission and vision of the organization and the strategic goals as defined for that budget period. Not all capital requests will be funded; funding depends on the amount of monies allocated for the capital budget and the total amount of monies requested by various areas.

 ## THE FUTURE RELATED TO INFUSION THERAPY

Infusion nurses see unmet needs and better ways to provide care on a daily basis. It is important that this information be used to develop research projects, publications, and improved technology.

RESEARCH PROJECTS

New research is needed as well as investigation of current literature to ensure that there is sound evidence for practice. Funding is available through grants and scholarships from professional organizations, foundations, and industry. Resources are also available for research program development through training programs and classes, health care medical libraries, and mentors in professional and health care organizations.

PUBLICATIONS

The infusion programs and practice can be positively impacted through publications. Infusion nurses need to share practice information through professional journals, books, newsletters, and presentations at professional meetings as well as taking advantage of computer-based learning.

TECHNOLOGY

The role of technology has played a major role in the success of infusion-related programs. One example is the use of peripherally inserted central catheters (PICCs). Infusion nurses recognized the need to assess and determine appropriate equipment at the onset of patient care. This decreased the number of venipunctures while decreasing cost of the procedure, and increasing patient satisfaction. Nurses recognized that they could provide services in a more cost-effective manner and became a valuable asset to the patient and health care facility, both from a clinical and from a financial viewpoint.

Technology continues to have a positive impact on infusion practices daily. Often this change results from infusion nurses' attempts to better meet the needs of their patients and the medical community. Infusion nurses continue to design a variety of products, as they work with health care facilities, professional organizations, industry, and, at times, their own health care companies. The products include infusion-related medical equipment, peripheral and central venous access devices (VAD), trays, and accessories. For example, infusion nurses were responsible for adapting VAD systems from continuous set-ups to intermittent devices.

Infusion nurses need to continue to offer information through surveys and for industry-related product development. Involvement also should include the development of educational materials and programs. As end-users, the input from infusion nurses impacts infusion-related technology and thus the quality of products available in the health care environment.

SERVICES

The future will continue to move forward in relation to infusion-related services. As mentioned earlier, much progress has been made since the onset of providing basic venipuncture procedures. Nurses own and manage companies that provide infusion services in a variety of settings, and this should continue to expand. Nurses will continue to play a valuable role in providing education and services in specialty practice areas involving medication delivery (e.g., biologicals, pain control). As a service to other nurses, infusion nurses need to continue to develop and provide educational programs and training opportunities.

MARKETING

Infusion nurses create new products and services. However, many times these are not shared with others. Often after expounding the many facets of infusion therapy to other medical and nonmedical professionals, the reply comes, "I have never heard of infusion therapy. Why do you not let people know who you are and what you do—there is such a need?"

Now and in the future, nurses need to be more cognizant of marketing who they are, what they do, and what their impact is on the business and health care environment, as well as their services to the public.

 ## SUMMARY

Historically, infusion teams began by initiating venipunctures for routine patient procedures requiring infusion therapy, primarily on the day shift. Some teams tended to stagnate in this mode. Other teams went a step further and took into account the infusion needs over a 24-hour period. As a result, hours of service were expanded, patient satisfaction was increased, and complications were minimized or eliminated. Infusion needs were recognized outside of initial hospitalization with the creation of outpatient and home care services.

The future of health care, including infusion therapy, is based on the quality of care provided, patient outcomes, customer satisfaction, and third-party reimbursement. To attain success, all members of the health care team must continually monitor and make appropriate changes in the day-to-day care provided to maintain cost-effectiveness and achieve national quality benchmarks.

Earlier information was provided on the validation of infusion teams. Often the focus is on the initiation of infusion programs. However, success is measured by longevity, which is determined through outcomes, customer satisfaction, staff encouragement, and reimbursement. To be successful, infusion programs cannot remain stagnant.

Infusion nurse leaders must continue to investigate the needs of patients, medical practices, and health care organizations and provide evidence-based practice to meet those needs. The nurses involved in the practice of infusion therapy are certainly among the best to help leaders determine practice needs and use the findings to assist in developing the policies, procedures, and technology required to provide efficient and effective infusion therapy. At the same time, the financial aspect of infusion therapy and health care must be given high priority to make infusion therapy a viable option for the patient, provider, and private and third-party payers.

 REFERENCES

Castro AG, Layman E: Principles of healthcare reimbursement, Chicago, 2006 *Am Health Inform Manag Assoc*, 1-15, 2006.

Centers for Medicare & Medicaid Services (CMS): *OASIS user manual*, 2007. Accessed 6/23/08 from http://www.cms.hhs.gov/HomeHealth QualityInits/14.HHQIOASISUserManual.asp.

Centers for Medicare & Medicaid Services (CMS): *Durable medical equipment center*, 2008a. Accessed 6/23/08 from http://www.cms. hhs.gov/center/dme.asp.

Centers for Medicare & Medicaid Services (CMS): *Home health PPS—overview*, 2008b. Accessed 6/23/08 from http://:www.cms.hhs. gov/HomeHealthPPS/.

Harvard Business Essentials: *Finance for managers*, Boston, 2002, Harvard Business School.

Infusion Nurses Society: *Infusion therapy team implementation module*, Norwood, Mass, 2005, Author.

National Home Infusion Association (NHIA): *Does Medicare cover home infusion therapy?* Accessed 6/23/08 from http://www.nhianet. org/faqs.cfm.

Niedzwiecki MH: The revenue cycle: what it is, how it works, and how to enhance it, *AORN* 84:578-601, 2006.

Siciliano G: *Finance for non-financial managers*, New York, 2003, McGraw-Hill.

Thorwarth WT: From concept to CPT to compensation: how the payment system works, *J Am Coll Radiol* 1:48-53, 2004.

10 ANATOMY AND PHYSIOLOGY RELATED TO INFUSION THERAPY

Lynn C. Hadaway, MEd, RN, BC, CRNI®

Knowledge of the anatomy and physiology of the skin, peripheral vasculature, and cardiopulmonary and neurological systems is crucial for the safe administration of any parenteral therapy. Many factors related to these body functions can encumber or increase the success of infusions. Conversely, parenteral therapy administration can have a detrimental effect on the anatomy and physiological function of all body systems. Our goal of this chapter is to consider all pertinent factors in an effort to manage the risk of parenteral therapy and ensure a positive outcome for the patient.

When an IV device is inserted, the skin is the first organ affected. Skin serves several functions: it is a mechanical barrier against microorganisms and radiation, provides sensory and temperature regulation, and helps maintain fluid and electrolyte balance. Breaking this natural barrier increases the risk of infection. The use of antiseptic solutions, stabilization devices, and dressing materials can affect the skin's natural composition of bacteria, oils, and sweat. Factors such as age, chronic disease, and the environment can produce changes in the skin, making entry through the skin a difficult process.

Vascular anatomy is of primary importance when locating and cannulating veins or arteries. Both the insertion site and the location of the catheter tip are important considerations. Extreme variations in pH, osmolarity, volume, and rate can alter the risk of complications if consideration is not given to the size of the vessel lumen and the amount and type of blood flow. Fluid volume status and general cardiopulmonary condition can limit the volume and rate of infusion and lead to a negative patient outcome when not monitored closely.

The neurological system affects all other systems and can influence the success or failure of any parenteral therapy. The close proximity of peripheral veins and nerves leads to risk of nerve damage with routine venipuncture. The sensory receptors in the skin, the innervation of the walls of veins and arteries, the systemic responses evoked by emotion and pain, and the use of the epidural space for infusions necessitate knowledge of the central nervous system.

Finally, variation in personal technique used for insertion, infusion, injection, and withdrawal is another vital component affecting anatomy and physiology. The impact of differences in catheter types and components and solution composition can be evaluated and monitored more easily than the nuances of individual technique. A thorough working knowledge of the anatomy and physiology of multiple body systems, combined with a carefully crafted expertise, is necessary to ensure positive patient outcomes.

INTEGUMENT AND CONNECTIVE TISSUE

The integument, or skin, is a highly specialized organ that protects the body from its environment. It ranges in thickness from 1.5 to 4.0 millimeters (mm), with the thickest skin appearing on the palms of the hands and plantar aspect of the feet (Standring, 2005). Skin functions as a protective barrier between the body and environmental elements such as microbial invasion and mechanical, chemical, and ultraviolet radiation damage. Skin also synthesizes vitamin D, cytokines, and other growth factors; is under the influence of hormones; and assists with control of body temperature (Standring, 2005).

Skin is divided into two layers: the epidermis and the dermis. Lying immediately under the dermis is the hypodermis, which is composed of adipose tissue. This layer cushions and protects the underlying structures and acts as insulation for the body (Figure 10-1).

Loose connective tissue lies under the skin and is composed of several types of fibers and cells. Its primary functions include providing structure and defense. Superficial veins for venipuncture lie in this layer of loose tissue.

STRUCTURE AND FUNCTION
Epidermis

The epidermis is composed of five layers of squamous cells (Figure 10-2). From deepest to most superficial, the basal layer is closest to the dermis and contains interlocking ridges to maintain the integrity of the two structures. The prickle cell layer (stratum spinosum) contains Langerhans cells and a few lymphocytes. The granular layer (stratum granulosum) provides

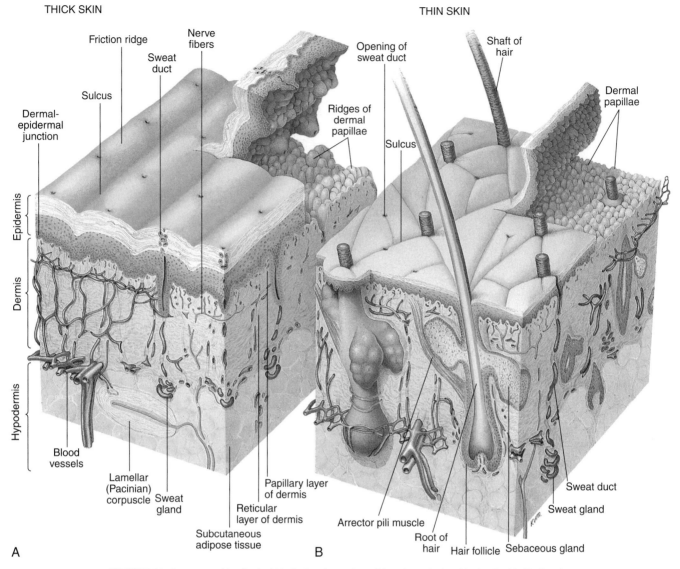

FIGURE 10-1 Anatomy of the skin. **A,** Thick skin, found on surfaces of the palms and soles of the feet. **B,** Thin skin, found on most surface areas of the body. (From Thibodeau GA, Patton KT: *Anatomy & physiology,* ed 6, St Louis, 2007, Mosby.)

the principle barrier to prevent penetration by gases or liquids. The clear layer is only present in hairless skin of the palm and soles of the feet. The cornified layer (stratum corneum) is the most superficial layer with depths ranging from a few cells in thin skin to more than 50 cells in normal skin (Standring, 2005). These layers represent different stages of the maturation process. Individual cells are constantly maturing, moving upward to the surface and being replaced by new cells from the base. Loss of skin cells is only perceptible when it is excessive, such as peeling or scaling associated with certain skin disorders. Stressful agents such as prolonged exposure to sunlight, habitual pressure, and abrasion cause thickening of the cornified layer and can be measured by ultrasound (Matsumura and Anathaswamy, 2002; Lopez et al, 2004). This may explain difficult venipunctures in some patients, especially those who are manual laborers or others whose lifestyle involves excessive exposure to sunlight.

Keratins, a large group of filament proteins in all epithelial cells, change as the cells mature and move upward through the layers. These proteins are a group of more than 50 distinct gene

sequences in humans, and mutations can be the cause of several skin disorders (McLean, 2003).

Three other types of cells can be found in the epidermis: Langerhans cells, melanocytes, and Merkel cells. Langerhans cells are found in an extensive network throughout the epidermis. Their function is to detect antigens, react to inflammatory signals from the other keratinocytes, and then migrate to the nearest lymph nodes. Migration of Langerhans cells to lymph nodes has been demonstrated after mechanical tape stripping and exposure to antigens, but no such migration was seen after stripping and exposure to nonantigenic solutions. There is a growing body of information linking the loss of the skin's barrier function to the development of atopic dermatitis and allergies (Callard and Harper, 2007).

Melanocytes contain melanin, the pigment that imparts color to the skin. Variation in color depends on the number and composition of melanocytes and on genetic, hormonal, and environmental factors. Melanin protects the skin from sun damage and is a scavenger for free radicals that can also cause cellular damage (Standring, 2005). Little is known about the

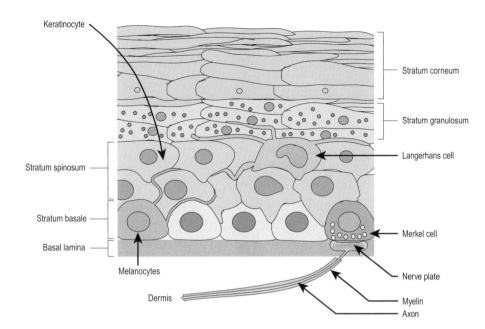

FIGURE 10-2 Layers and features of the epidermis. (From Kierszenbaum A: *Histology and cell biology: an introduction to pathology,* ed 2, St Louis, 2007, Mosby.)

physiology of Merkel cells, yet they are located close to sensory nerve endings in the epidermis and create and release numerous peptides (Boulais and Misery, 2007).

Dermis

The dermis, the thickest layer of the skin, is composed of dense connective tissue with varying amounts of elastin fibers, collagen fibers, blood, and lymphatic vessels. Collagen is the largest component of the dermis and provides mechanical or tensile strength. Sebaceous glands, sweat glands and ducts, hair follicles, and arrector pili muscles surrounding hair follicles are also located in the dermis (see Figure 10-1).

The dermis is divided into the papillary and reticular layers. The papillary layer is immediately under the epidermis and serves to anchor the epidermis mechanically and support it metabolically. Fingerlike projections, known as rete ridges, extend into the base of the epidermis to mate with the rete pegs in the epidermis and enhance the bond between the two layers. The reticular layer is the deepest and is characterized by dense, irregular, connective tissue. This type of connective tissue is formed by strong collagen fiber bundles arranged in a multilayered network, providing the ability to stretch. Elastin fibers are usually thinner and have almost perfect recoil.

The hair bulb, responsible for generating the growth of hair, is located in the dermis and is surrounded by the hair follicle. Arrector pili muscles extend at an angle from the follicle into the dermis. When these muscles are stimulated by cold or emotion, the hair shaft is pulled upward and the skin appears dimpled. Sebaceous glands are located in the angle between the muscle and follicle and the muscular action expresses sebum, the secretion from the sebaceous glands. Sebum passes through a duct, into the hair follicle, and onto the skin surface. The function of sebum, composed of glycerides, cholesterol, and wax esters, is to lubricate and protect the hair and skin and contribute to body odor.

Sweat glands and ducts arise from the dermis and communicate with the skin surface. The greatest number is located on the face and hands with the fewest number on the surfaces of the extremities. These glands secrete a clear, odorless, hypotonic fluid containing urea, lactate, immunoglobulin, and other proteins as well as ions such as sodium, chloride, calcium, and bicarbonate. Secretion is stimulated by temperature elevation and emotional stimulation, with as much as 10 L of sweat produced daily (Standring, 2005).

Superficial fascia or hypodermis

Continuing downward to the next layer, the superficial fascia is a layer of loose connective tissue (see Figure 10-1). This layer contains the same collagen and elastin fibers as the dermis. Adipose tissue or fat cells are located in this layer, where they serve as energy stores and thermal insulation. A large variety of defensive cells similar to those found in the blood are found in this tissue. Among all these important components lie the superficial veins used for peripheral venipuncture.

Blood vessels, lymphatics, and nerves

The skin does not have a great metabolic demand, yet the amount of blood flow far exceeds nutritional requirements and is equal to approximately 5% of cardiac output (Standring, 2005). Blood is supplied to the skin by a direct cutaneous network of vessels arising from the muscles and superficial fascia (Figure 10-3). Arterioles supply sweat and sebaceous glands and hair follicles; capillaries loop upward to the base of the epidermis through the rete ridges; and venules pass back through the dermis to join small veins in the superficial fascia. The skin is also served by a large number of small lymphatic vessels beginning in the papillary dermis. There are numerous anastomoses at all levels that are responsible for moving lymphocytes, Langerhans cells, and macrophages to lymph nodes (Standring, 2005).

Cutaneous circulation serves as a thermoregulator. Blood flow to the skin is 10 times greater than its nutritional requirements. In response to the need for heat loss or conservation, cutaneous blood flow can be increased or decreased by 20 times the normal capacity. Cold conditions can quickly

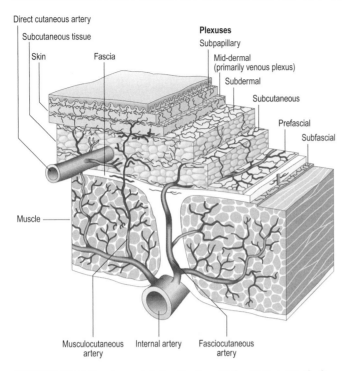

FIGURE 10-3 Vascular supply to the skin. (From Mathes SJ, Hentz VR: *Plastic surgery,* ed 2, Philadelphia, 2006, Saunders.)

TABLE 10-1	Anatomical and Physiological Changes Related to Aging
Location	**Changes**
Epidermis	Flattening of projections between the two layers; widening space between keratinocytes; slower maturation of keratinocytes; decreased thickness of layer
Dermis	Decreased thickness of layer; thicker and calcified elastin fibers, sometimes with complete fragmentation; decrease in total amount of collagen; reduction in vascular network around hair follicles and glands; decreased number of blood vessels and shorter capillary loops; decreased amount of mucopolysaccharides, resulting in changes in turgor; decreased number of nerve endings; decreased number of sweat glands and sweat production
Cells	Decreased number of melanocytes, resulting in decreased protection from ultraviolet light; decreased number of mast cells and reduction in histamine release

cause vasoconstriction, making venipuncture difficult, yet heat application rapidly causes vasodilation (Standring, 2005).

The extensive nerve supply in the skin acts as a sensory organ and regulator of response to mechanical, thermal, painful, or noxious stimuli. Sensory receptors in the form of free nerve endings provide needed information about the external environment. Encapsulated mechanoreceptors are found in the deep dermal layer and respond to weight, pressure, and vibration.

AGE-RELATED CHANGES

The normal physiological process of aging can have a distinct effect on the appearance and performance of the skin. An environmental source of skin changes is habitual sun exposure, called *photoaging,* and is considered to be preventable damage (Matsumura and Anathaswamy, 2002).

Changes in the appearance of skin attributed to age include wrinkling, dryness, and looseness. These effects can be found in all layers and cells of the skin (Table 10-1). Such changes indicate that the skin has a continually decreasing capability to respond to forces and strain, becoming more rigid and inflexible. The common clinical picture of these problems as related to parenteral therapy includes bleeding from venipuncture sites, shearing of skin layers when tape or dressing materials are removed, and excessive skin dryness with the use of alcohol and other antiseptic agents.

Photoaging from exposure to the sun differs with the length of exposure, gender, and individual differences in the skin. However, the same problems are seen as those that occur with the normal aging process.

ROLE IN INFECTION PREVENTION

Normal resident flora on human skin includes four bacterial groups and a fungal group. Coryneforms and staphylococci are the major bacterial groups, with *Micrococcus* and *Acinetobacter*

as the minor bacterial group. *Acinetobacter* species can easily be found in the antecubital fossa. *Malassezia* is the primary fungus found on skin. Microorganisms are found in pilosebaceous ducts and on the skin surface in microcolonies. These colonies are larger in men than in women and are found in different quantities depending on the type of skin. For instance, the dry skin of the forearm may have only 100 organisms per colony, whereas the shoulder area may have colonies containing 10^5 organisms (Matsumura and Anathaswamy, 2002). Factors affecting the growth of skin microorganisms include the amount and type of nutrients such as lipids, adherence properties of the flora, and humidity at the skin surface. Presence of water at the skin surface leads to rapid microbial growth in short periods. The three most important factors in infection prevention are immunocompetence, nutritional status, and the maintenance of an intact integument. Therefore careful attention must be given to the condition of the skin under dressings, the patient's response to various antiseptic solutions and dressing materials, and the number of venous, arterial, or epidural cannulations with the necessary break in the skin.

The skin's primary function in the prevention of infection is as a mechanical barrier to the invasion of pathogenic organisms. Chemical barriers include sebaceous secretions that have antibacterial and antifungal fatty acids; the role of circulating immunoglobulins, cellular immunity, and delayed hypersensitivity; and the acidic pH of the skin (usually between 3 and 5) (Matsumura and Anathaswamy, 2002). The inflammatory process and subsequent infections are influenced by these factors.

WOUND HEALING

Because initiating any parenteral therapy requires breaking the skin, it is appropriate to consider the process for the healing of that wound. The anatomy of skin has been presented from the outer surface inward. However, to understand the process of restoring the dermis and epidermis after injury, it is necessary to discuss the repair of the dermis and the regeneration of the epidermis.

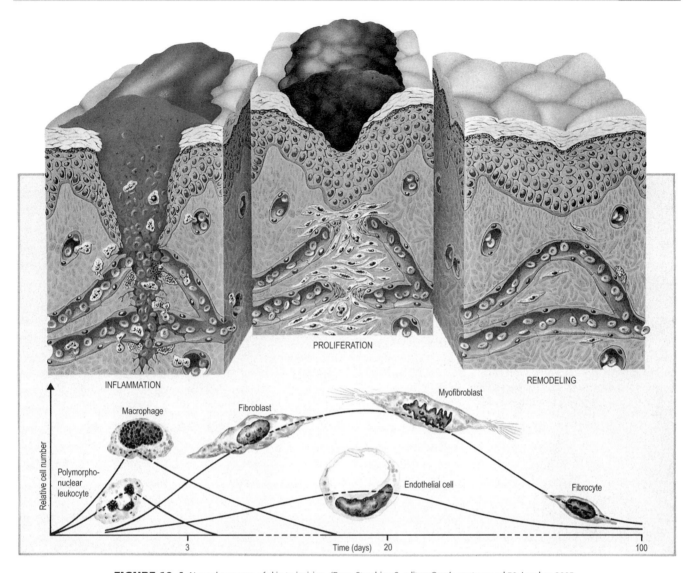

FIGURE 10-4 Normal response of skin to incision. (From Standring S, editor: *Gray's anatomy,* ed 39, London, 2005, Churchill Livingstone.)

Immediately after any wound is sustained, the initial phase is one of inflammation in response to stimulation of platelets and mast cells (Figure 10-4). Bleeding is controlled by activation of the complex clotting cascade and the activation of platelets. The permeability of local blood vessels increases and causes plasma proteins to leak into the wound, forming an extravascular clot. Neutrophils, which control bacteria, and monocytes enter the wound. Monocytes become macrophages and have a phagocytic action; in addition, they release chemicals necessary for granulation.

The second phase, proliferation or granulation, is characterized by the formation of a large number of capillaries through the process of angiogenesis. These are embedded in a thick matrix of fibronectin, a glycoprotein that acts like glue. Macrophages are present in this stage and act to debride the wound. Collagen is synthesized, which adds more strength to the tissue.

Within a few hours after injury, the epidermis begins to regenerate new epithelial cells. Keratinocytes use a "leapfrog" action, moving over each other to reach the bed of the wound. They then stop moving and begin to divide, forming new epidermal cells. This process seals and protects the healing wound

and severs the connection between the underlying clot and wound surface.

Two factors may inhibit the healing process at this point. The presence of anti-inflammatory steroids prevents macrophages from entering the wound, thus slowing the formation of granulation tissue. A lack of ascorbic acid (vitamin C) can interfere with the production of collagen.

The final stage of dermal repair is remodeling. Granulation tissue, containing a large number of cells and blood vessels, is gradually replaced with scar tissue, which contains fewer cells and vessels. Fibronectin is removed and replaced with randomly crosslinked collagen fibers. Over time these fibers become more organized, and the tensile strength of the new tissue improves, although it may not regain its original tensile strength (Standring, 2005).

Healing of wounds is delayed when there is excessive or prolonged bleeding during the initial injury. Red blood cells and fibrin must be removed before the repair begins. Lack of oxygen in the tissue causes vasoconstriction and decreases the deposit of cells necessary for the inflammatory process. Improper nutrition and underlying diseases such as diabetes also slow wound healing.

NEUROLOGICAL SYSTEM

The human nervous system acts as an information loop containing billions of neurons and hundreds of thousands of synaptic connections. When changes in the environment are picked up by the sensory organs of the body, information is fed back to the controlling organ, or brain, which coordinates this with numerous other pieces of information, decides what response to make, and then communicates that response back to the body.

The system can be studied in many ways. Distinct functional divisions of the nervous system include the following: (1) the sensory ability to transmit information from tactile, visual, and auditory receptors; (2) the motor functions, controlling all skeletal and smooth muscles; and (3) the autonomic system, which controls glands and smooth muscles. Anatomic divisions are the central system, composed of the brain and spinal cord, and the peripheral system, composed of 12 cranial and 31 spinal nerves.

INFORMATION PROCESSING

The nervous system processes enormous amounts of information in a manner that produces correct responses. While much sensory information (such as how clothing contacts the body) is unimportant, significant information is channeled and processed to produce the desired response.

Information travels from one neuron to the next through two types of synapses (Figure 10-5). Chemical synapses, the type found in most human central nervous system tissue, secrete a neurotransmitter. There are more than 40 neurotransmitters but the most common ones are acetylcholine, norepinephrine, epinephrine, histamine, γ-aminobutyric acid, glycine, serotonin, and glutamate (Guyton and Hall, 2006). Electrical synapses conduct electricity through open fluid channels between nerve cells. Chemical synapses send signals in only one direction, from the presynaptic neuron to the postsynaptic neuron, but electrical synapses transmit in either direction.

Chemical neurotransmitters can be divided into two groups. Small-molecule, rapidly acting transmitters are released within a millisecond or less, producing the acute responses of the nervous system. Neuropeptides are slow-acting transmitters, such as hormones, that act in the hypothalamus and pituitary glands, the gastrointestinal tract, or brain. Examples of neuropeptides are vasopressin, oxytocin, insulin, glucagon, angiotensin II, bradykinin, and substance P (Guyton and Hall, 2006).

Synaptic transmission is affected by special factors. Fatigue can occur when the firing rate is very rapid at first, and then becomes progressively slower over the next few seconds. Serum pH and low oxygen levels also produce changes. Acidosis and hypoxia decrease synaptic transmission, while alkalosis increases the excitability of neurons (Guyton and Hall, 2006).

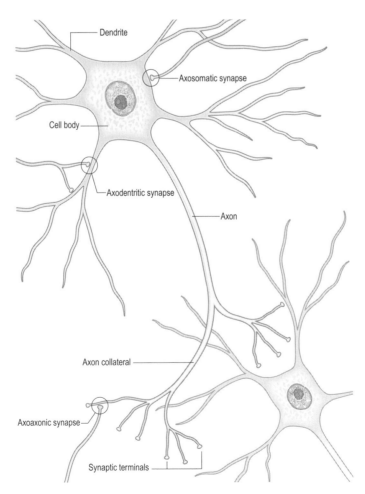

FIGURE 10-5 Structure of a typical neuron. (From Standring S, editor: *Gray's anatomy,* ed 39, London, 2005, Churchill Livingstone.)

FUNCTIONAL DIVISIONS
Sensory receptors

There are five types of sensory receptors (mechanoreceptors, thermoreceptors, nociceptors, electromagnetic receptors, and chemoreceptors), with corresponding stimuli for each (Table 10-2). Except for electromagnetic receptors, all have an effect on parenteral therapy. Many types of stimulation, such as heat, light, cold, pressure, and sound, must be processed appropriately. All these variations in modalities of sensation are transmitted along different afferent fibers, ending at a specific point in the central nervous system. This is called the *labeled line principle* (Guyton and Hall, 2006), which means that pain receptors transmit a painful response whether it is caused by puncture, crushing, or electricity. The sensation of touch is transmitted along a single path, no matter how the stimulation occurs.

The sensation of pain can have a profound impact on parenteral therapy. Pain can be felt quickly or slowly. Fast pain is felt within 0.1 second after stimuli, but slow pain takes seconds to be felt and may increase over minutes (Guyton and Hall, 2006). Pain receptors in skin, subcutaneous tissue, and vessel walls are free nerve endings. Fast pain is associated with skin punctures, cuts, or electrical shock. Slow pain is more intense, occurring over a prolonged period, and is usually associated with tissue destruction that can occur with catheter complications such as thrombophlebitis, infiltration and extravasation. Mechanical, thermal, and chemical stimuli can activate pain receptors. Fast pain is evoked primarily by mechanical and thermal means,

whereas slow pain is associated with all three stimuli. Histamine, bradykinin, potassium ions, serotonin, acetylcholine, and proteolytic enzymes can stimulate pain receptors. Bradykinin and potassium ions appear to be responsible for producing pain following tissue damage. Pain from ischemia is probably related to the formation of large amounts of lactic acid produced from anaerobic metabolism (Guyton and Hall, 2006). Phlebitis, infiltration, and extravasation injuries produce the tissue damage involving these chemicals.

Motor function

Sensory information comes from all areas of the nervous system into the spinal cord, brain stem, and cerebrum where it produces muscular functions transmitted to the body along efferent nerve fibers. Specific areas of the cerebral cortex and brain stem control motor functions. The pyramidal tract (or corticospinal tract) is the principal pathway for the transmission of impulses from the motor cortex through the brain stem and down the spinal cord. Other pathways for impulses include the mesencephalon (midbrain) and the cerebellum. The term *extrapyramidal motor system* has been used clinically to describe those motor functions outside the pyramidal system. Because there are many functions and pathways included in this term, it is difficult to use it for physiological purposes. However, the term *extrapyramidal side effects* is used to describe uncoordinated motor movements of the neck, jaw, and extremities that are associated with the administration of some types of medications.

TABLE 10-2 **Sensory Receptors and Related Parenteral Therapy Procedures**

Type of receptor	Sensation	Effect of parenteral therapy
Mechanoreceptor	Skin tactile sensibilities	Palpation for veins and arteries; application of antiseptic solutions and dressings; removal of tape and dressings
	Deep tissue sensibilities	Puncture of vein or artery; tight or constricting dressing
	Arterial pressure control through baroreceptor or pressure receptor system in all large arteries	Excessive infusion of intravenous solution, increasing circulating blood volume, and activating pressure receptors
	Hearing	None
	Equilibrium	None
Thermoreceptor	Cold, warmth	Application of heat or cold to treat phlebitis, infiltration, or extravasation
Nociceptor	Pain	Puncture of vein or artery for insertion of any catheter; puncture of lumbar area for epidural catheter insertion; removal of dressings; infusion of irritating medications subcutaneously; application of extreme heat or cold
Electromagnetic receptor	Vision	None
Chemoreceptor	Decreased arterial pressure stimulates receptors in aorta and carotid arteries to respond to low oxygen levels and increased carbon dioxide levels	Inadequate amount of solution infused, resulting in decreased circulating blood volume
	Osmotic changes in blood	Infusion of extremely hypertonic or hypotonic solutions
	Taste	Dysgeusia, or alteration in taste, produced by many IV medications
	Smell	None

Autonomic nervous system

The autonomic nervous system regulates the body's internal organs and controls such functions as glandular secretions, arterial blood pressure, sweating, and body temperature. Perhaps the most astonishing factor about this system is the speed with which changes occur. The heart rate can double within 3 to 5 seconds, the blood pressure can drop enough to cause fainting within 4 to 5 seconds, and sweating can occur within seconds (Guyton and Hall, 2006). The two major divisions of the autonomic nervous system are the sympathetic and parasympathetic, both of which send signals to specific organs (Figure 10-6). There is also a system of visceral or enteric reflexes that receives subconscious sensory signals from the viscera, sending back a reflex response to control that specific organ. The vagus nerves (cranial nerve X) contain about 75% of all parasympathetic nerve fibers, extending to the thoracic and abdominal areas of the body.

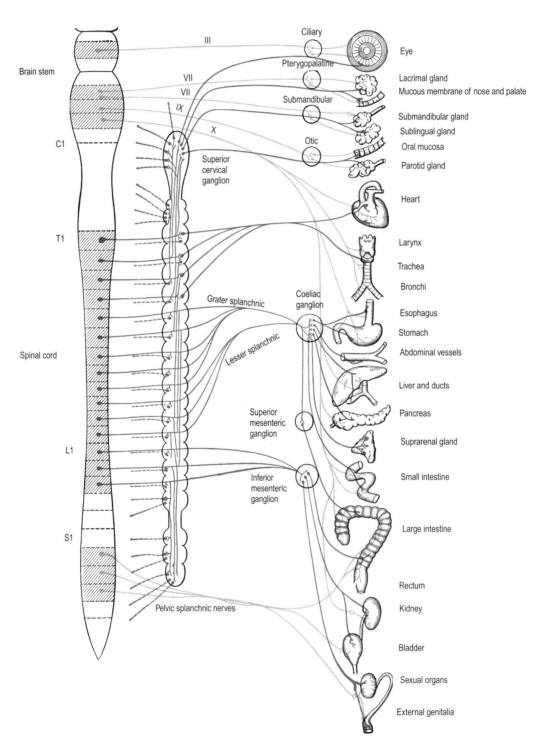

FIGURE 10-6 Autonomic nervous system. (From Standring S, editor: *Gray's anatomy,* ed 39, London, 2005, Churchill Livingstone.)

Synaptic transmission involves primarily acetylcholine (known as cholinergic fibers) and norepinephrine (known as adrenergic fibers). Virtually all parasympathetic nerve endings secrete acetylcholine, and almost all sympathetic nerves secrete norepinephrine.

Sympathetic stimulation may cause excitation in some organs but has an inhibitory effect on others. The same can be said for the parasympathetic system. Also, the two systems may work in a reciprocal arrangement, with one causing excitation and the other producing inhibition. For example, sympathetic stimulation increases the rate and force of heart contraction, and parasympathetic stimulation has the opposite effect. Systemic blood vessels, especially in the skin of extremities, are constricted by sympathetic stimulation, thus increasing the difficulty of peripheral venipuncture. Parasympathetic stimulation has no effect on blood vessels except for those in the face that react in the form of a blush (Guyton and Hall, 2006). Table 10-3 provides a list of autonomic effects on various body organs.

Numerous intravenous medications act on the autonomic nervous system. Adrenergic or sympathomimetic drugs stimulate organs that respond to the sympathetic system and include epinephrine, methoxamine, phenylephrine, isoproterenol, and albuterol. Other drugs block adrenergic activity, including reserpine, phentolamine, propranolol, and metoprolol. Parasympathomimetic drugs include pilocarpine and methacholine, while atropine and scopolamine block cholinergic activity.

ANATOMIC DIVISIONS
Central nervous system

The spinal cord extends from the medulla oblongata and occupies about two thirds of the length of the vertebral column. In most adults, the cord terminates between the first and second lumbar vertebrae. The cord is enclosed within three protective layers. The pia mater is the most proximal to the cord, the arachnoid mater is next, and the dura mater is the most distal. Between the pia and arachnoid mater is the subarachnoid space, which contains cerebrospinal fluid. The subdural space lies between the arachnoid and dura mater and does not contain fluid. The subdural space below the level of the cord can be used for the epidural infusion of medication, such as that used for pain management.

Peripheral nervous system

Twelve pairs of cranial nerves and 31 pairs of spinal nerves compose this system. Cranial nerves originate at the base of the brain and have four functions: motor, somatic sensory, special senses, and parasympathetic.

Of primary importance for parenteral therapy is the vagus nerve, which has the longest course of any cranial nerve. It descends behind the internal jugular vein, crosses the subclavian artery, and enters the thorax where it passes behind the brachiocephalic vein and superior vena cava (Figure 10-7). Numerous branches extend to the pharynx, larynx, heart, lungs, esophagus, stomach, liver, pancreas, spleen, small intestines, and kidneys. Six branches of the vagus nerve innervate the heart. Venipuncture of the internal jugular vein can result in damage to the vagus nerve (Nakayama et al, 1994).

The phrenic nerve arises from the cervical area of the neck and descends into the thorax where it serves as the motor nerve to the diaphragm. The right phrenic nerve follows the right brachiocephalic vein and superior vena cava while the left phrenic nerve lies close to the left subclavian artery, left brachiocephalic vein, and aortic arch (see Figure 10-7). Numerous reports link right phrenic nerve damage to both left- and right-sided insertions of central venous catheters. Paralysis of the diaphragm results, although shoulder pain is the most frequent initial symptom (Rigg et al, 1997; Aggarwal et al, 2000; Takasaki and Arai, 2001; Reeves and Anderson, 2002; Mandala et al, 2004).

The brachial plexus arises from cervical and thoracic spinal nerves, passing posteriorly to the clavicle in close proximity to the subclavian artery and vein. There are two large branches of this plexus: the supraclavicular and infraclavicular (Figure 10-8). These branches bifurcate into smaller nerves that serve the muscles and cutaneous areas of the shoulder, chest, and upper and lower arm. The close proximity of this group of nerves to the puncture sites of the subclavian vein makes damage to the nerves and ultimately the areas served by that nerve a real possibility.

The median, ulnar, and radial nerves are all branches of the brachial plexus. The median nerve passes laterally to the brachial artery and then crosses the artery, descending medially into the antecubital fossa and then into the forearm and palm of the hand. Branches of the median nerve can be superficial in the volar aspect or palm side of the wrist (Figure 10-9). Veins in this area appear to be good for cannulation, but venipuncture is usually painful in this area because of the close proximity of the nerve.

Multiple intersections between the cephalic vein and the sensory branches of the radial nerve were found when researchers dissected the forearm and wrists of 33 cadavers at the origin of the cephalic vein (Figure 10-10) (Vialle et al, 2001). The researchers suggest that to avoid nerve damage from venipuncture in the cephalic vein of the lower forearm, the insertion site should be at least 12 centimeters (cm) above the level of the styloid process at the distal end of the radius. Other reports of peripheral nerve damage resulting from venipuncture include the medial and lateral antebrachial cutaneous nerves in the antecubital fossa (Rayegani and Azadi, 2007), the posterior interosseous nerve branching from the radial nerve in the antecubital fossa (Ragoowansi, Kirkpatrick, Moss, 1999), the anterior interosseous nerve branching from the median nerve at the antecubital fossa (Zubairy, 2002; Puhaindran and Wong, 2003), and radial nerve injury in the wrist (Stahl, Kaufman, Ben-David, 1996; So et al, 1999; Boeson, Hranchook, Stoller, 2000).

In the lower extremity, the sacral plexus arises from the sacral vertebrae and descends the leg in much the same manner as the brachial plexus in the arm (Figure 10-11). Of particular importance is the medial plantar nerve, which passes on the medial aspect of the foot near the ankle. The saphenous nerve passes close to the saphenous vein on the anterior aspect of the foot. When the foot of an infant is used for venipuncture, with subsequent immobilization of the joint, the nerves can be damaged if adequate padding and range-of-motion exercises are not used.

THE THORACIC CAVITY

The borders and boundaries of the thorax help determine the optimal locations for catheter insertion and catheter tip placement. The presence of any catheter and the solutions infused can affect the physiology of the heart and lungs, in addition to the anatomy of the vessels.

TABLE 10-3 Autonomic Effects on Various Organs of the Body

Organ	Effect of sympathetic stimulation	Effect of parasympathetic stimulation
Eye		
Pupil	Dilated	Constricted
Ciliary muscle	Slight relaxation (far vision)	Constricted (near vision)
Glands		
Nasal	Vasoconstriction and slight secretion	Stimulation of copious
Lacrimal		secretions (containing many
Parotid		enzymes for enzyme-secreting glands)
Submandibular		
Gastric		
Pancreatic		
Sweat	Copious sweating (cholinergic)	Sweating on palms of hands
Apocrine	Thick, odoriferous secretion	None
Vasculature		
Blood vessels	Most often constricted	Most often little or no effect
Heart		
Muscle	Increased rate	Slowed rate
	Increased force of contraction	Decreased force of contraction (especially of atria)
Coronaries	Dilated (beta$_2$-adrenergic); constricted (alpha-adrenergic)	Dilated
Lungs		
Bronchi	Dilated	Constricted
Blood vessels	Mildly constricted	Dilated
Gut		
Lumen	Decreased peristalsis and tone	Increased peristalsis and tone
Sphincter	Increased tone (most times)	Relaxed (most times)
Liver	Glucose released	Slight glycogen synthesis
Gallbladder and bile ducts	Relaxed	Contracted
Kidney	Decreased output and renin secretion	None
Bladder/Genitourinary System		
Detrusor	Relaxed (slight)	Contracted
Trigone	Contracted	Relaxed
Penis	Ejaculation	Erection
Systemic Arterioles		
Abdominal viscera	Constricted	None
Muscle	Constricted (alpha-adrenergic)	None
	Dilated (beta$_2$-adrenergic)	
	Dilated (cholinergic)	
Skin	Constricted	None
Blood		
Coagulation	Increased	None
Glucose	Increased	None
Lipids	Increased	None
Other		
Basal metabolism	Increased up to 100%	None
Adrenal medullary secretion	Increased	None
Mental activity	Increased	None
Piloerector muscles	Contracted	None
Skeletal muscle	Increased glycogenolysis	None
	Increased strength	
Fat cells	Lipolysis	None

From Guyton A, Hall J: *Textbook of medical physiology*, ed 11, Philadelphia, 2006, Saunders.

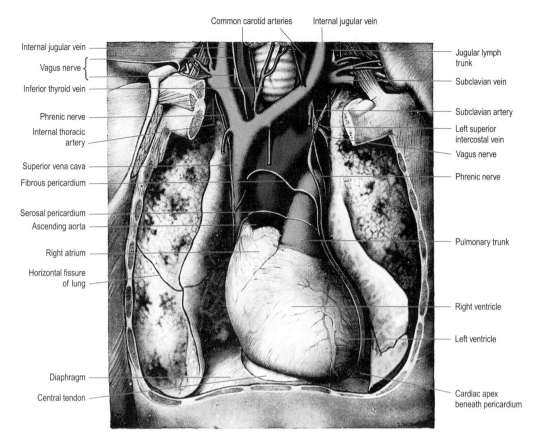

Common carotid arteries   Internal jugular vein

Internal jugular vein

Vagus nerve

Inferior thyroid vein

Phrenic nerve

Internal thoracic artery

Superior vena cava

Fibrous pericardium

Serosal pericardium

Ascending aorta

Right atrium

Horizontal fissure of lung

Diaphragm

Central tendon

Jugular lymph trunk

Subclavian vein

Subclavian artery

Left superior intercostal vein

Vagus nerve

Phrenic nerve

Pulmonary trunk

Right ventricle

Left ventricle

Cardiac apex beneath pericardium

FIGURE 10-7   Dissection that displays the heart, great vessels, and lungs. (From Standring S, editor: *Gray's anatomy*, ed 39, London, 2005, Churchill Livingstone.)

BONY THORAX

A framework of bone and cartilage surrounds the vital respiratory and circulatory structures of the thorax. The vertebrae of the spinal column form the posterior aspect. On the anterior aspect, the clavicles lie horizontally, connecting with the sternum to create the upper border.

The first rib curves from the first thoracic vertebra to the upper border of the sternum. This junction is difficult to palpate because the clavicle joins the sternum immediately in front of and superior to it (Figure 10-12). The costoclavicular ligament connects the first rib with the lower border of the clavicle close to the sternum. Motion of the sternoclavicular joint is involved with all shoulder movement. The first rib moves with respiration.

Subclavian vein cannulation in the medial aspect or close to the junction of the clavicle and first rib can have a negative outcome. Known as the *pinch-off syndrome*, the scissorlike action of these bones can sever the catheter, causing a catheter emboli (Pittiruti et al, 2000; Sarzo et al, 2004; de Graaff, Bras, Vos, 2006; Surov, Jordan, Burke, et al, 2006; Nuss et al, 2008). Positioning the patient in the Trendelenburg position with a rolled towel or sheet between the scapulas helps open the angle of these bones. When the patient is moved from this position, the angle is closed. The minimal clinical problem is compression of the catheter, causing difficult infusion. Irritation to the tunica intima of the vein could compound the problem, with the possibility of development of a thrombosis. Using a more lateral venipuncture location, at the axillary

vein, and then advancing into the central system can eliminate this problem.

The nerves and vascular structures in the thoracic outlet can be compressed by changes in normal anatomy caused by posture, physical activity, chronic illness, and occupation. Pain, muscle weakness and atrophy, and sensory changes result from these thoracic outlet syndromes. Arterial compression causes pallor of the fingers, while venous compression leads to edema and cyanosis. Venous cannulation can increase the risk of thrombosis in these patients (Urschel and Kourlis, 2007).

The kidney-shaped opening formed by the first rib, sternum, and vertebra is the *thoracic inlet*. It measures about 5 cm from front to back and about 10 cm from side to side, and is angled downward toward the anterior side (Standring, 2005). This small opening must accommodate many important structures, including the subclavian arteries and veins, carotid arteries, internal jugular vein, thymus gland and its muscles and nerves, trachea and esophagus, part of the brachial nerve plexus and vagus nerve, and the upper part of the pleura and apex of the lungs. Venous catheters inserted, terminating, or passing through the veins in this area could lead to complications affecting all these structures.

The sternum lies in the center of the anterior chest and is divided into three sections (Figure 10-13). Moving from top to bottom, the first section or manubrium is broad and thick and narrows toward the lower side. This section can be used for intraosseous infusion during emergencies in adults (Koschel, 2005). The midsection or body is long, narrow, and thin. The xiphoid process is the smallest section, extending into the epigastric region.

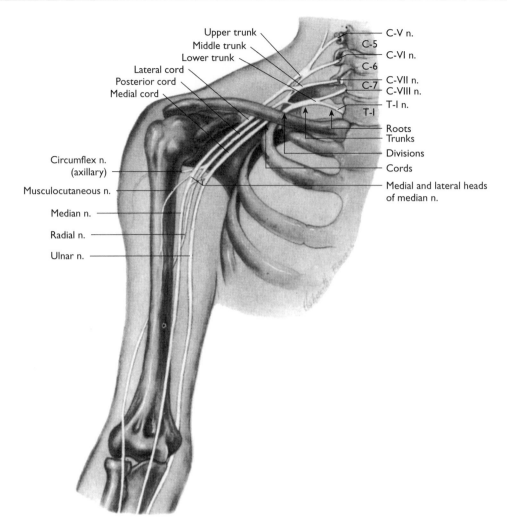

FIGURE 10-8 Brachial plexus and its skeletal relations. (From Jacob SW, Francone CA: *Elements of anatomy and physiology,* ed 2, Philadelphia, 1989, Saunders.)

There are 12 pairs of ribs encircling the thorax from the vertebrae to the sternum (see Figure 10-13). The upper seven pairs, known as true ribs, connect to the sternum by costal cartilages. Thoracic mobility and elasticity are directly related to the structure of this costal cartilage found between the ribs and sternum. The remaining five ribs are called false ribs, with the eighth, ninth, and tenth ribs attaching to the costal cartilage immediately above it. The eleventh and twelfth ribs are floating ribs without any attachment on the anterior side.

RESPIRATORY ANATOMY

The next layer of the thorax consists of the pleurae, or sacs, that cover the lungs. There are two layers of pleurae. The parietal pleura lines the internal surface of the ribs and costal cartilage, vertebrae, diaphragm, mediastinum, and lung apices. The visceral pleura adheres closely to all lung surfaces. Both pleurae easily slide over each other with the space between them called the pleural cavity. The elastic recoil of the lungs is opposed by the outward pull of the chest wall, thus creating negative pressure in this pleural space. Trauma, such as puncture during the insertion of a central venous catheter, results in air, fluid, blood, or lymph fluid accumulating in this space.

The mediastinum separates the lungs and can be divided into four parts (Figure 10-14). The superior mediastinum contains the internal thoracic arteries and veins; brachiocephalic veins and upper half of the superior vena cava; aortic arch; brachiocephalic, left common carotid, and subclavian arteries; left superior intercostal vein; vagus, cardiac, phrenic, and left recurrent laryngeal nerves; and the trachea, esophagus, thoracic duct, and superficial part of the cardiac plexus.

The anterior mediastinum extends between the sternum at the fourth costal cartilage to the pericardium, and contains loose connective tissue, ligaments, lymph nodes, and branches of the internal thoracic artery.

The middle mediastinum contains the heart, ascending aorta, lower half of the superior vena cava, azygos vein, tracheal bifurcations, and both main bronchi. The posterior mediastinum contains the pulmonary vessels, nerves, esophagus, thoracic duct, and lymph nodes.

The lungs sit on either side of the heart and are free inside the pleural cavity (Figure 10-15). Their only attachment is the heart, trachea, and pulmonary ligaments. In healthy adults, lungs are dark gray in color, feel spongy, and can float in water.

The trachea is a flexible tube made of cartilage and muscle tissue and is about 10 to 11 cm long. It extends from the larynx

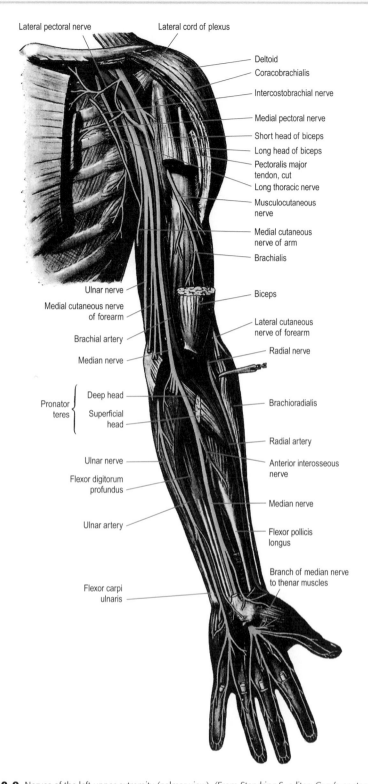

FIGURE 10-9 Nerves of the left upper extremity (palmar view). (From Standring S, editor: *Gray's anatomy,* ed 39, London, 2005, Churchill Livingstone.)

at the sixth cervical vertebra to the fifth thoracic vertebra where it divides into the right and left bronchi (see Figure 10-15). The carina, or the point where the left and right bronchi divide, is an important marker for assessing the proper location of a central venous catheter tip (Stonelake and Bodenham, 2006; Ryu et al, 2007). The bronchi continue to divide into bronchioles and then into alveoli, which are balloonlike structures where gas exchange takes place.

RESPIRATORY FUNCTION

The blood flows into the lungs through the pulmonary arteries, which carry deoxygenated blood. Pulmonary arteries and arterioles are short segments of vessels with large diameters. They have thin walls and are capable of distention, thus allowing for a large blood volume capacity. They follow the path of the bronchi, branching into smaller arterioles with a network of

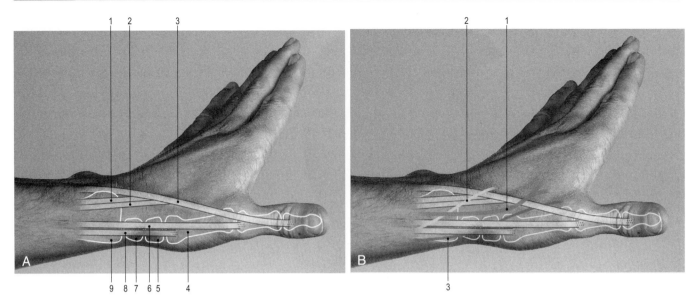

FIGURE 10-10 Radial aspect of the distal forearm and wrist. (From Lumley JSP: *Surface anatomy,* ed 4, London, 2008, Churchill Livingstone.)
PART A: 1. Tendon of extensor carpi radialis brevis. 2. Tendon of extensor carpi radialis longus. 3. Tendon of extensor pollicis longus. 4. First metacarpal. 5. Trapezium. 6. Tendon of extensor pollicis brevis. 7. Scaphoid. 8. Tendon of abductor pollicis longus. 9. Radial styloid.
PART B: 1. Cephalic vein. 2. Radial nerve. 3. Radial artery.

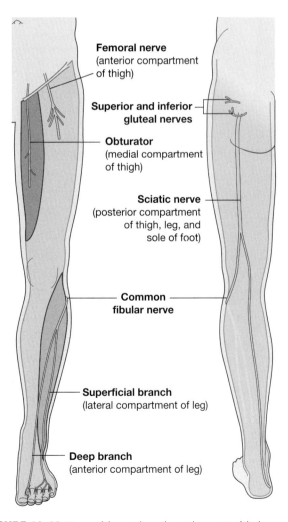

Femoral nerve
(anterior compartment
of thigh)

Superior and inferior
gluteal nerves

Obturator
(medial compartment
of thigh)

Sciatic nerve
(posterior compartment
of thigh, leg, and
sole of foot)

Common
fibular nerve

Superficial branch
(lateral compartment of leg)

Deep branch
(anterior compartment of leg)

FIGURE 10-11 Nerves of the anterior and posterior aspects of the lower extremity. (From Drake RL, Vogl W, Mitchell AMW: *Gray's anatomy for students,* London, 2005, Churchill Livingstone.)

capillaries surrounding each alveolus. The venous side of this same pathway, carrying oxygenated blood, follows the path of bronchioles, and becomes larger as it returns to the pulmonary veins. These veins are short and their ability to distend is about the same as that of the veins in the systemic circulation.

IV solutions contain many types of particulate matter. Undissolved drug particles, precipitate from incompatible drugs, rubber cores of vials or solution containers, glass particles from ampules, and plastic particles from administration sets make up this particulate matter. The most likely place for these particles to accumulate during intravenous infusion is the microcirculation of the lungs. The average diameter of pulmonary capillaries is about 5 micrometers (μm); the capillaries' small diameter acts as a trap for infused particles and requires red blood cells to change shape in order to pass through them (Guyton and Hall, 2006).

Clinical outcomes associated with infusion of particulate matter include pulmonary granulomas found on autopsy, local tissue infarction, and other forms of pulmonary dysfunction. An animal study demonstrated that particulate matter in antibiotic infusions lead to greater compromise of capillary perfusion in ischemic tissue, not normal tissue. This suggests that critically ill patients could suffer greater compromise to pulmonary function if receiving infusions containing large amounts of particulate matter. Filtration is the recommended method for removing these harmful insoluble particles at present (Lehr, Brunner, Rangoonwala et al, 2002; Kuramoto, Shoji, Nakagawa, 2006; Yorioka, Oie, Oomaki et al, 2006).

Gas exchange

Because the lungs expand and contract like balloons, pressures inside the chest are of great importance. The negative pressure in the pleural space becomes more negative during inspiration. Alveolar pressure, or the pressure inside the alveoli, is equal to atmospheric pressure when no air is moving in or out of the lungs and the glottis is open. When the alveolar pressure

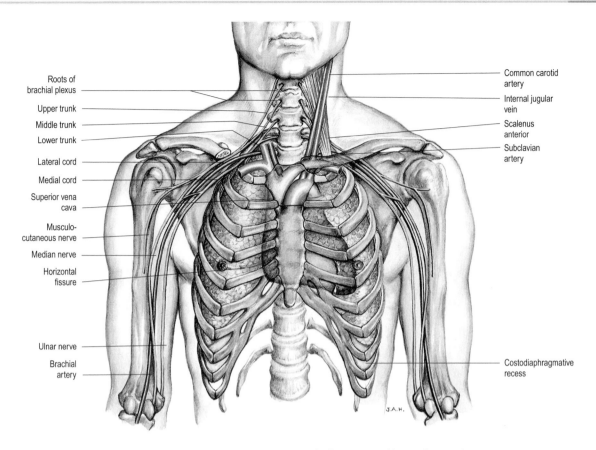

Roots of
brachial plexus

Upper trunk

Middle trunk

Lower trunk

Lateral cord

Medial cord

Superior vena
cava

Musculo-
cutaneous nerve

Median nerve

Horizontal
fissure

Ulnar nerve

Brachial
artery

Common carotid
artery

Internal jugular
vein

Scalenus
anterior

Subclavian
artery

Costodiaphragmative
recess

J.A.H.

FIGURE 10-12 Anterior view of the thorax, root of neck, and axilla. (From Standring S, editor: *Gray's anatomy,* ed 39, London, 2005, Churchill Livingstone.)

falls, inspiration occurs. With about 500 mL of air inside, the pressure rises above atmospheric pressure and expiration occurs. The Valsalva maneuver increases the chest pressure by holding air in the lungs against a closed glottis.

To prevent an air embolus, positive pressure in the chest is necessary when manipulating any catheter whose tip lies within the thorax. Inserting the catheter, changing administration sets, inadvertently disconnecting the tubing, and removing the catheter can place the patient at risk for an air embolus.

Gases, such as oxygen, carbon dioxide, and nitrogen, dissolved in water or body fluids exert the same pressure and movement as in the gaseous state. Gas molecules in the alveoli are still in the gaseous state, whereas gas molecules in the blood are dissolved. Transfer of the molecules occurs because of the partial pressure exerted by each gas. The partial pressure of oxygen in its gaseous state inside the alveoli is greater than the partial pressure of oxygen in the blood, so this pressure forces oxygen to move into the pulmonary membrane and into the capillary. The same is true for carbon dioxide—its partial pressure is greater in the blood so the transfer is in the opposite direction, from the blood across the membrane and into the alveolar sac.

Although the respiratory membrane is extremely thin, it is composed of several layers (Figure 10-16). The capillary is so small that a red blood cell must squeeze through the lumen, with the gases diffusing directly into and out of each red cell without passing through plasma. Although this individual unit is extremely small, there are about 300 million alveoli in both lungs. The surface area of the respiratory membrane covers about 70 m^2 in a normal adult (Guyton and Hall, 2006). With

gaseous exchange over such a large area, the speed of diffusion is understandable.

THE HEART

The heart lies at an oblique angle in the middle mediastinum between each lung. About one third of the heart lies to the right of the midline in the chest.

Heart wall

The heart is enclosed in a protective sac, called the *pericardium,* that extends between the second and sixth costal cartilages. The great vessels leading away from and into the heart are also enclosed in the pericardium (see Figure 10-7).

The pericardium has two layers: an outer fibrous layer and an inner serous layer. The fibrous layer is composed of strong collagen fibers and covers the aorta, superior vena cava, right and left pulmonary arteries, and the four pulmonary veins. This fibrous layer is actually a continuation of the adventitia of the great vessels and is not attached to the heart itself.

The serosal pericardium is further divided into the parietal and visceral layers. The parietal layer lies next to the fibrous pericardium, and the visceral layer or epicardium covers the heart. Between these two layers is a thin film of fluid that allows the heart to move. Vascular access devices within the great vessels and heart inside the pericardium have the potential to erode through the wall. The following two clinical conditions can occur: (1) pericardial effusion, with fluid leaking between the layers of the pericardium, or (2) cardiac

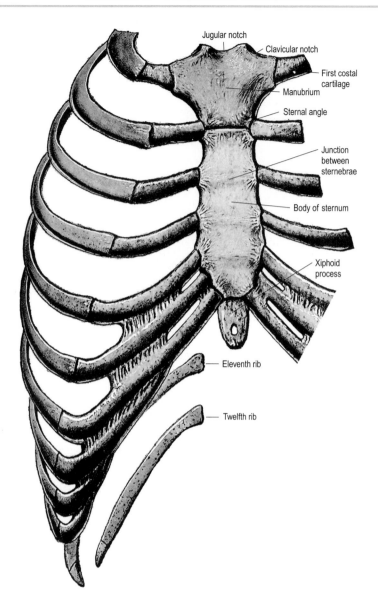

FIGURE 10-13 The sternum and costal cartilages, anterior aspect. (From Standring S, editor: *Gray's anatomy*, ed 39, London, 2005, Churchill Livingstone.)

tamponade, with the blood and fluid exerting pressure on the heart.

The endocardium is the innermost layer of the heart and is composed of a single layer of endothelial cells. This is a continuation of the same endothelial layer as that found on the internal surface of all arteries and veins.

Right side of the heart

The superior and inferior vena cava join the atrium of the right side of the heart on the posterior aspect. The superior vena cava returns blood from the upper part of the body and has no valve. The inferior vena cava returns blood from the lower part of the body, is larger than the superior vena cava, and has a semilunar valve near the opening into the atrium. Approximately 80% of blood flow moves through the atria without muscular contraction of the atria. The remaining 20% of blood flow moves to the ventricles because of atrial contraction; thus inadequate atrial contraction may remain unnoticed with normal physical activity (Guyton and Hall, 2006). A groove in the heart's exterior,

known as the sulcus terminalis, indicates the point where the vein becomes the atrium. This groove corresponds to the internal crest of the right atrium where the sinoatrial node is located.

Cardiac function

Cardiac output, the quantity of blood pumped into the aorta each minute, is regulated by changes in the volume of blood flowing into the heart and by the autonomic nervous system's control of the heart. *Venous return* is the amount of blood flowing into the right atrium each minute. The heart has a unique ability to pump out all that is returned, avoiding any pooling of blood in the veins. This is known as the *Frank-Starling mechanism*. For this reason, the heart can adapt easily to normal changes such as increased exercise. The force of the contractions increases as the heart chambers stretch to accommodate larger volumes. Stretching the right atrium also stretches the sinoatrial node, which signals an increase in the heart rate. It also initiates a nervous reflex that passes to the brain and back to the heart through the sympathetic nerves

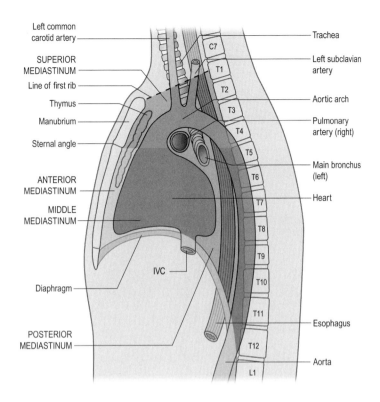

FIGURE 10-14 The major divisions of the mediastinum. (From Standring S, editor: *Gray's anatomy,* ed 39, London, 2005, Churchill Livingstone.)

and the vagus nerve to increase the rate. Cardiac contractions also require a delicate balance of potassium and calcium ions in the extracellular fluids, and can be altered from increased or decreased body temperature.

Cardiac conduction system

The impulse for cardiac contraction begins in the sinoatrial or S-A node (Figure 10-17). The impulse spreads through all the atrial muscle fibers until it reaches the atrioventricular or A-V node, located on the posterior wall of the right atrium near the tricuspid valve. The A-V bundle leads to the ventricles, allowing for impulse conduction in a one-way direction. The S-A node acts as the heart's pacemaker because it can fire impulses faster than the other components of the electrical system. Catheters passing the S-A node can be detected by changes in the P wave on an electrocardiograph (Gebhard et al, 2007).

THE GREAT VESSELS

The pulmonary vessels, the superior and inferior vena cava, and the aorta are considered to be the great vessels of the thorax (Figure 10-18).

The superior vena cava begins where the left and right brachiocephalic veins join. It is about 7 cm long, extending from the inferior border of the first costal cartilage behind the sternum to the level of the third costal cartilage, where it joins the right atrium. The lower half is inside the fibrous pericardium from the level of the second intercostal cartilage.

A variation of the anatomy of the superior vena cava can lead to the creation of a right and left location, or the superior vena cava being exclusively on the left side of the mediastinum. Known as a persistent left superior vena cava (PLSVC), this congenital anomaly occurs in 0.3% of healthy individuals, and in 2% to 4.4% of those with other cardiac anomalies (Miraldi et al, 2002). In the early embryo stages, the bilateral cardinal veins drain the head, neck, and arm into the right atrium. As the cardiovascular system develops, the left cardinal vein disappears to form the coronary sinus, the primary vessel for returning blood from the cardiac muscle to the heart. Failure of this change leaves a left superior vena cava, which is usually draining into the coronary sinus and then into the right atrium. Most people with this anomaly have a normal right superior vena cava and have no pathological problem; however, the left superior vena cava can join the left atrium, resulting in mild cyanosis (Miraldi et al, 2002). Absence of the right superior vena cava has also been reported when the insertion of a central venous catheter was reported to be an arterial placement (Azocar et al, 2002; Kamola and Seidner, 2004). The decision to allow a catheter to remain in a PLSVC depends upon angiographic documentation of blood flow into the right versus the left atrium (Shyamkumar and Brown, 2007).

The inferior vena cava returns blood from the lower half of the body. It passes through the diaphragm at the level of the eighth and ninth thoracic vertebrae, and then ascends to join the right atrium on the lower posterior side. The intrathoracic portion is short and covered by the fibrous pericardium; however, this is the preferred tip location for central venous catheters inserted via the femoral vein (Lynch et al, 2002).

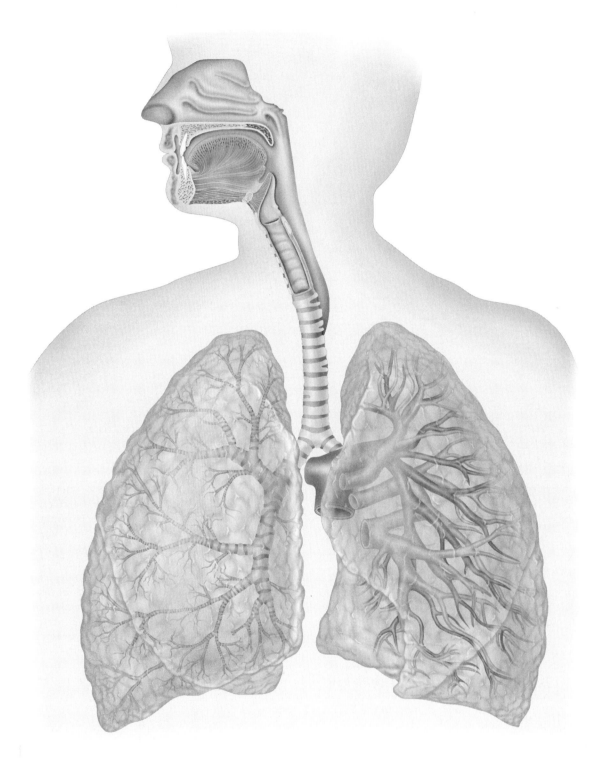

FIGURE 10-15 The respiratory tract. (From Standring S, editor: *Gray's anatomy,* ed 39, London, 2005, Churchill Livingstone.)

The pulmonary artery carries deoxygenated blood from the right ventricle to the lungs. It is about 5 cm long and is entirely within the pericardium. It branches to the right and left pulmonary arteries, usually following the path of the bronchi. After oxygenation, blood is returned to the left atrium through the pulmonary vein.

After passing through the left side of the heart, blood is pumped to the body through the aorta. It leaves the left ventricle on the lower side and ascends to the second left costal cartilage. The ascending aorta is enclosed in the fibrous pericardium. It continues into the aortic arch lying in the superior mediastinum and is very visible on chest radiographs. The

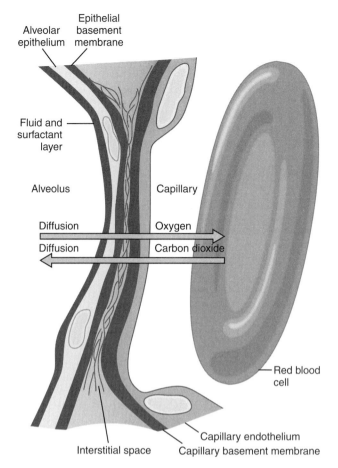

FIGURE 10-16 Ultrastructure of the alveolar respiratory membrane, shown in cross-section. (From Guyton AC, Hall JE: *Textbook of medical physiology*, ed 11, Philadelphia, 2006, Saunders.)

brachiocephalic arteries, left common carotid artery, and left subclavian arteries branch from the top of the aortic arch, although there can be many variations of this pattern. The descending aorta lies in the posterior mediastinum and extends from the fourth to the twelfth thoracic vertebra.

OTHER THORACIC STRUCTURES
Thymus gland

Consisting of two lobes, this endocrine gland lies primarily in the superior and anterior mediastinum. Its size varies with age, being larger in children and adolescents. Thymus-processed lymphocytes or T lymphocytes are created in the bone marrow, and then migrate to the thymus gland where each cell develops its reactivity for specific antigens. Additionally, the thymus gland ensures that these lymphocytes will not react to the body's own protein or other self-antigens. Most of this cell processing happens immediately before and for a few months after birth.

Thoracic duct

The lymph channels throughout the body drain excessive fluid and large particles that cannot be absorbed into the bloodstream. The thoracic duct connects the lymph system and bloodstream and is located in the base of the neck (Figure 10-19). The most common site for this junction is near the convergence of the left internal jugular and left subclavian veins. Variations

include termination into the left internal jugular vein, the left subclavian vein, or the left brachiocephalic vein. Insertion of central venous catheters in this region could damage the thoracic duct, leading to leakage of lymph fluid or chyle into the pleural space or from the puncture site. There is a smaller lymphatic trunk on the right side.

PERIPHERAL VASCULAR SYSTEM

For oxygen and carbon dioxide to be transferred at the cellular level, blood must reach all tissues of the body through an immense network of interconnecting tubes. Anatomical names for these tubes, based on size and structure, include arteries, arterioles, capillaries, venules, and veins. They may also be described in functional terms as vessels of distribution (arteries), resistance (arterioles), exchange (capillaries), capacitance (venules), or reservoir (veins). Small venules act as exchange vessels and larger venules act as reservoirs.

BLOOD VESSEL STRUCTURE

The walls of all arteries and veins are arranged in three layers: the tunica intima (innermost layer), tunica media (middle layer), and tunica adventitia (outer layer) (Figure 10-20). These layers have structural differences determined by the location and function of each vessel (Table 10-4).

The tunica intima is made up of a single layer of smooth, flat endothelial cells that lie along the length of each vessel, subendothelial connective tissue, and a basal lamina or basement membrane. The tunica media contains smooth muscle and other fibrous tissue, and is arranged around the circumference of the vessel. The tunica adventitia is connective tissue whose fibers are arranged along the length of the vessel. There is much variation in these tunicas, depending on the type of vessel.

All blood vessels, lymphatic vessels, and the heart are lined with endothelium, which is a single layer of flat, smooth cells with a thickness ranging from 0.2 μm up to 3 m (Standring, 2005). These cells are arranged along the length of the vessel and are firmly attached to each other at their edges. This layer of cells rests on a basement membrane to provide additional support. Each cell is linked together to form occluding or tight junctions, which prevent the leakage of fluids and cells from the vessel. Capillary walls are characterized by a thin endothelial structure, the presence of more junctions between cells, and fenestrations or openings in the cells, which allow for the rapid transfer of fluid and other substances. Biochemical mediators such as histamine, serotonin, leukotrienes, prostaglandins, and bradykinin alter vascular permeability by creating a separation of these cells.

Smooth muscle in the tunica media is composed of long, tapered spindles of muscle fibers. These spindles are arranged in bundles or layers around the circumference of the vessel and contract together as a single unit. Each bundle is closely arranged so that their cell membranes adhere in numerous places. The action potential for each bundle stimulates the remaining ones by communicating gap junctions through which ions flow freely. Smooth muscles of blood vessels are capable of maintaining contraction or a state of tension for lengthy periods. Several other differences exist between the function of smooth muscles and skeletal muscles. Compared to skeletal muscles, the force of contraction is greater in smooth muscles

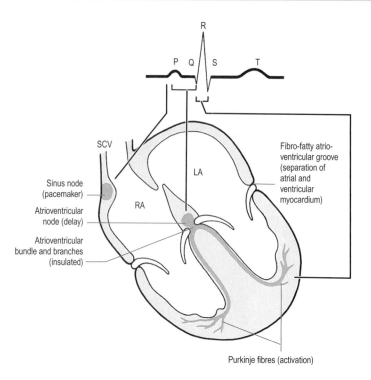

FIGURE 10-17 The basic conduction system of the heart. (From Standring S, editor: *Gray's anatomy,* ed 39, London, 2005, Churchill Livingstone.)

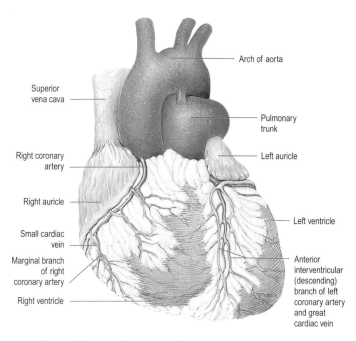

FIGURE 10-18 The heart and great vessels. (From Standring S, editor: *Gray's anatomy,* ed 39, London, 2005, Churchill Livingstone.)

and less energy is required to maintain contraction. Also, smooth muscles can shorten by two thirds during contraction, thus allowing the vessel lumen to change from very large to extremely small. This strong venous contraction could make it difficult to remove some midline and peripherally inserted central catheters.

The stress-relaxation phenomenon of smooth muscles is another important aspect of blood vessel physiology. When a tourniquet is placed on the extremity to distend peripheral

veins, the elastic tissue in the vessel wall allows immediate distention. This is followed by elongation of smooth muscle fibers to accommodate the increased volume collecting in the veins. The pressure increases quickly and then returns toward the normal level, even with the increased volume. When the tourniquet is removed, the volume and pressure suddenly fall, and within several minutes, the normal pressure is reestablished. Knowledge of this process is crucial when timing the removal of a tourniquet and advancing long catheters into the

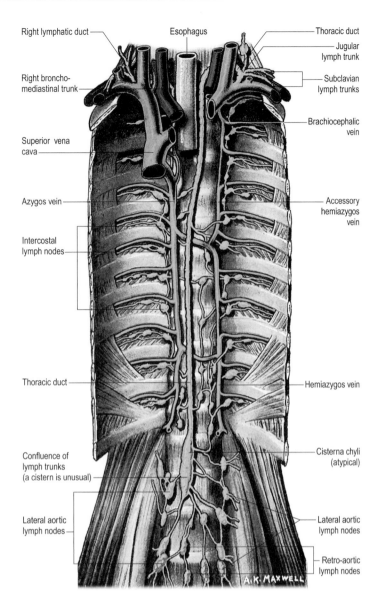

Right lymphatic duct

Esophagus

Thoracic duct

Jugular
lymph trunk

Right broncho-
mediastinal trunk

Subclavian
lymph trunks

Brachiocephalic
vein

Superior vena
cava

Azygos vein

Accessory
hemiazygos
vein

Intercostal
lymph nodes

Thoracic duct

Hemiazygos vein

Confluence of
lymph trunks
(a cistern is unusual)

Cisterna chyli
(atypical)

Lateral aortic
lymph nodes

Lateral aortic
lymph nodes

Retro-aortic
lymph nodes

A.K. MAXWELL

FIGURE 10-19 The thoracic and right lymphatic ducts. (From Standring S, editor: *Gray's anatomy,* ed 39, London, 2005, Churchill Livingstone.)

vein. Obstruction may be encountered if not enough time has elapsed to allow equilibrium to return.

Another characteristic of smooth muscles is excitation by stretch. When smooth muscles have been excessively stretched, the muscles contract to automatically resist that stretch. This explains what happens when a tourniquet has been left in place for an extended period and the veins can no longer be palpated.

Stimulation of the tunica media by trauma or changes in temperature and pressure can lead to vascular spasm. If an artery is affected, the result is an interruption in the flow of blood to the area served by that artery, with possible necrosis of that tissue. When this occurs in a vein, the outcome is not as negative, but the patient experiences pain at the site from a change in the blood flow.

The aorta, the major branches of the aorta, and the pulmonary arteries are elastic arteries. The flow of blood is rapid and under high pressure; so these vessels need to be composed of a large amount of elastic tissue. This allows for a high degree of

distensibility, especially during ventricular systole when blood is forced into these arteries. Medium and small arteries are muscular arteries, containing more muscular tissue, and are capable of controlling blood flow by constriction and dilation. Distention and recoil keep blood flowing during diastole in a smooth yet pulsatile manner.

As arteries branch and become smaller in diameter, they are known as *arterioles.* They further subdivide into terminal arterioles and metarterioles. All are considered resistance vessels. On the capillary end of each metarteriole is a precapillary sphincter, which controls the flow of blood through the capillary bed.

The venous side of the circulation is known for its compliance or the ability to increase in volume with a given increase in pressure. The amount of elastic tissue found in the wall of the vessel is the primary reason for the difference in compliance or capacitance. About three times more of the circulating volume of blood is located on the venous side than the arterial side. Because of the ability of the venous walls to distend about 6 to 10

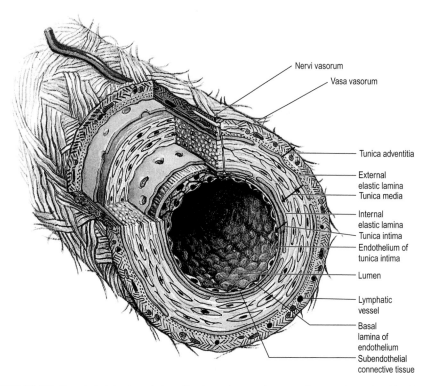

FIGURE 10-20 The principal structure of a large blood vessel as seen in a muscular artery. (From Standring S, editor: *Gray's anatomy,* ed 39, London, 2005, Churchill Livingstone.)

TABLE 10-4 **Structural Differences in Blood Vessels in Arterial and Venous Walls**

Layer	Arteries	Arterioles (lumen diameter <0.5 mm)	Capillaries	Venules	Veins
Tunica intima	Elastic arteries—elongated endothelial cells, multiple layer subendothelial tissue, and fenestrated elastic membrane; thicken with age and fatty deposits; contain baroreceptors and chemoreceptors Muscular arteries—thinner, allowing diffusion of metabolites; contain other afferent nerve fibers	Thin layer of endothelial cells with basal lamina	Single cell layer of endothelium and thin basal lamina	Endothelial layer and basal lamina	Endothelial layer of shorter, broader cells and basal lamina
Tunica media	Elastic arteries—thicker with more elastic and fibrous tissue arranged in circular bands; respond to pumping action of heart Muscular arteries— large mass of smooth muscle fibers controlling constriction and relaxation	Decreasing amounts of elastin; muscle cells form communicating (gap) junctions, allowing diffusion of ions and electrical stimulation	No middle layer	Small venules—no middle layer Larger venules—thin layer of smooth muscle	Thick layer of connective tissue with elastin fibers and smooth muscle fibers, although thinner than same layer in arteries
Tunica adventitia	Elastic arteries—layer of collagen and elastic fibers, mast cells, nerve bundles and lymphatic vessels, and vasa vasorum Muscular arteries—contain collagen and elastin; contain vasa vasorum, lymphatic channels, and both efferent and afferent nerve fibers	Fine collagen fibers; contain vasa vasorum, lymphatic channels, and efferent nerve fibers	Thin reticular tissue with occasional fibroblasts and mast cells	Thin fibrous tissue	Loose connective tissue, with elastin fibers; contain vasa vasorum and afferent and sympathetic nerves

times more than the arterial walls, a small increase in pressure results in a much larger quantity of blood in any vein. The same pressure increase in a corresponding artery would not result in a volume increase.

Blood is supplied to the vessel walls by the vasa vasorum, a dense capillary network within the tunica adventitia of each vessel. This capillary network may be a branch of the artery it serves or may be from a distant artery. In veins, this network may penetrate to the tunica media.

Sympathetic nerves are located in the adventitia of large arteries and veins. A steady flow of impulses is sent from the vasomotor center in the medulla and pons of the brain to maintain the vasomotor tone, which is a partial state of contraction of all vessels. Norepinephrine, the neurotransmitter at the synapse of these sympathetic nerves, acts on the alpha-adrenergic receptors of the smooth muscles in the vessels to cause contraction. This state of contraction supports the arterial pressure and keeps blood moving back to the heart. There are no nerve endings in vessels that directly cause vasodilation. Instead, a decrease in the impulses causing vasomotor tone leads to vasodilation. Also located in the intima and adventitia of systemic arteries are afferent peripheral nerves. Some of these may carry pain impulses, whereas others are baroreceptors and chemoreceptors (see Table 10-2).

Valves are found in veins but not in arteries. Valves are semilunar folds, extending from the tunica intima into the lumen of the vein (Figure 10-21). They are composed of collagen and elastin fibers covered with endothelial cells. Usually, valves are arranged in pairs, but there can be three folds or leaflets together as well as a single leaflet at other locations. Valves can be found in most veins, except for extremely small or large ones. They can be found at bifurcations or where two veins unite. However, there is little or no documentation about any specific locations for valves within the superficial veins used for venipuncture, probably because of the great variations among individuals. On the proximal side of each valve the vein wall expands, creating a sinus above each valve. When veins are distended, such as with the application of a tourniquet, venous blood flow is temporarily stopped. This creates a pooling of blood in these sinuses and yields a "knotted" appearance externally.

The purpose of valves is to keep blood moving toward the heart by way of the muscle pump, sometimes called the *venous pump* (Figure 10-22). With the contraction of each muscle during movement, pressure is applied to the vein, forcing blood back toward the heart. This pumping action opens the proximal valve and closes the distal valve, preventing a backward flow. Venous blood flow in all extremities is against gravity, resulting in a great rise in venous pressure if this pumping system fails. When valves become damaged or incompetent, pressure rises in the distal end of the extremity. The pooling of blood in capillaries causes fluid to leak outside the circulatory system, resulting in edema and a decreased blood volume. This muscle pump may have an impact on catheters made of soft, flexible material, causing them to migrate out of the vein. This may occur more often with patients in the alternative care setting who are engaged in normal activities of daily living. Catheter compression also leads to the expulsion of the locking fluid from the lumen with subsequent reflux of blood into the lumen when the compression is relieved.

The normal pattern of blood flow is through the aorta, which branches into smaller arteries, but there are some deviations from this pattern. Rather than ending in an arteriole, two arteries may anastomose and bypass the capillary bed. This occurs in some arteries in the brain, intestines, and joints. An arteriovenous anastomosis is a small artery and vein connected together. These may be found in mucous membranes and deep

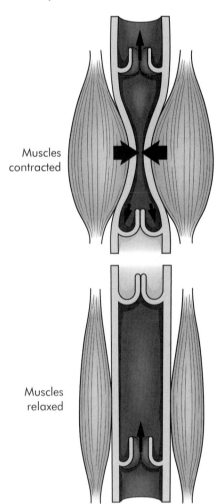

FIGURE 10-22 Muscle pump. (From Huether SE, McCance KL: *Understanding pathophysiology,* ed 4, St Louis, 2008, Mosby.)

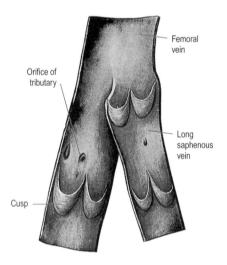

FIGURE 10-21 Venous valves of the upper portion of the femoral and long saphenous veins. (From Standring S, editor: *Gray's anatomy,* ed 39, London, 2005, Churchill Livingstone.)

in the dermis of the hands and feet. The venous side is affected by the higher pressure from the arterial side, and may result in unsuccessful venipuncture attempts in this area.

ENDOTHELIAL CELL FUNCTION

Important functions of endothelial cells include control of blood flow to the tissues, angiogenesis, thrombosis development, response to inflammation, and response to injury that leads to formation of atherosclerosis. Endothelial cells of small arteries and arterioles release *endothelium-derived relaxing factor* (EDRF), which is mostly composed of nitric oxide and has a half-life of 6 seconds (Guyton and Hall, 2006). The demand for more blood by tissue produces shear stress. The viscous nature of blood drags against the vessel wall, causing the endothelial cells to warp or change shape in the direction of the blood flow. This stress releases nitric oxide, which leads to relaxation of the blood vessels and increases the blood flow in upstream arteries. *Endothelin* is a peptide derived from endothelial cells that produces strong vasoconstriction with very small quantities. It is released from the cells after injury to blood vessels as a mechanism to prevent excessive bleeding (Loesch, 2005; Guyton and Hall, 2006).

Angiogenesis or the growth of new blood vessels is caused by other peptides including *vascular endothelial growth factor (VEGF)*, *fibroblast growth factor*, and *angiogenin*. These peptides cause a new vessel to develop from other small vessels. The basement membrane of an endothelial cell dissolves, followed by new endothelial cells quickly developing in a stream flowing outward through the vessel wall. These new cells form a cord that folds over to form a tube. This tube connects with another tube budding from another nearby vessel to form a capillary loop, and blood begins to flow through it. With substantial blood flow through this loop, smooth muscle cells invade and this loop grows into a new arteriole or venule or even a larger vessel. This phenomenon causes the creation of collateral circulation around an area of arterial or venous obstruction. This occurs rapidly with about half of the tissue's blood flow needs met within 1 day and all tissue needs met within a few days (Guyton and Hall, 2006). Angiogenesis related to VEGF is a major factor in many diseases such as cancer, eye disorders, and rheumatoid arthritis. Currently, a humanized monoclonal antibody to VEGF is available for treating metastatic colorectal cancer, and it is possible that future medications based on VEGF will be used to treat ischemic heart disease (Holmes and Zachary, 2005).

Several mechanisms prevent clot formation. The surface of the endothelial layer is smooth, allowing for blood to flow uninterrupted. A glycocalyx or mucopolysaccharide layer is absorbed to the surface of endothelial cells to repel platelets and other clotting factors. *Thrombomodulin* is a protein bound to the endothelial surface that binds thrombin. The thrombomodulin-thrombin complex slows the clotting process, along with activating protein C, another anticoagulant. Damage to the endothelial layer roughens the surface and causes the loss of the glycocalyx. This loss activates factor XII and platelets, triggering the intrinsic clotting cascade (Guyton and Hall, 2006).

Endothelial cells play an active role in the process of resolving acute inflammation and their failure can be associated with chronic inflammation. Leukocytes must adhere to the endothelial cells, which then allow the leukocytes to pass through the vein wall to the site of inflammation. The endothelial cells contract during this process, resulting in increased permeability and fluid leakage. These cells also produce endothelin-1, angiotensin II, and inflammatory cytokines such as interleukin-1 that increase permeability of the vascular wall. It then must reverse course upon resolution of the inflammation to prevent excessive fluid extravasation. When diseases such as hypertension or diabetes have altered the functionality of endothelial cells, these normal changes may not occur, thus promoting chronic inflammation (Kadl and Leitinger, 2005; Khazaei et al, 2008).

Hypercholesterolemia and cigarette smoking also contribute to endothelial dysfunction by enhancing the proinflammatory and prothrombotic state, allowing monocytes to adhere and penetrate the vascular wall. These conditions along with increased levels of C-reactive protein lead to atherosclerotic plaque. Additionally, plaque rupture is aggravated by overproduction of fibrinolytic agents such as plasminogen activator inhibitor-1 (Khazaei et al, 2008).

An additional iatrogenic cause of endothelial damage can be the introduction of microbubbles through the infusion of solutions. Although we have long known about the dangers of large venous air emboli, we now have an appreciation for the results of small bubbles that had previously been regarded as "harmless." Bubbles can be caused by turbulent fluid flow in IV administration sets and catheters or by warming of solutions being infused. Small bubbles are more buoyant and are easily carried by fluid flow, thus allowing them easier passage into the bloodstream. These bubbles float in the bloodstream until they become trapped in small capillaries, where the normal force of blood flow compresses the bubbles against the endothelial cells and causes detachment of the endothelial cells. Tissue ischemia is seen above and below the site of the bubble in the capillary, in addition to changes in pressure inside the vessel and the interstitium. Animal studies have demonstrated repeated air emboli lead to thickening of pulmonary arteries and pulmonary hypertension (Barak and Katz, 2005). Activation of complement proteins, enhancement of the inflammatory reactions, and increased platelet aggregation and clotting are also associated with microbubbles. The limited clinical information associated with microbubbles is derived from the study of decompression sickness associated with extreme sports such as diving. Mild complaints include joint pain and skin rash, while more severe forms include headache, blurred vision, paresthesias, convulsions, and death. Lung function changes attributed to microbubbles in divers include thickening of bronchiole walls and loss of lung elasticity. Large amounts of microbubbles can easily be produced from cardiopulmonary bypass, hemodialysis, mechanical heart valves, and very high infusion flow rates in shock-trauma situations and major surgeries. Prevention by trapping these bubbles in an in-line filter appears to be the most effective method, although current filters may not meet the demands of these high-flow clinical situations (Barak and Katz, 2005; Barak Nakhoul, and Katz, 2008).

Numerous other factors that promote coagulation or induce fibrinolysis can be found in the endothelium, including tissue plasminogen activator, plasminogen activator inhibitor, and von Willebrand factor (Guyton and Hall, 2006). Damage to these cells is the beginning of the inflammation process of phlebitis and of the clotting process that can cause thrombosis. The endothelial cells of veins and arteries can be damaged by the following:

- Rapid catheter advancement
- Catheter advancement without anchoring the skin and vein by holding traction on the skin

- Insertion of catheter too large for lumen of vein
- Insertion of catheter close to area of joint flexion without adequate support from arm boards
- Inadequate catheter stabilization, allowing for motion of catheter
- Inadequate skin preparation, allowing for invasion of microorganisms
- Nonocclusive, dirty, or wet dressing, allowing for invasion of microorganisms
- Location of catheter tip that causes impingement of tip on vein wall
- Infusion of particulate matter
- Infusion of hypertonic or hypotonic solutions
- Infusion of solution with an extremely high or low pH
- Rapid infusion of quantities too large for vessel lumen to accommodate

LOCATION OF IMPORTANT ARTERIES

The axillary artery extends from the first rib to the lateral edge of the chest in the axilla. The axillary sheath is a neurovascular bundle containing the axillary artery, axillary vein, and parts of the brachial nerve plexus controlling the arm. The continuation of the axillary artery is the brachial artery, which moves down the arm to immediately below the elbow. There it divides into the ulnar artery, on the medial side of the arm, and the radial artery, on the lateral side of the arm (see Figures 10-9 and 10-12).

Although the radial artery is smaller than the ulnar artery, it is preferred for arterial puncture for blood withdrawal and catheter insertion because it is more superficial and can be stabilized for easier entry. It is imperative that Allen's test be performed to assess the collateral circulation. This is done by locating and compressing both arteries and noting the blanching that occurs. When only the ulnar artery is released, color should return to the entire hand, indicating the ability of this artery to supply blood to the whole hand. If this positive assessment cannot be made, another site should be chosen.

Unintentional intra-arterial injection can have a devastating impact on the patient, involving both acute and chronic problems. The antecubital fossa is known as a high-risk area because veins and arteries are located very close to each other. The first complaints appear within seconds and range from mild irritation to intense pain distal to the injection site. Tingling and burning are followed by involuntary muscle contractures and weakness, along with changes in the skin such as flushing or mottling. Signs of vascular compromise appear within 7 to 10 days and include pain, absence of peripheral pulses, cyanosis, and paralysis, often indicting the beginning of compartment syndrome. Tissue necrosis, complex regional pain syndrome, and even amputation can be the clinical outcomes. A short peripheral catheter may show pulsatile blood backflow; however, this may not be obvious in a longer central venous catheter. Pressure transduction or blood gas analysis may be the only methods to confirm arterial placement (Sen ,Chini, Brown, 2005). Although these may require more time, it is well worth the investment to avoid the ruinous outcomes that could occur.

LOCATION OF IMPORTANT VEINS

Systemic veins can be divided into three types: superficial, deep, and perforating veins. Deep veins accompany arteries, usually of the same name, known as *venae comitantes*. Deep

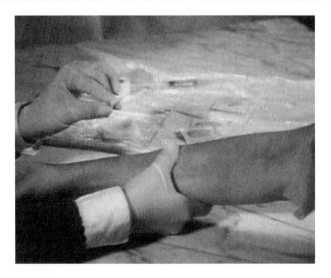

FIGURE 10-23 Holding traction on the skin over a vein during complete catheter advancement will secure the vein and prevent damage to the endothelium of the vein.

veins, arteries, and nerves are enclosed in a protective sheath of connective tissue. Superficial veins, best suited for venipuncture, lie in loose connective tissue under the skin. This location allows for easy movement of these veins. Therefore, during any attempt to cannulate a vein, some method must be used to anchor the vein. Without securing the vein, puncture and advancement of the catheter result in unnecessary damage to the endothelium of the vein and could lead to phlebitis. Using one hand to hold traction on the skin over the vein during complete catheter advancement secures the vein (Figure 10-23). Perforating veins connect deep and superficial veins and can be found near the origin of the cephalic vein in the wrist, and in numerous locations connecting the deep brachial veins of the upper arm with superficial veins (Figure 10-24).

The primary veins used to initiate IV therapy are the superficial veins in the hand and forearm. Both upper extremities should be assessed carefully (Table 10-5). Small digital veins line the borders of the fingers and unite on the back of the hand to form the dorsal venous network (Figure 10-25). On the lateral aspect of the wrist, proximal to the thumb, the cephalic vein rises from the dorsal veins. Close to this area are perforating veins, which pierce the deep fascia and connect the superficial veins with the deeper veins of the hand. The cephalic vein at this location is large enough for the insertion of a catheter, but there are several points to consider. The motion of the wrist may increase the patient's general discomfort, and irritation to the tunica intima results from movement of the catheter. Also, there are three long tendons that control the motion of the thumb. Although the vein is superficial to these tendons, slight movement of the thumb during the venipuncture procedure could easily obscure the vein (see Figure 10-10). The cephalic vein moves up the lateral aspect of the arm into the antecubital fossa. There may also be a network of veins on the lateral forearm that forms the accessory cephalic, joining the cephalic vein at or above the antecubital fossa (see Figure 10-24).

Moving medially across the palmar side of the forearm, the median vein ascends from the superficial palmar veins. In the wrist, these veins may appear to be suitable for venipuncture but are usually situated between two branches of the median nerve. This results in extremely painful venipuncture and should be avoided (see Figure 10-9).

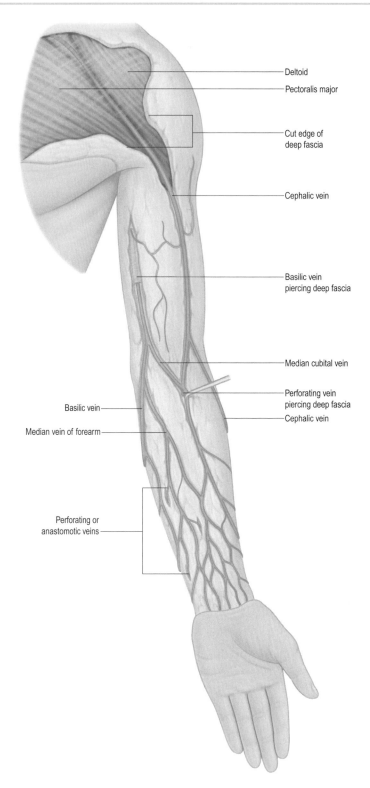

Deltoid

Pectoralis major

Cut edge of
deep fascia

Cephalic vein

Basilic vein
piercing deep fascia

Median cubital vein

Perforating vein
piercing deep fascia

Cephalic vein

Basilic vein

Median vein of forearm

Perforating or
anastomotic veins

FIGURE 10-24 Superficial veins of the upper extremity. (From Standring S, editor: *Gray's anatomy,* ed 39, London, 2005, Churchill Livingstone.)

The basilic vein is on the posterior-medial aspect of the forearm. Although it is usually a large vein, it may have been overlooked, and venipuncture may be awkward. This vein can be easily palpated and punctured when the patient's arm is placed across the chest, with the nurse on the opposite side of the patient from the arm being examined (Figure 10-26).

The radial and ulnar veins parallel the arteries of the same name. There is communication between the deep and superficial veins, and the muscle pump can be used to distend the superficial veins. Instructing the patient to open and close the hand helps force blood from the deep veins into the superficial veins, thus distending them for easier palpation and puncture.

The median vein joins the basilic vein slightly below the antecubital fossa on the medial aspect (see Figure 10-24). On some patients, this vein may be located too far to the posterior aspect of the elbow, making venipuncture difficult. Palpation

TABLE 10-5 **Short Peripheral Catheter Insertion Sites for Children and Adults**

Site	Advantages	Disadvantages
Dorsal venous network of hand	Most distal site, allowing successive sites in a proximal location; can be visualized and palpated easily; easily accessible	Should be stabilized on arm board; smaller than veins in forearm; diminished skin turgor and loss of subcutaneous tissue in geriatric patients; excessive subcutaneous fat in infants; limited ability to use hand may present problems for patients at home
Cephalic vein	Large vein; easy to stabilize; easily accessible for caregiver and patient; may be palpated above antecubital fossa	May be obscured by tendons controlling thumb; puncture sites directly in wrist and antecubital fossa can increase complications because of joint motion; damage to radial nerve
Accessory cephalic vein(s)	Medium to large vein(s); easy to stabilize; can be palpated easily	Valves at junction of cephalic vein may prohibit catheter advancement; length of vein may be too short for catheter; may not be located on children
Median vein	Medium vein; easy to stabilize; easily accessible for caregiver and patient	Puncture in wrist may be excessively painful because of close proximity of nerve; may be slightly more difficult to palpate and visualize
Basilic vein	Large vein; can be palpated easily; may be available after other sites have been exhausted	More difficult to access because of location; may be difficult for patient to access and observe site; puncture site directly in antecubital fossa may result in increased complications because of joint motion; cannot be palpated above antecubital fossa
External jugular vein	Large vein; easily accessible for emergency situations	Increased complications because of motion of neck; occlusive dressing difficult to maintain; torturous pathway; very close to transverse cutaneous and auricular nerves
Dorsal venous network on foot	Easily accessible	May not be easily palpated because of age or disease-related changes; higher incidence of complications related to impaired circulation; difficult to stabilize joint; greatly limits ability to walk
Medial and lateral marginal veins of foot	May be large; usually easy to palpate and visualize	Higher incidence of complications related to impaired circulation; difficult to stabilize joint; greatly limits ability to walk
Great and small saphenous veins	Large veins; usually easy to palpate and visualize	Higher incidence of complications related to impaired circulation; located close to perforating veins connecting to deep veins of leg

of this vein should begin on the distal end in the forearm and the course of the vein followed to evaluate its location.

In the antecubital fossa, the cephalic vein communicates with the basilic vein by the median cubital vein (see Figure 10-24). Perforating veins communicate with the deep veins where the median cubital vein enters the basilic vein. Variations in the median cubital vein may be seen. Some patients may have two branches of this vein: one angling toward the basilic, known as the *median basilic vein,* and the second one angling from the center of the fossa toward the cephalic, known as the *median cephalic vein.* Because of variations and the close proximity of nerves, careful evaluation and assessment of each patient is important before performing venipuncture in this area.

The upper part of the arm has three veins of importance (Figure 10-27). The cephalic vein continues upward lateral to the biceps muscle. The basilic vein is medial to the biceps and extends to the superior axilla, where it becomes the axillary vein. The paired brachial veins are located deep in the arm as a vena comitans in the sheath with the brachial artery (Figure 10-28).

The distal end of the axillary vein can be considered as the beginning of the veins in the shoulder area. The axillary vein is classified as a deep vein; it extends from the lateral aspect of the chest in the axilla to the lateral border of the first rib. The axillary vein receives the brachial vein at its midpoint and the cephalic vein near the border of the rib. The cephalic vein can also have variations in its path. It may only join the axillary vein, only connect with the external jugular vein in the

neck, or branch into two smaller veins connecting with the axillary and external jugular veins (Figure 10-29). There are 3 suprascapular veins and several other veins joining the axillary vein in this area, and as many as 40 valves can be documented in this region (Agur, 1999). For this reason, peripherally inserted central catheters (PICCs) can take several wayward paths, and the actual tip location can be confirmed only by chest radiography.

There are four jugular veins draining the head and face, with three of them located superficially (see Figure 10-29). The external jugular vein is on the outer border of the neck. The posterior external jugular vein drains the occipital region and the anterior jugular vein drains the face, with both joining the external jugular at the base of the neck. The external jugular joins the subclavian vein at its midpoint. The internal jugular vein is a deep vein covered by the muscles of the neck. It joins the subclavian vein at its proximal end.

From the lateral edge of the first rib to the sternal edge of the clavicle, the continuation of the axillary vein is the subclavian vein. The vein angles upward as it arches over the first rib and passes under the clavicle, forming a narrow passage for the vein (see Figure 10-7). The apex of the lungs is also extremely close to the location of the subclavian vein, increasing the potential for pneumothorax when the subclavian is punctured. Table 10-6 lists locations for central venous cannulation.

At the top of the thoracic inlet, the internal jugular and subclavian veins join to create the brachiocephalic vein, also called the *innominate vein.* At this junction is the last venous valve before the heart. The left brachiocephalic vein, which is

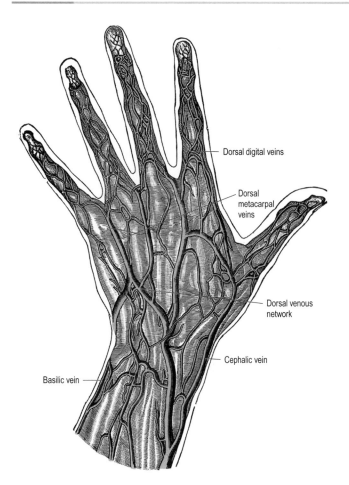

FIGURE 10-25 Veins of the dorsum of the hand. (From Standring S, editor: *Gray's anatomy*, ed 39, London, 2005, Churchill Livingstone.)

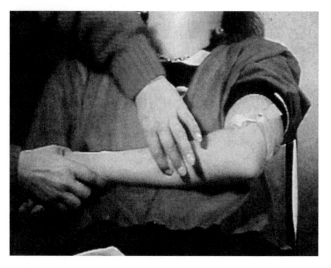

Figure 10-26 Palpation of the basilic vein with the patient's arm across the chest.

approximately 6 cm in length, is approximately twice as long as the right brachiocephalic vein (see Figure 10-7). The thoracic duct converges with the venous system in this area of the left side.

Other tributaries unite with the great thoracic veins and have been documented as aberrant locations for central venous catheters. The internal thoracic (mammary) vein joins the superior vena cava at the superior end. The left and right inferior thyroid veins join the respective brachiocephalic veins, draining the esophageal, tracheal, and laryngeal areas. The left superior intercostal vein joins the left brachiocephalic vein (see Figure 10-7). The azygos vein drains the spinal column and enters the posterior side of the superior vena cava immediately above the beginning of the pericardium (Figure 10-30).

In the lower extremity, the pattern of vascular distribution is similar to that of the upper extremity, with the superficial veins in the subcutaneous fascia and the deep veins accompanying the deeper arteries. The greatest difference is the presence of more valves in the lower extremity. The dorsal metatarsal veins form a network across the top of the foot. On the border of each foot lie the medial and lateral marginal veins. The great saphenous vein, the longest vein in the body, extends from the medial marginal vein in the foot up the medial aspect of the leg to the femoral vein in the inguinal area (Figure 10-31). The small saphenous vein arises from the lateral marginal vein at the ankle to above the knee, where it joins the popliteal vein.

The superficial veins are connected to the deep veins by perforating veins at the ankle, in the distal calf, and around the knee. These perforating veins have valves that prevent blood from flowing from the deep veins to the superficial veins. Muscular action pumps blood toward the heart. However, if the valves are not functioning properly, or during periods of muscle relaxation or atrophy, blood can move into the superficial veins. The increased pressure in the superficial veins causes fluid to leak into the subcutaneous tissue, with edema seen on examination. This increased pressure leads to blood stagnation and results in enlarged and torturous superficial veins called *varicosities*. Ulcerations can result from the damaged tissue and lack of circulation. Because of this process, the use of veins in the feet and ankles for the routine delivery of any IV therapy in adults is not recommended; however, veins of the feet and ankles are used in nonwalking infants.

SYSTEMIC BLOOD FLOW

Flow of any fluid is the amount of fluid that can pass a given point in a given period. For instance, the cardiac output of blood in an average resting adult is about 5 L/min. Blood circulates in a closed system and depends on more factors than the amount of blood pumped by the heart. These factors are the same as those for fluid flowing through any other closed system: the volume and properties of the fluid, pressures within the system and the resistance to those pressures, velocity or speed of flow, type of flow, and the ability of the system to comply with changes in demand.

BLOOD VOLUME AND DISTRIBUTION

Precise regulation of blood volume is the result of a complex interaction between cardiac output, excretion of excessive amount of fluids and electrolytes by the kidneys, and hormonal and nervous system factors. Inability of the heart to pump strongly enough to perfuse the kidneys, an increase in red cell production (polycythemia), and the creation of additional space for blood, such as during pregnancy or with large varicose veins, can increase the total volume of the system.

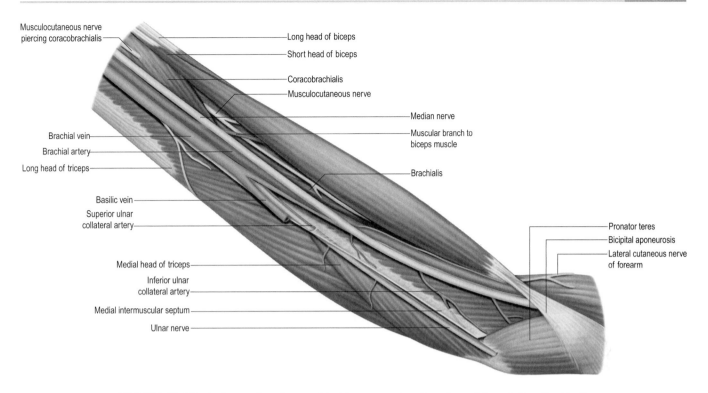

FIGURE 10-27 Muscles, vessels, and nerves of the left upper arm viewed from the medial aspect. (From Standring S, editor: *Gray's anatomy,* ed 39, London, 2005, Churchill Livingstone.)

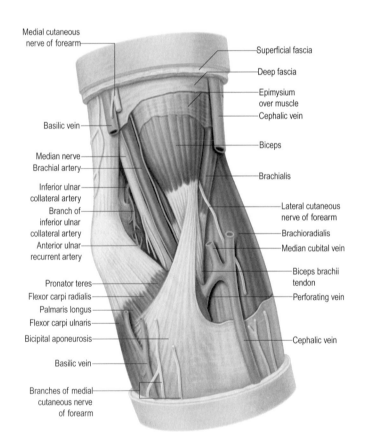

FIGURE 10-28 Anterior aspect of the left elbow, showing superficial structures. (From Standring S, editor: *Gray's anatomy,* ed 39, London, 2005, Churchill Livingstone.)

As illustrated in Figure 10-32, about 84% of blood volume is in the systemic circulation while the remaining 16% is in the pulmonary system. Note that the largest percentage, 64%, is found in the venous circulation and only 7% is in the capillaries (Guyton and Hall, 2006). The principal exchange of nutrients and waste occurs in the 10 billion capillaries in the whole body, equal to approximately 500 to 700 square meters (Guyton and Hall, 2006). Water and water-soluble substances such as sodium and glucose move by diffusion through channels or pores between the endothelial cells in the capillary wall. Lipid-soluble substances such as oxygen and carbon dioxide move by diffusion directly through the cell wall without having to move through these pores.

PHYSICAL PROPERTIES OF BLOOD

The viscosity of any fluid is defined as the degree of resistance to flow when pressure is applied. Viscosity of blood is primarily determined by the percentage of cells in blood (hematocrit). Friction from a high concentration of cells increases viscosity. Generally, the hematocrit ranges from 38% to 42%; its viscosity is about 3 times greater than that of water, and the viscosity of plasma proteins is about 1.5 times greater than that of water (Guyton and Hall, 2006). This means that it requires 3 times more force to move blood through a vessel than water. Many diseases, injuries, and fluid and nutritional imbalances can alter this normal value, with a corresponding increase in viscosity.

Two studies have identified a connection between phlebitis development and elevated hemoglobin levels in patients with short peripheral catheters. In a study of patients receiving infusion therapy for pneumonia, multivariate analysis showed that patients with higher hemoglobin levels had higher rates of phlebitis (Monreal et al, 1999b). The same results of higher

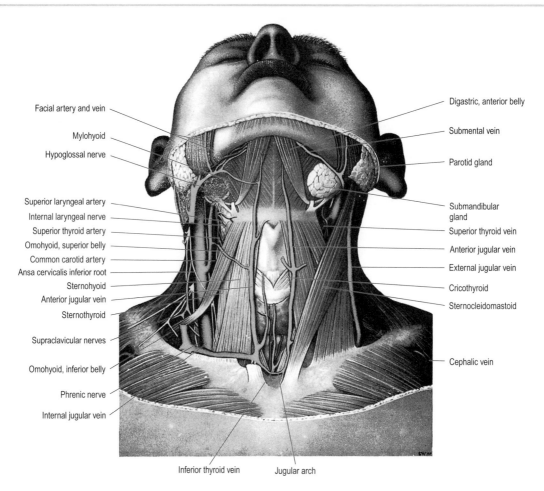

Facial artery and vein

Mylohyoid

Hypoglossal nerve

Superior laryngeal artery
Internal laryngeal nerve
Superior thyroid artery
Omohyoid, superior belly
Common carotid artery
Ansa cervicalis inferior root
Sternohyoid
Anterior jugular vein
Sternothyroid

Supraclavicular nerves

Omohyoid, inferior belly

Phrenic nerve

Internal jugular vein

Digastric, anterior belly

Submental vein

Parotid gland

Submandibular gland

Superior thyroid vein

Anterior jugular vein

External jugular vein

Cricothyroid

Sternocleidomastoid

Cephalic vein

Inferior thyroid vein   Jugular arch

FIGURE 10-29 Anterior view of the veins of the neck. (From Standring S, editor: *Gray's anatomy*, ed 39, London, 2005, Churchill Livingstone.)

hemoglobin levels producing greater rates of phlebitis were also found in a study of postoperative patients (Monreal et al, 1999a). The researchers theorized that the higher hemoglobin levels produced a slower flow of blood, thus reducing the dilution of irritating medications.

Viscosity is affected by vessel diameter. The most rapid flow in large vessels is found in the center of the vessel, with the flow closest to the vessel wall being the slowest. As the velocity of flow decreases, the viscosity increases; therefore blood flowing through small vessels and capillaries has a higher viscosity.

The presence of catheters in vessels with a small lumen decreases the velocity of flow. Because the vessel diameter is reduced, the viscosity of blood would increase. Therefore it is important to use the smallest catheter in the largest possible vessel. This allows room for blood to flow adequately between the wall of the vein and the wall of the catheter. Knowledge of the patient's hematocrit level and careful attention to adequate hydration are also important.

PRESSURE AND RESISTANCE TO FLOW

Because of the pumping action of the heart, the greatest pressure, approximately 100 millimeters of mercury (mm Hg) on average, is found in the aorta; however, this pressure ranges from 120 mm Hg on systole to 80 mm Hg on diastole. From this point, the pressure gradually decreases until it reaches the junction of the vena cava and the right atrium, where it measures

0 mm Hg. In the capillary bed, the pressure ranges from 35 mm Hg on the arterial side to 10 mm Hg on the venous side, with a functional pressure in the capillary of about 17 mm Hg (Guyton and Hall, 2006). The difference in pressure, called a pressure gradient, causes the blood to flow. This pressure gradient forces blood to move through the vessels where it is met with vascular resistance. Fluid through any tube flows only because of the difference in pressure between the two ends. Known as Ohm's law, it applies to blood flow through vessels as well as fluid flow through the administration set (Figure 10-33).

Flow through a single vessel is most affected by the diameter of the vessel (Figure 10-34). When the diameter doubles, the flow rate increases 16 times, and with a fourfold increase in lumen diameter, the flow rate dramatically increases 256 times.

Force from this pressure is met by resistance from the vessel wall, or vasomotor tone. Resistance is controlled by the vasomotor center in the brain stem, which sends impulses to the sympathetic nerve endings located in all vessels except the metarterioles, precapillary sphincters, and capillaries.

Blood flow through the capillary bed is not constant, as in other vessels, but is intermittent and based on the needs of the tissue served. When the oxygen level in the tissue decreases, the precapillary sphincter opens, allowing flow to proceed. The primary purpose of the thin capillary membrane is allowing diffusion of substances through the membrane. Two opposing forces control the amount of molecular movement across the membrane: hydrostatic pressure and colloid osmotic pressure.

TABLE 10-6   Central Venous Insertion Sites in Children and Adults

Site	Advantages	Disadvantages
Basilic	Largest vein; straight pathway in upper arm and thorax	May be located too far to posterior side for sterile procedure and routine care; may only be able to palpate a short segment
Cephalic	Easily accessible for insertion and routine care; easy palpation and visualization above and below antecubital fossa	Smaller than basilic; pathway in upper arm and thorax is variable and unknown
Brachial		Smaller than basilic; requires use of ultrasound to locate and access; close to large nerves and artery
Subclavian		
Infraclavicular	Easily accessible for insertion; flatter surface to maintain occlusive dressing; more published studies using this site; some believe this site has better anatomical landmarks; preferred for children	Longer needle may be necessary to pass through skin; muscle compression of vein and catheter with possible fracture of catheter if insertion is made in a medial site
Supraclavicular	Shorter distance from skin to vein; easily accessible	Occlusive dressing may be difficult to achieve in hollow contour above clavicle
		Both sites associated with pneumothorax, hemothorax, hydrothorax, brachial nerve plexus injury, thoracic duct injury, and injury to other superior mediastinal structures
Jugular		
Internal	Larger vein diameter; multiple insertion sites; easily accessible; straighter path to superior vena cava	May damage carotid arteries
External	Superficial vein, usually visible and easy to palpate	Catheter tip location in superior vena cava not always as successful as internal jugular
	Both sites are associated with fewer complications than subclavian	Maintaining occlusive dressing on either is extremely difficult because of movement of neck and because of beard on male patients
Femoral	Alternative site in emergencies; tip location in large inferior vena cava	Occlusive dressing is extremely difficult with high infection rates associated with this site; associated with higher incidence of thrombosis and other serious complications

Hydrostatic pressure is created by fluid in the vessel and the interstitial space. Colloid osmotic pressure is the opposing force exerted by plasma proteins. Proteins do not pass through the capillary membrane easily, which results in a difference in protein concentration between the plasma and interstitial fluid, and this difference remains steady. The concentration of plasma proteins is normally about 7 g/dL, with the interstitial protein level about 3 g/dL (Guyton and Hall, 2006). Colloid osmotic pressure is also called *oncotic pressure* to distinguish it from the osmotic pressure of fluid moving from the interstitial space into each individual cell.

Interstitium is the space between cells, containing both solid structures and fluid. Strong collagen fiber bundles provide tensile strength, and proteoglycan filaments are thin molecules mostly composed of hyaluronic acid. Fluid in this space comes from capillaries and has the characteristics of gel. Hyaluronidase is the enzyme that breaks down these proteoglycan filaments, thus allowing solutions and medications to move more readily into the bloodstream. Hyaluronidase is used in conjunction with purposeful subcutaneous infusions or to treat inadvertent infiltration or extravasation injuries (Hadaway, 2007).

Four forces determine fluid flow between the blood and interstitial space (Figure 10-35). Fluid is forced out of the capillary by the capillary pressure, which is opposed by the interstitial fluid pressure trying to move fluid into the capillary. Plasma colloid osmotic pressure moves fluid into the capillary by osmosis, while interstitial fluid colloid osmotic pressure moves fluid into the interstitial space.

Each heartbeat sends blood into the arteries, known for their capacity to distend. The difference between the systolic pressure and the diastolic pressure is known as the pulse pressure. Stroke volume output, or the amount of blood pumped out of the heart with each beat, and the total distensibility of the arterial tree are the most important factors impacting the pulse pressure. Large amounts of blood pumped and loss of distensibility (such as that caused by atherosclerosis) increase pulse pressure.

Pressure in the peripheral veins is directly related to the pressure in the right atrium and to the heart's ability to pump blood out of the right atrium. Central venous pressure is the common measure of right atrial functionality.

Normally, the right atrial pressure is 0 mm Hg, approximately equal to the atmospheric pressure around the body. In a variety of clinical conditions, the right atrial pressure can range from as high as 30 mm Hg during cardiac failure or the transfusion of massive amounts of blood, to as low as −5 mm Hg when the blood flow to the heart has been altered by hemorrhage or some other severe impediment.

The internal jugular and subclavian veins are subject to compression from atmospheric pressure or their sharp angulation and thus offer resistance to blood flow. For this reason, small peripheral veins will have a pressure about 4 to 6 mm Hg greater than that of the right atrium while the patient is in a reclined position. As the right atrial pressure rises, the points of venous compression are opened, causing them to distend.

The weight of blood in the vessels causes hydrostatic or gravitational pressure. In the arm veins, this pressure is 35 mm Hg in the hand, decreasing to 8 mm Hg at the level of a midline catheter, and to 6 mm Hg at the venipuncture site for a subclavian catheterization (Figure 10-36).

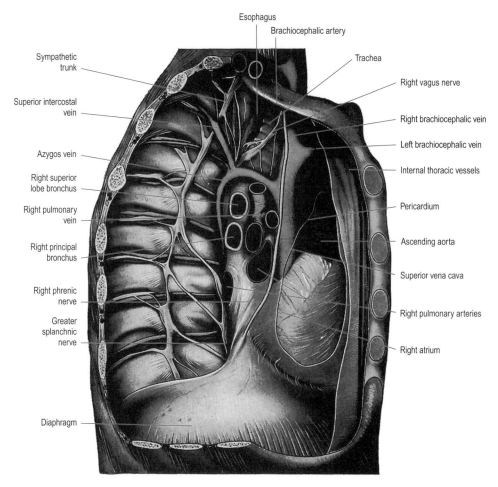

FIGURE 10-30 The right lateral aspect of the mediastinum. (From Standring S, editor: *Gray's anatomy,* ed 39, London, 2005, Churchill Livingstone.)

VELOCITY AND TYPES OF BLOOD FLOW

Velocity is the distance blood moves in a specific period. Normally, blood moves through the aorta at a rate of 33 cm/second, but in capillaries the velocity drops to 0.3 mm/second (Guyton and Hall, 2006).

Flow can be in two types or patterns: laminar or turbulent. In laminar flow, the blood moves in layers or concentric circles through the vessels (Figure 10-37). As blood moves through the vessels, the layer touching the vessel wall is slowed because of adherence to the wall. The next layer slides easily over the outer one, and the innermost layer moves easiest.

Turbulent flow is in all directions, flowing crosswise and lengthwise along the vessel (see Figure 10-37). This type of flow is created when the vessel's inner surface is rough, there is an obstruction or a sharp turn in the vessel, or the amount of flow has increased greatly. Large arteries such as the proximal aorta and pulmonary artery have the right conditions for turbulent flow.

CLOTTING PROCESS

The human body is normally quite efficient in hemostasis, or the prevention of blood loss. Hemostasis occurs in five stages: (1) vasoconstriction or vasospasm, (2) formation of a platelet plug, (3) activation of the clotting cascade, (4) formation of the clot, and (5) clot retraction and dissolution (Figure 10-38) (Guyton and Hall, 2006).

The first stage of the clotting process begins immediately after vessel injury when smooth muscle in the vessel wall contracts and reduces the blood flow from the vessel opening. The response of the smooth muscle comes from nerve reflexes and thromboxane released by platelets. A greater degree of trauma produces a greater vasospasm.

The second step is the formation of a platelet plug. Platelets are round disks usually only about 1 to 4 μm wide with a normal concentration of 150,000 to 300,000 per microliter (Guyton and Hall, 2006). Although they are not whole cells and cannot reproduce, they do contain several factors and enzyme systems that cause contraction. They also assist in the repair of damaged vessels by releasing a factor that causes growth of endothelial cells, smooth muscle cells, and fibroblasts. The platelet surface has a glycoprotein coat that prevents its adherence to intact endothelium, yet causes the platelet to adhere to damaged endothelial cells and the collagen in the other layers of the vessel wall. When platelets pass over a damaged portion of the vessel wall, they swell, change shapes, and release adenosine triphosphate and thromboxane that increase their stickiness. These changes attract more platelets, forming a loose plug that is capable of stopping blood loss in a small vessel opening.

The third step is the activation of the complex clotting cascade that results in the formation of a blood clot. Fibrin threads form and attach to the platelet plug. This meshwork attracts

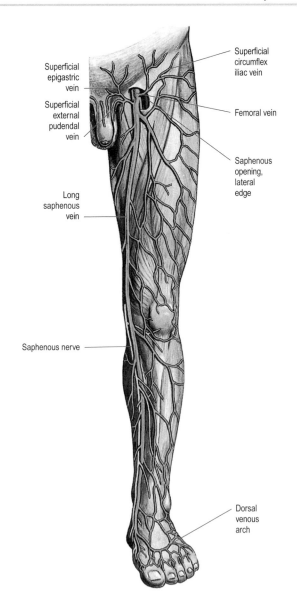

FIGURE 10-31 Veins of the lower extremity. (From Standring S, editor: *Gray's anatomy,* ed 39, London, 2005, Churchill Livingstone.)

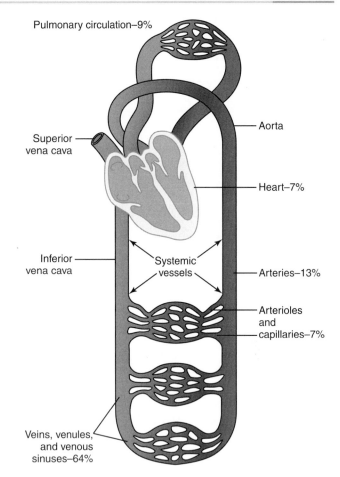

FIGURE 10-32 Distribution of blood in the different parts of the circulatory system. (From Guyton AC, Hall JE: *Textbook of medical physiology,* ed 11, Philadelphia, 2006, Saunders.)

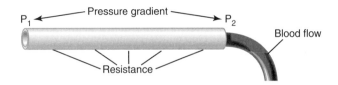

FIGURE 10-33 Interrelationships among pressure, resistance, and blood flow. (From Guyton AC, Hall JE: *Textbook of medical physiology,* ed 11, Philadelphia, 2006, Saunders.)

red blood cells, phagocytes, and microorganisms that tightly fill the vessel hole.

Fibrin, the end result of the clotting cascade, is not normally found in circulating blood. Blood coagulation is a battle between the components that promote clotting, called *procoagulants,* and those that prevent clotting, called *anticoagulants.* These two groups comprise more than 50 substances found in the blood. Normally, the anticoagulants are dominant, but at sites of vessel damage, the procoagulants become active and prevail over the anticoagulants.

The coagulation or clotting cascade acts in two different but interacting pathways: the extrinsic pathway, which starts with vessel or tissue damage; and the intrinsic pathway, which begins with the changes in the blood or blood coming into contact with collagen from a traumatized vessel wall. The extrinsic pathway includes tissue factor released from damaged tissue, factor VII, and activated factor X, which combines with phospholipids and factor V to form prothrombin activator. When the blood is traumatized or when blood contacts collagen in

the vascular wall, the intrinsic pathway begins by activating factor XII and platelet phospholipids. Through enzymatic actions, factor XII activates factor XI, then factor IX, and then factor X. With the help of factor V, platelets, and phospholipids, prothrombin activator is formed.

The end result of both pathways is the formation of prothrombin activator. With the help of calcium and prothrombin receptors on platelets, prothrombin activator converts prothrombin, a plasma protein, to thrombin.

The fourth stage is the formation of the clot. Thrombin, a protein enzyme, converts fibrinogen, a large protein made by the liver, to fibrin. Early in the formation, fibrin strands are loosely bound together and can be broken apart very easily. However, within minutes, fibrin-stabilizing factor is released from the platelets inside the clot to form a strongly bonded and cross-linked mesh of fibrin. Fibrin attaches to the vessel wall, closing the hole in the vascular wall. Within 1 hour, the clot retracts

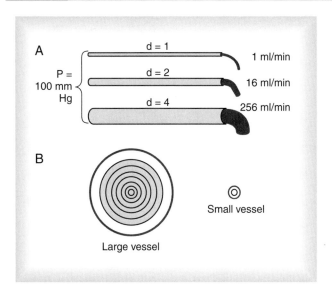

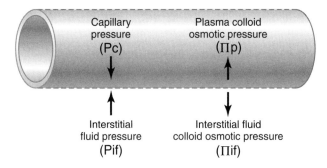

FIGURE 10-34 **A,** Demonstration of the effect of vessel diameter on blood flow. **B,** Concentric rings of blood flowing at different velocities. (From Guyton AC, Hall JE: *Textbook of medical physiology,* ed 11, Philadelphia, 2006, Saunders.)

FIGURE 10-35 Fluid pressure and colloid osmotic pressure forces at the capillary. (From Guyton AC, Hall JE: *Textbook of medical physiology,* ed 11, Philadelphia, 2006, Saunders.)

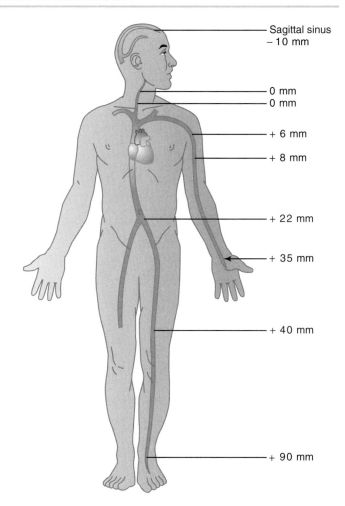

FIGURE 10-36 Effect of gravitational pressure on the venous pressures throughout the body in the standing person. (From Guyton AC, Hall JE: *Textbook of medical physiology,* ed 11, Philadelphia, 2006, Saunders.)

to force out serum with all the clotting factors removed. As the clot becomes smaller, the vessel edges are pulled together.

A blood clot continues to produce thrombin and attract platelets, causing it to grow. Within approximately 1 or 2 days, the clot stops growing and begins to break down. Tissue plasminogen activator (t-PA) is released from the injured tissue and endothelium. Plasminogen is converted to plasmin, an enzyme with action similar to that of digestive enzymes. Plasmin digests the fibrin and other components of the clot (Guyton and Hall, 2006).

As discussed previously, many factors on the endothelial surface act to prevent clotting. Venipuncture for all purposes disrupts the endothelium. Traumatic catheter advancement or catheters too large for the vein diameter also damage endothelium. The smooth surface of the endothelium is destroyed, bringing blood into contact with collagen in the subendothelial layer and initiating the intrinsic clotting cascade. Destruction of the endothelium also destroys the glycocalyx and thrombomodulin found on the cell surface. For these reasons, reducing catheter-related thrombosis requires proper choices of catheter size in relation to the vein diameter, the most skillful methods of nontraumatic catheter insertion, adequate catheter stabilization, and careful attention to the osmolarity, pH, and particulate matter of fluids and medications.

MECHANISMS OF DEFENSE

Intact skin, mucous membranes, and the biochemical barriers discussed earlier compose the first line of defense. During the delivery of all infusion therapy, skin is the first barrier to be breached. Inflammation is the body's response to injury from microorganisms, trauma, harmful chemicals, and temperature extremes. This process involves many types of cells and plasma proteins and begins within seconds after injury. Inflammation is not specific to the type of invader and proceeds with the same process regardless of the type of injury or the number of times cellular injury has occurred. Immunity is the human body's form of protection against all types of invading organisms, toxins, or other foreign substances.

INFLAMMATION

Cellular injury initiates the process of acute inflammation. Many aspects of infusion therapy begin with cellular injury. Venipuncture breaks the skin, subcutaneous tissue, and the vessel wall. The degree of cellular injury depends on the skill used to enter the vein and advance the catheter to the desired location. Using peripheral veins to insert midline and peripherally inserted central catheters increases the potential

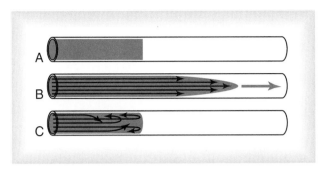

FIGURE 10-37 A, Two fluids before flow begins. **B,** The same fluids 1 second after flow begins. **C,** Turbulent flow with elements of the fluid moving in a disorderly pattern. (From Guyton AC, Hall JE: *Textbook of medical physiology,* ed 11, Philadelphia, 2006, Saunders.)

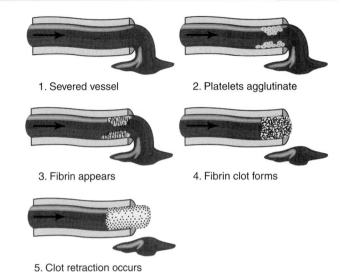

1. Severed vessel

2. Platelets agglutinate

3. Fibrin appears

4. Fibrin clot forms

5. Clot retraction occurs

FIGURE 10-38 Clotting process in a traumatized blood vessel. (In Guyton AC, Hall JE: *Textbook of medical physiology,* ed 11, Philadelphia, 2006, Saunders. Modified from Seegers WH: *Hemostatic agents,* Springfield, Ill, 1948, courtesy of Charles C Thomas, Publishers.)

for inflammation because longer vein sections can be injured. Injury to the skin surface can result from repeated application and removal of dressings and tape, rigid pieces of tubing anchored tightly to the skin, catheter migration into or out of the insertion site, and use of antiseptic agents. Rapid infusion of large volumes and infusion of solutions with extremes in osmolarity and pH through veins with small amounts of blood flow can injure the vein wall. Invasion of microorganisms is always a distinct possibility with any type of infusion therapy. Temperature changes and oxygen and nutrient deprivation also produce cellular injury. Classic signs and symptoms of inflammation include redness, heat, edema, pus formation, thrombus formation, and pain.

The sequence of events in the process of inflammation begins with contraction of the arterioles close to the injury followed by vasodilation, which increases blood flow to the area (Figure 10-39). Large quantities of fluid leak from capillaries, resulting in localized edema. Blood volume in the capillaries decreases and becomes more viscous. Neutrophils move into the area and stick to vessel walls. Endothelial cells lining capillaries and venules retract, creating space between the cells for more fluid to leak into the tissue. Vascular permeability continues through the acute phase, allowing fluids and cells to move to the injured tissue, where they stimulate and control inflammation.

Neutrophils constrict to the size of the pores of the capillary, allowing them to move into the tissue. This process is known as diapedesis. Enlarged neutrophils called macrophages are drawn to the injured area through a phenomenon known as chemotaxis. Neutrophils and macrophages then attach, engulf, and ingest the offending microorganisms or other agents, a process known as phagocytosis. Enzymes in the neutrophils and macrophages then digest the organisms and directly kill bacteria by the presence of bacteriocidal oxidizing agents.

Basophils in the blood and mast cells in the tissue are closely related cells involved in the inflammatory response. Both cells release heparin, histamine, bradykinin, and serotonin during the process of inflammation. Platelet aggregation occurs in the inflamed area to control bleeding from injured vessels.

IMMUNITY

The immune response can be divided into two types: innate or natural immunity and acquired immunity. Innate immunity is part of many other systems already discussed including phagocytosis, the natural protective barrier of the skin, and

acid secretions in the stomach destroying the oral ingestion of organisms. White blood cells and many chemical compounds of blood are constantly available for a "search and destroy" mission against invading agents. Natural immunity is present at birth and does not require any form of stimulation to create it. For instance, humans have a natural immunity to many animal diseases, such as cowpox and distemper.

Acquired or adaptive immunity develops following exposure to a foreign substance known as an *antigen*. Antigens include bacteria, fungi, parasites, viruses, pollens, foods, venoms, drugs, vaccines, transfusions, and transplanted tissue. Once the body has been challenged by these invaders, certain physiological and biochemical interactions lead to the maturation and activation of two types of immunocompetent cells—B and T lymphocytes. The cells are located in lymph nodes throughout the body, along with other lymphoid tissue in the spleen, gastrointestinal tract, thymus, and bone marrow.

Both types of lymphocytes are derived from pluripotent hematopoietic stem cells and look alike under a microscope, but they are processed in different methods. The thymus gland is responsible for processing T lymphocytes so that each cell is designated to react against a specific antigen. T lymphocytes are processed immediately before and for a few months after birth, and then they migrate to lymphoid tissue all over the body. The thymus is responsible for selecting and releasing only those cells that will not react with the body's natural antigens such as those found on red blood cells. This is known as cell-mediated immunity.

B lymphocytes are processed in the liver and bone marrow during mid-fetal and late-fetal life and after birth. While the whole cell of a T lymphocyte reacts against the antigen, a B lymphocyte secretes antibodies or large protein molecules that can destroy the antigen. B lymphocytes are more diverse, capable of forming millions of types of antibodies, and are known as humoral immunity.

Upon antigen exposure, certain T lymphocytes form activated T cells while certain B lymphocytes form antibodies. Each can only react to a designated antigen, but once the process begins, these cells can reproduce in large numbers.

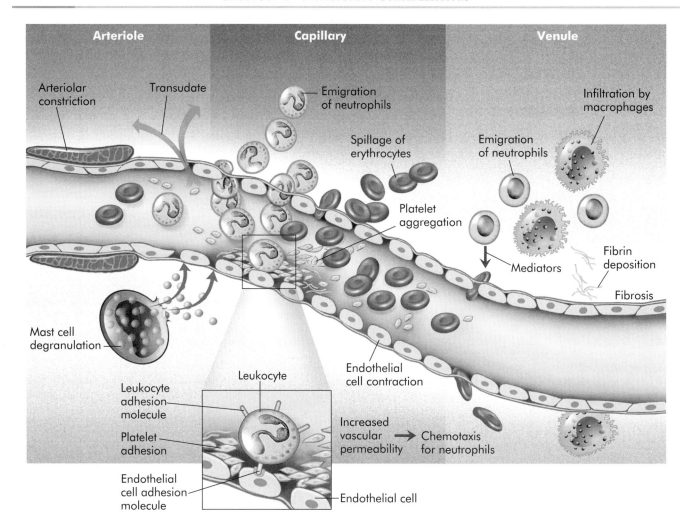

FIGURE 10-39 The sequence of events in the process of inflammation. (From Huether SE, McCance KL: *Understanding pathophysiology,* ed 4, St Louis, 2008, Mosby.)

Upon entry of an antigen, macrophages phagocytize it and present it to B lymphocytes, which enlarge and appear as lymphoblasts. Some lymphoblasts become plasmablasts and mature into plasma cells producing gammaglobulin antibodies. Rather than becoming plasma cells, a few lymphoblasts form new B lymphocytes with a specific "memory" for the antigen that started the process. These memory cells circulate to lymphoid tissue throughout the body and serve to create a very rapid antibody response upon subsequent exposure to the same antigen.

Antigens are complex, large-molecule proteins that are foreign to the host and whose structures match receptor sites on lymphocytes or antibody molecules (Figure 10-40). Antibodies are immunoglobulins (Ig) possessing a specific receptor site for a specific antigen. There are five classes of antibodies: IgG, IgA, IgM, IgE, and IgD. About 75% of the antibodies in a normal human are IgG (Guyton and Hall, 2006). IgE is of particular importance because it mediates allergic reactions.

Antibodies act in two ways. The first method occurs by a direct attack on the invading antigen, causing the antibodies to agglutinate or form large clumps, render the antigen insoluble, or lyse the antigen's membrane. The second method is activation of the complement system. This is a collection of about 20 proteins that are precursors to enzymes. When the antigen and antibody unite, a portion of the antibody is activated, which then binds with one of these proteins to begin a complex cascade of

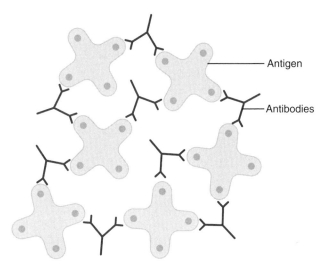

FIGURE 10-40 Binding of antigen molecules to one another by bivalent antibodies. (From Guyton AC, Hall JE: *Textbook of medical physiology,* ed 11, Philadelphia, 2006, Saunders.)

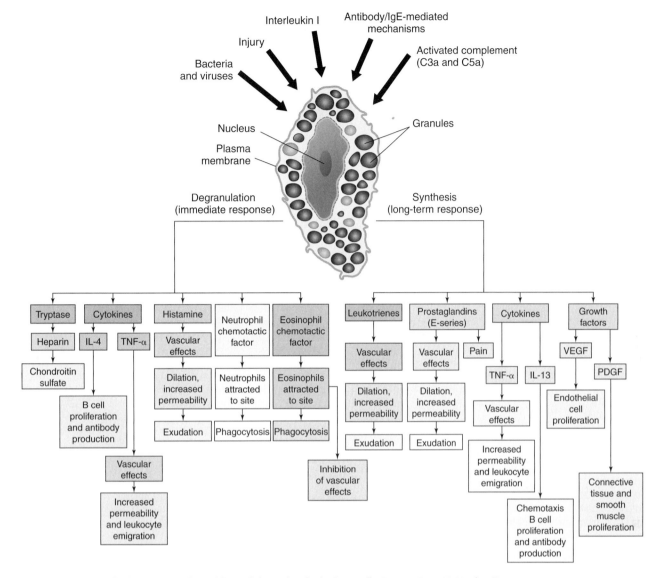

FIGURE 10-41 Effects of degranulation and synthesis of mast cells. (From McCance KL, Huether SE: *Pathophysiology: the biologic basis for disease in adults and children,* ed 5, St Louis, 2006, Mosby.)

reactions. Increasing amounts of these enzymes are produced, leading to many forms of tissue protection such as phagocytosis, chemotaxis, and activation of mast cells and basophils.

Mast cells are granular cells found in all connective tissue and are involved with inflammation and immunity. They originate in the bone marrow and are similar to basophils in the blood. They are the principal mediators of allergic reactions or immune hypersensitivity but may offer a protective function. They can be found in large numbers around blood vessels and nerves (Coleman, 2002; Nigrovic and Lee, 2005; Slominski, 2006).

When stimulated, mast cells release histamine, heparin, and numerous proteases, causing an immediate reaction. At the time of injury, the mast cell wall also releases arachidonic acid, which produces leukotrienes and prostaglandins. These substances act in the later stages of the event and are responsible for the prolonged signs and symptoms of the inflammatory reaction. Mast cells are the primary source for many cytokines and chemokines released when mast cells are activated by any means (Coleman, 2002).

Physical injury, chemical injury, IgE-mediated mechanisms, and activation of the complement system all stimulate mast cells

to release their granules (Figure 10-41). Physical injury includes trauma by catheter advancement, heat, ultraviolet light, and x-rays. Chemical injury comes from toxins, snake and bee venom, and drugs such as vancomycin, morphine, barbiturates, and many muscle relaxants used during anesthesia. Neuropeptides and tissue enzymes can also cause chemical injury.

 ## SUMMARY

Through this exploration of human anatomy and physiology, it is clear that many systems of the human body are involved with the delivery of infusion therapy. It is also quite amazing to understand how all these systems are so interdependent upon each other. We are breaching the first defense mechanism when we make a venipuncture, and then invading the complex circulatory system that traverses the entire body. To provide safe therapy and minimize the risk of infusion-related complications, it is necessary for each practitioner to appreciate the dependent nature of one system upon the other.

REFERENCES

Aggarwal S, Hari P, Bagga A et al: Phrenic nerve palsy: a rare complication of indwelling subclavian vein catheter, *Pediatr Nephrol* 14:203-204, 2000.

Agur A: *Grant's atlas of anatomy*, Baltimore, 1999, Williams & Wilkins.

Azocar R, Narang P, Talmor D et al: Persistent left superior vena cava identified after cannulation of the right subclavian vein, *Anesthes Analg* 95:305-307, 2002.

Barak M, Katz Y: Microbubbles: pathophysiology and clinical implications, *Chest* 128:2918-2932, 2005.

Barak M, Nakhoul F, Katz Y: Pathophysiology and clinical implications of microbubbles during hemodialysis, *Semin Dialysis* 21(3):232-238, 2008.

Boeson MB, Hranchook A, Stoller J: Peripheral nerve injury from intravenous cannulation: a case report, *AANA J* 68:53-57, 2000.

Boulais N, Misery L: Merkel cells, *J Am Acad Dermatol* 57:147-165, 2007.

Callard R, Harper J: The skin barrier, atopic dermatitis and allergy: a role for Langerhans cells? *Trends Immunol* 28:294-298, 2007.

Coleman JW: Nitric oxide: a regulator of mast cell activation and mast cell-mediated inflammation, *Clin Exp Immunol* 129:4-10, 2002.

de Graaff JC, Bras LJ, Vos JA: Early transection of a central venous catheter in a sedated ICU patient, *Br J Anaesthiol* 97:832-834, 2006.

Gebhard RE, Szmuk P, Pivalizza EG et al: The accuracy of electrocardiogram-controlled central line placement, *Anesthes Analg* 104:65-70, 2007.

Guyton A, Hall J: *Textbook of medical physiology*, ed 11, Philadelphia, 2006, Saunders.

Hadaway L: Emergency: infiltration and extravasation—preventing a complication of IV catheterization, *Am J Nurs* 107:64-72, 2007.

Holmes DI, Zachary I: The vascular endothelial growth factor (VEGF) family: angiogenic factors in health and disease, *Genome Biol* 6:209, 2005.

Kadl A, Leitinger N: The role of endothelial cells in the resolution of acute inflammation, *Antioxid Redox Signal* 7:1744-1754, 2005.

Kamola PA, Seidner DL: Peripherally inserted central catheter malposition in a persistent left superior vena cava, *J Infus Nurs* 27:181-184, 2004.

Khazaei M, Moien-Afshari F, Laher I: Vascular endothelial function in health and diseases, *Pathophysiology*, 2008.

Koschel MJ: Sternal intraosseous infusions: emergency vascular access in adults, *Am J Nurs* 105:66-68, 2005.

Kuramoto K, Shoji T, Nakagawa Y: Usefulness of the final filter of the IV infusion set in intravenous administration of drugs—contamination of injection preparations by insoluble microparticles and its causes, *Yakugaku Zasshi* 126:289-295, 2006.

Lehr HA, Brunner J, Rangoonwala R et al: Particulate matter contamination of intravenous antibiotics aggravates loss of functional capillary density in postischemic striated muscle, *Am J Respir Crit Care Med* 165:514-520, 2002.

Loesch A: Localisation of endothelin-1 and its receptors in vascular tissue as seen at the electron microscopic level, *Curr Vasc Pharmacol* 3:381-392, 2005.

Lopez H, Beer J, Miller S et al: Ultrasound measurements of skin thickness after UV exposure: a feasibility study, *J Photochem Photobiol, B* 73:123-132, 2004.

Lynch RE, Lungo JB, Loftis LL et al: A procedure for placing pediatric femoral venous catheter tips near the right atrium, *Pediatr Emerg Care* 18:130-132, 2002.

Mandala M, Ciano C, Ghilardi M et al: Acute dyspnea due to right phrenic palsy during infusional chemotherapy, *Ann Oncol* 15: 691-692, 2004.

Matsumura Y, Anathaswamy H: Short-term and long-term cellular and molecular events following UV irradiation of skin: implications for molecular medicine, *Expert Rev Mol Med* 4:1-22, 2002.

McLean W: Genetic disorders of palm skin and nail, *J Anat* 202: 133-141, 2003.

Miraldi F, di Gioia CR, Proietti P et al: Cardinal vein isomerism: an embryological hypothesis to explain a persistent left superior vena cava draining into the roof of the left atrium in the absence of coronary sinus and atrial septal defect, *Cardiovasc Pathol* 11: 149-152, 2002.

Monreal M, Oller B, Rodriguez N et al: Infusion phlebitis in post-operative patients: when and why, *Haemostasis* 29:247-254, 1999a.

Monreal M, Quilez F, Rey-Joly C et al: Infusion phlebitis in patients with acute pneumonia: a prospective study, *Chest* 115:1576-1580, 1999b.

Nakayama M, Fujita S, Kawamata M et al: Traumatic aneurysm of the internal jugular vein causing vagal nerve palsy: a rare complication of percutaneous catheterization, *Anesthes Analg* 78:598-600, 1994.

Nigrovic PA, Lee DM: Mast cells in inflammatory arthritis, *Arthritis Res Ther* 7:1-11, 2005.

Nuss R, Cole L, Le T et al: Pinch-off syndrome in patients with sickle cell disease receiving erythrocytapheresis, *Pediatr Blood Cancer* 50:354-356, 2008.

Pittiruti M, Cina A, Cotroneo A et al: Percutaneous intravascular retrieval of embolised fragments of long-term central venous catheters, *J Vasc Access* 1:23-27, 2000.

Puhaindran ME, Wong HP: A case of anterior interosseous nerve syndrome after peripherally inserted central catheter (PICC) line insertion, *Singapore Med J* 44:653-655, 2003.

Ragoowansi R, Kirkpatrick NW, Moss AL: Posterior interosseous nerve palsy after intravenous cannulation of forearm, *J R Soc Med* 92:411, 1999.

Rayegani SM, Azadi A: Lateral antebrachial cutaneous nerve injury induced by phlebotomy, *J Brachial Plex Peripher Nerve Inj* 2:6, 2007.

Reeves J, Anderson W: Permanent paralysis of the right phrenic nerve, *Ann Intern Med* 137:551-552, 2002.

Rigg A, Hughes P, Lopez A et al: Right phrenic nerve palsy as a complication of indwelling central venous catheters, *Thorax* 52:831-833, 1997.

Ryu HG, Bahk JH, Kim JT et al: Bedside prediction of the central venous catheter insertion depth, *Br J Anaesth* 98:225-227, 2007.

Sarzo G, Finco C, Zustovich F et al: Early rupture of subclavian vein catheter: a case report and literature review, *J Vasc Access* 5:39-46, 2004.

Sen S, Chini EN, Brown MJ: Complications after unintentional intra-arterial injection of drugs: risks, outcomes, and management strategies, *Mayo Clin Proc* 80:783-795, 2005.

Shyamkumar NK, Brown R: Double superior vena cava with a persistent left superior vena cava: an incidental finding during peripherally inserted central catheter placement, *Australas Radiol* 51(suppl): B257-259, 2007.

Slominski AT: Proopiomelanocortin signaling system is operating in mast cells, *J Invest Dermatol* 126:1934-1936, 2006.

So E, Sanders GM, Au TK et al: Radial nerve injury after intravenous cannulation at the wrist—a case report, *Ann Acad Med Singapore* 28:288-289, 1999.

Stahl S, Kaufman T, Ben-David B: Neuroma of the superficial branch of the radial nerve after intravenous cannulation, *Anesthes Analg* 83:180-182, 1996.

Standring S, editor: *Gray's anatomy*, ed 39, London, 2005, Churchill Livingstone.

Stonelake PA, Bodenham AR: The carina as a radiological landmark for central venous catheter tip position, *Br J Anaesth* 96:335-340, 2006.

Surov A, Jordan K, Buerke M et al: Atypical pulmonary embolism of port catheter fragments in oncology patients, *Support Care Cancer* 14:479-483, 2006.

Takasaki Y, Arai T: Transient right phrenic nerve palsy associated with central venous catheterization, *Br J Anesth* 87:510-511, 2001.

Urschel HC, Kourlis H: Thoracic outlet syndrome: a 50-year experience at Baylor University Medical Center, *Proc (Bayl Univ Med Cent)* 20:125-135, 2007.

Vialle R, Pietin-Vialle C, Cronier P et al: Anatomic relations between the cephalic vein and the sensory branches of the radial nerve: how can nerve lesions during vein puncture be prevented? *Anesthes Analg* 93:1058-1061, 2001.

Yorioka K, Oie S, Oomaki M et al: Particulate and microbial contamination in in-use admixed intravenous infusions, *Biol Pharm Bull* 29:2321-2323, 2006.

Zubairy A: How safe is blood sampling? Anterior interosseus nerve injury by venepuncture, *Postgrad Med* 78:625, 2002.

11 FLUIDS AND ELECTROLYTES

Judy Hankins, BSN, CRNI®*

The specialty practice of infusion therapy evolved from the need to provide blood, fluids, and electrolytes to maintain life. With all its intricacies, the body relies on water, one of the simplest elemental forms, to sustain life. Water makes up almost two thirds of an adult's body weight. The relationship and balance of water with electrolytes among the body's compartments determine human health and well-being.

The continuous biochemical processes of the body maintain the body in a state of equilibrium. Water moves between various spaces and compartments. This movement depends on the types and amounts of solutes in the body. The body strives to match daily excretion with intake. Any alteration in intake or excretion results in an imbalance. Recognition and prevention of, or interventions to correct, these imbalances are among the most important roles the nurse has when caring for the patient requiring infusion therapy.

It is important to understand the purpose that water serves in the human body. It does the following:

- Provides a medium for cellular metabolism
- Helps transport materials into and out of cells
- Is the solvent in which many of the solutes available for cell function are dissolved
- Helps regulate body temperature
- Maintains the physical and chemical consistency of intracellular and extracellular fluids
- Helps digest food through hydrolysis
- Provides a medium for excreting waste

It is estimated that a normal healthy person needs approximately 2600 mL of fluids daily to meet the body's water requirements. It has also been estimated that the absolute minimum amount of water required by that same healthy person is approximately 1500 mL/day. These facts demonstrate the importance of water in body function to prevent breakdown of the homeostatic regulating mechanisms. An alteration in the body's normal fluid and electrolyte balance not only affects functions within the fluid compartments but also can eventually affect every body system. Therefore it is vital to understand how water and electrolytes work within the homeostatic framework.

Illness or disease states can easily disrupt the delicate balance of body fluid and its solutes, and treating these imbalances can lead to further complications. With proper knowledge of the intravenous (IV) fluids and electrolytes that are administered daily, it is possible to prevent further complications. It is therefore imperative that the nurse responsible for delivering fluids, electrolytes, and other medications has a thorough working knowledge of normal fluid and electrolyte balances and movements within the body. Understanding the physiological effects of IV fluids and electrolytes in the presence of an imbalance is an important aspect of infusion therapy.

▌ TRANSPORT MECHANISMS

Understanding fluid and electrolyte therapy begins with understanding the intake, output, and utilization of water and electrolytes. Regulating mechanisms include osmosis, diffusion, filtration, and active transport, all of which affect the movement of water and electrolytes within the body. The cell membrane is selectively permeable to substances depending on the construction of the membrane and the ionic charge of particles or solutes attempting to move through it. Each cell is surrounded by a membrane, which is composed of phospholipids consisting of a hydrophilic head and a hydrophobic tail. The hydrophilic head faces the outside of the membrane, allowing for water retention and adhering to other cells. The lipid composition of the hydrophobic tail determines the fluid content of the cell membrane. The protein molecules in the membrane act as carriers to transport lipid-insoluble particles through the membrane while others form ion channels for the exchange of electrolytes (Baumberger-Henry, 2005).

REGULATING MECHANISMS
Osmosis

Osmosis is a passive transport mechanism that allows the movement of water freely through the semipermeable membrane (Figure 11-1). During osmosis, fluid moves in relation to the concentration of solutes; it moves through a membrane from an area of low solute concentration to an area of high solute concentration. This process continues until the solutions

*The author and editors wish to acknowledge the contributions made by Rose Anne Waldman Lonsway as co-author of this chapter in the second edition of *Infusion Therapy in Clinical Practice*.

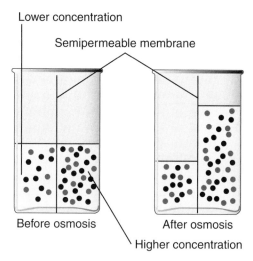

FIGURE 11-1 Osmosis through a semipermeable membrane. (Modified from Lewis, Heitkemper, Dirksen: *Medical-surgical nursing: assessment and management of clinical problems,* ed 6, St Louis, 2004, Mosby.)

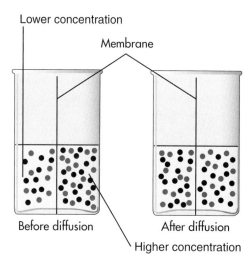

FIGURE 11-2 Diffusion. (Modified from Lewis SM et al: *Medical-surgical nursing: assessment and management of clinical problems,* ed 6, St Louis, 2004, Mosby.)

on both sides of the membrane are of equal concentration. Osmotic pressure or osmolality is the pressure exerted by the particles, ions, and molecules that moves the water from high concentration to a lower concentration to create an equal concentration (Chernecky, Macklin, Murphy-Ende, 2002). This is due to the number of particles versus the size of the particles, and is influenced primarily by sodium, the main extracellular electrolyte. The process of osmosis depends on how much of the membrane is involved and on certain characteristics of the solution—the temperature, solute solubility, and particularly the concentration.

The number of solutes in a solution is expressed by a unit of measurement called the *osmole (osm)*. *Osmolality* describes the number of osmoles per kilogram (kg) of water. The liter (L) is the usual unit of measure for water volume. Osmolality can be expressed as a total volume of 1 L of water plus a small volume occupied by the solutes in that liter of fluid. *Osmolarity* refers to the osmolar concentration in 1 L of solution (mOsm/L). Osmolality is expressed as osm/kg of water; osmolarity is expressed as osm/L. Osmolarity is usually used when referring to fluids outside the body and osmolality for describing fluids inside the body (see Chapter 13). Usually, there is little difference between these two measurements when expressed in clinical practice. The important fact to remember is that osmolality reflects the potential for water movement and water distribution between and within body fluid compartments.

Diffusion

Diffusion, a passive transport mechanism, is the random movement of molecules and ions from an area of higher concentration to an area of lower concentration in a solution, such as the exchange of oxygen and carbon dioxide between the alveoli and capillaries in the lungs (Figure 11-2). Several factors influence how diffusion occurs: membrane permeability, the size and number of the diffusing molecule or ion, and differences in electrical charges (positive and negative) of the ions involved. Temperature affects this process, with increased diffusion occurring as the temperature increases (Chernecky et al, 2002).

Filtration

Filtration is the movement together of solutes and water through selectively permeable membranes, always moving from an area of higher pressure to an area of lower pressure. Filtration involves the movement of solutes and water in relation to hydrostatic pressure. It differs from diffusion and osmosis in that diffusion and osmosis are a response to concentrations, and filtration is a response to pressure.

Hydrostatic pressure is generated by the action of the heart pumping blood to the capillaries and is opposed by oncotic pressure that moves the fluid, electrolytes, and waste back into the capillaries. Oncotic pressure is exerted mainly by plasma proteins, specifically albumin, because they are the only dissolved constituents in the plasma and interstitial fluids that do not readily pass through the capillary pores (Guyton and Hall, 2006). It is these proteins that are responsible for the osmotic pressure on both sides of the capillary membrane known as colloid osmotic pressure or oncotic pressure (different from the pressure exerted at the cell membrane). There is also a Donnan effect—caused by sodium, potassium, and other cations held in the plasma by the proteins—that impacts the colloid osmotic pressure (Guyton and Hall, 2006).

The movement of fluid into or out of the capillaries depends on the balance between opposing forces. These forces are referred to as *Starling forces* when they relate to the movement of water and solutes through capillaries. Again, it is oncotic pressure that opposes capillary hydrostatic pressure (Figure 11-3).

Active transport

With osmosis, diffusion, and filtration, fluids passively move from higher concentrations/pressures to lower concentrations/pressures to equalize the concentrations on either side of the semipermeable membrane. There are times when a higher concentration is required on one side of the membrane than on the other.

What makes the uneven concentrations possible is a process called active transport. The active transport process requires energy to move the molecules or ions "uphill" against osmotic pressure to an area of higher concentration (Elkin, Perry, Potter,

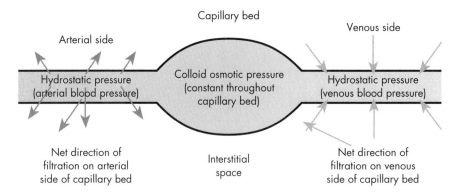

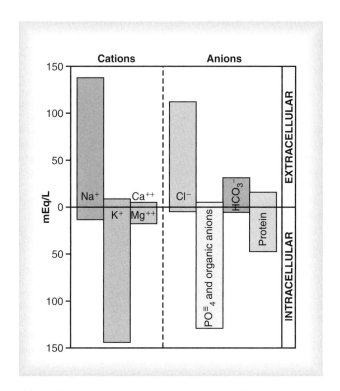

FIGURE 11-3 Filtration and hydrostatic pressure. (From Elkin MK et al: *Nursing interventions & clinical skills,* ed 4, St Louis, 2007, Mosby.)

2007). There are two types of active transport depending on the energy source: primary and secondary. The energy source for primary active transport is primarily adenosine triphosphate (ATP). The most familiar example of primary active transport is the sodium-potassium pump, allowing a higher concentration of potassium inside the cell while the sodium concentration is higher outside the cell.

There are two forms of secondary active transport including co-transport and counter-transport. With co-transport, the molecule or ion that has a higher concentration outside the cell creates a storehouse of energy that will be used for its transport into the cell. With appropriate conditions, the high concentrated molecules or ions may pull other substances through the cell membrane. The counter-transport process allows the transportation of molecules/ions in a direction opposite to the primary ion with both bound to the same carrier protein (e.g., sodium and calcium) (Guyton and Hall, 2006).

Ionization

An important factor in the movement of fluid in the body is the electrical charge of the particles, or solutes, found in a particular fluid. Solutes are chemical compounds that act in one of two ways when in solution: they either remain whole or develop an electrical charge when dissolved. Compounds that develop an electrical charge break into particles, called *ions,* in a process called *ionization.* Such chemical compounds are commonly known as *electrolytes.* Some electrolytes have a positive charge when placed in water, whereas others develop a negative charge. Ions are dissociated particles of an electrolyte, and they too carry either a positive charge (a cation) or a negative charge (an anion). Cations are electrolytes such as sodium, potassium, calcium, and magnesium. Examples of anions are chloride, bicarbonate, phosphate, and sulfate.

The number of electrically charged ions in a defined amount of fluid is measured as milliequivalents per liter (mEq/L) (*milliequivalent* refers to the chemical activity of an element). To achieve electrical balance, the number of cations and anions in a solution (expressed in milliequivalents) must always be equal. Milliequivalents are used as the measure of ions rather than milligrams because milligrams measure only the weight of the electrolyte. Weight gives no indication of the number of ions or the number of electrical charges contained (Figure 11-4) (Chernecky et al, 2002; Weinstein, 2007).

Other substances important in the homeostasis of fluids and electrolytes are glucose, protein, organic acids, oxygen, and carbon dioxide. Although these are not necessarily considered

FIGURE 11-4 Major cations and anions of the intracellular and extracellular fluids. The concentrations of Ca^{2+} and Mg^{2+} represent the sum of these two ions. The concentrations shown represent the total of free ions and complex ions. (From Guyton AC, Hall JE: *Textbook of medical physiology,* ed 11, Philadelphia, 2006, Saunders.)

charged particles, they are important in the body's state of balance.

HOMEOSTATIC MECHANISMS

There are many homeostatic mechanisms that help keep the volume and composition of body fluids within the narrow range defined as normal. Before discussing the regulating organs, there are two principles that are helpful to remember when considering homeostasis in the body.

The first principle states that the overall amount and composition of fluid within each compartment must remain stable and that each compartment must be electrically neutral—that is, the ions must be balanced between anions and cations. There should be no net electrical charge in any compartment at any given time. In addition to maintaining balance, the compartments are constantly exchanging and replacing individual ions. The work required to maintain this balance can use up to 20% of the body's ATP stores.

The second principle states that the osmolality among the intracellular, interstitial, and intravascular compartments needs to be equal. In osmosis, if there is a difference in the total number of active particles, the water moves into the compartment that contains the higher number of particles. A solution of higher osmolality has a lower water concentration (or higher particle concentration) than a solution of lesser osmolality.

REGULATORY ORGANS

Many organs, including the kidneys, heart and blood vessels, lungs, skin, adrenal glands, hypothalamus, pituitary gland, parathyroid gland, and gastrointestinal (GI) tract, are associated with maintaining the body's homeostasis.

The kidneys are considered the primary force in homeostasis because the kidneys' major function is to adjust the amount of water and electrolytes that leave the body to equal the amount that enters the body. The homeostasis is primarily due to the retention and excretion of sodium and water through the regulation of the glomerular filtration rate by the kidneys. There are a variety of hormonal factors involved in this regulation.

The hypothalamus secrets antidiuretic hormone (ADH) and stores it in the posterior pituitary gland. ADH is secreted in response to a decreased blood volume by increasing reabsorption of water through the kidney tubules, resulting in a decreased urine output. In reverse, as blood volume increases, ADH secretion is decreased and water is excreted through the kidneys.

The right atrium releases an atrial natriuretic peptide (ANP) hormone in response to atrial distention of the heart. ANP stimulates the kidney to initiate diuresis of water and sodium, resulting in a decreased intravascular volume (Elkin et al, 2007).

The renin-angiotensin-aldosterone system regulates sodium reabsorption in the renal tubules. The adrenal glands, positioned above the kidneys, consist of two different sections: the adrenal cortex and the adrenal medulla. The adrenal cortex secretes two mineralocorticoid hormones, aldosterone and cortisol, that affect homeostasis. Aldosterone acts on the kidney's tubular cells, is active in the reabsorption of sodium and water, and can decrease potassium excretion. An increase in the level of aldosterone results in the retention of sodium and the loss of potassium. When sodium is retained, water is also retained. A decreased secretion of aldosterone results in the excretion of sodium and water and the retention of potassium. Cortisol, among its many functions, helps regulate blood pressure by regulating the amount of vasoconstriction necessary to maintain a normal blood pressure. Aldosterone is considered the more powerful of the two hormones, but when cortisol is secreted in large quantities, it can also affect sodium and fluid retention and potassium excretion.

The parathyroid glands are attached to the lateral lobes of the thyroid gland and consist of four to five glands. Parathyroid hormone (PTH), secreted from the parathyroid glands, has an effect on calcium and phosphate concentrations and influences the reabsorption of calcium. An increase in the PTH level increases the serum calcium concentration and lowers the serum phosphate concentration. The reverse is also true; a decreased secretion of PTH lowers the serum calcium and elevates the serum phosphate concentrations. Decreased serum calcium levels stimulate the release of PTH, which in turn increases the serum calcium level. The thyroid gland, which secretes calcitonin, also has an effect on calcium levels in the body. If there is an increase in the serum calcium level, this causes an increased secretion of calcitonin. The effect of calcitonin on calcium is opposite that of PTH.

The heart and blood vessels also play a major role in fluid balance. The pumping action of the heart and the resulting circulation through the blood vessels allow blood to reach the kidneys in sufficient volume to regulate water and electrolytes. Circulation of blood through the kidneys also allows urine to form. Adequate renal perfusion is the foundation for adequate renal function. In addition, there are special stretch receptors in the blood vessels and atrium of the heart whose purpose is to react to hypovolemic states by stimulating fluid retention.

The lungs also contribute to homeostasis through the ventilatory process. Under the control of the medulla oblongata and in response to hydrogen level changes in the blood, the lungs act rapidly to correct metabolic acid-base disturbances. The lungs also regulate oxygen and carbon dioxide levels.

Other organs that affect fluid and electrolyte balance in the body are the skin and the GI tract. Because the skin communicates with our environment, it allows water to escape from the body through perspiration. The GI tract also plays a role in water absorption and reabsorption.

All the organs of homeostasis can be likened to a symphony. To make music, each musician needs to play his or her part in harmony with the other musicians. When they play together, beautiful music can be made. So it is with the organs of homeostasis. Through their interdependencies and interaction, they all work together to meet a common goal: the maintenance of a balanced state in the human body.

FLUID AND WATER MOVEMENT

FLUID COMPARTMENTS

The internal environment of the human body is largely composed of fluid, with water being the most abundant component. Approximately 60% of body weight in an adult is water. The amount of total body water as a percentage of body weight varies somewhat among individuals because of differences in the amount of adipose tissue, which contains little water. The total body water also varies for the young and old with a total of 75% to 80% for newborns and 45% for the older adult (Weinstein, 2007).

Body water is distributed between the intracellular, extracellular, and transcellular compartments. Intracellular fluid is the fluid content of all cells, and represents about two thirds of total body weight.

Extracellular fluid constitutes about one third of total body weight. The extracellular fluid compartment is divided into two separate areas. Fluid found in tissue spaces between blood vessels and cells of the body, including lymph fluid, is referred to as *interstitial fluid*. The other type of extracellular fluid is plasma, which accounts for approximately 5% of total body weight. Extracellular fluid serves two functions in the body. First, it provides a relatively constant environment for the cells. Second, it helps transport substances to and from the cells. Plasma is a highly specialized fluid in the body and contains red blood cells and protein in large amounts. Plasma proteins have a negative charge that increases the binding of sodium and potassium ions (Guyton and Hall, 2006).

Transcellular fluid is considered a component of the extracellular fluid compartment and is the product of cellular metabolism (Weinstein, 2007). The fluid that is contained in transcellular areas is specialized and is composed of cerebrospinal, pericardial, intraocular, peritoneal, or synovial fluid. GI fluid is also classified as transcellular. It is separated from the blood, but unlike the other fluid compartments, it is separated by capillary endothelial cells and epithelial tissue; therefore it is compartmentalized fluid.

Transcellular fluid is not usually considered when talking about fluid and electrolyte balance; however, because of the special attributes of transcellular fluids, physical symptoms are attributed to their loss.

Although intracellular and extracellular fluids contain the same types of anions and cations, the amounts in which they are found vary between the two compartments. The principal cation in intracellular fluid is potassium. Found in lesser amounts are magnesium, sodium, and calcium. The most prevalent anion in intracellular fluid is phosphate, with smaller amounts of bicarbonate and chloride. The fluid cation found in most abundance in extracellular fluid is sodium; present in much smaller amounts are potassium, calcium, and magnesium. The principal anion of extracellular fluid is chloride, with bicarbonate and phosphate found in smaller amounts.

Therefore major electrolytes in extracellular fluid are sodium as a cation and chloride as an anion. Sodium, chloride, and bicarbonate represent more than 90% of the total amount of solutes found in the extracellular space. Potassium is the major cation in cells, and magnesium is also found in high concentration. The anions in the intracellular compartment are phosphate, sulfate, bicarbonate, and proteinate (Figure 11-5).

MOVEMENT OF FLUIDS AND ELECTROLYTES

One way that water moves in the body is through osmotic pressure. The distribution of water in the body depends on electrolyte balance and on the distribution of electrolytes and fluids within the intracellular and extracellular compartments. Osmotic gradients are established and maintained by solutes. While water is largely unconfined, electrolytes are usually confined to their respective compartments.

Effects of body fluid concentration

If there is no water movement through a membrane because of an osmotic balance, the solutions on either side of the membrane are isotonic. That is, they exert the same amount of osmotic pressure on each side of the membrane, and they contain the same amount of osmotically active solutes. Isotonic osmolality is approximately 300 mOsm/L. Fluid containing a large number of solutes is considered hypertonic when compared with water containing no solute particles. Conversely, water is considered hypotonic when compared with a fluid containing many solute particles. *Osmotic pressure* refers to how strongly water can be pulled across a membrane; the strength or pressure of that pull depends on the amount of solutes or molecules in the solution.

Colloids

Electrolytes and other low-molecular-weight substances exert a normal osmotic pressure. Colloids, such as protein and albumin, are nondiffusible substances that have a higher molecular weight. Therefore they exert a higher osmotic pressure, the

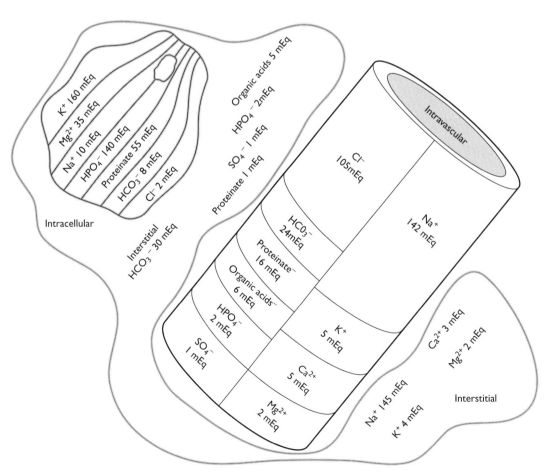

FIGURE 11-5 Anions and cations of intracellular, interstitial, and intravascular fluids.

colloid osmotic or oncotic pressure, which causes water to be pulled into the intravascular space.

Crystalloids

Diffusible substances are referred to as *crystalloids*. They are important in fluid balance because they can pass through capillary walls, which are the barriers between plasma and interstitial fluid. Crystalloids can expand both intravascular and interstitial spaces. Usually, only about 25% of crystalloids administered remain in the intravascular space, with the rest moving to the interstitial space. Examples of crystalloids are dextrose in water, electrolytes in water, and sodium chloride solutions. See the Focus on Evidence box for the use of crystalloids and colloids for fluid management.

Plasma

Because it contains protein, the plasma component of extracellular fluid responds in a special way to fluid balance. Proteins pull water into the intravascular space.

Sodium

Fluid balance is also regulated by the sodium concentration in plasma, and is minimally influenced by glucose and urea levels in plasma. Sodium and associated anions, primarily bicarbonate and chloride, contribute more than 94% of extracellular fluid solutes (Guyton and Hall, 2006). The osmotic pressure produced by sodium determines the state of cellular hydration. Osmosis occurs when the extracellular fluid contains an electrolyte content lower or higher than normal. For example, if plain water with no electrolyte content was injected into the bloodstream, the red blood cells in the plasma would absorb the water. This would cause the cells to swell and burst. If a solution with high sodium content were injected into the body, the red blood cells would lose water to the salt and the cells would shrink.

FOCUS ON EVIDENCE

Use of Crystalloids Versus Colloids for Fluid Management

- A meta-analysis of 63 eligible trials, 55 presenting mortality data, comparing colloids to crystalloids concluded there is no evidence that resuscitation with colloids reduces the risk of death compared with crystalloids in patients experiencing trauma or burns or following surgery (Parel and Roberts, 2007).

- A meta-analysis including 32 trials analyzed resuscitation and volume expansion in critically ill patients using human albumin. The conclusion revealed that for hypovolemic patients there was no evidence that albumin reduces mortality when compared with saline. Also, there was no evidence that albumin reduces mortality in critically ill patients with burns and hypoalbuminemia. There remains a possibility that there is a select group of critically ill patients in which albumin may be indicated (The Albumin Reviewers, 2004).

- A randomized, double-blinded study involving patients (n = 6997) admitted to the ICU compared the use of 4% albumin or normal saline. The conclusion was that the outcomes for both infusions were similar at 28 days (Finfer et al, 2004).

- In a post hoc study of critically ill patients with traumatic brain injury, fluid resuscitation with albumin was associated with a higher death rate than those resuscitated with saline (Myburgh et al, 2007).

Solute concentration

Solute concentration and the associated osmotic force affect body water distribution. As stated earlier, water moves from an area of lower solute concentration to an area of higher solute concentration, or an area of high osmolality. A change in the osmolality of one compartment always alters the osmolality of the other compartment; stated another way, a change in extracellular fluid compartment osmolality dictates a change in the osmolality of intracellular fluids. The body is striving for homeostasis, and there is water movement until the osmolality values of both compartments are relatively equal.

Fluid pressure

To understand the movement of fluids and solutes within the body, fluid pressures and the amounts of solutes and water in the various compartments must be considered. As water moves to achieve a state of equilibrium, so do pressures exerted on the fluids change to reach a state of equilibrium. There are four pressures to consider when studying water exchange between plasma and interstitial fluid. Movement is determined by blood hydrostatic and colloid osmotic pressures on one side of the capillary membrane and by interstitial fluid hydrostatic and colloid osmotic pressures on the other side. Blood hydrostatic pressure forces fluid out of the capillaries into the interstitial fluid on one side; however, blood colloid osmotic pressure draws fluid back into the capillaries. Interstitial fluid hydrostatic pressure forces fluids out of the interstitial space into the capillaries, and interstitial fluid colloid osmotic pressure moves fluid back out of the capillaries. The net effect is that two of these pressures exert a force in one direction, and two exert pressure in the opposite direction. The difference between these two sets of opposing pressures represents the net or effective filtration pressure. An increase in plasma volume causes an increase in hydrostatic pressure of the blood, which then affects the pressure gradient and the movement of fluid. This results in a condition known as *edema*. The lymphatic system has an impact on fluid pressure because of its removal of excess fluid and debris from the tissue into the blood circulation. This process creates a slight negative pressure in interstitial fluid (Guyton and Hall, 2006).

Hydrostatic pressure is comparable to the principle of filtration, which is the transfer of water-soluble substances from an area of high pressure to an area of low pressure. Fluid and water-soluble substances are moved by hydrostatic pressure in the vessels. Hydrostatic pressure can be exerted by the pumping action of the heart. The difference in arterial and venous pressures also plays a role in the movement of fluids. Hydrostatic pressure is greater than colloid osmotic pressure at the arterial end of a capillary, which causes fluids to move out of the vessel. Conversely, the osmotic force is greater than the hydrostatic pressure on the venous end of a capillary, enabling fluid to reenter a capillary on the venous end (Guyton and Hall, 2006).

Vascular effects

For the body to function correctly, there must be enough circulating fluid to support osmosis, diffusion, and filtration. Baroreceptors, or stretch receptors, located in the carotid sinuses and the aortic arch, respond to the amount of stretch in the vessel wall. The stretch depends on the volume of blood flowing through the vessel. If there is a drop in arterial pressure, these baroreceptors generate fewer impulses, which in turn causes an accelerated heart rate and an increase in blood pressure. The mechanism controlling water movement between fluid compartments is a rapid-response system. Its primary action is to maintain a normal blood volume, even at the expense of interstitial fluid volume. The interstitial space may expand by several liters over a long period without major changes in the intravascular or intracellular compartments.

Body fluid volume and composition

Age, gender, and the amount of adipose tissue all affect the amount of fluids in the human body. Women have less body fluid than men because men have less body fat. This gender difference in fluid amount is not seen until adolescence but remains throughout life. A newborn's fluid content is 70% to 80% of body weight. Premature infants have an even higher percentage of fluid, approximately 90% of their body weight. Infants are more susceptible to fluid volume deficit because their bodies have a higher fluid percentage and they have more extracellular fluid. More than half of the newborn's body fluid is extracellular fluid. In adults, extracellular fluid accounts for only one third of body fluid. Extracellular fluid is more readily lost from the body. By the end of the second year of life, the infant's total body fluid approaches that of the adult. The adult body composition of 40% cellular and 20% extracellular is reached by puberty. After the age of 40 years, the total fluid percentage of body weight begins to decrease for both men and women (Weinstein, 2007). After 60 years of age, the percentages decrease even more, because with aging there is a decrease of lean body mass and an increase in fat content. Therefore the body holds less water. Changes in fluid volume and composition throughout life are shown in Table 11-1.

Water regulation
Intake

The goal is to maintain a state of equilibrium between fluid compartments and between the body's daily fluid intake and output. The average healthy adult requires from 2000 to 2800 mL of fluid a day. Usually, 1000 to 1500 mL of this total is taken into the body in liquid form. Another 800 to 1000 mL comes from food eaten during the day. Oxidation in body tissues accounts for another 350 mL. Fluid loss amounts to approximately 2500 mL/day. When the body is functioning correctly, the intake is balanced by the output.

TABLE 11-1 Body Fluid Volume

Age	Approximate percentage
Infant (birth)	75-80
1 year	67
Adult	50-60
Older adult	45

Modified from Chernecky C, Macklin D, Murphy-Ende K: *Real world nursing survival guide: fluids & electrolytes*, Philadelphia, 2002, Saunders.

Mechanisms of intake. There are various ways to achieve intake and output of fluids and electrolytes. Water is taken into the body by food or drink. The liquid that is ingested is measured as part of intake. Liquid is also taken into the body through food. Water is formed by oxidation when food is broken down into energy by the body. Oxidation releases water for use in metabolism; approximately 350 mL of water comes from the oxidation process daily. Thirst is controlled by osmoreceptors found in the hypothalamus and by intravascular volume. Thirst is an even more important mechanism in supplying endogenous water to the body and is activated when the total body water content is decreased by about 2%. ADH plays an important role in preventing dehydration and therefore hypertonicity of body fluids.

Thirst mechanism. The thirst mechanism is activated when stimulated by osmoreceptors in the anterior hypothalamus, where antidiuretic hormone (ADH) is synthesized, and in the posterior pituitary gland, where ADH is released (Guyton and Hall, 2006). Plasma osmolality and sodium concentrations are usually kept within a narrow range. The upper limit of this range is determined by the osmotic threshold for thirst, referred to as the *threshold* for drinking (Guyton and Hall, 2006). When the sodium concentration increases by about 2 mEq/L above the normal level, the physical desire for water increases. The drinking mechanism is stimulated, creating a desire for water so that the extracellular fluid level returns toward normal as water is ingested. Through several processes, thirst is relieved almost immediately after drinking fluid. However, it may take 30 to 60 minutes before the fluid is distributed throughout the body (Guyton and Hall, 2006).

Output

The kidneys, in addition to excreting urine, can adjust the amount of water and electrolytes that leave the body so that it equals the amount of water and electrolytes that enter the body. They have a vital role in fluid and electrolyte balance and in acid-base balance. On average, the kidneys filter approximately 180 L of water in a 24-hour period (Guyton and Hall, 2006). This amount varies according to the fluid intake. The usual amount of fluid output through the kidney is approximately 60 mL/hour (1.5 L/day) (Elkin et al, 2007).

Perspiration. Water and electrolytes can be lost through the skin; these are referred to as *sensible losses*. Sensible losses, or perspiration, can account for up to 1 to 2 L/hour under hot, dry conditions or with heavy exercise, whereas average general loss is approximately 100 mL/day (Guyton and Hall, 2006). Perspiration is considered a hypotonic fluid; it contains chiefly sodium and potassium. Losses by perspiration vary according to environmental temperature. Body temperature and ambient room temperature also affect the amount of perspiration. The skin also loses water by evaporation, which can be up to 600 mL/day. Evaporation is considered an *insensible loss*.

Respiration. Approximately 300 mL of water is lost through the lungs in any 24-hour period. This is considered insensible water loss, and the amount lost varies according to the rate and depth of respiration. In addition, the lungs play a role in homeostasis because of their ability to eliminate about 13,000 mEq of hydrogen ions in 24 hours, which is significantly more than the kidneys excrete.

Gastrointestinal tract. Although the GI tract is responsible for 100 to 200 mL of fluid loss daily, it can actually filter up to 8 L of fluid in 24 hours. Much of this fluid, however, is reabsorbed through the small intestine. Greater losses can occur from adverse conditions such as diarrhea, vomiting, or fistula development.

Other mechanisms. Water and electrolytes can be lost through other mechanisms, such as from tears and through feces. Abnormal losses can occur from the use of strong diuretics, which deplete body fluids and electrolytes, or through wound drainage, fever, hyperventilation, mechanical ventilation, and GI tubes.

Antidiuretic hormone. The release of ADH in response to osmotic dehydration is affected by plasma osmolality. Osmoreceptors can detect very small changes in the concentrations of sodium and other solutes in plasma. Sodium concentration is the driving force in ADH secretion (Guyton and Hall, 2006). With a normal plasma osmolality, the secretion of ADH is low enough to permit maximum urinary output. If plasma becomes hyperosmolar, ADH is secreted to maintain maximum water retention in the kidneys, and solutes continue to be excreted in an effort to bring osmolality back to normal. The reverse is also true—in a hypoosmolar state, ADH secretion is diminished, allowing the excretion of water while solutes are retained by the kidney. This process returns the plasma to a more normal osmolality.

Effects of age on intake and output

When considering the intake of fluid into the body and the output of that fluid and associated electrolytes, the effect of age on homeostatic mechanisms should be considered. The elderly may experience up to a 50% reduction in kidney function, which results from a decrease in blood flow to the kidneys. There is also an inability to concentrate urine when the fluid intake is reduced, so the glomerular filtration rate is also decreased. This indicates that the elderly are more susceptible to drug toxicities because of decreased renal function. Cardiac output and stroke volume of the heart are lowered in the elderly. Glands may atrophy, which reduces the ability to eliminate fluid through perspiration and causes some control of body temperature to be lost. There is sometimes a loss of muscle tone of the intestinal tract. Thirst mechanisms may be diminished in the aging person, so the attempt to reach homeostasis based on thirst is then compromised.

Likewise, infants also require special consideration. There is proportionately more water in the extracellular compartment of an infant than in that of an adult. Therefore the infant is more vulnerable to fluid volume deficit. The infant may turn over half of its extracellular fluid daily, whereas adults may change only one sixth of their extracellular volume in the same 24-hour period. This means that the infant has less body fluid in reserve. Infants have a large amount of metabolic waste to excrete because their daily fluid exchange is up to two times greater per unit of body weight than that of an adult. Large volumes of urine are formed each day to excrete all the waste products. Infants have a proportionally higher body surface area than adults, so they have a greater fluid loss potential through their skin. Infants can also suffer greater losses from the GI tract in a relatively shorter period than adults.

FLUID DISORDERS

Homeostatic mechanisms of the body are complex and delicate. Generally, this system has the ability to maintain equilibrium, but sometimes these mechanisms fail and the body can be in a state of fluid deficit or excess.

Fluid volume excess

An increase in extracellular fluid volume is known as fluid volume excess or *hypervolemia*. The increased volume may occur in the extracellular and the intracellular compartments while the extracellular overload can be with the intravascular or interstitial fluids. Hypervolemia is generally the result of an increase in body sodium concentration, which in turn causes water retention. Hypervolemia may be classified as isotonic, hypotonic, or hypertonic. When both sodium and water are retained, the relative serum sodium concentration remains essentially normal (Pagana and Pagana, 2007). Once an imbalance develops, the body attempts to compensate. This occurs through the release of atrial natriuretic factor, which causes the kidneys to increase the rate of filtration and excretion of sodium and water. There is also a decrease in the aldosterone and ADH levels.

Cause

Fluid volume excess is related to an increase in sodium, water, or a combination of the two. Extracellular fluid overload may be due to an increased intake of sodium through diet or hypertonic fluid administration. It can also be caused by regulatory mechanisms. The kidneys, which help regulate sodium and water levels, may be diseased, leading to sodium and water retention. This is particularly true in the presence of a decreased output. Increased secretion of ADH and aldosterone results in fluid retention.

Another major organ that is a part of the normal regulatory system is the heart. In conditions such as congestive heart failure, the diseased heart cannot circulate the intravascular fluids adequately. This pseudointravascular deficit signals the kidneys to conserve sodium and water, leading to fluid volume excess.

A malfunctioning liver could lead to excessive fluid retention. In cirrhosis, for example, the retention is related to a decreased serum albumin level, which facilitates the loss of intravascular fluids into the interstitial space. Additional fluid may be lost into the peritoneal cavity because of hepatic venous obstruction. Again, this decreased intravascular volume signals the kidney to release more renin, which leads to an increase in the aldosterone level and results in sodium and water retention.

Hypervolemia may occur as a result of an excessive sodium and fluid intake. This is generally caused by the excessive administration of IV solutions, particularly those that contain sodium. Also, the excessive ingestion of sodium contained in food or medications may lead to fluid volume excess; this is especially true in those with a heart or kidney abnormality.

Other possible causes of hypervolemia are the administration of excessive doses of steroids and fluid volume shifts within the body. In the case of steroids, the increased fluid volume is related to sodium and water retention. A shift of interstitial fluid to plasma may occur with the treatment of burns. Often, initial burn treatment includes the administration of large amounts of IV solutions because of a fluid volume deficit. Several days later, there is a shift of fluid from the interstitial space back into the intravascular space, which could lead to hypervolemia.

Intracellular fluid overload may be related to an increased administration of hypotonic IV solutions including 0.45% sodium chloride. An isotonic solution, 5% dextrose in water, can also become hypotonic as the body rapidly absorbs the glucose. The overload may also be due to excessive use of free water from irrigation of enteral or nasogastric tubes. Other causes include the syndrome of inappropriate antidiuretic hormone (SIADH), with increased reabsorption of water, and psychogenic polydipsia, from excessive ingestion of water (Baumberger-Henry, 2005).

Assessment

The signs and symptoms of hypervolemia are related to the location and degree of fluid volume excess and to the rate of onset. A sudden, rapid onset results in more pronounced problems.

Probably the most visible characteristic is edema, which is increased fluid volume in the interstitial space. When edema is present, it is usually most visible in dependent areas, as well as around the eyes. The degree of edema may be determined by applying finger pressure around the ankle and sacral areas. Removing the finger leaves a small indention or pit as the fluid excess becomes more severe.

Weight gain usually accompanies the increased fluid volume. This would not occur, however, if the increase were a shift from another compartment. Weight gain is approximately 1 kg/1000 mL fluid increase (Chernecky et al, 2002).

Fluid may shift to another cavity in the body, primarily the abdominal cavity. Accumulation in the abdominal cavity, known as *ascites,* is often seen in patients with advanced renal or hepatic disease. It is noted by shortness of breath or decreased cardiac output caused by the increased pressure of the excessive fluid volume.

Another characteristic of hypervolemia is pulmonary edema, which can lead to moist rales, shortness of breath, and wheezing. There may be an increase in blood pressure, distention of the neck veins, slower emptying of the peripheral veins, and a more rapid and bounding pulse rate. Polyuria is present if the kidneys are functioning normally.

Laboratory findings reveal a decreased hematocrit and decreased blood urea nitrogen (BUN) value resulting from hemodilution. If the excessive volume is caused by water retention, the serum sodium level and osmolality decrease. In most cases, the urine specific gravity also decreases. Pulmonary congestion may be shown on chest x-ray examination. Because of a decrease in oxygen transport capabilities with pulmonary edema, the arterial blood gases may show a decreased Pao_2 and $Paco_2$ and an increased pH.

Treatment

Treatment of fluid volume excess depends on its cause. When the cause cannot be determined, it is necessary to treat the disorder symptomatically. This generally includes restriction of sodium and fluid intake, bed rest, and/or diuretic administration. The diuretic will depend on kidney function, degree of hypovolemia, and potency of the diuretic, and may need to be given by the IV route. There may be special requirements for some patients, such as paracentesis in the case of ascites. Dialysis may also be indicated in the presence of renal disease.

Sodium restriction may extend to the diet and to medications, particularly those containing a sodium salt. There are also a variety of over-the-counter preparations that contain sodium.

Nursing interventions should include monitoring vital signs, shortness of breath, cough, and body weight. Any continued presence of edema should be noted. Intake and output records and electrolyte levels should be monitored, particularly after diuretic administration.

Observations should be clearly documented, including the response to diuretics. All abnormal observations should be communicated to the physician.

Fluid volume deficit

Fluid volume deficit, or *hypovolemia,* occurs as a result of excessive but relatively equal fluid and electrolyte depletion in the extracellular compartment. The body attempts to compensate for the losses by stimulating thirst, increasing the heart rate, and releasing ADH and aldosterone. If the deficit is severe and not corrected in a timely manner, it could lead to renal failure and death. As with fluid volume excess, a fluid volume deficit can be classified as isotonic, hypotonic, or hypertonic (or osmolar). With isotonic deficit, the loss of water and solutes is equal. In a hypertonic deficit, the loss of fluid is greater than solute loss. Hypotonic deficits, which occur less often than the other types, exhibit a decreased concentration of solute (usually sodium and potassium) in the extracellular fluid (Guyton and Hall, 2006).

Cause

Hypovolemia may result from an abnormal loss of body fluids or inadequate fluid intake, which affects the fluid and electrolyte content. Fluid deficit may be caused by the loss of GI fluids. This may occur through vomiting, diarrhea, suctioning, and fistulas.

The skin is another mechanism for fluid loss. Under normal conditions, fluid is lost through the skin as a means of regulating body temperature. In the presence of a fever, however, there are abnormal, insensible fluid losses. Any type of trauma related to the skin, such as burns and cuts, also facilitates the abnormal loss of fluids. In the case of burns, fluid moves from the vascular to the interstitial space where it surrounds the burned area.

Excessive loss takes place through the renal system. This may be caused by polyuria related to administering osmotic diuretics or concentrated IV solutions and tube feedings. Polyuria may also occur with hyperglycemia and some renal disorders.

Trauma, surgery, and bleeding disorders may result in hemorrhage, which rapidly decreases the intravascular fluid volume. There may also be a decrease in the circulating volume because of *third spacing.* With this phenomenon, there is a shift of fluid from the circulating volume into a space where it cannot easily be exchanged with fluid in the extracellular space. Because third spacing is only a shifting of fluid, there is no actual fluid loss. The fluid deficit in this case is the result of the decreased circulating volume.

Finally, hypovolemia may occur because of a decreased fluid intake, particularly in the infant and older adult populations. Infants have a larger body surface area and tend to lose more fluid than adults. They depend on others to provide oral fluids. Older adults have a decreased sense of thirst and therefore are less likely to seek fluid replacement. The ability to replace fluid may be further complicated by decreased mobility. Patients who cannot respond to thirst (because they are confused or comatose, for example) are subject to fluid volume depletion.

Assessment

As with fluid volume excess, the signs and symptoms of hypovolemia are related to the degree of the deficit and how fast it occurs. There is a loss of weight as the fluid volume decreases, except in the case of third spacing.

Assessment reveals a decreased central venous pressure, flattened jugular vein while in the supine position, capillary filling time longer than 3 seconds, and slow filling of the hand veins (longer than 3 to 4 seconds) (Elkin et al, 2007). The lower circulating volume leads to decreased blood pressure and possibly postural hypotension. With less volume, there is decreased tissue perfusion, which creates a variety of problems, including muscle weakness, dizziness, lethargy, and confusion. As the body tries to maintain an adequate intravascular volume, the pulse rate increases and becomes weaker. The kidneys try to conserve fluid, so there is a decreased urine output.

Skin turgor should be checked by pinching the skin, which slowly returns to the normal position in the presence of hypovolemia. The tongue, which normally has one furrow, has several small furrows. The eyes appear sunken and the face has a pinched expression.

As fluid loss becomes more severe, the patient may go into shock. The extremities become cool and clammy, diaphoresis occurs, urinary output drops sharply, and the patient may become comatose.

Laboratory findings show an increased BUN level elevated out of proportion to the serum creatinine level (ratio greater than 20:1) (Smeltzer et al, 2008). This is the result of the kidneys conserving water and urea, which follows the water. The hematocrit also increases except when the deficit is caused by hemorrhage. With blood loss, red blood cells and serum are lost in equal amounts. However, as the body attempts to compensate for the fluid deficit, interstitial fluid shifts into the intravascular space and the hematocrit decreases. There is an increase in the urine specific gravity and osmolality. The electrolyte levels, serum osmolality, and acid-base balance vary according to the type of fluid lost and the causative factor.

Treatment

The treatment of hypovolemia includes correcting the cause of the deficit and returning the extracellular fluid to a normal level. If oral fluids cannot replace the deficit, IV therapy should be initiated based on physician orders, patient assessment, and established procedures. An isotonic electrolyte solution such as lactated Ringer's is generally used to initiate therapy for hypovolemia. The severity of the deficit generally dictates the administration rate. As the fluid is replaced, the IV solution may be changed to one that provides free water. This helps the kidneys excrete wastes.

If the deficit is severe enough, oliguria may be present. In this case, it is important to determine whether the cause is fluid volume deficit or renal disease. This may be accomplished through a fluid challenge test, in which the patient is monitored closely as IV solutions are administered. If the kidneys respond by producing urine, then oliguria is probably the result of fluid volume deficit. When there is no increase in urinary output, the cause of the oliguria is most likely related to renal failure or decreased cardiac function.

During treatment for fluid volume deficit, the patient must be monitored closely. This includes monitoring the urinary output, vital signs, hemodynamic pressures, and body weight. Monitoring laboratory test results can help maintain normal fluid and electrolyte levels. The rate of administration for IV solutions should be monitored to prevent fluid overload. Assessment findings need to be clearly documented and the physician notified of abnormal results.

ACID-BASE BALANCE

The body's complexity and delicate balance is also seen in the principles of acid-base balance. The body continually produces acids that are then neutralized and excreted to maintain homeostasis. Acid-base balance is primarily controlled by buffers, which act immediately; the respiratory system, which responds in minutes; and the renal system, which can take from hours up to 3 days (Baumberger-Henry, 2005; Elkin et al, 2007). It is imperative that this balance be maintained within a very narrow range, with a pH between 7.35 and 7.45. Any excess in either direction, without correction or intervention, can result in death.

To understand pH, and therefore acids and bases, one must first understand the function of hydrogen in pH. Certain characteristics of a solution are measured by its pH, which is the hydrogen ion concentration of the solution. Because this concentration is very small, it is generally expressed as a logarithm. For example, water has a pH of 7, which can be expressed as a negative logarithm, or 0.0000001 (10^{-7}). The logarithm makes it much easier to work with and conceptualize the pH value (Baumberger-Henry, 2005).

The concentration of hydrogen ions in a solution determines its acidity or alkalinity. If a solution is acidic, it has a low pH. If a solution is alkaline, it has a high pH. The normal pH range is 1 to 14, with 7 being approximately neutral. Water, with its pH of 7, is considered neutral because of the balance between the concentration of hydrogen ions (H^+) and hydroxyl (OH^-) ions. Hydroxyl ions are released when a base breaks apart in water, and hydrogen ions are released when an acid dissociates in water.

ACIDS

An acid is a chemical substance that dissociates and donates hydrogen ions to a solution or in combination with another substance. Acids can be classified as strong or weak. Strong acids such as hydrochloric acid (HCl) release hydrogen ions into solution and tend to remain dissociated in that solution. Weak acids such as carbonic acid (H_2CO_3) also give up hydrogen ions in solution, but not completely, as does the strong acid. Weak acids are only partially dissociated in acidic solutions.

Volatile acids are acids that can form a gas and are eliminated from the body as a gas; therefore they are excreted from the lungs. An example of a volatile acid is carbonic acid, which is a combination of carbon dioxide (CO_2) and water (H_2O). Nonvolatile or fixed acids cannot be converted into gas form. They are excreted by the kidneys in the urine and in small amounts in feces. Nonvolatile acids result from various metabolic processes. Some are produced in the form of uric acid, which is an organic acid. Some may be in the form of sulfuric and phosphoric acids. It is important to remember that any discussion of acids is a discussion of hydrogen ion concentration. To summarize, nonvolatile hydrogen ions are excreted through the renal system or the kidneys, and volatile hydrogen ions or acids are excreted through the lungs or respiratory system (Baumberger-Henry, 2005; Elkin et al, 2007).

Respiratory system influences

Most of the carbonic acid available in the body is found in conjunction with carbon dioxide gas. Therefore the pH of body fluids is affected by changes in the carbon dioxide concentration. When the concentration of carbon dioxide gas in body fluids is increased, the pH decreases. Conversely, when the concentration of carbon dioxide gas is decreased, the pH increases. The rate of alveolar ventilation is a major factor in the regulation of carbon dioxide concentration in the body. Alveolar hyperventilation causes carbon dioxide to be blown off through the lungs. In turn, the release of carbon dioxide through the lungs decreases its concentration in body fluids and increases the pH. On the other hand, alveolar hypoventilation causes the retention of carbon dioxide, which decreases the pH.

The respiratory feedback system is a rapid-response system that can begin to correct changes in pH within minutes, although it may take several hours to achieve. Therefore it is necessary for the third line of defense, the renal system, to take over against the pH changes when the buffer and respiratory feedback mechanisms are not sufficient by themselves.

BASES

A base is a chemical substance that, when dissociated in solution, can combine with a hydrogen ion. When the base combines with a hydrogen ion, it in effect removes the hydrogen from a solution. Examples of bases are bicarbonate and protein. Proteins can function as bases because they act as anions and easily bind or accept hydrogen ions. Bases may be strong or weak, just like acids. A strong base easily accepts hydrogen and removes it from solution. Hydroxyl ions (OH^-) are strong bases. Weak bases do not have the same affinity for hydrogen ions as strong bases and are only partially dissociated in alkaline solutions. Bicarbonate is considered a weak base.

In the human body, most of the acids and bases required for life are weak acids and weak bases. Strong acids and bases would allow sudden and dangerous changes in the pH of body fluids, whereas weak acids and bases allow for a greater degree of stabilization of pH. Weak acids or bases can neutralize strong acids or bases.

Normal response allows the kidneys to reabsorb and conserve bicarbonate and, when needed for acidosis, the kidneys can generate additional bicarbonate and eliminate excessive hydrogen ions (Elkin et al, 2007).

Renal system influences

Like the respiratory system, the renal system responds to changes in hydrogen ion concentration; however, it responds more slowly. It may take up to several days for the renal system to fully achieve its purpose in pH correction. The kidneys provide acid-base regulation through secretion of hydrogen into the urine or through reabsorption of filtered bicarbonate and production of new bicarbonate (H_2CO_3) from CO_2 and H_2O. Carbonic anhydrase catalyzes the dissociation of H_2CO_3, forming H^+ and HCO_3^-. The kidneys regulate excess acid by secreting hydrogen that has been buffered by phosphate and ammonia into the urine while preventing loss of bicarbonate in the urine by reabsorbing it from the distal renal tubules (Baumberger-Henry, 2005; Guyton and Hall, 2006).

BUFFERS

In addition to respiratory and renal system influences, there is a system of buffers that works to maintain acid-base balance. In the presence of an acid-base disturbance, there are three main mechanisms to regain homeostasis, and two have already been discussed. One is the increase in alveolar ventilation. This depends on the lungs and chemoreceptors and acts to reverse an alteration within 1 to 2 minutes. The second defense mechanism is hydrogen ion elimination coupled with increased bicarbonate reabsorption. This occurs in the kidneys and provides

the strongest defense against acid-base disturbances. However, it takes several hours to several days for the renal system to try to reestablish equilibrium. The third defense is a system of buffers. The buffer system begins immediately to equilibrate the hydrogen ion concentration.

A buffer protects the body against hydrogen ion concentration fluctuations. Buffers can inactivate excess hydrogen ions and hydroxyl ions. By doing so, they can maintain the pH within the normal range.

Carbonic acid-sodium bicarbonate buffer system

The carbonic acid-bicarbonate buffering system plays a major role in pH regulation with the respiratory and renal systems. Carbonic anhydrase, the enzyme that catalyzes the reaction, is found in the alveoli walls of the lungs and in epithelial cells in the renal tubules. The lungs excrete or retain carbonic acid or its component, carbon dioxide, and the kidneys excrete or retain sodium bicarbonate. This is the most important buffering system in the extracellular fluid. It can buffer up to 90% of the hydrogen ions contained in extracellular fluid, and has little effect on the cells.

Because of the effects of carbonic acid or sodium bicarbonate, the buffering must occur through the lungs or kidneys. This means that the pH can be moved up or down by the renal system, the respiratory system, or both, acting together. Carbonic acid and sodium bicarbonate are measured by their relative concentrations. The ratio between the two is 1:20, or 1 part of carbonic acid to every 20 parts of sodium bicarbonate. When monitoring acid-base balance, it is important to examine this ratio. When it is disturbed, the hydrogen balance in the body is also disturbed (Chernecky et al, 2002; Baumberger-Henry, 2005; Guyton and Hall, 2006; Elkin et al, 2007).

Phosphate buffer system

The phosphate buffer system operates at a slightly different pH than the carbonic acid-sodium bicarbonate buffer system. Phosphate buffer is more abundant in cells, so its role is more cellular than extracellular. It works mainly in the tubular fluid of the kidneys. This system can buffer strong acids and strong bases into weak acids and weak bases, so that the weakened state of the acids or bases has little effect on the pH of the blood.

Protein buffer system

Proteins can act as both intracellular (such as hemoglobin) and extracellular (such as globulins and albumin) buffers and as acids or bases, a property referred to as *amphoteric*. Since most proteins exist inside the cell, protein is primarily an intracellular buffering mechanism. Approximately 60% to 70% of the total chemical buffering of body fluids is inside the cells and is primarily attributable to proteins (Guyton and Hall, 2006). Their ability to behave as either acid or base depends on the pH of the solution, and makes proteins a powerful buffering agent. Proteins tend to buffer carbon dioxide quickly and bicarbonate more slowly, over several hours.

In addition, hemoglobin and oxyhemoglobin can act as a buffer system. This system works because of a reaction that occurs between hemoglobin and hydrogen ions in red blood cells. The red blood cell is permeable to bicarbonate ions. Therefore, when a hydrogen ion is bound by hemoglobin, a bicarbonate ion diffuses out of the red blood cell into the plasma. The bicarbonate ion is then exchanged for a chloride ion to maintain electrical neutrality.

Potassium-hydrogen exchange

Potassium and hydrogen are positively charged ions that move interchangeably in and out of the cells depending on excess. In the extracellular fluids, excess hydrogen will move inside the cell to act as a buffer and, at the same time, potassium will move into the extracellular fluid to restore the acid-base balance (Baumberger-Henry, 2005).

COMPENSATORY MECHANISMS

Compensatory mechanisms are activated in the presence of a hydrogen imbalance. There are three basic compensatory mechanisms. The first is the dilution of hydrogen in the extracellular fluid and the buffering systems discussed earlier. The second compensatory mechanism is the respiratory system, and the third is the renal system.

The goal of compensation is to return the pH to normal without overcompensating or correcting the pH past the point of normal. The normal range for pH is from 7.35 to 7.45. The absolute normal value is considered 7.4. By definition, acidemia is a condition in which hydrogen ion concentration is elevated in the blood. Stated another way, the blood could have an acid excess or a base deficit, reflected by a pH of less than 7.35. Alkalemia is a condition in which hydrogen ion concentration is decreased. Stated differently, the blood could have an acid deficit or a base excess, indicated by a pH greater than 7.45. Acidosis and alkalosis are the processes that result in acidemia or alkalemia. These terms may be used interchangeably.

BLOOD VALUES: MEASUREMENT AND INTERPRETATION

The evaluation of acid-base balance is based on various blood gas values. In addition to acid-base balance, these values are used to determine the level of oxygenation within the patient's body, both extracellularly and intracellularly. Usually, blood gases are measured from arterial blood, which provides information about the oxygenation status of the blood passing through the lungs. Occasionally, mixed venous blood is used rather than arterial blood to determine oxygen levels in the tissues. If the tissues are receiving adequate oxygen, this can mean that ventilation and circulation within the body are adequate to meet the patient's needs and establish acid-base balance.

The three variables monitored most often are the pH, $Paco_2$, and HCO_3^- levels. As stated earlier, pH measures the level of hydrogen ions present, which determines the alkalinity or acidity of the blood. As the hydrogen ion concentration decreases, the pH increases and vice versa.

The $Paco_2$, or Pco_2, is a measure of the ventilation capability. The P represents the pressure or tension exerted by the carbon dioxide (CO_2) gas. The a designates arterial blood. If it were a venous sample, the letter v would be substituted for a. When there is no P preceding the CO_2 level, it refers to the total CO_2 content rather than the amount of carbon dioxide in the blood as a gas. The total CO_2 content is the amount of CO_2 gas that can be obtained from plasma when a strong acid is added in a laboratory setting. The total CO_2 content consists of bicarbonate, carbonic acid, and dissolved carbon dioxide gas. Because the total CO_2 content measures the sum of bicarbonate,

carbonic acid, and dissolved CO_2, an elevation of the plasma CO_2 content indicates alkalosis. A decrease in plasma CO_2 content indicates acidosis (Baumberger-Henry, 2005).

By measuring the $Paco_2$, the presence of alkalosis and acidosis may be determined. When this value is lower than 35 millimeters of mercury (mm Hg), hypocapnia is present, indicating respiratory alkalosis. Conversely, when this value is greater than 45 mm Hg, hypercapnia is said to be present, indicating respiratory acidosis.

When discussing blood gases, consideration must be given to CO_2 and oxygen (O_2) concentrations in the blood. Pao_2 is the amount of pressure exerted by oxygen dissolved in arterial blood. Most oxygen carried by the blood is carried by hemoglobin. A small amount of oxygen is dissolved in plasma. Therefore there are three ways to measure oxygen in the blood. The first is oxygen content, defined as the number of milliliters of oxygen carried in 100 mL of blood. The Po_2, or the pressure exerted by oxygen dissolved in plasma, is the second measurement. The third is the oxygen saturation of hemoglobin.

Oxygen saturation is a measure of the percentage of oxygen that is carried on the hemoglobin in relation to the total amount of oxygen that the hemoglobin is able to carry. Oxygen saturation provides the closest estimate of the total amount of oxygen carried in the blood. The Po_2 is only the pressure exerted by the small amount of oxygen that is dissolved in the plasma. There is a relationship between the Po_2 and the O_2 saturation of hemoglobin. When the Po_2 in plasma is low, hemoglobin carries less oxygen. Conversely, when the Po_2 in plasma is high, the hemoglobin carries a great deal of oxygen. Measurement of the O_2 saturation can be accomplished through the use of a blood gas machine or through pulse oximetry, a noninvasive method.

The hemoglobin molecule has room to carry four molecules of oxygen. If all four oxygen receptor sites on the hemoglobin are filled, 100% O_2 saturation has been reached (Guyton and Hall, 2006). If three oxygen receptor sites are filled and one is not, 75% O_2 saturation has been reached. When measuring the arterial oxygen content, it is the sum of the oxygen chemically bound to hemoglobin and the oxygen dissolved in plasma that equals the Po_2. A normal O_2 saturation level is considered 95% or higher. The normal Pao_2 level is from 80 to 100 mm Hg in arterial blood.

The bicarbonate level is the concentration of bicarbonate in plasma that has been specially manipulated with oxygen at a $Paco_2$ of 40 mm Hg. This is done in a laboratory to saturate the hemoglobin fully and is called the *standard bicarbonate measure*. When this equilibration is performed, any abnormality remaining in the standard bicarbonate level is known to have a metabolic cause. A normal bicarbonate level is between 22 and 26 mEq/L. Other values used to evaluate blood gas status are base excess and anion gap.

The interpretation of blood gas results begins with three basic steps (see Table 11-2 for a list of normal blood gas values). The first step in the process is to look at the value of the pH. As stated earlier, 7.35 to 7.45 is a normal pH, with 7.4 being a midpoint. If the pH is lower than 7.35, an acidotic state exists in the body. If the pH is greater than 7.45, an alkalotic state exists. The second value to assess is the $Paco_2$, which has a normal value between 35 and 45 mm Hg. If the value of $Paco_2$ is below 35 mm Hg, a state of respiratory alkalosis exists. If the value is greater than 45 mm Hg, a respiratory acidosis exists. This is true because the $Paco_2$ is considered a respiratory measurement, and CO_2 is considered to act as an acid.

The third value to examine is the bicarbonate level. Again, the normal bicarbonate level is 22 to 26 mEq/L. A value lower than 22 mEq/L indicates metabolic acidosis, and a value higher than 26 mEq/L indicates metabolic alkalosis. The bicarbonate level reflects a metabolic response, which can also be referred to as *nonrespiratory* or *renal*.

There are several helpful hints to remember when interpreting blood gas values. Although it has already been stated, it should be noted that if a change in pH is mainly caused by a change in the bicarbonate level, the cause of the alteration is nonrespiratory or metabolic. If the change in pH is caused by changes in the Pco_2, the driving force behind the alteration is respiratory in nature. When the pH and Pco_2 move in opposite directions, the primary effect on the acid-base imbalance is the respiratory system. If the changes in pH and Pco_2 are in the same direction, there is a nonrespiratory or metabolic cause. Table 11-3 may be useful in making these determinations.

The body always tries to keep the ratio of bicarbonate to Pco_2 at 20:1. This indicates a ratio of alkali (bicarbonate) to acid (CO_2). When it remains at 20:1, the pH remains unchanged, or around the normal level. If the bicarbonate level increases, alkalosis is present, which causes the pH to rise. If the bicarbonate (base) level falls, there is an acidotic state and the pH falls. The change in this ratio is described as *base excess*.

Base excess is most descriptive of the concentration of bicarbonate in the blood and is generally only affected by metabolic processes. The normal base excess value is between +2 and −2. A positive base excess value signifies that there is too much base present and not enough acid. A negative value indicates too little base and too much acid. Therefore a positive base excess value reflects a metabolic alkalosis and a negative value indicates metabolic acidosis. Plasma proteins and hemoglobin may also be considered bases and can influence base excess, although to a smaller degree.

ACID-BASE ALTERATIONS
Respiratory acidosis

Respiratory acidemia occurs when an event causes the $Paco_2$ to rise above 45 mm Hg. This event is usually associated with a decreased ventilatory exchange, which results in the CO_2 level of the blood increasing because of an increase in the hydrogen ion concentration. The pH of the blood then decreases to below 7.35. Because of alveolar hypoventilation, CO_2 is not eliminated through the lungs. Various disease states and alterations can cause this acidotic state (Box 11-1).

The causes of respiratory acidosis may be acute or chronic. The differentiation between acute and chronic states of acidosis is usually attributed to how long the carbon dioxide retention has lasted. In the chronic state, $Paco_2$ levels can increase slowly, or they may remain stable over time, but elevated. In the acute state, there is a rapid or sudden rise in the CO_2 level with a previously normal acid-base balance. Generally, chronicity results from a disease or condition that in some way decreases or prevents the gaseous exchange that normally occurs between the blood and alveolar air or that causes obstruction. Obstruction prevents the exhalation of carbon dioxide by decreasing the surface area of the lung.

Assessment

Patients experiencing respiratory acidosis may exhibit headache, fatigue, drowsiness, blurred vision, tremors/muscle twitching, vertigo, irritability, and disorientation resulting from central nervous system depression. Other symptoms include dyspnea, hypoventilation, cardiac arrhythmias, and possibly cyanosis. In mild cases there may be flushed, warm skin, and in severe cases the lethargy may progress to coma. It is important to recognize that the clinical presentation between acute and chronic respiratory acidosis is slightly different. This

---

TABLE 11-2 **Normal Blood Gas Values***

Parameter	Arterial	Venous (mixed)
pH	7.35-7.45	7.33-7.43
O_2 saturation	≥95%	70-75%
Pao_2	80-100 mm Hg	35-40 mm Hg
$Paco_2$	35-45 mm Hg	41-51 mm Hg ($Pvco_2$)
HCO_3^-	22-26 mEq/L	24-28 mEq/L
Base excess	−2 to +2	0 to +4

*May vary slightly with the institution and geographic location.

TABLE 11-3 **Aid to Interpreting Blood Gas Values**

Respiratory Alterations

pH up	Pco_2 down
pH down	Pco_2 up

Metabolic Alterations

pH up	Pco_2 up
pH down	Pco_2 down

Box 11-1   CAUSES OF RESPIRATORY ACIDOSIS

- Depression of the respiratory center (medulla)
- Drug overdose
- Any medication or condition that causes respiratory depression
- Guillain-Barré syndrome
- Myasthenia gravis
- Chronic bronchitis
- Emphysema

- Pneumothorax
- Hemothorax
- Pulmonary fibrosis
- Acute alcoholism
- Burns of the respiratory tract
- Congestive heart failure
- Adult respiratory distress syndrome

is particularly noticeable in patients with chronic obstructive pulmonary disease (COPD).

Compensatory response

Patients with COPD gradually accumulate CO_2. Because the alteration occurs gradually, compensatory changes have already occurred when the Pa_{CO_2} level exceeds 50 mm Hg. The respiratory center and the medulla no longer use CO_2 to stimulate respiration. Hypoxia then becomes the major respiratory drive in place of the increased CO_2 concentration. In this chronic state, if a patient receives too much oxygen, the stimulus for respiration is then removed. The patient develops carbon dioxide narcosis because the lack of oxygen as the stimulus to breathe is compensated by the delivery of oxygen from an external source. In addition, because of the compensated state of chronic respiratory acidosis, blood gas results will show an elevated bicarbonate level in a patient with chronic alterations. When a state of respiratory acidosis exists, the body responds in various ways (Table 11-4). The initial response includes the initiation of buffering by noncarbonate buffers. In other words, hemoglobin and proteins in the extracellular fluid and phosphates, proteins, and lactate in the intracellular fluid are activated in an attempt to regulate and overcome the increase in hydrogen ions. The respiratory rate increases to try to "blow off" excess hydrogen ions as a byproduct of the breakdown of carbonic acid into water and CO_2. If the alteration is not corrected by this mechanism, other buffer systems go into effect. The kidneys secrete hydrogen ions and retain bicarbonate. Sodium is reabsorbed to maintain ionic balance. The buffer also increases the chloride shift in the blood because red blood cells release a greater number of chloride ions and exchange them for bicarbonate. This results in excess carbonic acid being neutralized, and the normal 20:1 ratio between sodium bicarbonate and carbonic acid is reinstated.

Nursing interventions

In the patient with respiratory acidosis, nursing assessment and monitoring should include the following: vital signs, skin color, skin temperature, moistness of mucous membranes, muscle strength, level of consciousness, and monitoring of laboratory values.

Respiratory alkalosis

Any disease process that reduces carbon dioxide content in the blood or Pa_{CO_2} results in respiratory alkalemia. The hydrogen ion concentration is decreased, which causes the pH to rise to a level above 7.45. Because the problem is respiratory in nature, the Pa_{CO_2} is lower than 35 mm Hg. The respiratory alkalosis is caused by hyperventilation, which comes from the alveolar level. The hyperventilation decreases the hydrogen ion concentration, resulting in the increased pH. Respiratory alkalosis can arise from several disorders and may be classified as acute or chronic (Box 11-2).

Assessment

Symptoms are related to central nervous system irritability because of decreased calcium levels secondary to the binding of calcium to protein (Baumberger-Henry, 2005). The patient with respiratory alkalosis presents with carpopedal spasms, hyperventilation, and dyspnea and may sigh frequently. Tachycardia, atrial arrhythmia, and possibly severe ventricular arrhythmia may follow respiratory alkalosis. Palpitations, syncope, substernal chest pain, and seizures have occurred after mechanical overventilation. Patients may state that they are lightheaded, complain of weakness and muscle cramps, and exhibit hyperactive deep tendon reflexes. They may possibly convulse if hypocalcemia is present.

Compensatory response

When the pH of the extracellular fluid reaches/exceeds 7.45, hydrogen ions are released from the intracellular compartment (Table 11-5). These ions are usually exchanged for potassium.

TABLE 11-4 Blood Gas Alterations in Respiratory Acidosis*

Parameter	Direction of change
pH	Down (<7.35)
Pa_{CO_2}	Up (>45 mm Hg)
HCO_3^-	Normal or up (>26 mEq/L)
Na^+	Normal (usually)
Cl^-	Down in compensation
K^+	Up

*Breathing pattern—hypoventilation.

Box 11-2 CAUSES OF RESPIRATORY ALKALOSIS

- Hyperventilation syndrome
- Trauma
- Infection, particularly encephalitis or meningitis
- Brain tumors (tumors may be malignant or nonmalignant)
- CVA (cerebrovascular accident)
- Pharmacological agents (salicylate poisoning, nicotine, aminophylline-type drugs, some catecholamines)
- Heat stroke
- Fever
- Gram-negative septicemia
- Exercise beyond the person's normal capabilities
- Carbon monoxide poisoning
- Hypotension
- Severe anemia

- Pneumonia
- Pulmonary edema
- Pulmonary emboli
- Mechanical overventilation
- Chronic respiratory alkalosis
- Recovery phase of CVA
- Recovery phase of central nervous system infections
- Central nervous system malignancies
- Severe ongoing anemia
- Heart conditions that cause cyanotic conditions
- Pregnancy
- Hepatic disease
- Treatment for metabolic acidosis

TABLE 11-5 Blood Gas Alterations in Respiratory Alkalosis*

Parameter	Direction of change
pH	Up (>7.45)
$Paco_2$	Down (<35 mm Hg)
HCO_3^-	Normal until compensation
Na^+	Normal
Cl^-	Up with compensation
K^+	Down
Ca^{2+}	Down

*Breathing pattern—hyperventilation.

TABLE 11-6 Blood Gas Alterations in Metabolic Acidosis

Parameter	Direction of change
pH	Down (<7.35)
$Paco_2$	Normal, until compensation occurs
HCO_3^-	Down (<20 mEq/L)
Na^+	Normal (unless diuresis)
K^+	Up or normal
Cl^-	Up, down, or normal

Production of lactate and other metabolic acids is increased to compensate for the alkalotic state. The body then initiates the same three compensatory mechanisms discussed earlier for respiratory acidosis.

The buffer system works in the plasma by increasing the plasma content of organic acids. These acids then combine with excess bicarbonate ions to provide neutralization and maintain the 1:20 ratio between carbonic acid and sodium bicarbonate.

The pulmonary system decreases the rate and depth of respiration to achieve an increase in the CO_2 level. This continues until the CO_2 concentration reaches a level that again stimulates respiration in the medullary centers and the baroreceptors. The change in respiration also causes excess hydrogen ions to be secreted to compensate for the decreased levels of carbonic acid in the plasma.

Hydrogen ions secreted above the needs of the compensatory mechanisms are excreted through the kidney. This also decreases the amount of ammonia that is produced, which allows for the retention of hydrogen ions until the 1:20 ratio of carbonic acid to sodium bicarbonate is reinstated.

Nursing interventions

Nursing interventions attempt to alleviate the underlying cause of hyperventilation. The cardiac, pulmonary, and neurological systems and fluid and electrolyte status must all be monitored.

Metabolic acid-base alterations

Metabolic acid-base alterations include any acid-base disturbance that is not caused by an alteration in the CO_2 level in the extracellular fluid. These metabolic alterations involve bicarbonate levels and base excesses. When metabolic processes lead to a buildup of acids or loss of bicarbonate, the bicarbonate values drop below the normal range, resulting in a negative base excess value. Conversely, when there is a loss of acid or an accumulation of excess bicarbonate, the bicarbonate levels rise, resulting in a positive base excess value. As stated earlier, base excess refers to bicarbonate. It may also include other bases in the blood such as plasma, protein, or hemoglobin. Metabolic alterations include metabolic acidosis and metabolic alkalosis.

Metabolic acidosis

Metabolic acidosis results from an accumulation of metabolic acids. Metabolic acids are also referred to as *fixed* acids and include all acids except carbonic acid, which is a respiratory

acid. Metabolic acidemia results when there is a decrease of bicarbonate concentration in the extracellular fluid to less than 22 mEq/L. A base deficit exists, and the pH is below 7.35. These values result from an increase in metabolic (fixed) acids (Table 11-6).

When discussing metabolic acidosis, it is important to understand the concept of the *anion gap*. Body fluids are essentially electrically neutral with the number of cations (positively charged ions) equaling the number of anions (negatively charged ions). The cation usually measured is sodium and the anions are usually chloride and bicarbonate. The anion gap, which is only a diagnostic concept calculated by the laboratory, is the difference between unmeasured cations and unmeasured anions in the blood. The major unmeasured cations include calcium, magnesium, and potassium and the unmeasured anions are albumin, phosphate, sulfate, lactate, and other organic anions (Guyton and Hall, 2006).

Metabolic acidemia can result from an increase of unmeasured anions, but it can also be caused by conditions that do not increase unmeasured ions. Therefore it is important to understand the difference to allow proper monitoring of the patient and anticipate potential problems. The use of a formula helps determine the amount of anion gap, which indicates which process is occurring. The anion gap is calculated by using the values of the serum sodium, chloride, and bicarbonate levels. The serum chloride and bicarbonate ion concentrations are added together and subtracted from the serum sodium concentration:

$$[Na^+] - ([Cl^-] + [HCO_3^-])$$

Usually the anion gap ranges between 8 and 16 mEq/L with the unmeasured anions exceeding the unmeasured cations. Anion gap normal values may vary because of differing electrolyte values and laboratory methods (Guyton and Hall, 2006; Pagana and Pagana, 2007).

There are four major mechanisms that allow metabolic acidosis to occur: (1) loss of base from the body fluids; (2) failure of kidneys to excrete metabolic acids; (3) excess formation of metabolic acids; and (4) ingestion/infusion of metabolic acids (Guyton and Hall, 2006). An increase in acid production may overwhelm body buffer systems as well as pulmonary and renal mechanisms.

High anion gap causes include starvation, diabetic ketoacidosis, renal failure, lactic acidosis (e.g., from heavy exercise), and drug use (e.g., methanol, ethanol, formic acid, paraldehyde, aspirin). Causes related to a normal anion gap include renal tubular acidosis and diarrhea (Elkin et al, 2007). It is believed that diarrhea is probably the most common cause of normal anion gap metabolic acidemia. With diarrhea, it is possible to lose large amounts of bicarbonate through the intestines.

Assessment

Metabolic acidosis results from an existing problem. In addition to the disease characteristics, patients with an alteration toward metabolic acidosis have tachypnea with deep respirations, Kussmaul's respirations (particularly when acidosis is severe), flushed skin, fatigue, weakness, malaise, anorexia, nausea, vomiting, abdominal pain, stupor, and coma. Sometimes headache, drowsiness, confusion, cardiac arrhythmias, hypotension, shock, and pulmonary edema are also present.

Compensatory response

Hemoglobin and phosphate buffers are predominant in the compensation for metabolic acidemia because bicarbonate ions are used to lower hydrogen ion concentration. The lungs compensate by increasing alveolar ventilation—blowing off carbon dioxide to reduce hydrogen ion levels. Because the cause of the alteration is nonrespiratory, the lungs' response is explained by the increased hydrogen ion concentration in the cerebrospinal fluid. Because the lungs cannot excrete fixed acids, the kidneys are the primary compensatory mechanism for correcting the alteration. The urinary buffers of ammonia and ammonium and the phosphate buffer system are called on, but it may be 24 hours before the renal system can begin to move the pH in the proper direction. It is estimated that 4 or 5 days may be needed for the entire acid load to be excreted.

Monitoring

Monitoring required for this condition includes assessing vital signs, intake and output, weight, skin color, temperature, GI function, muscle strength, and laboratory values. It may be necessary to institute seizure precautions and maintain bed rest if the acidosis is severe. The patient may need assistance in maintaining conscious orientation.

Metabolic alkalosis

A metabolic alkalemic state results from a process that increases bicarbonate ion concentration or decreases hydrogen ion concentration. The result of this alteration increases the pH to a level greater than 7.45. Metabolic alkalosis tends to occur less often than metabolic acidosis. The exception to this is the patient with nasogastric suctioning or fluid loss from the upper GI tract, such as vomiting. The bicarbonate concentration can increase either because of loss of hydrogen ions from the extracellular fluid or because of addition of bicarbonate to the extracellular fluid.

Metabolic alkalosis can develop from diuretic therapy, excessive ingestion of alkaline drugs, corticosteroid therapy, and severe hypocalcemia, and in the patient with vomiting or continuous nasogastric suction without proper electrolyte replacement. These alterations result in hydrogen ion loss and excess sodium bicarbonate levels, which affect the 1:20 ratio between carbonic acid and sodium bicarbonate and cause a base alteration.

Assessment

The patient may exhibit signs of confusion, irritability, disorientation, muscle cramps, hyperactive tendon reflexes, tetany, carpopedal spasms, polyuria, polydipsia, nausea, vomiting, diarrhea, or hypoventilation. Laboratory tests reveal decreased serum potassium and serum chloride levels, although the sodium level generally remains unchanged (Table 11-7).

TABLE 11-7 **Blood Gas Alterations in Metabolic Alkalosis**

Parameter	Direction of change
pH	Up (>7.45)
$Paco_2$	Normal (up when compensation occurs)
HCO_3^-	Up (>26-30 mEq/L)
Na^+	Normal
K^+	Down
Cl^-	Down

Compensatory response

Intracellular phosphates and proteins shift to the extracellular compartment. The phosphate and protein buffering systems provide hydrogen ions, which buffer excess bicarbonate ions. Alveolar hypoventilation occurs in an effort to retain carbon dioxide, thereby increasing the $Paco_2$. During compensatory efforts, a secondary respiratory acidosis may occur because of the retention of carbon dioxide and decreased oxygen intake. This results in hypoxia. The $Paco_2$ attempts to rise in relation to the increase in pH. This is necessary to reestablish the 20:1 ratio, enabling the pH to move back toward the normal range. The kidneys can excrete bicarbonate rapidly and therefore attempt to restore normal bicarbonate levels in the extracellular fluid. If chloride ions are unavailable, the bicarbonate may be reabsorbed. This is because sodium reabsorption requires a negatively charged ion, either chloride or bicarbonate. When there is not enough chloride, the kidney reabsorbs bicarbonate in its place.

Monitoring

The patient should continue to be monitored for vital signs, intake and output, weight, level of consciousness, and muscle strength, and laboratory values should be reviewed. Losses from the upper GI tract, such as from gastric suctioning or vomiting, should be monitored.

Mixed acid-base alterations

The preceding acid-base alterations are considered primary acid-base alterations. It is possible for patients to undergo single imbalances, but there are clinical conditions in which a patient may exhibit two primary acid-base disturbances concurrently. When a patient has an acid-base alteration, it is important to remember that as compensation occurs, more than one acid-base alteration may occur simultaneously. Mixed acid-base disorders can include combinations of respiratory acidosis, respiratory alkalosis, metabolic acidosis, or metabolic alkalosis. When the normal compensatory responses to one of these alterations fail, a mixed disturbance can occur. Mixed disturbances can also occur in various clinical circumstances. When dealing with mixed alterations, the arterial pH alone cannot give the total picture of the underlying pathophysiology. The pH provides information only on the current status of the hydrogen ion.

An example of a mixed acid-base alteration is metabolic acidosis and respiratory alkalosis. This condition can be associated with cardiac and pulmonary arrest, severe pulmonary edema, or poisoning. With this alteration the patient can exhibit a high, low, or normal blood pH. The pH level depends on the severity of the two primary disorders. The bicarbonate and $Paco_2$ values are usually low. The mixed alteration of metabolic acidosis and metabolic alkalosis is another condition in which there is little change in the blood pH. Conditions that may lead to metabolic acidosis and metabolic alkalosis are salicylate intoxication, sepsis, and severe liver disease. The mixed alteration of metabolic alkalosis and respiratory acidosis is usually evidenced by a high bicarbonate level and a high $Paco_2$. Conditions associated with this alteration are chronic pulmonary diseases such as COPD, particularly in a patient with chronic respiratory acidosis who has suddenly experienced improved ventilation.

The combination of metabolic alkalosis and respiratory alkalosis can result in severe alkalemia, which is associated with critical illness. Contributory conditions include severe liver disease coupled with vomiting, gastric suction, overinfusion of Ringer's lactate and bicarbonate, overuse of diuretics or steroids, and massive transfusion of citrated blood.

It may be difficult to recognize these mixed acid-base alterations without a systematic examination of the patient and laboratory data. It is helpful to follow the steps given earlier to evaluate blood gas results systematically. In mixed alterations, it is extremely important to apply the anion gap calculation and base excess measurements to understand both primary and complicated disturbances.

Compensation response

The last factor to consider in acid-base balance alterations is the degree of compensation present. Acid-base alterations can be uncompensated, compensated, fully compensated, or partially compensated. In some instances, they can also be considered corrected. An acid-base alteration is considered corrected when all the acid-base values (usually pH, $Paco_2$, bicarbonate) return to normal. This is accomplished by effecting a change in the acid-base component that is primarily affected (Table 11-8). Compensation occurs when the alteration in pH is returned toward normal by resolution of the component not primarily affected by the alteration. In other words, if the primary alteration is of respiratory origin, the compensatory system is metabolic.

An acid-base alteration is acutely uncompensated when there is an abnormal pH and a change in one blood value, either the respiratory or the metabolic value. In partial compensation, the pH has moved toward normal but has not yet achieved normality. All three values (pH, $Paco_2$, and HCO_3^-) remain abnormal. Compensation occurs more slowly than

changes credited to the buffering process. When an acid-base alteration is corrected, all values return to normal (Baumberger-Henry, 2005).

Reaching an understanding of alterations in acid-base balance is complex and sometimes confusing. The material presented in this section is an overview. For more in-depth information, it is recommended that further study be undertaken to fully understand the more complex principles and their applications (Baumberger-Henry, 2005; Guyton and Hall, 2006).

PRINCIPLES OF ELECTROLYTE THERAPY

ELECTROLYTES

As noted earlier, chemical compounds known as *electrolytes* dissociate in water to positive ions (cations) or negative ions (anions). Disorders of electrolytes can have profound effects on the body.

Sodium

Sodium is found mainly in the extracellular fluid and has a positive charge (cation). The normal value for serum sodium level is 135 to 145 mEq/L. The bile and saliva as well as intestinal, gastric, and pancreatic secretions contain high concentrations of sodium (Chernecky et al, 2002). The most important roles of sodium are in controlling water distribution and maintaining extracellular fluid volume, thus being responsible for the osmolality of the vascular fluids. This control is accomplished through the kidneys' excretion and conservation of sodium, which is primarily determined by water intake and excretion. Since the cell membrane is impermeable to sodium, it depends on the sodium-potassium pump for transportation in and out of the cells. Excess sodium triggers the thirst mechanism and the resulting fluid intake stimulates ADH secretion, leading to fluid retention and normalization of the serum sodium concentration. On the other hand, a decreased serum sodium level inhibits the secretion of ADH and allows for water diuresis, which results in equalization of the water and sodium levels. Other regulators include aldosterone, which causes conservation of sodium, thereby decreasing renal losses; and natriuretic hormone, which increases renal losses of sodium. When the intake and output do not balance or the internal control mechanism is not functioning properly, imbalances occur.

Hyponatremia
Once the serum sodium level falls below 135 mEq/L, homeostasis no longer exists. The sodium deficit is referred to as hyponatremia and can be classified as hypovolemic, hypervolemic, or hypo/hyperosmolar.

Cause
Sodium deficit, or hyponatremia, may be related to inadequate intake, water gain, sodium loss, shift of sodium into the cell, or shift of water from the cell. Usually, when losses occur, there is an approximately equal proportion of water and sodium or a slightly larger amount of water lost. However, because deficits lead to thirst and greater intake, the amount of water may exceed the amount of sodium. The continued use of certain diuretics, particularly thiazides, may lead to excessive losses of sodium.

TABLE 11-8	Direction of Compensation in Acid-Base Alterations		
Disturbance	**Primary effect**	**Compensation**	**Ph**
Metabolic acidosis	Low HCO_3^-	Low $Paco_2$	Toward high alkaline
Metabolic alkalosis	High HCO_3^-	High $Paco_2$	Toward low alkaline
Respiratory acidosis	High $Paco_2$	High HCO_3^-	Toward high alkaline
Respiratory alkalosis	Low $Paco_2$	Low HCO_3^-	Toward low acid

An increased extracellular fluid volume may be related to increased production of ADH, as found in the syndrome of inappropriate antidiuretic hormone (SIADH). SIADH, an example of hypoosmolar hyponatremia, can be caused by failure of the renal system to respond to ADH, neoplasms, central nervous system disorders, medications, or pulmonary disease. As water is retained, serum sodium is diluted. Psychogenic polydipsia, a psychiatric disorder, may occasionally initiate an excessive intake of fluids that the normal kidney may not be able to excrete. Edema may lead to dilution of the sodium content. Sodium deficits resulting from water gain may be caused by continued or excessive use of hypotonic or sodium-free IV solutions. Hyponatremia can also occur postoperatively as a result of the release of vasopressin.

Assessment

Assessment findings vary according to the classification and degree of the deficit and the rate of onset; a more rapid onset results in more severe symptoms. GI symptoms include anorexia, nausea, and vomiting. Many of these symptoms are caused by low serum sodium concentration, which allows water to be pulled into the cells. The major impact of this fluid shift is seen in the form of neurological effects, including muscular weakness and spasms, personality changes, irritability, headaches, and possibly eventual seizures and coma.

When the cause of hyponatremia is a decreased extracellular fluid volume, the symptoms are those of fluid volume deficit (elevated pulse rate, postural hypotension, decreased blood pressure). In contrast, when the causative factor is increased extracellular volume, the symptoms are those of fluid volume excess (increased blood pressure, rapid pulse rate, edema, weight gain, distended neck veins).

Laboratory findings show decreased serum osmolality and decreased serum and urine sodium levels, except in SIADH and adrenal insufficiency.

Correction

Hyponatremia is corrected by alleviating the underlying cause and replacing the sodium, preferably by oral replacement. Sodium may also be replaced through gastric tube feedings and IV solutions (e.g., 0.9% sodium chloride solution). When IV replacement is deemed necessary, the delivery rate depends on the severity and duration of symptoms as well as the extracellular fluid volume.

Deficits related to fluid gain may be treated with diuretics to help excrete the excess fluid. With severe hyponatremia, hypertonic saline solutions (3% or 5% sodium chloride) may be used in addition to loop diuretics. Caution must be exercised when hypertonic saline solutions are being administered to prevent intravascular fluid overload.

The treatment plan for hyponatremia resulting from SIADH involves removing the cause. If this is not possible, fluids need to be restricted and diuretics administered. Additional medications to inhibit the action of ADH may be used for patients requiring long-term therapy.

Hypernatremia

Sodium excess, or hypernatremia, occurs when the serum sodium level exceeds 145 mEq/L.

Cause

Accumulation of excessive amounts of sodium and an abnormal loss of water are causative factors for sodium excess. Excessive fluid volume may result from an increased intake or decreased loss of sodium. As the sodium level increases, thirst also increases and leads to fluid intake that normalizes the concentration. This mechanism generally prevents hypernatremia. However, there are some situations in which this process fails and the hypernatremia is caused by an inability to respond to thirst. This can happen with infants, older adults, and comatose patients who cannot obtain replacement fluids, or when there is a problem with the hypothalamus. It may also result from the administration of medications and sodium-containing IV solutions, particularly hypertonic saline.

Water loss may occur in many ways and for a number of reasons including use of medications, such as corticosteroids. Increased losses may occur through the skin because of fever or burns, in the lungs because of infections, and in the kidneys because of osmotic diuresis. Water may also be lost because of a lack of ADH or the kidneys' inability to respond to ADH, as in diabetes insipidus.

Assessment

Assessment of a patient with hypernatremia reveals thirst, dry and sticky mucous membranes, and a decrease in tears and saliva. The temperature is elevated, and the skin appears flushed. There may be problems with speech because the tongue is rough, red, dry, and swollen. The fluid status depends on the cause; water loss leads to symptoms of fluid volume deficit, and sodium gain leads to those of fluid volume excess.

Many of the symptoms are related to alterations in intracellular volume as fluid is drawn from the cells in an attempt to decrease the intravascular sodium concentration. Restlessness, weakness, and fatigue are early signs of a moderate sodium imbalance. As the imbalance becomes more severe, with increased cellular dehydration, the signs become more apparent. Dehydration of brain cells leads to agitation, seizures, and coma.

Laboratory findings show an elevated serum sodium level and serum osmolality. If the hypernatremia is the result of fluid loss, the central venous pressure is low. There is also an increased urine specific gravity and osmolality, with the exception of diabetes insipidus or osmotic diuresis, in which there is a decrease.

Correction

Correction of hypernatremia depends on the cause and is directed toward decreasing the sodium to normal levels. When the excess levels are caused by sodium gain, initial treatment is restricting sodium intake.

An excess in sodium resulting from fluid loss necessitates the restoration of the fluid volume through oral or IV solutions. Dextrose 5% in water or hypotonic saline may be given to correct the sodium imbalance. Caution must be exercised to prevent too rapid a correction or overcorrection, which might cause a shift of fluid into the cells and lead to cerebral edema, seizures, permanent neurological damage, or death (Baumberger-Henry, 2005). Diuretics may be used in conjunction with IV solutions to decrease the potential for overcorrection.

Treatment of diabetes insipidus depends on its type and primary problem. Measures include replacing ADH, administering diuretics, and restricting sodium intake.

Nursing interventions vary according to the cause and may include restricting sodium intake or initiating infusion therapy to improve the fluid volume deficit. Monitoring includes measuring intake/output, weight, and vital signs; determining laboratory values; observing neurological signs; and providing a safe environment in the presence of confusion, delirium, and seizures. During fluid replacement, any signs of cerebral edema should be reported immediately to the physician.

Potassium

Potassium is the main cation in the intracellular compartment. All but approximately 2% of potassium is located in the cells. The normal serum potassium level is 3.5 to 5.0 mEq/L while the intracellular concentration is approximately 150 mEq/L (Pagana and Pagana, 2007). Potassium is important in influencing neuromuscular function and in cell metabolism. It is continually moving into and out of the cells. The potassium-sodium pump helps keep most of the potassium in the cell and the sodium outside the cell. Acid-base balance also plays a role in maintaining potassium levels. Potassium tends to be pulled out of cells in the presence of acidosis and shifted back into cells with alkalosis.

The majority of potassium is excreted through the kidneys. The amount excreted is related to the serum level, the presence of aldosterone, and the rate of urine flow. The kidney does not control the excretion of potassium as closely as that of sodium, and potassium will continue to be excreted even without replacement.

Hypokalemia

Hypokalemia, or potassium deficit, occurs when the serum potassium level falls below 3.5 mEq/L.

Cause

The major cause of hypokalemia is potassium loss, which may occur for various reasons. The primary site for potassium loss is the renal system. Potassium loss is often associated with the use of diuretics and other drugs (e.g., amphotericin B, cisplatin, insulin), but GI disorders such as vomiting and diarrhea account for some depletion. Gastric suctioning and fistulas are also factors in developing potassium deficits. Losses may be excessive because of increased aldosterone levels, magnesium depletion, increased sweating, and osmotic diuresis.

The cause may stem from inadequate intake. Potassium must be replaced daily and as long as oral intake is not a problem, potassium levels are maintained easily through ingestion of a variety of foods. However, when intake by mouth is limited or not possible, the deficit can result from inadequate replacement in enteral or parenteral nutrition solutions.

The increased release of aldosterone and epinephrine may be triggered by physical or emotional stress. Aldosterone increases urinary excretion, taking potassium at the same time. The temporary shifting of potassium from the extracellular compartment into the cells may also be related to alkalosis, increased glucose and insulin levels, and the process of tissue repair from burns and trauma.

Assessment

Minor potassium deficits are often asymptomatic. Symptoms are generally focused on neuromuscular changes. With more severe deficits, there is a slowing of impulses required for the muscles and nerves to transmit signals. As a result, there may be fatigue, muscle weakness, leg cramps, paresthesias, and diminished deep tendon reflexes. There is decreased bowel motility, constipation, ileus, nausea, and vomiting.

Cardiac abnormalities are common in the presence of hypokalemia. Various atrial and ventricular arrhythmias may occur.

Electrocardiogram (ECG) changes may include flattened or inverted T waves, prominent U waves, and ST-segment depression. With potassium deficits, patients become more sensitive to cardiac toxicity in the presence of digitalis preparations (Baumberger-Henry, 2005; Pagana and Pagana, 2007).

Laboratory findings disclose a serum potassium level below 3.5 mEq/L. Arterial blood gas values often indicate metabolic alkalosis. Improper blood drawing techniques may provide inaccurate elevated levels. Potassium is found in urine samples, with the amount depending on the cause of the deficit. The ECG shows abnormal tracings, as described earlier.

Correction

The goal of treatment is to replace the potassium to achieve a normal level. Diet or potassium supplements, including chloride, bicarbonate, citrate, gluconate. and phosphate salts, may be used to treat mild to moderate deficits (Kraft et al, 2005). If oral intake is not possible or the deficit is severe, potassium is replaced through the IV route. IV preparations of potassium include potassium acetate, potassium phosphate, and potassium chloride, with the latter being the most frequently used. Because potassium is excreted by the kidneys, a non–potassium-containing solution should be used to provide hydration and determine renal function before administering any potassium preparations for dehydrated patients. Potassium must not be given by IV push and must be diluted and thoroughly mixed throughout the IV solution before it is administered. Generally, the final IV concentration should usually not exceed 40 mEq/L, with a flow rate not to exceed 20 mEq/hour except in cases of severe depletion, in which initial concentrations of 60 to 80 mEq/L may be given more rapidly. Premixed potassium chloride (KCl) boluses are available in single-use containers, which may decrease accidental overinfusion and ensure dispersion of the KCl throughout the solution. Caution should be exercised and ECGs monitored when rates exceed 20 mEq/hour because of the potential for cardiac side effects (McEvoy, 2007). In these situations, cardiac monitoring is recommended. An IV solution containing additional potassium may prove to cause pain in the area where it first enters the vein. This may necessitate decreasing the concentration or the flow rate.

Nursing interventions include establishing IV access and administering a properly diluted potassium admixture, as ordered. Questionable orders or laboratory findings should be referred to the physician before initiating therapy. Also, a new venipuncture site should be used if there is any concern about patency. During the administration of potassium-containing solutions, the patient should be observed for possible vascular intolerance. ECG readings, urine output, and serum potassium levels should continue to be monitored. All procedures and assessments should be properly documented.

Hyperkalemia

Hyperkalemia, or potassium excess, occurs when the serum potassium level exceeds 5.0 mEq/L.

Cause

The cause of hyperkalemia is primarily related to decreased excretion, increased intake, or shift of potassium from the cells. It is most often associated with renal disease leading to inadequate excretion. Potassium-sparing diuretics may lead to excessive fluid loss, leaving high potassium levels. Adrenal insufficiency and any condition causing a decreased aldosterone level may increase fluid excretion, leading to hyperkalemia.

The potassium excess may also result from the administration of certain medications, such as nonsteroidal anti-inflammatory agents in association with renal disease. Medications creating potassium excess in the absence of underlying renal disease include aminocaproic acid, epinephrine, heparin, and antineoplastic agents (Pagana and Pagana, 2007).

The administration of inappropriate amounts of potassium may lead to excesses. This may occur through oral intake as well as inadequate dilution or rapid infusion of potassium-containing solutions. Potassium administered by IV push leads to lethal results, so it should be avoided. Normally, the body can adapt to influxes of potassium, but factors affecting absorption or excretion may inhibit normalization of the levels.

Hyperkalemia may be caused by potassium shifting from the cells. This may result from cell breakdown, as in trauma, burns, or hemolysis; severe infections; or lysis of malignant cells (following chemotherapy). An excess may result when beta-adrenergic blockers interfere with potassium shifting into the cells. The conditions associated with cell breakdown often occur in conjunction with acidosis. Metabolic acidosis also enhances the movement of potassium from the cells as the positively charged hydrogen ion enters the cells. Hyperglycemia resulting from insulin deficiency may pull potassium from the cells as water moves out of the cells in an attempt to dilute the excessive intravascular glucose content. Because insulin forces potassium into the cells, insulin deficiency may lead to hyperkalemia.

When laboratory tests indicate a high serum potassium level without any clinical indicators, consideration should be given to the method of collecting the blood sample. Inaccurate high levels may occur because of the tourniquet being in place too long, hemolysis of blood cells, delayed separation of serum and cells, or drawing blood samples in close proximity to an infusing IV solution containing potassium.

Assessment

Assessment for hyperkalemia usually reveals altered cardiac or neuromuscular activity. Cardiac arrhythmias are probably the most prominent characteristics. With excessive potassium levels, initially there are high, peaked T waves. Progressively, there is a prolonged PR interval, followed by disappearance of the P wave, widened QRS complex and QT intervals, ventricular fibrillation, and, finally, possible cardiac standstill.

Excessive potassium levels alter the impulses needed to send messages to the nerves and muscles. This leads to fatigue, mental confusion, and paresthesias (of the face, tongue, hands, and feet), irritability, and GI hyperactivity, resulting in nausea, diarrhea, and abdominal cramping. Paralysis leads to respiratory arrest in the late stages of hyperkalemia.

Diagnostic findings reveal a serum potassium level above 5.0 mEq/L. Values indicative of metabolic acidosis are often seen with arterial blood gas studies. ECGs indicate the abnormal findings described earlier.

Correction

Quality patient care includes prevention through assessment for potential hyperkalemia. The treatment goal for hyperkalemia is to eliminate the cause of the excess and return the potassium level to within normal limits. Mild excesses may be treated by eliminating the cause. Slower but more permanent forms of treatment include cation exchange resins, hemodialysis, and peritoneal dialysis. Caution should be exercised with infusion therapy because of the potential for cardiac glucoside toxicity related to rapid lowering of potassium plasma levels

(McEvoy, 2007). Treatment of more excessive amounts may include the use of hypertonic glucose IV infusions (300 to 500 mL of 10% to 25%) and insulin (5 to 10 units/20 g of dextrose) given over 1 hour to shift potassium into the cells (McEvoy, 2007). Insulin helps move potassium into the cells, whereas glucose helps prevent hypoglycemia. The effect begins in 15 to 45 minutes and lasts for several hours (Kraft et al, 2005). Some clinicians recommend that insulin be given as a separate injection to prevent the insulin from adhering to the fluid container and administration set (McEvoy, 2007). Administering sodium bicarbonate intravenously also shifts potassium back into cells. An infusion of 40 to 160 mEq of sodium bicarbonate over 5 minutes has been recommended for plasma levels exceeding 6.5 mEq/L, and may be repeated every 10 to 15 minutes until ECG abnormalities are corrected (McEvoy, 2007). This usually takes effect in approximately 30 minutes and lasts for several hours (Kraft et al, 2005). Both therapies are temporary measures because they do not actually remove potassium from the body. When a more urgent response is needed for patients with ECG changes not receiving cardiac glycosides, an IV infusion of 1 to 2 g of calcium gluconate may be used. It acts within 1 to 2 minutes but lasts only 30 to 60 minutes. It is preferable not to use this form of therapy for patients receiving digitalis therapy. Again, the calcium is only a temporary measure, but it also helps counteract the adverse effects of potassium on the neuromuscular membranes.

Nursing interventions include monitoring the serum potassium level, cardiac function, intake and output, and signs and symptoms. IV access may be needed to administer solutions and medications and the site should be monitored for complications. When sodium- or calcium-containing medications are used, it is important to observe for imbalances of these electrolytes. Patients receiving digitalis should be monitored for digitalis toxicity if calcium gluconate is the treatment of choice.

Calcium

Calcium is the fifth most abundant substance in the body and the normal serum level of total calcium is 4.3 to 5.3 mEq/L, or 8.5 to 10.5 mg/dL. Calcium is important in the formation of teeth and bones, where approximately 99% of it is located. The remaining 1% is located in the cells and fluid compartments, mainly the extracellular compartment (Chernecky et al, 2002). It is also necessary for muscle contraction, including skeletal and cardiac muscles, and neural function, where it regulates cardiac contractions and transmission of nerve impulses and has a sedative effect on nerve cells. It is important for normal blood coagulation by stimulating thromboplastin release from platelets, and assists in the conversion of prothrombin to thrombin and of fibrinogen to fibrin (Chernecky et al, 2005). Calcium is a divalent cation and is available in ionized and nonionized forms. The ionized component is considered free calcium; it makes up slightly less than half of the total serum calcium level and conducts the physiological functions. Most of the remaining nonionized calcium is bound to protein, 41% to albumin and a small amount to globulin. A small percentage is chelated to nonprotein anions, including phosphate, citrate, and carbonate.

Calcium is regulated by PTH, which is released by the parathyroid gland, as well as by calcitonin from the thyroid gland. PTH, secreted in response to a low serum calcium level, promotes the transfer of calcium from bone to plasma. Thyrocalcitonin (TCT) is secreted in response to a high serum calcium level and works to reduce the level (Chernecky et al, 2002). PTH also controls kidney reabsorption and promotes intestinal absorption. Vitamin D is important in all of these processes (Baumberger-Henry, 2005).

The action of shifting calcium from plasma to bone is produced by calcitonin. Calcium is eliminated through urine, the GI tract, bone deposition, and sweat. It has a reciprocal relationship with phosphorus.

Hypocalcemia

A calcium deficit, or hypocalcemia, occurs as the serum calcium level drops below 4.5 mEq/L (8.5 mg/dL).

Cause

Calcium deficits may be related to reduced intestinal absorption, increased loss, altered regulation, and albumin, phosphorus, and magnesium imbalances.

The decreased intestinal absorption of calcium may be related to vitamin D deficiency, small bowel disease (in which most of the dietary calcium is absorbed), and decreased calcium intake. Intestinal surgery also affects calcium absorption.

Excessive losses of calcium may be caused by renal disease or the use of loop diuretics. When the kidneys are unable to excrete phosphorus, the levels increase, causing calcium levels to decrease. Calcium may also be lost through fistulas or damaged skin, as might occur with burns.

Because the parathyroid glands produce PTH, any damage to or surgical removal of these glands may lead to acute hypocalcemia and can be life-threatening. Because slightly less than half of ionized calcium is bound to albumin, any decrease in these albumin levels affects calcium levels. Hypoalbuminemia is often caused by malnutrition, particularly with alcoholics, and large volume infusions (Pagana and Pagana, 2007). Alkalosis may increase the amount of calcium bound to albumin. A large number of blood transfusions may cause a calcium level decrease as a result of free calcium being bound to citrate additives.

Medications that may decrease calcium levels include anticonvulsants, phosphates, cisplatin, calcitonin, heparin, loop diuretics, aspirin, and laxatives. Any medication that lowers magnesium levels may decrease calcium mobilization from bone.

Other electrolytes play a role in maintaining balanced calcium levels. Because of the reciprocal relationship of calcium and phosphorus, as the serum level for one goes up the other level goes down. Therefore excessive phosphorus levels result in deficient calcium levels. This may occur with extensive tissue damage, hypothermia, or cell destruction caused by cancer chemotherapy. Hypomagnesemia is also associated with calcium deficits. This is the result of impaired PTH secretion and decreased response to the hormone.

Assessment

Many of the symptoms associated with hypocalcemia are related to neuromuscular activity, such as tetany, convulsions, and numbness and tingling of the fingers, toes, and circumoral region. There may be muscle cramps and hyperactive deep tendon reflexes. Chvostek's sign is positive and is presented as unilateral twitching of the facial muscles by tapping the facial nerve just in front of the ear. Trousseau's sign is also positive and is apparent through the development of carpal spasm following inflation of a blood pressure cuff on the upper arm. Mental changes may include depression and confusion. As the deficits increase in severity, there may be respiratory effects, including

dyspnea and laryngeal muscle spasms. Cardiovascular findings may show arrhythmias and a prolonged QT interval as a result of elongation of the ST segment and possible development of a form of ventricular tachycardia (torsades de pointes). Bradycardia and asystole may occur (Elkin et al, 2007).

Hypocalcemia may cause dry skin, brittle nails, periodontal disease, and dry hair. Also, osteoporosis, increased peristalsis, and diarrhea may occur.

Laboratory test results show a decreased serum calcium level. There may also be other electrolyte imbalances, including excessively high phosphorus and abnormally low magnesium levels.

Correction

The goal of treatment should be to eliminate the cause of the deficit and return the serum calcium level to normal. Acute symptomatic hypocalcemia requires immediate treatment.

Calcium deficits necessitate the use of oral or, in emergency situations, IV administration of calcium. Calcium gluconate may be used for routine maintenance and calcium chloride should be restricted for more emergent situations. Calcium gluconate is the drug of choice for peripheral infusions. Calcium should not be administered in conjunction with phosphate because this will cause precipitate formation. For mild or moderate deficits, calcium gluconate 1 to 2 g may be mixed in 5% dextrose in water or 0.9% sodium chloride and infused over 30 to 60 minutes. The dose may be repeated until levels return to normal values. The initial calcium dose for emergency serum elevation is 1000 mg of calcium chloride or 3 g of calcium gluconate given over 10 minutes to control symptoms; and the effects last approximately 2 hours. For severe, acute deficits, a continuous infusion may be required at a rate of 0.8 to 1.5 mEq/min because of the potential for cardiac arrhythmias related to rapid infusions, and serum levels should be monitored every 6 hours (Kraft et al, 2005).

Calcium chloride ionizes more readily, providing three times more elemental calcium, and is therefore more potent and irritating to tissues than calcium gluconate (Kraft et al, 2005). IV infusion of both medications should be given slowly to prevent sensations of heat, tingling, hypotension, bradycardia, cardiac arrhythmias, and cardiac arrest (McEvoy, 2007). Both calcium preparations can cause tissue irritation and burning, and there may be necrosis and sloughing of tissue if IV extravasation occurs. Because of the potential side effects, a more diluted concentration of calcium gluconate is preferred to a direct IV injection.

Nursing interventions need to include ongoing monitoring of signs and symptoms, laboratory tests results, and ECG readings. Precautions related to respiratory problems and tetany should be exercised. Because of potential problems related to extravasation, the IV site should be monitored carefully.

Hypercalcemia

Hypercalcemia, or calcium excess, occurs when the serum calcium level exceeds 5.5 mEq/L (10.5 mg/dL).

Cause

The most common causes of hypercalcemia are malignancy and hyperparathyroidism, with other causes accounting for only a small percentage of the hypercalcemia-related cases (Kraft et al, 2005). Malignancy-related excesses may be related to lysis of the bone or production of a parathyroid hormone–like substance (Pagana and Pagana, 2007).

When hyperparathyroidism is present, there is an increase in the PTH level. This higher concentration causes an excessive amount of calcium to shift from the bone, an increase in retention of calcium by the renal system, and increased GI absorption.

Other causes include excessive administration of IV calcium and oral intake of calcium through milk and antacids. There may be a decrease in urinary excretion because of thiazide diuretics or renal failure. Hypercalcemia may follow prolonged immobilization as a result of the lack of weight-bearing bone stress, which is important for bone resorption and deposition (Baumberger-Henry, 2005). Finally, there may be an increase in the ionized portion of calcium because of acidosis.

Assessment

Assessment findings of hypercalcemia vary according to serum levels and rate of development. Symptoms are related to the effects of calcium on neuromuscular excitability and cell membrane permeability. This sedative action results in fatigue, muscular weakness, and depressed deep tendon reflexes. The neuromuscular effect also carries over to the GI tract, where there may be anorexia, nausea, vomiting, or constipation. As a result, the patient should be monitored for weight loss, dehydration, increased thirst, and hypoactive bowel sounds or paralytic ileus.

Excessive calcium levels can alter the kidneys' ability to concentrate urine, resulting in polyuria and fluid volume depletion. These adverse effects may lead to acute or chronic renal failure.

Cardiovascular findings include heart rate reduction, and disturbances in heart rate rhythm, myocardial muscle function, and systemic vasculature. Heart block may lead to asystole.

Hypercalcemia can produce mental changes, including confusion, depression, and memory impairment. If these symptoms are not corrected, they may lead to acute psychosis.

Laboratory findings show an increased serum calcium level. The ECG demonstrates a shortened QT interval and ST segment. The PR interval can be prolonged. Radiological findings may indicate bone changes and reduced bone density.

Correction

As with all imbalances, the treatment goal is directed at eliminating the cause and returning the calcium level to within normal limits. Mild hypercalcemia may be treated by decreasing or eliminating medications that might contribute to the excess, encouraging mobilization, and increasing fluid intake.

Hypercalcemia may become life-threatening and necessitates immediate treatment. Patients with normal renal and cardiac function initially receive a 0.9% sodium chloride solution at 200 to 300 mL/hour. The solution is given rapidly to provide sodium and intravascular volume, because patients often also have a fluid volume deficit. The saline solution helps dilute the calcium concentration and facilitates calcium excretion. Furosemide 40 to 100 mg is usually given every 4 hours in conjunction with saline infusions to help prevent fluid overload and further increase calcium excretion (Kraft et al, 2005). Once adequate fluid volume has been attained, slower infusions of 0.9% and/or 0.45% sodium chloride solutions may be given to increase calcium elimination. Caution should be exercised to prevent additional intravascular depletion.

Other measures, especially when related to malignancy, incorporate the use of bisphosphonates (including etidronate, pamidronate, and zoledronic acid) to inhibit bone resorption by action on osteoblast and osteoclast precursors. These have a limited role in acute treatment (Kraft et al, 2005). Other measures include the administration of calcitonin and glucocorticoids as well as the use of peritoneal dialysis or hemodialysis. Mithramycin (Plicamycin), a cytotoxic antibiotic, may be used to decrease bone resorption and should be used cautiously long term because of nephrotoxic and hepatotoxic side effects (Baumberger-Henry, 2005). Corticosteroids may be used to reduce intestinal calcium absorption and to decrease reabsorption by the renal system. However, the long-term side effects of glucocorticoid therapy also need to be considered.

Nursing interventions include ongoing monitoring of serum calcium levels, vital signs, ECGs, renal function, and neurological status. Following emergency treatment, caution should be taken to observe for signs of calcium, potassium, and magnesium deficits. The patient should be monitored for signs of fluid overload when large volumes of IV saline are being administered. Treatment for nausea and constipation may be needed. All information should be documented clearly and precisely, and the physician notified of any abnormal findings.

Magnesium

Magnesium is a cation that is located primarily in the bones (50% to 60%). The remainder of the magnesium in the body is located in the cells, where it is the second most abundant electrolyte, and approximately 1% is found in the extracellular fluid. Normal serum levels are 1.5 to 2.5 mEq/L. Like calcium, the serum levels do not accurately reflect the total amount of magnesium in the body. Because part of the magnesium, approximately one third, is bound to protein, serum albumin levels should be considered when making decisions related to imbalances. Most of the magnesium is bound to an adenosine triphosphate (ATP) molecule, which is the body's main energy source, and is important in phosphorylation (Pagana and Pagana, 2007). Magnesium is controlled mainly through renal excretion and distal small bowel absorption.

The role of magnesium is multifaceted and includes the activation of enzymes related to carbohydrate and protein metabolism. It is important in activating the sodium-potassium pump. Magnesium acts directly on the myoneural junction, affecting neuromuscular irritability and contractility. It acts on the skeletal muscle by depressing acetylcholine release at the synaptic junction. Magnesium assists with the contraction of the heart muscle and is a co-factor in the blood-clotting cascade (Chernecky et al, 2002). Magnesium levels and activity are interdependent with those of calcium (antagonist) and potassium.

Hypomagnesemia

Hypomagnesemia, or magnesium deficit, occurs when the serum magnesium level falls below 1.5 mEq/L. The deficit is often found in the critically ill patient and may be mistaken for hypokalemia. Hypomagnesemia has been observed frequently in critically ill patients, leading to an increased death rate (Kraft et al, 2005).

Cause

Magnesium deficit may result from decreased intake, abnormal absorption, increased output, or chronic alcoholism. A decreased intake may be related to prolonged malnutrition, prolonged administration of magnesium-deficient, sodium-rich IV or parenteral nutrition solutions, and occasionally a diet deficient in magnesium.

Decreased uptake of magnesium may occur with any problem related to the lower GI tract because this is where most of the absorption takes place. This may occur in the presence of inflammatory bowel disease or following surgical procedures involving the lower GI tract. Absorption may be impacted in bulimia with the binging and purging.

Individuals suffering from alcoholism often experience semi-starvation, leading to reduced intake of magnesium-containing foods. Impaired renal function allows for increased losses and intestinal malabsorption, which decrease the utilization of the electrolyte. In addition, there may be emesis and intermittent diarrhea, which increase the losses. During alcohol withdrawal, excessive loss may occur as glucose moves into the cells (Chernecky et al, 2002).

Other causes include refeeding following prolonged malnutrition because magnesium is pulled from intravascular fluid and deposited into new cells. Some medications, such as amphotericin B, insulin, diuretics, laxatives, aminoglycoside antibiotics, and cisplatin, may cause deficits. Increased elimination through prolonged diarrhea, intestinal fistulas, vomiting, and prolonged nasogastric suctioning may lead to magnesium deficits. Magnesium deficits may also be caused by impaired renal reabsorption, trauma, infection, sepsis, pancreatitis, burns, and surgical procedures.

Assessment

Symptoms related to hypomagnesemia are most often manifested through neuromuscular changes, and their severity is directly related to the level of the deficit. Symptoms include increased reflexes, weakened skeletal muscles, tremors, convulsions, and tetany. Chvostek's and Trousseau's signs are positive. Paresthesias may be present. Increased nerve transmission may lead to mood changes ranging from apathy and depression to extreme agitation and hallucinations. Breathing may be compromised as a result of the effect on respiratory muscles.

Hypomagnesemia may result in various cardiac arrhythmias, such as supraventricular tachycardia and ventricular fibrillation. This deficit may increase the potential for digitalis toxicity related to an increased retention of the drug.

Gastrointestinal manifestations include dysphagia, nausea, and vomiting leading to anorexia.

Laboratory findings include magnesium levels below 1.5 mEq/L and low levels of calcium and potassium. ECG changes include prolonged PR and QT intervals, widened QRS complex, depressed ST segment, and inverted T waves.

Correction

The goal of treatment is to eliminate the cause and correct the deficit. The aggressiveness of treatment is directly related to the severity of the deficit. Mild deficiencies may be treated with diet or oral supplements, whereas more severe deficits may necessitate intramuscular or IV administration of magnesium.

Magnesium sulfate is usually the drug of choice, particularly for more severe deficits. The dosage, which varies according to the severity of the deficit, may be given intramuscularly or intravenously. Dosing for a mild to moderate deficit is 8 to 32 mEq (up to 1 mEq/kg) and that for a severe deficit is 32 to 64 mEq (up to 1.5 mEq/kg). The maximum infusion rate for doses greater than 6 g should be 8 to 12 hours. For asymptomatic patients, the maximum rate should not exceed 12 g over 12 hours. The concentration should be 20% or less. For some conditions with severe symptoms (e.g., preeclampsia and eclampsia), doses may be 5 g administered over 4 to 5 minutes (Kraft et al, 2005). Other suggested IV dosing is 5 g in 5% dextrose in water or 0.9% sodium chloride, to be infused over 3 hours (McEvoy, 2007).

Nursing interventions should include monitoring of serum magnesium levels, at least daily during repletion, and urinary output because magnesium is eliminated by the kidneys. Calcium and phosphorus levels should also be checked. There should be periodic checks of the knee-jerk reflexes because these disappear before respiration becomes depressed. Vital signs should be monitored and preparations made to counteract depressed respirations in case of magnesium excess, including artificial ventilation and IV calcium administration. Seizure precautions should also be exercised. All procedures and responses to therapy should be clearly and precisely documented.

Hypermagnesemia

Hypermagnesemia, or magnesium excess, usually occurs when the serum magnesium level exceeds 2.5 mEq/L. Hypermagnesemia occurs on an infrequent basis.

Cause

Hypermagnesemia usually results from decreased output or increased intake. The major cause of decreased output is renal disease. However, even when there is decreased output, it is often also associated with additional intake, such as magnesium-containing medications or IV solutions. Patients with endocrine disturbances such as hypothyroidism or hyperparathyroidism may have excess magnesium.

Antacids and laxatives are examples of medications that, if used excessively, may lead to hypermagnesemia. The use of enemas and continuous or large doses of magnesium to treat eclampsia or delay delivery may also increase magnesium levels.

Assessment

Usually a mild deficit is asymptomatic. As the deficit increases, there may be nausea and vomiting. There may be a decrease in muscle cell activity attributable to a blockage of acetylcholine release at the myoneural junction where the muscle fibers and nerves meet (Chernecky et al, 2002). This may lead to increased muscle weakness, paralysis, and depressed deep tendon reflexes. Respiratory muscles may be depressed, leading to respiratory arrest in the presence of excessively high levels.

As the serum levels increase, so do the cardiovascular indicators. Small increases may result in flushing and a sensation of skin warmth caused by peripheral vasodilation. With more severe increases, the pulse rate may decrease, which could lead to complete heart block.

Laboratory findings show an increased serum magnesium level. ECG readings may show an increased PR interval and prolonged QT and QRS intervals. ECG tracings in the presence of excessively high levels may indicate heart block and cardiac arrest.

Correction

Treatment should be directed at eliminating the cause and returning magnesium levels to within normal limits. Magnesium-containing foods and medications should be eliminated, if possible. Moderate excesses may be treated by the IV administration of 0.45% sodium chloride solution and diuretics to help the kidneys excrete the excess magnesium. The kidneys need to be functioning properly before initiating this form of therapy.

For more severe excesses, IV calcium doses of 500 to 1000 mg may be administered through a central venous access device over 5 to 10 minutes, and repeated until the patient is symptom free. Calcium gluconate 1 to 3 g may be infused intravenously via a peripheral catheter over 3 to 10 minutes (Kraft et al, 2005). This antagonizes the action of the magnesium but is only a temporary measure. Again, diuretics may be administered if kidney function is adequate. Dialysis may be indicated in the presence of renal impairment.

Nursing interventions include monitoring serum magnesium levels, patellar reflexes, and vital signs. Precautions should be exercised, including having equipment and medication available in the event of respiratory or cardiac arrest. Patients and families should be instructed in regard to the excessive use of over-the-counter magnesium-containing medications. All procedures, including the administration of IV solutions and medications, and observations, particularly those related to the deep tendon reflexes and respirations, should be relayed to the physician and accurately documented.

Phosphorus

Phosphorus is found in the intracellular and extracellular fluids and is the primary anion in the intracellular compartment. Most phosphorus is located in the teeth and bones, with only a small amount in the soft tissue. Like calcium and magnesium, serum levels do not necessarily reflect the true levels of the total body content. Most phosphorus is in the form of phosphate, and the two terms are often used interchangeably. Normal serum phosphorus levels range from 1.8 to 2.6 mEq/L, or 2.7 to 4.5 mg/dL, and vary according to gender, age, and diet.

The metabolism and homeostasis of phosphorus are related to those of calcium. They have an inversely proportional relationship, and both are controlled by the parathyroid glands. Both electrolytes need vitamin D for absorption from the GI tract.

Phosphorus is important in carbohydrate, protein, and fat metabolism. It is necessary for nerve and muscle function and for the maintenance of the acid-base balance, in which it is the primary urinary buffer. Phosphorus, bound to ATP, is used to form energy-storing substances required in all physiological, homeostatic, and metabolic functions (Chernecky et al, 2002; Kraft et al, 2005). It is also essential in the functioning of red blood cells and the utilization of vitamin B. It is important for conversion of glycogen to glucose.

Hypophosphatemia

Hypophosphatemia, or phosphorus deficit, results when the serum phosphorus level falls below 1.8 mEq/L (2.7 mg/dL).

Cause

Hypophosphatemia may result from increased losses or utilization, decreased intestinal absorption, or intracellular shifts. Increased losses of phosphorus may be the result of glycosuria, hypokalemia, hyperparathyroidism, or hypomagnesemia. The use of diuretics (thiazides) increases the elimination of phosphorus.

Problems related to the GI tract, such as diarrhea, vomiting, vitamin D deficiencies, and lack of absorption, lead to phosphorus deficits. Continuous use of antacids leads to phosphorus binding.

Transient intracellular shifts play a major role in phosphorus deficits. The administration of concentrated glucose solutions increases insulin production, which causes phosphorus to shift into the cells. Shifts may also be related to an increased intracellular pH, as with prolonged respiratory alkalosis. Additionally, critically ill intensive care unit (ICU) patients may be at risk because of malnutrition, inadequate stores and/or replacement, alkalosis, diabetic ketoacidosis, and GI losses (Kraft et al, 2005). Malnourished patients may develop phosphorus deficits as calories are provided for nourishment. Because of poor nourishment and GI problems such as diarrhea and vomiting, the alcoholic patient may also experience hypophosphatemia.

Assessment

As with most electrolyte imbalances, symptoms related to hypophosphatemia are related to the severity of the deficit and whether it is acute (sudden decrease) or chronic (gradual decrease). Symptoms include those related to the neurological system, such as confusion, seizures, coma, paresthesias, weakness, numbness, and ataxia. Weakness may lead to difficulty speaking, breathing, and swallowing.

Cardiovascular findings are related to decreased respiratory function and include myocardial dysfunction and chest pain. If prolonged, arrhythmias may develop. Platelet dysfunction may result in bruising and bleeding. The GI disturbances include nausea, vomiting, or ileus. Other symptoms include long bone pain and fractures.

Diagnostic findings show a decreased serum phosphorus level, and possibly decreased serum potassium and magnesium levels. Levels of calcium and alkaline phosphatase will be elevated.

Correction

The treatment goal is to eliminate the cause of the deficit and help return the phosphorus level to within normal limits. The best treatment is preventing the imbalance by not using phosphorus-binding medications, such as antacids, particularly if there is increased potential for phosphorus deficits.

Mild to moderate deficits may be treated through diet and oral supplements. More severe deficits may necessitate IV supplements, such as sodium phosphate or potassium phosphate, with the sodium preparation being the drug of choice unless there is simultaneous hypokalemia. The medication may be given over 4 to 6 hours to minimize side effects. Laboratory follow-up should be done 2 to 4 hours following administration (Kraft et al, 2005). The IV site should be monitored closely because potassium phosphate can cause necrosis and sloughing of tissue.

Hyperphosphatemia

Hyperphosphatemia, or phosphorus excess, occurs when the serum phosphorus level exceeds 2.7 mEq/L (4.5 mg/dL).

Cause

Hyperphosphatemia is most often related to renal disease (acute and chronic). It might also be caused by increased intake, destruction of cells, trauma, infections, hemolysis, and shifts from cells to the extracellular fluid.

In renal failure, the diseased kidney cannot excrete phosphorus, which leads to excessive levels. Increased intake may be the result of laxatives containing phosphate, vitamin D excess, or phosphorus supplements.

Shifts may occur from cells being damaged, as with chemotherapy, releasing phosphorus. Respiratory acidosis may also cause an intracellular to extracellular shift.

Assessment

Most symptoms of hyperphosphatemia are related to hypocalcemia. Chvostek's and Trousseau's signs are positive. There may be anorexia, nausea, vomiting, tachycardia, and muscle spasm, pain, or weakness. Irritability and apprehension may be present. When excess levels of phosphorus are sustained for prolonged periods, precipitation of calcium phosphate may occur in areas other than the bones.

Laboratory findings reveal an increased serum phosphate level, above 2.7 mEq/L, and decreased calcium level. Monitoring should also include uric acid levels. Other tests, such as creatinine and PTH levels, may be performed to help determine the cause.

Correction

Treatment is directed toward identifying and alleviating the cause. Nursing interventions include monitoring serum phosphorus and calcium levels. Patient and family education is directed at avoiding foods and medications that contain high phosphorus levels. Oral phosphate binders, available as calcium, magnesium, or aluminum salts, should be used cautiously to prevent side effects (Kraft et al, 2005). Precautions should be exercised in the event of hypocalcemic tetany, such as monitoring for seizures, confusion, and laryngeal muscle spasms. When kidney function is normal, IV saline infusions may be used to increase excretion. Phosphorus can be forced into the cells when used in conjunction with insulin. Dialysis may be necessary with abnormal renal function.

Chloride

Chloride is the major anion in the extracellular fluid. Extracellularly, chloride is found in gastric secretions, pancreatic juices, and bile (Baumberger-Henry, 2005). Chloride helps maintain serum osmolarity, acid-base balance, and the balance of cations, including sodium, potassium, and calcium, in the intracellular and extracellular fluids. In the GI system, it joins with hydrogen to make hydrochloric acid to aid in digestion (Baumberger-Henry, 2005). The kidneys and GI tract are the major regulators of chloride levels, and normal values are 98 to 110 mEq/L.

Hypochloremia

Hypochloremia, a chloride deficit, occurs when the chloride level falls below 98 mEq/L.

Cause

Hypochloremia can occur following GI losses, including vomiting, fistulas, and prolonged nasogastric suctioning. Chloride can also be lost when diuretics are used. The deficit could be related to excessive intake of water in the body. A deficit may occur as a result of decreased intake, orally or intravenously.

Assessment

The symptoms are related to changes in other electrolytes or pathophysiological processes. Laboratory findings include a serum chloride level below 98 mEq/L and alterations in other electrolyte levels (depending on the cause) and acid-base balance.

Correction

Treatment should be directed toward eliminating the cause as well as monitoring and replacing the appropriate electrolytes.

Hyperchloremia

Hyperchloremia, chloride excess, occurs when the level exceeds 106 mEq/L.

Cause

The causative factors include sodium excess and bicarbonate deficit. Other causes include hyperparathyroidism or hyperaldosteronism (Baumberger-Henry, 2005). Excessive chloride

intake, orally or intravenously with hypertonic solutions, followed by water loss may be the causative factor.

Assessment

Symptoms are related to the causative factor. Laboratory findings disclose a high serum chloride level, as well as alterations for other electrolytes or acid-base balance.

Correction

Elimination of the cause is the first priority. The intake/output of chlorides should be monitored along with the serum levels of chloride and other electrolytes. All pertinent information should be documented appropriately. In acidotic states, bicarbonate may be administered. Lactated Ringer's may be given IV to increase the bicarbonate level, allowing the liver to convert the lactate to bicarbonate. Thus the bicarbonate could potentially bind with sodium, allowing chloride to be excreted (Baumberger-Henry, 2005).

 SUMMARY

Under normal conditions, the body maintains a state of equilibrium, or homeostasis. This balanced state is achieved through various checks and balances. The preceding information describes this delicate process and the imbalances that may occur when the body cannot function properly. Correction of the imbalance may be as simple as eliminating the cause, or as complex as initiating life-support measures including the use of IV fluids and medications.

Part of the homeostatic mechanism involves the maintenance of fluid balance. Water travels throughout the various body compartments. Fluid shifts are an attempt to balance fluid intake and output and are affected by the solutes contained within the various compartments, preexisting medical conditions, intake volume, and the environment. The crucial role of water has been discussed in detail throughout this chapter. Alterations in fluid volume can lead to imbalances and complications. Fluid volume also affects the concentration of solutes, and any imbalances may precipitate various side effects.

Equally important to fluid balance is electrolyte balance. Electrolytes have a direct impact on the movement of solutions and thus on the maintenance of fluid balance. These ions affect the functioning of all major systems, including the cardiovascular, renal, and neurological systems. The body generally maintains the proper types and concentrations of electrolytes to ensure normal activity. Abnormal concentrations can lead to ill effects, with severe excesses and deficits possibly leading to death.

It is important that the nurse be knowledgeable about normal fluid and electrolyte levels and their importance to the overall maintenance of homeostasis. It is also important to recognize abnormal findings and to understand their impact on the body. When recognized and treated promptly, most imbalances can be resolved and the body returns to a normal state.

The nurse also needs to be familiar with proper treatment modalities, which help ensure that appropriate equipment and supplies are available. This familiarity allows the nurse to question possible incorrect treatment orders or laboratory findings. Knowledge of normal and abnormal findings related to fluid and electrolyte balance, along with expertise in infusion therapy, helps ensure prompt, quality patient care.

REFERENCES

Baumberger-Henry M: *Quick look nursing: fluid and electrolytes*, Boston, 2005, Jones and Bartlett.

Chernecky C, Macklin D, Murphy-Ende K: *Real world nursing survival guide: fluids & electrolytes*, Philadelphia, 2002, Saunders.

Elkin MK, Perry AG, Potter PA: *Nursing interventions & clinical skills*, ed 4, St Louis, 2007, Mosby.

Finfer S, Bellomo R, Boyce N et al: A comparison of albumin and saline for fluid resuscitation in the intensive care unit, *New Engl J Med*, 350:2247-2256, 2004.

Guyton AC, Hall JE: *Textbook of medical physiology*, ed 11, Philadelphia, 2006, Saunders.

Kraft MD, Btaiche IF, Gordon SS et al: Treatment of electrolyte disorders in adult patients in the intensive care unit, *Am J Health-Syst Pharm* 62:1663, 2005.

Lewis SM, Heitkemper MM, Dirksen SR et al: *Medical-surgical nursing: assessment and management of clinical problems*, ed 6, St Louis, 2004, Mosby.

McEvoy GK: *AHFS drug information 2007*, Bethesda, Md, 2007, American Society of Health-System Pharmacists.

Myburgh J, Cooper J, Finfer S et al: Saline or albumin for fluid resuscitation in patients with traumatic brain injury, *New Engl J Med* 357:874-884, 2007.

Pagana KD, Pagana TJ: *Diagnostic and laboratory test reference*, ed 8, St Louis, 2007, Mosby.

Parel P, Roberts I: Colloids versus crystalloids for fluid resuscitation in critically ill patients, *Cochrane Database Systemat Rev*, Issue 4, Article No. CD000567, DOI: 10.1002/14651858.CD000567.pub3, 2007.

Smeltzer, SC, Bare, SC, Hinkle, JL et al: *Brunner & Suddarth's textbook of medical-surgical nursing*, ed 11, New York, 2008, Lippincott Williams & Wilkins.

The Albumin Reviewers (Alderson P, Bunn F, Li Wan Po A et al): Human albumin solution for resuscitation and volume expansion in critically ill patients, *Cochrane Database Systemat Rev*, Issue 4, Article No. CD001208, DOI: 10.1002/14651858.CD001208.pub2/, 2004.

Weinstein SM: *Plumer's principles & practice of intravenous therapy*, ed 8, Philadelphia, 2007, Lippincott Williams & Wilkins.

12 INFECTION PREVENTION AND CONTROL

Mary McGoldrick, MS, RN, CRNI®*

Healthcare–associated infections are 1 of the top 10 leading causes of death in the United States (CDC, 2008b). In American hospitals alone, health care–associated infections account for an estimated 1.7 million infections and 98,987 associated deaths each year. Of these infections, 14% or 30,665 deaths were caused by or associated with a bloodstream infection (Klevins et al, 2007). Hospital-acquired infections are an emerging national issue with many states enacting laws requiring hospitals to publicly report their rates of infections. Given that the cost of care for a patient with a catheter-related bloodstream infection is $45,000 (CDC, 2002b), these infections could cost up to $2.3 billion on an annual basis. On October 1, 2008, as part of the Centers for Medicare & Medicaid Services' (CMS) Deficit Reduction Act (DRA) of 2005, Medicare reimbursement to hospitals for preventable vascular catheter–related infections will end.

Venous access devices (VADs) are an integral component of providing venous access in the management of patients that are critically and chronically ill, and continue to be used in the inpatient and outpatient settings. However, VADs disrupt the integrity of the skin, making infection with bacteria and/or fungi possible. Infection may spread to the bloodstream (bacteremia), and hemodynamic changes and organ dysfunction (severe sepsis) may ensue, possibly leading to death. Approximately 90% of catheter-associated bloodstream infections occur with central venous catheters (CVCs) (Mermel, 2000). Almost half (48%) of all patients in an intensive care unit (ICU) have central venous catheters, which accounts for approximately 15 million central venous catheter-days per year in ICUs alone. Studies of catheter-related bloodstream infections that control for the underlying severity of illness suggest that attributable mortality for these infections is between 4% and 20%. In addition, healthcare-associated bloodstream infections prolong hospitalization by a mean of 7 days. Estimates of attributable cost per bloodstream infection are between $3700 and $29,000 (Soufir et al, 1999).

DEFINITIONS

To understand the principles of infection prevention and control, it is important to understand some key concepts. The following infection control terms are briefly defined and discussed.

An *infection* is the transmission of microorganisms into a host after evading or overcoming defense mechanisms, resulting in the organism's proliferation and invasion within host tissue(s). Host responses to infection may include clinical symptoms or may be subclinical, with manifestations of disease mediated by direct organism pathogenesis and/or a function of cell-mediated or antibody responses that result in the destruction of host tissues (Siegel et al, 2007).

Colonization is the proliferation of microorganisms on or within body sites without a detectable host immune response, cellular damage, or clinical expression. In many instances, the terms colonization and carriage are synonymous. The presence of a microorganism within a host may occur with varying duration, but may become a source of potential transmission (Siegel et al, 2007). Colonization also refers to the persistent presence of microorganisms at a particular site. Certain species of bacteria form colonies on the surface of the skin or in certain regions of the body. For example, the colonization of *Escherichia coli* is

*The author and editors wish to acknowledge the contributions made by Kathryn Carlson, Maxine B. Perdue, and Judy Hankins as authors of this chapter in the second edition of *Infusion Therapy in Clinical Practice*.

considered normal in the bowels; however, its presence in the bladder is not considered normal and can result in a urinary tract infection. Likewise, *Staphylococcus aureus* found in the nares or on the epidermal surface of the skin is considered normal; however, its presence in the bloodstream can contribute to bacteremia.

Bacteria entering the blood can cause serious problems called a bloodstream infection or bacteremia. A *bacteremia* is a bloodstream infection that is identified by a positive blood culture. Bacteremias are commonly classified as primary and secondary. A primary bloodstream infection has no identified underlying source, but is usually associated with the use of IV devices. A secondary bloodstream infection arises from an existing infectious source. This is also called hematogenous seeding from a distant site of infection. Central venous and arterial catheters can be colonized from remote, unrelated sites of infection. Most fungal vascular access infections appear to be the result of hematogenous seeding from another site of infection. An example is a patient with burns or an intraabdominal wound infection being at risk for developing a secondary bloodstream infection. Signs and symptoms of bacteremia include fever, chills, hypotension, and a positive blood culture.

Sepsis, or *septicemia,* is a systemic infection in the circulating blood caused by pathogenic microorganisms or their toxins. Septicemia can occur when microorganisms migrate into the bloodstream and cause a profound systemic reaction. Intravascular device–related septicemia is often caused by *Staphylococci* (especially coagulase-negative *Staphylococci), Trichophyton beiglii, Corynebacterium* species, *Candida* species, *Fusarium* species, or *Malassezia furfur* (Bennet and Brachman, 1998).

Septicemia is a serious, life-threatening infection that gets worse very quickly. Septicemia can begin with spiking fevers, chills, rapid breathing, and rapid heart rate and the person will appear very ill. The symptoms can rapidly progress to shock with decreased body temperature (hypothermia), falling blood pressure, confusion or other changes in mental status, and blood clotting problems that lead to petechiae and ecchymosis. There also may be decreased or no urine output. Septicemia is not common, but when it does occur the effects can be devastating. Septicemia can rapidly lead to adult respiratory distress syndrome (ARDS), septic shock, and death. Septic shock has a high death rate, exceeding 50%, and the outcome depends on the type of organism involved, and how quickly the patient is hospitalized (National Library of Medicine, 2008). Nurses must be aware of the patient's history, possible risk factors, and the clinical signs and symptoms of septicemia, and implement prompt interventions when septicemia is suspected.

Phlebitis is an inflammation of the vein. Since phlebitis is an inflammatory process and not an infectious process it is addressed in Chapters 23 and 25, which discuss the complications associated with peripheral and central venous catheters.

IMMUNE SYSTEM AND SUSCEPTIBILITY TO INFECTION

The body's normal defense system includes the skin; the lining of the nose, mouth, and gastrointestinal tract; and certain blood cells (i.e., leukocytes or white blood cells) that are part of the immune system. All of these systems work to protect the body from microorganisms that cause infections. When a venipuncture is performed, the body's first line of defense, the skin, is broken, providing a mode of entry for many microorganisms such as fungi, bacteria, and viruses. The immune system, which is a complex network of cells and organs, responds to this invasion of microorganisms.

Leukocytes (white blood cells) are an important component of the immune system. Neutrophils and lymphocytes compose 80% to 90% of the total white blood cell (WBC) count. Granulocytes and monocytes are the foundation of the body's nonspecific immune response. Neutrophils, referred to as polymorphonuclear leukocytes, are the body's first line of defense against infection. Segments are mature neutrophils. When infections occur, the bone marrow releases immature neutrophils (sometimes identified as bands) that, together with mature neutrophils, engulf and destroy bacteria. This phenomenon is referred to as a shift to the left. Polymorphonuclear leukocytes can destroy invading bacteria and remain in the peripheral blood for 6 to 10 hours before moving into tissue, performing their function, and dying (Gaynes et al, 1991). Neutrophils are the first cells to appear in large numbers within exudates in the initial inflammation stages.

The next leukocyte in the line of defense is the monocyte cell, also referred to as a macrophage. Neutrophils and monocytes engulf and partially digest, or phagocytize, invading antigens. Monocytes are slower to respond to infections and inflammatory diseases and respond late in the acute phase of infection, but once activated, they are stronger than neutrophils, ingesting larger particles of debris and continue to function during the chronic phase.

Lymphocytes have the ability to recognize specific antigens from any foreign living organism, such as viruses, fungi, and bacteria. An increase in the number of lymphocytes (lymphocytosis) occurs in viral infections. Lymphocytes can be divided into two main subgroups: T cells and B cells. B cells produce immunoglobulins, and T cells are responsible for effector and regulatory functions. Cell-mediated immunity is the responsibility of the effector T cells. This includes defense against intracellular bacterial or fungal infections, cytolysis of virus-infected cells, allograft rejection, graft-versus-host reaction, and certain types of tumor immunity (Gaynes et al, 1991). Regulatory T cells moderate the functions of effector T cells and B cells by inducing or suppressing proliferation and differentiation of these cells.

There are four subsets within the T cell system: (1) helper/inducer T lymphocytes (CD4 cells) induce other T cells, and helper B cells produce antibodies. Interleukin-2 (IL-2), a growth factor produced by T cells, stimulates the proliferation and differentiation of activated T cells. IL-1, a cytokine released by macrophages, stimulates CD4 cells to produce IL-2 (Gaynes et al, 1991); (2) delayed hypersensitivity T lymphocytes produce chemotactic lymphokines in response to particulate and soluble antigens. One of the chemotactic lymphokines macrophage-activating factor, induces membrane alterations that cause clumping and immobilization of cells. This factor, interferon, has several functions, including inhibiting tumor cell growth; (3) cytotoxic T lymphocytes destroy antigen-specific target cells on contact; (4) suppressor T lymphocytes (CD8) consist of three cells—inducer, effector, and transducer—that regulate humoral and cell-mediated responses (Gaynes et al, 1991).

Eosinophils and basophils are other types of WBCs. During allergic reactions and parasitic conditions, as well as after

TABLE 12-1 White Blood Cell Differential Values*

Cell type	Normal range (Cells/mm³)
Granulocytes	
Neutrophils (total)	1.8-7.7 × 10⁹/L
Eosinophils	0-0.45 × 10⁹/L
Basophils	0-0.1 × 10⁹/L
Agranular (Mononuclear)	
Lymphocytes	1.0-4.8 × 10⁹/L
Monocytes	0-0.8 × 10⁹/L

*The values listed are for adults and may vary depending on the lab's reference ranges.

TABLE 12-2 Levels of Neutropenia

Absolute neutrophil count (Cells/μL)	Risk for infection
1500-2000	No increased risk
1000-1500	Slightly increased risk
500-1000	Moderately increased risk
Less than 500	Severely increased risk

From Family Care Research Program. Accessed at http://www.cancercare.msu.edu/patientscaregivers/symptoms/neutropenia.htm.

radiation exposure, the number of eosinophils increases. When there is an increase in the levels of steroids, either during periods of stress or when administered parenterally, the number of eosinophils and basophils decreases.

The normal WBC count ranges from 4.1 to 10.9 × 10⁹/L (Gaynes et al, 1991; Jarvis et al, 1991). The WBC differential sorts the WBCs into its different types, and then counts each type and reports the percentage of each type. This information can indicate infectious processes, as well as the patient's risk for infection. The normal values for a WBC differential are listed in Table 12-1.

Neutropenia refers to a decrease in the absolute neutrophil count (ANC). The neutrophil count is an absolute count, which means it is the actual number of neutrophils in a measured amount of blood (cells per microliter [μL]). The ANC is calculated by adding the percentage of neutrophils together with the percentage of bands (if present) and multiplying by the total WBC count percentage. Table 12-2 contains values of absolute neutrophil counts and correlates these values with the patient's risk for infection.

In patients with neutropenia, the risk for infection has been linked to both the magnitude and duration of neutropenia. The depth of neutropenia is the most important factor, with an ANC of less than 500 μL being associated with a substantial risk for infection. The highest risk, however, is an ANC of less than 100 μL. In addition, patients with prolonged neutropenia (i.e., more than 7 days) are at higher risk for infection than patients who recover their granulocyte count in less than 1 week (Friese et al, 2006).

INDICATIONS OF INFECTION

FEVER

Body temperature is maintained within narrow limits by the hypothalamic temperature regulatory center in the brain. Fever (core body temperature elevated above normal) is often a sign of infection. When proper antibiotic therapy and host defenses work together to eradicate an infection, fever usually resolves; body temperature response is therefore a good measure of the effectiveness of antibiotic therapy. Exogenous chemicals, including antimicrobials and other medications, can sometimes cause fever. Concurrent corticosteroids, acetaminophen, aspirin, or other nonsteroidal anti-inflammatory drugs act as antipyretics; they may mask a fever and can complicate the monitoring of antimicrobial therapy.

The idea of using a designated temperature for fever is controversial, especially as many elderly persons have minimal or no temperature increase, and not all health care providers perform routine temperature checks on every patient in the absence of direct indications. However, for surveillance purposes, fever needs to be specified. Therefore fever is present when the patient's temperature is 2.4° F greater than the baseline temperature. This is important to note since normal temperature in the elderly is usually lower than 98.6° F and an elderly patient can be running a fever at 99.0° F (Association for Professionals in Infection Control and Epidemiology, 2008). The CDC surveillance definitions located in Boxes 12-1 and 12-2 also contain specific fever parameters to be used in surveillance activities based on the patient's age and care settings.

Another indicator of infection and response to antimicrobial therapy is the peripheral leukocyte count (WBC count). The WBC count is typically elevated in response to an acute bacterial infection. Because of the short life span of leukocytes, the WBC count usually drops rapidly during successful treatment. Patients with low leukocyte counts (neutropenia) may respond poorly to therapy for infection. Similarly, patients with other defects in humoral or cellular immunity may have impaired neutrophil function and be at risk for bacterial and fungal infections despite normal leukocyte counts. Noninfectious causes of elevated leukocyte counts include myeloproliferative disorders, trauma, acute myocardial infarction, and corticosteroid or lithium therapy.

INFECTION IN THE NEUTROPENIC PATIENT

Patients who are immunocompromised are at greater risk for developing an intravascular device–related infection. Infection is a frequent problem in patients with neutropenia, with sepsis being the most common cause of chemotherapy-induced death (Rosenthal, 2001). The usual signs and symptoms of infection (i.e., erythema, pain, redness, drainage, pulmonary infiltrates, or pyuria) are not present in the patient with neutropenia. This may be attributable to the patient's lack of polymorphonuclear neutrophils, which normally would be recruited to the site(s) of infection to incite the inflammatory response. Therefore a neutropenic patient with an indwelling venous access device may not trigger the "usual" signs of infection (i.e., erythema, drainage at the exit site). The hallmark of infection in the neutropenic patient is fever. Sometimes an infection will develop without a fever, and the patient may have a sudden onset of weakness, hypotension, or confusion (Rosenthal, 2001). The presence of febrile neutropenia is a medical emergency that often results in hospitalization. Febrile neutropenia has been defined by

Box 12-1 CLASSIFICATION OF PRIMARY BLOODSTREAM INFECTIONS

Primary bloodstream infections are classified according to the criteria used, either as laboratory-confirmed bloodstream infection (LCBI) or as clinical sepsis (CSEP).

LABORATORY-CONFIRMED BLOODSTREAM INFECTION (LCBI)

The LCBI criteria 1 and 2 may be used for patients of any age, including patients ≤1 year of age, whereas LCBI criterion 3 may only be used for patients ≤1 year of age. LCBI must meet one of the following three criteria:

Criterion 1:

Patient has a recognized pathogen cultured from one or more blood cultures (i.e., a positive blood culture is when at least one bottle from a blood draw is reported by the laboratory as having grown organisms)
   and
organism cultured from blood is not related to an infection at another site. (See notes 1 and 2.)

Criterion 2:

Patient has at least *one* of the following signs or symptoms: fever (>38° C), chills, or hypotension
   and
signs and symptoms and positive laboratory results are not related to an infection at another site
   and
common skin contaminant (i.e., diphtheroids [*Corynebacterium* spp.], *Bacillus* [not *B. anthracis*] spp., *Propionibacterium* spp., coagulase-negative staphylococci [including *S. epidermidis*], *viridans* group streptococci, *Aerococcus* spp., *Micrococcus* spp.) is cultured from two or more blood cultures drawn on separate occasions. (See notes 3 and 4.)

Criterion 3:

Patient ≤1 year of age has at least *one* of the following signs or symptoms: fever (>38° C, rectal), hypothermia (<37° C, rectal), apnea, or bradycardia
   and
signs and symptoms and positive laboratory results are not related to an infection at another site
   and
common skin contaminant (i.e., diphtheroids [*Corynebacterium* spp.], *Bacillus* [not *B. anthracis*] spp., *Propionibacterium* spp., coagulase-negative staphylococci [including *S. epidermidis*], *viridans* group streptococci, *Aerococcus* spp., *Micrococcus* spp.) is cultured from two or more blood cultures drawn on separate occasions. (See notes 3, 4, and 5.)

Notes:

1. In criterion 1, the phrase "one or more blood cultures" means that at least one bottle from a blood draw is reported by the laboratory as having grown organisms (i.e., a positive blood culture).
2. In criterion 1, the term "recognized pathogen" does not include organisms considered common skin contaminants (see criteria 2 and 3 for a list of common skin contaminants). A few of the recognized pathogens are *S. aureus*, *Enterococcus* spp., *Escherichia coli*, *Pseudomonas* spp., *Klebsiella* spp., and *Candida* spp.
3. In criteria 2 and 3, the phrase "two or more blood cultures drawn on separate occasions" means (1) that blood from at least two blood draws was collected within 2 days of each other (e.g., blood draws on Monday and Tuesday or Monday and Wednesday would be acceptable for blood cultures drawn on separate occasions, but blood draws on Monday and Thursday would be too far apart in time to meet this criterion), and (2) that at least one bottle from each blood draw is reported by the laboratory as having grown the same common skin contaminant organism (i.e., is a positive blood culture). (See note 4 for determining sameness of organisms.)
    a. For example, an adult patient has blood drawn at 8 AM and again at 8:15 AM of the same day. Blood from each blood draw is inoculated into two bottles and incubated (four bottles total). If one bottle from each blood draw set is positive for coagulase-negative staphylococci, this part of the criterion is met.
    b. For example, a neonate has blood drawn for culture on Tuesday and again on Saturday and both grow the same common skin contaminant. Because the time between these blood cultures exceeds the 2-day period for blood draws stipulated in criteria 2 and 3, this part of the criteria is not met.
    c. A blood culture may consist of a single bottle for a pediatric blood draw because of volume constraints. Therefore to meet this part of the criterion, each bottle from two or more draws would have to be culture-positive for the same skin contaminant.
4. There are several issues to consider when determining sameness of organisms.
    a. If the common skin contaminant is identified to the species level from one culture, and a companion culture is identified with only a descriptive name (i.e., to the genus level), then it is assumed that the organisms are the same. The speciated organism should be reported as the infecting pathogen (see examples below).

Culture	Companion culture	Report as
S. epidermidis	Coagulase-negative staphylococci	*S. epidermidis*
Bacillus spp. (not *anthracis*)	*B. cereus*	*B. cereus*
S. salivarius	*S. viridans*	*S. salivarius*

(Continued)

Box 12-1   CLASSIFICATION OF PRIMARY BLOODSTREAM INFECTIONS—cont'd

b. If common skin contaminant organisms from the cultures are speciated but no antibiograms are done or they are done for only one of the isolates, it is assumed that the organisms are the same.

c. If the common skin contaminants from the cultures have antibiograms that are different for two or more antimicrobial agents, it is assumed that the organisms are not the same (see table below).

d. For the purpose of NHSN antibiogram reporting, the category interpretation of intermediate (I) should not be used to distinguish whether two organisms are different.

Organism name	Isolate A	Isolate B	Report as
S. epidermidis	All drugs **S**	All drugs **S**	Same
S. epidermidis	OX **R**	OX **S**	Different
	Cefaz **R**	Cefaz **S**	
Corynebacterium spp.	Pen G **R**	Pen G **S**	Different
	Cipro **S**	Cipro **R**	
Streptococcus viridans	All drugs **S**	All drugs **S**	Same
		Except Erth **R**	

5. For patients <1 year of age, the following temperature equivalents for fever and hypothermia may be used:
Fever: 38° C rectal/tympanic/temporal artery = 37° C oral = 36° C axillary
Hypothermia: 37° C rectal/tympanic/temporal artery = 36° C oral = 35° C axillary

CLINICAL SEPSIS (CSEP)

The CSEP definition may be used only to report a primary BSI in neonates and infants (i.e., patients ≤1 year of age) and must meet the following criteria:

Criterion:

Patient ≤1 year of age has at least one of the following clinical signs or symptoms with no other recognized cause: fever (>38° C, rectal), hypothermia (<37° C, rectal), apnea, or bradycardia
   and
blood culture *not* done or *no* organisms detected in blood
   and
no apparent infection at another site
   and
Physician Institutes treatment for sepsis

From the Centers for Disease Control and Prevention, 2008. Accessed 7/2/08 from http://www.cdc.gov/ncidod/dhqp/nhsn.html.

---

the National Comprehensive Cancer Network (NCCN) as the presence of fever (>38.3° C at a single reading or ≥38.0° C over 1 hour) and severe neutropenia (ANC <500 μL or <1000 μL and a predicted decline to ≤500 μL over the next 48 hours) (NCCN, 2006). Initial infections in the neutropenic patient are typically bacterial, and involve gram-positive organisms such as *Staphylococcus aureus* and gram-negative organisms such as *Pseudomonas aeruginosa, Escherichia coli, Klebsiella,* and *Serratia* species (Rosenthal, 2001). The majority of infections occurring in immunocompromised patients result from colonization of organisms from within the patient's own mouth or intestinal tract.

PREVENTION OF CATHETER-ASSOCIATED INFECTIONS

The incidence of catheter-associated infections can be reduced by implementing policies and procedures that are based on evidence from authoritative bodies such as the Centers for Disease Control and Prevention (CDC), the National Quality Forum (NQF), the Institute for Healthcare Improvement (IHI), and from professional nursing organizations, such as the Infusion

Nurses Society (INS) that has developed the *Infusion Nursing Standards of Practice* (INS, 2006).

PRINCIPLES OF ASEPSIS

Adhering to the principles of aseptic technique can decrease the risk of catheter-associated infection. Aseptic technique should be maintained for the insertion and care of all intravascular catheters. Appropriate aseptic technique does not necessarily require sterile gloves; a new pair of disposable nonsterile gloves can be used in conjunction with a "no-touch" technique for the insertion of peripheral venous catheters (CDC, 2002b). Discussion as to when sterile and nonsterile gloves should be worn and hand hygiene performed is noted within the infection prevention discussion that follows. The Infusion Nurses Society's policy and procedure on how to perform aseptic technique is noted in Box 12-3.

INSTITUTE FOR HEALTHCARE IMPROVEMENT'S CENTRAL LINE BUNDLE

The Institute for Healthcare Improvement (IHI), an independent not-for-profit organization, led the improvement of health care by formulating care bundles. Care bundles are

Box 12-2   APIC-CDC HICPAC SURVEILLANCE DEFINITIONS IN HOME HEALTH CARE AND HOME HOSPICE INFECTIONS

LABORATORY-CONFIRMED BLOODSTREAM INFECTION (LCBSI) (must meet one of the following three criteria):

Criterion 1:

- Patient has a recognized pathogen cultured from one or more blood cultures *and*
- Organism cultured from blood is *not* related to an infection at another site.

Criterion 2:

- Patient has at least one of the following three signs or symptoms: fever (≥100.4° F [(≥38° C]), or chills, or hypotension *and*
- Signs and symptoms and positive laboratory results are *not* related to an infection at another site *and*
- Common skin contaminant (e.g., diphtheroids [*Corynebacterium* spp.], *Bacillus* [not *B. anthracis*] spp., *Propionibacterium* spp., coagulase-negative staphylococci [including *S. epidermidis*], *viridans* group streptococci, *Aerococcus* spp., *Micrococcus* spp.) is cultured from *two* or more blood cultures drawn on separate occasions.

Criterion 3:

- Patient aged <1 year has at least one of the four following signs or symptoms: fever (≥100.4° F [(≥38° C]) rectal/tympanic/temporal artery, (≥37° C oral), (≥36° C axillary); or hypothermia (<98.6° F [<37° C]) rectal/ tympanic/temporal artery, (≥36° C oral), (≥35° C axillary); or apnea; or bradycardia *and*
- Signs and symptoms and positive laboratory results are *not* related to an infection at another site *and*
- Common skin contaminant (e.g., diphtheroids [*Corynebacterium* spp.], *Bacillus* [not *B. anthracis*] spp., *Propionibacterium* spp., coagulase-negative staphylococci [including *S. epidermidis*], *viridans* group streptococci, *Aerococcus* spp., *Micrococcus* spp.) is cultured from *two* or more blood cultures drawn on separate occasions.

CLINICAL SEPSIS (CSEP) (must meet the criteria below):

- Must have at least one of the following clinical signs with no other recognized cause: fever, or hypotension (systolic pressure <90 mm Hg), or hypothermia, or apnea, or bradycardia *and*
- Meets all of the following:
Blood culture not done or no organisms detected in blood.
No apparent infection at another site.
Physician institutes treatment for sepsis.
Hospital admission for clinical sepsis and/or death attributable to clinical sepsis.

Association for Professionals in Infection Control and Epidemiology (Feb 2008): *APIC-CDC HICPAC surveillance definitions in home health care and home hospice infections.* Accessed 7/2/08 from http://www.apic.org/AM/Template.cfm?Section=Guidelines&CONTENTID=10427&TEMPLATE=/CM/ContentDisplay.cfm.

groupings of best practices that when applied together result in better outcomes when followed for every patient, every single time. When a bundle element is missed, the patient is at much greater risk for serious complications. The central line bundle is a group of five evidence-based interventions for patients with intravascular central catheters to prevent catheter-associated bloodstream infections that include the following:

1. Hand hygiene
2. Maximal barrier precautions
3. Chlorhexidine skin antisepsis
4. Optimal catheter site selection, with the subclavian vein as the preferred site for nontunneled catheters
5. Daily review of line necessity, with prompt removal of unnecessary lines (IHI, 2008)

Hospitals that have implemented the central line bundle have demonstrated striking reductions in the rate of central line infections. A statewide effort in Michigan to implement the central line bundle resulted in a 66% reduction in catheter-related bloodstream infection rates over an 18-month period (Pronovost et al, 2006). In another study, Berenholtz et al demonstrated that ICUs that implemented multifaceted interventions similar to the central line bundle nearly eliminated catheter-related bloodstream infections (Berenholtz et al, 2004).

NATIONAL QUALITY FORUM SAFE PRACTICES

The National Quality Forum (NQF) has endorsed 30 "safe practices" that should be universally used in health care settings to reduce the risk of harm resulting from processes, systems, or environments of care and to improve care. Of the 30 safe practices, safe practice number 20 requires adherence to effective methods for preventing central venous catheter–associated bloodstream infections and also suggests that the requirements be specific in policies and procedures. NQF safe practice number 20 includes *all* of the following elements:

- Wash hands or use an alcohol-based hand rub before and after insertion or care of the central line.
- Use maximal barrier precautions in preparation for line insertion, including each of the following: cap, mask, sterile gown, sterile gloves, and large sterile sheet.
- Perform skin antisepsis, preferably using 2% chlorhexidine-based preparation before catheter insertion; chlorhexidine may be contraindicated for use in very low birth weight (VLBW) infants.
- Select the optimal catheter site for each patient; for the prevention of infection, the subclavian vein is the preferred site for nontunneled catheters in adults. The optimal catheter site selection for the infant or child is specific to his or her size, condition, and accessibility factors.

Box 12-3   ASEPTIC TECHNIQUE

POLICY

Aseptic technique is described as performing procedures in a manner that will minimize the chance of contamination or introduction of pathogens.

Aseptic technique shall be an integral component of every infusion-related procedure.

PROCEDURE

1. Hand Hygiene
   - Wash hands using the appropriate antiseptic soap or solution before and after all patient contact.
2. Site Preparation
   - Use antiseptic solution to prepare skin before venipuncture. Recommended solutions include:
     - Alchol
     - Chlorhexidine gluconate
     - Povidone-iodine
     - Tincture of iodine
3. Use of Personal Protective Equipment (PPE)
   - Don cap, mask, gown, protective eyewear, and gloves, as needed.
4. Site Care and Maintenance
   - Inspect site routinely for signs of catheter-associated complications.
   - Rotate peripheral venous access sites routinely.
   - Change administration sets and site dressing routinely.
   - Maintain closed system on infusion administration systems.
5. Equipment and Supplies
   - Inspect all solution containers for integrity before initiation of therapy.
   - Check expiration dates.
   - Inspect all administration sets, add-on devices, and junction securement devices before use to ensure protective coverings are intact and product integrity is not compromised.
   - Visually inspect vascular access device (VAD) before insertion.
   - Routinely cleanse durable medical equipment (DME) with disinfectant that is effective in preventing cross-contamination.

From Infusion Nurses Society: *Polices and procedures for infusion nurses*, ed 3, Norwood, Mass, 2006, Author.

- Replace the catheter site dressings as specified by Centers for Disease Control and Prevention (CDC) guidelines.
- Perform daily assessment of central line necessity, and promptly remove unnecessary lines (NQF, 2006).

GENERAL INFECTION PREVENTION STRATEGIES
Hand hygiene

Hand hygiene is an important activity to prevent cross-contamination and a health care–associated infection resulting from the insertion or ongoing care and maintenance of a venous access device. The health care workers' (HCWs) hands are the greatest potential source for transmission of potentially infectious organisms to other patients. The following are Category IA, IB and IC recommendations that are strongly recommended or required for implementation by the CDC's *Guideline for Hand Hygiene in Health-Care Settings* and the National Quality Forum's endorsed *Safe Practices for Better Healthcare*. These recommendations are designed to improve hand hygiene practices and to reduce the transmission of pathogenic microorganisms to patients and personnel in health care settings:

1. Indications for handwashing and hand antisepsis
   A. When hands are visibly dirty or contaminated with proteinaceous material or are visibly soiled with blood or other body fluids, wash hands with either a non-antimicrobial soap and water or an antimicrobial soap and water (IA).
   B. If hands are not visibly soiled, use an alcohol-based hand rub for routinely decontaminating hands in all other clinical situations described below in items IC – H (IA). Alternatively, wash hands with an antimicrobial soap and water in all clinical situations described below in items IC – H (IB).
   C. Decontaminate hands before having direct contact with patients (IB).
   D. Decontaminate hands before donning sterile gloves when inserting a central intravascular catheter (IB).
   E. Decontaminate hands before inserting peripheral vascular catheters, or other invasive devices that do not require a surgical procedure (IB).
   F. Decontaminate hands after contact with a patient's intact skin (IB).
   G. Decontaminate hands after contact with body fluids or excretions, mucous membranes, nonintact skin, and wound dressings if hands are not visibly soiled (IA).
   H. Decontaminate hands after removing gloves (IB).
   I. Before eating and after using a restroom, wash hands with a non-antimicrobial soap and water or with an antimicrobial soap and water (IB).
2. Hand hygiene technique
   A. When decontaminating hands with an alcohol-based hand rub, apply product to palm of one hand and rub hands together, covering all surfaces of hands and fingers, until hands are dry (IB). Follow the manufacturer's recommendations regarding the volume of product to use.
   B. When washing hands with soap and water, wet hands first with water, apply to hands an amount of product recommended by the manufacturer, and rub hands together vigorously for at least 15 seconds, covering all surfaces of the hands and fingers. Rinse hands with water and dry thoroughly with a disposable towel. Use towel to turn off the faucet (IB). Avoid using hot water, because repeated exposure to hot water may increase the risk of dermatitis (IB).
3. Selection of hand hygiene agents
   A. Provide personnel with efficacious hand hygiene products that have low irritancy potential, particularly when these products are used multiple times per shift (IB).
   B. To maximize acceptance of hand hygiene products by HCWs, solicit input from these employees regarding the feel, fragrance, and skin tolerance of any products under consideration. The cost of hand hygiene products should not be the primary factor influencing product selection (IB).
   C. Do not add soap to a partially empty soap dispenser. This practice of "topping off" dispensers can lead to bacterial contamination of soap (IA).

4. Skin care
   A. Provide HCWs with hand lotions or creams to minimize the occurrence of irritant contact dermatitis associated with hand antisepsis or handwashing (IA).
   B. Solicit information from manufacturers regarding any effects that hand lotions, creams, or alcohol-based hand antiseptics may have on the persistent effects of antimicrobial soaps being used in the institution (IB).
5. Other aspects of hand hygiene
   A. Do not wear artificial fingernails or extenders when having direct contact with patients at high risk (e.g., those in intensive care units or operating rooms) (IA).
   B. Wear gloves when contact with blood or other potentially infectious materials, mucous membranes, and nonintact skin could occur (IC).
   C. Remove gloves after caring for a patient. Do not wear the same pair of gloves for the care of more than one patient, and do not wash gloves between uses with different patients (IB) (CDC, 2002a).

In addition, the CDC's *Guidelines for the Prevention of Intravascular Catheter-Related Infections* requires that hand hygiene be performed before and after palpating catheter insertion sites, as well as before and after inserting, replacing, accessing, repairing, or dressing an intravascular catheter (CDC, 2002b).

 ## PERIPHERAL VENOUS CATHETER

SKIN ANTISEPSIS

When the skin is prepared for the insertion of a peripheral intravenous catheter, cleaning an area 2 to 4 inches in diameter is generally considered safe and acceptable. When tincture of iodine is used for skin antisepsis before catheter insertion, it should be removed with alcohol because it may cause skin irritation (INS, 2006). The catheter insertion site should not be palpated after the skin has been cleansed with the antiseptic unless palpated with sterile gloves.

SITE CARE

A transparent, semipermeable dressing over a peripheral intravenous catheter should be changed when the catheter is replaced and immediately if the integrity of the dressing is compromised (INS, 2006). When the dressing is replaced, touch contamination of the catheter insertion site should be avoided.

INSERTION SITE

In adults, an upper extremity site should be selected for the insertion of a peripheral venous catheter, rather than a lower extremity site. If a peripheral venous catheter is inserted in a lower extremity site, it should be moved to an upper extremity site as soon as possible. In pediatric patients, the hand, the dorsum of the foot, or the scalp can be used as the catheter insertion site (INS, 2006).

Peripheral intravenous catheters should be selected on the basis of the intended purpose and duration of use, known complications (e.g., phlebitis and infiltration), and experience of individual clinicians. Steel needles for the administration of fluids and medication that might cause tissue necrosis if extravasation occurs should be avoided (CDC, 2002b). A peripheral venous access device should never be readvanced (INS, 2006).

Prophylactic topical antimicrobial or antiseptic ointment or cream should not be routinely applied to the insertion site of a peripheral venous catheter (CDC, 2002b).

The peripheral venous catheter insertion site should be inspected visually and palpated for tenderness only through the intact dressing (if the patient has no signs or symptoms of an infection). If there is tenderness, fever without an obvious source, or symptoms of a local or bloodstream infection, the dressing should be removed and the site directly inspected. Gauze and opaque dressings should not be removed if the patient has no clinical signs of infection.

The peripheral venous catheter should be removed if the patient develops signs of phlebitis (e.g., warmth, tenderness, erythema, and palpable venous cord), infection, or a malfunctioning catheter. Peripheral venous catheters should be removed at least every 72 hours (INS, 2006) or up to 96 hours (CDC, 2002b), and immediately upon suspected contamination, complication, or therapy discontinuation in adults to prevent phlebitis. If sites for venous access are limited and no evidence of phlebitis or infection is present, peripheral venous catheters can be left in place for longer periods, although the patient and the insertion site should be closely monitored and appropriate information documented. Peripheral venous catheters may be left in place in children until the intravenous therapy is completed or unless complications (e.g., phlebitis and infiltration) occur (CDC, 2002b). Injection caps or valves on peripheral short venous catheters should be changed when the catheter is replaced (CDC, 2002b).

ADMINISTRATION SET

The primary administration set change shall coincide with the peripheral catheter change and with initiation of a new container of solution. The secondary set change will coincide with the change of the primary administration set and with the initiation of a new container of solution. Primary intermittent administration sets shall be changed every 24 hours and immediately upon suspected contamination, or when the integrity of the product or system has been compromised (INS, 2006).

MIDLINE CATHETER

A midline catheter is considered a peripheral venous catheter as it does not enter a central vein. It is inserted 3 to 8 inches via the antecubital fossa with the distal tip dwelling in the proximal basilic or cephalic veins at or below the axillary level and distal to the shoulder (CDC, 2002b; INS, 2006). A midline catheter should be selected when the duration of intravenous therapy will likely exceed 6 days. A midline catheter should not be routinely replaced to reduce the risk of infection (CDC, 2002b).

 ## CENTRAL VENOUS CATHETER INFECTION PREVENTION STRATEGIES

MAXIMAL BARRIER PRECAUTIONS

Maximal barrier precautions should be used to reduce the chance of catheter contamination and a subsequent catheter-associated bloodstream infection. For the individual placing the central line and for those assisting in the procedure, maximal barrier precautions means strict compliance with hand hygiene and wearing a cap, mask, sterile gown, and sterile gloves. The cap should cover all hair and the mask should cover the nose and mouth tightly. For the patient, applying maximal barrier precautions means covering the patient from head to toe with a sterile drape, with a small opening for the site of insertion (CDC, 2002b; INS, 2006; NQF, 2006; IHI, 2008).

PREINSERTION VENOUS ACCESS DEVICE INFECTION PREVENTION STRATEGIES
Skin preparation

If excess hair needs to be removed from the skin before skin antisepsis for the insertion of a catheter, the hair should be removed with scissors or an electric clipper. Shaving with a razor is not recommended because it may cause microabrasions that can damage skin integrity, which can increase the risk of infection. Removing the hair by using a depilatory is not recommended because of the potential for an allergic reaction (INS, 2006).

Skin antisepsis

Cleansing and antisepsis of the skin at the catheter insertion site are among the most important measures for preventing a catheter-associated infection. Before a venous access device is inserted, all surface dirt on the skin should be removed. Otherwise, the antiseptic solution may not be effective as it cannot penetrate the surface dirt. Once the skin is cleaned, an appropriate antiseptic should be applied to the skin before the catheter is inserted and during dressing changes using aseptic or sterile technique as appropriate. A 2% chlorhexidine-based preparation for performing skin antisepsis (CDC, 2002b; INS, 2006; NQF 2006) or formulations containing a combination of alcohol (ethyl or isopropyl alcohol) and povidone-iodine are preferred. Tincture of iodine and povidone-iodine, as single agents or in combination, used individually or in a series, may also be used (CDC, 2002b; INS, 2006). Alcohol should not be applied after the application of povidone-iodine or tincture of iodine (INS, 2006).

Chlorhexidine skin antisepsis has been proven to provide better skin antisepsis than other antiseptic agents such as povidone-iodine solutions (Maki, Ringer, Alvarado, 1991; Chaiyakunapruk et al, 2002). Except for chlorhexidine, the antiseptic agent should be applied to the insertion site and wiped outward in a circular motion. Chlorhexidine should be applied in a back and forth motion for at least 30 seconds. Excess antiseptic should not be blotted or wiped off (CDC, 2002b; INS, 2006; IHI, 2008). When alcohol is used to perform skin antisepsis, the catheter itself should not be cleaned with the alcohol as it can compromise the catheter's material over time.

The use of chlorhexidine gluconate in infants weighing <1000 grams has been associated with contact dermatitis and should be used with caution in this patient population (INS, 2006). It may be contraindicated for use in very low birth weight (VLBW) infants (NQF, 2006). The CDC does not recommend the use of chlorhexidine sponge dressings in neonates aged less than 7 days or of gestational age <26 weeks (CDC, 2002b).

For neonates, isopropyl alcohol or products containing isopropyl alcohol are not recommended for access site preparation. Povidone-iodine or chlorhexidine gluconate solutions are recommended, but require complete removal after the preparatory procedure with sterile water or sterile 0.9% sodium chloride (USP) to prevent product absorption (INS, 2006).

A single-unit container or packet of the skin antiseptic agent is recommended (INS, 2006). Before puncturing the site, the selected antiseptic agent should be allowed to remain on the insertion site and air dry completely on the skin, which may take up to 2 minutes or longer (CDC, 2002b; INS, 2006). In addition, do not palpate the insertion site after the application of the antiseptic agent, unless sterile technique is maintained. An organic solvent, such as acetone and acetone-based products, should not be applied to the skin before the insertion of catheters and during dressing changes (CDC, 2002b; INS, 2006).

Optimal catheter site selection

It is generally not within the scope of practice for a nurse to insert a central line in a location other than the upper extremity; however, in collaboration with other members of the health care team, it is important for the nurse to be aware that in adults, the subclavian vein is the preferred catheter insertion site for nontunneled catheters (rather than a jugular or a femoral site) and is based solely on the lower risk of infection (NQF, 2006; IHI, 2008). However, subclavian catheter placement may have other associated risks. The central line bundle requirement for optimal site selection suggests that other factors (e.g., the potential for mechanical complications, such as pneumothorax, subclavian artery puncture, subclavian vein laceration, subclavian vein stenosis, hemothorax, thrombosis, air embolism, catheter misplacement, and catheter-operator skill) be considered in the final placement selection. When an insertion site other than the subclavian is selected, this aspect of the bundle is considered met if there is dialogue among the clinical team members as to why the site (other than the subclavian) was selected and their rationale. This discussion and rationale should also be documented (IHI, 2008). The optimal catheter site selection in the pediatric patient will need to be specific to the size of the infant or child, the child's condition, and accessibility factors (NQF, 2006). Catheters used for hemodialysis and pheresis should be placed in a jugular or femoral vein rather than a subclavian vein to avoid venous stenosis, if catheter access is needed. During the catheter insertion, a sterile sleeve should be used to protect pulmonary artery catheters during insertion, and arterial or venous cutdown procedures should not be routinely used as the method to insert a central venous catheter (CDC, 2002b).

Central venous catheter selection

The catheter selected should have the minimum number of ports or lumens essential for the management of the patient, and the insertion technique selected should be that with the lowest risk for complications (infectious and noninfectious) for the anticipated type and duration of infusion therapy. Recent guidelines from the Infectious Diseases Society of America (IDSA) and the Society for Healthcare Epidemiology of America (SHEA) recommend use of antimicrobial or antiseptic-impregnated central venous catheters only if hospital units or patient populations have a high CLABSI rate despite implementation of basic, comprehensive practices or in patients with limited venous access and a history of infections or those who are at heightened risk for severe consequences from an infection such as those patients with recently implanted intravascular devices (Marschall, Mermel, Classen et al, 2008).

The comprehensive strategy should include the following three components: (1) the education of the person(s) inserting and maintaining catheters, (2) the use of maximal sterile barrier precautions, and (3) the use of 2% chlorhexidine preparation for skin antisepsis during central line insertion (CDC, 2002b). A totally implantable access device should be used for patients who require long-term, intermittent vascular access. A patient requiring dialysis should have a cuffed central venous catheter selected if the period of temporary access is anticipated to be prolonged (e.g., >3 weeks). However, a fistula or graft should be used instead of a central venous catheter as a permanent access for dialysis.

POSTINSERTION VENOUS ACCESS DEVICE INFECTION PREVENTION STRATEGIES
Daily review of central line necessity

Any intravascular catheter is to be promptly removed when it is no longer essential (CDC, 2002b). To ensure that the central line is removed in a timely manner, reviewing the medical necessity of the central line should be performed on a daily basis (NQF, 2006; IHI, 2008). The purpose of the daily review is to prevent any unnecessary delays in promptly removing a central line that is no longer clearly needed for the patient's care. This daily review is applicable to the acute care setting, and may be considered in other care settings, such as ambulatory or home care. Many times, central lines remain in place simply because they provide reliable venous access and/or because health care personnel have not considered removing them. The risk of infection clearly increases over time as the central line remains in place, and the risk of infection decreases when the line is removed.

Catheter replacement

Central venous or arterial catheters should not be replaced solely for the purpose of reducing the incidence of infection. A short-term central venous catheter should be replaced if purulence is observed at the insertion site, which indicates infection. Guidewire techniques are not to be used to replace catheters in patients suspected of having a catheter-related infection (CDC, 2002b). A guidewire exchange should be used to replace a malfunctioning nontunneled catheter only if no evidence of infection is present and a new set of sterile gloves is put on before handling the new catheter.

Administration set replacement

An administration set includes the area from the spike of tubing entering the fluid container to the hub of the vascular access device. However, a short extension tube might be connected to the catheter and should be considered a portion of the catheter to facilitate aseptic technique when changing administration sets. Administration sets, including secondary sets and add-on devices, should be of Luer-Lok™ design and replaced no more frequently than 72-hour intervals, unless a catheter-associated infection is suspected or documented (CDC, 2002b; INS, 2006) or when the integrity of the product or system has been compromised (INS, 2006). INS makes a separate and distinct recommendation for administration set changes to be done every 24 hours for primary intermittent infusions (Gorski, 2008). The CDC does not make this distinction. It is important to recognize that when an intermittent infusion is repeatedly disconnected and reconnected for the infusion, there is much more manipulation of the tubing and

the catheter/injection cap or valve. Frequent changes increase the risk for contamination and potential catheter-associated bloodstream infection. The problem is further compounded by documentation of poor practices. The Institute for Safe Medication Practices (ISMP) (ISMP, 2007) documents the problems of failure to place a sterile cap on the end of the reused administration set for the intermittent infusion and failure to disinfect the injection cap/valve when accessing the infusion for flushing or medication administration. Tubing used to administer blood, blood products, or lipid emulsions (those combined with amino acids and glucose in a 3-in-1 admixture or infused separately) should be replaced within 24 hours of initiating the infusion. If the solution contains only dextrose and amino acids, the administration set does not need to be replaced more frequently than every 72 hours. Tubing used to administer propofol infusions should be replaced every 6 or 12 hours, depending on its use, per the manufacturer's recommendation (CDC, 2002b).

Needleless systems

Blunt cannulas used to access needleless devices should be removed immediately after use, and a new, sterile, blunt cannula should be aseptically attached. For systems without a blunt cannula, a compatible sterile covering device should be aseptically attached after each intermittent use. Administration sets and needleless devices should be aseptically maintained between medication dosages (INS, 2006).

Dressing changes

Skin surface moisture is another important property of infection control. Studies have concluded that the collection of moisture enhances the proliferation of microorganisms, so it is essential to maintain a dry, sterile, and intact site dressing. Catheter site care should consist of sterile cleansing of the catheter-skin junction with an appropriate antiseptic solution, application of a new stabilization device, and application of a sterile dressing. Dressings should be changed on midline (peripheral) catheters and tunneled, nontunneled, or implanted central venous catheter exit sites no more often than every 7 days (CDC, 2002b; INS, 2006), until the insertion site has healed. An exception is in pediatric patients, because in this patient population the risk for dislodging the catheter outweighs the benefit of changing the dressing (CDC, 2002b). A dressing should also be placed over the noncoring needle placed in an implanted port and the dressing changed every 7 days. When a dressing is needed over a tunneled central venous catheter, either a sterile gauze dressing or a sterile, transparent, semipermeable dressing may be used (CDC, 2002b; INS, 2006). If the patient is not immunosuppressed and healing at the insertion site is complete, site care for tunneled catheters may be limited to daily inspection and cleansing with soap and water while bathing.

A transparent, semipermeable dressing over a central venous catheter should be changed at least every 7 days (INS, 2006); when it becomes damp, loosened, or soiled; when inspection of the site is necessary; and at each hemodialysis session (CDC, 2002b). Gauze dressings should be changed every 48 hours (INS, 2006); when they become damp, loosened, or soiled; and when inspection of the site is necessary. However, there is an exception in pediatric patients because in this patient population the risk for dislodging the catheter outweighs the benefit of changing the dressing (CDC, 2002b). A gauze dressing is preferable to a transparent, semipermeable dressing if the patient is diaphoretic, or if the site is bleeding or oozing. If a gauze dressing is used, a transparent, semipermeable dressing is to be placed over the gauze dressing to maintain the integrity of the gauze and secure the dressing. When a transparent dressing is placed over a gauze dressing covering the exit site to maintain the integrity of the gauze dressing, it is considered a gauze dressing and should be changed every 48 hours. When a gauze dressing is placed under a noncoring needle to stabilize the needle and a transparent, semipermeable dressing is placed over the port access site, it is considered a transparent, semipermeable dressing and should be changed every 7 days (INS, 2006). Some well-healed exit sites of long-term cuffed and tunneled central venous catheters may not require dressings (CDC, 2002b). In a study of 78 patients with cancer, there were no significant differences in sepsis rates among patients with newly inserted tunneled central venous catheters and who were randomized either to a gauze dressing or to no dressing starting at 21 days after catheter insertion (Olson et al, 2004). Topical antibiotic ointment or creams should not be used on the catheter insertion site (except when using dialysis catheters) because of their potential to promote fungal infections and antimicrobial resistance. The catheter site should be monitored visually or by palpation through the intact dressing on a regular basis, depending on the clinical situation of individual patients. If patients have tenderness at the insertion site, fever without obvious source, or other manifestations suggesting local or bloodstream infection (BSI), the dressing should be removed to allow thorough examination of the site (CDC, 2002b).

Chlorhexidine-impregnated dressing

A chlorhexidine-impregnated dressing (e.g., protective disk with chlorhexidine gluconate) may be considered for placement at the catheter-skin junction to protect the extraluminal pathway to help eliminate or reduce the incidence of infection. In one multicenter study, a chlorhexidine-impregnated sponge dressing placed over the site of short-term arterial and central venous catheters reduced the risk for catheter colonization and catheter-related bloodstream infection, with no adverse systemic effects (Maki et al, 2000). In a meta-analysis of eight randomized controlled trials, the use of BIOPATCH™ in dressings for CVCs (and epidural catheters) was associated with a significant reduction in bacterial colonization at the intravascular catheter exit site and there was a somewhat lower, but nonsignificant reduction in infections (Kwok et al, 2006). Chlorhexidine sponge dressings should not be used in neonates aged less than 7 days or of gestational age less than 26 weeks (Garland et al, 2001; CDC, 2002b). When a chlorhexidine-impregnated dressing is used under a semipermeable transparent dressing, it should be placed at the catheter-skin junction and replaced at the same time as the dressing (e.g., minimally every 7 days). The 2008 IDSA/SHEA guidelines recommend use of chlorhexidine-impregnated sponge dressings as a special approach only if hospital units or patient populations have a high CLABSI rate despite implementation of basic, comprehensive practices or in patients with limited venous access and a history of infections or those who are at heightened risk for severe consequences from an infection such as those patients with recently implanted intravascular devices (Marschall et al, 2008).

Catheter stabilization device

A catheter stabilization device prevents the inadvertent movement of the venous access device at the point of insertion (i.e., the catheter-skin junction), which prevents catheter migration. In one small randomized controlled trial, there were fewer overall complications in the group of patients whose peripherally inserted central catheters (PICCs) were secured using a manufactured securement device as compared to standard securement with sutures, and there was a significant finding of fewer bloodstream infections in the securement device group (Yamamoto et al, 2002).

Stabilization of the catheter has the following results:
- It lowers the risk for mechanical phlebitis from the lack of pistoning movement.
- It lowers the risk of catheter-related infection from pathogens on the skin migrating into the catheter tract during catheter movement.
- It lowers the risk of the loss of venous access.

The catheter stabilization device should be used in a manner that does not interfere with assessment and monitoring of the access site, or impede vascular circulation or the delivery of the prescribed therapy. The catheter stabilization device should be changed using aseptic technique (because of its proximity to the catheter-skin junction) when catheter site care is performed (INS, 2006). Another accepted method of venous access device stabilization is the use of sterile tape and surgical strips. However, they can loosen from patient activity or moisture accumulation under the dressing material, resulting in catheter movement and problems associated with catheter movement.

Injection or access cap

Access device injection or access caps should be of a Luer-Lok™ design. Before the system is accessed, contamination risks can be minimized by aseptically cleaning the injection or access port using a twisting, turning, and scrubbing motion, similar to "juicing an orange," with 70% alcohol or povidone-iodine. While there are no published guidelines addressing duration of the scrub, in an in vitro study four different brands of needleless injection caps were inoculated with bacteria and subsequently disinfected for 15 seconds with either 70% alcohol or 3.15% chlorhexidine/70% alcohol; both solutions were found to be effective in disinfection (Kaler, 2007).

The CDC recommends that injection caps not be changed more frequently than every 72 hours or according to manufacturers' recommendations (CDC, 2002b); however, the INS standards recommend that the injection cap on a midline catheter or central venous catheter be changed when the catheter dressing is changed, any time the injection cap is removed from the catheter, if residual blood remains in the injection port, or whenever contamination occurs (INS, 2006).

ADDITIONAL INFECTION PREVENTION MEASURES

FILTERS

In-line filters reduce the incidence of infusion-related phlebitis; however, data do not support their efficacy in preventing infections associated with intravascular catheters and infusion systems. Therefore the CDC does not recommend the routine use of in-line filters for infection control purposes (CDC, 2002b). However, in-line filters should be used to remove particulate matter that could result in an obstruction to the vascular or pulmonary system. For non–lipid-containing solutions that require filtration, a 0.2-micron filter containing a membrane that is air-eliminating and bacteria- and particulate-retentive should be used. For lipid infusions or total nutrient admixtures that require filtration, a 1.2-micron filter containing a membrane that is bacteria- and particulate-retentive and air-eliminating should be used. Blood and blood by-product filters appropriate to the therapy should be used to reduce particulate matter, microaggregates, or leukocytes in infusions of blood or blood components. For intraspinal infusions, a 0.2-micron filter that is surfactant-free, particulate-retentive, and air-eliminating should be used. The filter should be located as close to the patient as possible and changed at the same frequency in which the IV administration set is changed (INS, 2006).

REPLACEMENT OF PARENTERAL FLUIDS

Lipid-containing solutions (e.g., 3-in-1 solutions) should be infused within 24 hours. The infusion of lipid emulsions alone should be completed within 12 hours of hanging the emulsion. However, if volume considerations require more time, the infusion should be completed within 24 hours. The infusion of blood or other blood products should be completed within 4 hours of hanging the blood. The CDC has no recommendations for the hang times of other parenteral fluids (CDC, 2002b).

UMBILICAL CATHETERS

Umbilical artery catheters or umbilical venous catheters should be removed as soon as possible when no longer needed or when any sign of vascular insufficiency to the lower extremities is observed; these catheters should not be replaced if any signs of catheter-associated bloodstream infection, vascular insufficiency, or thrombosis are present. The umbilical venous catheters should be replaced only if the catheter malfunctions. Optimally, umbilical artery catheters should be left in place less than 5 days. Umbilical venous catheters can be used up to 14 days if managed aseptically. The umbilical insertion site should be cleansed with an antiseptic before catheter insertion; tincture of iodine should be avoided (i.e., because of the potential effect on the neonatal's thyroid) while other iodine-containing products (e.g., povidone-iodine) can be used. Topical antibiotic ointment or creams should not be used on the umbilical catheter insertion site because of the potential to promote fungal infections and antimicrobial resistance. Low doses of heparin should be added to the fluid infused through umbilical arterial catheters (CDC, 2002b).

PRESSURE MONITORING SYSTEMS

Peripheral arterial catheters should not be routinely replaced to prevent a catheter-associated infection. Disposable or reusable transducers and assemblies should be used whenever possible and replaced at 96-hour intervals. If the use of a disposable transducer is not feasible, the reusable transducer should be sterilized according to the manufacturers' instructions. Other components of the system (including the tubing, continuous-flush device, and flush solution) should be replaced at the time the transducer is replaced. All components of the pressure monitoring system (including calibration devices and flush solution) should be kept sterile with the number of manipulations of and entries into the pressure monitoring system minimized. A closed-flush system (i.e., continuous flush) rather than an open system (i.e., one that requires a syringe and stopcock) should be used to maintain the patency of the pressure monitoring catheters. When the pressure monitoring system is accessed through a diaphragm rather than a stopcock, the diaphragm should be wiped with an appropriate antiseptic before accessing the system. Solutions containing dextrose or parenteral nutrition fluids should not be administered through the pressure monitoring circuit (CDC, 2002b).

SAFE WORK AND INJECTION PRACTICES

Preventing exposure to bloodborne pathogens while providing infusion therapy is paramount in protecting both the patient and the nurse. The CDC and the Occupational Safety and Health Administration (OSHA) recommend the application of standard precautions by health care workers at all times to prevent the transmission of bloodborne pathogens. That is, all blood and body fluids from all patients should be treated as being potentially infected with the hepatitis B virus (HBV), hepatitis C virus (HCV), human immunodeficiency virus (HIV), and other bloodborne pathogens (OSHA, 1991). The prevention of needlesticks and other sharps-related injuries is an essential component of standard precautions. Injuries attributable to needlesticks and other sharps have been directly associated with transmission of HBV, HCV, and HIV to health care personnel. The federal Needlestick Safety and Prevention Act, signed into law in November 2000, authorized OSHA's revision of its bloodborne pathogens standard. The revision more explicitly requires the use of safety-engineered sharp devices so that needles and other sharps will be handled in a manner that prevents injury to the nurse and others who may encounter the device during or after a procedure (OSHA, 2000).

PREVENTION OF MUCOUS MEMBRANE CONTACT

Exposure of mucous membranes of the eyes, nose, and mouth to blood and body fluids has been associated with the transmission of bloodborne viruses and other infectious agents to health care personnel. The prevention of mucous membrane exposures has always been an element of standard precautions for routine patient care and is subject to OSHA bloodborne pathogen regulations. Safe work practices, in addition to wearing personal protective equipment (PPE), should be implemented to protect the mucous membranes and nonintact skin from contact with potentially infectious material. Safe practices include careful donning of PPE before patient contact and keeping gloved and ungloved hands that are contaminated from touching the mouth, nose, eyes, or face.

OSHA requires health care workers to use protective barriers such as gloves, masks, protective eyewear, and fluid-impervious gowns whenever there is a risk of exposure to blood or body fluids. Gloves can reduce the infusion nurse's risk of infection, but they offer little protection from needlestick injuries. To protect against needlesticks, the use of needleless systems, safety syringes, and cannulas is required. Needles should never be recapped, bent, or broken. After use, needles and syringes should

---

Box 12-4   SAFE INJECTION PRACTICES

1. Use aseptic technique to avoid contamination of sterile injection equipment.
2. Do not administer medications from a syringe to multiple patients, even if the needle or cannula on the syringe is changed. Needles, cannulae, and syringes are sterile, single-use items; they should neither be reused for another patient nor be used to access a medication or solution that might be used for a subsequent patient.
3. Use fluid infusion and administration sets (i.e., intravenous bags, tubing, and connectors) for one patient only and dispose appropriately after use. Consider a syringe or needle/cannula contaminated once it has been used to enter or connect to a patient's intravenous infusion bag or administration set.
4. Use single-dose vials for parenteral medications whenever possible.
5. Do not administer medications from single-dose vials or ampules to multiple patients or combine leftover contents for later use.
6. If multidose vials must be used, both the needle or cannula and the syringe used to access the multidose vial must be sterile.
7. Do not keep multidose vials in the immediate patient treatment area and store in accordance with the manufacturer's recommendations; discard if sterility is compromised or questionable.
8. Do not use bags or bottles of intravenous solution as a common source of supply for multiple patients.

From the U.S. Public Health Service, U.S. Department of Health and Human Services, Centers for Disease Control and Prevention, Atlanta, Ga. Siegel JD, Rhinehart E, Jackson M, Chiarello L, Healthcare Infection Control Practices Advisory Committee: *Guidelines for isolation precautions: preventing transmission of infectious agents in healthcare settings*, June 2007. Accessed at http://www.cdc.gov/ncidod/dhqp/pdf/guidelines/Isolation2007.pdf.

---

be disposed in an impervious, puncture-resistant container located as close as possible to the patient's care area.

SAFE INJECTION PRACTICES

Four large outbreaks of HBV and HCV among patients in ambulatory care facilities in the United States identified a need to define and reinforce safe injection practices (Siegel et al, 2007). The primary breaches in infection control practice that contributed to these outbreaks were the reinsertion of used needles into a multiple-dose vial or solution container (e.g., saline bag) and the use of a single needle/syringe to administer intravenous medication to multiple patients. In one of these outbreaks, preparation of medications in the same workspace where used needles/syringes were dismantled also may have been a contributing factor. These and other outbreaks of viral hepatitis could have been prevented by adherence to basic principles of aseptic technique for the preparation and administration of parenteral medications.

Whenever possible, use of single-dose vials is preferred over multiple-dose vials, especially when medications will be administered to multiple patients. Outbreaks related to unsafe injection practices indicate that some health care personnel are unaware of, do not understand, or do not adhere to basic principles of infection control and aseptic technique. Therefore, to ensure that all health care workers understand and adhere to recommended practices, principles of infection control and aseptic technique need to be reinforced in training programs and incorporated into institutional polices that are monitored for adherence. The recommendations listed in Box 12-4 apply to the use of needles, cannulas that replace needles, and, where applicable, intravenous delivery systems.

 ## IV-RELATED INFECTIONS

PATIENT RISK FACTORS

Risk factors related to IV infections can be divided into those related to the patient and those related to the venous access device. There are many risk factors that increase a patient's susceptibility to developing an IV-associated infection. These include,

but are not limited to, the following: neutropenia; diminished granulocyte function; immunosuppression and immunodeficiency; burns; presence of concurrent infection; severe underlying illness; age less than 6 months or greater than 65 years; and the presence of an indwelling medical device.

SKIN COLONIZATION AS A RISK FACTOR

The microbes colonizing the skin surrounding the insertion site are the source of most catheter-related bloodstream infections (Mermel, 2000). Studies of a variety of catheters indicate that heavy cutaneous colonization of the insertion site is a strong predictor of catheter-related infections. Burn patients who have a large population of microorganisms on the skin surface also experience very high rates of catheter-related infections (Bennet and Brachman, 1998).

Studies also indicate that the skin at the insertion site is the most common source of colonization and infection for vascular catheters that have been in place for less than 10 days. The organisms migrate from the skin through the insertion site along the external catheter surface, and colonize the distal intravascular tip of the catheter. This colonization leads to bloodstream infection. Skin-related microorganisms causing catheter-related bloodstream infections include *Staphylococcus epidermidis, S. aureus, Bacillus* species, and *Corynebacterium* species. Microorganisms on the hands of health care personnel inserting or caring for catheters, including *Pseudomonas aeruginosa, Acinetobacter* species, *Stenotrophomonas maltophilia, Candida albicans,* and *Candida parapsilosis,* can cause infection (Raad, 1998). The hands of health care workers contain two different type of flora: resident and transient. Transient flora is loosely attached to the skin and can be readily removed with soap, water, and mechanical friction or an alcohol-based hand rub product, thereby preventing the transfer of microorganisms (CDC, 2002a).

Skin temperature plays an important role in infection; the higher the skin's temperature, the greater the occurrence of microbial growth. The skin on the upper and lower extremities has a lower temperature than that on the trunk and neck. Most central venous catheters are inserted into the trunk, which has a higher temperature and thus a greater potential for microbial growth. Peripheral sites rarely have more than 50 to 100 colony-forming units (CFUs) of bacteria per 10 cm^2 of skin, whereas the skin on the neck and chest has greater than 1000 to 10,000 CFUs/cm². This reduced amount of skin flora may play a role in the lower rates of catheter-related septicemia reported for peripherally inserted central catheters (PICCs) and midline catheters.

IV PRODUCT AND CATHETER-RELATED CONTAMINATION

Despite improved catheter technology (i.e., antibiotic-impregnated catheters, cuffs, and dressing materials) catheter-related infections continue to occur when the IV infusion system becomes contaminated. Contamination can occur by intrinsic or extrinsic means.

INTRINSIC CONTAMINATION

Intrinsic contamination is contamination that occurs in IV fluids and products at any time during the manufacturing or sterilization process before reaching the health care organization. After the IV fluid or product has been sterilized, any damage to the IV fluid or product container provides an entry point for microorganisms. Entry points can result from a damaged port seal, a crack in a bottle, or a hole in a plastic IV bag. A defect in the fluid container may occur during the manufacturing or sterilization process. For example, if no seal is placed or if a seal is positioned incorrectly on the port of an IV bag, fluid contamination may result.

The product may also become contaminated during sterilization or during storage and delivery. Contamination during storage can occur at the manufacturing site, the wholesaler, the health care facility, or an alternative care setting, including the patient's home. Products are delivered in a variety of ways and to numerous sites before reaching the patient, and product contamination can occur at any time along the way. Contamination of infusates is the most common cause of epidemic device-related bloodstream infections. Causative organisms for fluid-related contamination include the following: tribe Klebsielleae (*Enterobacter cloacae, Enterobacter agglomerans, Serratia marcescens,* and *Klebsiella* species); *Burkholderia cepacia, Burkholderia acidovorans,* and *Burkholderia pickettii; Citrobacter freundii* and *Flavobacterium* species; and *Candida tropicalis* (Bennet and Brachman, 1998). In addition to the IV fluids and equipment, contaminated antiseptic solutions can also cause infections.

Although intrinsic contamination does not often occur, when it does occur, its effects can be far-reaching because of the large volumes of product that are produced and processed at one time. Also, if a contaminant is introduced into the fluid at the manufacturing level, there is more time for the microorganism to proliferate. To prevent an intravascular infection and prevent the IV fluid or product from reaching the patient, the infusion nurse should carefully complete the following steps:

- Check bottles and containers carefully for cracks, including cracks that may be hidden by the label.
- Check the neck of the bottle to ensure that all the closure components are intact.
- Inspect the IV bags for puncture holes by squeezing the container and rotating the bag.
- Observe fluid containers for droplet formation on the bag's surface.

- Inspect all protective coverings and seals of entry ports to ensure proper fit.
- Inspect the clarity of the solution.
- Check the manufacturer's expiration date to ensure that it has not been surpassed.

If there is any question about the sterility or integrity of the IV solution or product, it should not be used. If intrinsic contamination is suspected, the nurse manager, pharmacist, manufacturer, and the U.S. Food and Drug Administration (FDA) should be notified immediately. Samples of the affected product with the same lot number should be made available for inspection and analysis.

EXTRINSIC CONTAMINATION

Many extrinsic sources exist that can contaminate the IV fluid, product, insertion site, or catheter, all of which are considered crucial areas for the prevention of IV-related infections. Extrinsic contamination can occur in whatever setting infusion therapy is provided (e.g., the hospital, ambulatory infusion clinic, or the patient's home). Extrinsic contamination should not be permitted to occur. Examples of extrinsic contamination that can be prevented include the following:

- IV fluids or medications can become contaminated during the admixture procedure by not using a laminar flow hood or by using hoods with expired certification.
- Incorrect use of admixing equipment, such as needles, syringes, or calibrating devices, may result in contaminated products.
- Improper refrigeration of admixed IV solutions increases the rate of proliferation of microorganisms and the potential risk and severity of infection. Because products may be prepared in large numbers in IV admixture programs, the potential for patient exposure to contamination is high.
- Contamination can occur from improper technique, such as when adding medications to the IV fluid container already in use, while administering intermittent medications, or by the failure to maintain a sterile, closed infusion system.
- Damage during delivery and storage of the product allows microorganisms to enter the sterile container.
- Contamination of the administration set can occur when the administration set is added to the fluid container if the set's spike comes in contact with the outside of the IV container port.
- When add-on devices are attached (e.g., filters, stopcocks, extension sets), equipment contamination can occur.
- Inadequate site preparation, touch contamination of the needle or cannula, and improper application of the dressing during the venipuncture and port-a-cath access procedure can cause contamination.
- IV pathway contamination can occur when additional solutions or medications are connected, when air is removed from the line, or when there is accidental separation of the line at any connection.
- Contamination can occur if the hub of the catheter is not cleaned with alcohol before flushing the catheter or attaching the administration set.
- Soiled or damp dressings that have not been changed can cause contamination.

• Tubing left in place longer than the recommended hang time, including blood sets, provides a source for microorganisms to proliferate.

BIOFILM AND INFECTION

Biofilm provides a habitat or a reservoir for microorganisms in which they are protected from harmful conditions; therefore biofilm serves as a reservoir for microorganisms that can infect the patient. If a biofilm is present, there is always a risk that cells can detach and then can cause an infection (Flanders and Yildiz, 2004). Studies show that most indwelling vascular catheters have microorganisms imbedded in a biofilm layer, and this can occur as early as 24 hours after insertion (Raad, 1998). There are four phases of the biofilm life cycle, including: (1) adhesion, (2) aggregation/colonization, (3) exopolysaccharide encasement, and (4) detachment and dispersal. It is in this last phase that the microorganisms embedded in the biofilm detach and enter the bloodstream, possibly resulting in an infection. Biofilm is the source of infection when the numbers of cells released overwhelm the host's defense mechanisms (Donlan and Costerton, 2002). Infection can only occur when microorganisms are present; however, the presence of microorganisms does not always lead to an infection. Even with antibiotic treatment, microorganisms may survive because of the protective properties of the biofilm (Flanders and Yildiz, 2004). The link between biofilm and infection is that biofilm provides a sustained reservoir for microorganisms that, after detachment, can infect the host (Purevdorj-Gage and Stoodley, 2004). Anti-infective technology may reduce the amount of biofilm and enhance lumen patency. Antimicrobial agent combinations (including chlorhexidine-silver sulfadiazine, rifampin-minocycline, and silver-platinum) are impregnated in nontunneled central venous catheters, with the rifampin-minocycline combination available in peripherally inserted central catheters (Hadaway, 2006).

CATHETER SURFACE CHARACTERISTICS

The physical characteristics of the catheter's surface, the surface characteristics of adherent bacteria, the presence of host-derived proteins, and the intrinsic phenotypic charges of adherent bacteria that form the biofilm determine the adherent nature of microorganisms (Figure 12-1). For microorganisms to adhere to a catheter, there must be an interaction with the catheter's physical characteristics. Examples of catheter characteristics that allow for such interaction include irregular surfaces and charge differences. An example of bacteria surface characteristics is hydrophobicity. Hydrophobic staphylococcal organisms adhere well to some surfaces, such as polyvinyl chloride, silicone, and polyethylene, but not so well to polyurethane or Teflon polymers (Raad, 1998).

Catheter design and composition contribute to the risk of infectious complications. Catheter size has an obvious impact; the larger the catheter, the larger the venipuncture site through the skin and vessel and the greater the injury to tissue. With a larger catheter, it is more difficult to stabilize and maintain an intact dressing. It is recommended that the smallest gauge catheter of the shortest length possible be used to administer the prescribed therapy.

Multilumen catheters may increase a patient's risk for infection. Patients who require multilumen catheters are often critically ill, require parenteral nutrition, may be immunocompromised, and have extended hospitalizations. When treating such patients, it is important to reduce the number of catheter manipulations as much as possible, to adhere to strict aseptic technique, to maintain a closed system, and to designate each lumen of a multilumen catheter for a specific purpose. Colonization of microorganisms on the catheter hub is an important source of pathogens causing catheter-associated infections (Bennet and Brachman, 1998).

Catheter composition has also been suggested as a possible factor in IV-related infections. Most central venous catheters are composed of polyvinylchloride or a silicone elastomer. Both

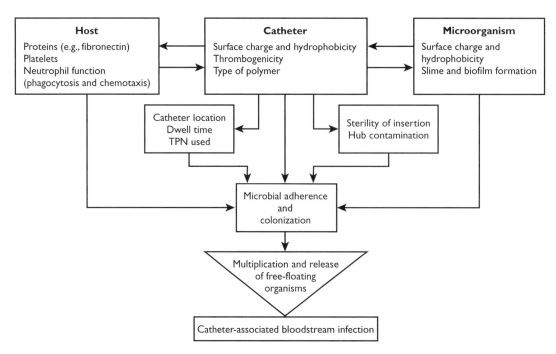

Figure 12-1 Pathogenesis of vascular catheter–associated colonization and infection. *TPN,* Total parenteral nutrition.

materials are soft and flexible. Polyvinylchloride, polyethylene, and silicone catheters have been reported to have a higher incidence of coagulase-negative *Staphylococcus* colonization than polytetrafluoroethylene (Teflon) or polyurethane catheters. Microscopic examination of infected central venous catheters has shown heavy colonization on the external surface. Studies have shown that coagulase-negative *Staphylococcus,* the predominant aerobic species on human skin, is the most common agent of catheter-associated bacteremia (Bennet and Brachman, 1998). Polyurethane and silicone elastomer catheters have been associated with decreased thrombogenicity (Linder et al, 1984).

Antimicrobial-impregnated catheters (chlorhexidine and silver sulfadiazine) have been shown to reduce the rate of central venous colonization (Collin, 1999). Also, there were fewer removals or exchanges of these catheters, and the extending protective effects decreased patient risk and hospital cost. Another study found that using coated triple-lumen catheters (chlorhexidine and silver sulfadiazine) reduces the incidence of significant growth on the tip or intradermal segments but has no effect on the incidence of catheter-related bacteremia (Heard et al, 1998). Chlorhexidine and silver sulfadiazine–impregnated catheters are considered when there is a high rate of infection despite adherence to other strategies (Mermel, 2000; Marschall et al, 2008). A tissue-interface barrier has been developed to help protect against extraluminal microbial migration. This device consists of a detachable cuff made of biodegradable collagen to which silver ions are chelated (Bennet and Brachman, 1998). The cuff is attached to the central venous catheter before insertion. After insertion, the subcutaneous tissue grows into the cuff, creating a physical and chemical barrier against pathogen migration.

Several of the protein components of a thrombus have been shown to increase the adherence of *S. aureus, S. epidermidis,* and *Candida* species to central venous catheters. In turn, thrombus formation is associated with catheter-associated bloodstream infections. Prophylactic use of warfarin and heparin has reduced thrombus formation, but the reduction in catheter-associated bloodstream infection varies by study (Mermel, 2000).

FLUSHING THE CATHETER

Solutions that are used to flush venous access devices may reduce the development of or proliferation of intraluminal biofilm, which can ultimately reduce the patient's risk for infection. Primarily VADs are flushed to prevent thrombosis. Fibrin deposits and thrombi in catheters also may serve as a central point for microbial colonization of the VAD. Catheter thrombosis appears to be one of the most important factors associated with infection of central venous catheters and implanted ports. Thus the use of anticoagulants (e.g., heparin) or thrombolytic agents may have a role in the prevention of catheter-associated bloodstream infections. In a peripheral-short catheter, flushing with 0.9% sodium chloride (USP) at established intervals may be used in lieu of heparin for maintaining catheter patency and reducing phlebitis (INS, 2006). The routine use of heparin to maintain catheter patency, even at doses as low as 250 to 500 units/mL, has been associated with thrombocytopenia and thromboembolic and hemorrhagic complications.

Indwelling central venous catheters (e.g., Hickman and Broviac catheters, PICC, ports) should be routinely flushed with an anticoagulant. The lowest amount and concentration should be used to maintain catheter patency. Catheters with a valve at the proximal or distal tip of the catheter are flushed with 0.9% sodium chloride (USP) solution only and do not require routine flushing with an anticoagulant.

A peripheral venous heparin lock should be routinely flushed with a preservative-free 0.9% sodium chloride (USP) solution. Consideration may be given to the use of a heparin flush solution in low doses (1 to 10 units/mL of heparin) in neonates and pediatric patients because of their tiny veins and the small-gauge catheter used. Isotonic solutions of heparin 0.5 unit/mL should be used for umbilical artery catheters (INS, 2006). If blood has been withdrawn from the catheter, the catheter should be flushed with 0.9% sodium chloride (USP) in sufficient amounts to remove residual blood from the catheter's lumen(s) before the final flushing with the appropriate solution.

The amount of flush solution used is also a consideration in maintaining catheter patency. The flushing volume should be equal to two times the volume capacity of the catheter, in extension and needle-free systems (INS, 2006). For example, if the volume of a peripheral venous catheter and the extension loop is 1.5 mL, the minimum amount needed to flush the catheter is 3 mL. During flushing, the turbulence of the manual flush may reduce the intraluminal biofilm; however, further studies are needed. The positive pressure exerted should be maintained during and after the administration of the flush, to prevent reflux of blood into the catheter lumen, unless a positive-pressure injection valve is in place. If resistance is met during the attempt to flush the catheter, no further flushing attempts should be made because this could result in a clot dislodging into the vascular system or catheter rupture.

ENDOGENOUS SOURCES OF MICROORGANISMS

Healthcare–associated infections may be caused by microorganisms from either endogenous or exogenous sources. Endogenous sources are body sites, such as the skin, nose, mouth, GI tract, or vagina, that are normally inhabited by microorganisms. An endogenous infection is caused by the patient's own flora. For example, the microorganisms from endotracheal secretions may colonize a central venous access device inserted into the subclavian or jugular vein of an intubated patient. The microorganism *S. aureus* appears to be dependent on the presence of preabsorbed plasma or tissue. Other organisms, such as *S. epidermidis,* adhere only to fibronectin and not to other receptors of the patient's protein. Because many tissue proteins are an integral part of thrombus formation, the presence of a thrombus on the catheter surface appears to promote microorganism adherence leading to catheter infections (Bennet and Brachman, 1998).

EXOGENOUS SOURCES OF MICROORGANISMS

Exogenous sources of microorganisms result from the transmission of microorganisms from a source other than the patient. Exogenous sources are those external to the patient, such as health care personnel, visitors/family members, medical equipment and invasive devices, intravenous infusate, or the patient's environment. Extraluminal and intraluminal pathways are significant sources of catheter-associated bloodstream infection. One study of 1263 short-term, nontunneled, noncuffed central venous catheters showed that 26% of the infections were found to be intraluminally acquired, 45% were extraluminally acquired, and the other 29% were undetermined (Safdar and Maki, 2004).

INFECTION PREVENTION AND CONTROL IN THE ALTERNATIVE CARE SETTING

Vascular access devices are commonly used in alternative care settings such as skilled nursing facilities, physicians' offices, and ambulatory infusion centers, and in patients' homes. The same basic principles for infection prevention and control as well as standards of practice apply in the home (Rhinehart and McGoldrick, 2006) or alternative care setting. Few studies are available about vascular access device infection rates or catheter care protocols in alternative care settings. It is generally believed that the at-home risk factors for developing a catheter-associated infection are somewhat reduced. Studies documenting the rate or risk of infection for patients receiving home infusion therapy are cited in the Focus on Evidence box. A study that analyzed the outcomes of central venous catheters in home infusion patients found that bloodstream infection rates were lower than those of the acute care setting, and typically occurred after the first 30 days the catheter was inserted. This underscores the need for vigilance in maintaining aseptic technique in routine catheter care and management (Moureau et al, 2002). Similar findings were identified in Gorki's 7-year study in which the home care infection incidence rates for patients with central venous access devices were reviewed. It was noted that most infections were identified 25 days after

FOCUS ON EVIDENCE

Low Incidence of Infection in the Home Care Setting

- In a systematic review of 200 studies that prospectively examined risk of BSIs in patients with all types of vascular access catheters, 15 studies were analyzed that included patients with PICCs; 9 studies addressed analysis of PICCs in the outpatient (which included home care) setting. Among inpatients and outpatients with PICCs, the pooled mean of BSIs per 1000 device days was 1.1 (95% CI 0.9-1.3). The inpatient rate was 2.1 BSIs per 1000 device days (95% CI 1.0-3.2) and the outpatient rate was half the rate, at 1.0 BSI per 1000 device days (95% CI 0.8-1.2) (Maki, Kluger, Crnich, 2006).

- A prospective study was undertaken to identify infectious complications among 300 patients receiving home infusion therapy through either peripheral or central venous catheters. There were 6 cases of bacteremia, defined as positive blood cultures in patients with either catheter site inflammation or no inflammation elsewhere in the body, attributed to the catheter. The rate was expressed as 6.0 infections per 10,000 home catheter days; per data provided in the study, when expressed per 1000 home catheter days, the rate would be 0.59 (Graham et al, 1991).

- A prospective, cohort observational study was performed to evaluate bloodstream infection rates for patients receiving home infusion therapy via either a central or a peripheral IV catheter. A total of 827 patients were followed over a 1-year period in 2 different sites. There were 69 BSIs that occurred over 69,532 catheter days, calculations yielding a BSI rate of 0.99 infection per 1000 catheter days. Significant risk factors for BSIs were identified and included bone marrow transplantation, total parenteral nutrition, multilumen catheter, history of previous BSI, and receiving infusion therapy outside of the home such as in a physician's office or outpatient clinic (Tokars et al, 1999).

- A retrospective, descriptive study was conducted to describe the type and rate of central venous catheter and midline catheter related complications. Data were obtained from a national home care database including 50,470 patients (primarily adult; 14% pediatric) receiving home infusion therapy over an 18-month period. Catheter infection was defined by documentation of laboratory findings such as positive blood and catheter cultures. The overall infection rate for all types of catheters was 0.26 infection per 1000

catheter days. PICCs were the most common type of catheter used (51%) and had the lowest incidence of BSIs as compared to other central venous catheter types at 0.11 infection per 1000 catheter days. The majority of catheter-related BSIs (65%) occurred more than 30 days after catheter placement (Moureau et al, 2002).

- A retrospective cohort study (n = 279 patients who underwent 307 courses of IV antimicrobial therapy) examining adverse events associated with home intravenous antimicrobial therapy among older versus younger adults found an overall bacteremia rate of 0.43 per 1000 antimicrobial days; there was no significant difference in bacteremia rates between adults 60 years and older versus those younger than 60 (Cox et al, 2007).

- In a letter to the editor addressing the preceding study, the Minnesota Visiting Nurse Agency submitted their complication rates for 63 patients who received home IV antimicrobial therapy during 2006 and reported no episodes of either bacteremia or local site related infections (Brooks and Meyers, 2008).

- A descriptive, retrospective review of medical records for patients with a central venous access device at a single home care agency was conducted over a 7-year period. Data were collected on 551 catheters representing 20,879 home catheter days. PICCs were the most common type of catheter (49.5%). Catheter infection was validated by a blood culture finding of bacteremia or by the presence of a central venous access device and at least two additional criteria including fever, local pain and redness at the exit site, hypotension, WBC >10,000/mm³, or physician validation of infection with initiation of treatment or catheter removal. There was a cumulative rate of 0.77 systemic infection per 1000 catheter days. Total parenteral nutrition as the infusate was a statistically significant risk factor associated with systemic catheter-related infections (Gorski, 2004).

- In a retrospective medical record review of 67 home care patients with either a peripheral or a central venous catheter, an infection rate of 1.25 infections per 1000 home catheter days was found. Included were local site infections, defined as purulence at the exit site, and CRBSIs according to the definition by the CDC (White and Ragland, 1993).

admission to home care, with the author concluding that most of the infection transmissions occurred from the introduction of bacteria through the catheter hub, since by day 25 patients were independent in their infusion therapy (Gorski, 2004). Also, a limited number of outbreaks in home care, all involving home infusion therapy, have been reported in the literature (Danzig et al, 1995; Kellerman et al, 1996; Do et al, 1999). Further research is needed to describe infection risks for patients having their central line management in the home and other alternative care settings.

 ## SURVEILLANCE IN INFUSION THERAPY

Surveillance activities should be conducted in ICUs and other patient populations and care settings where infusion therapy is provided to monitor trends in the rates, to identify lapses in infection prevention and control practices, and to implement action plans to improve these practices. Collecting data is the only way to know whether a change represented an improvement. For organizations that provide infusion therapy, two measures are of interest. These two measures are: (1) the rate of bloodstream infections associated with the use of a central line and (2) assessment of how well the CVC insertion team is adhering to the central line bundle.

SURVEILLANCE DEFINITIONS

Infusion nurses should be aware of the difference between a surveillance definition and clinical definition of an infection. The surveillance definition for a central line–associated bloodstream infection (CLABSI) includes all bloodstream infections (BSIs) that occur in patients with central venous catheters (CVCs) when other sites of infection have been excluded. The surveillance definition overestimates the true incidence of catheter-related bloodstream infection (CRBSI) because not all BSIs originate from a catheter. Some bacteremias are secondary BSIs from undocumented sources of infection (e.g., postoperative surgical site infection, intra-abdominal infection, pneumonia, or urinary tract infections). Therefore surveillance definitions are really definitions for catheter-associated BSIs. A more rigorous definition may only include BSIs for which other sources of infection were excluded by clinical record review, and where a culture of the catheter tip demonstrated substantial colonies of an organism identical to those found in the bloodstream. Such a clinical definition would focus on catheter-associated BSIs (CDC, 2008b).

SOURCE OF INFECTION

During patient surveillance activities, the health care organization will attempt to identify the source of the infection reported and determine if the infection was acquired from any of the following:

- Care or services received under the direction of the health care organization
- The community
- Care received during a recent hospitalization or from care rendered in another health care setting

These infections are called either healthcare–associated or community-associated. The term "associated" is preferred over the term "acquired" as often the geographic location of where the infection was acquired is uncertain. Sometimes an infection is called a nosocomial infection as the infection can be directly linked to an infection that developed during or as a result of an admission to an acute care facility (e.g., hospital) and the infection was not incubating at the time of admission.

DEFINITIONS

A health care–associated infection (HAI) is a localized or systemic condition resulting from an adverse reaction to the associated presence of an infectious agent(s) or its toxin(s) that:

- occurs in a patient in a health care setting (e.g., a hospital or outpatient clinic)
- was not found to be present or incubating at the time of admission unless the infection was related to a previous admission to the same setting
- meets the criteria for a specific infection site as defined by the CDC, if the setting is a hospital (Horan and Gaynes, 2004)

An infection that is associated with a complication or an extension of an infection that is already present on admission is not considered a HAI, unless a change in pathogen or symptoms strongly suggests the acquisition of a new infection. In addition, colonization and inflammation are not considered an infection. Colonization is the presence of microorganisms on skin, on mucous membranes in open wounds, or in excretions or secretions, but the microorganisms are not causing adverse clinical signs or symptoms. Inflammation is the tissue's response to injury or stimulation by noninfectious agents, such as chemicals. A community-acquired infection is an infection that occurs outside of a hospital or health care facility in an otherwise relatively healthy person that has not been recently (within the past year) hospitalized or had a medical procedure performed (such as dialysis, surgery, or catheter insertion) (CDC, 2008a).

 ## DEFINITION OF A CENTRAL LINE–ASSOCIATED BLOODSTREAM INFECTION

A central line is an intravascular catheter that terminates at or close to the heart or in one of the great vessels. The central line is used for infusion, withdrawal of blood, or hemodynamic monitoring. The following are considered great vessels for the purpose of reporting central line infections and counting central line-days in the CDC's National Healthcare Safety Network's (NHSN) system: aorta, pulmonary artery, superior vena cava, inferior vena cava, brachiocephalic veins, internal jugular veins, subclavian veins, external iliac veins, and common femoral veins. In neonates, the umbilical artery/vein is considered a great vessel. Neither the insertion site location nor the type of device should be used to determine if a line qualifies as a central line. The device must terminate in one of these vessels or in or near the heart to qualify as a central line. An introducer is considered an intravascular catheter. Pacemaker wires and other nonlumened devices inserted into central blood vessels or the heart are not considered central lines, because fluids are not infused, pushed, or withdrawn through such devices. A permanent central line is a tunneled catheter, which includes certain dialysis catheters and implantable catheters and ports, whereas a temporary central line is one that is not tunneled. An umbilical catheter is a central line inserted through the umbilical artery or vein in a neonate. There is no minimum period of time that the central line must be in place in order for the BSI to be considered central line–associated (CDC, 2008).

PRIMARY BLOODSTREAM INFECTION

Central line–associated bloodstream infections (CLABSIs) can be prevented through proper management of the central line. An estimated 200,000 CLABSIs occur in U.S. hospitals each year (CDC, 2008b). Specifically, these are primary bloodstream infections that are associated with the presence of a central line or an umbilical catheter in neonates at the time of or before the onset of the infection. Primary bloodstream infections are usually serious infections that typically caused a prolongation of hospital stay and increased cost and risk of mortality. A CLABSI is a primary bloodstream infection (BSI) in a patient that had a central line within the 48-hour period before the development of the BSI. If the BSI develops within 48 hours of discharge from a location, it is associated with the discharging location.

Primary bloodstream infections are classified according to the criteria used, either as laboratory-confirmed bloodstream infection (LCBI) or as clinical sepsis (CSEP). CSEP may be used to report only a primary BSI in neonates (<30 days old) and infants (<1 year old). Organisms cultured from blood should be reported as a BSI-LCBI when no other site of infection is evident. To accurately compare a health care organization's infection rate to published data, or to other organizations, comparable definitions should be used. Refer to Box 12-1 for the CDC's surveillance definitions for most health care settings and refer to Box 12-2 for the APIC-CDC HICPAC's surveillance definitions specific for the home care setting.

SECONDARY BLOODSTREAM INFECTION

A secondary bloodstream infection is a culture-confirmed BSI associated with a documented HAI at another site. If the primary infection is cultured, the secondary BSI must yield a culture of the same organism and exhibit the same antibiogram as the primary HAI site. For example, if a blood culture is positive in a patient with a nosocomial urinary tract infection (UTI) and organisms and antibiograms of both blood and urine specimens are identical, infection is reported as a UTI with secondary BSI. Secondary BSI is not reported separately. If, on the other hand, an organ/space surgical site infection (SSI) is identified by computerized tomography (CT) scan, no culture is used to meet the criteria for surgical site infection-gastrointestinal tract (SSI-GIT), and a blood culture grows *Bacteroides fragilis,* then the SSI-GIT is recorded as an SSI with a secondary BSI. The pathogen for the SSI is recorded as *Bacteroides fragilis* (CDC, 2008b).

In addition to clinical signs and symptoms, the definition of catheter-associated bloodstream infection should include positive blood culture results with cultures drawn from two separate sites. One culture specimen should be drawn through the IV catheter and a second obtained through a percutaneous blood draw. If both cultures grow the same organism (i.e., genus and species) with the same antibiotic sensitivity pattern, the infection can be considered a catheter-associated bloodstream infection. Catheter tips should not be routinely cultured.

Purulent phlebitis confirmed with a positive semiquantitative culture of a catheter tip, but with either negative or no blood culture, is considered a cardiovascular system infection-arterial or venous infection (CVS-VASC), not a BSI (CDC, 2002b).

COLLECTING THE SURVEILLANCE DATA

Data should be collected on BSIs that are central line–associated. Collecting these data requires active, prospective surveillance of central line–associated infections that occur while a patient is receiving care from the health care organization. Laboratory-based surveillance should not be used alone, unless all possible criteria for identifying an infection are solely determined by laboratory evidence. Surveillance data are collected by seeking out infections and screening from a variety of data sources. These data sources may include, but not be limited to, the following: laboratory results, reports from staff, clinical record documentation, admission/discharge/transfer data, and pathology databases. Retrospective chart reviews should be used only when patients are discharged before all of the information can be gathered (e.g., laboratory results). Any trained person may report the infection, but for accuracy and consistency the data should be collected at the same time each day and the infection preventionist must make the final determination as to when the surveillance definition for a CLABSI has been met (CDC, 2008b).

COLLECTING THE DENOMINATOR DATA

To calculate the central line device days, for each day of the month, at the same time each day, the number of patients who have a central line in place should be recorded. The CLABSI data should be expressed as the number of catheter-associated BSIs per 1000 catheter-days for both adults and children and stratified by birth weight categories for neonatal ICUs to facilitate comparisons with national data in comparable patient populations and health care settings (CDC, 2008). The parameter of 1000 central venous catheter days is more useful than the rate expressed as the number of catheter-associated infections per 100 catheters (or percentage of catheters studied). This is because it accounts for BSIs over time, and adjusts the risk for the number of days the catheter is in use. The CLABSI rate per 1000 central line-days is calculated by dividing the number of CLABSIs by the number of central line-days and multiplying the result by 1000 as follows:

$$\frac{\text{Total number of CLABSI cases}}{\text{Total number of central line-days}} \times 1000$$

$$= \text{CLABSI rate per 1000 catheter days}$$

 ## CENTRAL LINE INSERTION PRACTICES' ADHERENCE MONITORING

The CDC, IHI, and NQF recommend the implementation of evidence-based central line insertion practices, also referred to as the central line bundle, known to reduce the risk of subsequent central line–associated bloodstream infection. Data demonstrate improvement in outcomes when all five components of the central line bundle are followed; therefore compliance with the entire central line bundle should be measured, not just parts of the bundle. Despite the scientific evidence supporting these measures, reports suggest that adherence to these practices remains low in U.S. hospitals. Therefore surveillance data should be collected that demonstrate how well the CVC insertion team is adhering to the central line bundle.

The Institute for Healthcare Improvement recommends that acute care providers start data collection in one intensive care unit or even a random sample within one unit initially. The purpose of the data collection is for improvement within that unit and not for hospital-wide infection surveillance. Surveillance activities may also occur in any type of patient care location where central lines are inserted. Surveillance data may be collected for insertion practices during a month when concomitant CLABSI surveillance is being conducted, or insertion practice data may be collected during a month when no CLABSI surveillance is being conducted or in locations where CLABSIs are not monitored (e.g., emergency department, operating room).

Organizations participating in the CDC's National Healthcare Safety Network (NHSN) may use the Central Line Insertion Practices Adherence Monitoring Form (form JJ CDC 57.75) to collect and report central line insertion practices for every central line insertion occurring during the month selected for surveillance. The form includes information pertaining to demographics of the patient, information pertaining to the inserter, information on maximal sterile barriers used, the reasons for central line insertion, skin antisepsis, hand hygiene practice before insertion, type of central line and insertion site, and use of a guidewire. These data will be used to calculate adherence to recommended catheter insertion practices. The CDC's adherence rate for specific insertion practices is calculated by dividing the number of central line insertions during which the recommended practice was followed by the total number of central line insertions and multiplying the result by 100 (CDC, 2008b). Other organizations may also calculate the reliability of bundle compliance using the IHI formula as follows:

1. Pick a day and select all patients with central lines and check for compliance with all elements of the central line bundle.
2. Review the data collection cards used, either all cards or a random sample if the sample size is large. Check the cards for compliance with all elements of the central line bundle.
3. Calculate the score: 100% of the elements of the bundle must be met to be in full compliance. Otherwise, the case is not in compliance as there is no partial compliance. For example, if there are 7 patients with central lines, and 6 have all 5 bundle elements completed, then 6/7 (86%) are in compliance with the central line bundle. If all 7 had all 5 elements completed, compliance would be 100%. If all 7 were missing even a single item, compliance would be 0%.

$$\frac{\text{Number with ALL 5 elements of central line bundle}}{\text{Number with CVCs on the day of the sample}} \times 100$$
$$= \text{Reliability of bundle compliance}$$

4. State the level of compliance with the central line bundle as a percentage (IHI, 2008).

Obviously the targeted goal for the data analysis is 100%. Consideration should also be given to linking the adherence to the central line bundle insertion practices to the patient's outcomes and the incidence of central line–associated bloodstream infections. This can be accomplished by generating a line graph of patients in whom a central line was inserted, linking the actual compliance with the central line bundle to any information on a patient's subsequent CLABSI, and comparing those outcomes to other patients who did not have a CLABSI during the surveillance time period.

 PATIENT AND CAREGIVER EDUCATION

In all health care settings, patient education is an important tool for preventing catheter-associated complications. The importance of patient and caregiver education, specifically hand hygiene and manipulation of the catheter tubing and other supplies, is imperative in preventing infection in the alternative care setting. Information regarding catheter management should be individualized to meet the patient's needs but should remain consistent with the established policies and procedures of the health care organization and the *Infusion Nursing Standards of Practice.*

In home care, patients and caregivers are taught to set-up and self-administer intravenous therapies, often via central venous access devices. The patient or caregiver responsible for administering IV therapy and manipulating venous access devices must be well trained and competent. Patient and caregiver education should include a hands-on demonstration and practice with actual items that the patient or caregiver will be expected to use, all under the direct observation of nursing staff. The compounding facility, in conjunction with nursing staff, is responsible for initially ensuring that the patient and/or caregiver understands, has mastered, and is capable of and willing to comply with the responsibilities of self-administering the IV medication in the home. The patient's or caregiver's competence should be assessed on initiation of infusion therapy and throughout the course of care to include a hands-on demonstration of skills. This demonstration of skills is to ensure that the patient and/or caregiver can correctly and consistently accomplish the following:

- Describe the therapy involved, including the disease or condition for which the medication is prescribed, the goals of therapy, expected therapeutic outcome, and potential side effects of the medications to be infused.
- Inspect all medications to be infused, devices, equipment, and supplies on receipt to ensure that the proper temperatures were maintained during transport and that goods received showed no evidence of defects or deterioration.
- Handle, store, and monitor all medications to be infused and related supplies and equipment in the home, including all special requirements.
- Visually inspect all medication, devices, and other items the patient or caregiver is required to use immediately before administration in a matter to ensure all items are acceptable for use. For example, all medications to be infused must be free from cracks, leaks, particulate matter, precipitate, haziness, discoloration, or other deviations from normal expected appearance, and the immediate packages of sterile devices must be completely sealed with no evidence of tampering.
- Check labels immediately before administration to ensure the right drug, dose, patient, and time of administration.
- Clean the in-home preparation area, scrub hands, use proper aseptic technique, and manipulate all containers, equipment, apparatus, devices, and supplies used in conjunction with administration.

- Employ all techniques and precautions associated with medication administration; for example, preparing supplies and equipment, handling of devices, priming the tubing, and discontinuing an infusion.
- Care for catheters, change dressings, and maintain site patency as indicated.
- Monitor for and detect occurrences of therapeutic complications such as infection, phlebitis, electrolyte imbalance, and catheter misplacement.
- Respond immediately to emergency or critical situations such as catheter breakage or displacement, tubing disconnection, clot formation, flow obstruction, and equipment malfunction.
- Know when to seek and how to obtain professional emergency services or professional advice.
- Handle, contain, and properly dispose of wastes such as needles, syringes, devices, biohazardous spills or residuals, and infectious substances (U.S. Pharmacopeial Convention, 2008).

In addition, the patient and caregiver should be taught how to self-monitor for signs and symptoms of the following:

- A local catheter-associated infection and to assess for redness, swelling, drainage, and/or tenderness at the catheter exit site or along the subcutaneous tunnel (in a tunneled central venous access device).
- Catheter-associated sepsis and to monitor for the sudden onset of fever, chills, and hypotension, or a more insidious onset with signs and symptoms of low-grade fever, headache, malaise, and/or elevated blood glucose level if self-monitoring blood glucose level with an in-home glucose monitoring device (Gorski, 2005).

PATIENT SAFETY

Patients may also be at higher risk for infection when nursing is understaffed and overtime hours are increased in the acute care setting. Hospitals that have higher staff levels and better working conditions are safer for elderly intensive care unit patients. A review of outcomes data for more than 15,000 patients in 51 U.S. hospital intensive care units showed that those with high nursing staffing ratios (the average was 17 registered nurse hours per patient day) had a lower incidence of central line–associated bloodstream infections, a common cause of mortality in intensive care settings. Higher levels of overtime hours were associated with higher rates of infection (Stone et al, 2007).

The Joint Commission's 2009 National Patient Safety Goals (i.e., NPSG.07.04.01) also include a goal that accredited health care organizations are required to implement best practices or evidence-based guidelines to prevent central line–associated bloodstream infections. This requirement covers short- and long-term central venous catheters and PICCs and can be viewed at http://www.jointcommission.org/PatientSafety/NationalPatientSafetyGoals.

STAFF COMPETENCIES

The principles of infection control provide the foundation for the delivery of infusion therapy. Infection prevention begins with being knowledgeable about the risk factors that can

Box 12-5   NURSING DIAGNOSES

- Patient or caregiver knowledge deficit related to set-up and self-administration of home infusion therapy
- Patient or caregiver knowledge deficit related to care and maintenance of venous access device and self-monitoring activities and actions to take for complications of IV therapy
- Patient or caregiver knowledge deficit related to care and maintenance of venous access device and self-monitoring activities for complications
- Patient or caregiver knowledge deficit related to disposal of medical waste and contaminated supplies
- Patient or caregiver knowledge deficit related to principles of asepsis and how to effectively perform hand hygiene
- Potential for skin and soft tissue infection at exit site of venous access device
- Potential for primary bloodstream infection related to the use of a central venous access device

PATIENT OUTCOMES

Infection prevention and control is important in ensuring positive outcomes for IV therapy. Patient outcomes include the following:

- The patient will exhibit no signs or symptoms of infusion-related infections throughout the course of infusion therapy.
- The patient and caregiver will verbalize the signs and symptoms of infection and state to whom to report these signs and symptoms of infections, as well as verbalize strategies to prevent an infection.
- The home care patient and/or caregiver will successfully perform a return demonstration of effective hand hygiene and the skills to aseptically set-up and administer home infusion therapy.

predispose a patient to an intravascular device–related infection. Nurses involved in maintaining vascular access devices must have the knowledge and competency to identify nursing diagnoses (Box 12-5), initiate appropriate care protocols, implement nursing actions that prevent complications, make appropriate nursing interventions if complications occur, and evaluate patient outcomes. One of the most important skills is effectively performing hand hygiene. A competence assessment form to evaluate the nurse's competence in hand hygiene is listed in Figure 12-2.

SUMMARY

Central line–associated bloodstream infections can be prevented, but it is going to take a focused, team effort to accomplish a targeted goal of zero CLABSIs. Preventing CLABSIs begins with the individuals inserting the central line and continues through to the nurse providing care in the home setting who will continue the patient's education, continue to assess the patient's knowledge and competence, and provide ongoing catheter care and maintenance activities as needed. It is important that we slow down and focus on the goal of ensuring that preventable infections do not occur.

HAND HYGIENE MONITORING TOOL

Employee name:_____   Date:_____

Washes Hands with Plain or Antimicrobial Soap and Water (Observation and/or Question and Answer Session)	Met	Not met
When hands are visibly dirty or contaminated with proteinaceous material or are visibly soiled with blood or other bodily fluids.		
Before eating and after using the restroom.		
When potential for exposure to spore-forming organisms is strongly suspected/proven (i.e., patient with *Clostridium difficile*-associated disease).		
Uses Alcohol-based Hand Rub or Antimicrobial Soap and Water (Observation and/or Question and Answer Session)	Met	Not met
Uses an alcohol-based hand rub routinely if hands are not visibly soiled. Alternatively, washes with antimicrobial soap.		
Before handling medication.		
Before preparing food.		
Before having direct contact with patients.		
Before handling an invasive device (regardless of whether gloves are worn) and inserting an invasive device.		
If moving from contaminated-body site to clean-body site during care.		
After contact with patient's intact skin (e.g., after taking a pulse, etc.).		
After contact with body fluids or excretions, mucous membranes, nonintact skin, and wound dressings if hands are not visibly soiled.		
After contact with objects in the immediate vicinity of the patient.		
After removing gloves.		
Demonstrates Hand Hygiene Technique: Using Alcohol-based Hand Rub (Observation)	Met	Not met
Applies alcohol-based hand rub in sufficient quantity and rubs the hands together.		
Covers all surfaces of the hands and fingers with the product.		
Rubs the hands together covering all surfaces until the hands are dry.		

(Continued)

Figure 12-2 Hand hygiene competence assessment form. (From McGoldrick M: *Hand hygiene, home care infection prevention and control program,* Saint Simons Island, Ga, 2007, Home Health Systems Inc. Used with permission. www.homecareandhospice.com/resources.)

HAND HYGIENE MONITORING TOOL

Employee name:_____   Date:_____

Demonstrates Hand Hygiene Technique: Using Antimicrobial Soap and Water (Observation)	Met	Not met
Wets the hands with water. Avoids using hot water to reduce the risk of dermatitis.		
Applies the amount of soap necessary to cover all surfaces in an amount recommended by the manufacturer.		
Vigorously rubs the hands together for a minimum of 15 seconds covering all surfaces of the hands and fingers.		
Rinses the hands with water to remove residual soap.		
Pats the hands dry with a disposable towel.		
Turns off the faucet using a towel or "no-hands technique".		
Discards the disposable towel without re-wiping hands.		
Home Care Hand Hygiene Products and Supplies (Direct Observation in Bag/Vehicle)	Met	Not met
Liquid antibacterial soap: Present and not expired.		
Alcohol-based hand rub: Present and not expired, stored at proper temperature.		
Paper towels: Present and in sufficient quantity.		
Skin lotion/cream: Present (if moisturizer/emollient not present in product).		
Other Hand Hygiene Considerations (Direct Observation and Question and Answer)	Met	Not met
Artificial nails or extenders absent.		
Natural nail tips ¼" or less.		
Nail polish not chipped or worn (if applicable).		
Minimal jewelry and rings present.		

☐   Successful completion: All items met and no follow-up actions required at this time.
☐   Follow-up action required:

Observer's signature:_____   Date:_____

Employee's signature:_____   Date:_____

Figure 12-2, cont'd Hand hygiene competence assessment form.

REFERENCES

Association for Professionals in Infection Control and Epidemiology (Feb 2008): *APIC-CDC HICPAC surveillance definitions in home health care and home hospice infections.* Accessed 7/2/08 from http://www.apic.org/AM/Template.cfm?Section=Guidelines.

Bennet JV, Brachman PS: *Hospital infections,* Philadelphia, 1998, Lippincott-Raven.

Berenholtz SM, Pronovost PJ, Lipset PA et al: Eliminating catheter-related bloodstream infection in the intensive care unit,, *Crit Care Med* 32:2014-2020, 2004.

Brooks B, Meyers R: Safety and efficacy of home intravenous therapy, *J Am Geriatr Soc* 56(1):177, 2008.

Centers for Disease Control and Prevention: *The National Healthcare Safety Network Manual: patient safety component protocols,* Jan 2008b. Accessed 7/2/08 from http://www.cdc.gov/ncidod/dhqp/pdf/nhsn/.

Centers for Disease Control and Prevention: Guideline for hand hygiene in health-care settings. Recommendations of the Healthcare Infection Control Practices Advisory Committee and the HICPAC/SHEA/APIC/IDSA Hand Hygiene Task Force, *MMWR* 51(RR-16): 33-36, 2002a.

Centers for Disease Control and Prevention: Guidelines for the prevention of intravascular catheter-related infections. Recommendations of the Hospital Infection Control Practices Advisory Committee (HICPAC), *MMWR* 51(RR-10):1-36, 2002b.

Centers for Disease Control and Prevention (CDC). (2008a). Community-associated MRSA. http://www.cdc.gov/ncidod/dhqp/ar_mrsa_ca_public.html. Accessed on June 1, 2008.

Chaiyakunapruk N, Veenstra DL, Lipsky BA et al: Chlorhexidine compared with povidone-iodine solution for vascular catheter-site care: a meta-analysis, *Ann Intern Med* 136:(11)792-801, 2002.

Collin GR: Decreasing catheter colonization through the use of an antiseptic-impregnated catheter, *Chest* 115:1632, 1999.

Cox AM, Malani PN, Wiseman SW et al: Home intravenous antimicrobial infusion therapy: a viable option in older adults, *J Am Geriatr Soc* 55:(5)645-650, 2007.

Danzig L, Short L, Collins K et al: Bloodstream infections associated with a needleless intravenous infusion system in patients receiving home infusion therapy, *J Am Med Assoc* 23:1862-1864, 1995.

Do AN, Banerjee R, Barnett B et al: Bloodstream infection associated with needleless device use and the importance of infection control practices in home health care setting, *J Infect Dis* 179: 442-448, 1999.

Donlan RM, Costerton JW: Biofilms: survival mechanisms of clinically relevant microorganisms, *Clin Microbiol Rev* 15:(2)167-193, 2002.

Flanders JR, Yildiz FH: Biofilms as reservoirs for disease, In Ghannoum M, O'Toole GA, editors: *Microbial biofilms* (pp 314-331), Washington, DC, 2004, ASM Press.

Friese C, Giblin J, Donohue R et al: *Applying evidence to practice: recent advances in the management of chemotherapy-induced neutropenia,* 2006, Plainfield, NJ: ArcMesa Educators.

Garland JS, Alex CP, Mueller CD et al: A randomized trial comparing povidone-iodine to a chlorhexidine gluconate-impregnated dressing for prevention of central venous catheter infections in neonates, *Pediatrics* 107:1431-1436, 2001.

Gaynes RP, Martone WJ, Culver DH et al: Comparison of rates of nosocomial infections in neonatal intensive care units in the United States, *Am J Med* 91:(suppl 3B)S192-S196, 1991.

Gorski L: Central venous access device outcomes in a homecare agency: a 7 year study, *J Infus Nurs* 27:(2)104-111, 2004.

Gorski L: *Home infusion therapy,* Sudbury, Mass, 2005, Jones and Bartlett.

Gorski L: Speaking of standards: standard 48: administration set change, *J Infus Nurs* 31:(5)267-268, 2008.

Graham DR, Keldermans MM, Klemm LW et al: Infectious complications among patients receiving home intravenous therapy with peripheral, central, or peripherally placed central venous catheters, *Am J Med* 91:(suppl 3B)95S-100S, 1991.

Hadaway L: Technology of flushing vascular access devices, *J Infus Nurs* 29:(3)137-145, 2006.

Heard S, Wagle M, Vijayakumar E et al: Influence of triple-lumen central venous catheters coated with chlorhexidine and silver sulfadiazine on the incidence of catheter-related bacteremia, *Arch Intern Med* 1:(58)81, 1998.

Horan TC, Gaynes R: Surveillance of nosocomial infections, In Mayhall CG, editor: *Hospital epidemiology and infection control* (pp 1659-1702), Philadelphia, 2004, Lippincott Williams & Wilkins.

Infusion Nurses Society: Infusion nursing standards of practice, *J Infus Nurs* 29(suppl 1S), 2006.

Institute for Healthcare Improvement: 5 Million Lives Campaign. *Getting started kit: prevent central line infections how-to guide,* Cambridge, Mass, 2008, Author. Accessed 6/5/08 at www.ihi.org.

Institute for Safe Medication Practices: *Failure to cap IV tubing and disinfect IV ports place patients at risk for infections,* 2007. Available at http://www.ismp.org/newsletters/acutecare/articles/20070726.asp.

Jarvis WR, Edwards JR, Culver DH et al: Nosocomial infection rates in adult and pediatric intensive care units in the United States, *Am J Med* 91:(suppl 3B):S185-191, 1991.

Kaler W: Successful disinfection of needleless access ports: a matter of time and friction, *J Assoc Vasc Access* 12:(3)140-142, 2007.

Kellerman S, Shay D, Howard J et al: Bloodstream infections in home infusion patients: the influence of race and needleless intravascular access devices, *J Pediatr* 129:711-717, 1996.

Klevins RM, Edwards JR, Richards CL et al: Estimating healthcare-associated infections and deaths in U.S. hospitals, 2002, *Public Health Rep*160-166. 122(March/April), 2007.

Kwok M, Ho KM, Litton E: Use of chlorhexidine-impregnated dressing to prevent vascular and epidural catheter colonization and infection: a meta-analysis, *J Antimicrob Chemother* 58:281-287, 2006.

Linder LE: Material thrombogenicity in central venous catheterization: comparison between soft, antebrachial catheters of silicone elastomer and polyurethane, *J Parenter Enteral Nutr* 8:399, 1984.

Maki DG, Kluger DM, Crnich CJ: The risk of bloodstream infection in adults with different intravascular devices: a systematic review of 200 published prospective studies, *Mayo Clin Proc* 81:1159-1171, 2006.

Maki DG, Mermel LA, Klugar D et al: *The efficacy of a chlorhexidine impregnated sponge (Biopatch) for the prevention of intravascular catheter-related infection—a prospective randomized controlled multicenter study [abstract].* Presented at the Interscience Conference on Antimicrobial Agents and Chemotherapy, Toronto, Ontario, Canada, 2000, American Society for Microbiology.

Maki DG, Ringer M, Alvarado CJ: Prospective randomized trial of povidone-iodine, alcohol, and chlorhexidine for prevention of infection associated with central venous and arterial catheters, *Lancet* 338(8763):339-343, 1991.

Marschall J, Mermel LA, Classen D et al: Strategies to prevent central line-associated bloodstream infections in acute care hospitals, *Infect Control Hosp Epidemiol* 29(suppl1), S22-S30, 2008.

McGoldrick M: *Home care infection prevention and control program,* 2008. Accessed 11/2/08 from www.HomeCareandHospice.com.

Mermel LA: Prevention of intravascular catheter-related infections, *Ann Intern Med* 132(5):391-402, 2000.

Moureau N, Poole S, Murdock M et al: Central venous catheters in home infusion care: outcomes analysis in 50,470 patients, *J Vasc Intervent Radiol* 13(10):1009-1016, 2002.

National Comprehensive Cancer Network (NCCN): *Fever and neutropenia,* March 2006. Accessed 6/5/08 at http://www.nccn.org.

National Library of Medicine: *Septicemia,* 2008. Accessed 6/2/08 at http://www.nlm.nih.gov/medlineplus/ency/article/001355.htm.

National Quality Forum (NQF): *Safe practices for better healthcare, update 2006,* 2006. Accessed 6/6/08 at http://www.qualityforum.org/projects/completed/safe_practices.

Occupational Safety and Health Administration: *Occupational safe exposure to bloodborne pathogens: final rule,* Washington, DC, 1991, Department of Labor, Docket No. H-370.

Occupational Safety and Health Administration: *Needlestick safety and prevention act of 2000*. Nov 2000, *Pub. No* 106-430:114. Stat. 1901.

Olson K, Rennie RP, Hanson J et al: Evaluation of a no-dressing intervention for tunneled central venous catheter exit sites, *J Infus Nurs* 27:37-44, 2004.

Pronovost P, Needham D, Berenholtz S et al: An intervention to decrease catheter-related bloodstream infections in the ICU, *New Engl J Med* 355(26):2725-2732, 2006 (erratum in New *Engl J Med* 356[25]:2660, 2007).

Purevdorj-Gage LB, Stoodley P: Biofilm structure, behavior, and hydrodynamics, In Ghannoum M, O'Toole GA, editors: *Microbial biofilms* (pp 160-173), Washington, DC, 2004, ASM Press.

Raad I: Intravascular-catheter-related infections, *Lancet* 351:893, 1998.

Rhinehart E, McGoldrick M: *Infection control in home care and hospice*, Sudbury, Mass, 2006, Jones and Bartlett.

Rosenthal P: Complications of cancer and cancer treatment, In Lenhard R, Osteen R, Gansler T, editors: *Clinical oncology* (p 241), Atlanta, Ga, 2001, American Cancer Society.

Safdar N, Maki D: The pathogenesis of catheter-related bloodstream infection with noncuffed short-term central venous catheters, *Intens Care Med* 30(1):62-67, 2004.

Siegel JD, Rhinehart E, Jackson M, Chiarello L, Healthcare Infection Control Practices Advisory Committee: *Guidelines for isolation precautions: preventing transmission of infectious agents in healthcare settings, June 2007*. Accessed 6/4/08 at http://www.cdc.gov/ncidod/dhqp/pdf/isolation2007.pdf.

Soufir L, Timsit JF, Mahe C et al: Attributable morbidity and mortality of catheter-related septicemia in critically ill patients: a matched, risk-adjusted, cohort study, *Infect Control Hosp Epidemiol* 20(6): 396-401, 1999.

Stone PW, Mooney-Kane C, Larson E et al: Nurse working conditions and patient safety outcomes, *Medical Care* 45:(6)571-578, 2007.

Tokars JI, Cockson ST, McArthur MA et al: Prospective evaluation of risk factors for bloodstream infection in patients receiving home infusion therapy, *Ann Intern Med* 131(5):340, 1999.

U.S. Pharmacopeial Convention: *U.S. Pharmacopeia 27. Chapter <797> Pharmaceutical compounding—sterile preparations. Revision bulletin*, Rockville, Md, 2008, Author. Accessed 6/4/08 at www.usp.org.

White MC, Ragland KE: Surveillance of intravenous catheter-related infections among homecare clients, *Am J Infect Control* 21:231-236, 1993.

Yamamoto AJ, Solomon JA, Soulen MC et al: Sutureless securement device reduces complications of peripherally inserted central venous catheters, *J Vasc Intervent Radiol* 13:(1)77-81, 2002.

13 PARENTERAL FLUIDS

Lynn Phillips, MSN, RN, CRNI®*

Fluids and electrolytes play an important role in maintaining homeostasis. When imbalances occur, parenteral fluids are the most common intravenous (IV) agents used for correction. IV solutions are also used to provide nutrients or act as a vehicle for medication administration.

To provide infusion therapy safely, the infusion nurse should be aware of the patient's physical status and clinical picture, and understand the legal implications of treatment. Determination of the type of fluid needed is based on the nursing assessment, laboratory findings, and the purpose for which it is being prescribed. To act properly on the authorized prescriber's order, the nurse must be familiar with the various IV solutions, including their uses, components, and potential complications. This information should be incorporated into a plan of care or clinical pathway. This care plan should also include applicable nursing diagnoses with measurable outcomes. With careful organization and a strong database, the delivery of infusion therapy should be a safe and effective treatment modality.

PHYSIOLOGY RELATED TO DELIVERY OF PARENTERAL SOLUTIONS

The human body is a contained fluid environment of water and electrolytes. The human body is approximately 60% water by weight; of this, 40% of body weight is water contained in cells (intracellular water) and 20% is water outside cells (extracellular water). The usual blood volume of the human body is 7% to 8% of the total body weight (Beck, 2003).

WATER

The cell wall separates the intracellular compartment from the extracellular compartment. The capillary endothelium and the walls of arteries and veins divide the extracellular compartment into the intravascular and interstitial compartments. Water

moves freely through cell and vessel walls and is distributed through all these compartments (Grocott, Mythen, and Gan, 2005).

Holliday and Segar (1957) established that regardless of age, to dissolve and eliminate metabolic wastes all healthy persons require approximately 100 milliliters (mL) of water per 100 calories metabolized. This means that a person who expends 1800 calories of energy requires approximately 1800 mL of water for metabolic purposes. The metabolic rate increases with fever; it rises approximately 12% for every 1° C (7% for every 1°F) increase in body temperature. Fever also increases the respiratory rate, resulting in additional loss of water vapor through the lungs (Porth, 2007). Water and solute depletion may occur because of either decreased intake (e.g., fasting before surgery, anorexia, or altered consciousness level) or increased losses (e.g., diarrhea, vomiting, or pyrexia). There are two main physiological mechanisms that assist in regulating body water: thirst and antidiuretic hormone (ADH). Thirst is primarily a regulator of water intake and ADH a regulator of water output. Both mechanisms respond to changes in extracellular osmolality and volume (Porth, 2007).

OSMOSIS AND OSMOTIC PRESSURE

Osmosis is a process by which a solvent, usually water, moves through a semipermeable membrane from a solution of lower concentration to a solution of higher concentration. The osmotic pressure exerted by particles in a solution is determined by the number of particles per volume of fluid versus the mass or size of the particles (Phillips, 2005). The osmotic pressure at the cell membrane differs from that at the capillary membrane. At the capillary membrane, the pressure is referred to as oncotic pressure, while at the cell membrane the pressure is referred to as osmotic pressure (Hankins, 2006). Because proteins are the only dissolved substances in the plasma and interstitial fluid that do not diffuse readily through the capillary membrane, the colloid osmotic pressure is influenced by proteins. The concentration of proteins in plasma is two to three times greater than the concentration of proteins found in the interstitial fluid. Only those substances that do not pass through the semipermeable membrane exert osmotic pressure,

*The author and editors wish to acknowledge the contributions made by Judy Hankins and Carolyn Hedrick as authors of this chapter in the second edition of *Infusion Therapy in Clinical Practice*.

and proteins are the only substances that do not readily penetrate the pores of the capillary membrane. Therefore proteins in the extracellular fluid spaces are responsible for the osmotic pressure at the capillary membrane.

In a healthy person, the net intracapillary pressures are more than the interstitial pressures, and this results in a pressure gradient that produces a slow continuous flow of fluid from capillary lumen to interstitium. This tissue space, or interstitial fluid, drains via the lymphatic system back into the systemic circulation. In disease, all these factors can be altered, often resulting in an increase in the loss of fluid from the circulation (Grocott et al, 2005). Starling (1896) formulated the Law of Capillaries, which states that equilibrium exists at the capillary membrane when the fluid leaving the circulation and the amount of fluid returning to circulation are exactly equal.

Capillary pressure tends to force fluid and dissolved substances through the capillary pore into the interstitial spaces. Colloid osmotic pressure tends to cause fluid to move via osmosis from the interstitial spaces into the blood, thus preventing a significant loss of fluid volume (Hankins, 2006). The volume of distribution of infused fluids is dictated by their solute content. In turn, the plasma volume expansion effect is directly related to the volume of distribution:

$$\text{Plasma volume expansion} = \frac{\text{Volume infused}}{\text{Volume of distribution}}$$

Infusion of isotonic crystalloid (e.g., 0.9% sodium chloride or lactated Ringer's solution) will expand all the components of the extravascular volume, and 20% of the volume infused will remain in the intravascular space. Infusion of an "ideal colloid," containing large molecules that do not escape from the circulation, will expand the intravascular volume by 100% of the volume infused (Grocott et al, 2005). To rationally prescribe fluid replacement, it is important to identify which compartment is depleted.

The osmotic activity of a solution may be expressed in terms of either its osmolarity or its osmolality. Osmolarity refers to the osmolar concentration in 1 liter (L) of solution (mOsm/L) and osmolality is the osmolar concentration in 1 kilogram (kg) of water (mOsm/kg of H_2O). Osmolarity is usually used when referring to fluids outside the body and osmolality for describing fluids inside the body. Because 1 L of water weighs 1 kg, the terms osmolarity and osmolality are often used interchangeably (Porth, 2007). The term osmolality will be used in this chapter. Extracellular osmolality is primarily determined by the sodium level because it is the main solute found in extracellular fluid. A rough estimation of extracellular osmolality can be made by multiplying the plasma sodium concentration by 2 (Porth, 2007).

TONICITY

A change in water content causes cells to swell or shrink. The term tonicity refers to the tension or effect that the osmotic pressure of a solution, with impermeable solutes, exerts on cell size because of water movement across the cell membrane. Tonicity is determined solely by effective solutes such as glucose that cannot penetrate the cell membrane, thereby producing an osmotic force that pulls water into or out of the cell, causing it to change size.

Solutions to which body cells are exposed can be classified as isotonic, hypotonic, or hypertonic depending on whether they cause cells to swell or shrink. Cells placed in an isotonic solution, which has the same effective osmolality as intracellular fluids (280 to 295 mOsm/L), neither shrink nor swell. When cells are placed in hypotonic solution, which has a lower effective osmolality than intracellular fluids, they swell as water moves into the cell, and when they are placed in a hypertonic solution, which has a greater effective osmolality than intracellular fluid, they shrink as water is pushed out of the cell.

ASSESSMENT OF FLUID REQUIREMENTS

To understand the use of parenteral solutions the nurse must understand two important concepts: (1) the rationale for the authorized prescriber's order of infusion therapy, and (2) the type of solution ordered, together with the composition and clinical use of that solution (Phillips, 2005). Objectives or rationales for administration of IV solutions fall into three broad categories:

1. Maintenance therapy for daily body fluid requirements
2. Replacement therapy for existing losses
3. Replacement therapy for ongoing losses

These three objectives differ with regard to the time necessary to complete the IV solution administration. The following factors affect the choice of objective in prescribing a parenteral solution and the rate of administration determined by the authorized prescriber: patient's renal function, daily maintenance requirements, existing fluid and electrolyte imbalance, clinical status, and disturbances in homeostasis as a result of parenteral therapy (Metheny, 2000).

MAINTENANCE THERAPY

Water has the priority in maintenance therapy. The body needs water to replace insensible loss, which can occur as perspiration from the skin and moisture from respirations. The average adult loses 500 to 1000 mL of water over 24 hours through insensible loss. Water is also an important dilutor for waste products excreted by the kidneys. In addition, an individual's fluid requirements are based on age, height, weight, and amount of body fat.

Maintenance therapy provides nutrients that meet the daily needs of a patient for water, vitamins, electrolytes, glucose, and protein, with water having priority. The typical patient profile for maintenance therapy is an individual who is allowed nothing by mouth (NPO) or whose oral intake is restricted for any reason. Remember that insensible loss is approximately 500 to 1000 mL every 24 hours. Maintenance therapy should be 1500 mL per square meter (m^2) of body surface area over 24 hours (Metheny, 2000). For example, a man weighing 85 kg (187 lb) has a body surface area of 2 m^2; 1500 times 2 equals 3000; therefore he needs 3000 mL of fluids for maintenance therapy. Balanced solutions for maintenance therapy include water, daily needs of sodium and potassium, and glucose.

REPLACEMENT THERAPY FOR EXISTING LOSSES

Replacement therapy is necessary to take care of the fluid, electrolyte, or blood product deficits of patients in acute distress; this type of therapy is supplied over a 48-hour period. The following are examples of conditions of patients needing replacement infusion therapy (and their replacement requirements):

- Hemorrhage (for replacement of cells and plasma)
- Low platelet count (for replacement of clotting factors)

- Vomiting and diarrhea (for replacement of losses of electrolytes and water)
- Starvation (for replacement of losses of water and electrolytes) (Phillips, 2005)

Replacement therapy has a twofold rationale. The first rationale is to restore fluid loss when the previous output exceeded intake. After kidney status has been considered, a hydrating solution (e.g., 5% dextrose in 0.2% sodium chloride) is administered. This restores an adequate output of urine and then allows electrolytes to be replaced. The other rationale for replacement therapy is to restore present fluid and electrolyte losses, such as loss of intestinal fluid through continuing diarrhea. A solution such as lactated Ringer's injection can be used to replace this type of loss. Replacing continuing losses prevents acidosis and alkalosis.

When the maintenance of body requirements cannot be met, the authorized prescriber should institute replacement therapy. The authorized prescriber must determine the losses and calculate replacement over a 48-hour period. Assessment of kidney function is the first step in determining appropriate replacement therapy. Patients requiring replacement therapy, except those in shock, require potassium. Patients under stress from tissue injury, wound infection, or gastric or bowel surgery also require potassium. Adequate replacement is achieved using 20 mEq/L of potassium (Metheny, 2000). A key nursing assessment before beginning replacement therapy is validation of kidney function before administering potassium in replacement therapy.

REPLACEMENT THERAPY FOR ONGOING LOSSES

Therapy for concurrent losses is achieved on an ongoing daily basis. Critical evaluation of concurrent losses of fluids and electrolytes is done at least every 24 hours. Accurate documentation of intake and output is extremely important in this type of fluid and electrolyte management. Restoration of homeostasis depends on the nursing assessment of intake of IV solutions, as well as on the documentation of all body fluid losses. The types of clinical patients who require 24-hour evaluation are those with draining fistulas, abscesses, nasogastric tubes, burns, and abdominal wounds. The fluid and electrolyte management of these patients cannot be completed in 48 hours. Therefore maintenance therapy and replacement therapy do not meet these patients' needs. A day-by-day restoration of vital fluids and electrolytes is necessary. With these types of patients, you will see frequent changes in the types of solutions ordered, in the amounts of electrolytes ordered based on laboratory test results, and in the rate of infusion. Restoration of electrolyte imbalance is imperative for proper homeostatic management therapy. The type of restoration fluid ordered depends on the type of fluid that is being lost. For example, excessive loss of gastric fluid must be replaced by solutions that include sodium, potassium, and chloride.

NURSING FOCUSED ASSESSMENT

Assessment of a patient for delivery of parenteral solutions includes collecting a nursing history, performing a focused physical assessment, monitoring pertinent laboratory tests, and evaluating intake and output. The purpose of this assessment is to identify patients at risk for or already experiencing alterations in fluid and electrolyte balance.

Nursing history related to fluid and electrolyte balance includes questions about the patient's medical history, current health concerns, food and fluid intake, fluid elimination, medications, and lifestyle. Physical assessment correlates data with the nursing history and laboratory studies. Focused assessment would include, but not be limited to, the following:

- *Skin*: Assess for color, temperature, moisture content, continuity, turgor, and edema.
- *Mucous membranes*: Inspect the tongue and buccal mucosa; assess the color, moisture, and continuity of mucous membranes.
- *Cardiovascular system*: Pulse, blood pressure, and respiration are all affected by fluid and electrolyte status. Assess for orthostatic hypotension, capillary refill, and venous filling.
- *Respiratory system*: Assess respiratory rate, depth, and pattern, as well as breath sounds.
- *Neurological system*: Level of consciousness provides cues to fluid and electrolyte as well as acid-base balance.
- *Vital signs*: All of the vital signs are affected by fluid, electrolyte, and acid-base balance.

In addition to the systems' assessment listed, the nurse will need to track vital sign changes, monitor daily weights, and record intake and output. The intake and output record should be a standard nursing order on all patients receiving intravenous solutions. Accuracy is of utmost importance; therefore all liquids (intake or output) should be measured carefully and should be estimated when they cannot be measured. Monitoring for signs and symptoms of fluid volume overload includes assessment of lungs, symptoms of fluid volume excess, vital signs, and laboratory values. These are independent nursing actions, and they do not require an authorized prescriber's order (Heitz and Horne, 2005).

The next important aspect of determining fluid needs is the review and interpretation of a patient's laboratory findings. The two systems that have the most direct impact on fluid and electrolyte balance are the renal and cardiovascular systems. Therefore tests that reflect the proper functioning of the kidneys and heart require consistent and close scrutiny. Box 13-1 summarizes laboratory findings for monitoring effective parenteral fluid therapy.

Box 13-1   SUMMARY OF LABORATORY VALUES NEEDING EVALUATION DURING PARENTERAL FLUID THERAPY

Test	Clinical considerations
Blood urea nitrogen (BUN)	Renal function assessment during replacement therapy
Creatinine	Renal function assessment during replacement therapy
Specific gravity	Urine concentration reflects fluid volume concentrations
Urine osmolarity	Reflects fluid volume changes
Serum electrolytes	Reflect deviations from normal
Complete blood count (CBC)	CBC screening for hemoglobin, hematocrit, red blood cells, white blood cells, and platelets before replacement of these components or when expanding ECF
Blood gases	Evaluation of acid-base status
Coagulation studies	Evaluation needed before use of plasma volume expanders
Serum glucose	Monitor osmotic diuresis
Lactate dehydrogenase	Monitor cellular enzyme associated with carbohydrate metabolism

PATIENT OUTCOMES

Expected outcomes with the infusion of parenteral solutions include:

- The patient's intake and output remains adequate for effective fluid and electrolyte replacement.
- The patient's hemodynamic measurements remains stable or returning to stability.
- The patient's physical signs and symptoms of imbalance returns to normal for patient.
- The patient's laboratory measurements remains within normal limits or returns to normal.
- The patient remains free of complications associated with colloid administration (e.g., allergic reaction, anaphylactoid reaction, electrolyte imbalances).
- The patient's hemodynamic parameters improve.

The Infusion Nurses Society (INS, 2006) identifies standards of practice for infusion nursing while the Centers for Disease Control and Prevention (CDC, 2002) provides guidelines for the implementation of care related to infusion therapy. The *Infusion Nursing Standards of Practice* provides measurable components that assist the clinician when establishing nursing competencies and evaluation of patient outcomes related to delivery of parenteral therapy (INS, 2006).

TYPES AND CHARACTERISTICS OF INTRAVENOUS SOLUTIONS

CRYSTALLOID SOLUTIONS

Crystalloids are materials capable of crystallization (i.e., have the ability to form crystals). Crystalloids are solutes that, when placed in a solution, mix with and dissolve into the solution and cannot be distinguished from the resultant solution. Because of this, crystalloid solutions are considered true solutions that are capable of diffusing through membranes. Crystalloid solutions contain electrolytes as dissolved particles in solution that diffuse readily between compartments. To expand the vascular space to a degree equal to that resulting from colloid solutions, crystalloids must be given in three to four times their volume. Types of crystalloid solutions include dextrose solutions, sodium chloride solutions, balanced electrolyte solutions, and alkalizing and acidifying solutions (Phillips, 2005).

IV crystalloid solutions will be distributed to the compartment that contains similar sodium concentration and fluid volume. Crystalloid solutions are rated, before infusion, according to their comparative tonicity to plasma. Their composition dictates fluid movement within and between compartments. Crystalloid solutions are further divided into isotonic, hypotonic, and hypertonic categories.

Initial and therapeutic responses

Crystalloid administration can be divided into two phases: the initial response and the therapeutic response. The initial response is the immediate reaction that occurs when the IV solution is introduced into the circulation. As the solution enters the bloodstream, it immediately contacts red blood cells (RBCs) and the cells of the vein intima. Hypotonic and hypertonic solutions change the immediate surroundings of the red blood cells (Humes, 2000). Extremely hypertonic solution may cause shrinkage of the RBC. As red blood cells move toward a more isotonic environment, they regain their original shape (Hill and Petrucci, 2004).

Hypotonic solutions will cause absorption of water into the intravascular cells (Humes, 2000; Metheny, 2000). The cells will return to their normal shape as they move into a more isotonic environment, as do the cells bathed in hypertonic solutions.

Compared to the initial response of RBCs, the initial response of crystalloid therapy to the vein intima may be as dramatic but is not life-threatening. The intima, at the point of fluid injection, will be repeatedly subjected to the fluid. Hypotonic fluids will cause the endothelial cells to swell while hypertonic solutions will draw fluid from the endothelial cells, causing them to shrink. The risk of cellular dehydration increases as the tonicity of fluid increases. The administration of hypertonic saline or dextrose preparations greater than 10% through small veins is associated with phlebitis, as a result of this cellular dehydration (Cook, 2003).

The therapeutic response of crystalloid administration occurs as the fluid disperses through the extracellular fluid (ECF) and intracellular fluid (ICF). The therapeutic response is predictable and is the reason one fluid is chosen over another.

The therapeutic response to isotonic solutions when administered by the intravenous route results in the tonicity of the plasma remaining unchanged. The solutions 0.9% sodium chloride and lactated Ringer's remain isotonic even after they disperse into the interstitial spaces; therefore the tonicity of the interstitial space is unchanged. The interstitial space is three times as large as the intravascular space; 75% of the fluid will be dispersed interstitially and 25% will remain in the plasma (Jordan, 2000).

The solution of 5% dextrose in water is considered isotonic in the initial response but the mechanics are different than with isotonic electrolyte solutions. Dextrose in water is an electrolyte-free solution. As the fluid disperses through the ECF, the dextrose is absorbed into the cells to be used for energy. What is left is free water that dilutes the osmolality of the ECF (Porth, 2007). The cells are suddenly suspended in a hypotonic environment and osmosis will occur, with the cells absorbing the fluid until the two compartments are isotonic. The intracellular compartment is two thirds the size of the ECF compartment; 67% of the water will enter the cells and 33% will remain in the ECF. The dispersion of 1 L of 5% dextrose in water will divide the 1000 mL into 667 mL intracellularly, approximately 250 mL into the interstitial space, and 83 mL into plasma. Hypertonic dextrose solutions alter the initial response because the solutions are irritating to the vein intima; however, the therapeutic response is the same in dextrose solution with higher dextrose concentrations (Humes, 2000).

Many crystalloid solutions are made up of a combination of dextrose and electrolyte solutions, most of which are hypertonic initially. The therapeutic response to these fluids can be predicted based on the tonicity of the solution. Once the cells use the dextrose, the remaining sodium chloride and electrolytes will be dispersed as isotonic electrolyte solution, hydrating only the ECF compartment.

Isotonic crystalloid solutions

Isotonic solutions have an osmolality of 250 to 375 mOsm/L. Blood and normal body fluids have an osmolarity of 280 to 295 mOsm/L. These fluids are used to expand the extracellular fluid (ECF) compartment. Infused isotonic solution is distributed between the intravascular space and interstitial space, with very little moving into the cell. Approximately 20% of the isotonic crystalloid solution volume remains in the intravascular compartment and 80% moves into the interstitial space. The concentration of sodium within the isotonic solution determines the distribution time in which the solution remains in the intravascular space. This influences the choice of isotonic solution selected for replacement or maintenance therapy (Cooper and Moore, 2000).

Many isotonic solutions are available. Examples include 0.9% sodium chloride, lactated Ringer's solution, and 5% dextrose in water. Dextrose 5% solution becomes hypotonic when dextrose is metabolized. The solution should be used cautiously in patients with renal and cardiac disease because of the increased risk of fluid overload (Kraft, 2000). Isotonic solutions are commonly used to treat fluid loss, dehydration, and hypernatremia (sodium excess).

Hypotonic crystalloid solutions

Hypotonic solutions have fewer electrolytes and a lower osmolarity than isotonic solutions. Hypotonic fluids have an osmolarity lower than 250 mOsm/L. By lowering serum osmolarity, the crystalloid solutions shift out of blood vessels into cells and interstitial spaces. These solutions only increase the intravascular volume by approximately 8% with the remaining 92% distributing evenly between the interstitial space and intracellular space (Cooper and Moore, 2000). The resulting osmotic pressure gradient draws water into the cells from the ECF, causing the cells to swell. Hypotonic solutions hydrate cells and can deplete the circulatory system. Water moves from the vascular space to the intracellular space when hypotonic fluids are infused.

Hypotonic solutions are used for patients who have hypertonic dehydration, require water replacement, and have diabetic ketoacidosis after initial sodium chloride replacement (Kraft, 2000). Examples of hypotonic solutions include 0.45% sodium chloride (half-strength saline), 0.33% sodium chloride, and 2.5% dextrose in water. The use of hypotonic solutions for patients with low blood pressure will further a hypotensive state (Phillips, 2005).

Hypertonic crystalloid solutions

Hypertonic solutions have a higher osmolality than isotonic solutions as a result of a greater number of electrolytes pulling water from the intracellular space and interstitial space into blood vessels, increasing intravascular volume. Hypertonic fluids have an osmolarity of 375 mOsm/L or higher. The resulting osmotic pressure gradient draws water from the intracellular space, increasing extracellular fluid volume. These fluids are used to replace electrolytes, to treat hypotonic dehydration, and for temporary treatment of circulatory insufficiency and shock. Examples of hypertonic fluids include 5% dextrose in 0.45% sodium chloride, 5% dextrose in 0.9% sodium chloride, 5% dextrose in lactated Ringer's, and 10% dextrose in water.

Hypertonic solutions are irritating to the vein walls and should be given slowly to prevent circulatory overload. Some hypertonic solutions are contraindicated in patients with cardiac or renal disease because of the increased risk of congestive heart failure and pulmonary edema.

pH

The pH of a crystalloid solution reflects the degree of acidity or alkalinity of a solution. Blood pH is not a significant problem for routine parenteral therapy. Normal kidneys can achieve an acid-base balance as long as enough water is supplied. The United States Pharmacopeia (USP) standards require that solution pH must be slightly acidic (a pH of between 3.5 and 6.2). Many solutions have a pH of 5.0. The acidity of solutions allows them to have a longer shelf life.

DEXTROSE SOLUTIONS

Dextrose solutions contain carbohydrates and can be administered by the parenteral route as dextrose, fructose, or invert sugar. Dextrose is the most commonly administered carbohydrate. The percentage solutions express the number of grams of solute per 100 g of solvent. Thus 5% dextrose in water (D_5W) solution contains 5 g of dextrose in 100 mL of water.

Dextrose is a non-electrolyte, and the total number of particles in a dextrose solution does not depend on ionization. Dextrose is thought to be closest to the ideal carbohydrate available because it is well metabolized by all tissues. The tonicity of dextrose solutions depends on the particles of sugar in the solution. Dextrose 5% in water is rapidly metabolized and has no osmotically active particles after it is in the plasma. The USP pH requirements for dextrose fall between 3.5 and 6.5 (Metheny, 2000).

Dextrose in water is available in various concentrations including 2.5%, 5%, 10%, 20%, 30%, 40%, 50%, and 70%. Dextrose is also available in combination with other types of solutions. The 5% and 10% concentrations can be given peripherally. Concentrations higher than 10% are given through central veins. A general exception is the administration of limited amounts of 50% dextrose given slowly through a peripheral vein for emergency treatment of hypoglycemia (usually 3 mL/min) (Phillips and Kuhn, 1999).

More concentrated dextrose solutions, 20% to 70%, are hypertonic, and range from 1010 to 3530 mOsm/L. When these solutions are being administered, consideration should be given to the possibility that tolerance to glucose may be compromised by sepsis, stress, hepatic and renal failure, and by some medications, such as steroids or diuretics. Refer to Table 13-1 for a comparison of dextrose solutions.

Major uses

Dextrose solutions provide calories for energy, sparing body protein and preventing ketosis, which occurs when the body burns fat. Dextrose also makes it easier for potassium to move from the extracellular to the intracellular compartment; therefore it can be effective in treating hyperkalemia when given as a 10% concentration. Dextrose solutions also provide free water for the kidneys, helping them excrete solutes, and improve liver function (glucose is stored in the liver as glycogen). Concentrations of 2.5% and 5% dextrose are used to treat a dehydrated patient and to decrease sodium and potassium levels; they are also suitable diluents for many medications (Cook, 2003). The more concentrated solution of 10% dextrose is also used to correct hypoglycemia. Dextrose 20% to 70% with electrolytes can provide long-term nutrition as parenteral nutrition.

TABLE 13-1 Dextrose Solutions

Solution	Osmolarity	pH	Dextrose (g/100 mL)	Cal/100 mL
2.5% Dextrose/water	Hypotonic	4.5	2.5	8
5% Dextrose/water	Isotonic (hypotonic when infused)	4.8	5	17
10% Dextrose/water	Hypertonic	4.7	10	34
20% Dextrose/water	Hypertonic	4.8	20	68
50% Dextrose/water	Hypertonic	4.6	50	170
70% Dextrose/water	Hypertonic	4.6	70	237

The maximum rate at which dextrose can be infused without producing glycosuria is 0.5 g/kg of body weight/hour. Dosage and constant infusion rate of intravenous dextrose must be selected with caution in pediatric patients, particularly neonates and low birth weight infants, because of the increased risk of hyperglycemia/hypoglycemia (Hospira, 2006).

Complications

There may be complications related to administering dextrose solutions intravenously, including electrolyte imbalances, venous irritation or phlebitis, dehydration, hyperglycemia, and agglomeration. Dextrose solutions can be dangerous if infused too freely, because of the lack of electrolytes (Metheny, 2000). Vein irritation, vein damage, and thrombosis may result when hypertonic dextrose solutions are administered in a peripheral vein. Vein irritation may occur because of the slightly acidic pH (3.4 to 4.0) of the solution.

The use of 5% dextrose in water for hydration should be monitored closely, particularly if used past the initial stage of treatment. It can also lead to water intoxication, which may be signaled by rapid weight gain, thirst, diluted urine, nonpitting edema, arrhythmias, and low sodium levels. If this process is not corrected, symptoms of cerebral intracellular fluid excess (hyponatremic encephalopathy), including seizures, coma, and death, will occur when water shifts into the brain cells (Kee, Paulanka and Purnell, 2004). Women that are premenopausal should be evaluated carefully while receiving dextrose solutions. Researchers (Ayus and Arieff, 1990) believe that physiological responses in premenopausal women place them at higher risk for hyponatremic encephalopathy because estrogen stimulates ADH release and antagonizes the brain's ability to adapt to swelling. In men, androgens suppress ADH release and enhance the brain's ability to adapt to swelling.

Solutions of 20% to 70% dextrose infused rapidly act as an osmotic diuretic and pull interstitial fluid into plasma, causing severe cellular dehydration. Any solution of dextrose infused rapidly can place the patient at risk for dehydration and hyperosmolar coma. To prevent this adverse reaction, infuse the dextrose solution at the prescribed rate.

Hypertonic dextrose solutions are contraindicated for patients with preexisting conditions such as anuria, intraspinal/intracranial hemorrhage, delirium tremens (in the presence of dehydration), diabetic coma, and known allergies to corn or corn products.

Before any medication is added to a dextrose solution, compatibility information should be checked. Dextrose may also affect the stability of admixtures. A pharmacist should be contacted for additional information about questionable admixtures. In

TABLE 13-2 Sodium Chloride Solutions

Solution	Osmolarity	pH	Sodium (mEq)	Chloride (mEq)
0.2% Sodium chloride	Hypotonic	4.5	34	4
0.45% Sodium chloride	Hypotonic	5.6	77	77
0.9% Sodium chloride	Isotonic	6.0	154	154
3% Sodium chloride	Hypertonic	6.0	513	513
5% Sodium chloride	Hypertonic	6.0	855	855

addition, dextrose cannot be mixed with blood components because it causes hemolysis (i.e., agglomeration) of the cells.

Sudden discontinuation of any hypertonic dextrose solution may leave a temporary excess of insulin. To prevent hyperinsulinism, infuse an isotonic dextrose solution (5% to 10%) to wean the patient off hypertonic dextrose. The infusion rate should be gradually decreased over 48 hours.

SODIUM CHLORIDE SOLUTIONS

Sodium controls water distribution and is the major cation found in extracellular fluid. Various IV solutions are available to supplement sodium intake, with pH values ranging from 4.5 to 7. The concentrations of sodium chloride contained in solution have a range from 0.25% to 5%, the most common percentages of sodium chloride being 0.25%, 0.45%, 0.9%, 3%, and 5%. The 0.45% sodium chloride solution is hypotonic, with 1000 mL containing 77 mEq of sodium and 77 mEq of chloride. It provides sodium, chloride, and free water and is used primarily as a hydrating solution. It may also be used to treat hyperosmolar diabetes or assess renal function status. Sodium chloride solution is available as an isotonic solution containing 154 mEq of sodium and 154 mEq of chloride per liter. This 0.9% sodium chloride solution closely approximates the osmotic pressure of body fluids. It does not enter the intracellular fluid compartment but does expand the extracellular fluid. Refer to Table 13-2 for comparison of sodium chloride solutions.

Major uses

There are many clinical uses of sodium chloride solutions, including treatment of shock, hyponatremia, use with blood transfusions, resuscitation in trauma situations, fluid challenges, metabolic alkalosis, hypercalcemia, and fluid replacement in diabetic ketoacidosis. Some medications require this isotonic solution as a diluent to ensure stability. Many protocols advocate the use in shock of 0.9% sodium chloride solution, which has been shown to be as effective as 4.5% human albumin in adults admitted to intensive care units (Finfer et al, 2004; Molyneux and Maitland, 2005).

Sodium chloride solutions provide ECF replacement when chloride loss is greater than or equal to sodium loss (e.g., a patient undergoing nasogastric suctioning). Sodium chloride solutions can be used to treat patients with metabolic alkalosis in the presence of fluid loss (the 154 mEq of chloride helps compensate for the increase in bicarbonate ions). Additional uses of sodium chloride include treating patients with sodium depletion and initiating or terminating blood transfusions.

There are currently three primary indications for the use of hypertonic sodium chloride in critically ill patients: hyponatremic states, volume resuscitation in shock, and brain injury (Johnson and Criddle, 2004). Hypertonic (3%) sodium chloride has also been used as emergent treatment of exercise-associated hypotonic encephalopathy (Siegel, 2007). Refer to the Focus on Evidence box for the use of hypertonic sodium chloride.

Complications

Sodium chloride solution should be used cautiously in patients with congestive heart failure, edema, renal insufficiency, or hypernatremia because it replaces ECF and can lead to fluid overload (Phillips, 2005). Rapid infusion rates or continuous administration of only 0.9% sodium chloride solutions may lead to hypernatremia and fluid overload, potentially leading to all the problems associated with these conditions, including peripheral edema, acid-base imbalances, and electrolyte dilution. Other electrolytes, especially potassium, may be depleted by the continuous infusion of isotonic sodium chloride. Problems related to nutritional status can occur if dextrose is not included in replacement sodium chloride solutions.

Infusion of more than 1 L of isotonic (0.9%) sodium chloride per day may supply more sodium and chloride than normally found in serum, and can exceed normal tolerance, resulting in hypernatremia. This may also cause a loss of bicarbonate ions, resulting in an acidifying effect. Infusion of sodium chloride

---

FOCUS ON EVIDENCE

Use of 3% Sodium Chloride to Treat Hypotonic Encephalopathy

- A recent evidence-based consensus statement concluded that both excessive fluid consumption and a decrease in urine formation contribute to the dilutional effect in hyponatremia that can lead to life-threatening and fatal cases of pulmonary and cerebral edema. Strategies for prevention and treatment include use of intravenous hypertonic solutions, such as 3% sodium chloride, to reverse the symptoms related to moderate and life-threatening hypotonic encephalopathy (Hew-Butler et al, 2005).
- Researchers reported an inverse relationship between the serum concentration of sodium and intracranial pressure; higher sodium levels are associated with improved control of intracranial pressure and decreased requirement for other therapy (Simma et al, 1998).

---

solutions without additional electrolytes may cause low potassium levels (i.e., hypokalemia).

There are two hypertonic sodium-containing solutions: 3% and 5%. The 3% sodium chloride solution contains 513 mEq/L of sodium and the same amount of chloride and has an osmolarity of approximately 1025 mOsm/L. The 5% solution has 855 mEq/L of sodium and an equal amount of chloride and has an approximate osmolarity of 1710 mOsm/L. The rapid or continuous use of hypertonic 3% or 5% sodium chloride IV solutions may result in hyperchloremia or hypernatremia. Excessive amounts, of chloride may lead to the loss of bicarbonate with an acidifying effect (Heitz and Horne, 2005).

Nurses should follow steps to ensure safe administration of hyperosmolar sodium chloride solutions by checking serum sodium levels before and during administration. Administer this solution only in intensive care settings. Monitor aggressively for signs of pulmonary edema. Only small volumes of hyperosmolar fluids are usually administered and a volume-controlled device or electronic infusion pump should be used (Heitz and Horne, 2005).

COMBINATION DEXTROSE AND SODIUM CHLORIDE SOLUTIONS

Dextrose and sodium chloride injection (USP) provide electrolytes and calories and are a source of water for hydration. Solutions that contain dextrose and sodium chloride provide more water than is required for excretion of salt and are useful as hydrating fluids. Table 13-3 lists the common hydrating solutions.

Hydrating fluids are used to assess the status of the kidneys. Carbohydrates in hydrating solutions reduce the depletion of nitrogen and liver glycogen and are also useful in rehydrating cells. When sodium chloride is infused, the addition of 100 g of dextrose prevents formation of ketone bodies. Dextrose prevents catabolism, which is the breakdown of chemical compounds by the body. Carbohydrates and sodium chloride fluid combinations are best used when there has been an excessive loss of fluid through sweating, vomiting, or gastric suctioning (Phillips, 2005).

The administration of a hydrating solution at a rate of 8 mL/m^2 of body surface per minute for 45 minutes is considered a fluid challenge. When urinary flow is established, it indicates that the kidneys have begun to function; the hydrating solution may then be replaced with a specific electrolyte solution. If the urinary flow is not restored after 45 minutes, the rate of infusion should be reduced and monitoring of the patient should continue without administration of electrolyte additives, especially potassium (Metheny, 2000).

Major uses

Combination dextrose and sodium chloride solutions temporarily treat patients with circulatory insufficiency and shock caused by hypovolemia in the immediate absence of a plasma expander. They provide early treatment of burns, along with plasma or albumin, and help replace nutrients and electrolytes. Combination solutions act to hydrate cells and promote diuresis, and are frequently ordered when checking kidney function before replacement of potassium.

Subcutaneous dextrose with 0.45% sodium chloride or 5% dextrose with 0.33% sodium chloride can be used effectively for the treatment of dehydration by hypodermoclysis or for subcutaneous fluid infusion in the elderly. Research by Slesak

TABLE 13-3 Common Combinations of Dextrose and Sodium Chloride Solutions

Solution	Osmolarity	pH	Dextrose (g/100 mL)	Cal/100 mL	Sodium (mEq)	Chloride (mEq)
2.5% Dextrose and 0.45% sodium chloride	Isotonic	4.5	2.5	8	77	77
5% Dextrose and 0.25% sodium chloride	Isotonic	4.6	5	17	34	34
5% Dextrose and 0.45% sodium chloride	Hypertonic	4.6	5	17	77	77
5% Dextrose and 0.9% sodium chloride	Hypertonic	4.4	5	17	154	154

et al (2003) in a randomized controlled trial concluded that both rehydration by subcutaneous route and rehydration by IV infusion were equally well accepted by geriatric patients, similarly feasible, and comparatively safe and effective (Turner and Cassano, 2004).

Complications

Complications related to dextrose and sodium chloride solution infusions include hypernatremia, acidosis, circulatory overload, and electrolyte imbalance, especially potassium. Additionally, these solutions require cautious administration in patients with cardiac, renal, or liver disease (Phillips, 2005).

BALANCED ELECTROLYTE SOLUTIONS

There are many combinations of balanced electrolyte fluids on the market today with a wide array of electrolyte combinations. Special fluids for maintenance needs are available from manufacturers, or fluids are formulated to replace specific body fluids. Each manufacturer usually affixes its own trade name to these solutions, making it necessary to refer to these fluids by the number of cations in the solution. For example, 1 L of electrolyte #48 contains 25 mEq of sodium, 20 mEq of potassium, and 3 mEq of calcium with addition of equal numbers of anions (e.g., chloride, phosphate, and a bicarbonate precursor) (Metheny, 2000).

Maintenance solutions approximate normal body electrolyte needs. Replacement solutions contain one or more electrolytes in amounts higher than those found in normal body fluids. Balanced solutions also may contain lactate or acetate (yielding bicarbonate), which helps to combat acidosis and provide a truly "balanced solution."

The use of the various electrolyte combinations often depends on the experience of the authorized prescriber and on solution availability. The patient's clinical picture, including laboratory test results, should be assessed when selecting the appropriate solution. Electrolyte solutions are generally isotonic until dextrose is added, which increases tonicity of the solution. Some calories (170 cal/L) may be provided in addition to electrolytes by using 5% dextrose in lactated Ringer's. The inclusion of dextrose changes the concentration and makes it a hypertonic solution (527 mOsm/L) with a pH of about 4.9. Consideration should be given to conditions and diseases affected by dextrose administration. All multiple electrolyte formulations contain sodium, potassium, and chloride. Some may also contain calcium, magnesium, or acetate. Refer to Table 13-4 for a comparison of balanced electrolyte solutions.

Ringer's injection and lactated Ringer's

The most frequently prescribed balanced electrolyte solution, lactated Ringer's, carries the same name regardless of commercial supplier. This solution is considered a near-physiological solution. The electrolyte content of lactated Ringer's solution is similar to that of plasma, and includes sodium, potassium, calcium, and chloride. Lactate, an organic ion, has been added as a buffer and is metabolized to produce bicarbonate, which is normally found in extracellular fluid. Lactated Ringer's is an isotonic solution with a pH of about 6.6.

Ringer's injection is an isotonic solution with a pH of 5.0 to 7.5. The electrolyte content of Ringer's injection approximates that of plasma and includes sodium, 147 mEq/L; potassium, 4 mEq/L; calcium, 4 mEq/L; and chloride, 155 mEq/L.

Major uses

Multiple electrolyte fluids are recommended for use in patients with trauma, alimentary tract fluid losses, dehydration, sodium depletion, acidosis, and burns.

Lactated Ringer's solution provides electrolytes and is used to treat hypovolemia. When oral intake is limited or absent or when losses are abnormally high, lactated Ringer's does not provide adequate electrolytes for maintenance therapy. Lactated Ringer's does not provide magnesium; therefore it may need to be supplemented in specific clinical cases. Ringer's injection is used to replace electrolytes and to provide water for hydration and is often used to replace extracellular fluid losses.

Complications

Even though the content is similar to that of plasma, continual delivery of only Ringer's injection or lactated Ringer's may lead to complications. The solutions contain potassium and calcium, but the amount is not adequate for maintenance or replacement if there is inadequate intake or abnormal loss of these electrolytes. Rapid administration may lead to excessive amounts of electrolytes. Administration of only this type of fluid could result in a calorie deficit. Ringer's injection may also cause fluid overload, which could dilute the electrolytes. As with any type of fluid, this could also cause fluid overload, leading to pulmonary edema.

Ringer's injection and lactated Ringer's also are available with dextrose added. Lactated Ringer's plus 5% dextrose provides the same electrolytes as Ringer's injection plus 5 g of dextrose (170 cal/L). Lactated Ringer's with 5% dextrose has an osmolality of 561 mOsm/L, making it a hypertonic solution, and its pH

TABLE 13-4 Comparison of Balanced Electrolyte Solutions

Solutions	mOsm*	pH	Dextrose (g)	Cal/100 mL	Na+ (mEq)	Cl− (mEq)	K+ (mEq)	Ca2+ (mEq)	Mg2+ (mEq)	Phosphate (mEq)	Lactate (mmol/L)
Lactated Ringer's	Isotonic	6.5	0	0	130	109	4	3	0		28
Ringer's injection	Isotonic	5.5	0	0	147	156	4	4	0		0
5% D/electrolyte #48 injection†	Isotonic	5.0	5	18	25	24	20	0	3	3	23
5% D/electrolyte #75 injection†	Hypertonic	5.0	5	0	40	48	35	0	0	15	20

*D, dextrose; mOsm, osmolality.
†Baxter Healthcare Systems.

is approximately 4.3. It has the same applications as Ringer's injection, plus the ability to provide calories. Before Ringer's injections are used, each solution component should be considered. For example, because the solution contains potassium, precautions need to be exercised when treating patients with cardiac or renal disorders. If the solution contains dextrose, caution should be exercised if the patient has diabetes mellitus.

Clinical evaluation and periodic laboratory tests are important to ascertain fluid balance, electrolyte levels, and acid-base status. The type and volume of fluid administered depend on the patient's age, weight, and condition.

The complications produced by Ringer's injection are also applicable for lactated Ringer's solutions. These include overhydration, electrolyte excess (particularly sodium), electrolyte dilution, and calorie depletion. Excessive administration may lead to metabolic alkalosis. Lactated Ringer's solution is contraindicated in patients with hepatic disorders because lactate is metabolized in the liver. A different solution should be considered in the presence of lactic acidosis because the body's buffering system can be overloaded.

ALKALIZING SOLUTIONS

Sodium bicarbonate solution is an alkalizing agent and a sodium salt. The 5% sodium bicarbonate solution dissociates to provide the bicarbonate ion, which is the principal buffer in extracellular fluid. Bicarbonate helps maintain osmotic pressure and acid-base balance. It contains 0.595 mEq each of sodium and bicarbonate ions per milliliter and the osmolarity is 1190 to 1203 mOsm/L. Sodium bicarbonate is physically and/or chemically incompatible with many drugs, especially calcium, and compatibility information should be checked before admixing. The administration of sodium bicarbonate increases plasma bicarbonate concentration and may increase plasma pH until the body compensates and returns the level to a normal value (Metheny, 2000).

Major uses

Sodium bicarbonate is used to treat metabolic acidosis associated with many diseases, including severe renal disease, uncontrolled diabetes, and cardiac/circulatory diseases. It is administered in the treatment of severe hyperkalemia, in which it alkalinizes the plasma and results in a temporary shift of potassium into the cells. The sodium in the solution also antagonizes the cardiac effects of the potassium.

Complications

Metabolic alkalosis, hypocalcemia, and hypokalemia may occur following the rapid or excessive administration of sodium bicarbonate. There may be water and sodium retention leading to hypernatremia, particularly when there is a preexisting condition such as renal or cardiac disease. The fluid overload may lead to electrolyte imbalances. Extravasation may cause chemical cellulitis, necrosis, ulceration, or sloughing.

Patients with metabolic and respiratory alkalosis are not good candidates for sodium bicarbonate therapy. It is also contraindicated in the presence of hypocalcemia or hypochloremia. Caution should be exercised when cardiac or renal problems exist.

PREMIXED SOLUTIONS

A large number of premixed IV solutions are available. These solutions have many advantages over manually prepared admixtures. Premixed solutions have been sterilized after the admixture procedure and therefore have a longer shelf life. There is no difficulty in selecting the correct diluent, and the pH has been adjusted to improve stability. Finally, the correct amount of medication has been added to the proper volume and type of IV solution. Premixed solutions decrease the amount of time needed to get the fluid to the patient, which is particularly important in emergency situations.

There are also disadvantages in using premixed IV solutions. The wrong amount of medication may be used if a particular admixture comes in more than one dosage or if there are multiple types that are premixed and the wrong medication or solution is used. Premixed IV solutions can also cost more.

The number of premixed medications available is increasing. Potassium chloride comes in several concentrations and in various IV solutions. Its use depends on the patient's history, physical assessment, and laboratory findings. Before any of the potassium-containing solutions are administered, it is important to establish good renal function. Complications are related to the content of the particular fluid. Rapid infusion or continual administration may lead to hypervolemia, electrolyte excess (particularly potassium), or electrolyte dilution. Using only one type of solution over an extended period may result in electrolyte depletion and, if no source of nutrients is available, calorie depletion. The patient should be monitored carefully for electrolyte imbalances during the course of treatment.

Other medications premixed in IV solutions include heparin sodium, theophylline, lidocaine hydrochloride, nitroglycerin, dobutamine hydrochloride, and dopamine hydrochloride. There are also a variety of medications that are premixed in small volumes of IV solutions, including antibiotics and histamine antagonists. In addition to premixed products, there are also products that allow the medication container to be attached directly to the IV solution. Just as for premixed potassium solutions, it is important to review the patient's history, physical assessment, and laboratory findings. The nurse should be familiar with complications related to the particular medication and the base IV solution to which it has been added. The pharmacy department should be contacted if information is unclear or unfamiliar.

COLLOID SOLUTIONS

Solutions used to expand the intravascular space are known as colloids, or plasma expanders. The increase in volume is accomplished by these solutions pulling fluid from the interstitial spaces. Plasma expanders include albumin, dextran, mannitol, hetastarch and pentastarch, and gelatins.

Ideal colloid solutions would include the following advantages:

- Distributed to intravascular compartment only
- Readily available
- Long shelf life
- Inexpensive
- No special storage or infusion requirements
- No special limitations on volume that can be infused
- No interference with blood grouping or crossmatching
- Acceptable to all patients and no religious objections to its use

For more than 70 years colloids have been used to maintain intravascular volume after blood loss from surgery or from other causes of shock. There are four general types of colloid products available for clinical use: albumin is the predominant plasma protein and remains the standard against which other colloids are compared; dextran and hetastarch, both of which have been widely used as a plasma volume expander; and gelatin, which is new in the U.S. market.

Colloids have various nononcotic properties that may influence vascular integrity, inflammation, and pharmacokinetics. All colloids affect the coagulation system, with dextran and starch solutions having the most potent antithrombotic effects. Colloids restore intravascular volume and tissue perfusion more rapidly than crystalloids in all shock states, regardless of vascular permeability (Martin and Matthay, 2004).

Controversy exists regarding the appropriate choice of resuscitation fluid for the trauma victim with mild to moderate hemorrhage. The focus of this controversy centers primarily on the effect the colloid administered has on the lungs. Most studies have compared a single colloid versus crystalloid therapy or compared two colloids; therefore the choice of the "best" colloid is elusive. There does not seem to be a study that demonstrates improved survival or reduced risk of acute complications with a specific therapy. Cost of the solutions makes the starches, dextrans, and gelatins compare favorably with albumin. Crystalloid therapy remains the least expensive method of plasma volume expansion. Results from studies yield similar clinical outcomes with colloid and saline for fluid resuscitation (Roberts and Bratton, 1998; Kelley, 2005; Hankins, 2006). The controversy over the type and method of fluid to be used in

resuscitation of the acutely injured patient is well documented. Both crystalloid and colloid fluids are capable of restoring circulating volume (Jordan, 2000). Refer to Table 13-5 for a comparison of common crystalloid and colloid solutions and their maximum volume expansion.

Crystalloid fluids used for trauma resuscitation include lactated Ringer's solution and 0.9% sodium chloride. Crystalloid fluids fill both the interstitial and the intravascular spaces. Advantages of crystalloid fluid include cost-effectiveness, nonallergenic properties, and reduced viscosity, leading to improved microcirculation.

At present isotonic sodium chloride is recommended as the first-line fluid in resuscitation of hypovolemic trauma patients (Revell, Porter, and Greaves, 2002).

Specific indications for colloid products include hypoproteinemia, malnourished states, patients requiring plasma volume expansion who cannot tolerate large amounts of fluid, and orthopedic and reconstructive procedures requiring prevention of thrombus formation (Roberts and Bratton, 1998).

Albumin

Albumin is a natural plasma protein pooled from human blood and blood-related products, and is available in 5% and 25% concentrations. It contains 130 to 160 mEq of sodium per liter. It plays an important role in regulating plasma volume and tissue fluid balance. The administration of albumin causes fluid to be pulled from the interstitial space into the intravascular space. Because it is a plasma protein, there may be a slight increase in the plasma protein volume. The 5% solution is isotonic. The 25% solution is hypertonic, and in a well-hydrated patient, each volume (amount given) draws about 3.5 volumes of additional fluid into circulation within 15 minutes (McEvoy, 2007).

Major uses

Albumin is used for plasma volume expansion in treating shock or impending shock related to a circulatory volume deficit. Albumin is used widely in the management of medical and surgical conditions. The 5% solution is generally used to treat hypovolemia, and the 25% solution is usually reserved for treatment when there are fluid and sodium restrictions.

Complications

The potential for complications should be considered if cardiac, hepatic, or renal disease is present. These systems may be unable to handle the increased intravascular volume if they are impaired. The increased circulating volume may result in fluid overload and lead to further complications. Anemia may occur if large volumes of albumin alone are used to replace blood loss.

FOCUS ON EVIDENCE

Colloid Versus Saline Use in Fluid Resuscitation

- One of the largest prospective clinical studies to date, the SAFE (Saline versus Albumin Fluid Evaluation) trial randomized a heterogeneous group of 7000 critically ill patients requiring fluid resuscitation to receive isooncotic albumin or isotonic crystalloid. Over 28 days, mortality was 21% and did not differ according to treatment assignment (Finfer et al, 2004).

TABLE 13-5 Comparison of Common Colloid and Crystalloid Solutions

Solution	Molecular weight	Osmolality	Max vol. expansion* (%)	Duration of expansion vol. (hr)	Side effects
Albumin 4%, 5%	69	290	70-100	12-24	Allergic reactions
Albumin 20%, 25%	69	310	300-500	12-24	Allergic reactions
Starches *Hetastarch* 3%, 6%, 10%	450	300-310	100-200	8-36	Renal dysfunction
Starches *Pentastarch* 10%	280	326	100-200	12-24	Renal dysfunction
Dextrans 10% Dextran 40 3% Dextran 60 6% Dextran 70	40 70	280-324 280-324	100-200 80-140	1-2 <8-24 }	Anaphylactoid reactions Anaphylactoid reactions
Gelatins Succinylated and crosslinked: 2.5%, 3%, 4% Urea-linked: 3.5%	30-35	300-350	70-80	<4-6	High calcium content (urea-linked forms)
Crystalloids 0.9% NaCl	0	285-308	20-25	1-4	Hyperchloremic metabolic acidosis
Crystalloids Ringer's lactate	0	250-273	20-25	1-4	Hyperkalemia

*Max volume expansion is expressed as a percentage of administered volume (Vol.).
Adapted from American Thoracic Society Documents (Martin GS, Matthay MA): Evidence-based colloid use in the critically ill: American Thoracic Society Consensus Statement, *Am J Respir Crit Care Med* 170(11):1247, 2004. Accessed at http://ajrccm.atsjournals.org/cgi/content/full/170/11/1247.

The rapid influx and excretion of fluid may dilute or deplete electrolytes. The serum protein concentration and hematocrit level should be monitored because these levels may be decreased. Symptoms of allergic reactions may be present. Bleeding may occur postoperatively or posttraumatically as the intravascular volume and pressure increase. Albumin is contraindicated in patients with severe anemia, cardiac failure, or known hypersensitivity. Angiotensin-converting enzyme (ACE) inhibitors should be withheld for at least 24 hours before administering large amounts of albumin because of an increased risk of atypical reactions (e.g., flushing, hypotension) (McEvoy, 2007).

Dextrans

Dextran fluids are polysaccharides that behave as colloids. They are available as low-molecular-weight dextran (dextran 40) and high-molecular-weight dextran (dextran 70). High-molecular-weight dextrans, dextran 70 and dextran 75, are available with average molecular weights of 70,000 and 75,000, respectively. Dextran 70 is more effective than dextran 40 as a substitute for plasma expansion. It is important to monitor the patient's pulse, blood pressure, and urine output every 5 to 15 minutes for the first hour of administration of dextran and then every hour after that. Dextran should be administered at a rate of 20 mL/kg of body weight over 24 hours to prevent hypersensitivity reactions and decrease the risk of bleeding (Phillips and Kuhn, 1999).

Dextran fluids are used for plasma substitution or expansion. An advantage of dextran use is that the intravascular space is expanded in excess of the volume infused. Dextran solutions have effects similar to those of human albumin for expanding intravascular volume.

Major uses

High-molecular-weight dextran is used to treat shock or impending shock related to trauma, surgery, burns, or hemorrhage (McEvoy, 2007). Dextran solutions should not be used as substitutes for blood and blood products. However, they may be used on short notice if there is no time for crossmatching or if blood or blood products are unavailable.

Low-molecular-weight dextran is used for early fluid replacement and to treat shock related to vascular volume loss such as that produced by burns, hemorrhage, surgery, and trauma (Gahart and Nazareno, 2008). Because of its action in preventing sludging of blood, low-molecular-weight dextran is used to help prevent venous thrombosis and pulmonary embolism during surgical procedures.

Complications

An anaphylactoid reaction is rare but may be fatal. Hydration status is important because limited intake may deplete tissue fluids and excessive fluids may dilute electrolytes. Circulatory overload may occur, leading to various congestive states. Dextran can have an adverse effect on hepatic function. Higher dosages may increase bleeding times. Because of the expansion of vascular volume, the hematocrit and plasma protein may be diluted. Blood should be drawn before dextran administration because dextran may interfere with laboratory testing, depending on the test method or the agent used in the testing process.

Low-molecular-weight dextran should not be given to patients with cardiac or renal disease caused by possible overload problems and is contraindicated in the presence of thrombocytopenia, hypofibrinogenemia, and hypersensitivity to dextran. Dehydrated patients should receive fluids before and during dextran infusion to prevent tissue dehydration. Caution should be used when active hemorrhage is present. Patients should be monitored for pulse, blood pressure, central venous pressure (if possible), and urine output. Rates may need to be slowed and the patient monitored for circulatory overload if the central venous pressure is not being monitored.

Mannitol

Mannitol is a hexahydroxy alcohol substance that is available in concentrations of 5%, 10%, 15%, 20%, and 25%, and is classified as an osmotic diuretic. This solution is limited to the extracellular space, where it draws fluid from the cells as a result of its hypertonicity (275 to 1375 mOsm/L). It is usually dosed by kilograms of body weight. Mannitol increases the osmotic pressure of the glomerular filtrate, thereby inhibiting reabsorption of water and electrolytes. Administration of this solution causes excretion of water, sodium, potassium, chloride, calcium, phosphorus, magnesium, urea, and uric acid (Deglin and Vallerand, 2008; Gahart and Nazareno, 2008).

Major uses

It is used to promote diuresis in patients with oliguric acute renal failure, to promote excretion of toxic substances in the body, to reduce excess cerebrospinal fluid (CSF), to reduce intraocular pressure, and to treat intracranial pressure and cerebral edema (Phillips, 2005).

Complications

Fluid and electrolyte imbalances are the most common and severe complications. Administration of mannitol can reduce excess CSF within 15 minutes. Mannitol may induce dehydration and result in hyperkalemia and hypernatremia. It is irritating to the vein intima and may cause phlebitis. Extravasation of mannitol may lead to skin irritation and tissue necrosis (Deglin and Vallerand, 2008). Mannitol may interfere with laboratory tests. Use caution when administering mannitol to patients with impaired cardiac or renal function. It is contraindicated in the presence of anuria, severe pulmonary and cardiac congestion, and intracranial bleeding.

The infusion nurse needs to monitor the administration of mannitol for crystal formation. It is recommended that an in-line filter be used during administration of 15%, 20%, and 25% solutions (Deglin and Vallerand, 2008).

Hydroxyethyl starches

Hetastarch is a synthetic polymer with colloidal properties similar to those of human albumin. It has an approximate pH of 5.5 and an osmolarity of 310 mOsm/L. It is available in a 6% concentration in 0.9% sodium chloride. The colloidal osmotic effect pulls fluid from the cells into the intravascular space, thus increasing the volume in this area. Maximum volume expansion occurs shortly after completion of the infusion. The duration of effect depends on the preadministration plasma volume, distribution of the hetastarch in body water, and renal function status. The molecules in this solution vary in size. The smaller hetastarch molecules (hydroxyethylated glucose) are excreted rapidly, but it may take 2 weeks or longer for the larger molecules (starch) to be degraded sufficiently for elimination. Hetastarch does not interfere with blood typing and crossmatching, as do other colloidal solutions.

Pentastarch is another polydisperse formulation of hydroxyethyl starch with a lower molecular weight. Pentastarch has a greater colloid osmotic pressure than hetastarch. This leads to greater expansion of the intravascular space, nearly twice that of the volume infused. A randomized clinical trial of 10% pentastarch (London, Ho, and Triedman, 1989) found that pentastarch over 5% albumin may provide greater plasma volume expansion for the volume infused, with faster onset and more rapid elimination, than albumin or hetastarch.

In 2007 the FDA approved Voluven, a 6% hydroxyethyl starch injection, for the prevention and treatment of dangerously low blood volume (McEvoy, 2007).

Major uses

The hydroxyethyl starches are used for early fluid replacement and to treat shock related to a decreased circulating volume resulting from trauma, burns, hemorrhage, and surgery. Hydroxyethyl starches are also used with leukopheresis to help increase the yield of granulocytes by centrifugal means (McEvoy, 2007).

Complications

The administration of hetastarch may produce a severe anaphylactoid reaction. It may interfere with platelet function and increase bleeding times. As with any volume expander, the danger of fluid overload is always a possibility. This may lead to disorders related to congestion, dilution, or depletion of electrolytes; dehydration of peripheral tissue; electrolyte excess; and a decrease in the hematocrit, platelet counts, hemoglobin, and plasma protein levels. Hetastarch is contraindicated in patients with liver disease and severe cardiac and renal disorders, particularly when oliguria or anuria is present. It also should not be used in the presence of bleeding disorders. The patient should be evaluated clinically and laboratory tests monitored regularly. Partially used containers should be discarded because hetastarch does not contain preservatives.

Gelatins

Gelatin is the name given to the proteins formed when the connective tissues of animals are boiled. They have the property of dissolving in hot water and forming a jelly when cooled. Gelatin is thus a large-molecular-weight protein formed from hydrolysis of collagen. Several modified gelatin products are available; they have been collectively called the new-generation gelatins. There are three types of gelatin solutions currently in use: succinylated or modified fluid gelatins (e.g., Gelofusine, Plasmagel, Plasmion); urea-crosslinked gelatins (e.g., Polygeline); and oxypolygelatins (e.g., Gelifundol). Gelatins are supplied as a 3.5% solution of degraded gelatin polypeptides crosslinked via urea bridges with electrolytes. Gelatins have no preservatives and have a recommended shelf life of 3 years when stored at temperatures less than 30° C. They are rapidly excreted by the kidney following infusion. Gelatins (GEL) have the advantage of their unlimited daily dose recommendation and minimal effect on hemostasis (Van der Linden et al, 2005).

Major uses

Gelatins are used for replacement of intravascular volume resulting from acute blood loss. They are also used in priming heart-lung machines.

Complications

Gelatins are associated with anaphylactoid reactions and may also cause depression of serum fibronectin levels. Urea-linked gelatin has much higher calcium and potassium levels than succinylated gelatin (Kelley, 2005). Concerns have been raised about the risks associated with bovine-derived gelatin because of the association between new-variant Creutzfeldt-Jakob disease and bovine spongiform encephalitis. There are no known cases of transmission involving pharmaceutical gelatin preparations, but awareness of this issue is important (Marwick, 1997; Grocott et al, 2005).

SUMMARY

Parenteral fluid administration has many facets in maintaining homeostasis and is not without its complexities and complications. These concerns challenge the nurse who is caring for the patient with potential imbalances. The nurse, by effectively evaluating the many nursing considerations involved in fluid administration, can help ensure positive outcomes for patients receiving parenteral fluids.

REFERENCES

Ayus J, Arieff A: Symptomatic hyponatremia: making the diagnosis rapidly, *J Crit Care* 5(8):846-856, 1990.

Beck DE: Fluids, electrolytes and dehydration, *United Ostomy Assoc* 40(2):66-67, 2003.

Centers for Disease Control and Prevention: Guidelines for the prevention of intravascular catheter-related infections, *MMWR* 51(RR-10):1-29, 2002.

Cook LS: IV fluid resuscitation, *J Infus Nurs* 26(5):296-303, 2003.

Cooper A, Moore M: Clinical update. IV fluid therapy: part 2: fluid selection, *Austral Nurs J* 6:(7)23-26, 2000.

Deglin JH, Vallerand AH: *Davis's drug guide for nurses*, ed 11, Philadelphia, 2008, FA Davis.

Finfer S, Bellomo R, Boyce N et al: A comparison of albumin and saline for fluid resuscitation in the intensive care unit, *New Eng J Med* 350:2247-2256, 2004.

Gahart L, Nazareno AR: *2008 Intravenous medications*, ed 24, St Louis, 2008, Mosby.

Grocott M, Mythen MG, Gan TJ: Perioperative fluid management and clinical outcomes in adults, *Int Anesthes Res Soc* 100:1093-1106, 2005.

Hankins J: The role of albumin in fluid and electrolyte balance, *J Infus Nurs* 29:(5)260-265, 2006.

Heitz U, Horne MM: *Pocket guide to fluid, electrolyte, and acid-base balance*, ed 5, St Louis, 2005, Mosby.

Hew-Butler T, Ayus JC et al: Consensus statement of the 1st international exercise-associated hyponatremia consensus development conference, Cape Town, South Africa, 2005, *Clin J Sport Med* 15:208-213, 2005.

Hill JW, Petrucci RH: *General chemistry: an integrated approach*, ed 3, Upper Saddle River, NJ, 2004, Prentice Hall.

Holliday MA, Segar WE: The maintenance need for water in parenteral fluid therapy, *Pediatrics* 19:823-832, 1957.

Hospira: *20%, 30%, 40%, 50%, and 70% dextrose injection*, USP, 2006 (website). Accessed 1/8/08 at www.hospira.com.

Humes HD: *Kelley's textbook of internal medicine*, ed 4, Philadelphia, 2000, Lippincott Williams & Wilkins.

Infusion Nurses Society: Infusion nursing standards of practice, *J Infus Nurs* 29(1S), 2006.

Johnson AL, Criddle LM: Pass the salt: indications for and implications of using hypertonic saline, *Crit Care Nurs* 24:(5)36-48, 2004.

Jordan KS: Fluid resuscitation in acutely injured patients, *J Intraven Nurs* 23(2):81-87, 2000.

Kee JL, Paulanka BJ, Purnell LD: *Fluids and electrolytes with clinical applications: a programmed approach*, ed 7, Florence, KY, 2004, Thomson Delmar Learning.

Kelley DM: Hypovolemic shock: an overview, *Crit Care Nurs Q* 28(1): 2-19, 2005.

Kraft PA: The osmotic shift, *J Intraven Nurs* 23(4):220-224, 2000.

London MJ, Ho JS, Triedman JK: A randomized clinical trial of 10% pentastarch (low molecular weight hydroxyethyl starch) versus 5% albumin for plasma volume expansion after cardiac operations, *J Thorac Cardiovasc Surg* 97(5):785-797, 1989.

Martin GS, Matthay MA: Evidence-based colloid use in the critically ill. Consensus conference statement subcommittee of the American Thoracic Society Critical Care Assembly, *Am J Respir Crit Care Med* 170(11):1247-1259, 2004.

Marwick C: BSE sets agenda for imported gelatin, *JAMA* 51:989, 1997.

McEvoy GK: *AHFS drug information 2007*, Bethesda, Md, 2007, American Society of Health System Pharmacists.

Metheny NM: Fluid and electrolyte balance. In Metheny NM, editor: *Nursing considerations*, ed 4 (pp 169-171), Philadelphia, 2000, Lippincott Williams & Wilkins.

Molyneux EM, Maitland K: Intravenous fluids—getting balance right, *New Engl J Med* 353(9):941-944, 2005.

Phillips LD: *Manual of I.V. therapeutics*, ed 4, Philadelphia, 2005, FA Davis.

Phillips LD, Kuhn M: *Manual of I.V. drugs*, ed 2, Philadelphia, 1999, J.B. Lippincott.

Porth CM: *Pathophysiology: concept of altered health states*, ed 6, Philadelphia, 2007, Lippincott Williams & Wilkins.

Revell M, Porter K, Greaves I: Fluid resuscitation in prehospital trauma care: a consensus view, *Emerg Med J* 19(6):494-499, 2002.

Roberts JS, Bratton SL: Colloid volume expanders: Problems, pitfalls and possibilities, *Drugs* 55(5):621-630, 1998.

Siegel AJ: Hypertonic (3%) sodium chloride for emergent treatment of exercise-associated hypotonic encephalopathy. Conference paper, *Sport Med* 37(94-95):459-462, 2007.

Simma B, Burger R, Falk M et al: A prospective, randomized and controlled study of fluid management in children with severe head injury: lactated Ringer's versus hypertonic saline, *Crit Care Med* 26:1256-1270, 1998.

Slesak G, Schnurle JW, Kinzel E et al: Comparison of subcutaneous and intravenous rehydration in geriatric patients: a randomized trial, *J Am Geriatr Soc* 51:155-160, 2003.

Starling EH: On the absorption of fluids from the connective tissues spaces, *J Physiol* 19:312-326, 1896.

Turner T, Cassano AM: Subcutaneous dextrose for rehydration of elderly patients—an evidence-based review, 2004, *BMC Geriatr* 4:2, 2004. Accessed 1/10/08 at www.pubmedcentral.nih.gov/article.

Van der Linden PJ, Hert SG, Cromheecke S et al: Hydroxyethyl starch 130/0.4 versus modified fluid gelatin for volume expansion in cardiac surgery patients: the effects on perioperative bleeding and transfusion needs, *Int Anesthes Res Soc* 101:629-634, 2005.

14 BLOOD COMPONENT THERAPY

Nancy L. Trick, RN, CRNI®*

This chapter provides a foundation on which to construct a broader understanding of the more encompassing subject of transfusion therapy. The topics addressed here are not intended to be all-inclusive of the discipline of transfusion therapy, nor are they offered as a "how to" manual. They are intended to establish a firm theoretical footing and a practical framework on which the practitioner may build.

It was fewer than 200 years ago that James Blundell performed the first blood transfusion to save a life. Since then, because of the incredible advances in knowledge and technology that have been made in blood group identification, collection, fractionation, storage, and transmissible disease testing, transfusion medicine has evolved into a specialty of its own. This specialty has made advances in new surgical procedures possible and has supported the ever-changing approaches to cancer chemotherapy.

Blood component therapy has advanced so far so fast and is so common in today's medicine that there could be a tendency to approach this familiar therapy with some complacency. Therefore it should be remembered that blood infusion is a "living transplant" that carries with it significant risks, only a few of which are avoidable. Consequently, this effective and readily accessible therapy should be used prudently; the potential benefit should always outweigh the potential for harm. Furthermore, it is the practitioner's duty in transfusion therapy to be knowledgeable in the application of this therapy and to be familiar with its possible untoward effects and their appropriate interventions.

DONOR TESTING

The American Red Cross began testing for syphilis in the United States in 1948, and since 1985 has been testing for HIV/AIDS. All blood donated for the purpose of homologous transfusion must be subjected to a number of tests (Table 14-1).

ABO AND RH TYPING

ABO forward typing is the process in which red blood cells are mixed with a known antibody (anti-A or anti-B). This process identifies the antigens present on the red blood cells by the visually apparent agglutination of the cells when an antibody combines with the corresponding antigen (e.g., anti-A with antigen A).

ABO reverse typing tests serum for the presence of predicted ABO antibodies by adding red blood cells of a known ABO type.

The Rh factor is the red cell antigen D. Rh typing is accomplished by testing red cells against anti-D serum. If agglutination occurs, the red cells possess the D antigen and the blood is Rh positive. Some people demonstrate a weak expression of the D antigen (formerly referred to as D^U). In the past, laboratory testing to identify this weak D antigen included the indirect antiglobulin test. However, that test is no longer necessary in most cases because licensed anti-D reagents are sufficiently potent to identify patients with a weak expression of the D antigen as Rh positive. These individuals are considered Rh positive as donors and recipients.

Additional testing for red cell antigens is not recommended or encouraged by the AABB, formerly known as the American Association of Blood Banks.

SCREENING FOR UNEXPECTED ANTIBODIES

Unexpected antibodies are those other than anti-A or anti-B. Many blood banks screen all donated units for clinically significant antibodies rather than limiting their search to the donor group most likely to harbor them. The most likely donors of blood with unexpected antibodies are those with a history of pregnancy or previous transfusion. In general, clinically significant antibodies are those known to have caused hemolytic disease of the newborn, a frank hemolytic transfusion reaction, or unacceptably short survival of transfused red blood cells (Roback et al, 2008).

*The author and editors wish to acknowledge the contributions made by Jean A. Weir as author of this chapter in the second edition of *Infusion Therapy in Clinical Practice*.

242

TABLE 14-1 Testing of Donor Blood

Test	To determine
ABO—forward typing	Presence of antigen A or B on RBC
ABO—reverse typing	Presence of antibody A or antibody B in plasma
Rh typing:	
With anti-D sera	Presence of D antigen on RBC
With anti-D sera or with indirect antiglobulin test	Presence of weak D antigen
Screen for unexpected antibodies	Presence of antibodies other than anti-A and anti-B
Screen for transmissible disease:	
Serologic test for syphilis	*Treponema* infection
Hepatitis B surface antigen	Infectivity for hepatitis B
Hepatitis C (anti-HCV)	Infectivity for hepatitis C
Hepatitis B core antibody	May indicate HBV carrier
Alanine aminotransferase*	Indicates liver damage
Human immunodeficiency virus (HIV):	
Enzyme-linked immunosorbent assay	Presence of antibody to HIV-1 and HIV-2
HIV antigen	Presence of antibody to HIV virus
Human T-cell leukemia/ lymphoma virus I (HTLV-I)	Presence of antibody to HTLV-I/II

HBV, hepatitis B virus; *RBC,* red blood cell.
*No longer required but included by many centers.

TABLE 14-2 Anticoagulants-Preservatives

Anticoagulant-Preservative	Composition	Shelf life provided (days)
CPD	Citrate, phosphate, and dextrose	21
CPDA-1	CPD plus adenine	35
Additive systems	CPD plus various preservative combinations	35–42

- Test for the presence of the antibody to the human T-cell lymphotropic viruses 1 and 2 (HTLS-1/2). (See Adverse Effects later in this chapter.)

Donor screening

Donors are required to answer questions that may have a bearing on the safety of their blood. For example, donors with a history of intravenous drug abuse are routinely deferred. Since November 1999, the FDA has requested the blood industry to defer potential donors who had lived in European countries with reported or suspected cases of bovine spongiform encephalopathy (BSE), the "mad cow disease," and who therefore might be carriers of the BSE agent.

Donor lists

Blood collection centers must keep current a list of deferred donors and use it to make sure that they do not collect blood from anyone on the list. Donated blood must be quarantined until it is tested and shown to be free of infectious agents. To ensure a safe blood supply, blood collection centers must investigate manufacturing problems, correct all deficiencies, and notify the FDA when product deviations occur in distributed products.

SCREENING FOR TRANSMISSIBLE DISEASE

All donor blood must be tested to detect units that might transmit disease (Klein and Anstee, 2005). Components and whole blood units must not be used for transfusion unless all tests are nonreactive, are negative, or have values within normal limits.

- Test for syphilis using a serological test as required by the U.S. Food and Drug Administration (FDA).
- Test for the presence of the hepatitis B surface antigen to identify hepatitis B infectivity.
- Test for the presence of the antibody for hepatitis C virus (HCV).
- Test for the presence of the hepatitis B core antibody. This component of the hepatitis B virus (HBV) testing may indicate an HBV carrier state.
- Alanine aminotransaminase (ALT) is a serum enzyme that, if elevated, can signal liver malfunction. This test is no longer required by the AABB, but many blood centers still perform it.
- Test for the presence of the antibody to human immunodeficiency viruses 1 and 2 (anti–HIV-1/2). A positive result using the standard screening methods necessitates a repeat standard screen and then a confirming screen using a more specific assay. In addition to this enzyme-linked immunosorbent assay (ELISA) to detect antibody, all blood must be tested for the presence of HIV (HIV-1 antigen test).

 BLOOD STORAGE AND PRESERVATION

Because blood is a living tissue at the time of its harvest from a donor and because it must remain healthy during its storage, substances are added to meet two conditions necessary for successful shelf life:

1. A food source must be provided to maintain adequate nutrition to the stored cells.
2. Anticoagulation must be achieved to ensure that the blood remains in its liquid cellular state for the duration of the storage period.

Several anticoagulants-preservatives are available from which to choose. All of them provide the aforementioned necessary conditions for shelf life, but they differ in the length of storage time that they provide (Table 14-2).

CPD (citrate-phosphate-dextrose) and CPDA-1 (citrate-phosphate-dextrose-adenine) differ in composition by just one substance—adenine. However, the addition of adenine extends the shelf life by 14 days and is of great significance to a blood transfusion service whose concern revolves around adequate blood reserves and their ability to supply upon demand.

CPDA-1 is considered the anticoagulant-preservative of choice for whole blood and is also used when the donated unit may be processed into separate components.

The additive solutions, commonly called *adenine-saline*, are approved by the FDA for the extended storage of red blood cells. These solutions differ in composition by manufacturer. However, there is a limited menu from which these compounds are made. They contain various combinations of 0.9% sodium chloride, adenine, dextrose, phosphate, citrate, and mannitol. These additives allow red cells to be stored for up to 42 days. The additive solutions, which are secondary or "add-on" solutions, are used only with red cells that were harvested in a primary anticoagulant-preservative such as CPD. The red cells are then separated and mixed with the additive solutions.

ANTICOAGULANTS AND PRESERVATIVES

The following is a brief summary of the substances that preserve blood:

- *Citrate:* Sodium citrate by itself, or sometimes in combination with citric acid, achieves anticoagulation by inhibiting several calcium-dependent steps in the coagulation cascade. It also slows the process of glycolysis, which is the conversion of glucose to lactic acid and adenosine triphosphate (ATP) through various metabolic pathways (Embden-Meyerhof, Krebs cycle, and the electron transport system). Slowing glycolysis allows adequate amounts of ATP to continue to be produced and the limited supply of sugar in the stored cells to be preserved.
- *Phosphate:* Inorganic phosphate acts as a buffer that helps maintain the pH.
- *Dextrose:* When sugars were first investigated as possible participants in blood preservation, red blood cells were thought to be impermeable to them. Therefore it was theorized that sugar would act as a colloid to protect the cells against hemolysis. It was soon recognized that red blood cells are permeable to dextrose and that this was an excellent food source for the stored cells (Klein and Anstee, 2005). Dextrose is a deterrent to hemolysis, but not because of a colloidal action. It supplies the food from which ATP, the principal intracellular energy-storage compound, is formed. Adequate supplies of ATP are necessary for the continued integrity of the cell.
- *Adenine:* Although other factors appear to be involved, the ATP content of stored red blood cells generally can be equated with their viability (i.e., their capacity to survive in the recipient's bloodstream after transfusion). In the 1950s, it was shown that the ATP content of stored cells could be restored by adding adenosine, which consists of adenine and the five-carbon sugar ribose. However, because of its toxicity, adenosine was never used in transfusion practice. Later it was discovered that adding adenine by itself accomplishes the same positive result of restoring ATP levels in stored red cells (Klein and Anstee, 2005).
- *Mannitol:* Mannitol, which appears to reduce hemolysis by its effect as an osmotic stabilizer, is found in at least one of the additive systems.

REJUVENATION OF RED CELLS

Red cells that have been stored up to 3 days beyond their expiration dates can be incubated (at 37° C for 1 hour) in FDA-approved solutions containing inosine, pyruvate, phosphate, adenine, and sometimes glucose. This incubation will increase the cellular levels of ATP and 2,3-diphosphoglycerate (2,3-DPG). These rejuvenated cells may be washed and used within 24 hours, or they may be glycerolized and frozen for extended storage (Roback et al, 2008).

IMMUNOHEMATOLOGY

Immunology is the scientific discipline that deals with the immune system and immune response (antibody response to antigenic stimulus). Immunohematology narrows the view of immunology to focus specifically on the antigens and antibodies of the blood.

The antigens of the blood, called *agglutinogens*, are found as integrated parts of the red cell membrane, as components of the white cells, and as soluble substances in the plasma. The largest group of agglutinogens, which numbers more than 400 belonging to 24 known systems, is associated with red cells.

The first set of red cell antigens discovered, those of the ABO system, was identified by Landsteiner at the turn of the twentieth century. The ABO system is the most important of the known antigen systems and is the foundation for determining compatibilities in transfusion therapy.

THE ABO SYSTEM

There are four blood types in the ABO system: A, B, AB, and O. The name of the blood type is determined by the name of the antigen on the red cell. The type of antigen present on the red cell is an inherited characteristic; the A and B genes are equally dominant, and the O gene is recessive (Table 14-3).

The A and B genes dictate the presence of A and B antigenic determinant sites, respectively. Although the O gene is inactive and does not code for any of the erythrocyte alloantigens, blood group O erythrocytes do exhibit an antigenic glycoprotein on their surface—the H antigen. This glycoprotein is not the product of the O gene, as evidenced by its presence on red blood cells of all types.

The relationship between the A, B, and H antigens can be explained as follows. During the synthesis of the blood group molecules, the H antigen is synthesized first; thus the H antigen is present on all red cells. If the A gene is present, it will code for a transferase (enzyme), which will facilitate the attachment of the sugar *N*-acetylgalactosamine to the H antigen. This chemical complex is the antigenic determinant for blood group A.

TABLE 14-3 **ABO Blood Groups**

Possible genotypes	Phenotype	Blood group	Red blood cell antigen	Plasma antibody
OO	O	O	Neither A nor B	A and B
AA or AO	A	A	A	B
BB or BO	B	B	B	A
AB	AB	AB	A and B	Neither A nor B

TABLE 14-4 Summary of Compatibilities

Component	Compatibilities	
Whole blood	Give type-specific blood only	
Packed red cells (stored, washed, or frozen/washed)	**Donor**	**Recipient**
	O	O, A, B, AB
	A	A, AB
	B	B, AB
	AB	AB
Fresh-frozen plasma	**Donor**	**Recipient**
	O	O
	A	A, O
	B	B, O
	AB	AB, B, A, O
Platelets	RBC: ABO and Rh compatible *preferred*	
	Donor	**Recipient**
	O	O, A, B, AB
	A	A, AB
	B	B, AB
	AB	AB
Cryoprecipitate	Plasma: ABO compatible *preferred*	
	Donor	**Recipient**
	O	O
	A	A, O
	B	B, O
	AB	AB, B, A, O

Similarly, the B gene will code for a different transferase that will allow for the attachment of an alternate sugar group, D-galactose, which will complete the antigenic determinant for blood type B. Group O individuals do not possess either enzyme system, and thus group O erythrocytes possess only the unmodified H antigen on their surface (Smith, 2001; Roback et al, 2008). The antibodies of the ABO system occur naturally (i.e., without direct antigen stimulation) and are called *isohemagglutinins*. They are complete, and in the presence of red cells that exhibit the corresponding antigen; they can cause agglutination in a 0.9% sodium chloride medium. The antibody that agglutinates type A is called *antibody A* (anti-A), and the corresponding antibody for antigen B is called *antibody B* (anti-B).

This adversarial relationship between antigen and the corresponding antibody is the basis for understanding compatibilities within the ABO system. The antigens are located on the cells, and the antibodies reside in the plasma. If a unit of red cells is to be administered it should be thought of as an antigen and should be given only to a recipient who does not exhibit the corresponding antibody. Conversely, plasma should not be given to a recipient who possesses the corresponding red cell antigen (Table 14-4).

THE RH SYSTEM

The Rh system is complex and extensive. Because nearly 50 Rh antigens have been identified, a complete discussion of this system is not included here. Sufficient for the topic of routine transfusion therapy are the unmodified terms of Rh+ (Rh positive) and Rh– (Rh negative), which respectively refer to the presence or absence of the red cell antigen D.

The blood recipient who carries antigen D (Rh positive) may receive products that are either Rh+ or Rh–. However, a recipient who is Rh negative should receive only blood products that are Rh negative. This is especially true for Rh-negative women of childbearing age who might become sensitized to the D antigen, which could raise the potential for complications in subsequent pregnancies.

THE HLA SYSTEM

The HLA blood grouping system consists of a series of highly immunogenic antigens that can be found predominantly on the cells of the leukocyte family. These antigens exist on the surface of the lymphocytes, granulocytes, monocytes, and platelets. Although the HLA antigens and their precipitated antibodies are best known for their role in transplantation rejection, they also contribute to several of the complications of transfusion therapy, including the following:

- Febrile nonhemolytic reaction (FNH)
- Immune-mediated platelet refractoriness
- Transfusion-related acute lung injury (TRALI)
- Transfusion-associated graft-versus-host disease (TA-GVHD)

PREPARATION AND CLINICAL APPLICATION OF BLOOD COMPONENTS

WHOLE BLOOD

Whole blood requires no processing beyond collection into an anticoagulated closed collection system and testing. It is stored at 1° to 6° C with the satellite pack attached. If packed cells are needed at any time during the shelf life of the blood, this satellite pack will allow for their separation within a closed system. However, because whole blood transfusions are rarely used except to treat massive blood loss, most homologous donations are not stored as whole blood but are separated into components soon after donation. Autologous donations, which are planned to be transfused back to the donor within the shelf life period for refrigerated blood, are stored whole. These units are often given as whole blood. They can be spun down and given as packed cells if the donor-recipient does not need or cannot tolerate the additional volume that the plasma represents.

Clinical applications for the administration of whole blood include the following:

- When increased oxygen-carrying capacity and volume expansion are needed
- When active bleeding has resulted in a 25% to 30% blood volume loss
- When exchange transfusion is performed

Although whole blood may be appropriate for the preceding clinical situations, it is not always readily available. Therefore the use of packed red cells in combination with asanguineous solutions has become the standard when replacement therapy is needed in surgery or trauma cases (Klein, Spahn, and Carson, 2007; Roback et al, 2008).

PACKED RED BLOOD CELLS

Packed red blood cells are prepared by separating the plasma from the cellular portion of a unit of whole blood. This can be done any time before the expiration date. Cells can be separated from plasma by centrifuge, which causes a rapid separation, or by sedimentation, in which cells will settle to the bottom of an upright container and the plasma will concentrate on top. Once separation has occurred, 200 to 250 mL of plasma can be manually expressed into the attached satellite bag.

The shelf life of a unit of packed red blood cells (PRBCs) is the same as that for the unit of whole blood from which it was obtained, but it can be extended if an additive system is mixed with the cells at the time of their separation (see previous discussion under Anticoagulants and Preservatives). These additive solutions, which must be added within 72 hours of the blood donation, extend the shelf life of the packed cells from 35 to 42 days.

PRBCs are used for routine blood replacement during surgery and to increase the oxygen-carrying capacity (i.e., the red blood cell mass) in patients with symptomatic anemia that cannot be treated with pharmaceuticals.

MODIFIED PACKED RED BLOOD CELLS
0.9% sodium chloride–washed red blood cells

The 0.9% sodium chloride washing of red blood cells (RBCs) is carried out in the blood bank using automated or semiautomated equipment. The washed cells are suspended in sterile 0.9% sodium chloride solution. The processed product has a hematocrit of 70% to 80%. This process removes platelets and cellular debris, diminishes plasma to trace levels, and reduces the number of leukocytes. It should be noted that the leukocytes are not eliminated, so this component does contain viable lymphocytes and it can precipitate the graft-versus-host response. Stored packed cells may be washed at any time during the shelf life. However, because the washing is performed in an open system, their shelf life at 1° to 6° C is only 24 hours after washing. This limited shelf life is imposed because of concerns for bacterial contamination; washed red cells are not considered free from the risk of disease transmission.

Washed packed cells are used for patients with recurrent or severe allergic reactions thought to be related to one or more plasma proteins and for neonatal and intrauterine transfusions.

Frozen-deglycerolized packed cells

Two decades ago, there were many reasons for freezing blood, but they have diminished over time because of improved technologies. Today, blood is frozen for one reason: long-term storage. For autologous blood, this extended storage capacity means that blood can be stored well beyond the 42-day shelf life afforded by refrigeration. This permits scheduling of elective surgical procedures well in advance and allows the donation of enough blood to provide for the safety of autologous transfusion.

In addition to its application in autologous transfusion, blood is frozen to maintain stores of rare blood types. AABB's *Standards for Blood Banks and Transfusion Services* allows frozen blood intended for routine transfusion to be stored for up to 10 years (AABB, 2008). A policy should be developed if rare frozen units are to be retained beyond this time.

Blood that is to be frozen may be collected in CPD or CPDA-1 solutions and stored as whole blood. It can also be stored as packed cells with or without an additive system. Most often, blood is glycerolized and frozen within the first 6 days after donation. Glycerol is added to the cells before freezing because it is a cryoprotective agent that prevents cell dehydration and mechanical damage from ice formation. Although the first 6 days after donation is the usual window in which to freeze blood, red cells nearing the end of their shelf life may be rejuvenated for up to 3 days after expiration and then frozen. PRBCs preserved in adenine-saline solutions may be frozen up to 42 days after donation. These options help eliminate unnecessary waste of valuable blood stores. Frozen blood is maintained at −65° C or colder (Roback et al, 2008).

When a unit of frozen blood is needed, it is first thawed in a water bath (37° C) or a dry warmer (37° C). It is then washed to remove the glycerol, which is hypertonic to the blood. The washing process used to deglycerolize red cells is the same as that used to process washed red cells.

As with 0.9% sodium chloride–washed packed cells, there are concerns for bacterial contamination with frozen-deglycerolized cells. This product must be infused within 24 hours of processing. Also, as is true with washed packed cells, frozen-deglycerolized cells are not considered free from the risk of disease transmission. Clinical applications for frozen-deglycerolized red blood cells are the same as those for washed PRBCs.

Leukocyte-filtered red blood cells

Leukocyte-filtered RBCs, also known as *leukocyte-reduced RBCs*, are indicated for patients who have experienced repeated febrile nonhemolytic reactions associated with the transfusion of red cells or platelets (see discussion under Adverse Effects: Acute Effects). They should also be used as prophylaxis against alloimmunization in selected patients who are expected to receive long-term blood component therapy and for recipients who are at risk for post-transfusion cytomegalovirus (CMV) infection.

Leukocyte-reduced packed cells can be prepared in the blood bank by centrifugation and filtration and by automated 0.9% sodium chloride washing of liquid or previously frozen blood. In the past, frozen and washed packed cells, which have a 95% to 99% reduction in leukocytes, were considered the components of choice when white blood cell reduction was indicated. However, the newer generations of leukocyte filters, which are more efficient in terms of leukocyte reduction and less costly, have made leukocyte-filtered components the products of choice. The cells may be filtered during the initial processing of red cells before storage or during transfusion using an in-line filter (Dzik et al, 2000; Nordmeyer, Forestner, and Wall, 2007; Roback et al, 2008). The AABB *Technical Manual* states that in all clinical applications of leukocyte-reduced products, prestorage leukocyte-filtered components are recommended over those that are filtered during transfusion (Dzik et al, 2000; Nordmeyer et al, 2007; Roback et al, 2008).

Clinical applications for leukocyte-reduced red blood cells include the following:

- Patients with repeated febrile nonhemolytic transfusion reactions
- Patients at risk for HLA alloimmunization who may face hemotherapy
- Patients at risk for post-transfusion CMV infections

GRANULOCYTES

Granulocytes are usually prepared by leukopheresis. This blood component also contains other leukocytes, platelets, and some red cells in 200 to 300 mL of plasma. They should be transfused as soon as possible after collection but may be stored at 20° to 24° C without agitation for up to 24 hours (Roback et al, 2008).

The use of granulocyte transfusion in adults is rare. When this therapy is used, the recipient is usually severely neutropenic with documented infection that is unresponsive to aggressive antibiotic therapy. The candidate for granulocyte transfusion should meet the following three conditions:

1. Neutropenia (granulocyte count less than 500/μL)
2. Fever for 24 to 48 hours, unresponsive to appropriate antibiotic therapy, or bacterial sepsis unresponsive to antibiotics or other modes of therapy
3. Myeloid hypoplasia

In the pediatric population, granulocyte transfusion has been used in conjunction with antibiotic therapy for severe bacterial neonatal sepsis. Although controversy surrounds this choice of therapy, there appear to be clinical situations in which granulocyte transfusion can supplement antibiotics. The AABB (Roback et al, 2008) states that pediatric candidates for granulocyte transfusion are infants with *all* of the following conditions:

- Strong evidence of bacterial septicemia
- An absolute neutrophil count below 3000/μL
- A diminished marrow storage pool

Granulocytes should come from CMV-negative donors because they cannot be given though a leukocyte filter to reduce the risk of CMV transmission. Granulocytes should also be irradiated to reduce the risk of GVHD.

FRESH-FROZEN PLASMA

Fresh-frozen plasma (FFP) is prepared by removing the plasma from a unit of whole blood and freezing it within 6 hours of collection. The storage time for FFP is 1 year at 18° C or colder. This component, if kept frozen and then thawed in a warm water bath (30° to 37° C) just before use, is an excellent source of all clotting factors, including the labile factors V and VIII and fibrinogen. The activity of these labile factors is lost when plasma is stored in the nonfrozen state (Roback, et al, 2008).

FFP is indicated when clotting factors are needed for which a concentrate is not available, in the presence of severe liver disease where limited synthesis of plasma coagulation factors may be suspected, and when needed to counteract the effects of warfarin therapy (Box 14-1).

Box 14-1   CLINICAL APPLICATIONS FOR FRESH-FROZEN PLASMA

- For patients with active bleeding who have multiple coagulation factor deficiencies secondary to liver disease
- For patients with disseminated intravascular coagulation and evidence of demonstrated dilutional coagulopathy from large-volume replacement
- For patients with congenital factor deficiencies for which there are no concentrates (e.g., factors V and XI)
- For warfarin reversal

PLATELET CONCENTRATES

Platelet concentrates can be prepared by two methods: as single units from multiple donors or as multiple units from a single donor.

Multiple donors, single units

To prepare a single unit of platelet concentrate from multiple donors, a donated unit of whole blood that is less than 6 hours old and stored at room temperature is centrifuged to isolate the platelet-rich plasma. The platelet-rich plasma is then centrifuged at 20° C to separate the platelet concentrate from the now platelet-poor plasma. Fifty to seventy milliliters of plasma are allowed to remain with the platelet concentrate. After this second centrifugation, that which remains is a single unit of random-donor platelet suspended in plasma. The plasma will ensure that the platelets are kept at a pH of 6 or higher to maintain their viability during the 5-day storage period at 20° to 24° C.

Single donor, multiple units

Plateletpheresis is the harvesting of multiple units of platelets from a single volunteer donor. The quantity taken from a single donor is equal to approximately 6 units of random-donor platelets. The platelets are harvested by automated machines called *cell separators*. These separators isolate the blood component to be harvested as a concentrate, and those components not needed are returned to the donor.

Although plateletpheresis is an efficient way to obtain platelets, there are two reasons why this method is not used exclusively. First, there are several risks to the donor, including allergic reactions, chills, syncope, and citrate toxicity. The citrate toxicity is related to the anticoagulation of the donor blood, which is necessary before the blood is processed through the cell separator (Klein and Anstee, 2005). This anticoagulation, in varying amounts, is ultimately infused along with the returned components to the donor. The second reason that plateletpheresis is limited in its use is concern over its cost-versus-benefit ratio.

Single-donor platelets were traditionally used for patients who needed repeated platelet infusions and were at risk for alloimmunization to foreign leukocyte antigens (HLAs) present on leukocytes and platelets. Laboratory leukoreduction has made significant improvements in reducing the risk of alloimmunization.

Refractoriness is the state of being inadequately responsive to platelet transfusions. This occurs in about 20% to 70% of multitransfused thrombocytopenic patients and is more likely to be seen in patients being treated for malignant hematopoietic disorders (Roback et al, 2008).

There are both nonimmune reasons and immune-response causes for refractoriness. Some of the nonimmune causes of platelet refractoriness are active bleeding, sepsis, splenomegaly, disseminated intravascular coagulation (DIC), and antibiotic therapy. Of the possible immune-response causes, the presence of antibodies in the recipient to multiple HLAs is the most common precipitating factor. As explained earlier, alloimmunization to HLA is a direct result from previous exposure to white blood cells through transfusions. Therefore it has been recommended that all blood components containing white blood cells that are to be used for recipients requiring long-term transfusion support should be leukocyte reduced by filtration (Dzik et al, 2000). This would limit exposure to foreign HLAs and reduce the risk for alloimmunization and the majority of immune-response refractoriness. When these antibodies are known to be present, one approach is to transfuse multiunit platelets from a single donor.

The most suitable single-donor platelet preparation in cases of known HLA sensitization is the HLA-matched product, obtained by plateletpheresis from a volunteer donor who is HLA-matched to the recipient. Although this is a limited match (the donor and recipient have only some HLA antigens in common), this product is the most appropriate for the patient who has demonstrated unresponsiveness to platelet concentrates. HLA-matched platelets should be irradiated to prevent TA-GVHD (see Adverse Effects later in this chapter).

In addition to the HLA-matching approach to providing platelets in refractoriness, a second option is pretransfusion platelet crossmatching. This approach is predictive and can therefore avoid subsequent platelet transfusion failures. However, platelet crossmatching is not without shortcomings. When 70% or more of the donors are reactive to the recipient, finding enough compatible donors can be a problem (Roback et al, 2008).

TABLE 14-5   Factor VIII Complex

Factor	Activity
VIII:C	Procoagulant
VIII:Ag	Immune reactant antigen
VIII:vWF	von Willebrand's factor: required for normal platelet function

CRYOPRECIPITATE (CRYOPRECIPITATED ANTIHEMOPHILIC FACTOR)

Cryoprecipitate is used to treat hypofibrinogenemia and factor XIII deficiency. Cryoprecipitated antihemophilic factor is prepared by slowly thawing a unit of FFP at 4° to 6° C and then recovering the cold precipitated protein by centrifugation. Once harvested, cryoprecipitate can be refrozen at −18° C or colder and stored for 1 year. This component is a rich source of the entire factor VIII complex, factor XIII, fibronectin, and fibrinogen—and it is the only source of concentrated fibrinogen (Table 14-5) (Box 14-2).

ADMINISTRATION OF BLOOD COMPONENTS

Administering a blood component is the last step in the process of matching a donor component with a recipient. Remembering that the most common causes of fatal transfusion reactions are improperly labeled blood samples, mislabeled component units, and misidentified recipients, it is clear that most fatal transfusion errors are clerical rather than laboratory failures. The transfusionist is the last person in the administration process with the opportunity to note a clerical error. Therefore the transfusionist should be attentive to every detail of the administration procedure and guard against the relaxed approach that so often accompanies familiarity.

Policies and procedures for the administration of blood components vary greatly among providers of this therapy, but their purpose, which is to ensure precision and safety, is universal (Box 14-3). Therefore those who administer transfusion therapy should be knowledgeable of policy and adhere strictly to the procedures embraced by their particular organization or home care provider.

Box 14-2   MAJOR INHERITED COAGULOPATHIES

HEMOPHILIA A (CLASSIC HEMOPHILIA)

This gender-linked inherited disorder is manifested in males but is transmitted by female carriers. The clotting factor deficiency in classic hemophilia is factor VIII:C. Commercial factor VIII concentrates provide factor VIII:C. In the past, cryoprecipitate was used to treat this deficiency. Today, it is used only if commercial virus-inactivated concentrates are unavailable.

VON WILLEBRAND'S DISEASE

This condition, the most common of the inherited coagulopathies (Table 14-6), is not gender linked and affects both sexes. All three of the measurable activities of the factor VIII complex are deficient in von Willebrand's disease. However, it is the deficiency of factor VIII:vWF that is responsible for the capillary defect seen in this coagulopathy. von Willebrand's factor is necessary for normal platelet function, and thus a diminished level of this factor will result in platelet dysfunction characterized by capillary defect.

Mild cases of von Willebrand's disease can be treated with DDAVP (desmopressin acetate), which is a synthetic analog of vasopressin. DDAVP appears to cause the release of endogenous stores of high-molecular-weight von Willebrand's factor from the vascular subendothelium.

More severe cases of this disease are treated with virus-inactivated commercially prepared factor VIII concentrates. Although not all commercial concentrates contain therapeutic levels of vWF, there are a limited number that meet this need. If the appropriate commercially prepared product is unavailable, severe cases may be treated with cryoprecipitate or fresh-frozen plasma. In this situation, cryoprecipitate would be the component of choice because of its higher concentration of vWF.

HYPOFIBRINOGENEMIA

This deficiency may be inherited or acquired as part of the disseminated intravascular coagulation (DIC) syndrome. Cryoprecipitate is the only source currently available with concentrated fibrinogen.

FACTOR XIII DEFICIENCY

This clotting factor is also called the *fibrin stabilizing factor*. A deficiency of this factor leads to bleeding, poor wound healing, and an increased incidence of spontaneous abortion. Intravenous supplementation of factor XIII is accomplished by the use of cryoprecipitate.

TABLE 14-6 Inherited Coagulopathies

Type	Also known as	Factor deficiency
Hemophilia A	Classic hemophilia	VIII:C
Hemophilia B	Christmas disease	IX
von Willebrand's disease	Vascular hemophilia or angiohemophilia	VIII:C VIII:Ag VIII:vWF

Table 14-7 presents a detailed summary of blood components, including their preparation, indications for use, blood type compatibility, administration, and special considerations.

BLOOD COMPONENT THERAPY IN SEVERE SEPSIS AND SEPTIC SHOCK

In 2002 the European Society of Intensive Care Medicine, the International Sepsis Forum, and the Society of Critical Care Medicine collaborated with the aim of improving the diagnosis, survival, and management of patients with severe sepsis or septic shock through a systematic process or bundled model of patient care management. In 2004 this collaborative initiative resulted in the development and publication of the *Surviving Sepsis Campaign: Guidelines for Management of Severe Sepsis and Septic Shock,* inclusive of blood administration (Dellinger et al, 2008). The guidelines are available at the National Guideline Clearinghouse (www.guideline.gov). Refer to the Focus on Evidence box for recommendations for blood administration for severe sepsis.

SPECIAL EQUIPMENT

BLOOD WARMERS

Blood warming during transfusion is recommended in limited situations. Blood can be warmed by any of several commercial instruments that are designed for this purpose. Most of these instruments consist of dry heating blocks or controlled water baths that surround a portion of the infusion administration set downstream from the blood supply and immediately before the infusion site.

Blood warming should not be attempted with uncontrolled measures such as holding the unit of blood under hot water or warming it in a microwave oven. Such severe treatment of the blood cells can result in hemolysis or severe reactions. The AABB states that warming devices must not raise the temperature of the blood to a level that causes hemolysis (Roback et al, 2008). A warning system must be established to detect temperatures that exceed the manufacturers' designated temperature limit. Blood can be warmed safely using a setpoint of 42° C to prevent hemolysis secondary to warming (Smith, 2001).

All blood warmers are designed to help transfer heat. The efficiency of this heat transfer depends on the following factors:
- The temperature of the heating element (flat bed or water bath)
- The surface area of the heating element

Box 14-3   BASIC GUIDELINES FOR BLOOD ADMINISTRATION

- Gloves should be worn when handling blood products.
- Blood should not be out of controlled refrigeration for longer than 30 minutes before being initiated as a transfusion.
- Blood should not be stored in non–blood bank refrigerators because they are subject to vast fluctuations in temperature.
- No intravenous solution other than 0.9% sodium chloride should be added to or administered simultaneously with blood.
- A blood administration set should not be affixed ("piggy-backed") into a main line that has been used for any solution other than 0.9% sodium chloride.
- All blood components must be filtered using in-line or add-on filters that are appropriate for the component or specifically requested by a physician's order.
- A new administration set and filter should be used for each transfusion. A blood filter should not be used for more than 4 hours.

FOCUS ON EVIDENCE

Guidelines for Blood Product Administration in Severe Sepsis

- Once tissue hypoperfusion has resolved and in the absence of extenuating circumstances (e.g., myocardial ischemia, severe hypoxemia, acute hemorrhage, cyanotic heart disease, or lactic acidosis), it is recommended that red blood cell transfusion occur when the hemoglobin level decreases to <7.0 g/dL (<70 g/L) to target a hemoglobin level of 7.0 to 9.0 g/dL (70 to 90 g/L) in adults.
- It is recommended that erythropoietin not be used as a specific treatment of anemia associated with severe sepsis, but may be used when septic patients have other accepted reasons for administration of erythropoietin, such as renal failure–induced compromise of red blood cell production.
- It is recommended that fresh-frozen plasma not be used to correct laboratory clotting abnormalities in the absence of bleeding or planned invasive procedures.
- The guideline committee recommends against antithrombin administration for the treatment of severe sepsis and septic shock.
- In patients with severe sepsis, it is recommended that platelets should be administered when counts are <5000/mm³ (5 × 10⁹/L) regardless of apparent bleeding. Platelet transfusion may also be considered when counts are 5000 to 30,000/mm³ (5 to 30 × 10⁹/L) and there is a significant risk of bleeding. Higher platelet counts (≥50,000/mm³ [50 × 10⁹/L]) are typically required for surgery or invasive procedures.

Dellinger RP et al: Surviving sepsis campaign: international guidelines for management of severe sepsis and septic shock, *Intensive Care Med* 34(1):17-60, 2008.

- The diameter and the surface area of the administration set being used to deliver the blood
- The length of time the blood being infused remains in contact with the heat source

If any of these factors (temperature, surface area, or contact time) are changed, the efficiency of the heat transfer is altered. Therefore, when rapid infusion is necessary, the transfusionist needs to be aware that increasing the infusion rate reduces the time in contact between the blood and the heating element and the efficiency of the heat transfer.

TABLE 14-7 Summary of Blood Components

Component	Preparation/composition	Use/Indications	ABO/Rh compatibility		Administration	Special consideration
Whole blood	RBCs WBCs Plasma Platelets (WBCs, platelets, and some clotting factors not viable after 24 hr of storage)	Increase RBC mass Increase volume	Donor O A B AB Rh+ Rh−	Recipient O A B AB Rh+ Rh−, Rh+	1. Transfuse through a blood filter. 2. Should infuse within 4 hr.	1. One unit of whole blood will increase Hct by 3%; will increase Hgb by 1 g/dL. 2. Availability of packed RBCs has made use of whole blood obsolete in most cases. 3. Never infuse blood with anything except 0.9% sodium chloride.
Red blood cells (RBCs): packed	RBCs WBCs Platelets Minimal plasma	Increase RBC mass and oxygen-carrying capacity	Donor O A B AB Rh+ Rh−	Recipient O, A, B, AB A, AB B, AB AB Rh+ Rh−, Rh+	1. Transfuse through a blood filter. 2. Should infuse within 4 hr.	1. Hct of product is 60-80%. 2. One unit of RBCs will increase Hct by 3%; will increase Hgb by 1 g/dL. 3. Never infuse packed RBCs with anything except 0.9% sodium chloride.
RBCs: leuko-cyte- reduced	RBCs Negligible WBCs Minimal plasma and platelets	Same as packed RBCs plus: to decrease risk for alloimmunization (HLA) and disease transmission (CMV)	Same as packed RBCs		If not processed in blood bank, use in-line or add-on leukocyte-reduction filter.	1. Leukocyte-reduction filter for RBCs is *not* interchangeable with a leukocyte-reduction filter for platelets. 2. Other considerations are same as above for packed RBCs.
RBCs: 0.9% sodium chloride washed	RBCs Minimal WBCs 99% plasma proteins removed No platelets	Same as for packed RBCs plus: Decrease risk for alloimmunization to leukocyte or HLA antigens; however, *not* component of choice for this purpose Reduce incidence of urticarial and anaphylactic reactions to plasma	Same as packed RBCs		Same as packed RBCs	1. Units must be given within 24 hr of 0.9% sodium chloride washing. 2. Never infuse RBCs with any IV fluid or medications except 0.9% sodium chloride. 3. Does contain viable lymphocytes and can induce GVHD.
RBCs: frozen-deglycerolized	Same as washed RBCs	Same as packed RBCs plus: Prolonged blood storage Autologous blood Rare blood types	Same as packed RBCs		Same as packed RBCs	1. Blood may be frozen up to 10 yr. 2. Once blood has been thawed and deglycerolized, it must be transfused within 24 hr.
Fresh-frozen plasma	Plasma with all clotting factors	Treatment of some coagulation disorders Reversal of warfarin in patients who require emergency invasive procedures	Donor O A B AB Rh+ Rh−	Recipient O A, O B, O AB, O, A, B Rh+, Rh− Rh−, Rh+	Transfuse through a blood filter.	1. Must be infused within 24 hr of thawing. 2. May be stored for up to 1 yr at −18° C.

TABLE 14-7 **Summary of Blood Components—cont'd**

Component	Preparation/ composition	Use/Indications	ABO/Rh compatibility	Administration	Special consideration
Platelets: random donor	Platelets Plasma Small numbers of RBCs and WBCs	To control or prevent bleeding associated with deficiencies in platelet number or function Not usually effective in conditions of rapid platelet destruction (e.g., ITP and DIC)	ABO/Rh compatibility is preferred (because of RBCs in product), but not mandatory; an Rh— female in child-bearing years should receive Rh— platelets; if she receives Rh-positive platelets, titers should be monitored and/or consideration given for administration of Rh immune globulin	1. Transfuse through a blood filter. 2. Once individual units are pooled, they should be infused within 6 hr. 3. Concentrates may be infused individually or pooled immediately before administration.	1. Prophylactic pretransfusion medications (e.g., an antihistamine and/ or acetaminophen) may be given to decrease incidence of chills, fever, and allergic reactions. 2. Repeated transfusions may lead to alloimmunization to HLA and other antigens and result in development of a "refractory" state manifested by unresponsiveness to platelet transfusion. 3. A leukocyte-reduction filter for platelets may be used. 4. One unit of platelets should increase platelet count of a 70-kg adult by 5000/μL.
Platelets: apheresed	Platelets (1 unit approximately equivalent to 6 random-donor units) Some RBCs, WBCs, and plasma	Same as random-donor platelets May be used in non-refractory patients to limit multiple random donor exposures, especially in long-term hemotherapy	Same as random-donor platelets	Same as random-donor platelets	1. Prophylactic pretransfusion medications may be given. 2. A leukocyte-reduction filter for platelets may be used.
Platelets: HLA-matched	Same as apheresed platelets but with some donor HLA antigens in common with recipient	Same as random-donor platelets Used for patients who are unresponsive to random-donor platelet concentrates as a result of HLA alloimmunization May be used in patients being considered for future transplant	Same as random-donor platelets	Same as random-donor platelets	1. Prophylactic pretransfusion medications may be given. 2. A leukocyte-reduction filter for platelets may be used. 3. Advance scheduling to obtain HLA-matched platelets is usually required. 4. A blood sample for HLA typing should be done before immunosuppressive therapy is started. Leukopenia can make HLA typing difficult.

(Continued)

TABLE 14-7 Summary of Blood Components—cont'd

Component	Preparation/ composition	Use/Indications	ABO/Rh compatibility		Administration	Special consideration
Granulocytes	Granulocytes, varying amounts of leukocytes, platelets, and some RBCs in 200–300 mL of plasma Should come from CMV-negative donor Should be irradiated	Treatment of patients with severe neutropenia with serious infection unresponsive to antibiotic therapy *Adults*: rarely used *Pediatrics*: some applications	Donor O A B AB Rh+ Rh—	Recipient O, A, B, AB A, AB B, AB AB Rh+ Rh—, Rh+	1. Transfuse through blood filter. 2. Do *not* use leukocyte-reduction filter. 3. Transfuse ASAP after collection.	1. Use of pretransfusion medication strongly urged (e.g., antihistamines, acetaminophen, steroids, meperidine). 2. Prophylactic use is *not* appropriate.
Cryoprecipitate	Factor VIII; von Willebrand's factor; factor XIII; fibrinogen (suspended in plasma and frozen)	Treatment of deficiencies in factor XIII and fibrinogen If factor VIII concentrates unavailable, may be used for hemophilia A and severe von Willebrand's disease	Donor O A B AB Rh+ Rh— Cryoprecipitate contains a small amount of plasma and no RBCs; plasma compatibilities are preferred but not required	Recipient O A, O B, O AB, O, A, B Rh+, Rh— Rh—, Rh+	1. Transfuse through blood filter. 2. May be infused as single units or pooled.	1. 0.9% sodium chloride may need to be added to each bag of cryoprecipitate to facilitate recovery of product. (There are only 10-15 mL of cryo/plasma in each bag.) 2. Cryoprecipitate must be infused within 6 hr of thawing or 4 hr of pooling.
Factor VIII concentrate	Lyophilized concentration of factor VIII, trace amount of other plasma proteins This product is virus inactivated	Factor VIII deficiency (hemophilia A) Some of the newer concentrates can be used in von Willebrand's disease	Not required		1. Quantity of factor VIII present in each vial noted as International Units (IU). 2. Reconstituted with sterile diluent. 3. IV injected using filter needle or given by IV drip using a component recipient set.	1. May be used prophylactically before therapeutic procedures. 2. Risk of transmission of infectious disease is reduced.
Factor IX concentrate	Lyophilized concentration of factor IX; virus inactivated	Factor IX deficiency (hemophilia B), also known as *Christmas disease*	Not required		1. Quantity of factor IX present in each vial noted as activity units. 2. Reconstituted with sterile diluent. 3. IV injected using filter needle or given IV drip using a component recipient set.	1. Risk of transmission of infectious disease is reduced.
Albumin	Available as a 5% or 25% solution.	5% is used for volume expansion when crystalloid solutions are not adequate	Not required		1. 5% solution is isotonic. 2. 25% solution is hypenteric, will increase circulating volume by 3-4 times infused volume. Infuse slowly.	1. Does not transmit viral diseases because of extended heating period during processing.
Immune serum globulin: nonspecific	IgG antibodies	Provide passive immune protection Treatment of immunodeficiency disorders	Not required		May be given IM or IV, but various preparations are route of administration specific.	1. IM injections may be painful. Warm compresses may alleviate discomfort. 2. There is a possibility of hypersensitivity and anaphylactic reactions.

TABLE 14-7 Summary of Blood Components—cont'd

Component	Preparation/ composition	Use/Indications	ABO/Rh compatibility	Administration	Special consideration
Immune serum globulin: Rh immune globulin	IgG anti-D	Administered to Rh− patients who have been exposed to Rh(D) antigens through transfusions or pregnancy May be given antepartum to prevent sensitization to Rh(D) in Rh woman carrying an Rh+ fetus May be given before amniocentesis	Not required	Administered IM	1. Should be given within 72 hr of exposure for maximum effect. 2. IM injections may be painful. Warm compresses may alleviate discomfort. 3. Antepartum administration at 28 weeks.
Immune serum globulin: hepatitis B immune globulin	High titers of hepatitis B antibody	Provides passive immunity following exposure to hepatitis B virus	Not required	Administered IM	1. Should be given as soon as possible after exposure for maximum effect. 2. If given more than 7 days after exposure, its value is questionable. 3. IM injections may be painful. Warm compresses may alleviate discomfort.

CMV, cytomegalovirus; *DIC,* disseminated intravascular coagulation; *GVHD,* graft-versus-host disease; *Hct,* hematocrit; *Hgb,* hemoglobin; *IM,* intramuscular; *ITP,* idiopathic thrombocytopenia; *IV,* intravenous; *WBCs,* white blood cells.

Indications for blood warming

Multiple trauma/massive blood loss

Hypothermia is a serious threat for the patient who has lost large quantities of blood and requires multiple transfusions of refrigerated blood. A decrease in body temperature can precipitate cardiac arrhythmias and cardiac arrest (Klein and Anstee, 2005). Therefore, when large quantities of blood are to be infused very rapidly, blood warming is indicated. This is especially true if the infusion is through a central catheter. However, the present generation of blood warmers has been criticized for slow heat transfer and suboptimal flow rates. This has led to the use of blood warmers that use higher temperatures and positive-pressure-pump administration. An alternative technique, called *rapid admixture,* has been used in emergency departments (Smith, 2001). This technique involves keeping 0.9% sodium chloride intravenous (IV) solution stored in a clinical incubator at 70° C. When needed, the warmed bag of 0.9% sodium chloride (250 mL) is connected directly to the unit of packed cells to be infused, and the 0.9% sodium chloride is squeezed into the blood bag. This warms the blood to 37° C in less than 1 minute.

Cold agglutinin disease

Cold-loving autoantibodies correspond to the carbohydrate antigens I and i, which are found on red blood cells (Ness and Krustall, 2004). Many otherwise normal individuals have some anti-I in their serum, which can be demonstrated when tests are done at 4° C. This antibody, if present, is usually found at low titers and does not cause hemolysis. However, cold agglutinin hemolysis occurs both as a self-limited syndrome in association with certain infectious diseases and as a chronic illness, often without cause. Sometimes, however, it is seen to accompany lymphoma and other reticuloendothelial malignancies. The anti-I titers seen in cases of hemolysis are high, and red cell destruction can occur either extravascularly within the phagocytic cells or intravascularly, leading to hemoglobinemia.

The trigger for the activation of anti-I to bind with the antigen on the red blood cell, and thus cause hemolysis, is exposure to cold temperatures. Therefore recipients of blood transfusion who are known to carry a significant titer of anti-I should be transfused using an in-line blood warmer.

Pediatric application for blood warming

In pediatrics, blood warming should be used for exchange transfusions in infants and for blood infusion rates exceeding 15 mL/kg/hr in children (King, 2008).

SPECIALIZED BLOOD FILTERS

Blood filters are used to eliminate blood clots and cellular debris that occur during storage of the blood component. The size of the particles being filtered out is determined by the micron pore size of the filter. A standard blood filter of 170 microns will trap particles that are 170 microns or larger. However, microaggregates, which consist of degenerating platelets, leukocytes, and fibrin strands, range in size from 20 to 160 microns (Dzik et al, 2000; Roback et al, 2008). Some of these microaggregates, which form in blood after 5 days or more of storage, can pass through standard blood filters without difficulty. Therefore, when it is deemed medically necessary to eliminate debris smaller than 80 to 170 microns, specialized filters have to be used (Dzik et al, 2000).

Microaggregate filters

Microaggregate filters eliminate debris as small as 20 microns. They are used often during large-volume replacement in massive trauma. The use of these specialized filters is not considered warranted in routine transfusion therapy (Dzik et al, 2000; Roback et al, 2008).

Leukocyte-reduction filters

Leukocyte-reduction filters were first developed in Europe in the 1970s. The original filter material was cotton wool, which was later replaced by cellulose acetate fibers. Today, the most widely used leukocyte-reduction filters are of a flatbed, multilayered design and use polyester fibers to form the filter network. This latest generation of prestorage leukocyte-removing filters reliably reduces the number of leukocytes by 99.9% (Dzik et al, 2000; Roback et al, 2008).

One of the reasons for using leukocyte-reduction filters is to circumvent or prevent HLA alloimmunization. The minimum dose of white blood cells capable of stimulating antibody production is unknown. Although using leukocyte-filtered components will not completely eliminate the risk for alloimmunization, the filtered product nonetheless carries the lowest level of residual leukocytes. Another reason for using the filters is to reduce the risk for CMV transmission. Transfusion-associated CMV infections have been linked to the transfused peripheral blood leukocytes in which the virus established latent infection.

Prestorage filtration to reduce leukocytes has been advocated for the following reasons:
- To reduce the risk for transfusion-associated viral disease where the virus is known to have a latent phase in the white blood cells (some herpesviruses and some human T-cell lymphotropic viruses)
- To reduce the risk for febrile and allergic transfusion reactions; during storage, leukocytes degranulate and fragment, releasing substances that promote such reactions (Roback et al, 2008)
- To produce superior-quality packed cells that are leukocyte-reduced and free of microaggregates

 ADVERSE EFFECTS

From the standpoint of disease transmission, blood component therapy has never been safer than it is today. With new technologies in filtration, cell separation, and cell salvaging for autotransfusion, never have so many options been available for hemotherapy, and never has the therapy been used as often as it is today. Widespread use, however, is a double-edged sword. Blood component therapy can deliver great therapeutic benefit, but it is also known to carry significant risks, not all of which are preventable. The balance between risk and benefit should always be weighted toward therapeutic benefit.

The adverse effects of blood transfusion can be classified as immunologic or nonimmunologic, depending on whether the immune system is triggered. These classifications may be further divided into categories of acute and delayed effects. Acute effects are those that happen within the first 24 hours of transfusion. Delayed effects are those that appear beyond the acute time frame.

ACUTE EFFECTS

Acute adverse effects of blood transfusion can be immunologic or nonimmunologic (Table 14-8).

Immunologic classification

Intravascular hemolysis

The cause of intravascular hemolysis, a potentially fatal reaction, is ABO incompatibility. Because mortality has been associated with intravascular hemolysis, rapid recognition and immediate intervention can avoid the need for dialysis in the face of renal failure.

Improved compatibility testing and technology that identifies and links donated blood with laboratory test results and the intended recipient have dramatically reduced the risk of acute hemolytic hemolysis; however, it has not been eliminated. Acute hemolytic transfusion reactions and related mortality are now estimated at approximately 1 in 76,000 and 1 in 1.8 million units transfused, respectively (King, 2008). In the most recent analysis of transfusion-related deaths reported by the Food and Drug Administration (FDA), 7% were attributed to ABO-associated hemolytic reactions and an additional 20% to non-ABO antibodies. It cannot be overstated that every step of policy and procedure for identifying blood samples, recipients, and donor components for transfusion should be taken with strict attention to detail. Extra steps should be taken if a hemolytic reaction is suspected (Box 14-4) (Roback et al, 2008).

Extravascular hemolysis

Extravascular hemolysis is caused by the presence of antibodies to blood group systems other than ABO, such as Rh, Kidd, Kell, or Duffy. These antibodies do not cause immediate hemolysis within the vascular tree, but they bind with the corresponding antigen-carrying red cells. These cells are then seen as "defective" by the body and are destroyed extravascularly. This hemolysis is not as rapid as that seen in ABO incompatibility, and the symptoms are usually less dramatic. The post-transfusion direct antiglobulin test will be positive because the red cells are coated with antibodies in vivo.

Febrile nonhemolytic reaction

A *febrile nonhemolytic (FNH) reaction* is a temperature rise of 1° C or more occurring in association with transfusion and without any other explanation (Roback et al, 2008). A common cause for this event is an antigen-antibody response involving HLA antigens on donor white cells in conflict with antibodies in the recipient. The outward appearance of this reaction, which can include significant temperature increases often accompanied with rigors, can be dramatic and unnerving to the blood recipient. However, the signs and symptoms of this reaction are usually self-limiting.

FNH reactions usually are seen in recipients who have a history of multiple transfusions or multiple pregnancies and who have developed a significant HLA antibody titer. For

TABLE 14-8 Acute Adverse Effects

Reaction/complication	Etiology	Signs and symptoms	Treatment
Immunologic Response			
Intravascular hemolysis	ABO incompatibility, red cell infusion	Fever Low back pain Pain at IV site Hypotension Renal failure	Support blood pressure Maintain urine output Dialyze for renal failure
Extravascular hemolysis	Non-ABO incompatibility (e.g., Rh, Kidd, Kell)	Fever Anemia Increased bilirubin Positive DAT	Geared to symptomatology, which can resemble intravascular hemolysis, but seldom as severe
Febrile nonhemolytic (FNH)	Antibody to donor leukocytes	Fever Chills Rigors	Antipyretics With history of FNH: pretreat with antipyretics
Transfusion-related acute lung injury (TRALI)	Anti-HLA antibodies, neutrophil antibodies	Acute respiratory insufficiency Chills Fever Cyanosis Hypotension	Respiratory support IV steroids
Urticaric/allergic	Antibodies against foreign plasma protein	Urticaria	Oral or intramuscular antihistamines Temporarily stop infusion and resume after resolution of symptoms
Secondary response: anaphylaxis	Antibody to donor plasma, usually anti-IgA	Flushing Dyspnea Hypotension	Blood pressure support (low-dose dopamine) Epinephrine
Nonimmunologic Response			
Bacterial contamination	Most severe: gram-negative psychrophilic organisms (endotoxin-producing)	Fever Shock DIC Renal failure	High-dose antibiotics Blood pressure support Steroids

*DAT, direct antiglobulin test; DIC, disseminated intravascular coagulation; IV, intravenous.

Box 14-4   IF HEMOLYTIC REACTION IS SUSPECTED

- STOP THE TRANSFUSION. Take down the blood and all administration sets involved. Attach a new container of 0.9% sodium chloride (using all new administration equipment) to the IV catheter and keep the IV open.
- Notify the physician and the blood bank immediately.
- Check the blood bag compatibility tag, label, and patient identification for clerical errors.
- Send anticoagulated and clotted blood samples, a blood transfusion reaction form (if applicable), and the blood bag to the blood bank. The blood bank may also request a fresh urine sample.
- The physician may order blood urea nitrogen, creatinine, and coagulation studies.

individuals who have experienced two or more of these reactions, leukocyte-filtered products should be considered for future transfusions.

Transfusion-related acute lung injury

Transfusion-related acute lung injury (TRALI) has been estimated to occur after approximately 1 in every 5000 blood component transfusions. Mortality has been reported as high

as 15%. A record review of recipients of blood from an implicated donor indicates that TRALI remains underdiagnosed, especially in the intensive care setting (Goldman et al, 2005; Nordmeyer et al, 2007; Alter and Klein, 2008). Despite its increasing recognition, much about transfusion-related acute lung injury and its pathogenicity remains poorly understood. It is an uncommon complication of allogenic blood transfusion and considered to be the second or third leading cause of death related to transfusion. The U.S. code of federal regulations requires that the Food and Drug Administration (FDA) be informed when a transfusion is considered to be fatal. In cases reported to the FDA between 2001 and 2003, TRALI was the leading cause of transfusion fatalities in the average of all key cases reported and accounted for 16.3% of transfusion deaths (Goldman et al, 2005; Nordmeyer et al, 2007; Alter and Klein, 2008). Pulmonary symptoms, including anaphylactic and allergic reactions as well as circulatory overload, hemolytic transfusion reactions, and bacterial contamination, typically manifest within 6 hours and most often within 1 to 2 hours of the transfusion of a plasma-containing blood product (Roback et al, 2008). TRALI is caused by acquired leukocyte antibodies (anti-HLA or neutrophil antibodies). The offending antibodies can be found in the donor plasma, and the donor group with the highest potential for harboring these leukocyte antibodies is multiparous women. There appear to be two mechanisms by which this immune response precipitates symptoms of acute respiratory insufficiency disproportionate to the volume of blood infused and without evidence of heart failure:

1. The leukocyte antigen-antibody reaction produces white cell aggregates large enough to be trapped in the pulmonary microvasculature, producing transient changes in vascular permeability with resultant pulmonary edema (Roback et al, 2008).
2. The immune response may activate complement, which ultimately leads to the release of histamine and serotonin. Both histamine and serotonin, which participate in smooth muscle constriction and increased vascular permeability, could be active contributors to respiratory distress and pulmonary edema.

A lack of understanding of TRALI can lead to misdiagnosis and underreporting of the condition. TRALI may be misidentified as circulatory overload and non–transfusion-related acute respiratory distress syndrome (ARDS), or in less severe cases febrile or allergic reactions. All patients with TRALI require supplemental oxygen and more than 70% require mechanical ventilation. Most cases resolve within 4 days of transfusion, and 90% of all patients recover (AABB, 2008; Roback et al, 2008). The application of consistent transfusion guidelines may decrease unnecessary transfusions. Additionally, many investigators, transfusion medicine professionals, and the AABB advocate temporary disqualification of donors implicated in TRALI reactions until leukocyte antibody testing can be performed. Efforts to further define the effects of TRALI are needed, so that clinicians can accurately diagnosis and treat this life-threatening syndrome (see Table 14-8 for the signs, symptoms, and appropriate interventions).

Urticaria

Urticaria, an acute hypersensitivity reaction, is usually seen after a transfusion with plasma or with blood components that are accompanied by a large volume of plasma (whole blood or platelet concentrates). The cause of this reaction is thought to be a foreign plasma protein to which the recipient responds with an allergic display.

If the signs and symptoms do not broaden beyond simple urticaria, the physician may opt to interrupt the transfusion long enough to administer an antihistamine by IV injection, wait for the symptoms to recede, and proceed slowly with the transfusion. If a patient has a history of multiple allergic reactions to transfusions, pretreatment with an antihistamine may be appropriate.

Anaphylaxis

Anaphylaxis, the secondary or anamnestic response, almost always occurs in individuals who have been sensitized (carry an antibody titer) to a foreign protein. The anaphylactic reaction occurs quickly and can proceed to life-threatening shock. The following features of the anaphylactic reaction distinguish it from other acute responses:

- Occurs after the infusion of only a few milliliters of blood or plasma
- Occurs in the absence of fever

The array of symptoms that may accompany the secondary response includes respiratory distress, bronchospasm, abdominal cramps, nausea, vomiting, diarrhea, shock, and loss of consciousness (Roback et al, 2008).

Some of these reactions occur in IgA-deficient recipients who, through previous transfusion or pregnancy, have developed an anti-IgA titer. When these individuals are given blood products that contain IgA, the secondary response may be precipitated.

It is possible to obtain blood components from donors who are IgA deficient. Most authorities recommend that these components be reserved for individuals in whom anti-IgA has been identified and who have had previous documented anaphylactic reactions (Roback et al, 2008). If IgA-deficient donor blood is unavailable, frozen-deglycerolized or washed cells may be used.

Nonimmunologic classification

Marked fever with shock

Marked fever with shock is caused by bacterial contamination of donated blood, which can occur at any time during harvesting and processing. Mesophilic (warm-loving) organisms proliferate best in components that are stored at room temperature, whereas psychrophiles (cold-loving) multiply best in refrigerator temperatures. Gram-negative psychrophiles are responsible for the most clinically dramatic and life-threatening septicemic transfusion reactions. These severe reactions are characterized by high fevers, hypotension, DIC, and renal failure. Averting a fatal outcome requires that these reactions receive immediate intervention with high-dose IV antibiotics combined with treatment for shock.

Nonimmune hemolysis

Most cases of nonimmune hemolysis are related to improper handling of the blood product during processing, storage, or administration. Nonimmune hemolysis can result from the following:

- Red cell exposure to nonisotonic IV solutions
- Improper storage such as nonglycerolized freezing or overheating

Mechanical stress resulting from the following:

- Less-than-adequate gauge of the infusion catheter
- Roller pump for infusion (cardiac bypass)
- Improperly set pressure (psi) on the infusion pump
- Improperly inflated or positioned blood bag pressure cuff

Miscellaneous adverse effects
Circulatory overload

Post-transfusion congestive heart failure usually is seen in individuals who are already cardiac or pulmonary decompensated. However, high infusion rates or large-volume replacement can precipitate decompensation in those who are borderline unstable.

Hypothermia

Hypothermia is seen with rapid infusion of large volumes of refrigerated blood and can result in cardiac arrest (see Blood Warmers under Specialized Equipment).

Citrate overload (hypocalcemia)

Citrate is metabolized by the liver, and blood recipients with liver impairment may be unable to handle the high citrate load that accompanies large-volume transfusion. As the plasma level of citrate rises, it binds with free calcium and a secondary hypocalcemia results. Depending on the severity of the calcium deficit, the calcium may be replaced by oral supplement or intravenous infusion.

DELAYED EFFECTS

Immunologic classification

Transfusion-associated graft-versus-host disease (TA-GVHD)

A well-recognized but rare complication of transfusion therapy is transfusion-associated graft-versus-host disease (TA-GVHD). It is most often caused by the infusion of immunocompetent lymphocytes into a severely immunosuppressed recipient. Historically, patients who have been viewed at highest risk for TA-GVHD are those whose immune systems are suppressed for one of the following reasons:

- Congenital immunodeficiency
- HIV infection
- Premature birth
- Immune suppression secondary to aggressive chemotherapy or radiation therapy in ongoing cancer treatments, or intentional immune suppression in transplantation

Once infused, the immunocompetent lymphocytes engraft, multiply, and turn against the "foreign tissues" of the recipient-host. The resulting clinical picture of this immune response is dramatic, including fever, hepatitis, bone marrow suppression, and overwhelming infection progressing to an often fatal outcome. TA-GVHD has a 90% to 100% mortality rate.

TA-GVHD can be prevented by pretransfusion irradiation of all blood products containing lymphocytes. This radiation does not kill the donor lymphocytes, but it renders them incapable of replication in the recipient and thus eliminates an essential step in the graft-versus-host response.

When irradiation of red blood cells is indicated, it is usually carried out as close to the time of transfusion as possible. Any unit of cells that is properly typed and crossmatched to the recipient is appropriate for this purpose, without regard for its length of time in storage. Mature red blood cells are seen as relatively resistant to radiation damage.

Prestorage irradiation of packed cells has never been seen as optimal but has been recognized as necessary in situations in which immediate pretransfusion irradiation is not an option. There are two ways to accomplish the irradiation of PRBCs and their subsequent storage to meet the need for delayed infusion:

1. The cells can be irradiated and stored in their liquid state at 4° C. This preparation expires on the original expiration date for the component or 28 days from the date of irradiation, whichever comes first.
2. The red cells may be irradiated immediately after donation, stored in the liquid state for up to 6 days, and then frozen for future use.

A number of cases of TA-GVHD have been recognized in immunocompetent patients who received directed-donation transfusions from blood relatives. The cause of this immune response seems to be in the similar genetics shared by the donor and recipient. The donor lymphocytes are sufficiently similar not to be recognized as "foreign" by the recipient. However, with engraftment and proliferation of these donor cells, which are sufficiently dissimilar not to recognize the recipient as "self," the immune system is triggered and the natural cascade of events leads to the graft-versus-host response. For this reason, the AABB recommends the irradiation of all donations from blood relatives.

The AABB's *Standards for Blood Banks and Transfusion Services* recommends irradiation of cellular components in the following situations:

- For patients identified as at risk for TA-GVHD
- Transfusion of HLA-selected products
- Transfusion of cellular components between blood relatives

Post-transfusion thrombocytopenic purpura

Post-transfusion thrombocytopenic purpura is a rare event related to a platelet-specific antibody. It is seen almost exclusively in multiparous women. The development of this antibody is most likely a result of sensitization during pregnancy of an antigen-negative woman, producing a discernible antibody titer. This entity can also be seen in men and women who were sensitized by previous transfusion. Regardless of the method of sensitization, post-transfusion purpura is not common; 98% of the population carries the antigen, leaving only 2% of the population at risk (Roback et al, 2008).

When an antibody-positive individual is transfused with antigen-positive platelets, the donor platelets will be destroyed. In some recipients, their own antigen-negative platelets will also be destroyed, leading to a clinical picture of severe thrombocytopenia. Although this condition is usually self-limiting, it can be severe enough to warrant exchange plasmapheresis and/or treatment with intravenous immunoglobulin. Continued infusion of platelets appears to be an ineffective treatment because the transfused platelets are destroyed as rapidly as they are given. Following recovery, the AABB recommends that future transfusions be done with washed PRBCs or with components from antigen-negative donors (Roback et al, 2008).

Nonimmunologic classification

Transmitted disease

In the United States approximately 14 million units of whole blood are donated each year. The responsibility for ensuring the safety of each unit is left up to the more than 3000 blood collection centers, which collect and process each unit. The Food and Drug Administration ensures those 3.5 million patients who receive a blood transfusion each year are protected by a series of safeguards.

Diseases transmitted through blood transfusion are not limited to those with a viral cause, although viruses seem to be the center of attention. Diseases caused by bacteria and protozoa are also transmitted by transfusion.

Bacterial infection

Bacterial contamination of a donated unit of blood can have several causes: (1) preexisting donor infection, (2) contamination during the phlebotomy procedure, or (3) contamination during processing.

An opportunity for contamination exists during the acquisition of the donor unit. A small percentage of percutaneously acquired blood samples are contaminated, primarily with components of the normal skin flora. These organisms belong to a group called *mesophiles,* which have an optimal growth temperature range of 30° to 44° C. They do not survive refrigerator temperatures (4° to 6° C) well and are therefore not associated with post-transfusion bacteremias traceable to refrigerated components.

Platelets that are stored at room temperature pose a higher risk for harboring and transmitting mesophiles. Although few in number, cases of post-transfusion septicemia resulting from platelet concentrates that have been contaminated with normal skin flora have been documented. *Staphylococcus epidermidis* and diphtheroid bacilli are the most common isolates from platelet concentrates, but many other organisms have been linked to post-platelet transfusion septic incidents. However, bacterial counts are usually low in the contaminated units, and clinically recognized septicemia from platelet transfusion is rare.

Psychrophiles are the opposite of mesophiles. Psychrophiles have optimal growth temperature around 29° C. However, they can tolerate low temperatures and will proliferate at a substantial rate even at 0° C. Psychrophilic organisms, which are primarily pseudomonads, present a challenge to blood banks and transfusion therapists. In addition to their ability to survive refrigerator temperatures, pseudomonads can use citrate as their carbon source. The combination of the citrate-based anticoagulant-preservative system and the refrigerator temperatures under which blood is stored provides a suitable environment for these gram-negative organisms to flourish.

Transfusion-associated gram-negative sepsis, although extremely rare, has a potentially fatal outcome. The rapidly progressing clinical picture demands immediate intervention and symptoms usually include high fever, shock, DIC, and renal failure. Treatment may include high-dose antibiotics and therapy to combat shock.

Syphilis. At one time, syphilis was a notable post-transfusion complication as it is bloodborne and sexually transmitted. However, syphilis is now rarely seen secondary to blood transfusion, for the following two reasons:

1. All donated units are serologically tested for syphilis (mandated by FDA).
2. *Treponema pallidum* is not likely to survive temperatures of 4° to 6° C for more than 72 hours.

Protozoal infection

Malaria. There are four species of malarial plasmodia in humans: *Plasmodium vivax, P. ovule, P. malariae,* and *P. falciparum.* The clinical presentation of the diseases produced and the incubation periods differ by species. However, all share a life cycle stage in which the parasites reside within the host erythrocytes. During this erythrocyte cycle, the disease can be transmitted through blood transfusion.

Malaria parasites survive for at least 1 week at room temperature or at 4° C. They can survive cryopreservation with glycerol and subsequent thawing. Any component that contains red cells can transmit infection (Roback et al, 2008).

The known source of post-transfusion malaria is asymptomatic carriers who donate blood. Because there is no practical screening test to identify such donors, deferral of prospective donors is based on their medical and travel histories (Roback et al, 2008). The AABB's *Standards for Blood Banks and Transfusion Services* defers donation of red cells from persons who have had malaria in the preceding 3 years. Casual travelers to areas in which malaria is endemic are deferred for 1 year (AABB, 2008). The occurrence of post-transfusion malaria in the United States is estimated to be 1 in 4 million transfused units (Roback et al, 2008).

Babesiosis. As with malaria, the causative agent of babesiosis is a protozoan, *Babesia microti.* This parasite, which is found mostly on the northeast coast of the United States with a concentration on Cape Cod and the islands of Massachusetts, has the northern deer tick as its vector. The clinical picture resulting from this infection can range from the mild febrile event seen in most cases, to a severe and even fatal outcome, which has occurred when the infection is superimposed on immunosuppression or splenectomy.

Although not common, babesiosis can be transmitted via blood transfusion for the following three reasons:

1. *Babesia microti* has an intraerythrocytic phase in its life cycle.
2. The parasite can survive up to 35 days at 4° C.
3. An individual infected with this parasite can be asymptomatic and donate blood.

Symptoms of transfusion-transmitted babesiosis are often so mild that the true nature of the infection goes undiagnosed; this may explain the small number of cases in the United States. Persons with a history of babesiosis are indefinitely deferred from donating blood because lifelong parasitemia can follow recovery from symptomatic disease. No screening test to detect asymptomatic carriers is currently available for the *Babesia* species.

Chagas' disease. Chagas' disease—or American trypanosomiasis—is a life-threatening cardiac disease endemic to South and Central America. The agent of Chagas' disease is the protozoan *Trypanosoma cruzi,* which is a flagellate transmitted by blood-sucking insects. This parasite invades the macrophages of the host and spreads throughout the body. A small percentage of those infected develop symptoms of an acute illness, but most infected individuals remain asymptomatic. Chagas' disease is considered life-threatening throughout its three phases: acute, latent, and chronic. In the acute phase, mortality is most often secondary to congestive heart failure. In the chronic phase, death is often a result of lethal arrhythmias.

The characteristic of Chagas' disease that makes it a concern for transmission by blood transfusion is its high incidence of asymptomatic infection. This disturbing lack of symptoms is true during the acute and latent phases of the illness. There are screening tests for the antibody to *T. cruzi;* however, posttransfusion Chagas' disease is rare in the United States.

Viral infections

The identification of HIV and the recognition of its impact on hemotherapy have renewed interest in post-transfusion disease of viral cause. The three virus groups of greatest concern in blood component therapy are the primary hepatic viruses, herpesviruses, and human T-cell lymphotropic viruses.

Primary hepatic viruses. The Public Health Service has recommended an approach to blood safety in the United States. U.S. blood donations have been screened for antibodies to HIV-1 since March 1985 and HIV-2 since June 1992. In 1996 the p24 antigen test was added. Blood and blood products that test positive for HIV are safely discarded and are not used for transfusions. At present, transfusion-associated hepatitis incidence is so low that it has to be mathematically modeled, and the risk of hepatitis C is calculated to be 1 case in every 1.5 million to 2 million exposures, a remarkable incidence compared with the 30% rate that prevailed in 1970 and the 10% rate in 1980 (Stillman and McLaughlin, 2006).

The hepatitis virus family consists of six identified human pathogens: hepatitis A, hepatitis B (HBV), hepatitis C (HCV), hepatitis D (or delta agent), hepatitis E, and hepatitis G. Of these, only HBV and HCV are associated with posttransfusion disease. With stringent procedures and more restrictive policies regarding blood donation, the estimated current risk of posttransfusion for HBV and HCV is 1:220,000 units and 1:1,800,00 units, respectively (Roback et al, 2008).

HBV belongs to a group of viral agents called the *hepadnaviruses,* which are DNA viruses that attack liver cells. This intact virion has three areas of antigenic capability: (1) hepatitis B surface antigen, which is incorporated into the outer shell or envelope; (2) hepatitis B core antigen, which is the protein of the nucleocapsid; and (3) the poorly understood hepatitis B core-related antigen, which is thought to be part of the virion core. The host response to each of the hepatitis B antigens is to produce distinct antibodies to each.

An estimated 70,000 to 80,000 people are infected with HBV every year in the United States. Most of those infections are in young people with behavioral risk factors. The chronically infected asymptomatic carrier of HBV is of concern in blood banking. Healthy-appearing individuals can be infected with and infectious for HBV. However, posttransfusion hepatitis B, which was once a common and greatly feared event with potentially fatal consequences, has been significantly reduced because of advancements in screening technology for detecting infectious donors. However, transfusion-related hepatitis B has not been eliminated (Stillman and McLaughlin, 2006).

HCV infection usually presents a significantly less dramatic clinical picture than HBV. Many HCV infections are detected only through liver function studies. Most individuals infected with HCV become chronic carriers, with approximately 85% having persistent serologic evidence of the presence of the virus for years. At least 50% of these carriers have evidence of liver disease, but most HCV-infected individuals remain asymptomatic (Roback et al, 2008). As with hepatitis B infection, the asymptomatic chronic carrier is the primary concern in blood banking. HCV is responsible for 90% to 95% of all transfusion-related hepatitis (Stillman and McLaughlin, 2006).

Routine screening for the antibody to hepatitis C (anti-HCV) began in 1990 for all donated bloods.

Herpesviruses. The human herpesvirus family includes herpes simplex 1 and 2, varicella-zoster virus, CMV, and Epstein-Barr virus. All members of this family are known to establish latent infection with the potential for reactivation after varying periods of time. The ability to establish latency categorizes the herpesviruses as persistent infections. The ability to establish persistence is the hallmark of most transfusion-transmitted viruses. However, although all members of this virus family show persistence, not all members are a risk for post-transfusion infection. The only herpesvirus of significant concern in transfusion therapy is cytomegalovirus (CMV).

CMV has worldwide distribution. The prevalence of anti-CMV ranges from 50% to 80% among healthy blood donors in the U.S. population (AABB, 2008; Roback et al, 2008) Although most people infected with CMV are asymptomatic, this virus is known to be a common cause of congenital viral infection, an etiologic agent for a mononucleosis-like syndrome, and a significant pathogen in bone marrow, liver, and heart transplantation patients.

CMV is one of the infectious agents most often transmitted by blood transfusion. This is probably attributable to the fact that prospective blood donors can be infected with CMV and be infectious without knowing it. This lack of awareness is explained by the following facts about CMV:

- CMV infections, both primary and recurrent, are largely asymptomatic.
- Viremia occurs in both primary and recurrent infections.
- Most importantly, sites of latency for CMV include one or more of the peripheral blood leukocytes.

Despite CMV's high potential for involvement in post-transfusion infection, the transfusion of blood from a sero-positive donor to a seronegative recipient does not result in an automatic post-transfusion infection. Studies of the transmissibility of CMV by blood transfusion consistently show that only some seropositive donors transmit the virus. Although approximately 50% of blood donors can be expected to be CMV seropositive, it is estimated that less than 1% of seropositive cellular components are able to transmit the virus (Roback et al, 2008; Snyder et al, 2008).

Asymptomatic infection with no known sequelae is the outcome of most transfusion-associated CMV infections. Therefore blood with a reduced risk for transmitting CMV is not necessary in the immunocompetent recipient, with one exception. Because cytomegalovirus can be transmitted perinatally, a seronegative expectant mother requiring a transfusion should be given CMV-negative blood (Roback et al, 2008). Infants infected with CMV in utero may develop a variety of congenital abnormalities, including deafness and mental retardation.

The immunocompromised individual is at much greater risk for significant morbidity and even mortality from transfusion-associated CMV infection. Recipients who should be protected from the risk of CMV transmission include the following (Roback et al, 2008):

- Low-birth-weight premature infants born to a seronegative mother
- Seronegative recipients of any organ transplant, including bone marrow, from a seronegative donor
- Recipients of intrauterine transfusions
- Seronegative individuals who are candidates for autologous or allogenic marrow transplant

Blood components appropriate for transfusion to those at risk for post-transfusion CMV infection include blood and blood components from CMV-negative donors and leukocyte-filtered cellular blood components.

Human T-cell lymphotropic viruses. Human T-cell lymphotropic viruses (HTLVs) are retroviruses and can cause persistent, permanent infection. Because they appear to target the T-lymphocyte, they are candidates for transmission by blood transfusion even when latent.

HTLV type I (HTLV-I) was the first of this virus family to be identified. It was isolated by Robert Gallo and associates in 1978 from an American man with T-cell leukemia, and it was the first human retrovirus found to have a causal association with a malignant disease, adult T-cell lymphoma-leukemia (Sayers, 1996). In addition, HTLV-I is associated with the neurological condition HTLV-associated myelopathy (HAM), also referred to as *tropical spastic paraparesis*. This condition occurs in a small minority of persons harboring the virus (often above 1%) (Roback et al, 2008).

Donor screening for anti-HTLV-I in the United States began in 1988. At that time, the confirmed rate of positive tests was approximately 1 in 5000 units collected. A tenfold reduction in that rate has occurred since screening began and seropositive donors have been eliminated from the donor pool (AABB, 2008).

HTLV type II was isolated in 1982 from a man with hairy cell leukemia. However, no causal relationship to that disease has ever been established. HTLV-II has a strong genetic sequence resemblance to HTLV-I (Sayers, 1996; Roback et al, 2008); antibodies to both show marked cross-reactivity in tests with viral lysates (Roback et al, 2008). The only disease associated with HTLV-II is HAM, which is more often associated with HTLV-I (Schreiber et al, 1996; Roback et al, 2008).

For both HTLV-I and HTLV-II, infection and seropositivity are lifelong. However, infection does not present as an acute event, and with the exception of the development of adult

T-cell lymphoma-leukemia or HAM, most infected individuals are unaware of the infection (Roback et al, 2008). The current combined risk for transfusion-transmitted HTLV-I/II infection is approximately 1:2,993,000 units of blood (AABB, 2008; Roback et al, 2008).

Human immunodeficiency viruses. HIV type 1 (HIV-1) and HIV type 2 (HIV-2) are the causative agents of AIDS. AIDS was recognized in 1981, and its causative organism was isolated in 1983 to 1984. The French group that claimed to have discovered this virus called it *lymphadenopathy I,* and the American group that made the same claim called it *human T-cell lymphotropic virus III* (HTLV-III). In the spring of 1985, routine testing for the antibody to HTLV-III was begun on all blood donations. In 1986 an international committee recommended the common name of human immunodeficiency virus. The subsequent discoveries of at least two types and multiple subtypes of HIV led to the current classification system of human immunodeficiency viruses.

HIV-2, which was isolated in 1985, was found to be endemic in many countries of West Africa but seldom seen elsewhere (Murphy et al, 1997; Roback et al, 2008). The first case of HIV-2 infection seen in the United States was in 1988 in a recent immigrant from West Africa. The diseases caused by HIV-1 and HIV-2 are very similar. However, HIV-2 appears to have a longer incubation period and a lower incidence of progression to AIDS (Busch, 2008). In 1991 the combination antibody tests for HIV-1/HIV-2 were instituted in the U.S., providing a better surveillance of HIV-2.

AABB's *Standards for Blood Banks and Transfusion Services* (AABB, 2008) requires that all units of blood and components be nonreactive for anti-HIV-1, HIV-2, HIV-1, and RNA1 before they are issued for transfusion. Since the implementation of donor screening, only 49 transfusion-associated cases have been identified, primarily from window period donations before the introduction of nucleic acid screening tests for HIV RNA in 2000. No cases have been attributed to clotting factor concentrates after the introduction of virocidal treatments in the early 1980s. The current risk of transfusion-transmitted HIV is estimated to be 1 case per 2.3 million transfusions (Roback et al, 2008).

▌AUTOLOGOUS BLOOD TRANSFUSION

Autologous blood transfusion (also known as *autotransfusion*) is the collection and reinfusion of the patient's own blood for the purpose of intravascular volume replacement (O'Brien, George, and Holmberg, 1992). This procedure's historical roots can be traced to 1818, when an Englishman, James Blundell, salvaged vaginal blood from patients with postpartum hemorrhage. By swabbing the blood from the bleeding site and rinsing the swabs with 0.9% sodium chloride, he found that he could reinfuse the result of the washings. This unsophisticated method resulted in a 75% mortality rate but marked the start of autologous blood transfusion (Martine, Harris, and Johnson, 1989). In the early 1900s, others tried autotransfusion (during limb amputation, ruptured ectopic pregnancies, splenectomies, and neurosurgery) with varying degrees of success. The interest in autotransfusion dwindled during World War II because there was a large pool of donors. After the war, blood testing, typing, and crossmatching techniques were improved, making blood banks the answer

---

Box 14-5	ADVANTAGES OF AUTOLOGOUS BLOOD TRANSFUSION

- Reassures patients concerned about blood risk
- Prevents transfusion-transmitted disease
- Prevents red cell alloimmunization
- Provides compatible blood for those with alloantibodies
- Supplements the blood supply
- Prevents some adverse transfusion reactions

---

to the increased demand for blood (Martine et al, 1989). In 1970 Klebanoff brought modern credibility to the concept of autotransfusion with his report of a roller pump system for retrieving blood, a system that was used successfully in Vietnam (Nicholson, 1988).

The National Blood Policy, published in 1974, provided for the increased use of autotransfusion throughout the country. Its four goals were to maintain the following: (1) an adequate blood supply; (2) availability of blood to all people; (3) efficient utilization of blood; and (4) the highest standards of transfusion therapy with the safest blood (Martine et al, 1989).

In response to increasing public and professional awareness and concern about potential infectious disease complications of homologous blood transfusion, interest in alternative transfusion programs increased in the early 1980s (Peterson, 1992). Autologous blood represents the safest possible blood for transfusion (Box 14-5).

There are four categories of autotransfusion available: (1) preoperative autologous blood donation, (2) perioperative isovolemic (normovolemic) hemodilution, (3) intraoperative cell salvage, and (4) postoperative blood salvage.

PREOPERATIVE AUTOLOGOUS BLOOD DONATION

The most widely available autologous option is the preoperative collection, storage, and reinfusion of donated blood, sometimes referred to as *predeposit donation.* Patients scheduled for elective surgical procedures who anticipate the need for blood replacement should be considered candidates for this option.

The ideal donor-patient is in good health, is afebrile, and has 4 to 6 weeks until surgery. The hemoglobin concentration should be no less than 110 g/L (11 g/dL). The packed cell volume, if substituted, should be no less than 0.33 (33%) (Dzik et al, 2000). Patients with active infection or who may be bacteremic are not eligible because bacteria may proliferate while collected blood is stored.

An important aspect of patient management for those participating in predeposit programs is iron replacement. The requesting physician should prescribe supplemental iron as soon as surgery is scheduled. Insufficient iron is often the limiting factor in collecting multiple units of blood over a short time (Roback et al, 2008).

The preferred phlebotomy schedule is weekly, with the last unit drawn no less than 72 hours before surgery. The amount of blood harvested at each session is determined by the donor's age, weight, and medical history. The donated blood is usually stored in the liquid state at 1° to 6° C for 35 to 42 days, depending on the anticoagulant-preservative system used. If a longer storage period is necessary, the blood may be frozen. In addition, autologous blood that has not been frozen at the time of donation can be rejuvenated and subsequently frozen when it reaches its expiration date. This practice prevents autologous blood from being discarded when surgery is delayed.

The FDA requires testing of all autologous donations for syphilis, HIV-1 antigen, HIV-2 antibodies, antibodies to hepatitis C, hepatitis B surface antigen, and hepatitis B core antibody. Because autologous donors may not meet the strict requirements for allogenic donors, the donated autologous units are discarded if they are not used by the donor (Roback et al, 2008). The AABB's *Standards for Blood Banks and Transfusion Services* requires that the use of autologous blood be reserved for use of the donor (AABB, 2008).

PERIOPERATIVE ISOVOLEMIC (NORMOVOLEMIC) HEMODILUTION

Hemodilution is an option for patients who can tolerate rapid withdrawal of blood before surgery. This procedure involves collecting up to 2 L of blood in CPD or CPDA-1 immediately before surgery, usually after anesthesia has been induced, and replacing the blood with a sufficient volume of crystalloid or colloid solution to attain normovolemic hemodilution. The blood collected at the start of the procedure is stored at room temperature in the operating room. Because the blood is fresh and kept at room temperature, the platelets and clotting factors remain viable. Blood stored at room temperature should be transfused within 8 hours. If the surgical procedure is expected to last longer than 8 hours, the blood should be stored in monitored refrigeration. Refrigerated blood should be transfused within 24 hours (Roback et al, 2008).

The rationale for hemodilution is based on studies done in the early 1970s that demonstrated that isovolemic hemodilution, using dextran and crystalloid, lowers blood viscosity and that maximum oxygen delivery is attainable when the hematocrit is lower than 30%. The studies suggested that the viscosity-lowering effect of hemodilution leads to an increase in cardiac output and perfusion and that this increase easily compensates for the lower oxygen-carrying capacity of the diminished supply of red blood cells (Peterson, 1992).

The application of this option has obvious limitations. First, the patient on whom this procedure is done must be able to tolerate a significant blood loss before the surgery is begun. Second, because the amount of blood that can safely be withdrawn is limited, it may not be adequate to meet the volume replacement required. In such cases, homologous blood is used as a supplement. Therefore, like predeposit autologous transfusion, hemodilution may reduce but does not always eliminate the need for homologous blood use.

INTRAOPERATIVE AUTOTRANSFUSION/ INTRAOPERATIVE CELL SALVAGE

Intraoperative autotransfusion (IAT) is the collection of shed blood from the surgical field and its subsequent reinfusion to the patient. It can be used in cardiac, vascular, and selected trauma surgeries, and in liver transplants and orthopedic procedures. IAT is especially useful when preoperative donation is impossible or inadequate. The rule of thumb in IAT is that a return of 3 units makes it cost-effective. However, many argue that any cost using this method is offset by the reduced risk of autologous transfusion versus homologous transfusion.

Numerous blood-collection and cell-processing machines are available. The objective is the same for all: collect, in some

cases process, and return the patient's blood. If processing machinery is used, the blood shed from the surgical field is suctioned off and anticoagulated through a dual-lumen catheter that terminates in a collection reservoir. When the volume in this reservoir reaches the optimal level for processing, the blood is washed, spun, and returned to the patient.

IAT should not be used in certain situations. Because neither filtration nor washing can completely remove bacteria from blood, salvage is not attempted if the operative field has gross bacterial contamination. In addition, IAT is not usually used if a collagen hemostatic agent has been placed in the wound. These powerful agents, which activate the clotting cascade when in contact with red blood cells, have a molecular size similar to that of red cells and may not be eliminated by cell washing. Also, because malignant cells cannot be removed from salvaged blood, IAT is usually contraindicated in cancer resections. Returning salvaged blood could result in the seeding of malignant cells to other areas.

POSTOPERATIVE BLOOD SALVAGE

Postoperative salvage is the collection of shed blood from the postoperative surgical wound for reinfusion to the patient. Continuous and intermittent techniques and equipment are available for salvaging blood lost after surgery. These methods are usually used to collect blood lost from chest tubes or joint cavities. Because anticoagulation is not used, this blood is defibrinated and contains high titers of fibrinogen-fibrin degradation products. Such collections may be processed using cell-washing techniques before reinfusion, or they may be reinfused without processing. In either case, they must be filtered, and microaggregate filtration is preferred when cell washing has not been used. Because of the opportunity for contamination of these collections, it is recommended that shed blood collected under postoperative or posttraumatic conditions be reinfused within 6 hours of the initiation of the collection.

 SUMMARY

Transfusion therapy is a commonly ordered treatment for many reasons and yet it has the potential to cause harm to the patient. Therefore it cannot be taken lightly. The patients of today are knowledgeable consumers. Through media coverage they have been made aware of the potential diseases that can be transmitted through blood transfusions and are not afraid to question the health care practitioner. The nurse administering any blood

PATIENT OUTCOMES

Expected outcomes with transfusion therapy include:
- The component is appropriate for the patient as ordered.
- The component is typed and crossmatched as required or ordered.
- The patient receives the correct component through proper identification according to procedure.
- The patient will be monitored for transfusion-related reactions and interventions will be initiated immediately as needed.
- The patient's laboratory results will demonstrate improvement based on the component administered.

or blood components should have thorough knowledge of all aspects of transfusion therapy from collection to postinfusion complications.

 REFERENCES

Alter HJ, Klein HG: Blood: the hazards of blood transfusion in historical perspective, *Blood* 112:(7)2617–2626, 2008.

American Association of Blood Banks: *Standards for blood banks and transfusion services*, ed 25, Bethesda, Md, 2008, Author.

Busch M: Transfusion-associated AIDS, In Rossi EC, editor: *Principles of transfusion medicine*, ed 4, 2008, Bethesda, Md: Wiley-Blackwell.

Dellinger RP et al: Surviving sepsis campaign: international guidelines for management of severe sepsis and septic shock, *Intensive Care Med* 34(1):17–60, 2008. Retrieved 12/8/08 from http://www.guideline.gov/summary/summary.aspx?doc_id=12231&nbr=006316&string=Sepsis+AND+Campaign#s23.

Dzik S, Abuchon J, Jeffries L et al: Leukocyte reduction of blood components: public policy and new technology, *Transfusion Med Rev* 14:34–52, 2000.

Goldman M, Webert K, Arnold D et al: Proceedings of a consensus conference: towards an understanding of TRALI, *Transfusion Med Rev* 19:2–31, 2005.

King K, editor: *Blood transfusion therapy: a physician's handbook*, ed 9, 2008, Bethesda, Md, AABB.

Klein HG, Anstee D: *Mollison's blood transfusion in clinical practice*, ed 11, 2005, London, Blackwell.

Klein H, Spahn D, Carson J: Red blood cell transfusion in clinical practice, *Lancet* 370:415–426, 2007.

Martine E, Harris A, Johnson N: Autotransfusion systems (ATS), *Crit Care Nurs* 9(7):65, 1989.

Murphy EL, Fridey J, Smith JW et al: HTLV-II infected blood donors: the REDS investigators, *Neurology* 48:315, 1997.

Ness PM, Kruskall MS: *Hematology: basic principles and practices*, ed 3, 2004, Churchill Livingstone.

Nicholson E: Autologous blood transfusion, *Nursing Times* 84(2):33, 1988.

Nordmeyer D, Forestner J, Wall M: Advances in transfusion medicine, *Adv Anesthesia* 25:41–58, 2007.

O'Brien T, George JR, Holmberg SD: Human immunodeficiency virus type 2 infection in the United States; epidemiology, diagnosis, and public health implications, *JAMA* 267:2775, 1992.

Peterson K: Nursing management of autologous blood transfusion, *J Intrav Nurs* 15:(3)128, 1992.

Roback J et al editors: *Technical manual*, ed 16, Bethesda, Md, 2008, American Association of Blood Banks.

Sayers M: Cytomegalovirus and other herpesviruses. In Peltz LD, et al, *Clinical practice of transfusion medicine*, ed 3, New York, 1996, Churchill Livingstone.

Schreiber GB, Bush MP, Kleinman SH et al: The risk of transfusion transmitted viral infections: the retrovirus epidemiolgy donor study, *New Engl J Med* 334:1685, 1996.

Stillman C, McLaughlin N: Transfusion-related acute lung injury, *Blood Rev* 20(8):139–159, 2006.

Smith CE: Principles of fluid warming in trauma, *Semin Anesthesia, Periop Med Pain* 20(1):51–59, 2001.

Snyder E, Solheim B, Barbara J et al: *Rossi's principles of transfusion medicine*, ed 4, St. Louis 2008, Mosby.

15 PHARMACOLOGY

Michelle S. Turner, PharmD, BCPS and Judy Hankins, BSN, CRNI®*

The intravenous (IV) route is a common route of drug administration in many health care settings. IV drugs were once reserved for emergency situations or critically ill patients. They are now routinely used throughout the hospital, as well as in outpatient, long term care, and home care settings. Many of the quality initiatives as well as quality core measures include medication administration (e.g., pneumonia, acute myocardial infarction [MI], heart failure, and surgical infection prevention). There is a great deal of interest in safe medication administration, including The Joint Commission's National Patient Safety Goals.

With the dramatic increase in the use of the IV route for drug delivery, nurses have assumed increased responsibility. Nurses administer IV drugs, monitor patients' responses to pharmacological agents, and instruct patients regarding the prescribed drug therapy. Nurses must therefore have a thorough understanding of the principles of IV drug administration. This knowledge is necessary for the safety of both patients and health care workers to ensure quality patient outcomes.

It is the intent of this chapter to broaden the nurse's knowledge regarding IV drug therapy. Because of the breadth of the subject, this chapter has been divided into four sections. In the first, the nurse's role in IV drug administration is reviewed. Specific consideration is given to legal aspects of IV drug administration and application of the nursing process. The second section discusses the various aspects of IV drug delivery. Commonly used equipment is described, as well as the different modes of IV drug administration. The third section discusses drug dosage and flow rate calculations. The greatest emphasis is placed on the fourth section, where the different classifications of IV drugs are presented and the drug most representative of each classification is examined in detail.

CONSIDERATIONS FOR INTRAVENOUS DRUG ADMINISTRATION

The administration of IV medications has increased dramatically, with some medications only being manufactured for IV infusion. The IV route for drug administration offers many

advantages including the following: the IV route is ideal for patients who are unable to tolerate, use, or absorb drugs via the gastrointestinal (GI) tract; the IV route may eliminate pain or trauma at the delivery site; IV infusion provides rapid delivery/utilization and better control of administration rates. The increased need for drug-related education goes hand-in-hand with the increased use of IV drugs and the nursing role. This education is provided in schools of nursing; from health facility courses, computer-based learning, webcasts, and manuals/books; as well as through one-on-one information-sharing with pharmacists.

NURSING RESPONSIBILITIES

The determination of who may administer IV drugs is based on the Nurse Practice Act. Each state has such an act, but most only broadly define the scope of professional nursing responsibilities. This differs for a licensed practical nurse (LPN) in that several states have established boundaries in which the LPN may practice.

In addition to the Nurse Practice Act, health care facilities have established policies regarding nursing responsibilities. Although these policies cannot exceed the limits established by the Nurse Practice Act, they may clarify or place further restrictions on nursing functions. For example, institutional guidelines for IV drug administration define who may administer certain drugs and in what areas the drug can be used.

A third set of criteria regarding IV drug administration is contained in the *Infusion Nursing Standards of Practice* (INS, 2006a). This document provides an emphasis on evidence-based practice and research and includes information to measure the quality of IV nursing care, including IV drug administration. Because the standards are meant to protect the public and define nursing accountability, they are the basis for the development of IV policies in all practice settings in which IV drugs are administered.

LEGAL CONSIDERATIONS

To legally administer an IV drug, or any drug, the medication must be prescribed by a physician or appropriate licensed professional. However, it is the nurse's responsibility to ensure that the order is complete, correct, appropriate, and valid. The

*The author and editors wish to acknowledge the contributions made by Jean B. Douglas and Carolyn Hedrick as authors of this chapter in the second edition of *Infusion Therapy in Clinical Practice*.

nurse needs to be familiar with information related to the use of investigational drugs and controlled substances. To provide quality, safe medication delivery, basic knowledge related to medications and administration is needed along with knowing how to correctly respond to medication errors.

A complete order must contain the name of the drug (generic or trade), dosage, route of administration, frequency or time of administration, date and time the order was written, and signature as well as the reason for as-needed (PRN) orders. On some occasions, a verbal or telephone order may be needed. For these orders, the signature of the nurse is required and the prescriber should co-sign the order within 24 hours. Drug orders may be standing, PRN, or single dose, which could include a "stat" or "now" request.

A correct and appropriate order is one that is indicated and proper for the patient's condition. Indications for each drug classification and specific drugs are discussed later in this chapter. Determination of the appropriateness of the order is based on the nursing assessment of the patient and requires knowledge of pharmacokinetics and pharmacodynamics. Pharmacokinetics focuses on the effects of the body on the drug; pharmacodynamics involves the effects of the drug on the body.

A valid medication order requires that the order be written and signed by the physician or other authorized health care professional. Although verbal orders are acceptable in some situations, the order is not legally finalized until it is countersigned by a licensed physician or appropriate licensed professional.

There are additional legal considerations regarding controlled substances. Controlled substances are prescription drugs that, because of their high potential for drug dependence or abuse, are covered by the Controlled Substances Act of 1970. The Act established five categories of controlled substances, known as *schedules,* based on potential for abuse and dependence and the medical indications for the drug's use (Elkin, Perry, and Potter, 2007). Many of the IV drugs administered for pain control are Schedule II drugs, which have specific prescription and record-keeping requirements. The result of failing to follow established policies could be loss of professional license as well as fines and imprisonment.

Another area that has legal implications is the administration of investigational drugs. Informed consent must be obtained from all patients and/or families participating in clinical drug trials. This means that the patient must be supplied information by the principal investigator regarding the risks, benefits, expected effects on the disease process, and alternatives to the investigational therapy before consenting to participate in the trial. In addition, the clinical trial must be approved by the appropriate institutional committee, and drug information must be readily available for the nurse administering the drug. All documentation must meet the guidelines of the study and information returned according to established times.

Legal consideration must also be given to the occurrence of medication errors. Errors may be associated with prescribing and dispensing the drug, but they more commonly occur because of failure to follow safe administration procedures. The traditional five rights of medication administration specifying that the *right* dose of the *right* drug must be administered to the *right* patient at the *right* time by the *right* route should now include a sixth right, *right* documentation. Errors have resulted because of the "look alike" generic names (e.g., the cephalosporin antibiotics) (Box 15-1), failure to identify the patient appropriately, administering the drug by an incorrect route, illegible writing,

Box 15-1 LOOK-ALIKE/SOUND-ALIKE MEDICATIONS

acetohexamide	acetazolamide
amphotericin lipid	amphotericin conventional
Ativan (lorazepam)	Xanax (alprazolam)
atracurium	cisatracurium
carboplatin	cisplatin
Cipro IV	heparin IV
dobutamine	dopamine
Doxil	doxorubicin
doxorubicin conventional	doxorubicin liposomal
epinephrine	phenylephrine; ephedrine
hydralazine	hydroxyzine
hydromorphone	morphine
methocarbamol	metronidazole; methyldopa
quinidine	quinine
Taxol	Taxotere

TABLE 15-1 Do Not Use Abbreviations

Use	Do not use	Reason
Units	U or u	Mistaken as a "0," "4," or "cc"
0.1 mg	.1 mg	No leading zero results in easily missed decimal point (i.e., 10 times the dose)
0.1 mg or 1 mg	.10 mg or 1.0 mg	Trailing zero results in easily missed decimal point (i.e., 10-100 times the intended dose)
mcg or micrograms	μg	Mistaken for mg
Morphine sulfate	MS	Mistaken for MSO_4 and $MgSO_4$
Morphine sulfate	MSO_4	Mistaken for MS and $MgSO_4$
Magnesium sulfate	$MgSO_4$	Mistaken for MS and MSO_4
International unit	IU	Mistaken for IV and 10
Daily	Q.D.	Mistaken for Q.O.D. The period after the Q can be mistaken for an "I"
Every other day	Q.O.D.	Mistaken for Q.D. The period after the Q can be mistaken for an "I" and the "O" can be mistaken for "I"
Left ear	AS	Confused with left eye (OS)
Right ear	AD	Confused with right eye (OD)

improper abbreviations (Table 15-1), range orders, and the physician's failure to specify the route. Errors may be documented by manually completing paper forms or by populating data in computer-based programs. The programs should be nonpunitive and include follow-up, education, trending, reporting to appropriate individuals/committees, and practice change. The person discovering the error is responsible for documentation.

NURSING PROCESS

The administration of IV drugs requires proper application of the nursing process. The patient must be assessed, the drug therapy planned and implemented, the patient outcomes evaluated, and the plan of care reviewed and revised based on the evaluation. These basic steps are interrelated and are essential to ensure that drug therapy results in the desired patient outcomes.

Assessment

Patient assessment begins with a review of the patient's health history followed by talking with the patient, family, or significant others (Box 15-2). Where language barriers are present, it is important to have an interpreter. Printed material in various languages is also helpful for understanding and compliance.

During the questioning, it is particularly important to obtain information about known allergies to drugs, foods, and environmental factors. There are cross-sensitivities between many drugs, so an allergy to one may result in similar effects with another. A primary example is the possible cross-sensitivity between penicillins and cephalosporins.

Assessment should also include the patient's lifestyle, resources, and knowledge level. This is particularly important in home care and should include the family or other caregiver as well as the patient. Specific factors to consider are the patient's and family's daily schedules and the physical and human resources available. The ability to comprehend information may influence adherence to the drug regimen.

The last area to be assessed is patient-related factors that may alter the patient's response to the drug. These include genetic factors, preexisting conditions, and age. Genetic factors, such as the absence of a specific enzyme, may affect the drug's action within the body. Preexisting renal, liver, and cardiovascular disease may impair the metabolism or elimination of the drug. Age is also a predictor of drug response. For example, children do not have the mature physiological mechanisms needed for adult dosages, whereas physiological changes in older adults tend to extend the effects of drugs within the body. In addition, drug interactions and incompatibilities with other medications and with body fat may negatively affect the drug response.

Planning

A comprehensive assessment helps develop and follow a plan of care specific to the patient and the drug therapy. Once the plan has been identified, the patient's plan of care may be established. The care plan should include short- and long-term

goals, and it should focus on actions to achieve the desired patient outcomes.

An important feature to consider when planning care for the patient is the time-response nature of drug action. Although the drug may be administered as a single dose, it is more common for it to be administered repeatedly. Repeated administration at regular intervals causes the plasma concentration of most drugs to reach a constant concentration in the blood. More drugs are being developed that require fewer doses over a 24-hour period. If plans are not made to administer the drug at the scheduled times, the plateau may not be reached, seriously affecting the effectiveness of the drug therapy.

Another time-response factor to consider when planning the patient's care is the therapeutic drug concentration range. Whereas a plateau is achieved with a fixed dosing schedule, there are still peaks and troughs in the drug plasma concentration. The peak concentration occurs immediately after IV administration, and the trough level is the minimum concentration present immediately before administration of the next scheduled dose. Several drugs have a relatively narrow margin of safety, meaning that there is little difference between concentrations that produce therapeutic responses and those that cause serious adverse effects. When such drugs are prescribed, arrangements must be made to determine whether the drug levels are within a therapeutic range. The most important aspect of this planning is ensuring that blood samples are drawn appropriately in conjunction with a scheduled dose. For example, the administration of gentamicin requires that a trough specimen be drawn before the scheduled dose and that a peak specimen be obtained following infusion.

A third time-response aspect to consider is the plasma half-life of the drug. *Half-life* refers to the amount of time required for the elimination processes to reduce the blood concentration of the drug by 50% (Dipiro et al, 2002). For example, many IV drugs are eliminated by the kidneys. Because renal impairment may increase the half-life of such drugs, planning should include verification that reduced dosages have been prescribed.

Implementation

Important facets of implementing drug therapy are medication reconciliation before beginning treatment and at discharge, patient education before administration and discharge, drug administration, and documentation. Because of differences among health care settings, these facets may not receive equal attention. In home care, greater emphasis is placed on patient education to prepare the patient for the self-administration of medication. This differs from the hospital setting, where IV drugs are usually administered by the nurse. Regardless of the setting, documentation plays a vital role because it validates that the actions have been implemented as well as the outcomes.

Evaluation

Evaluation of the drug therapy determines the drug's effectiveness and may suggest beneficial modifications of the patient's plan of care. A therapeutic response is desired because it signifies that the intended effects of the drug have been produced. However, there may be an ineffective or toxic response. An ineffective response may indicate that less than the minimum required dose has been administered or that other factors have interfered with the action of the drug. For example, a patient

TABLE 15-2   Untoward Drug Responses

Response	Effects	Example
Tolerance	Increasing amounts of drug needed to produce same therapeutic response	Patient receiving morphine infusion over 2 weeks has decreasing relief from pain
Tachyphylaxis	A rapidly developing tolerance occurring after very few doses	Has been reported with sodium nitroprusside
Accumulation	Amount of drug builds up in body, resulting from input exceeding output	May occur when usual adult dosage of gentamicin is administered to patient with renal impairment
Idiosyncrasy	Unpredictable response that differs in quality from expected response but not caused by hypersensitivity	Aplastic anemia develops in 1 in 40,000 patients who receive chloramphenicol
Drug allergy	Adverse response to a drug resulting from previous exposure to that or a related drug and mediated by an antigen-antibody reaction; hypersensitivity	Reaction that occurs when penicillin is given to patient with penicillin allergy
Dependence	Continued administration of drug required to prevent withdrawal syndrome	Patient receiving hydromorphone for cancer pain has visible tremors, restlessness, and profuse perspiration when a dose is withheld

who experiences only slight relief from pain after the administration of morphine has an ineffective response. In contrast, a toxic response is an exaggeration of the usual pharmacological actions of the drug or the appearance of signs and symptoms related to drug toxicity. For example, the toxic response to digoxin is typically evidenced by the clinical symptoms of anorexia, nausea, and vomiting.

The patient should also be evaluated for unexpected and undesired effects of the drug. Although these responses are often called *side effects*, this term is misleading. Side effects are therapeutically undesirable, but are an unavoidable secondary effect of the normal action and therapeutic dose of the drug. An example is the loss of potassium from the body after the administration of furosemide. *Untoward drug responses*, also known as *adverse effects*, are undesired and unexpected responses. Table 15-2 describes several potential untoward drug responses.

Untoward effects may be caused by the interaction of the drug with other drugs within the body. Drug-drug interactions may be *potentiative*, meaning one drug intensifies the effects of the other drug, or *inhibitory*, meaning one drug reduces the effects of the other drug; or the drug combination may produce a new response that neither drug used alone would produce. Potentiative and inhibitory interactions may be beneficial or detrimental. Sulbactam and ampicillin illustrate a beneficial potentiative interaction that increases ampicillin's therapeutic action. A detrimental potentiative interaction occurs with warfarin and aspirin, which increases the risk of bleeding.

A beneficial inhibitory interaction occurs between morphine and naloxone when treating overdoses, reversing the toxicity of the opioid analgesic (Gahart and Nazareno, 2008). A detrimental inhibitory interaction occurs between terbutaline and propranolol, which causes a reduction in bronchial dilation (McEvoy, 2007). An example of a drug-drug interaction resulting in a new response is the combination of disulfiram (Antabuse) and alcohol, which causes hazardous effects that do not occur when either drug is used alone (McEvoy, 2007).

DRUG ADMINISTRATION

The nurse's role in IV drug administration is determined by the health care setting. In the inpatient setting, the nurse may be responsible for drug preparation and administration, whereas home care usually requires the nurse to educate the patient or family in self-administration techniques. Before initiating any infusion, the nurse must identify the patient, order, and drug/IV solution; practice appropriate hand hygiene; and select correct supplies/equipment. The nurse should also understand the drug's therapeutic effects and be able to recognize side effects/adverse reactions. Use of aseptic technique throughout the process as well as appropriate documentation is paramount. The first dose of medication is preferably administered in the hospital or in the presence of a physician (INS, 2006b). Barcoding of solutions/medications, patient identification bands, and caregiver identification are making drug administration safer for the patient and provide improved processes for the health care employee.

DRUG PREPARATION

Generally, IV drugs and admixtures are prepared in a centralized pharmacy, where there is greater assurance of accuracy and sterility. No matter where the drug is prepared, appropriate manufacturing practices, such as those described in the *USP <797> Guidelines*, must be met. These guidelines include directions related to the areas of facility, preparation, personnel, and products. Cleaning, environmental testing, and expiration/end-of-use information have been defined in these guidelines. The admixture process may be performed by technicians employed by the pharmacy, working under the direction of the pharmacist. In emergencies or when medication must be prepared immediately before administration, nurses may also prepare IV drugs.

Laminar flow hood

When IV drugs are prepared in the pharmacy, they are usually prepared under a laminar flow hood. The design of the laminar flow hood decreases the possibility of airborne contaminants entering the IV solution. Air enters the back of the hood, and is circulated through filters before it is directed into the work area in uniform, parallel streams. Either a horizontal or a vertical laminar flow hood may be used; however, vertical models are recommended for preparing cytotoxic agents.

Drug containers

IV drugs are available in various containers, including ampules, vials, partially filled solution containers, additive piggyback vials, and premixed admixtures. Ampules pose the greatest risk because of the possibility of particulate contamination. Glass fragments may enter the ampule when it is broken open; the related risks are reduced when the drug is drawn up with a filter needle and infused through a standard needle. Vials pose another risk of particulate contamination because of the potential risk of *coring;* when the needle is introduced through the stopper of the vial, the needle bevel may cut away fragments of the seal.

Partially filled containers and additive piggyback vials, often referred to as *minibags* or *minibottles,* are potential sources of particulate matter. This may be the result of incomplete reconstitution of the powdered drug or precipitates formed by the physical incompatibility of the admixture. Partially filled containers of 50 to 150 mL of 0.9% sodium chloride or 5% dextrose in water (D_5W) require that a liquid form of the drug be added to the container. In an additive piggyback vial, the drug is in powdered form, which must be reconstituted with a small volume of diluent.

Premixed admixtures are prepared by the manufacturer and require no further preparation other than providing proper labeling. However, they are sometimes available in frozen form, which must be restored to room temperature before administration. Cefazolin is an example of an admixture available in frozen form. It is generally recommended that frozen admixtures not be warmed by placing them in a water bath or exposing them to microwave radiation. Special units are available for rapidly thawing premixed frozen minibags, but the preferred method is to allow the admixture to thaw at room temperature.

Diluents

Another consideration for the preparation of IV drugs is the diluent used to reconstitute the drug. Diluents with bacteriostatic properties, such as bacteriostatic sodium chloride, contain benzyl alcohol as a preservative. Although this bacteriostatic agent is desirable in most situations, it is contraindicated for neonates and for the administration of intraspinal or epidural drugs (McEvoy, 2007). In addition, certain drugs, such as amphotericin B, are incompatible with preservatives and must be reconstituted with sterile water for injection (McEvoy, 2007).

DRUG COMPATIBILITY AND STABILITY
Drug incompatibility

Incompatibility is an undesirable reaction that occurs between the drug and the solution, the container, or another drug. The three types of incompatibilities associated with IV drugs are physical, chemical, and therapeutic. A *physical incompatibility* refers to a visible reaction, such as a color change, haze, turbidity, precipitate, or gas formation, occurring within the drug. The largest number of physical incompatibilities involve precipitate formation, such as that seen when diazepam is added to D_5W.

Chemical incompatibility involves the chemical degradation of the drug, and is the result of hydrolysis, reduction, oxidation, or decomposition. It differs from physical incompatibility in that the reaction may not be visible (Weinstein, 2007). Such a reaction may occur when penicillin is added to a very acidic or alkaline solution.

Therapeutic incompatibility, which occurs within the patient, is the result of the overlapping effects of two drugs administered concurrently. Although the effects may not be evident until the patient's response to the drug therapy has been evaluated, knowledge of potential incompatibilities may prevent their

TABLE 15-3 **Factors That Affect Drug Stability**

Factor	Effect	Example
Number of additives	The greater the number of drugs contained in the admixture, the greater the chance of one of the drugs becoming unstable	Multiple additives in PN solution
Dilution	Limited amounts of a drug are stable in the solution, whereas large doses may be unstable	Only limited amounts of heparin and hydrocortisone are stable in amphotericin solution
Time	The length of time the drug is in solution may affect stability	Ampicillin is stable for only 4 hr when added to D_5W
Light	Some drugs are sensitive to light, and exposure may result in degradation of the drug	Exposure of levarerenol may result in degradation of drug
Temperature	Lower temperatures usually extend the stability of the drug	Cephalothin is stable for only 6 hr at room temperature, but up to 48 hr when refrigerated
Order of additives	The order in which drugs are added to a solution affects compatibility and stability	Addition of lipids to PN solution
Container	The composition of the container may affect the stability of the drug	Potency of insulin reduced by at least 20% when added to a plastic container

D_5W, 5% dextrose in water; *PN,* parenteral nutrition.

occurrence. Examples of therapeutic incompatibility were previously discussed as part of the evaluation of drug interactions.

Drug stability

Stability, on the other hand, refers to the length of time the drug retains its original properties and characteristics. One of the most important factors in drug stability is the solution's hydrogen ion concentration, or pH. Most drugs are stable over a narrow range of pH values. This means that they are unstable in either very acidic (pH below 4) or alkaline (pH above 8) solutions. The concept of stability is best characterized by penicillin. This drug is most stable in a slightly acidic environment (pH of 6.5) but deteriorates if added to a very acidic or alkaline solution. Additional factors that affect drug stability are listed in Table 15-3.

METHODS OF IV DRUG ADMINISTRATION

The mode of IV drug administration depends on the drug used, the patient's condition, and the desired effects of the drug. The mode of administration is specified by the physician or other qualified provider. Each of the four primary modes of administration—continuous infusion, intermittent infusion, direct injection, and patient-controlled analgesia—has advantages and disadvantages.

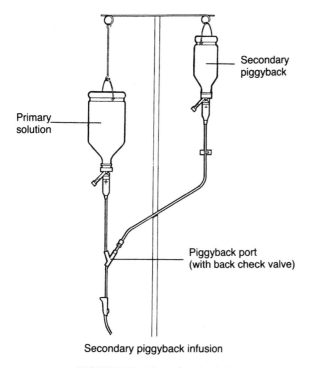

FIGURE 15-1 Secondary piggyback.

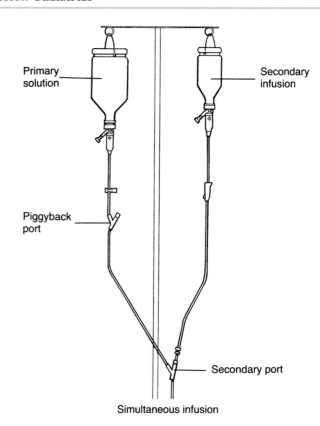

FIGURE 15-2 Simultaneous infusion.

Continuous infusion

Continuous infusion refers to the admixture of the drug in a large volume of solution that is infused continuously over several hours to several days. The solution container is connected to an administration set, and the drug (in solution) is infused through the venous access device. Depending on the potency, an electronic infusion control device may be used to deliver the drug accurately at the prescribed rate of flow.

Continuous infusion is used when the drug must be highly diluted, constant plasma concentrations of the drug must be maintained, or large volumes of fluids and electrolytes must be replaced. Examples are infusions of nitroprusside or potassium chloride. Disadvantages associated with continuous infusion are possible fluid overload and potential incompatibilities between the infusion and other IV drugs administered through the same venous access device. Patient comfort issues and mobility should also be considered.

Intermittent infusion

For an *intermittent infusion,* the drug is added to a small volume of fluid (25 to 250 mL) and infused over 15 to 90 minutes at prescribed intervals. Advantages of the intermittent mode are the ability of the drug to produce peak blood concentrations at periodic intervals, decreased risk of fluid overload, and greater convenience for the patient. However, there are disadvantages. The increased concentration of the drug in the intermittent solution may cause venous irritation, the drug may be less effective than if administered by continuous infusion, and additional equipment is required. IV antibiotics are generally administered using this mode.

Intermittent infusions may be administered in various ways. One of the most common methods is for the drug to be given as a piggyback infusion through the established pathway of the primary solution (Figure 15-1). Although the primary infusion is interrupted during the piggyback infusion, the drug from the intermittent infusion container mixes with the primary solution below the piggyback injection port. Hence, if this method is used, the drug and the primary solution should be compatible.

A second way to administer intermittent infusions is simultaneous infusion. With this method, the drug is administered as a secondary infusion concurrently with the primary infusion (Figure 15-2). Rather than connecting the intermittent infusion at the piggyback port, it is attached to the lower secondary port. One of the major disadvantages of this method is the tendency for blood to back up into the tubing once the secondary infusion has been completed, possibly occluding the venous access device. This does not occur with the piggyback method because hydrostatic pressure closes the back check valve (incorporated into the administration set) once the intermittent infusion is completed. Although drug incompatibility is a possibility with both methods, it is a greater risk with a simultaneous infusion.

A third method is the use of a volume control set. Although it was originally designed to control the fluid volume delivered to the patient, a drug may be added to a small amount of solution in the volume control set and infused at the desired rate (Figure 15-3). This method shares many of the disadvantages previously discussed. However, it is still used in some pediatric settings because it limits the amount of fluid the child receives.

The fourth method for administering intermittent infusions is directly into the venous access device. The device must be one that is intended for intermittent administration, such as a peripheral heparin or saline lock or a long-term, centrally placed catheter. The drug is added to a minibag or minibottle and infused intermittently. Between doses, the drug container and administration set are eliminated. This

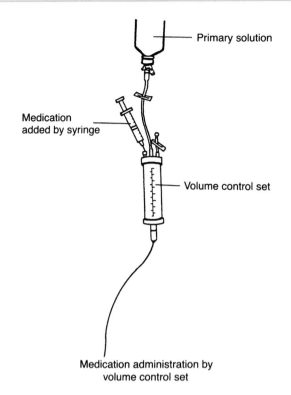

FIGURE 15-3 Volume control set.

method is generally preferred because it decreases the risk of fluid overload, and affords greater freedom of movement for the ambulatory patient. However, failure to promptly remove the empty drug container and administration set and flush the venous access device may result in occlusion of the venous access device.

Technological developments have produced alternatives for the administration of intermittent doses. One manufacturer has introduced a system whereby the drug is supplied in a powdered form that is attached between the primary solution and the infusion set. Once the drug vial is connected, the solution flows from the primary container through the drug vial and to the patient. Although the use of this system eliminates the costs associated with preparing and administering the drug by the traditional piggyback method, it is applicable only to situations in which the drug and primary solution are compatible.

A second innovation has been the introduction of intermittent doses of drugs that are activated at the time of use. Rather than preparing and refrigerating the drug before administration, the pharmacy simply dispenses the drug vial attached to a small container of solution. Immediately before administering the drug, the nurse activates the system by removing the barrier between the drug and the solution. Although this has proven cost-effective, errors have been reported because of failure to remove the barrier and activate the system.

The third major innovation is the result of the space program and is based on elastomeric technology. The system consists of an elastomeric drug container that is specially designed to establish a set delivery rate. Once the pharmacist fills the system with the drug, it may be infused at the preset rate by opening the slide clamp on the tubing attached to the container. An advantage of this system is that neither gravity nor electronic assistance is required for precise delivery of the drug. However,

not all drugs may be administered with an elastomeric container. Because of the expense, it is usually reserved for the home setting.

Finally, drug delivery systems containing dual compartments, one for fluid and one for powdered medication, are available. To reconstitute, at the time of administration the "hanger tab end" is rolled toward the port end, which is pointing downward, until the seal between the diluent and powder opens, releasing the diluent into the drug chamber. The container is agitated until the drug is completely dissolved. This system also offers the advantages of longer end-of-use (expirational) datings and eliminates need for refrigeration. With the advantages, comes the disadvantage of an increased cost (Figure 15-4).

Systems that offer premixed drugs that are enclosed in a single container offer some advantages. The diluent and drug are measured and verified in a single sterile container by the manufacturer. These systems decrease the risks of incorrect drugs/diluents, volume of drug/diluent, and labeling, and of contamination during processing.

Direct injection

Direct injection, also known as *IV push* or *bolus,* is the administration of a drug directly into the venous access device or through the proximal injection port on a continuous infusion set. The purpose is to achieve rapid serum concentrations, but this may be accompanied by a greater risk of adverse effects. Instead of regulating the rate of administration by the infusion rate, direct injection requires only the time it takes to push the plunger of the syringe. Many drugs have maximum rates at which they may be administered, so the rate of the injection must be timed and the drug injected in increments. Because the drug may be incompatible with the infusing solution or heparin may be present in the intermittent device, the venous access device should be flushed with 0.9% sodium chloride before and after injecting the drug.

Direct injections may require that the drug be drawn into a syringe before administration or that the drug be available in a prefilled syringe. There are a variety of systems available to allow for direct injections. Some include prefilled syringes that are added to syringe holders, which may or may not be included in the packaging. Others require removing an affixed plunger from the outside of the syringe and attaching it at the plunger end of the prefilled syringe.

A needleless system is mandated to prevent needlestick injuries and inadvertent puncture of the tubing or device.

Patient-controlled analgesia

A fourth mode of administration is patient-controlled analgesia (PCA), which promotes patient comfort through the self-administration of analgesic agents. With this method, an electronic pump (PCA pump) is programmed to administer a small bolus of the drug when activated by the patient. The bolus amount and the time between doses (lock-out interval) are predetermined by the physician and programmed into the pump by the nurse. At the end of a shift, the nurse can review the infusion history to determine the amount of drug received as well as the number of unsuccessful attempts, possibly indicating inadequate pain control. Technological advances have added features to the pump, permitting both continuous infusion and patient-controlled doses.

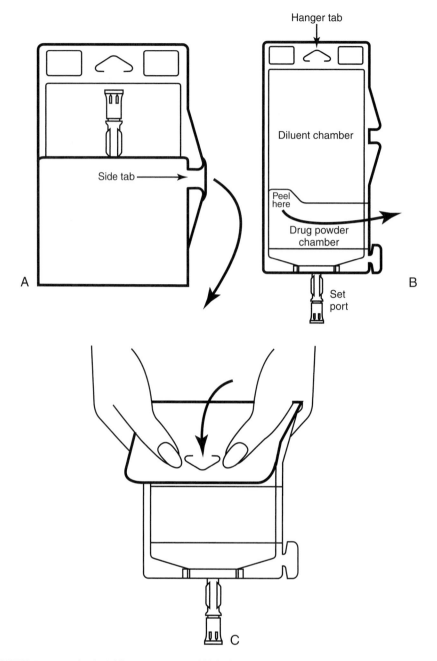

FIGURE 15-4 Duplex drug delivery system. **A,** Unfold duplex container. **B,** Inspect diluent and powder chambers. **C,** Activate: fold container just below the diluent meniscus and squeeze folded diluent's chamber to release diluent into powder chamber. Agitate mixture until completely dissolved. (Used with permission from B. Braun Medical, Inc., Bethlehem, Pa.)

CALCULATIONS

A physician or authorized prescriber is responsible for prescribing patient medications, but the nurse must ensure that the medication order is accurate and will be safe for the patient. This section primarily focuses on a variety of calculations that will help ensure the ordered medication can be administered correctly.

METRIC SYSTEM

The metric system is universally accepted by the medical profession. It provides the most accurate means for calculating drug dosages. The effects of a drug administered directly into

the vascular system may be immediate, so accuracy is very important. The precise measurements attainable by using the metric system make it preferable to the apothecary and household measuring systems. Box 15-3 lists common abbreviations used in the metric system, and Box 15-4 provides conversions among metric units.

DRUG DOSAGE DETERMINATION

In determining dosages, most nurses are familiar with either the ratio-proportion or the formula method. Each method is reviewed here; however, readers should use their preferred method.

Box 15-3 METRIC SYSTEM ABBREVIATIONS

WEIGHT
Kilogram = kg
Gram = g
Milligram = mg
Microgram = mcg

LENGTH
Centimeter = cm
Millimeter = mm

VOLUME
Liter = L
Milliliter = mL
Cubic centimeter = cc

Box 15-4 METRIC CONVERSION FACTORS

WEIGHT

Kilogram	×	1000	=	1000 grams
1 gram	×	1000	=	1000 milligrams
1 milligram	×	1000	=	1000 micrograms
1 microgram	÷	1000	=	0.001 milligram
1 milligram	÷	1000	=	0.001 gram
1 gram	÷	1000	=	0.001 kilogram

VOLUME

1 liter	×	1000	=	1000 milliliters
1 milliliter	÷	1000	=	0.001 liter

Ratio-proportion method

To use this method effectively, it must be remembered that a ratio is a comparison between two related items, and a proportion is the equality of two ratios.

When setting up a proportion, start with what you know about the drug from the label: the strength of the drug on hand (H) and volume of the drug on hand (V). Place this information in the form of a ratio (H:V) on the left of the equal sign (=). The ratio for the dose desired is the relationship of the dose ordered (D) and the amount to give (G), and this is placed on the right of the equal sign:

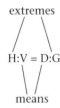

extremes

$$H:V = D:G$$

means

Thus the strength on hand (H) is related (:) to the volume (V) as (=) the dose ordered (D) is related (:) to the amount to give (G).

For an answer to be correct, the product of the means must equal the product of the extremes. The extremes are always the two outside numbers.

Example: A vial contains clindamycin phosphate, 600 mg/4 mL. What volume must be given to administer 300 mg?

$$H(mg):V(mL) = D(mg):G(mL)$$

$$600:4 = 300:X$$

$$600X = 1200$$

$$X = 2 \text{ mL of clindamycin phosphate}$$

Formula method

The terminology applied to the ratio-proportion method remains the same for the formula method; the equation, however, is changed to the following:

$$\text{Amount to give (G)} = \frac{\text{Dose ordered (D)}}{\text{Strength on hand (H)}} \times \text{Volume (V)}$$

Example: A vial contains clindamycin phosphate, 600 mg/4 mL. What volume must be given to administer 300 mg?

$$X = \frac{300}{600} \times 4 \text{ mL} = \frac{1200}{600} = 1200 \div 600$$

$$= 2 \text{ mL of clindamycin phosphate}$$

FLOW RATE DETERMINATION

To administer an IV solution accurately, the flow rate must be regulated carefully. Flow rates may be expressed in the form of an infusion over a period of hours, milliliters per hour or milliliters per minute, or number of drops per minute. The responsibility for administering the solution rests on the nurse, who should evaluate the available administration sets and select the one most appropriate for administering the solution. Criteria for administration set selection include its ability to deliver the required flow rate. When calculating the flow rate, it is important to know that the exact amount of solution in a manufacturer's container is unknown as there is an acceptable range of overfill allowed.

Milliliters per hour

Several formulas provide the information necessary for the delivery of a precise flow rate; however, the three-step method is the most complete.

Three-step method

The *three-step method* is a comprehensive flow rate calculation because it determines the rate in milliliters per hour and milliliters per minute, as well as the number of drops per minute for solution administration.

Example: A physician has ordered 3000 mL of solution to be administered over 24 hours.

Step 1: Determine the flow rate per hour.

Formula Method

Total volume ÷ Administration time = Milliliters per hour (hr)

$$3000 \text{ mL} \div 24 \text{ hr} = 125 \text{ mL/hr}$$

Step 2: Determine the rate per minute.

Formula Method

Milliliters per hour ÷ Minutes per hour (60)
= Milliliters per minute

$$125 \text{ mL} \div 60 \text{ min} = 2.08 \text{ mL/min}$$

Step 3: The administration set drop factor is 15 drops (gtt)/mL. Determine the number of drops per minute.

Formula Method

Milliliters per minute × Drop factor = Drops per minute

$$2.08 \text{ mL} \times 15 \text{ gtt} = 31.2 \text{ gtt/min (rounded to 31 gtt/min)}$$

An infusion at a rate of 31 gtt/min administers the 3000 mL over 24 hours.

Length of administration and flow rate

The hours for administration are based on milliliters per hour. On occasion, it may be necessary to determine the hours required for an infusion. The calculation can be completed through the use of simple arithmetic.

Formula Method

Volume to be infused (mL) ÷ mL/hr = Number of hours

DRUG CLASSIFICATIONS

Drug reference books generally list medications alphabetically, even when a classification system is used. Such a system aids the nurse in clinical practice, but it is not conducive to learning. To help the nurse understand the wide array of IV drugs discussed in this chapter, a prototype approach is used. The drugs are divided into different categories: antibiotics, other anti-infective drugs, central nervous system (CNS) drugs, cardiovascular drugs, hematological agents, agents for electrolyte and water balance, gastrointestinal (GI) drugs, hormones and synthetic substitutes, immune modulators, respiratory smooth muscle relaxants, and vitamins. The drug most representative of each classification is examined in detail. Additional drugs related to the prototype, including antidotes, are then discussed in terms of their differences and similarities or their relationship to the prototype.

Drug dosages vary widely, even among the prototype and its related drugs. Inclusion of dosing information on all the drugs discussed would require more pages than are allotted for this chapter. Therefore drug dosing is discussed only when pertinent to understanding administration of the drugs and their potential side effects. Information on dosing schedules for each drug is available in *American Hospital Formulary Service Drug Information* (McEvoy, 2007) and in *Drug Facts and Comparisons* (Wickersham, 2007). These were the primary references consulted for specific drug information, although additional references may be cited to explain the various drug classifications.

ANTIBIOTICS

Antibiotics are used to treat infection and represent the largest category of commonly used IV medications. Antibiotics may be categorized as either bactericidal or bacteriostatic. *Bactericidal agents* can destroy the organism by lysis of the cell wall or by prevention of its intact formation. *Bacteriostatic agents* inhibit growth of the organism by inhibiting protein synthesis. Although bacteriostatics may eliminate the organism in high concentrations, they usually depend on the patient's immune system to eradicate the organism once its growth has been inhibited. Sometimes combinations of antibiotics with differing mechanisms of actions are used for synergistic effects.

Antibiotics also have differing pharmacokinetic and pharmacodynamic profiles. Pharmacokinetics is the effects the body has on the drug, and pharmacodynamics refers to the effects the drug has on the body. Pharmacokinetic parameters such as volume of distribution and elimination half-life influence the dose of a drug and how often it must be administered. Pharmacodynamics examines different drug exposure measurements to determine which measurement is most closely tied to efficacy. Examples include time above minimum inhibitory concentration (MIC) and peak to MIC ratio, with minimum inhibitory concentration being the lowest concentration of antibiotic that will inhibit growth of the organism. Time and peak are specific to the concentrations of antibiotic achieved. Knowledge of which pharmacodynamic parameter is most optimal for the selected antibiotic combined with its pharmacokinetic profile often yields a customized regimen for the patient.

The primary contraindication for antibiotics is a known sensitivity to the drug. A patient with a history of hypersensitivity reactions to a certain antibiotic should be considered allergic to all antibiotics within the same class. For example, a patient who has a known sensitivity to penicillin is also considered allergic to aminopenicillins. In addition, there is evidence of a cross-sensitivity among antibiotics that are structurally similar, such as penicillins and cephalosporins. Therefore cephalosporins are used cautiously in patients who are sensitive to penicillin.

One of the major disadvantages of antibiotics is that their prolonged use may result in a bacterial or fungal superinfection. A *superinfection* occurs when the normal flora of the body is altered by an antibiotic, allowing the proliferation of bacteria or fungi that are resistant to the antibiotic.

Since antibiotics have been overused for decades, some are proving ineffective against resistant strains of bacteria. Whenever available, the clinician should check sensitivity data prepared by the clinical laboratory before selecting a specific antibiotic.

Penicillins

The penicillins include natural and semisynthetic antibiotics produced or derived by the fermentation of certain strains of the fungus *Penicillium*. Penicillins are still some of the most important antibiotics because of their relatively low cost, low toxicity, and good clinical efficacy in the treatment of many infections.

Natural penicillins

The mechanism of action of the natural penicillins is bactericidal. These agents disrupt the synthesis of the bacterial cell wall, making the organism osmotically unstable. Instability of the cell wall causes it to lyse, and the organism is destroyed. Since the cell walls of gram-positive bacteria are relatively permeable to most penicillins, these drugs are generally effective against such organisms. However, gram-negative bacteria have an outer membrane around the cell wall that decreases accessibility to the natural penicillins.

Prototype: penicillin G potassium

Penicillin G is indicated for the treatment of severe infections caused by some gram-positive and anaerobic organisms. Since it exerts specific antibiotic action against these organisms and is relatively nontoxic to the host, penicillin G is generally considered the drug of choice for many streptococcal, pneumococcal, and spirochetal infections.

Penicillin G may be administered as an intermittent infusion, although because of its short half-life it may also be administered continuously. Adverse reactions are rare and are usually limited to hypersensitivity reactions. The manifestations of a hypersensitivity reaction may be varied and can be divided into four basic types (Goldman and Ausiello, 2008).

The most common hypersensitivity reactions are dermatological reactions. Symptoms include urticarial, erythematous, or maculopapular rash accompanied by pruritus. These reactions are delayed, occurring 48 hours or more after the administration of penicillin G.

The second type of hypersensitivity reaction is serum sickness–like reactions. These reactions are usually evident 6 to 10 days after the initiation of therapy, and are characterized by fever, malaise, urticaria, arthralgia, myalgia, lymphadenopathy, and splenomegaly. Although the reaction may be severe, it is usually short-lived and disappears within days or weeks after discontinuing the drug.

The third type of reaction includes hematological reactions, such as hemolytic anemia, agranulocytosis, and leukopenia. Typically, this type of reaction is associated with large doses of penicillin G. A positive direct antiglobulin (Coombs') test occurs in up to 3% of patients (McEvoy, 2007) receiving large doses, and a small number of these patients develop hemolytic anemia during or after penicillin therapy. Once the drug is discontinued, the hemoglobin concentration and reticulocyte count return to pretherapy levels, although the Coombs' test may not revert to negative for 3 months or longer.

The fourth and most serious type of hypersensitivity reaction is anaphylaxis. Although anaphylaxis is reported in less than 0.05% of patients receiving penicillin, it has been fatal in 5% to 10% of reported cases (McEvoy, 2007). Anaphylactic reactions to penicillin typically occur within 30 minutes of administration. These reactions are characterized by laryngeal edema, bronchospasm, stridor, cyanosis, and circulatory collapse. Treatment includes immediate discontinuation of the drug and emergency measures such as maintaining a patent airway and administering epinephrine, oxygen therapy, and corticosteroids.

Penicillin interacts with several other antibiotics. Aminoglycosides are physically and chemically incompatible with penicillin, and are inactivated if administered in the same IV container or administration set. However, it is not uncommon for aminoglycosides and penicillins to be used concomitantly because of their differing mechanisms of action. Penicillins and cephalosporins have similar mechanisms of action and are customarily not used together.

Related drugs

Penicillin G is commercially available as a potassium or sodium salt. Both are readily soluble in water and are considered aqueous, crystalline penicillins, but penicillin G potassium is usually preferred. The administration of either form requires special consideration because every 1 million units of penicillin G potassium contains 1.7 mEq of potassium and every 1 million units of penicillin G sodium contains 2 mEq of sodium.

Penicillinase-resistant penicillins

The critical component of the natural penicillins is the β-lactam ring incorporated into the penicillin molecule. Some strains of bacteria produce an enzyme known as penicillinase, which destroys the ring. Thus the organism is considered penicillin resistant. To overcome this resistance, the penicillinase-resistant penicillins have been developed. These antibiotics are used exclusively to treat penicillinase-resistant organisms such as *Staphylococcus aureus* and *Staphylococcus epidermidis*. Their mechanism of action, contraindications, and precautions are similar to those of the natural penicillins.

Prototype: nafcillin sodium

Nafcillin sodium (Unipen) is mainly indicated for the treatment of infections caused by penicillinase-producing staphylococci. It is also used preoperatively to reduce the incidence of staphylococcal infections associated with certain surgical procedures. Nafcillin is commonly given as an intermittent infusion, although it may also be administered as a continuous infusion.

Certain strains of staphylococci are resistant to all penicillinase-resistant penicillins and are often termed "methicillin-resistant" because of the historical fact that methicillin previously was the penicillinase-resistant penicillin used for resistance testing. These resistant strains are prevalent in both the hospital and the community and are being reported with increasing frequency.

The side effects of nafcillin are similar to those associated with the use of penicillin G, with hypersensitivity reactions being the most common adverse effects reported. One of the more common hypersensitivity reactions linked to nafcillin is acute interstitial nephritis that manifests both systemically (fever, rash) and locally in the kidneys (hematuria, proteinuria). In rare instances, transient neutropenia, leukopenia, granulocytopenia, and thrombocytopenia have been reported. Generally, these hematological effects are not evident until more than 10 days after the initiation of therapy and resolve within 2 to 7 days once the drug is discontinued. Rarely, nafcillin causes transient asymptomatic elevations of serum alkaline phosphatase, alanine aminotransferase, and aspartate aminotransferase levels.

Related drugs

An additional penicillinase-resistant penicillin is oxacillin sodium (Bactocill). Oxacillin is similar to nafcillin, but nafcillin is more likely to cause phlebitis than other penicillinase-resistant penicillins. However, oxacillin may cause more adverse hepatic effects than nafcillin.

Aminopenicillins

Aminopenicillins have a free amino group added to the penicillin nucleus, which increases their bactericidal effectiveness against gram-negative bacteria. However, they are deactivated by penicillinase-producing organisms.

Prototype: ampicillin sodium

Ampicillin sodium (Omnipen-N) is highly effective in the treatment of severe infections caused by *Salmonella, Shigella, Proteus mirabilis,* and *Escherichia coli.* Ampicillin is also used for treatment of susceptible enterococcal and streptococcal infections. Although ampicillin may be administered by direct injection, it is generally administered as an intermittent infusion. Concentrated doses of ampicillin are stable for 4 hours in 5%

dextrose in water and 5% dextrose in 0.45% sodium chloride, but potency is extended to 8 hours when added to 0.9% sodium chloride without dextrose. When the drug is further diluted in a minibag or minibottle, stability may be extended up to 48 hours.

Adverse reactions to ampicillin are similar to those of penicillin G. Ampicillin sodium may also produce a distinct, nonimmunological reaction characterized by a generalized erythematous, maculopapular rash similar to measles. The rash typically occurs 3 to 14 days after the initiation of therapy and generally disappears despite the continuation of therapy. It is more common in patients with mononucleosis and is not indicative of a hypersensitivity to penicillin. Hematological effects such as neutropenia, agranulocytosis, and thrombocytopenia have also been reported, but these are usually reversible once the drug is discontinued.

Because of the probability of patients with infectious mononucleosis developing a rash during therapy, ampicillin is generally not prescribed to patients with this disease. In addition, the potential for ampicillin rash is increased for patients receiving allopurinol and ampicillin concomitantly.

Related drugs

Ampicillin sodium-sulbactam sodium (Unasyn) is a combination of ampicillin and sulbactam that prevents inactivation of the drug by β-lactamase-producing organisms. It is primarily indicated in the treatment of skin and skin structure, intra-abdominal, and gynecological infections.

Extended-spectrum penicillins

As a result of the structural differences in the side chains of the extended-spectrum penicillins, they have a wider spectrum of activity than the other penicillins. Specifically, the extended-spectrum penicillins are effective against gram-negative organisms, including *Pseudomonas*. Like the natural penicillins, the extended-spectrum penicillins are ineffective against penicillinase-producing organisms.

Prototype: piperacillin sodium

Piperacillin sodium (Pipracil) is bactericidal against several gram-negative, gram-positive, and anaerobic organisms. It is used for treatment of bacterial septicemia, febrile neutropenia, and infections of the respiratory, genital, and urinary tracts.

Piperacillin may be administered by direct injection, intermittent infusion, or continuous infusion. However, administration should not exceed the recommended rates. Too rapid infusions of extended-spectrum penicillins and higher-than-normal dosages have resulted in seizures. Other side effects of piperacillin are similar to those of penicillin G and include dermatological and hematological reactions, thrombophlebitis, and anaphylaxis.

Drug interactions associated with piperacillin are similar to those of the other penicillins. There may also be an increased risk of bleeding in patients who are receiving anticoagulants.

Related drugs

Another extended-spectrum penicillin includes ticarcillin disodium (Ticar). Piperacillin sodium-tazobactam sodium (Zosyn) and ticarcillin disodium-clavulanate potassium (Timentin) are co-formulated with a β-lactamase inhibitor that expands the activity of the extended-spectrum penicillin. These drugs are usually selected based on laboratory sensitivity data and availability.

Cephalosporins

Cephalosporins are bactericidal antibiotics that share a close structural similarity with the penicillins. Therefore they have similar mechanisms of action, side effects, and contraindications. Cephalosporins are classified by their spectrum of activity, or *generation*.

First-generation cephalosporins

First-generation cephalosporins are active against susceptible gram-positive bacteria, such as *S. aureus* and *S. epidermidis,* and some gram-negative organisms. As a result of their low cost, they are the preferred drugs for most gram-positive infections.

Prototype: cefazolin sodium

Cefazolin sodium (Kefzol) is effective in the treatment of serious infections of the soft tissue, respiratory tract, genitourinary tract, and cardiovascular system. It may be administered as a direct injection or as an intermittent infusion. The primary route of elimination for cefazolin is the kidney; therefore patients with renal impairment require a dosage reduction.

Although cefazolin is considered relatively nontoxic, allergic reactions have been reported in up to 5% of patients receiving the drug. These reactions are similar to those associated with penicillin G and range from a mild rash to anaphylaxis. Nephrotoxicity has been reported, but it is rare and more likely to occur in geriatric patients or in those with renal impairment.

There are few reported drug interactions involving cefazolin. However, the concurrent use of nephrotoxic drugs such as aminoglycosides and cefazolin may increase the risk of renal toxicity.

Second-generation cephalosporins

The second-generation cephalosporins have greater gram-negative activity than the first-generation drugs, but they are less effective against gram-positive organisms. Their mechanism of action, side effects, contraindications, and precautions are similar to those of cefazolin.

Prototype: cefoxitin sodium

Cefoxitin sodium (Mefoxin) is indicated for the treatment of serious infections of the respiratory and genitourinary tracts, gynecological infections, and septicemia. Cefoxitin also has increased activity against anaerobic bacteria, making it an option for treatment of intra-abdominal infections. Since it is excreted by the kidneys, a reduced dosage of cefoxitin is indicated in patients with renal impairment.

Related drugs

Additional second-generation cephalosporins are cefotetan disodium (Cefotan) and cefuroxime sodium (Zinacef). Second-generation cephalosporins are often used for surgical prophylaxis.

Third-generation cephalosporins

Third-generation cephalosporins are more active against gram-negative organisms, but are less effective against gram-positive organisms. An important characteristic of this category of drugs is their ability to cross the blood-brain barrier when the meninges are inflamed. Third-generation cephalosporins share many of the characteristics of the first- and second-generation drugs.

Prototype: cefotaxime sodium

Cefotaxime sodium (Claforan) is indicated for the treatment of bacteremia, meningitis, and serious infections of the respiratory and genitourinary tracts. It is usually administered by intermittent infusion but may also be given by direct injection.

Related drugs

Related third-generation drugs include ceftizoxime sodium (Cefizox) and ceftriaxone sodium (Rocephin). Ceftriaxone is generally preferred for home care because it requires only a single daily dose. Ceftazidime (Fortaz) also has activity against *Pseudomonas aeruginosa*.

Fourth-generation cephalosporins

Fourth-generation cephalosporins, like the third generations, have an expanded spectrum of activity against gram-negative bacteria compared with the first- and second-generation drugs. Activity is improved in vitro against *Pseudomonas aeruginosa* and certain Enterobacteriaceae, as well as gram-positive bacteria.

Prototype: cefepime

Cefepime (Maxipime) is used for the treatment of uncomplicated and complicated urinary tract infections, uncomplicated skin and skin structure infections, moderate to severe pneumonia caused by susceptible organisms, and febrile neutropenia.

Carbapenems

Carbapenems are β-lactam derivatives that inhibit cell wall synthesis, resulting in bactericidal activity. The carbapenems are resistant to β-lactamases and therefore have one of the broadest spectra of activity. Carbapenems are effective against many gram-positive, gram-negative, and anaerobic organisms and are therefore useful for treatment of polymicrobial infections.

Prototype: imipenem-cilastatin sodium

Imipenem-cilastatin sodium (Primaxin) is used for treatment of lower respiratory tract, urinary tract, intra-abdominal, gynecological, and skin and soft tissue infections. Doses are diluted in 100 mL of IV solution and administered over 30 to 60 minutes. Imipenem-cilastatin requires dose adjustment for renal insufficiency.

Adverse effects include gastrointestinal effects such as nausea, vomiting, and diarrhea. Hypersensitivity reactions have been reported, and since imipenem is a β-lactam derivative there is a slight potential for cross-reactivity in patients allergic to penicillins or cephalosporins. Adverse CNS effects including seizures may occur with imipenem therapy. Imipenem is nephrotoxic when administered alone and therefore it is coformulated with cilastatin, a substance with no antimicrobial activity that prevents the metabolism of imipenem in the renal tubules.

Related drugs

Meropenem (Merrem) is a synthetic carbapenem with a similar spectrum of activity as imipenem. It is used for treatment of intra-abdominal infections, bacterial meningitis, respiratory tract infections, and febrile neutropenia. Doripenem (Doribax) is the newest carbapenem and is similar to meropenem. Both meropenem and doripenem report seizures as an adverse effect, but the risk of seizures with these two agents is felt to be less than that with imipenem. Ertapenem (Invanz) has a slightly narrower spectrum of activity than the other carbapenems, lacking activity against *Pseudomonas aeruginosa* and *Acinetobacter*. It is often used in the outpatient setting since its long half-life allows for once-daily administration.

Aminoglycosides

Aminoglycosides are bactericidal antibiotics that are effective against several gram-negative organisms. Their name is derived from the amino sugars contained within their chemical structure.

Prototype: gentamicin sulfate

Gentamicin sulfate (Garamycin) is well distributed throughout all body fluids, achieves peak plasma concentrations within 30 minutes to 2 hours of administration, and maintains serum levels for up to 12 hours. It is often administered concurrently with a penicillin because the two drugs have synergistic bactericidal effects. Gentamicin is effective in the treatment of serious infections of the respiratory, urinary, and GI tracts; septicemia; and infections of the skin and soft tissue.

The most significant side effects associated with gentamicin are ototoxicity (associated with high peak plasma levels) and nephrotoxicity (associated with high trough levels). It has been suggested that this is the result of accumulation of the drug intracellularly in the inner ear and kidneys. Otic effects are manifested by vestibular symptoms (such as dizziness, nystagmus, vertigo, and ataxia) or auditory symptoms (such as tinnitus and hearing impairment). Nephrotoxicity is evidenced by increased blood urea nitrogen and serum creatinine levels and decreased creatinine clearance and urine specific gravity. Both ototoxicity and nephrotoxicity are more likely to occur in geriatric patients, patients with renal impairment, patients receiving high dosages or extended length of therapy, and patients receiving other ototoxic or nephrotoxic drugs. However, symptoms are usually reversible once the drug is discontinued.

Gentamicin may produce dose-related and self-limiting neuromuscular blockade. Symptoms range from general muscular weakness to seizures and a myasthenia gravis–like syndrome. Gentamicin may also provoke hypersensitivity reactions such as rash, urticaria, stomatitis, pruritus, fever, and eosinophilia.

There is a narrow margin between therapeutic and toxic concentrations of gentamicin. Therapeutic drug monitoring should be implemented to assess both peak and trough concentrations. Target peak concentrations can range from 4 to 12 mcg/mL depending on the infection. It is desirable to avoid peak serum concentrations of greater than 12 mcg/mL and trough levels above 2 mcg/mL. Monitoring of gentamicin serum levels requires that the trough sample be drawn 30 minutes before a scheduled dose, the dose be administered as scheduled, and the peak sample be drawn 30 to 60 minutes after completion of the scheduled dose.

Once-daily dosing of aminoglycosides has been recommended for patients without serious infections, severe renal dysfunction (creatinine clearance below 40 mL/min), or impaired host defenses. This dosing regimen achieves therapeutic effects by using the postantibiotic effect (the drug continues to eradicate bacteria for some time after the drug has cleared from the body) and reduces adverse effects. Higher concentrations are associated with increased bactericidal effects and reduction in resistance. Once-daily dosing also allows the body more time to clear the aminoglycoside, yielding reduced toxicity. Because of the larger total daily dosage, the infusion time should be extended to 60 minutes.

For serious enterococcal infections, an aminoglycoside antibiotic is added to the penicillin to eradicate the infection. Using the aminoglycoside adds synergy to the penicillin, which is often inadequate therapy when used alone.

Related drugs

Aminoglycosides similar to gentamicin include amikacin sulfate (Amikin), kanamycin sulfate (Kantrex), and tobramycin sulfate (Nebcin). These drugs are usually reserved for the treatment of gentamicin-resistant infections.

Tetracyclines

Tetracyclines were the first broad-spectrum antibiotics developed. They are considered bacteriostatic but may have bactericidal activity in high concentrations. Although IV tetracycline is no longer available commercially, there are other tetracycline antibiotics that may be administered intravenously.

Prototype: doxycycline hyclate

Doxycycline hyclate (Vibramycin) is indicated for infections caused by susceptible organisms such as *Rickettsiae, Chlamydia,* and *Mycoplasma,* and as a substitute when penicillin therapy is contraindicated. Doxycycline is usually administered by intermittent infusion in 100 to 200 mL of fluid over 1 to 4 hours.

The most common side effects of doxycycline are dose-related effects on the GI tract. Manifestations include nausea, vomiting, diarrhea, and anorexia. Other adverse effects include hypersensitivity reactions and blood dyscrasias. In addition, the administration of doxycycline may cause venous irritation and thrombophlebitis, requiring that the IV site be rotated more frequently than every 72 hours. Photosensitivity reactions may occur, resulting in exaggerated sunburn on areas of the body exposed to the sun. Although it is not a significant risk for hospitalized patients, home patients should be alerted to this potential reaction.

Related Drugs

Tigecycline (Tygacil) is the first member of the glycylcycline class, and is structurally related to the tetracyclines. It has a broad spectrum of activity including gram-positive, gram-negative, and anaerobic organisms. Tigecycline is approved for treatment of complicated skin and skin structure infections and intra-abdominal infections, and has activity against resistant organisms such as methicillin-resistant *Staphylococcus aureus* (MRSA) and vancomycin-resistant *Enterococcus* (VRE). It is administered over 30 to 60 minutes in 100 mL of fluid.

The most common adverse effects reported with tigecycline are gastrointestinal, including nausea, vomiting, and diarrhea. Nausea and vomiting affect a significant portion of patients who receive tigecycline, with rates reported to exceed 20% (McEvoy, 2007). Other adverse effects include hepatic enzyme elevation and local injection site reactions.

Macrolides

Like the tetracyclines, the macrolides are generally bacteriostatic but may have bactericidal activity when administered in high concentrations. The only macrolide administered intravenously is erythromycin lactobionate, but a macrolide subclass of azalide antibiotics have experienced increased use because of better patient tolerance.

Prototype: erythromycin lactobionate

Erythromycin lactobionate (Erythrocin) is primarily indicated for staphylococcal, pneumococcal, and streptococcal infections and in the treatment of legionnaires' disease. It may also be used as an alternative for patients allergic to penicillin. Although erythromycin may be administered as a continuous infusion, it is generally given as an intermittent infusion in 100 to 250 mL of fluid over 20 to 60 minutes. The infusion time may be extended if the patient experiences venous discomfort during administration.

Erythromycin is relatively free from serious side effects. However, the patient must be monitored for hearing loss secondary to IV erythromycin. The most common complaint is localized venous irritation during administration, which may be minimized by slowing the infusion rate, further diluting the medication, and rotating the site more often. Mild allergic reactions such as urticaria and rash have also been reported.

Since erythromycin is unstable if the pH is lower than 5.5, 1 mL of sodium bicarbonate (e.g., Neut) may be added to acidic solutions such as D_5W to increase its stability. When erythromycin is in solution for only a short period, as with an intermittent infusion activated at the time of use, such buffering is considered unnecessary.

Increased serum levels of cyclosporine, digoxin, carbamazepine, and theophylline may occur with the administration of erythromycin. Serum levels of these drugs may be tested to monitor therapy.

Azalide subclass
Prototype: azithromycin

Azithromycin (Zithromax) is used for treatment of respiratory tract infections caused by organisms such as *Haemophilus influenzae, Chlamydiae, Mycoplasma, Streptococcus,* and *Legionella.* This drug may be used if the patient is known to be allergic to penicillin. This drug is administered by IV infusion in 250 to 500 mL of solution to give a concentration of 1 to 2 mg/mL over 1 hour. Azithromycin is well tolerated, but hypersensitivity reactions have been reported. Few drug interactions have been reported with azithromycin.

Quinolones

The quinolones are usually bactericidal in action. These antibiotics have activity against gram-positive and gram-negative organisms, and some quinolones also have antipseudomonal activity. Resistant strains of *Pseudomonas, Neisseria gonorrhoeae,* and *E. coli* have emerged where fluoroquinolones have been used excessively.

Prototype: ciprofloxacin

Ciprofloxacin (Cipro) should be diluted to a concentration of 1 to 2 mg/mL and infused over 60 minutes. A large vein is recommended for administration to lessen venous irritation. Hydration is recommended to prevent crystalluria. For patients with renal or hepatic impairment, dosages should be adjusted and monitored through the course of treatment. Central nervous system (CNS) reactions have been reported, ranging in severity from insomnia to manic reactions and toxic psychosis. Infrequent adverse effects include hypersensitivity reactions, photosensitivity, and tendon rupture.

Related drugs

Levofloxacin (Levaquin) and moxifloxacin (Avelox) are quinolones that are used in ambulatory settings and hospitals because of their once-daily administration regimen and ability to penetrate soft tissues as well as the respiratory tract. Dosage adjustment in those with renal impairment is necessary for levofloxacin.

Miscellaneous antibiotics

Some antibiotics do not belong to a specific classification. Because they share common properties with all antibiotics, only their unique characteristics are discussed here.

Aztreonam

Aztreonam (Azactam) is the first drug in a new class of antibiotics known as monobactams. Aztreonam has a similar mechanism of action as other β-lactams and has activity against gram-negative organisms. However, aztreonam differs structurally from β-lactams and has a very low rate of cross-sensitivity with penicillins and cephalosporins. Given the probability of cross-sensitivity is not as great and typically does not result in a serious, life-threatening allergic reaction, aztreonam may still be indicated for patients with a β-lactam allergy.

Chloramphenicol sodium succinate

Chloramphenicol is a bacteriostatic antibiotic that may be bactericidal when used in high concentrations. Although different forms of the drug are available for oral and topical administration, only the sodium succinate salt of chloramphenicol may be administered intravenously. Chloramphenicol sodium succinate (Chloromycetin) is reserved for serious infections caused by susceptible organisms such as *Rickettsia, H. influenzae, Bacillus anthracis,* and *Salmonella typhi.* It is reserved for use when less toxic agents are ineffective or contraindicated. Regardless of the indication, the preferred method of administration is by intermittent infusion.

Although chloramphenicol is associated with fewer minor side effects than other antibiotics, it is more likely to cause serious and potentially fatal adverse reactions. Most notable are its hematological effects, which may lead to two types of bone marrow depression. The first is rare, irreversible, and not dose related, and results in aplastic anemia, with a mortality rate that exceeds 50% (McEvoy, 2007). The second and more common type is dose related; it is usually reversible once the drug is discontinued. Symptoms include reticulocytopenia, anemia, leukopenia, and thrombocytopenia. Because of the possibility of hematological effects, a serum level should not exceed 5 to 20 mcg/mL, and laboratory values should be monitored carefully.

Clindamycin phosphate

Clindamycin phosphate (Cleocin) is a bacteriostatic antibiotic that is effective against anaerobic and aerobic organisms. It is chemically unrelated to penicillin, so it is useful in penicillin-sensitive patients. Side effects associated with clindamycin are diarrhea, pseudomembranous colitis, and a generalized rash. Because hypotension and cardiopulmonary arrest have been reported following too rapid administration of the drug, it is recommended that clindamycin be administered by intermittent infusion over a minimum of 10 minutes.

Colistimethate sodium

Colistimethate sodium is inactive until hydrolyzed in solution to colistin. Colistin is a bactericidal compound that has activity against gram-negative organisms. Due to serious side effects, such as nephrotoxicity and neurotoxicity, colistin use had decreased with the development of safer alternatives such as the carbapenems. However, due to increasing antibiotic resistance colistin is again being employed as a treatment for highly resistant gram-negative infections. Its adverse effect profile warrants close monitoring of renal function and neurological status.

Daptomycin

Daptomycin (Cubicin) is a bactericidal antibiotic used for treatment of gram-positive infections. It has activity against *Staphylococcus aureus* and *Enterococci,* including MRSA and VRE. Daptomycin is inactivated by lung surfactant and therefore cannot be used for the treatment of pneumonia or other lung infections. Daptomycin can cause skeletal muscle pain and increased creatine kinase (CK) levels. It is recommended to monitor CK levels weekly while receiving daptomycin. Daptomycin is often used in patients with serious infections who cannot receive vancomycin.

Linezolid

Linezolid (Zyvox) is a bacteriostatic antibiotic with activity against gram-positive organisms, including MRSA and VRE. It has good tissue penetration and is often used for treatment of serious, hospital-acquired pneumonias. Linezolid can cause myelosuppression, especially in patients who receive linezolid for more than 2 weeks. It is recommended to monitor a complete blood count (CBC) at least weekly while receiving linezolid therapy.

Quinupristin/dalfopristin

Quinupristin/dalfopristin (Synercid) is a combination of two semisynthetic streptogramin antibiotics: quinupristin and dalfopristin in a ratio of 30:70. Quinupristin/dalfopristin inhibits protein synthesis in the ribosomes and is converted to several major active metabolites in the body. It has activity against *Enterococcus faecium, S. aureus,* and *Streptococcus pyogenes,* including MRSA and VRE. Because the drug has a postantibiotic effect against certain organisms, dosing regimens of every 8 to 12 hours may be used. The drug is compatible only with D$_5$W. Because D$_5$W flushes are not commercially available, a container of D$_5$W must be used to flush the line. Quinupristin/dalfopristin is stable for only 5 hours at room temperature; this extends to 54 hours when stored under refrigeration. Major side effects reported are inflammation, edema, pain at the infusion site, and arthralgias. It has been reported that if the dose is reduced, the arthralgias will improve. Because of the 25% incidence of venous intolerance, it is recommended that a central line or a peripherally inserted central catheter be used to administer this drug. Quinupristin/dalfopristin requires larger infusion volumes because of phlebitis: 100 mL for central lines and 250 mL for peripheral lines. Increasing the infusion volume to 500 mL may help with the venous irritation. The use of hydrocortisone or diphenhydramine hydrochloride does not decrease the phlebitis.

Vancomycin hydrochloride

Vancomycin hydrochloride (Vancocin) is a bactericidal antibiotic. It is considered the drug of choice for methicillin-resistant staphylococcal infections and for staphylococcal infections in patients who are allergic to penicillin. The two most serious side effects of vancomycin are ototoxicity and nephrotoxicity. In addition, rapid administration results in hypotension and a transient reddish blotching caused by histamine release (red man syndrome). This reaction can be avoided if vancomycin is administered over a minimum of 60 minutes.

OTHER ANTI-INFECTIVE AGENTS

Since antibiotics are primarily effective against bacterial organisms, other agents are required to treat infections caused by fungi, viruses, and protozoa. Categories of drugs discussed in this section include antifungal agents, antiviral agents, and antiprotozoal drugs. Although sulfonamide combination products have antibacterial activity, they have been included in this section because of their unique properties.

Antifungal agents

Systemic fungal infections, although rare, are difficult to treat and are more common in immunosuppressed patients. Such infections may be treated with antifungal agents that act by binding to sterols in the membrane of the fungal cell. Once the drug binds to the cell membrane, the cell no longer has a protective barrier, the cellular constituents are lost, and the cell is destroyed. Bacteria do not contain sterols in their cell membranes; therefore antifungal agents are not active against these organisms.

Amphotericin B deoxycholate

Amphotericin B deoxycholate (Fungizone) is used for treating progressive and potentially fatal infections such as aspergillosis, blastomycosis, coccidioidomycosis, cryptococcosis, and histoplasmosis.

Common infusion-related side effects of amphotericin include headache, chills, fever, malaise, anorexia, nausea, and vomiting. Antipyretics, antihistamines, and antiemetics may provide symptomatic relief when administered before or during therapy, and hydrocortisone may be added to the infusion to decrease the severity of febrile reactions. Another expected reaction to amphotericin is thrombophlebitis at the injection site, but the incidence may be decreased by the addition of 500 to 1000 units of heparin to the infusion.

The selective binding of amphotericin to sterols accounts for the toxicity of the drug. Some body cells, such as kidney cells, contain sterols that bind to the drug, making the cell subject to alterations in cellular permeability. Some degree of nephrotoxicity occurs in more than 80% of patients receiving amphotericin and may be manifested by elevated blood urea nitrogen (McEvoy, 2007) and creatinine levels, hypokalemia, and hypomagnesemia. To decrease these nephrotoxic effects, a sodium load of 0.9% sodium chloride by direct IV may be administered immediately before each dose of amphotericin.

Amphotericin may also bind with sterols in the cellular membrane of erythrocytes. Consequently, a reversible, normocytic, normochromic anemia occurs in most patients receiving amphotericin. Cardiovascular toxicities such as hypotension, ventricular fibrillation, and cardiac arrest are rare but may occur with rapid infusion of the drug.

Precautions regarding the administration of amphotericin may include infusing the drug over a minimum of 4 hours to reduce the incidence of infusion reactions and monitoring the injection site for signs of phlebitis. However, more rapid infusion rates may be used if the patient's renal function is normal. Throughout therapy, the patient's serum electrolyte levels and renal function require monitoring, and the patient should be assessed for symptoms of electrolyte imbalance.

Related drugs

Amphotericin B lipid complex (Abelcet), amphotericin B liposomal (AmBisome), and amphotericin B cholesteryl sulfate (Amphotec) are newer agents that may be infused more quickly than amphotericin B deoxycholate (Fungizone) (over 2 hours initially and shorter for the next therapy, if tolerated). These agents have been reported to be less nephrotoxic and are generally reserved for patients who cannot tolerate amphotericin B deoxycholate.

Azoles

The azole class of antifungal agents is commonly used for treatment of candidiasis. Selected azoles are also effective for other fungal infections such as cryptococcosis, coccidioidomycosis, blastomycosis, histoplasmosis, and aspergillosis. In general, the azoles are better tolerated than amphotericin B.

Prototype: fluconazole

Fluconazole (Diflucan) is indicated for the treatment of serious systemic candidal infections and cryptococcal infections. Fluconazole is generally well-tolerated. Common adverse events include nausea and vomiting, headache, and abdominal pain. Serious hepatic reactions and exfoliative skin disorders may also occur but are less likely. With serious, life-threatening infections, patients are usually given a loading dose to elevate serum levels. Fluconazole, as with all azoles, is an inhibitor of the cytochrome P450 enzyme system that can lead to an increase in serum levels of drugs metabolized by this system.

Related drugs

Voriconazole (VFEND) has a similar mechanism of action as fluconazole, and it has increased activity against *Aspergillus*. An adverse reaction unique to voriconazole is a change in color vision or visual perception, which usually resolves with discontinuation of therapy. The IV formulation contains cyclodextran to improve solubility, as voriconazole can accumulate in patients with decreased renal function. Therefore the IV formulation should not be used in patients with a creatinine clearance less than 50 mL/min.

Echinocandis

The echinocandins are a newer class of antifungal agents. They are primarily used for treatment of candidal infections.

Prototype: caspofungin acetate

Caspofungin acetate (Cancidas) is indicated for treatment of invasive candidal infections. It may also be used for aspergillosis when patients are intolerant of other therapies such as voriconazole or amphotericin B. A loading dose of 70 mg is administered on day 1 of therapy, followed by 50 mg daily. Common adverse effects include phlebitis, diarrhea, and vomiting. Unlike the azoles, caspofungin does not affect the cytochrome P450 enzyme system and therefore has minimal drug interactions.

Related drugs

Anidulafungin (Eraxis) and micafungin (Mycamine) are similar to caspofungin in activity and adverse effect profile.

Antiviral agents

Treatment for viral diseases is generally less effective than that for bacterial infections. Agents capable of killing the virus can also kill the host cells; therefore antiviral therapy is limited to inhibiting the viral replication process. In addition, viral infections often progress without clinical signs or symptoms early in the course of illness, when the drugs might be most effective.

Prototype: acyclovir sodium

Acyclovir (Zovirax), indicated in the treatment of herpes simplex and varicella-zoster infections, is one of the most common and useful antiviral agents. Acyclovir is activated by an enzyme produced by the virus, resulting in the inhibition of DNA production within the virus, thus preventing viral replication.

Each acyclovir dose is administered over at least 1 hour since rapid administration may result in precipitation of the drugs in renal tubules. Acyclovir crystals may occlude the renal tubules; therefore adequate hydration and urine output must be maintained before and during the infusion. The more common side effects associated with acyclovir are headache and thrombophlebitis.

Other antiviral agents

Other antiviral agents include ganciclovir sodium (Cytovene), zidovudine (AZT), foscarnet (Foscavir), and ribavirin (Vibrazole). Ganciclovir is structurally and pharmacologically related to acyclovir, and is indicated in the treatment of cytomegalovirus in immunosuppressed patients, particularly those infected with human immunodeficiency virus (HIV). Because of its mutagenic potential, guidelines for handling cytotoxic agents must be followed when preparing and administering ganciclovir. Zidovudine is an antiviral agent effective against human immunodeficiency virus, and is the only HIV agent available in an IV formulation. The primary use for IV zidovudine is to prevent transmission of HIV from mother to baby in the peripartum period. The most serious side effects of zidovudine are hematological effects, nausea, and headache. Ribavirin has broad antiviral activity and is therefore used for a variety of viral illnesses, including adenovirus infections and viral hemorrhagic fevers. Foscarnet is effective against herpes viruses including cytomegalovirus. Foscarnet causes nephrotoxicity to some degree in almost all patients who receive the drug, and many require dosage adjustment.

Antiprotozoal drugs

The two drugs identified for their antiprotozoal activity, metronidazole and pentamidine, also have properties that make them effective against certain other organisms.

Prototype: metronidazole

Metronidazole (Flagyl) is a bactericidal agent that is effective against protozoa and specific anaerobic bacteria. Indications include serious intra-abdominal, gynecological, and lower respiratory tract infections and *Clostridium difficile* infection. Although metronidazole may be given as a continuous infusion, it is typically administered as an intermittent infusion over a minimum of 1 hour.

The most common side effects of metronidazole are nausea, anorexia, headache, and an unpleasant metallic taste. Peripheral neuropathy, characterized by tingling, numbness, or paresthesia of the extremity, has been reported but is reversible once the drug is discontinued. If alcohol is ingested while receiving metronidazole, disulfiram-like reactions, such as flushing, headache, nausea, sweating, and abdominal cramps, may occur. Patients with hepatic dysfunction require a lower dosage.

Related drugs

Another antiprotozoal agent is pentamidine isethionate (Pentam). It is specifically indicated in the treatment of *Pneumocystis jiroveci* pneumonia if the patient does not respond to trimethoprim-sulfamethoxazole. Severe hypotensive reactions may occur, particularly if pentamidine is administered over less than 60 minutes. Other adverse reactions include nephrotoxicity, hypoglycemia, leukopenia, and thrombocytopenia.

Trimetrexate

Trimetrexate is used to treat moderate to severe *P. jiroveci* pneumonia in immunosuppressed patients, including those with HIV. It is a dihydrofolate reductase inhibitor, and many of its adverse effects are due to its activity on the folic acid pathway (neutropenia, thrombocytopenia, anemia). To lessen the incidence of adverse effects, leucovorin should be administered concomitantly and for 72 hours after the last dose of trimetrexate.

Sulfonamide combination products

Sulfonamides are broad-spectrum antimicrobial agents that have been used for more than 50 years. Although their general use has declined with the introduction of penicillins and cephalosporins, they remain an inexpensive and effective antibacterial therapy. Sulfonamides are usually bacteriostatic; they act by depriving the bacteria of folate products required for DNA synthesis. This inhibits the growth and reproduction of the microorganism. Body cells, unlike bacterial cells, do not synthesize their own folic acid and are unaffected by the drugs.

Sulfonamides are associated with numerous adverse reactions that involve nearly every body system. Because sulfonamide combination products contain a sulfonamide in addition to another drug, all precautions applicable to sulfonamides apply to the combination products.

Prototype: trimethoprim-sulfamethoxazole

Trimethoprim-sulfamethoxazole (Bactrim, Septra) is a combination of sulfamethoxazole and trimethoprim at a fixed 5:1 ratio, which produces bactericidal effects. It is used in the treatment of severe urinary tract infections, *P. jiroveci* pneumonia, and many other uncommon infections.

Since it contains a sulfonamide, trimethoprim-sulfamethoxazole is associated with three major types of side effects. First are hypersensitivity reactions, which range from rash to anaphylaxis. Second, sulfonamides may crystallize in the renal tubules, causing renal damage. The risk is reduced by maintaining adequate hydration and urinary output or by reducing the dosage. Third, sulfonamides may have a toxic effect on the bone marrow, resulting in aplastic anemia, thrombocytopenia, and agranulocytosis. Overall, the most common side effects of trimethoprim-sulfamethoxazole are nausea, vomiting, and rash.

Sulfonamides bind to the plasma proteins, either displacing or being displaced by other protein-bound drugs. They potentiate the effects of warfarin and phenytoin but are inhibited by alkalinizing agents and thiopental. In addition, sulfonamides can be cross-sensitized with other drugs containing a sulfa structure, such as thiazide diuretics and oral hypoglycemics. Dosages must be reduced for patients with moderate to severe renal dysfunction.

CENTRAL NERVOUS SYSTEM AGENTS

The central nervous system (CNS) is biologically complex and susceptible to interference by many pharmacological agents. Because the CNS controls multiple physiological functions, drugs that act centrally may have secondary effects on other body systems. There are many ways of classifying CNS drugs, but one of the most useful is according to their mechanism of action.

Analgesics

Analgesics are administered to relieve pain. Narcotic agonist analgesics may cause stupor or insensibility, also known as *narcosis*. These drugs are often referred to as *opiate agonists* because they are chemically related to morphine, which is derived from the opium poppy (Katzung, 2007).

Narcotic analgesics

Although the narcotic analgesics vary in potency, they share several common properties. In addition to pain relief, narcotic analgesics act as agonists on specific opiate receptors, share the major side effect of respiratory depression, and cause drowsiness. Repeated administration may produce tolerance to the drug or the phenomenon of cross-tolerance, which occurs when tolerance to the action of one narcotic also confers tolerance to the action of a different narcotic.

Prototype: morphine sulfate

The prototype of all narcotic analgesics is morphine sulfate. By binding to the opiate receptors, morphine relieves severe pain and inhibits the perception of pain. It may also alter the patient's mood, producing a feeling of euphoria. The primary indications for morphine are severe pain and apprehension associated with coronary occlusion, chronic pain associated with malignancies, and postoperative pain.

Although morphine may be administered by slow, direct injection or continuous infusion, it may also be administered as a patient-controlled analgesic (PCA). Using a PCA pump, the patient may self-administer frequent, small doses based on requirements for pain relief and the program prescribed for the PCA device.

The major side effect of morphine is respiratory depression. Patients with impaired respiratory function or those receiving morphine by rapid injection are at greatest risk. Other adverse effects of morphine include hypotension, miosis, drowsiness, and sedation. Minor side effects such as pruritus, nausea, vomiting, and constipation are more common.

The contraindications for morphine are based on its pharmacological effects. Because morphine may produce respiratory depression, it is generally contraindicated in patients with poor pulmonary function, such as those with emphysema and asthma, and in patients with closed head injuries. Morphine also produces spasmogenic effects on the smooth muscle of the GI and genitourinary tracts and should be used with caution in patients with disorders affecting these systems.

The action of morphine may be potentiated by other drugs that have similar effects. A reduced dosage of both drugs may be indicated. Drugs that cause sedation or CNS depression should be used with caution in combination with morphine.

Related drugs

The other narcotic analgesics are related to morphine but differ in terms of analgesic potency. Hydromorphone hydrochloride (Dilaudid) is approximately 5 times as potent as morphine, whereas meperidine hydrochloride (Demerol) has an analgesic potency equivalent to 20% that of morphine and a shorter duration of action.

Antagonists

Naloxone (Narcan) is a narcotic antagonist that blocks the opiate receptors, thus inhibiting or reversing the narcotic effects. Naloxone is specifically used to counteract opiate-induced respiratory depression and narcotic overdose. The usual dosage is 0.4 to 2 mg administered as a direct injection. Potential adverse reactions include nausea, vomiting, tremor, and hyperventilation.

Nalmefene (Revex) is similar in activity to naltrexone, but has a longer duration of activity.

Mixed opiate agonist-antagonists

Mixed opiate agonist-antagonists behave as agonists when administered to a patient who has not previously received a narcotic analgesic. In this manner, the drugs interact with the receptors and alter the function of the cells to produce effects similar to those of the narcotic analgesics. However, when mixed opiate agonist-antagonists are administered to a patient who is receiving a narcotic analgesic, they produce an antagonistic effect and inhibit the response to the narcotic analgesic. Mixed opiate agonist-antagonists are also called *opiate partial agonists* because their actions are similar to those of opiate agonists, but only under specific conditions (Katzung, 2007; Goldman and Ausiello, 2008).

Prototype: buprenorphine hydrochloride

The prototype of the mixed opiate agonist-antagonists is buprenorphine hydrochloride (Buprenex). When administered as a narcotic agonist, buprenorphine is 30 times more potent than morphine. It is therefore indicated for the relief of moderate to severe pain, especially in patients with a hypersensitivity to narcotic analgesics. Although buprenorphine produces an antagonistic effect approximately three times greater than that of naloxone, it is rarely used clinically to reverse the effects of opiates.

The major side effect associated with buprenorphine is excessive sedation. Other effects on the nervous system include dizziness, vertigo, headache, confusion, euphoria, and insomnia. Nausea, vomiting, and respiratory depression have also been reported after buprenorphine administration.

Related drugs

Related opiate partial agonists are nalbuphine hydrochloride (Nubain) and pentazocine lactate (Talwin). The mechanism of action, indications, and side effects of both drugs are similar to those of buprenorphine. However, respiratory depression associated with nalbuphine does not increase with increasing doses, as occurs with buprenorphine.

Butorphanol (Stadol) is a synthetic partial opiate agonist analgesic. It is structurally related to morphine but pharmacologically similar to nalbuphine and pentazocine.

Sedatives, hypnotics, and anxiolytics

Several CNS depressants cause drowsiness (sedatives), induce sleep (hypnotics), or relieve anxiety (anxiolytics). These drugs may be chemically classified as barbiturates, which produce CNS depression ranging from sedation to anesthesia; benzodiazepines, which relieve anxiety without causing ataxia or sleep; and miscellaneous CNS agents that produce antiemetic and sedative or anxiolytic effects.

Barbiturates

Barbiturates make up the traditional group of CNS depressants. They can produce varying levels of CNS depression ranging from mild sedation and hypnosis to coma and death. Generally, barbiturates share the same pharmacological effects, side effects, contraindications, and drug interactions.

Prototype: phenobarbital sodium

Phenobarbital sodium (Luminal) is primarily used as an anticonvulsant for management of tonic-clonic and partial seizures, and may also be used for its sedative effects. It inhibits abnormal electrical activity in the brain without producing marked sedation, and is useful in both pediatric and adult patients.

Phenobarbital is administered by direct injection; too rapid administration of phenobarbital may cause respiratory depression, apnea, laryngospasm, and hypotension. The most common side effects of phenobarbital are excessive sedation and ataxia; fever and rash may also occur. In addition, phenobarbital may cause pain or thrombophlebitis at the injection site.

Phenobarbital may potentiate the effects of other CNS depressants and the adverse effects of antidepressants. Since phenobarbital stimulates the hepatic metabolizing enzymes, it increases the metabolism of corticosteroids and digoxin; therefore increased dosages of these drugs may be required. It also inhibits the effectiveness of doxycycline, propranolol, oral anticoagulants, and theophylline.

Related drugs

Other barbiturates that may be administered intravenously are pentobarbital sodium (Nembutal) and thiopental sodium (Pentothal). These drugs differ primarily in their onset and duration of action. Thiopental is an ultrashort-acting barbiturate used primarily for its anesthetic effect. Pentobarbital is a short-acting barbiturates used for preanesthetic sedation and to control status epilepticus or other acute seizures.

Benzodiazepines

Benzodiazepines differ from barbiturates chemically but share many of the same indications. Often, benzodiazepines are preferred to barbiturates because they have a greater margin of safety and are less likely to interact with other drugs and to cause physical dependence. Benzodiazepines have four basic actions: they reduce anxiety, produce sedation, relax muscle spasticity, and act as anticonvulsants.

Prototype: diazepam

Diazepam (Valium) depresses the autonomic, central, and peripheral nervous systems. For this reason, IV diazepam is indicated for the emergency treatment of status epilepticus or recurrent seizures, the treatment of acute alcohol withdrawal, the treatment of skeletal muscle spasm, and the relief of apprehension before electric cardioversion, endoscopy, or surgery.

Because of several reports of precipitation of the drug when diluted, the preferred method of diazepam injection is by direct injection into the vein. When direct IV injection is not feasible, diazepam should be injected into the administration set as close to the vein site as possible. If this alternative method is used, the IV catheter should be flushed with 0.9% sodium chloride before and after the administration of diazepam. The manufacturers state that diazepam may form a precipitate when mixed with other solutions, including sodium chloride, so the possibility of precipitate formation still exists when flushing the catheter. Nonetheless, most clinicians agree that this risk of precipitation is lower than if diazepam is mixed with other medications in the administration set.

The most common adverse reactions to diazepam are the results of CNS depression and include drowsiness, ataxia, confusion, syncope, and vertigo. Anticholinergic side effects, or atropine-like reactions, may also occur and result in blurred vision, mydriasis, and dry mouth. Other adverse reactions, such as apnea, hypotension, or bradycardia, are rare and are generally associated with rapid administration of the drug.

As a result of the possibility of anticholinergic effects, diazepam is contraindicated in patients with acute narrow-angle glaucoma. It is also contraindicated for patients with acute alcohol intoxication whose vital signs are depressed and for patients with known hypersensitivity to the benzodiazepines.

Diazepam is potentiated by other drugs that produce similar CNS depression and by cimetidine. In addition, diazepam potentiates the effects of narcotics, barbiturates, antihistamines, and phenothiazines. When diazepam is administered concurrently with levodopa, the antiparkinsonian effects of levodopa may be inhibited.

Related drugs

The three other benzodiazepines that are most commonly administered by the IV route are chlordiazepoxide hydrochloride (Librium), lorazepam (Ativan), and midazolam hydrochloride (Versed). Chlordiazepoxide is primarily used for acute or severe agitation and acute alcoholism withdrawal, and lorazepam is used as a preanesthetic medication for adult patients. Midazolam is a short-acting benzodiazepine that has been effective in producing conscious sedation for endoscopic and cardiovascular procedures in healthy adults. Since hypoxia or cardiac arrest may occur after midazolam is given, administration of the drug should be limited to settings in which respiratory and cardiac function may be monitored continuously.

Antagonists

Flumazenil (Romazicon) is a benzodiazepine receptor antagonist indicated for the reversal of the sedative effects of benzodiazepines. The duration and degree of reversal correspond with the dose of flumazenil administered and the resultant plasma concentration. The usual initial dosage is 0.2 mg administered by direct injection over 15 seconds; additional doses may be administered at 30-second intervals up to a cumulative dose of 3 mg. The onset of action is usually evident within 1 to 2 minutes after the injection is completed. Adverse effects include cutaneous vasodilation, dizziness, visual disturbances, and pain at the injection site.

Miscellaneous central nervous system agents

Two other CNS drugs, droperidol and dexmedetomidine, are often administered intravenously. Rather than reviewing their drug classifications, only information specific to these drugs is discussed here.

Droperidol

Droperidol (Inapsine) is a butyrophenone derivative. The primary indications of this drug are for preoperative sedation and for reduction of the incidence of nausea and vomiting during surgical and diagnostic procedures. Cases of QT-interval prolongation and torsades de pointes have been reported with droperidol. The manufacturer recommends all patients should have an electrocardiogram (ECG) performed before droperidol administration. Because of the potential for serious adverse events, droperidol is reserved for patients who do not respond to other treatment options.

Dexmedetomidine hydrochloride

Dexmedetomidine hydrochloride (Precedex) is an alpha$_2$-receptor agonist that produces sedative effects. It is used for preoperative sedation as an adjunct to anesthesia. Dexmedetomidine is administered by slow, continuous IV infusion with dose titrations to desired sedative response. Unlike many other sedative agents, dexmedetomidine does not provide amnestic effect. Common adverse effects are hypotension and bradycardia.

Anticonvulsants

Epilepsy is a neurological disorder characterized by a recurrent pattern of abnormal neuron discharges within the brain. The result is a sudden loss of consciousness, inappropriate behavior, and/or involuntary body movements. Seizures may be classified as partial, with electroencephalogram (EEG) changes confined to one area of the brain, or generalized, involving the symmetrical distribution of abnormal brain discharges. Status epilepticus results when several generalized seizures with convulsions occur successively without intervals of restored consciousness or normal muscle activity. Although anticonvulsants suppress the start or reduce the spread of seizures, they do not treat the underlying cause of the seizures. Therefore the type of seizure, not the underlying cause, determines the drug of choice.

Many of the drugs previously discussed have anticonvulsant properties. Phenobarbital is indicated for the treatment of generalized and partial seizures, and diazepam is the drug of choice for status epilepticus. Two additional categories of drugs, hydantoins and magnesium sulfate, are also indicated in the management of seizure activity.

Hydantoins

Hydantoins are used to treat tonic-clonic and complex partial seizures. Their principle feature is the ability to control seizures without causing sedation.

Prototype: phenytoin sodium

Phenytoin sodium (Dilantin) is a hydantoin derivative. Although it is used primarily for its anticonvulsant features, it also has antiarrhythmic properties similar to those of procainamide. The primary indications for phenytoin are the control of clonic-tonic and psychomotor seizures.

The preferred method for administering phenytoin is by direct IV injection at a rate not exceeding 50 mg/min. Since phenytoin precipitates if the pH is altered, the administration set and catheter must be cleared by flushing with 0.9% sodium chloride before and after administration. This prevents phenytoin from mixing with other drugs. Solutions of 0.9% sodium chloride can be used to infuse phenytoin in concentrations of 100 mg per 25 to 50 mL of diluent. When this alternative mode of administration is used, it is recommended the drug be infused through an in-line 0.22-micron filter.

When phenytoin is administered as an anticonvulsant, the most common side effects involve the CNS. Sluggishness, ataxia, nystagmus, confusion, slurred speech, dizziness, nervousness, and fatigue may occur. Gingival hyperplasia and excessive growth of the gums may also occur with extended therapy. Because of its antiarrhythmic properties, phenytoin is associated with adverse cardiovascular effects. Hypotension may occur with too rapid administration of the drug, whereas phenytoin toxicity may result in cardiovascular collapse. In addition, status epilepticus may result from abrupt withdrawal of the drug.

There is a narrow therapeutic margin associated with phenytoin. Acceptable plasma levels range from 10 to 20 mcg/mL, and signs of toxicity occur once plasma levels exceed 20 mcg/mL. Symptoms of toxicity include nystagmus, ataxia, dysarthria, tremors, and slurred speech.

The major contraindication for phenytoin is hypersensitivity to hydantoins. Because of its effects on cardiac electrical activity, phenytoin should not be administered to patients with sinus bradycardia, sinoatrial block, second- or third-degree heart block, or Adams-Stokes syndrome.

Related drugs

Fosphenytoin (Cerebyx), a prodrug of phenytoin, can be administered more rapidly than phenytoin. However, fosphenytoin must be converted to phenytoin in the body, yielding a similar onset of action. It is associated with less infusion-related problems as compared to phenytoin.

Miscellaneous anticonvulsants

Magnesium sulfate is a CNS depressant that exhibits anticonvulsant properties when administered parenterally. As such, magnesium sulfate is indicated for the prevention and control of seizures associated with severe preeclampsia or eclampsia. The primary adverse reaction associated with magnesium sulfate is magnesium intoxication. Symptoms of hypermagnesemia begin at serum magnesium concentrations of 4 mEq/L and include the absence of the knee-jerk reflex, hypotension with signs of tetany, hyperthermia, circulatory collapse, and depression of CNS and cardiac function. Levetiracetam (Keppra) is used for partial seizures in combination with other agents. Common adverse effects are somnolence and fatigue, coordination difficulties, and behavioral changes. Valproate sodium (Depacon) is used for simplex or complex absence seizures. It also is effective in treating bipolar disorder, schizophrenia, and migraine headaches. Adverse effects include injection site reactions, nausea, vomiting, anorexia, sedation, and drowsiness.

CARDIOVASCULAR AGENTS

Drugs that alter cardiovascular function have a variety of actions. They can affect cardiac strength and rhythm, counteract hypotension, control hypertension, and improve blood flow. Since a comprehensive discussion of these agents is beyond our scope here, the focus is on the major categories of cardiovascular agents. The sympathetic nervous system plays a major role in cardiovascular function, and drugs acting on the CNS are discussed in this section.

Drugs acting through adrenergic receptors

Adrenergic receptors on the target cells within the sympathetic nervous system mediate the response of neurotransmitters (for example, norepinephrine and epinephrine). Drugs that elicit biological responses similar to those produced by activation of the sympathetic nervous system are known as *sympathomimetics;* drugs that inhibit the effects of sympathetic stimulation are called *sympatholytics.* Since sympathomimetics mimic the sympathetic nervous system and provoke a response in the adrenergic receptors, they are also known as *adrenergic agonists.* In contrast, sympatholytics block the sympathetic nervous system and inhibit the adrenergic response, so they are referred to as *adrenergic blocking agents* (Katzung, 2007).

Cardiovascular drugs that elicit or inhibit the adrenergic response are also classified according to the subtype of adrenergic receptor site stimulated. There are four major subtypes of adrenergic receptors: alpha$_1$, alpha$_2$, beta$_1$, and beta$_2$. Alpha$_1$-adrenergic receptors mediate the typical sympathetic responses such as mydriasis and vasoconstriction, whereas alpha$_2$-adrenergic receptors provide a negative feedback to inhibit release of norepinephrine. Beta$_1$-adrenergic receptors mediate cardiac stimulation, but beta$_2$-adrenergic receptors mediate noncardiac responses, such as bronchodilation and vasodilation. Cardiovascular drugs that stimulate (or inhibit) both alpha- and beta-adrenergic receptors are considered totally nonselective; the drugs are highly selective if they stimulate (or inhibit) only one subtype of alpha- or beta-adrenergic receptor.

Alpha-beta-adrenergic agonists

The alpha-beta-adrenergic agonists act on the alpha- and beta-adrenergic receptors. Because these drugs are nonselective, they imitate almost all actions of the sympathetic nervous system.

Prototype: epinephrine hydrochloride

Epinephrine hydrochloride (Adrenalin) is the least selective adrenergic agonist and is identical to the epinephrine synthesized within the body. It acts on the cardiovascular system by strengthening the force of cardiac contraction, increasing the contraction rate, and usually increasing cardiac output. Epinephrine elevates the systolic blood pressure and may also affect diastolic blood pressure. Epinephrine also relaxes bronchial smooth muscle, and it inhibits histamine release as well as antagonizes the action of histamine. As a result of these effects, epinephrine is considered the drug of choice for anaphylactic shock and is also used in cardiac resuscitation. It is also the antidote of choice for allergic reactions. The usual dosage for cardiac resuscitation is 0.5 to 1.0 mg of a 1:10,000 solution by direct injection; this may be repeated every 3 to 5 minutes, as required.

Since epinephrine stimulates both the alpha- and the beta-adrenergic receptors, it may produce side effects in any patient receiving the drug. These are often transitory and include anxiety, dizziness, pallor, and palpitations. More serious side effects, such as cerebrovascular hemorrhage, fibrillation, severe headache, hypotension, pulmonary edema, and tachycardia, are associated with overdose or too rapid injection of the drug.

Epinephrine interacts with many drugs because of its mechanism of action. It is potentiated by anesthetics and antihistamines but antagonized by adrenergic blockers.

Related drugs

Norepinephrine bitartrate (Levophed) is pharmacologically equivalent to the sympathetic neurotransmitter norepinephrine. It is an agonist for the alpha- and beta$_1$-adrenergic receptors but has almost no effect on beta$_2$-adrenergic receptors. Since it is more selective, the actions of norepinephrine are more limited than those of epinephrine. Norepinephrine is primarily used as a vasopressor agent to raise the blood pressure in acute hypotensive states. Because of its potent vasoconstrictor effects, severe tissue necrosis can result from extravasation of this drug into the surrounding tissue. Metaraminol bitartrate (Aramine) also primarily stimulates alpha-adrenergic receptors, and also has activity on beta$_1$-adrenergic receptors, producing vasoconstriction and cardiac stimulation. It is less potent than norepinephrine, but has similar side effects and precautions.

Alpha-adrenergic agonists

The alpha-adrenergic agonists mimic the action of naturally occurring norepinephrine on the alpha-adrenergic receptors. The primary effect of these drugs is vasoconstriction.

Prototype: phenylephrine hydrochloride

Phenylephrine hydrochloride (Neo-Synephrine) produces vasoconstriction, which results in elevation of the systolic and diastolic blood pressures. Therefore phenylephrine is used for the treatment of hypotension and shock.

Phenylephrine may be administered as a direct injection in emergency situations; however, it is most effective when used as a continuous infusion. Doses are titrated to the desired blood pressure response. As with norepinephrine, infiltration of phenylephrine may result in tissue necrosis and sloughing.

Beta-adrenergic agonists

Drugs that act only on the beta-adrenergic receptors are used primarily to stimulate the heart or dilate the bronchi. When the mechanism of action is limited to only the beta$_1$-adrenergic receptors, the primary effect is cardiac stimulation. If the drugs act on the beta$_2$-adrenergic receptors, bronchodilation and vasodilation result.

Prototype: dopamine hydrochloride

Dopamine hydrochloride is a selective beta$_1$-adrenergic agonist indicated for the correction of hemodynamic imbalances. It produces a positive inotropic effect by stimulating cardiac contractile force and is sometimes classified as an inotropic agent. Since dopamine increases cardiac output, blood pressure, and urine output, it is administered as an adjunct in the treatment of shock. The patient's response must be monitored carefully based on these effects, and the administration rate must be adjusted accordingly.

Dopamine is administered by continuous infusion using an electronic infusion device. The usual initial dosage is 2 to 5 mcg/kg/min. The dosage is then gradually increased by 5 to 10 mcg/kg/min in 10- to 30-minute increments and titrated based on the patient's response to treatment. Blood pressure should be monitored closely. As with norepinephrine, there is a risk of tissue necrosis if the drug infiltrates into surrounding tissue.

The side effects of dopamine are associated with its cardiac effects. Tachycardia, vasoconstriction, and a widened QRS complex may occur. Other side effects include nausea, vomiting, headache, and dyspnea. The rate of infusion should be immediately decreased and the physician notified if there is a disproportionate rise in diastolic blood pressure, an increasing degree of tachycardia, or a decreased urinary output.

Related drugs

Dobutamine hydrochloride (Dobutrex) is a selective beta$_1$-adrenergic agonist that stimulates cardiac contractile force (positive inotropic effect), with less alteration in heart rate than dopamine. Following stabilization of the patient in the hospital, dobutamine can be continued in the home under closely supervised conditions for patients with advanced heart failure.

Isoproterenol hydrochloride (Isuprel) differs from dopamine in that it stimulates both beta₁- and beta₂-adrenergic receptors to produce cardiac and bronchial effects. The primary indications for isoproterenol are the treatment of atrioventricular (AV) heart block and bronchospasm.

Beta-adrenergic blockers

Beta-adrenergic blockers bind with the beta-adrenergic receptors to prevent the action of the naturally occurring beta-adrenergic receptor agonists (norepinephrine and epinephrine). Most beta-blockers are nonselective in that they do not differentiate between beta₁- and beta₂-adrenergic receptors. In contrast, cardioselective beta-blockers produce their antiarrhythmic and antihypertensive effects by inhibiting only the beta₁-adrenergic receptors. Since the cardioselective blockers have no effect on the beta₂-adrenergic receptors that mediate bronchial dilation, they are generally safer for patients who have accompanying respiratory disease.

Prototype: esmolol hydrochloride

Esmolol hydrochloride (Brevibloc) is a fast-acting nonselective beta-blocker indicated for the treatment of acute episodes of supraventricular or sinus tachycardia and atrial flutter or fibrillation. Because of its short half-life, esmolol must be administered by continuous infusion. Doses are titrated to the desired response. Adverse effects are extensions of the drug's pharmacological effects with the most common side effect of hypotension.

Related drugs

Propranolol hydrochloride (Inderal) is a nonselective beta-adrenergic blocker that acts on both beta₁- and beta₂-adrenergic receptors. Because of its negative chronotropic effects, propranolol is indicated in the management of tachyarrhythmias, and it can also produce decreases in blood pressure. In contrast, metoprolol tartrate (Lopressor) is a cardioselective beta-blocker. The IV formulation is used to slow heart rate in patients with tachyarrhythmias and in patients with acute myocardial infarction. Labetalol (Normodyne) primarily acts via nonselective beta-adrenergic receptor blockade, and it also has selective alpha₁-adrenergic receptor antagonism. It produces a vasodilatory effect and is used for management of hypertension.

Alpha-adrenergic blockers

The alpha-adrenergic blockers prevent the naturally occurring alpha-adrenergic receptor agonists (epinephrine and norepinephrine) from binding to the alpha-adrenergic receptor sites.

Phentolamine mesylate

Phentolamine mesylate (Regitine) blocks the alpha-adrenergic receptors and antagonizes responses to epinephrine and norepinephrine. Because of its ability to reduce blood pressure, phentolamine is primarily indicated for the treatment of hypertensive episodes associated with pheochromocytoma. If extravasation of catecholamines occurs, phentolamine may be administered subcutaneously into the tissue to counteract the catecholamine effect.

Drugs affecting cardiac strength and rhythm

When the heart loses its ability to contract with normal strength, drugs are administered to strengthen the cardiac contraction. Such drugs include the beta-adrenergic receptor agonists (see previous discussion), cardiac glycosides, and miscellaneous inotropic agents. In contrast, alterations in cardiac rate or rhythm require the administration of antiarrhythmics.

Cardiac glycosides

Cardiac glycosides act directly on the myocardium to increase cardiac contractility and alter electrical impulse generation and conduction. This results in slower, stronger contractions, with increased cardiac output.

Prototype: digoxin

Digoxin (Lanoxin) is indicated in the treatment of congestive heart failure and supraventricular tachyarrhythmias, including atrial fibrillation. Effects begin within 5 to 30 minutes of administration and last up to 3 days.

Digoxin has a narrow margin of safety. Dosages must be individualized because a therapeutic dose for one patient may be toxic to another. Whereas the first signs of toxicity may be detected on ECG monitoring, the most common clinical symptoms are nausea, vomiting, and anorexia. Patients may also experience blurred vision, disturbed color vision, headache, confusion, and diarrhea.

Many drugs interact with digoxin:

- Drugs that alter serum electrolyte levels, such as potassium-sparing diuretics, can affect the intensity of the response to digoxin.
- Autonomic agents can alter the effects of digoxin on cardiac conductivity.
- Drugs that affect the metabolism or excretion of digoxin, such as phenytoin, quinidine, or verapamil, may require adjustment of the digoxin dosage to maintain therapeutic effects.

Antidote

Digoxin immune Fab (Digibind) contains antidigoxin antibodies that bind to the digoxin molecules, rendering them unable to exert their toxic effects. Because it is obtained from sheep serum, digoxin immune Fab is potentially allergenic.

Miscellaneous inotropic agents

Other inotropic agents enhance the strength of cardiac contraction but differ from cardiac glycosides and beta-adrenergic receptor agonists in their mechanism of action. Inamrinone lactate (Inocor) and milrinone lactate (Primacor) produce inotropic and vasodilator effects through inhibition of phosphodiesterase. These drugs are mainly indicated for the short-term management of congestive heart failure in patients who have been unresponsive to conventional therapies.

Antiarrhythmics

Antiarrhythmics are administered to prevent or stop an irregular heart rate or rhythm. Because there is no universal antiarrhythmic, no single prototype can be identified. For purposes here, antiarrhythmics are grouped according to their mechanism of action and the most common drugs for each group are discussed. Because of the cardiac effects of these drugs, IV administration requires continuous ECG and blood pressure monitoring.

Class Ia

Some antiarrhythmics decrease the transport of sodium through the cardiac tissue and slow conduction through the AV node. This prolongs the refractory period and decreases the automaticity of the heart; therefore these drugs are indicated for the treatment of supraventricular arrhythmias, such as atrial fibrillation and flutter. Examples of such drugs are quinidine gluconate and procainamide hydrochloride (Pronestyl).

Quinidine gluconate. Quinidine is indicated for the management of atrial fibrillation and flutter. It has also been used to treat Wolff-Parkinson-White syndrome, which is characterized by supraventricular tachycardia. Since quinidine acts by decreasing AV node conduction, adverse effects include AV block. Other adverse reactions include acute hypotension, diaphoresis, tinnitus, and visual disturbances. In rare instances, ventricular tachycardia and fibrillation have occurred. Caution should be exercised in patients who need digoxin. Although this drug interaction can vary among patients, digoxin dosage should be reduced if quinidine is added.

Procainamide hydrochloride. Procainamide hydrochloride (Pronestyl) is similar to quinidine but has a more rapid onset of action and is less likely to cause hypotension or cardiac depression. Procainamide acts by slowing the heart rate and conduction, decreasing myocardial irritability, and prolonging the refractory period, and it is indicated for the emergency treatment of ventricular and supraventricular arrhythmias. Side effects of procainamide are usually dose related and are similar to those associated with quinidine. Caution should be used in patients requiring amiodarone because high procainamide levels may result.

Class Ib

Class Ib antiarrhythmics shorten the refractory period, especially in the Purkinje fibers and the ventricular myocardium. By acting preferentially on areas of the myocardium in which impulse conduction rates and automaticity are abnormal, these drugs promote uniform conduction rates throughout the heart. As a result, ventricular excitability is reduced without a reduction in the force of the ventricular contractions. The best known example of this group is lidocaine. Phenytoin, an anticonvulsant, also belongs in this group.

Lidocaine hydrochloride. Lidocaine hydrochloride is used for treatment of ventricular arrhythmias and ventricular tachycardias, especially following a myocardial infarction. The usual bolus dose is 50 to 100 mg administered at a rate not exceeding 25 mg/min. If the desired response is not achieved, a second dose (e.g., 25 to 50 mg) may be given 5 to 10 minutes later. Patients should not receive more than 200 to 300 mg within the first hour. After the bolus dose is administered, a continuous infusion of 1 to 4 mg/min is initiated to maintain a therapeutic serum level between 1.5 and 5 mcg/mL. Dosage should be reduced for patients with congestive heart failure or liver disease. Greater than recommended doses and too rapid administration rates are likely to cause excessive cardiac depression and CNS stimulation.

Lidocaine has a relatively low margin of safety. Serum levels above 6 mcg/mL are usually toxic and may suppress AV transmission, resulting in partial or complete heart block. In addition, high serum levels may produce adverse CNS effects. Sedation and drowsiness are associated with therapeutic blood levels. Higher levels may cause unconsciousness, generalized convulsions, and respiratory arrest. However, more common side effects (even at therapeutic blood levels) include apprehension, blurred vision, lightheadedness, tinnitus, and numbness.

Lidocaine is potentiated by beta-adrenergic blockers and phenytoin. The concomitant administration of these drugs with lidocaine may result in cardiac depression and an increased likelihood of excessive CNS effects.

Phenytoin sodium. Phenytoin sodium (Dilantin) is chemically unrelated to lidocaine, but the two drugs are similar in their antiarrhythmic actions. As discussed earlier, phenytoin is an effective anticonvulsant. However, it may be used for the treatment of digitalis-induced arrhythmias because it normalizes AV conduction and suppresses ectopic pacemakers. Adverse reactions and side effects of phenytoin are similar to those of lidocaine. Too rapid administration or toxic serum levels may cause severe depression of cardiac contractility, severe hypotension, and excessive CNS effects.

Class Ic

Class Ic antiarrhythmics also affect sodium channels in the heart and include flecainide and propafenone, which are not available as parenteral agents.

Class II

Antiarrhythmic effects are also produced by the beta-adrenergic receptor blockers. As discussed earlier, beta-adrenergic blockers inhibit the cardiac response from sympathetic nerve stimulation. They slow the heart rate by inhibiting AV conduction, reduce the force of cardiac contractility, and decrease arterial pressure and cardiac output. Beta-adrenergic blockers are particularly effective in the management of arrhythmias caused by excessive sympathetic cardiac stimulation or sympathomimetic drugs. Propranolol hydrochloride (Inderal), esmolol hydrochloride (Brevibloc), and metoprolol tartrate (Lopressor) are beta-adrenergic blockers used to manage arrhythmias involving increased sympathetic cardiac stimulation.

Class III

Class III antiarrhythmic agents affect potassium channels in the heart to lengthen the effective refractory period. Amiodarone (Cordarone) is the most commonly used class III agent; however, it also has properties of class I, II, and IV antiarrhythmics. Amiodarone is effective for supraventricular and ventricular arrhythmias. It is commonly administered as a 150-mg bolus given over 10 minutes, followed by an infusion of 1 mg/min for 6 hours, and then decreased to 0.5 mg/min.

The most common adverse effect observed with IV amiodarone is hypotension. The drug has worsened existing arrhythmias or caused new arrhythmias in 2% to 5% of patients (McEvoy, 2007). Few data are available on drug interactions with parenteral amiodarone therapy. Since this drug has a long half-life, the potential exists for drug interactions not only with concomitantly administered drugs, but also with drugs administered after amiodarone has been discontinued.

Ibutilide (Corvert) prolongs repolarization and the effective refractory period in both atrial and ventricular cardiac tissue. The drug has negligible direct effects on heart rate, cardiac contractility, or blood pressure. Ibutilide is used IV for rapid conversion of recent-onset atrial flutter or fibrillation to sinus rhythm. However, like other agents, it can cause potentially fatal arrhythmias. In addition, concomitant administration of other antiarrhythmics can cause prolonged refractoriness of cardiac tissue.

Class IV

Calcium channel blockers slow electrical impulse conduction rates and increase the cellular refractory period by blocking the influx of calcium into the cells. This action reduces conduction of the impulse through the SA and AV nodes, prolongs the refractory period in the AV node, and reduces ventricular rates. A common calcium channel blocker is diltiazem hydrochloride (Cardizem).

Diltiazem hydrochloride. Diltiazem hydrochloride (Cardizem) is effective in the treatment of supraventricular tachyarrhythmias and temporary management of a rapid ventricular rate in atrial flutter or fibrillation. Diltiazem has a frequency-dependent effect on the AV node in which it is able to selectively decrease heart rate in the presence of tachyarrhythmias, but has little effect on normal heart rate. Potential side effects include hypotension, nausea, dizziness, and headache.

Verapamil hydrochloride (Isoptin) is also in this group and inhibits the cardiac conduction system primarily at the AV node. When verapamil is administered, potential drug interactions must be considered. Patients receiving digoxin and verapamil may warrant a digoxin dose reduction.

Adenosine (Adenocard) is most similar to class IV antiarrhythmics. However, it exerts its activity on adenosine-sensitive potassium channels that inhibit the sinus and AV nodes. It is used to terminate supraventricular tachyarrhythmias. A 6-mg dose is given by rapid injection (over 1 to 3 seconds); if there is no response within 1 to 2 minutes, a 12-mg bolus may be given. A brief sinus pause may be observed after administration of adenosine.

Vasodilating agents

A vasodilating agent relaxes blood vessels, causing them to widen and increase blood flow to the heart muscle and surrounding tissue. The vasodilating agent nitroglycerin is used to control blood pressure in cardiovascular procedures; to treat ischemic pain, congestive heart failure, or pulmonary edema associated with acute myocardial infarction; and to control blood pressure during surgical procedures.

Prototype: nitroglycerin

Nitroglycerin is used during severe hypertension or myocardial infarction. An IV infusion dosage up to 100 mcg/min may be required, with effective dosages ranging from 5 to 100 mcg/min. Hypotensive effect is usually seen within 2 to 5 minutes. Nitroglycerin readily migrates into many plastics and manufacturers' instructions for dilution, dosage, and administration must be followed carefully. Headache, the most common adverse effect, is relieved by reducing the dosage or adding analgesics. Nitrate ions released during metabolism of nitroglycerin can oxidize hemoglobin to methemoglobin. Tolerance has developed following high or sustained plasma drug concentrations but does not occur in all patients.

Antihypertensives

To manage essential hypertension, these drugs are usually administered orally. IV administration is typically reserved for subacute or acute hypertensive emergencies. Discussion of antihypertensive agents in this section focuses on drugs used to treat severe and abrupt increases in blood pressure and is limited to those not previously discussed.

Methyldopate hydrochloride

Methyldopate hydrochloride (Aldomet) is a centrally acting antihypertensive that depresses sympathetic nervous system activity through alpha-adrenergic receptors in the CNS. IV methyldopate is indicated for the treatment of hypertensive crises.

The usual dosage of methyldopate is 250 to 500 mg administered over 30 to 60 minutes as an intermittent infusion every 6 hours. The patient's blood pressure needs to be monitored carefully throughout the therapy and the dosage withheld if the blood pressure is not within the limits established by the physician. Potential side effects include drowsiness, dizziness, dry mouth, sedation, and postural hypotension.

Hydralazine hydrochloride

Hydralazine hydrochloride (Apresoline) is a potent antihypertensive drug that lowers the blood pressure by relaxing the smooth muscle of the arteries and arterioles. For this reason, it is sometimes classified as a vasodilator. The primary uses of hydralazine are for the treatment of severe essential hypertension and to promote vasodilation in cardiovascular shock.

Hydralazine is administered as a direct injection at a rate not exceeding 10 mg/min. The usual dosage is 10 to 20 mg, but the dosage may be increased gradually as required to a maximum dosage of 300 to 400 mg in 24 hours.

As with methyldopate, the patient's blood pressure must be monitored carefully. Potential side effects include headache, tachycardia, palpitations, paresthesia, and postural hypotension. The peripheral vasodilation produced by hydralazine may stimulate the carotid sinus reflex, thus increasing the heart rate and cardiac output.

Sodium nitroprusside

Sodium nitroprusside (Nipride) is a vasodilator that produces effects similar to those of hydralazine. Nitroprusside is administered as a continuous infusion by an electronic infusion device at a usual starting dose of 0.3 mcg/kg/min. Sodium nitroprusside is converted to thiocyanate before it is excreted in the urine, and cyanide poisoning may occur if the recommended maximum dose of 10 mcg/kg/min is exceeded or in patients with impaired hepatic or renal function. Other potential side effects include abdominal pain, dyspnea, diaphoresis, palpitations, headache, and muscle twitching.

The potency of nitroprusside can be affected by exposure to light, so the solution container (and sometimes the administration set) should be covered with aluminum foil or an opaque material to protect the drug from light.

Diazoxide

Another potent vasodilator, diazoxide (Hyperstat) acts by relaxing the smooth muscle of the peripheral arterioles. Because the drug is administered as a single dose, it is preferred when an infusion pump and titration monitoring are not immediately available.

Enalaprilat

Enalaprilat (Vasotec) lowers the blood pressure by interrupting the renin-angiotensin-aldosterone system. It acts by inhibiting angiotensin-converting enzyme, which inhibits formation of the vasoconstrictor angiotensin II, and by indirectly reducing the blood levels of aldosterone. As a result, the peripheral arterial resistance is reduced and the blood pressure is lowered. Enalaprilat is administered as a direct injection over 5 minutes. Adverse reactions include headache, dizziness, hypotension, rash, hyperkalemia, and cough.

Nicardipine

Nicardipine (Cardene) is a calcium channel blocker that can be given intravenously to manage hypertensive crises. Headache is the most common adverse effect. Nicardipine has a negative inotropic effect and caution should be used when administering to patients with congestive heart failure.

HEMATOLOGICAL AGENTS

When a blood vessel wall is injured or severed, the body activates processes to maintain hemostasis. This protective mechanism is accomplished by means of a clotting cascade that is activated through a series of intrinsic and extrinsic factors. Although coagulation is usually the desired reaction, there are several clinical situations in which hemostasis must be inhibited or the coagulation process reversed. Hematological agents such as anticoagulants and thrombolytics, respectively, are the drugs indicated for such situations.

Anticoagulants

Anticoagulants interfere with the coagulation pathway to prevent clot formation. They are effective in decreasing the risk of clot formation and preventing the enlargement or fragmentation of blood clots; however, anticoagulants do not have clot-dissolving properties.

Prototype: heparin sodium

The prototype for parenteral anticoagulants is heparin sodium. Heparin works in conjunction with antithrombin III to neutralize thrombin and activated coagulation factors IX, X, XI, and XII. Heparin therapy is indicated for the prophylaxis and treatment of venous thrombosis and pulmonary emboli; prevention of coagulation during arterial and cardiac surgery and hemodialysis; prevention of embolism associated with prosthetic heart valves and atrial fibrillation; and treatment of acute myocardial infarction, acute coronary syndrome, and cerebral embolism.

To achieve a constant degree of anticoagulation, the preferred mode of IV administration of heparin is by continuous infusion. However, heparin may be administered by intermittent injection with the dosage adjusted according to coagulation times. The most common laboratory test for monitoring heparin action is the activated partial thromboplastin time (aPTT). A baseline aPTT is measured before heparin therapy is initiated. Because heparin prolongs the aPTT in a dose-dependent manner, the therapeutic range for the aPTT during heparin therapy is 1.5 to 2.5 times the control value. The anti-Xa assay is more specific than the aPTT and can also be used to monitor heparin, with a usual therapeutic goal of 0.3 to 0.7 unit/mL.

As a result of the pharmacological action of heparin, the major adverse effects are bleeding and hemorrhage. The frequency and severity of these effects may be minimized with careful monitoring of the aPTT or anti-Xa concentration during therapy. Whereas bleeding may occur at any site, the most common locations are the GI and urinary tracts and mucosal surfaces such as the nasal passages and gums. Epistaxis, hematuria, or tarry stools may be the first signs of complications.

A more uncommon adverse reaction to heparin is thrombocytopenia. The patient's platelet count must be monitored closely because a paradoxical reaction resulting in platelet aggregation, or white clot syndrome, may occur. Other side effects related to heparin therapy are rare but include hypersensitivity reactions, alopecia, and osteoporosis.

Heparin is contraindicated in patients with active bleeding, blood dyscrasias, history of bleeding disorder, or known hypersensitivity to the drug. In disease states that increase the risk of hemorrhage, such as aneurysm or hemophilia, heparin should be used with extreme caution. If heparin is administered with thrombolytic agents or antiplatelet drugs, the risk of hemorrhage may be increased.

Heparin may also be used to maintain the patency of venous access devices designed for intermittent use. The usual concentration of the heparin flush is 10 or 100 units of heparin per 1 mL of 0.9% sodium chloride. The amount of solution depends on the device to be flushed but should be enough to reach the tip of the catheter. The intervals between flushes are determined by the type of device and the frequency of use. Generally, a heparin flush is administered immediately following each IV medication or every 8 to 24 hours. Since heparin is incompatible with several other medications, the SASH technique should be used to instill the heparin flush. With this technique, the device is flushed with 0.9% sodium chloride (S), the medication is administered (A), the device is again flushed with 0.9% sodium chloride (S), and a heparin flush is administered (H).

Antidote

In the event of heparin overdose, protamine sulfate is administered to neutralize heparin's anticoagulant activity. Protamine molecules that have positive electrostatic charges combine with the negatively charged heparin molecules to form the protamine-heparin complex, which has no anticoagulant activity. The dosage of protamine is determined by the heparin dosage, and approximately 100 units of heparin are neutralized by 1 mg of protamine. Heparin has a short half-life, and blood concentrations of heparin decrease rapidly when the heparin infusion is stopped. Therefore the dose of protamine required decreases as the time from last heparin administration increases.

Side effects associated with the rapid administration of protamine include acute hypotension, bradycardia, dyspnea, and transient flushing. These effects are minimized when protamine is administered slowly and the total dosage for any 10-minute period does not exceed 50 mg. Hypersensitivity reactions are rare; cross-sensitivity is possible in persons allergic to fish because of the salmon origins of protamine.

Thrombolytic agents

In contrast to anticoagulants, which prevent the formation of clots or thrombi, thrombolytic agents promote thrombolysis. Thrombolytic agents act by dissolving the obstruction and preventing ischemic tissue damage in the organ involved when a thrombosis or embolism obstructs blood flow in organs such as the heart, lungs, or brain.

Prototype: alteplase

The prototype of the thrombolytic agents is alteplase (Activase). Alteplase is a recombinant form of human tissue-type plasminogen activator (t-PA) and works in a complex manner to combine with plasminogen found in the thrombi and convert it to plasmin. The plasmin in turn degrades fibrinogen and fibrin clots. Uses for alteplase include lysis of coronary artery thrombosis, acute ischemic stroke, cardiac arrest associated with acute massive pulmonary embolism, and deep vein and arterial thrombosis. Alteplase has also been used to clear totally or partially occluded catheters.

Since alteplase alters the normal hemostatic process, the major side effect is hemorrhage. Other adverse reactions include sensitivity reactions, ranging from urticaria to anaphylaxis. Alteplase is a recombinant product and some patients may develop antibodies to alteplase. Repeat administration of alteplase to patients previously exposed to the drug should be undertaken with caution. When the drug is used to lyse coronary artery thrombi, a reperfusion-induced arrhythmia may result. Major contraindications for alteplase are active internal bleeding, intracranial or intraspinal surgery, a recent cerebrovascular accident, severe uncontrolled hypertension, intracranial neoplasm, or a history of hypersensitivity to the drug.

Related drugs

There are two other thrombolytic agents that are similar to alteplase. Reteplase (Retavase) and tenecteplase (TNKase) are also biosynthetic forms of t-PA and exhibit actions similar to those of alteplase. Both reteplase and tenecteplase are used to lyse thrombi that are obstructing coronary arteries in the management of acute myocardial infarction.

Hemostatics

Hemostatics are indicated for the control of unexpected hemorrhagic episodes. Although all the drugs in this category arrest bleeding, each has a specific indication in clotting.

Prototype: aminocaproic acid

Aminocaproic acid (Amicar) is indicated in the treatment of excessive bleeding caused by overactivity of the fibrinolytic system. It inhibits plasminogen activator substances as well as plasmin. The primary indication for aminocaproic acid is systemic hyperfibrinolysis associated with cardiac surgery, aplastic anemia, or carcinoma of the lung, prostate, cervix, or stomach. It has also been effective in the treatment of overdosage of thrombolytic agents.

Adverse effects of aminocaproic acid are generally mild and disappear once the drug has been discontinued. They include nausea, cramping, diarrhea, dizziness, tinnitus, nasal stuffiness, headache, and rash. Bradycardia, hypotension, and cardiac arrhythmias are associated with rapid infusion of the drug but may be prevented if aminocaproic acid is administered as recommended.

Aminocaproic acid is contraindicated in those with disseminated intravascular coagulation unless the patient is receiving heparin concomitantly. It is also contraindicated in patients with active intravascular clotting.

Related drugs

The two related hemostatics antihemophilic factor (factor VIII) and factor IX complex (Profilnine) differ from aminocaproic acid in that they are used for the treatment of hemophilia. Antihemophilic factor is indicated in the treatment of a congenital deficiency of factor VIII associated with hemophilia A, whereas factor IX complex is used to prevent and control bleeding caused by hemophilia B. Both drugs are prepared from pooled plasma. Various processes are used in the manufacture of these products to reduce the viral infectious potential of these agents. A recombinant form of antihemophilic factor is available that does not use pooled plasma and therefore has a much lower associated risk of viral transmission. Patients may form antibodies against antihemophilic factor, which would preclude the use of both the human and the recombinant forms of the drugs. In these patients, anti-inhibitor coagulant complex (Felba VH) and factor VIIa (NovoSeven) are options for management of bleeding.

A third hemostatic is desmopressin acetate (DDAVP), which is used to manage spontaneous or trauma-induced bleeding in patients with hemophilia A or von Willebrand's disease. Desmopressin is a synthetic polypeptide that causes a dose-dependent increase in plasma factor VIII. This synthetic product may be preferred in patients with mild hemophilia because of the risks associated with antihemophilic factors prepared from pooled plasma. However, desmopressin is not indicated for use in patients with antihemophilic factor antibodies.

AGENTS FOR ELECTROLYTE AND WATER BALANCE

Fluid and electrolyte balance may be disturbed in many medical conditions and require intervention to restore equilibrium. To maintain homeostasis, drugs may be required to correct acid-base imbalances, mobilize fluid for excretion from the body, expand plasma volume, or replace or maintain electrolyte or fluid levels.

Agents used for acid-base imbalances

To preserve normal physiological processes, the pH of the body must be maintained within a narrow range of 7.35 to 7.45. The body works to maintain the pH of the extracellular fluid by various homeostatic buffering mechanisms. When these mechanisms fail, acidosis or alkalosis occurs.

Acidifying agents

Metabolic alkalosis may be caused by vomiting, excessive nasogastric suction, or overdiuresis. The cause of the alkalotic condition must be identified and treated, and acidifying agents may be administered to counteract the alkalosis.

Prototype: ammonium chloride

Ammonium chloride is indicated for the treatment of hypochloremia and metabolic alkalosis. In metabolic alkalosis, hypochloremia is usually present, resulting in an excess of bicarbonate. Once ammonium chloride is administered, it dissociates into an ammonium cation and a chloride anion. In the liver, the ammonium ions are converted to urea, freeing the hydrogen cations. The hydrogen cations then react with the excess bicarbonate to form water and carbon dioxide, which is excreted by the lungs. The chloride ions combine primarily with the sodium bases in the body, thus correcting the hypochloremic state.

The major side effects associated with ammonium chloride are caused by ammonia toxicity. These include bradycardia, disorientation, headache, pallor, sweating, irregular respirations, coma, metabolic acidosis, and calcium deficit resulting in tetany. Venous irritation and phlebitis may also occur after administration of the drug. To lessen the incidence of adverse effects, ammonium chloride is diluted to make a 0.2 mEq/mL solution and infused at a rate of 5 mL/min or less.

Alkalinizing agents

Acidosis occurs when the serum pH is lower than 7.35. The blood is acidic because of excess carbonic acid, which alters the bicarbonate to carbonic acid ratio. In this situation, alkalinizing agents are administered to buffer the excess acid and help return this ratio to normal.

Prototype: sodium bicarbonate

Sodium bicarbonate is indicated for the treatment of metabolic acidosis caused by circulatory insufficiency. It may also be used to treat hyperkalemia and salicylate or barbiturate poisoning. Calculation of the appropriate dosage is determined by the pH, $Paco_2$, calculated base deficit, and clinical response. Bolus doses are often used in acute situations. For less urgent situations, more dilute solutions of sodium bicarbonate are used and the rate of administration of the final concentration should not exceed 50 mEq/hour. In addition, the incompatibility of the drug with other drugs necessitates flushing the administration set with 0.9% sodium chloride before and after the administration of sodium bicarbonate.

Several side effects are associated with sodium bicarbonate. As a result of the hypertonicity of the drug, extravasation may result in chemical cellulitis, tissue necrosis, ulceration, or sloughing at the injection site. Rapid administration may cause alkalosis, hypokalemia, hypocalcemia, or cardiac arrhythmias resulting from an intracellular shift of potassium.

Diuretics

Diuretics increase the amount of fluid eliminated through the kidneys, thus decreasing the total volume of fluid in the body. This occurs primarily because of a natriuretic effect since diuretics increase the renal excretion of sodium. There are different classifications of diuretics, but the main types administered intravenously are the loop, thiazide, and osmotic diuretics.

Loop diuretics

Loop diuretics are so named because their primary site of renal action is in the ascending limb of the loop of Henle in the kidney. They inhibit the active reabsorption of sodium so that it is excreted in the urine, along with body water.

Prototype: furosemide

The prototype for the loop diuretics is furosemide (Lasix). Since furosemide is potent and has a rapid onset of action, it is indicated in the treatment of edema associated with congestive heart failure. Typically, the onset of action occurs within 5 minutes, and peak effects occur within 20 to 60 minutes. Other indications for furosemide include patients with acute pulmonary edema or nephrotic syndrome.

Since furosemide acts by inhibiting the reabsorption of water and electrolytes, major side effects are hyponatremia, potassium depletion, and hypovolemia, with resulting hypotension. Other side effects include tinnitus and hearing impairment if the drug is administered too rapidly or administered in conjunction with other ototoxic drugs. It is recommended that large doses of furosemide be administered by slow IV infusion rather than direct injection to reduce the ototoxic effects. Large doses should be infused at a rate not exceeding 4 mg/min; direct injections of 20 to 40 mg should be administered over 1 to 2 minutes.

The primary contraindication for furosemide is hypotension. Since it may decrease the plasma volume and produce a hypotensive effect, administration of the drug to a hypotensive patient may provoke an excessive reaction. Also, furosemide is a sulfonamide and should be used with caution in patients who report a sulfonamide allergy, although reports of cross-reactivity are infrequent.

Furosemide interacts with a number of other drugs, primarily because of its ability to reduce blood volume indirectly. Examples are the increased risk of nephrotoxicity from cephalosporins, excessive hypotensive effects with some antihypertensives, and ototoxicity or nephrotoxicity from aminoglycosides.

Related drugs

Three additional loop diuretics—bumetanide (Bumex), ethacrynic acid (Edecrin), and torsemide (Demadex)—are similar to furosemide. Approximately 1 mg of bumetanide is equal to 40 mg of furosemide. Ethacrynic acid is similar in potency to furosemide and is usually administered as a single dose of 100 mg. Ethacrynic acid is not chemically related to the sulfonamides and may be substituted for furosemide in patients with a known allergy to sulfonamides. Torsemide (Demadex) has a longer duration of action than furosemide. A 10-mg dose of torsemide is considered equivalent to furosemide 40 mg.

Thiazide diuretics

Thiazide diuretics enhance the excretion of sodium, chloride, and water by interfering with the reabsorption of sodium in the distal convoluted tubule in the kidney. Compared with loop diuretics, thiazides produce only modest diuresis.

Prototype: chlorothiazide sodium

Chlorothiazide sodium (Diuril) is indicated for the management of edema. Volume and electrolyte depletion may result from the administration of this drug, so many of the precautions discussed for the loop diuretics are pertinent to chlorothiazide. Oral administration is preferable to the IV route. However, chlorothiazide is the only non–loop diuretic available for IV use, and as such is often used in combination with loop diuretics when loop diuretics alone have failed. The purpose of this combination therapy is to produce diuretic synergy. Chlorothiazide is also structurally related to the sulfonamides, but reports of cross-sensitivity are rare.

Osmotic diuretics

Unlike loop diuretics and thiazides, osmotic diuretics do not inhibit the reabsorption of ions through the renal tubules. Rather, they exert diuretic effect through osmosis.

Prototype: mannitol

Mannitol (Osmitrol) induces diuresis by elevating the osmotic pressure in the renal tubules to hinder the reabsorption of water and electrolytes. It is primarily indicated for the treatment of oliguric acute renal failure following massive hemorrhage, severe trauma, and hemolytic transfusion reactions. Mannitol may also be used to reduce intracranial pressure, high intraocular pressure, and generalized edema and ascites.

The major side effects and contraindications for mannitol are the conditions for which loop diuretics and thiazides are indicated. Mannitol may increase blood volume and pressure, causing acute heart failure, pulmonary edema, or hypertensive crisis. Minor side effects are limited to chills, headache, and dizziness. Concentrated solutions of mannitol may precipitate when exposed to low temperatures. These solutions can be used if all crystals completely dissolve when the solution is warmed. The warmed solution should be cooled to body temperature before infusion.

Drug interactions with mannitol are rare. However, the therapeutic effect of drugs eliminated by the kidneys may be reduced as a result of increased diuresis.

Replacement solutions

Replacement solutions are indicated for specific fluid or electrolyte deficiencies. Since replacement solutions were discussed earlier with parenteral fluids, this section is limited to electrolyte supplements and volume expanders.

Electrolyte supplements

Electrolyte supplements are usually contained in electrolyte solutions and solutions of parenteral nutrition. However, there are situations in which additional supplements must be administered as a result of an electrolyte deficiency. Because calcium and potassium are the two most common electrolytes administered in this manner, both are discussed as prototypes.

Prototype: calcium gluconate

Calcium is a salt that is naturally present in the body. When there is a deficiency of calcium, tetany may ensue and a calcium supplement may be indicated. Other indications for calcium are as an antidote to magnesium intoxication (an increase in calcium provokes a reciprocal decrease in magnesium) and as adjunctive treatment in cardiac resuscitation.

Calcium gluconate may be administered by continuous infusion or by direct injection at a rate of 1 mL/min. Side effects associated with calcium administration include flushing, tingling, and bradycardia.

Although calcium gluconate is the most common calcium salt used, two other forms are available. Calcium chloride has three times the calcium content as calcium gluconate. Although all calcium salts may cause phlebitis, calcium chloride tends to be the most irritating.

Prototype: potassium chloride

Hypokalemia may be caused by diuretic therapy, vomiting, diarrhea, diabetic ketoacidosis, and metabolic acidosis. In these situations, the administration of potassium may be warranted. However, IV administration of potassium is not without risks. Precise measurement of the potassium deficiency is not possible; therefore too much potassium may be administered, resulting in hyperkalemia.

The IV administration of potassium requires that the drug be diluted in an appropriate volume of solution. Under no circumstances should potassium be administered undiluted as an IV injection; such administration results in cardiac arrest. Usual concentrations of potassium chloride range from 10 to 40 mEq/L. As a result of the venous irritation associated with the IV administration of potassium, it is recommended that the maximum peripheral concentration not exceed 40 mEq/L. If a central venous catheter is used, the concentration may be increased, up to 80 mEq/L. However, continuous cardiac monitoring is recommended for infusions given at a rate greater than 10 mEq/hour. Except in emergency situations, the rate of potassium chloride infusion should not exceed 20 mEq/hour.

Other potassium supplements are potassium acetate and potassium phosphate. Potassium acetate may be preferred for potassium deficiencies in patients with renal tubular acidosis because hyperchloremia is usually present. Potassium phosphate is indicated for specific intracellular deficiency not caused by alkalosis, and is primarily used for repletion of phosphate deficiency.

Volume expanders

Volume expanders increase the plasma volume and provide fluid replacement. These drugs produce a colloidal osmotic effect that draws water from the interstitial to the intravascular spaces.

Prototype: dextran 40

The primary indication for dextran 40 is as an adjunctive therapy in the management of shock resulting from hemorrhage, burns, trauma, and surgery. Dextran 40 is a low-molecular-weight polymer of glucose that increases plasma volume by one to two times its own weight. This means that each gram of dextran 40 holds 25 mL of water in the intravascular space.

Although the initial 500 mL of dextran 40 may be administered over 15 to 30 minutes, the remainder of the initial dose and subsequent daily doses should be evenly distributed over 8 to 24 hours. The patient's pulse, blood pressure, central venous pressure, and urine output should be monitored frequently during the first hour of the infusion and hourly thereafter. Dextran 40 does have antigenic properties, and allergic reactions ranging from mild urticaria to anaphylaxis may occur. Severe anaphylactoid reactions have been reported during the first minutes of the infusion.

Related drugs

Whereas dextran 40 has a low molecular weight, the colloidal properties of dextran 70 and hetastarch (Hespan) are approximately equal to those of human albumin. However, the indications, precautions, and side effects of dextran 70 and hetastarch are similar to those of dextran 40.

GASTROINTESTINAL AGENTS

Common disorders of the GI tract are nausea, vomiting, and peptic ulcers. The IV medications administered for these disorders are directed at controlling the symptoms rather than eliminating the underlying cause.

Antiemetics

Vomiting is a complex reflex initiated by the vomiting center in the medulla and affecting the smooth muscle of the upper alimentary tract. IV antiemetics act centrally to control or prevent this process.

5-HT$_3$ receptor antagonists

5-HT$_3$ (5-hydroxytryptamine$_3$) receptor antagonists block serotonin in the chemoreceptor trigger zone and on vagal nerve terminals to exert an antiemetic effect.

Prototype: ondansetron hydrochloride

Ondansetron hydrochloride (Zofran) is used for the prevention of nausea and vomiting associated with cancer, radiation, and surgical procedures. A single 4-mg dose is often effective for prevention of postoperative nausea and vomiting, while much higher doses are needed for chemotherapy-induced nausea, up to 32 mg/day. Doses of 4 mg may be given IV bolus; larger doses are infused over 15 minutes. Adverse effects are mild and include headache and diarrhea.

Related drugs

Other 5-HT$_3$ antagonists include granisetron hydrochloride (Kytril), dolasetron mesylate (Anzemet), and palonosetron hydrochloride (Aloxi). All have similar pharmacological and adverse event profiles as ondansetron.

Antihistamine/antiemetics

Antiemetics with antihistamine activity are thought to work in the chemoreceptor trigger zone to reduce nausea and vomiting.

Prototype: prochlorperazine edisylate

Prochlorperazine edisylate (Compazine) is a phenothiazine derivative with antihistamine activity. Prochlorperazine exerts antiemetic activity by blocking dopamine receptors in the chemoreceptor trigger zone. Doses range from 5 to 10 mg, and should not exceed 40 mg/day. Common adverse effects include drowsiness and anticholinergic effects. More serious, rare reactions are extrapyramidal symptoms (dystonia, restlessness, tremor) and neuroleptic malignant syndrome.

Related drugs

A related phenothiazine derivative is promethazine hydrochloride (Phenergan) that has potent sedative and antiemetic properties. Promethazine has similar side effects as prochlorperazine. The rate of administration of promethazine should not exceed 25 mg/min and it is recommended that it be administered through a free-flowing IV infusion to lessen the incidence of venous irritation. Promethazine has a low pH and therefore is highly caustic to tissues. Severe complications may occur if promethazine infiltrates or is administered by intra-artierial or subcutaneous routes.

Metoclopramide hydrochloride

Metoclopramide hydrochloride (Reglan) is a dopamine antagonist that also blocks serotonin receptors in the chemoreceptor trigger zone and augments the activity of acetylcholine in the gastrointestinal tract. It is primarily used for its prokinetic properties in gastric stasis situations. However, metoclopramide also has antiemetic properties and may be used for prevention of postoperative nausea and vomiting. Metoclopramide may be given as an IV infusion; however, it is most commonly administered as an IV injection with 10 mg of metoclopramide administered over 1 to 2 minutes. If it is administered too rapidly, metoclopramide causes intense anxiety, restlessness, and then drowsiness.

Adverse reactions associated with metoclopramide usually involve the CNS and include restlessness, drowsiness, and fatigue. Extrapyramidal reactions may also occur, especially in children or when large doses are administered. Once the drug is discontinued, the side effects usually disappear.

Histamine antagonists

Histamine stimulates gastric acid secretion by stimulating the H_2 receptors. H_2 antagonists block H_2 receptors and thereby decrease acid secretion.

Prototype: cimetidine hydrochloride

Cimetidine (Tagamet) was the first H_2 antagonist introduced. Because it inhibits gastric acid secretion, cimetidine is indicated for the treatment of duodenal ulcers, gastric ulcers, gastroesophageal reflux disease, and hypersecretory conditions. The usual dose is 300 mg every 6 hours, administered as a direct injection in 20 mL of 0.9% sodium chloride or as an intermittent infusion. When the prescribed dose is ineffective, the frequency of administration, not the amount, is increased. Continuous infusions of cimetidine may also be used as they provide more consistent pH control.

Cimetidine produces more side effects than the other H_2 blockers. With average doses, bradycardia, confusion, dizziness, delirium, hallucinations, diarrhea, muscular pain, or rash may occur. The rapid administration or overdosage of cimetidine may cause cardiac arrhythmia or hypotension. Therefore cimetidine should be administered over at least 5 minutes as a direct injection or over 15 minutes as an infusion.

Cimetidine interacts with a number of drugs because it inhibits the cytochrome P450 (drug-metabolizing) enzyme system in the liver. Increased plasma concentrations of warfarin, phenytoin, propranolol, lidocaine, metronidazole, and theophylline may occur if any of these drugs are administered concurrently with cimetidine therapy.

Related drugs

The related H_2 blockers are similar to cimetidine in that they share the same mechanism of action. However, they are more potent, have a longer duration of action, and are associated with a lower incidence of side effects and drug interactions. Ranitidine hydrochloride (Zantac) and famotidine (Pepcid) have similar uses and are more common selections for drug therapy from the H_2-blocker class.

Proton pump inhibitors

Proton pump inhibitors suppress gastric acid production by antagonizing the proton pump in the parietal cells.

Prototype: lansoprazole

Lansoprazole (Prevacid) is used for treatment of conditions where a decrease in gastric acid is desirable, such as duodenal and gastric ulcers, gastroesophageal reflux disease, hypersecretory conditions, and upper gastrointestinal bleeding. When administered intravenously, each 30-mg dose is diluted with a compatible solution and infused over 30 minutes. In active upper gastrointestinal bleeding, lansoprazole may be administered as a continuous infusion to provide more gastric acid suppression and thus better pH control. Proton pump inhibitors are not compatible with other medications and may not be administered with other drugs or diluents. Lansoprazole is well tolerated and adverse effects are usually mild, including nausea, diarrhea, abdominal pain, headache, and dizziness.

Related drugs

Pantoprazole (Protonix) is similar to lansoprazole in uses, adverse effects, and compatibility issues.

HORMONES AND SYNTHETIC SUBSTITUTES

The endocrine system controls homeostasis by releasing hormones. When there is hypoactivity of an endocrine gland, replacement therapy with a hormone or its synthetic analog is required.

Corticosteroids

Corticosteroids are hormones that are secreted by the adrenal cortex, or their synthetic analogs. In physiological doses, they replace deficient endogenous hormones; pharmacological doses may be used to decrease inflammation.

Prototype: hydrocortisone sodium succinate

Hydrocortisone sodium succinate (Solu-Cortef) is the drug of choice for replacement therapy in patients with adrenocortical insufficiency. Because of its anti-inflammatory effects, hydrocortisone is also indicated for acute hypersensitivity reactions and systemic lupus erythematosus relapse. In the treatment of neoplastic disease, hydrocortisone may be used alone as palliative treatment or in combination with cytotoxic and immunosuppressive drugs.

The adverse effects of hydrocortisone are generally associated with massive doses or long-term therapy. These include hyperglycemia caused by the drug's effects on glucose metabolism; cushingoid symptoms, characterized by a moon face and buffalo hump; and sodium retention with resultant edema. In addition, hydrocortisone depresses the immune response, increasing the susceptibility to infection. Because the usual signs of inflammation are masked, infections may be widely disseminated before they are recognized.

Related drugs
Two additional corticosteroids are administered for their anti-inflammatory effects. Dexamethasone sodium phosphate (Decadron) is 20 to 30 times as potent as hydrocortisone, whereas methylprednisolone sodium succinate (Solu-Medrol) is 5 times as potent.

Estrogens
Estrogens are potent female hormones capable of producing widespread effects on the body. Although they may be given as replacement therapy, IV administration is generally used for the palliative treatment of cancer.

Prototype: conjugated estrogens USP
Conjugated estrogens USP (Premarin) is a mixture of estrogens. The intravenous formulation is used to treat abnormal uterine bleeding caused by hormone imbalance. An initial dose of 25 mg is administered, and an additional dose may be repeated in 6 to 12 hours if needed. Since estrogens increase the body's ability to manufacture blood clotting factors, they are also used for management of uremic bleeding at a dose of 0.6 mg/kg daily for 5 days.

Insulin
Insulin acts as a catalyst in carbohydrate metabolism by facilitating the transport of glucose and promoting glucose utilization in the peripheral tissues. It also stimulates protein synthesis and inhibits the release of fatty acids from adipose cells. Although a number of forms of insulin are available, only regular insulin and insulin aspart (Novolog) are administered intravenously.

Prototype: regular insulin
Regular insulin is indicated for the emergency management of acute diabetic ketoacidosis and as an additive in solutions of parenteral nutrition. The dosage varies greatly based on the condition and response of the patient, but it generally ranges from 2 to 100 units/hour. Insulin may be administered by direct injection or continuous infusion. However, the potency of an insulin infusion may be reduced because of adsorption of the drug onto plastic IV solution containers or administration sets. The percentage of adsorption is inversely proportional to the concentration of insulin; the greater the concentration, the lower the percentage of adsorption.

Regular insulin may also be administered in combination with glucose for the treatment of hyperkalemia. This is done to facilitate a shift of potassium into the cells, thus lowering the plasma potassium level.

Because insulin is a hypoglycemic agent, the most common adverse reaction is hypoglycemia associated with overdosage. Symptoms range from clammy skin, drowsiness, and headache to disorientation, convulsions, and coma.

Antidote
The antidote for an insulin overdose is glucagon hydrochloride. Glucagon acts by converting glycogen to glucose in the liver. The action of the drug is prompt, with clinical response in 5 to 20 minutes.

Pituitary agents
The posterior pituitary gland synthesizes and releases two hormones: vasopressin and oxytocin. Vasopressin promotes water retention by the kidney and constriction of the peripheral vasculature; oxytocin stimulates the myometrium. The synthetic analogs of these hormones produce similar effects.

Vasopressin
Vasopressin (Pitressin) elicits all of the antidiuretic responses produced by endogenous vasopressin. The primary indication is in the treatment of diabetes insipidus to control polyuria and dehydration. Vasopressin has also been used as adjunctive therapy in the treatment of acute, massive hemorrhage caused by esophageal varices and peptic ulcer disease, by vasodilatory shock, and in resuscitation efforts. Adverse effects are usually associated with large doses and include increased blood pressure, bradycardia, heart block, and coronary insufficiency. For hemorrhage, vasopressin is administered as a continuous infusion at a rate of 0.2 to 0.4 unit/min; the rate may be progressively increased up to 0.9 unit/min. In Advanced Cardiac Life Support (ACLS) algorithms, vasopressin may be selected instead of one of the first doses of epinephrine, and a single dose of 40 units is administered. For vasodilatory shock, the usual dose is much lower, 0.03 to 0.04 unit/min. Patients with septic shock usually have a relative vasopressin deficiency. When vasopressin is replaced, vascular resistance and blood pressure improve, which in turn decreases the reliance on catecholamines to maintain adequate blood pressure. However, vasopressin may decrease blood flow to the heart, kidneys, and intestines, putting patients at risk for organ damage.

Desmopressin
Desmopressin (DDAVP) has a greater antidiuretic effect than vasopressin and also increases factor VIII activity. It is also used for treatment of diabetes insipidus at a dose of 2 to 4 mcg/day. Desmopressin also assists in the management of bleeding in patients with hemophilia A or von Willebrand's disease. A single dose of 0.3 mcg/kg is given by slow infusion before a procedure with bleeding risks. Side effects include tachycardia, facial flushing, and hypotension, especially with larger doses.

Oxytocin
Oxytocin (Pitocin) is a synthetic posterior pituitary hormone that produces rhythmic contraction of the uterine muscle. Because of this, oxytocin is used to induce labor or control postpartum bleeding. It is administered as an infusion with the rate precisely controlled by an electronic infusion device. Initial administration rates for the induction of labor are 0.5 to 1 milliunit/min, whereas control of postpartum bleeding requires an initial rate of 20 to 40 milliunits/min. Once the infusion is initiated, the rate may be titrated as needed. Adverse effects for the mother include anaphylaxis, cardiac arrhythmias, uterine rupture, and subarachnoid hemorrhage; bradycardia and hypoxia are possible fetal reactions.

IMMUNE MODULATORS
The immune system protects the body against foreign invaders. By distinguishing the body's own proteins from foreign proteins, it selectively attacks and destroys foreign substances that enter the body in a process known as the *immune response*.

FOCUS ON EVIDENCE

Use of Vasopressin for Shock Treatment

- Clinical interest in vasopressin was stimulated with the publication of case reports from Columbia University. Vasopressin was evaluated as an adjunctive agent to catecholamines in the treatment of septic shock at a dose of 0.03 to 0.04 unit/min. The researchers found that vasopressin improved mean arterial pressure in four of the five patients treated (Landry et al, 1997).
- A randomized, controlled trial involving 24 patients sought to evaluate the effects of a 4-hour infusion of vasopressin. Patients were randomized to receive either norepinephrine or vasopressin, and were to continue on any prestudy vasopressors. The vasopressin arm observed a statistically significant decrease in norepinephrine requirements and in urine output. Of note, the vasopressin was titrated in this study, and a median dose of 0.06 unit/min was reached (Patel et al, 2002).
- A small, randomized trial aimed to further explore these findings with vasopressin. Patients in this study were randomized to vasopressin or placebo, with the objective of comparing pressure response and catecholamine requirements between the groups. Vasopressin at a dose of 0.04 unit/min resulted in an observed improvement in mean arterial pressure and a decrease in catecholamines in the treatment group; however, this study only enrolled 10 patients and was not equipped to detect a statistical difference (Malay et al, 1999).
- A randomized trial of 48 patients evaluated vasopressin in combination with norepinephrine as compared to norepinephrine alone for vasodilatory shock. A slightly higher dose of 0.07 unit/min was chosen for this trial. As with the prior trials, vasopressin did improve mean arterial pressure, decrease heart rate, and decrease norepinephrine requirements (Dunser et al, 2003).
- With this information, some centers were using vasopressin as an adjuvant therapy in vasodilatory shock. A center in Austria published a retrospective review of their experience with vasopressin. The authors were able to review 316 patients, and found that vasopressin at 0.07 unit/min increased mean arterial pressure and decreased heart rate as compared to norepinephrine. This study, similar to the previous studies with vasopressin, was not equipped to evaluate mortality outcomes (Luckner et al, 2005).
- The compilation of the above data was unable to answer an important question with use of vasopressin in vasodilatory shock: Will the change in surrogate markers (mean arterial pressure, decreased catecholamine requirements) translate into a mortality benefit with vasopressin? Therefore the Vasopressin and Septic Shock Trial (VASST) was performed to evaluate vasopressin versus norepinephrine for management of septic shock. A total of 778 patients were enrolled, and patients randomized to vasopressin received 0.01 to 0.03 unit/min, titrated to a mean arterial pressure of 65 to 75 mm Hg. Open-label vasopressors could also be used. Vasopressin did decrease heart rate and norepinephrine requirements as compared to the norepinephrine arm. There was no difference in the mortality rate at 28 days: 35.4% for vasopressin versus 39.3% for norepinephrine (p value 0.26). The odds of death at 90 days and rate of organ dysfunction were also comparable between the groups. Of note, patients with cardiac abnormalities were excluded, and this is a subgroup where vasopressin may cause additional adverse events. Also, the mean arterial pressure at baseline was 72 mm Hg, which translates into evaluation of vasopressin as a catecholamine-sparing drug rather than as an adjunct to catecholamine-unresponsive shock. The dose of vasopressin selected in this study is lower than the dose most commonly used in clinical practice (0.04 unit/min), which may have an impact on clinical response (Russell et al, 2008).

However, there are certain situations in which the immune system may need to be enhanced or suppressed. Drugs that elicit such responses are classified as *immune modulators*.

Immunostimulants

Immunostimulants enhance the function of the immune system by producing immunity against certain diseases. Those administered intravenously accomplish this by transferring antibodies to the person who lacks endogenous active immunity. The result is a passive immunity against the infection.

Prototype: immune globulin IV

When immune globulin IV (Gamunex) is used for patients unable to produce adequate amounts of immunoglobulin G (IgG) antibodies, it provides immediate antibody levels for up to 3 weeks. Immune globulin is also used to provide immunity to susceptible patients who are allergic to a vaccine or when there is insufficient time for a vaccine to provide immunity. Since the drug is obtained from biological sources, wide ranges of allergic reactions are associated with immune globulin.

Immune globulin is administered as an infusion. Although the recommended administration rate is determined by the commercial product used, manufacturer recommendations must be followed. Too rapid injection of the drug may result in a hypotensive reaction.

Related drugs

$Rh_0(D)$ immune globulin (WinRho) suppresses the formation of anti-$Rh_0(D)$ antibodies in $Rh_0(D)$-negative individuals who are exposed to $Rh_0(D)$-positive blood. The most common use is in pregnancy when the mother is $Rh_0(D)$-negative and the fetus is $Rh_0(D)$-positive. It is also used for idiopathic thrombocytopenic purpura (ITP) and when incompatible blood products are transfused. The dose of $Rh_0(D)$ immune globulin is proportional to the amount of incompatible blood involved in the exposure.

Immunosuppressants

An active immune system is desirable for protection against infections and neoplasms. However, in situations such as organ transplants and autoimmune disorders, the immune response needs to be suppressed.

Prototype: cyclosporine

Cyclosporine (Sandimmune) is a potent immunosuppressant used to prevent organ rejection in patients who have received heart, kidney, or liver transplants. The IV formulation is reserved for patients who cannot tolerate oral administration because of the risk for anaphylaxis. Within 4 to 12 hours before transplantation, cyclosporine is administered as a continuous infusion over 2 to 6 hours. Maintenance doses are administered daily, and trough concentrations are monitored, as there is a narrow range between therapeutic and toxic concentrations. Possible adverse reactions include nephrotoxicity, tremor, and hypertension.

Related drugs

Antithymocyte globulin is used for the treatment of acute rejection of renal transplants. Since these products are derived from equine or rabbit sources there is risk for hypersensitivity reactions. Adverse effects are mainly flulike symptoms, allergic reactions, thrombophlebitis, and thrombocytopenia. Azathioprine sodium (Imuran) is an immunosuppressant used to prevent the rejection of a renal transplant. Side effects associated with azathioprine include leukopenia, thrombocytopenia, arthralgia, nausea, and vomiting. Tacrolimus (Prograf) is used for the prevention of liver or kidney transplant rejection. Similar to cyclosporine, the IV formulation has risk for anaphylaxis and is reserved for patients who cannot take oral medications. Basiliximab (Simulect) and daclizumab (Zenapax) are monoclonal antibodies used in combination with other immunosuppressants to prevent renal transplant rejection. These agents are a mixture of human and murine antibodies and thus have risk for anaphylactic reactions. Basiliximab may be administered IV bolus, but infusing the dose over 20 to 30 minutes decreases infusion-related reactions. Adverse effects are due to cytokine release and are flulike, including fever, chills, headache, and rigors.

Biological response modifiers

Infliximab (Remicade) is a monoclonal antibody that interferes with tumor necrosis factor alpha activity, thereby modifying its biological response. It is used to treat autoimmune diseases such as rheumatoid arthritis and Crohn's disease. Acute infusion reactions with infliximab occur in up to 22% of patients (McEvoy, 2007). Symptoms include urticaria, dyspnea, and hypotension. Infliximab should be administered over at least 2 hours, and a rate titration strategy may be used to lessen the incidence or severity of infusion reactions. Since infliximab modifies the body's immune response, patients may have an increased susceptibility to infection. Natalizumab (Tysabri) is a monoclonal antibody that affects the migration of T lymphocytes into the central nervous system. It is a treatment option for multiple sclerosis. Patients usually receive a 300-mg dose monthly, and each dose is infused over at least 1 hour. Of note, natalizumab has been linked to a rare viral infection of the brain, progressive multifocal leukoencephalopathy; therefore patients must be enrolled in a special registry program that mandates monitoring. A more extensive review of biologic therapy is presented in Chapter 16.

RESPIRATORY SMOOTH MUSCLE RELAXANTS

The smooth muscles of the trachea and bronchi are sensitive to various stimuli and may contract, causing a narrowing of the airways. When bronchospasm occurs, the patient experiences wheezing, coughing, dyspnea, and tightness of the chest. In such situations, drugs that relax the smooth muscles of the respiratory tract are indicated.

Prototype: theophylline

Theophylline may be classified as a bronchodilator because of its ability to open the bronchial passages or as a xanthine derivative because of its chemical structure. It is primarily indicated for the management of bronchial asthma and reversible bronchospasm associated with chronic bronchitis or emphysema.

The initial loading dose of theophylline is usually 4.6 mg/kg lean body weight infused over a minimum of 30 minutes. This is immediately followed by a continuous infusion of 0.2 to 0.7 mg/kg/hr. Since theophylline has a narrow therapeutic index, therapeutic drug monitoring is performed with a target serum concentration between 10 and 15 mcg/mL. Rapid infusion of theophylline or serum levels in excess of 20 mcg/mL may produce toxic reactions, such as anxiety, convulsions, ventricular fibrillation, and cardiac arrest.

Related drugs

Theophylline ethylenediamine (aminophylline) contains 79% theophylline and requires a minimum dilution of 25 mg/mL for administration.

VITAMINS

Vitamins may be administered in IV solutions to maintain optimal vitamin uptake following surgery, extensive burns, trauma, or severe infections. Examples of vitamin additives are thiamine hydrochloride (vitamin B_1), pyridoxine hydrochloride (vitamin B_6), folic acid as part of the vitamin B complex, ascorbic acid (vitamin C), and calcitriol (Calcijex) and paricalcitol (Zemplar) for vitamin D. These vitamins may also be administered as a multivitamin preparation (MVI-12), which contains vitamins A, C, D, and E and the B-complex vitamins.

Phytonadione (Mephyton) contains vitamin K_1 and is used to treat hypoprothrombinemia, most commonly caused by an overdose of warfarin. Because vitamin K_1 is essential for the production of clotting factors in the liver, the dosage and effects of phytonadione are patient-specific. It is recommended that the infusion rate of phytonadione not exceed 1 mg/min; higher rates are associated with the risk of anaphylaxis.

Iron replacement therapy

Iron may be replaced intravenously when iron stores in the body are significantly deficient. Iron is a hematinic used to replace the total body content of iron. Iron is needed for hemoglobin synthesis, oxygen transport, metabolism and synthesis of DNA, and various enzymatic processes. Iron loss in hemodialysis patients can occur because of increased iron utilization and blood loss. Hematological response to parenterally administered iron is no more rapid than that seen with orally administered iron, if absorption problems are absent.

Prototype: iron dextran

Iron dextran (InFeD) may be injected intravenously, undiluted, at a rate not exceeding 50 mg of iron per minute. A test dose is administered to patients who have never received iron dextran because of the risk of anaphylaxis. If no adverse reactions occur from the test dose, up to 100 mg of iron per day may be administered until the total calculated dose to replace iron stores has been given. Large doses, such as total dose infusions of iron in 250 to 1000 mL of 0.9% sodium chloride, may be associated with a higher incidence of adverse effects,

TABLE 15-4 Summary of IV Drugs

Category	Type	Prototype	Related drugs
Antibiotics			
Penicillins	Natural	Penicillin G potassium	Penicillin G sodium
	Penicillinase resistant	Nafcillin sodium (Unipen)	Oxacillin sodium (Bactocill)
	Aminopenicillins	Ampicillin sodium (Omnipen-N)	Ampicillin sodium/sulbactam sodium (Unasyn)
	Extended spectrum	Piperacillin sodium (Pipracil)	Ticarcillin disodium (Ticar)
			Piperacillin-tazobactam (Zosyn)
			Ticarcillin disodium-clavulanate potassium (Timentin)
Cephalosporins	First generation	Cefazolin sodium (Kefzol)	
	Second generation	Cefoxitin sodium (Mefoxin)	Cefuroxime sodium (Zinacef)
			Cefotetan disodium (Cefotan)
	Third generation	Cefotaxime sodium (Claforan)	Ceftriaxone sodium (Rocephin)
			Ceftazidime (Fortaz)
			Ceftizoxime sodium (Cefizox)
	Fourth generation	Cefepime (Maxipime)	
Carbapenems		Imipenem/cilastatin sodium (Primaxin)	Meropenem (Merrem)
			Doripenem (Doribax)
			Ertapenem (Invanz)
Aminoglycosides		Gentamicin sulfate (Garamycin)	Amikacin sulfate (Amikin)
			Kanamycin sulfate (Kantrex)
			Tobramycin sulfate (Nebcin)
Tetracyclines		Doxycycline hyclate (Vibramycin)	
	Glycylcycline	Tigecycline (Tygacil)	
Macrolides	Erythromycin	Erythromycin lactobionate (Erythrocin)	
	Azalide	Azithromycin (Zithromax)	
Quinolones		Ciprofloxacin (Cipro)	Levofloxacin (Levaquin)
			Moxifloxacin (Avelox)
Miscellaneous		Aztreonam (Azactam)	
		Chloramphenicol sodium succinate (Chloromycetin)	
		Clindamycin phosphate (Cleocin)	
		Colistimethate sodium	
		Daptomycin (Cubicin)	
		Linezolid (Zyvox)	
		Quinupristin/dalfopristin (Synercid)	
		Vancomycin HCl (Vancocin)	
Other Anti-Infectives			
Antifungals		Amphotericin B deoxycholate (Fungizone)	Amphotericin B lipid complex (Abelcet)
			Liposomal amphotericin B (AmBisome)
			Amphotericin B cholesteryl sulfate (Amphotec)
	Azoles	Fluconazole (Diflucan)	Voriconazole (VFEND)
	Echinocandins	Caspofungin acetate (Cancidas)	Micafungin sodium (Mycamine)
			Anidulafungin (Eraxis)
Antivirals		Acyclovir sodium (Zovirax)	Ganciclovir sodium (Cytovene)
			Zidovudine (AZT)
			Foscarnet (Foscavir)
			Ribavirin (Virazole)
Antiprotozoals		Metronidazole (Flagyl)	Pentamidine isethionate (Pentam)
		Trimetrexate	

(Continued)

TABLE 15-4 Summary of IV Drugs—cont'd

Category	Type	Prototype	Related drugs
Sulfonamide combination products		Trimethoprim-sulfamethoxazole (Bactrim, Septra)	
Central Nervous System Drugs			
Analgesic	Narcotics	Morphine sulfate	Hydromorphone HCl (Dilaudid)
			Meperidine HCl (Demerol)
			Antagonist: naloxone (Narcan)
			Nalmefene (Revex)
	Mixed narcotic agonist-antagonists	Buprenorphine HCl (Buprenex)	Nalbuphine HCl (Nubain)
			Pentazocine lactate (Talwin)
			Butorphanol (Stadol)
Sedatives, hypnotics, and anxiolytics	Barbiturates	Phenobarbital sodium (Luminal)	Thiopental sodium (Pentothal)
			Pentobarbital sodium (Nembutal)
			Methohexital sodium (Brevital)
	Benzodiazepines	Diazepam (Valium)	Chlordiazepoxide HCl (Librium)
			Lorazepam (Ativan)
			Midazolam HCl (Versed)
			Antagonist: flumazenil (Romazicon)
	Miscellaneous	Droperidol (Inapsine)	
		Dexmedetomidine HCl (Precedex)	
Anticonvulsants	Hydantoins	Phenytoin sodium (Dilantin)	Fosphenytoin sodium (Cerebyx)
	Magnesium sulfate	Magnesium sulfate	
		Levetiracetam (Keppra)	
		Valproate sodium (Depacon)	
Cardiovascular Drugs			
Drugs acting through adrenergic receptors	Alpha-/beta-adrenergic receptors	Epinephrine HCl (Adrenalin)	Norepinephrine bitartrate (Levophed)
			Metaraminol bitartrate (Aramine)
	Alpha-adrenergic agonists	Phenylephrine HCl (Neo-Synephrine)	
	Beta-adrenergic agonists	Dopamine HCl (Intropin)	Dobutamine HCl (Dobutrex)
			Isoproterenol HCl (Isuprel)
	Beta-adrenergic blockers	Esmolol HCl (Brevibloc)	Labetalol HCl (Normodyne)
			Metoprolol tartrate (Lopressor)
			Propranolol HCl (Inderal)
	Alpha-adrenergic blockers	Phentolamine mesylate (Regitine)	
Drugs affecting cardiac strength and rhythm	Cardiac glycosides	Digoxin (Lanoxin)	Antidote: digoxin immune Fab (Digibind)
	Miscellaneous inotropic agents	Inamrinone lactate (Inocor)	
			Milrinone lactate (Primacor)
	Antiarrhythmics	Class Ia	Quinidine gluconate
			Procainamide HCl (Pronestyl)
		Class Ib	Lidocaine HCl (Xylocaine)
			Phenytoin sodium (Dilantin)
		Class II	Beta-adrenergic blockers
		Class III	Amiodarone HCl (Cordarone)
			Ibutilide (Corvert)
		Class IV	Verapamil HCl (Isoptin)
			Diltiazem HCl (Cardizem)
Vasodilating agents		Nitroglycerin	

TABLE 15-4 Summary of IV Drugs—cont'd

Category	Type	Prototype	Related drugs
Antihypertensives		Methyldopa HCl (Aldomet)	
		Hydralazine HCl (Apresoline)	
		Nitroprusside sodium (Nipride)	
		Diazoxide (Hyperstat)	
		Enalaprilat (Vasotec)	
		Nicardipine (Cardene)	
Hematological Agents			
Anticoagulants		Heparin sodium	Antidote: protamine sulfate
Thrombolytic agents		Alteplase (Activase)	Reteplase (Retavase)
			Tenecteplase (TNKase)
Hemostatics		Aminocaproic acid (Amicar)	Antihemophilic factor (factor VIII)
			Factor IX complex (Profilnine)
			Anti-inhibitor coagulant complex (Felba VH)
			Factor VII$_a$ (Novo-Seven)
			Desmopressin acetate (DDAVP)
Agents for Electrolyte and Water Balance			
Agents for acid-base balance	Acidifying agents	Ammonium chloride	
Diuretics	Alkylating agents	Sodium bicarbonate	
	Loop diuretics	Furosemide (Lasix)	Bumetanide (Bumex)
			Ethacrynate sodium (Edecrin)
			Torsemide (Demadex)
	Thiazide diuretics	Chlorothiazide sodium (Diuril)	
	Osmotic diuretics	Mannitol (Osmitrol)	
Electrolyte supplements	Calcium	Calcium gluconate (Kalcinate)	Calcium chloride
	Potassium	Potassium chloride	Potassium acetate
			Potassium phosphate
Volume expanders		Dextran 40	Dextran 70
			Hetastarch (Hespan)
Gastrointestinal Drugs			
Antiemetics	5-HT$_3$	Ondansetron HCl (Zofran)	Granisetron (Kytril)
			Dolesetron mesylate (Anzemet)
			Palonosetron HCl (Aloxi)
	Antiemetic/Antihistamine	Prochlorperazine edisylate (Compazine)	Promethazine HCl (Phenergan)
			Metoclopramide HCl (Reglan)
Histamine (H$_2$) antagonists		Cimetidine HCl (Tagamet)	Famotidine (Pepcid)
			Ranitidine HCl (Zantac)
Proton pump inhibitors		Lansoprazole (Prevacid)	Pantoprazole (Protonix)
Hormones and Synthetic Substitutes			
Corticosteroids		Hydrocortisone sodium succinate (Solu-Cortef)	Dexamethasone sodium phosphate (Decadron)
			Methylprednisolone sodium succinate (Solu-Medrol)
Estrogens		Conjugated estrogens USP (Premarin)	
Insulin		Regular insulin	Antidote: glucagon
Pituitary agents		Vasopressin (Pitressin)	
		Oxytocin (Pitocin)	

(Continued)

TABLE 15-4 **Summary of IV Drugs—cont'd**

Category	Type	Prototype	Related drugs
Immune Modulators			
Immunostimulants		Immunoglobulin IV (Gamunex)	Rh$_0$(D) immune globulin (WinRho)
Immunosuppressants		Cyclosporine (Sandimmune)	Azathioprine sodium (Imuran)
			Antithymocyte globulin (Atgam)
			Tacrolimus (Prograf)
			Basiliximab (Simulect)
			Daclizumab (Zenapax)
Biological response modifiers		Infliximab (Remicade)	Natalizumab (Tysabri)
Respiratory Agents			
Smooth muscle relaxant		Theophylline	Theophylline ethylenediamine (aminophylline)
Vitamins			
Multivitamin preparations	Vitamin A	β-Carotene	
	Vitamin B$_1$	Thiamine	
	Vitamin B$_6$	Pyridoxine	
	B-complex vitamin	Folic acid	
	Vitamin C	Ascorbic acid	
	Vitamin D	Calcitriol (Calcijex)	Paricalcitol (Zemplar)
	Vitamin K$_1$	Phytonadione (AquaMEPHYTON)	
Iron	Iron replacement therapy	Iron dextran (Infed)	Sodium ferric gluconate complex in sucrose injection (Ferrlecit)
			Iron sucrose (Venofer)

including arthralgia, myalgia, and fever. Dilution with D$_5$W has caused more local pain and phlebitis than 0.9% sodium chloride.

Related drugs

Sodium ferric gluconate complex in sucrose injection (Ferrlecit) and iron sucrose (Venofer) are products used to replace iron in patients who cannot tolerate the iron dextran product. A test dose is not required for these agents, unlike iron dextran.

 SUMMARY

Table 15-4 presents a summary of the classifications of IV drugs discussed in this section.

 REFERENCES

Dipiro JT, Talbert RL, Yea GC et al: *Pharmacotherapy: a pathophysiologic approach*, ed 5, New York, 2002, McGraw-Hill.

Dunser MW, Mayr AJ, Ulmer H et al: Arginine vasopressin in advanced vasodilatory shock: a prospective, randomized, controlled study, *Circulation* 107:2313-2319, 2003.

Elkin MD, Perry AG, Potter PA: *Nursing interventions & clinical skills*, ed 4, St Louis, 2007, Mosby.

Gahart BL, Nazareno AR: *2008 Intravenous medications*, ed 24, St Louis, 2008, Mosby.

Goldman L, Ausiello D, editors: *Cecil medicine*, ed 23, Philadelphia, 2008, Saunders.

Infusion Nurses Society: Infusion nursing standards of practice, *J Infus Nurs* 29(1 suppl), 2006a.

Infusion Nurses Society: *Policies and procedures for infusion nursing*, ed 3, Norwood, MA, 2006b.

Katzung BG, editor: *Basic & clinical pharmacology*, ed 10, New York, 2007, McGraw-Hill Medical.

Landry DW, Levin HR, Gallant EM et al: Vasopressin pressor hypersensitivity in vasodilatory septic shock, *Crit Care Med* 25:1279-1282, 1997.

Luckner G, Dunser MW, Jochberger S et al: Arginine vasopressin in 316 patients with advanced vasodilatory shock, *Crit Care Med* 33:2659-2666, 2005.

Malay MB, Ashton RC Jr, Landry DW et al: Low-dose vasopressin in the treatment of vasodilatory septic shock, *J Trauma* 47:699-703, 1999.

McEvoy GK: *American Hospital Formulary Service drug information 2007*, Bethesda, Md, 2007, American Society of Health-System Pharmacists.

Patel BM, Chittock DR, Russell JA et al: Beneficial effects of short-term vasopressin infusion during severe septic shock, *Anesthesiology* 96:576-582, 2002.

Russell JA, Walley KR, Singer J et al: Vasopressin versus norepinephrine infusion in patients with septic shock, *New Engl J Med* 2358:877-887, 2008.

U.S. Pharmacopeial Convention: *U.S. Pharmacopeia 27. Chapter <797> Pharmaceutical compounding-sterile preparations. Revision bulletin*. Rockville, Md, 2008, Author.

Weinstein SM: *Plumer's principles & practice of intravenous therapy*, ed 8, Philadelphia, 2007, Lippincott Williams & Wilkins.

Wickersham RM, editor: *Drug facts and comparisons*, St Louis, 2007, Wolters Kluwer Health Inc.

CHAPTER

16 BIOLOGIC THERAPY

Cora Vizcarra, MBA, RN, CRNI®

B iologic therapy includes the use of agents derived from biological sources or of agents that affect biological responses. Primarily, these are products derived from the mammalian genome and represent the new "medicine cabinet" because of the modern genetic engineering techniques used in the creation of these agents (Oldham, 2003). Traditionally, biologic therapies were used to modify the body's immune responses. Although modulation of the immune response remains a main focus, the term "biotherapy" has replaced "immunotherapy" because the scope of the field has widened. Other names for biologic therapies include biologic agents, biologics, biologicals, and biological response modifier (BRM) therapy (Medicinenet, 2008). Biologics include a diverse range of products such as bacterial and viral vaccines; tissues; human blood and plasma and their derivatives; and certain products produced by biotechnology. These cells and biological molecules are extraordinarily specific in their interactions (Rieger, 2001). Because of this specificity, biotechnology's tools and techniques are precise and are tailored to operate in known, predictable ways. Biologic agents differ from most drugs as they are not small chemical compounds but are proteins structurally similar to autologous proteins. Biologic agents are not metabolized like drugs but are processed like other proteins in the body; thus adverse reactions might be different from those elicited by drugs (Pichler, 2006). The mechanisms of action of biologic agents involve the individual's own biological responses (Oldham, 2003). In this chapter, the discussion on biologic therapy will include immunoglobulin therapy and only biologic agents used in the treatment of select autoimmune disorders.

IMMUNE SYSTEM REVIEW

To understand how biologic agents interact with the immune system, it is important to recall how our immune system functions. There are two types of immunity—innate and adaptive immunity (Figure 16-1).

Innate immunity, also called nonspecific immunity, is the first line of defense against antigens, which are foreign substances that induce an immune response (Rieger, 2001). Innate immunity is present before exposure to an antigen and it is not enhanced by subsequent exposures. The first line of defense for the innate immune system includes mechanical barriers such as the intact skin and mucous membranes (Rieger, 2001). If these defenses fail, the innate immune system has other components as a second line of defense, including complement, phagocytes, and natural killer (NK) cells.

Adaptive immunity, also known as specific or acquired immunity, is characterized by specific recognition of foreign organisms and a memory response (Rieger, 2001). This allows the immune system to increase its ability to respond and defend the body with successive exposures to infectious organisms. There are two major branches of the adaptive immune responses—humoral immunity and cell-mediated immunity—depending on the components of the immune system involved in the response to the antigen.

Humoral immunity involves the production of antibody molecules in response to an antigen and is mediated by B lymphocytes. B lymphocytes, also called B cells, are specialized cells of the immune system and develop from the stem cells in the bone marrow. When matured, B lymphocytes can be found in the bone marrow, lymph nodes, spleen, some areas of the intestine, and, to a lesser extent, in the bloodstream. When B lymphocytes are stimulated by an antigen, they respond by maturing into another type of cell called plasma cells, the cells responsible for producing antibodies (Thibodeau and Patton, 2007).

Antibodies or immunoglobulins, produced by the plasma cells, interact with specific antigens to protect the host from potentially harmful substances. Each antibody consists of two identical heavy chains and two identical light chains, shaped to form a Y. The basic antibody structure is shown in Figure 16-2.

The tips of the Y's arms are called the variable region since these sections vary greatly from one antibody to another. These unique contours in the antigen binding site allow the antibody to recognize a matching antigen. The stem of the Y is called the constant region. This area is identical in all antibodies of the same class. It is this section that links the antibody to other participants in the immune defenses.

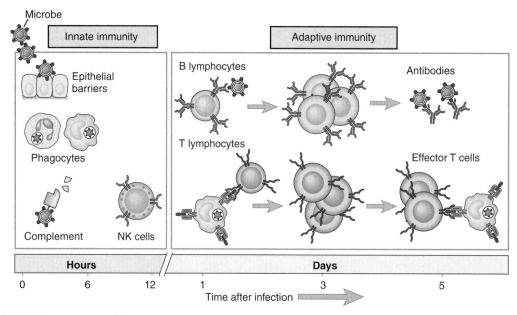

FIGURE 16-1 Innate and adaptive immunity. (From Thibodeau GA, Patton KT: *Anatomy & physiology,* ed 6, St Louis, 2007, Mosby.)

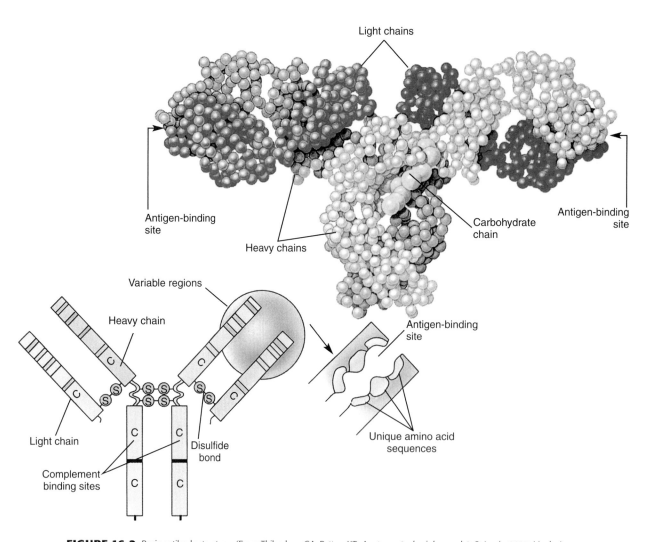

FIGURE 16-2 Basic antibody structure. (From Thibodeau GA, Patton KT: *Anatomy & physiology,* ed 6, St Louis, 2007, Mosby.)

There are five classes of antibodies or immunoglobulins: immunoglobulin gamma (IgG), immunoglobulin alpha (IgA), immunoglobulin delta (IgD), immunoglobulin epsilon (IgE), and immunoglobulin mu (IgM) (Thibodeau and Patton, 2007). The major immunoglobulin in the blood is IgG; it is produced in large quantities that exist for more than 1 month. IgG can enter into tissue spaces and works efficiently to coat microorganisms, speeding their destruction by other cells of the immune system. It is the only class of immunoglobulins that crosses the placenta and passes immunity from the mother to the newborn. IgA is shaped as a doublet guarding the entrance to the body; IgA is found in body fluids such as tears, saliva, and secretions of the respiratory and gastrointestinal tracts. IgD remains attached to B cells and plays a key role in initiating early B-cell response. IgE is normally present in only trace amounts in the blood and is responsible for the symptoms of allergy. IgM is a star-shaped cluster that remains in the bloodstream, where it is very effective in killing bacteria (Figure 16-3) (Thibodeau and Patton, 2007).

Cell-mediated immunity, on the other hand, involves the production of cytotoxic T lymphocytes, activated macrophages, activated NK cells, and cytokines in response to an antigen, and is mediated by T lymphocytes (Rieger, 2001). T lymphocytes, also called T cells, do not produce antibodies; instead, they directly attack foreign antigens such as viruses, fungi, or transplanted tissues and act as regulators of the immune system. Mature T lymphocytes leave the thymus and populate other organs of the immune system, such as the spleen, lymph nodes, bone marrow, and blood. T lymphocytes have molecules on their surfaces that are similar to antibodies and recognize antigens. T lymphocytes vary in types and functions. The killer or cytotoxic T lymphocytes perform the actual destruction of the invading microorganism, and also respond to foreign tissues in the body, such as a transplanted kidney. The killer T lymphocytes directly bind to their target and kill it. The helper T lymphocytes assist B lymphocytes in producing antibodies and assist the killer T lymphocytes in attacking foreign substances. The regulatory T lymphocytes suppress or turn off other T lymphocytes and act as a thermostat to the lymphocyte system. Natural killer (NK) cells come from the bone marrow and are present in low numbers in the bloodstream and in tissues. NK cells play an important role in killing cells infected with viruses and are believed to play a role in preventing cancer (Thibodeau and Patton, 2007).

Macrophages are large white blood cells found in many organs, including the lungs, kidneys, brain, and liver. Macrophages act like scavengers, removing debris and worn out cells from the body, and they also secrete monokines, a powerful chemical signal vital to the immune response. Cytokines are diverse and potent chemical messengers secreted by cells of the immune system. They are the chief communication signals of T cells, and encourage cell growth, promote cell activation, direct cellular traffic, and destroy target cells. Cytokines include interleukins, growth factors, and interferons. Interleukins serve as messengers between leukocytes and are also known as either lymphokines or monokines. When cytokines attract specific cell types to an area, they are called chemokines, and are released at the site of injury or infection where they attract other immune cells to the area to help repair damage and defend against infection. Interferons are naturally occurring cytokines that boost the immune system's ability to recognize cancer as a foreign invader (Thibodeau and Patton, 2007).

The major difference between humoral and cell-mediated immunity is that in cell-mediated immunity the immune response does not involve antibodies as it does in humoral immunity, but rather involves the activation of macrophages and NK cells, the production of antigen-specific cytotoxic lymphocytes, and the release of various cytokines in response to the antigen.

DISORDERS OF THE IMMUNE SYSTEM

The disorders of the immune system can be divided into two general categories: (1) excessive immune responses and (2) deficient immune responses. The category of excessive immune responses includes disorders in which the immune system is overfunctioning or hyperfunctioning. Examples include autoimmunity and hypersensitivity disorders. The category of deficient immune responses includes disorders in which the immune response is ineffective because of congenital, genetic, or acquired dysfunction. Examples include severe combined immunodeficiency (SCID) syndrome, DiGeorge syndrome, selective IgA deficiency, and the secondary immunodeficiencies associated with white blood cell malignancies. Human immunodeficiency virus/acquired immunodeficiency syndrome (HIV/AIDS) is a primary acquired immunodeficiency disorder (Copstead-Kirkhorn and Banasik, 2005).

In this chapter, the discussion will focus on disorders of the immune system treated with biologic agents and immune deficiency disorders treated with immunoglobulin.

AUTOIMMUNE DISORDERS

One of the most remarkable features of the immune system is its ability to distinguish between the self antigens, which are part of the host, and foreign antigens, which may present a threat to the host (Rieger, 2001). The immune system does not normally respond to self antigens. This immunological unresponsiveness to self antigens is called tolerance, and is important in understanding autoimmune disorders. The failure of this tolerance, because of the interaction of a wrong environment with the wrong genes, results in autoimmune disease (Mackay, 2000). Unfortunately, when a self antigen becomes immunogenic,

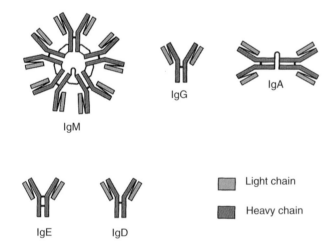

FIGURE 16-3 *Classes of antibodies. (From Thibodeau GA, Patton KT: Anatomy & physiology, ed 6, St Louis, 2007, Mosby.)*

Box 16-1 AUTOIMMUNE DISEASE BY MAIN TARGET ORGANS

Nervous system
- Multiple sclerosis
- Myasthenia gravis
- Guillain-Barré syndrome
- Autoimmune uveitis

GI system
- Crohn's disease
- Ulcerative colitis
- Primary biliary cirrhosis
- Autoimmune hepatitis

Blood/Blood vessels
- Autoimmune hemolytic anemia
- Pernicious anemia
- Autoimmune thrombocytopenia
- Temporal arteritis
- Antiphospholipid syndrome
- Vasculitides (Wegener's granulomatosis)
- Behçet's syndrome

Skin
- Psoriasis
- Dermatitis herpetiformis
- Pemphigus vulgaris
- Vitiligo

Endocrine glands
- Type 1 diabetes
- Grave's disease
- Hashimoto's thyroiditis
- Autoimmune oophoritis/orchitis
- Autoimmune adrenal gland disease

Musculoskeletal system
- Rheumatoid arthritis
- Systemic lupus erythematosus
- Scleroderma
- Polymyositis
- Ankylosing spondylitis
- Sjögren's syndrome

Data from *Understanding Autoimmune Disease* (website). Accessed 3/1/08 from http://www.nutritionadvisor.com/autoimmune-diseases.htm.

Box 16-2 PRIMARY AND SECONDARY IMMUNE DEFICIENCY TREATED WITH IMMUNOGLOBULIN THERAPY

Primary Immune Deficiency

Agammaglobulinemia (X-linked and autosomal form)

Hypogammaglobulinemia with impaired specific antibody production:
- Common variable immunodeficiency
- Hyper IgM syndromes
- Transient hypogammaglobulinemia

Normogammaglobulinemia with selective antibody deficiency:
- Wiskott-Aldrich syndrome
- Specific polysaccharide antibody deficiency and/or "lacunar" antibody deficiencies

Secondary Immune Deficiency

Chronic lymphocytic leukemia (CLL) with antibody deficiency and recurrent infection

Pediatric HIV infection

Hypogammaglobulinemia and/or specific antibody deficiency caused by chemotherapy and/or monoclonal antibody treatment

From The Immune Deficiency Foundation Nursing Advisory Committee: *IDF guide for nurses on immune globulin therapy for primary immunodeficiency diseases*, ed 2, Bethesda, Maryland, 2007, Immune Deficiency Foundation. Accessed 3/1/08 from http://www.primaryimmune.org/publications/book_nurse/Nurses_Guide.pdf.

it cannot be eliminated and the resulting inflammation becomes persistent and destructive. This is evident in autoimmune disorders such as rheumatoid arthritis, Crohn's disease, and psoriatic arthritis, just to name a few. Examples of autoimmune diseases by main target organs are listed in Box 16-1.

IMMUNE DEFICIENCY DISORDERS

When either part of the immune system is absent or its function is hampered, the result is an immune deficiency disease. An immune deficiency disease may be caused by an intrinsic (inborn) defect in the cells of the immune system, termed primary immune deficiency disease, or caused by an extrinsic environmental factor or agent, known as secondary immune deficiency disease. Primary immunodeficiency diseases are a group of disorders caused by basic defects in immune function that are intrinsic to, or inherent in, the cells and tissues of the immune system. There are more than 150 primary immunodeficiency diseases, ranging from common to rare, affecting a single cell or protein or more than one component of the

immune system (Immune Deficiency Foundation, 2007). Secondary immune deficiencies are conditions that impair immune function as a result of other processes. A number of physical, psychosocial, nutritional, environmental, and pharmacological factors can singly or in combination lead to the development of secondary immunodeficiency disorders (Copstead-Kirkhorn and Banasik, 2005). A list of primary and secondary immune deficiencies that may benefit from immunoglobulin therapy is presented in Box 16-2.

BIOLOGIC THERAPY FOR TREATMENT OF AUTOIMMUNE DISORDERS

There are a vast range of treatments available (Vizcarra, 2003) for traditional management of autoimmune disorders such as the following: rheumatoid arthritis, inflammatory bowel diseases such as Crohn's disease and ulcerative colitis, inflammatory skin conditions such as psoriasis, transplant-related diseases such as graft rejection, and neurological disorders such as multiple sclerosis. The traditional symptom-based treatment includes the use of anti-inflammatory drugs, corticosteroids, immunosuppressants, and even surgery, resulting in limited control and effectiveness often accompanied by safety and tolerability issues. It was this limitation and ineffective treatment partnered with the greater understanding of the underlying mechanisms of autoimmune disorders that facilitated the development of new biologic agents and revolutionized treatment (Olsen and Stein, 2004).

There are several biologic agents currently approved in the United States for the treatment of autoimmune disorders. Table 16-1 lists all types of biologic agents with approved indications related to the treatment of autoimmune disorders in the United States.

MONOCLONAL ANTIBODIES FOR AUTOIMMUNE DISORDERS

Monoclonal antibodies are produced using a technique developed by Kohler and Milstein in 1975 called hybridoma technique. This technique fuses an antibody-producing cell with a myeloma cell line, resulting in an "immortal hybrid" cell that produces a single antibody recognizing only a single antigen (Rieger, 2001). This technique made it possible to produce an unlimited batch of a pure monoclonal antibody that varied little and was highly specific for a single antigen (Rieger, 2001). The generic drug names of monoclonal antibodies end with the suffix "mab." The infixes preceding the suffix stem identify the target disease state and the product source. Thus, looking at the drug name rituximab, the "tu" indicates that the drug is for "tumor"; "xi" indicates that the drug is a chimeric monoclonal antibody, meaning derived from two or more genetically distinct sources; and "mab" indicates that the drug is a monoclonal antibody (American Medical Association, 2008).

The monoclonal antibody targeting tumor necrosis factor-alpha (TNFα), which is a key component in the development of various autoimmune disorders, includes anti-TNFα agents, also known as TNF antagonists, TNF inhibitors, TNF neutralizers, or TNF blockers. In certain autoimmune disorders such as rheumatoid arthritis (RA), Crohn's disease (CD), ulcerative colitis (UC), psoriasis, psoriatic arthritis, and ankylosing spondylitis, scientific evidence indicates that TNFα, a proinflammatory cytokine released by activated monocytes, macrophages, and T lymphocytes, is a central factor in the development of these diseases (Olsen and Stein, 2004). TNFα binds to its receptor cells, and the presence of TNFα in high concentration is responsible for inflammatory pathogenesis by mediating leukocyte recruitment and inflammation of the synovial membrane of the joint, intestinal mucosa, and skin (Papadakis and Targan, 2000; Feldmann and Maini, 2001). The TNFα antagonists work by impairing TNF binding to its receptors and lysing cells that express TNFα on their surface (Olsen and Stein, 2004). TNFα has been implicated in a wide spectrum of diseases beyond those previously mentioned, including sepsis, diabetes, cancer, osteoporosis, and multiple sclerosis (Chen and Goeddel, 2002). Examples of these agents are infliximab (Remicade, Centocor), adalimumab (Humira, Abbott), and certolizumab pegol (Cimzia, UCB). For the recommended dosing and administration of each agent, refer to Table 16-1.

Infliximab (Remicade, Centocor) is a chimeric human-murine (mouse) immunoglobulin gamma (IgG) monoclonal antibody composed of human constant and murine variable regions.

Infliximab binds specifically to TNFα and neutralizes its biological activity as a proinflammatory cytokine. By binding to the soluble and transmembrane forms of TNF, it inhibits the binding of TNFα to its receptors. Infliximab does not neutralize TNFβ, a related cytokine that uses the same receptors as TNFα. Infliximab is indicated for the treatment of rheumatoid arthritis, Crohn's disease in adults and children, fistulizing Crohn's disease, ankylosing spondylitis, psoriatic arthritis, ulcerative colitis, and plaque psoriasis.

Adalimumab (Humira, Abbott Labs) is a recombinant human IgG monoclonal antibody specific for human tumor necrosis factor (TNF). Adalimumab binds specifically to TNFα and blocks its interaction with the cell-surface TNF receptors. Adalimumab also modulates biological responses that are induced or regulated by TNF, including changes in the levels of adhesion molecules responsible for leukocyte migration. Adalimumab does not bind or inactivate TNFβ (lymphotoxin). Adalimumab is indicated for rheumatoid arthritis, juvenile idiopathic arthritis, psoriatic arthritis, ankylosing spondylitis, Crohn's disease, and plaque psoriasis.

Certolizumab pegol (Cimzia, UCB) is a recombinant, humanized antibody with specificity for human TNFα, conjugated to approximately 40-kilodalton (KDa) polyethylene glycol. Certolizumab pegol binds to human TNFα and selectively neutralizes TNFα for inhibition of human TNFα, but it does not neutralize lymphotoxin (TNFβ). Certolizumab is indicated for Crohn's disease in adults.

The monoclonal antibody targeting B cells used in the treatment of autoimmune disorders includes an agent such as rituximab (Rituxan, Biogen Idec/Genentech). Rituximab is genetically engineered chimeric murine-human monoclonal IgG directed against the CD20 antigen. Rituximab binds specifically to antigen CD20, a hydrophilic transmembrane protein located on pre-B lymphocytes and mature B lymphocytes. B cells are believed to play a role in the pathogenesis of rheumatoid arthritis (RA) and associated chronic synovitis. In this setting, B cells may be acting at multiple sites in the autoimmune/inflammatory process, including through production of rheumatoid factor (RF) and other autoantibodies, antigen presentation, T-cell activation, and/or proinflammatory cytokine production. The Fab domain (variable region) of rituximab binds to the CD20 antigen on B lymphocytes. The Fc domain (constant region) recruits immune effector functions to mediate B-cell lysis, which may include complement-dependent cytotoxicity (CDC), antibody-dependent cell-mediated cytotoxicity, and antibody induction of apoptosis in the B-cell lymphoma line. Rituximab is indicated for non-Hodgkin's lymphoma and rheumatoid arthritis. In this chapter, the discussion is limited to the use of rituximab for rheumatoid arthritis.

The monoclonal antibody targeting alpha₄-integrin (α₄-integrin) used in the treatment of autoimmune disorders includes an agent such as natalizumab (Tysabri, Biogen Idec/Elan Pharmaceuticals). Natalizumab is a recombinant humanized IgG monoclonal antibody that binds to α_4-integrin. Natalizumab binds to the alpha₄ subunit of α_4-integrin, β_1-integrin, and $\alpha_4\beta_7$-integrin expressed on the surface of all leukocytes except neutrophils, and inhibits the alpha₄-mediated adhesion of leukocytes to their counter-receptors. The receptors for the alpha₄ family of integrins include vascular adhesion molecule-1 (VCAM-1), which is expressed on activated vascular adhesion endothelium, and mucosal addressin cell adhesion molecule-1 (MAdCAM-1), which is present on vascular endothelial cells of the gastrointestinal tract. Disruption of these molecular interactions prevents the

TABLE 16-1 Biologic Agents in the United States Approved for Autoimmune Disorders

Name (Generic/Trade)	Mechanism of action	Approved indications	Recommended dosage (Initial)	Recommended dosage (Subsequent)	Comments
Abatacept/Orencia	Selective co-stimulation modulator; inhibits T-cell activation by binding to CD80 and CD86, thereby blocking interaction with CD28	Adult rheumatoid arthritis	*Adult:* <60 kg: 500 mg 60-100kg: 750 mg >100 kg: 1000 mg	Following initial dose, give at 2 and 4 weeks, then every 4 weeks	Administer as a 30-min infusion. Prepare vials using only silicone-free disposable syringe. Use sterile, nonpyrogenic, low protein binding filter.
		Juvenile idiopathic arthritis (pediatric patients 6 years of age and older)	*Pediatric:* <75 kg: 10 mg/kg ≥75 kg: follow adult dosing regimen, not to exceed maximum dose of 1000 mg	Following initial dose, give at 2 and 4 weeks, then every 4 weeks	Administer as a 30-min infusion. Prepare vials using only silicone-free disposable syringe. Use sterile, nonpyrogenic, low protein binding filter.
Adalimumab/Humira	Binds specifically to TNFα and blocks its interaction with p55 and p75 cell-surface receptors Lyses surface TNF-expressing cells in vitro in presence of compliment Does not bind or inactivate lymphotoxin (TNFβ)	Rheumatoid arthritis Psoriatic arthritis Ankylosing spondylitis	*Adult:* 40 mg every other week; some patients with RA not receiving methotrexate may benefit from increasing frequency to 40 mg every week	*Adult:* 40 mg every other week; some patients with RA not receiving methotrexate may benefit from increasing frequency to 40 mg every week	Administered by subcutaneous injection.
		Juvenile idiopathic arthritis	*For patients 4-17 yr, based on weight:* 15kg (33 lb) to <30 kg (66 lb): 20 mg every other week ≥30 kg (66 lb): 40 mg every other week	*For patients 4-17 yr, based on weight:* 15 kg (33 lb) to <30 kg (66 lb): 20 mg every other week	Administered by subcutaneous injection.
		Crohn's disease	*Adult:* 160 mg day 1 (given as four 40-mg injections in 1 day or as two 40-mg injections per day for 2 consecutive days)	Followed by 80 mg 2 weeks later (day 15); 2 weeks later (day 29) begin maintenance dose of 40 mg every other week	Administered by subcutaneous injection.
		Plaque psoriasis	*Adult:* initial dose of 80 mg	40 mg every other week starting 1 week after initial dose	Administered by subcutaneous injection.
Anakinra/Kineret	Blocks the biologic activity of IL-1 by competitively inhibiting IL-1 binding to IL-1 type 1 receptor, which is expressed in a wide variety of tissues and organs	Rheumatoid arthritis	100 mg/day Physician should consider a dose of 100 mg every other day for RA patients who have severe renal insufficiency or end-stage renal disease	100 mg/day Physician should consider a dose of 100 mg every other day for RA patients who have severe renal insufficiency or end-stage renal disease	Administered by subcutaneous injection. Administer dose at approximately same time every day.
Certolizumab pegol/Cimzia	Binds and inhibits human TNFα	Crohn's disease	*Adult:* 400 mg initially	At weeks 2 and 4; if response occurs, follow with 400 mg every 4 weeks	Administered by subcutaneous injection.

TABLE 16-1 Biologic Agents in the United States Approved for Autoimmune Disorders—cont'd

Name (Generic/ Trade)	Mechanism of action	Approved indications	Recommended dosage (Initial)	Recommended dosage (Subsequent)	Comments
Efalizumab/Raptiva	Binds to CD11a and inhibits binding of LFA-1 to ICAM-1, thereby inhibiting adhesion of leukocytes to other cell types	Plaque psoriasis	A single 0.7 mg/kg conditioning dose	Followed by weekly doses of 1 mg/kg (maximum single dose not to exceed total of 200 mg)	Administered by subcutaneous injection.
Etanercept/Enbrel	Binds specifically to TNF and blocks its interaction with cell-surface receptors	Rheumatoid arthritis Psoriatic arthritis Ankylosing spondylitis	*Adult:* 50 mg per week	*Adult:* 50 mg per week	Administered by subcutaneous injection.
		Juvenile idiopathic arthritis	*Pediatric (ages 2-17 yr):* 0.8 mg/kg per week up to maximum of 50 mg per week	*Pediatric (ages 2-17 yr):* 0.8 mg/kg per week up to maximum of 50 mg per week	Administered by subcutaneous injection. 50-mg prefilled syringe or autoinjector may be used for pediatric patients weighing 63 kg or more. 25-mg prefilled syringe is not recommended for pediatric patients weighing less than 31 kg.
		Plaque psoriasis	*Adult:* 50 mg given twice weekly (administered 3 or 4 days apart) for 3 months	Followed by a reduction to maintenance dose of 50 mg per week.	Administered by subcutaneous injection.
Natalizumab/Tysabri	Binds to alpha$_4$ subunit of $\alpha_4\beta_1$- and $\alpha_4\beta_7$-integrins expressed on surface of all leukocytes except neutrophils, and inhibits alpha$_4$-mediated adhesion of leukocytes to their counter-receptors	Relapsing form of multiple sclerosis	300 mg every 4 weeks	300 mg every 4 weeks	Administer intravenously over 1 hour. Only prescribers registered in MS Touch prescribing program may prescribe Tysabri.
		Crohn's disease	300 mg every 4 weeks	300 mg every 4 weeks	Administer intravenously over 1 hour. Only prescribers registered in CD Touch prescribing program may prescribe Tysabri.
Infliximab/Remicade	Neutralizes biological activities of TNFα by binding with high affinity to soluble and transmembrane forms of TNFα; inhibits binding of TNFα with its receptors Does not neutralize TNFβ, a related cytokine that uses same receptors as TNF	Rheumatoid arthritis	3 mg/kg as first infusion	Followed by 3 mg/kg at 2 and 6 weeks after first infusion and then every 8 weeks thereafter For patients with incomplete response, adjust dose up to 10 mg/kg or treat as often as every 4 weeks	Should be given in combination with methotrexate. Administered as an intravenous infusion over 2 hours.
		Ankylosing spondylitis	5 mg/kg	Followed by additional doses of 5 mg/kg at 2 and 6 weeks after first infusion, then every 6 weeks	Administered as an intravenous infusion over 2 hours.

(Continued)

TABLE 16-1 Biologic Agents in the United States Approved for Autoimmune Disorders—cont'd

Name (Generic/ Trade)	Mechanism of action	Approved indications	Recommended dosage (Initial)	Recommended dosage (Subsequent)	Comments
		Psoriatic arthritis	5 mg/kg	Followed by additional doses of 5 mg/kg at 2 and 6 weeks after first infusion, then every 8 weeks	
		Crohn's disease Fistulizing Crohn's disease	*Adult:* 5 mg/kg induction regimen at 0, 2, and 6 weeks	*Adult:* followed by maintenance regimen of 5 mg/kg every 8 weeks thereafter For adult patients who respond and then lose their response, consideration may be given to treatment with 10 mg/kg	Administered as an intravenous infusion over 2 hours. Patients who do not respond by week 14 are unlikely to respond with continued dosing and consideration should be given to discontinue Remicade.
		Pediatric Crohn's disease	*Pediatric:* 5 mg/kg induction regimen at 0, 2, and 6 weeks	Followed by maintenance regimen of 5 mg/kg every 8 weeks thereafter	Administered as an intravenous infusion over 2 hours.
		Ulcerative colitis	5 mg/kg	Followed by additional doses of 5mg/kg at 2 and 6 weeks after first infusion, then every 8 weeks thereafter	Administered as an intravenous infusion over 2 hours. Can be given with or without methotrexate.
		Plaque psoriasis	5 mg/kg	Followed by additional doses of 5 mg/kg at 2 and 6 weeks after first infusion, then every 8 weeks thereafter	Administered as an intravenous infusion over 2 hours.
Rituximab/Rituxan	Binds to CD20 antigen on B lymphocytes and recruits immune effector function to mediate B-cell lysis	Rheumatoid arthritis *Note:* rituximab is approved for NHL but not included in discussion of autoimmune disorders	Two, 1000-mg infusions separated by 2 weeks		Given in combination with methotrexate. Premedicate before each infusion. *First infusion:* initiate infusion at rate of 50 mg/hr. In absence of infusion toxicity, increase infusion rate by 50 mg/hr increments every 30 min, to maximum of 400 mg/hr. *Subsequent infusion:* initiate infusion at rate of 100 mg/hr. In absence of infusion toxicity, increase rate by 100 mg/hr increments at 30-min intervals, to maximum of 400 mg/hr. Interrupt infusion or slow infusion rate for infusion reactions. Continue infusion at half previous rate upon improvement of symptoms.

transmigration of leukocytes across the endothelium into inflamed parenchymal tissue. The specific mechanism by which natalizumab exerts its effects in multiple sclerosis and Crohn's disease has not been fully defined. Natalizumab is indicated as a monotherapy for the treatment of patients with relapsing forms of multiple sclerosis to delay the escalation of physical disability and reduce the frequency of clinical exacerbations. Because of the increased risk of progressive multifocal leukoencephalopathy (PML), an opportunistic viral infection of the brain that usually leads to death or severe disability, natalizumab is generally recommended for patients who have had an inadequate response to, or are unable to tolerate, alternate multiple sclerosis therapies. Natalizumab is also indicated for inducing and maintaining clinical response and remission in adult patients with moderately to severely active Crohn's disease, with evidence of inflammation, who have had an inadequate response to or are unable to tolerate conventional Crohn's disease therapies and inhibitors of TNFα. Because of the risk of PML, only prescribers, infusion centers, and pharmacies associated with infusion centers registered in the MS TOUCH or CD TOUCH prescribing programs are able to prescribe, distribute, or infuse natalizumab for either multiple sclerosis or Crohn's disease. In addition, natalizumab must be administered only to patients who are enrolled in and meet all the conditions of the TOUCH prescribing program (Natalizumab Prescribing Information, 2008).

Monoclonal antibodies targeting human CD11a used in the treatment of autoimmune disorders include efalizumab (Raptiva, Genentech). Efalizumab is an immunosuppressive recombinant humanized IgG monoclonal antibody that binds to human CD11a. CD11a, the alpha subunit of leukocyte function antigen-1 (LFA-1), is expressed on all leukocytes, and the binding with efalizumab decreases cell-surface expression of CD11a. Efalizumab inhibits the binding of LFA-1 to intercellular adhesion molecule-1 (ICAM-1), thereby inhibiting the adhesion of leukocytes to other cell types. Interaction between LFA-1 and ICAM-1 contributes to the initiation and maintenance of multiple processes, including activation of T lymphocytes, adhesion of T lymphocytes to endothelial cells, and migration of T lymphocytes to sites of inflammation, including psoriatic skin. Lymphocyte activation and trafficking to skin play a role in the pathophysiology of chronic plaque psoriasis. In psoriatic skin, ICAM-1 cell-surface expression is upregulated on endothelium and keratinocytes. Efalizumab is indicated for the treatment of adult patients with moderate to severe chronic plaque psoriasis who are candidates for systemic therapy or phototherapy (Efalizumab Prescribing Information, 2005).

OTHER BIOLOGIC AGENTS FOR AUTOIMMUNE DISORDERS

Aside from monoclonal antibodies, other biologic agents used in the treatment of autoimmune disorders include drugs such as abatacept (Orencia, Bristol Myers Squibb), etanercept (Enbrel, Amgen/Wyeth/Immunex), and anakinra (Kineret, Amgen). Refer to Table 16-1 for the recommended dosing and administration of these agents.

Abatacept (Orencia) is a soluble fusion protein that inhibits T-cell (T lymphocyte) activation by binding to CD80 and CD86, thereby blocking interaction with CD28. This interaction provides a co-stimulatory signal necessary for full activation of T lymphocytes. Activated T lymphocytes implicated in the pathogenesis of rheumatoid arthritis are found in the synovium of patients with RA. Abatacept is indicated for reducing signs and symptoms, inducing major clinical response, inhibiting the progression of structural damage, and improving physical function in adult patients with moderate to severely active rheumatoid arthritis who have had an inadequate response to one or more disease-modifying anti-rheumatic drugs (DMARDs) such as methotrexate or TNF antagonists (Abatacept Prescribing Information, 2008).

Etanercept (Enbrel) is a dimeric fusion protein form of the p75 TNF receptor that binds specifically to tumor necrosis factor (TNF) and blocks its interaction with cell-surface receptors. As previously mentioned, TNF is a naturally occurring cytokine that is involved in normal inflammatory and immune responses. It plays an important role in the inflammatory processes of RA, the polyarticular course of juvenile rheumatoid arthritis (JRA), ankylosing spondylitis, and plaque psoriasis. Etanercept inhibits binding of both TNFα and TNFβ to cell-surface receptors, rendering TNF biologically inactive. Etanercept is indicated for moderate to severely active RA, moderate to severely active polyarticular course JRA, psoriatic arthritis, ankylosing spondylitis, and moderate to severe plaque psoriasis (Etanercept Prescribing Information, 2008).

Anakinra (Kineret) is a recombinant, nonglycosylated form of the human interleukin-1 receptor antagonist (IL-1 RA). It blocks the biologic activity of IL-1 by competitively inhibiting IL-1 binding to the interleukin-1 type receptor (IL1RI), which is expressed in a wide variety of tissues and organs. IL-1 production is induced in response to inflammatory stimuli and mediates various physiological responses, including inflammatory and immunological responses. Anakinra is indicated for moderate to severely active rheumatoid arthritis, in patients 18 years of age or older who have failed one or more DMARDs. Anakinra can be used alone or in combination with DMARDs other than TNF blocking agents (Anakinra Prescribing Information, 2006).

ADVERSE EVENTS OF BIOLOGIC AGENTS

With biologic therapy, it is important to differentiate between target-related and agent-related adverse events. Target-related adverse events are common with biologic agents since the agent may alter the composition and functional integrity of the normal immune response, thereby predisposing the patient to certain adverse events, while the biologic agent itself is harmless (Pichler, 2006). In the treatment of autoimmune disorders, the use of monoclonal antibodies (TNFα antagonists in particular) is associated with a wide range of adverse events. Since the actions of the monoclonal antibodies affect the immune system and its components, adverse events may include infections, malignancies, injection site or infusion reactions, cardiac events, neurological events, hepatic involvement, hematological changes, and immune and autoimmune responses (Olsen and Stein, 2004). Table 16-2 is a summary of the adverse events reported in biologic agents used for the treatment of autoimmune disorders. It is important to refer to each of the product's prescribing information for more detailed discussion of the adverse events.

IMMUNOGLOBULIN THERAPY FOR IMMUNE DEFICIENCY

The use of immunoglobulin is based on either the principle of replacement for primary or secondary humoral antibody deficiency or the principle of immunomodulation for autoimmune or

TABLE 16-2 Adverse Events Associated with Biologic Agents for Autoimmune Disorders

Adverse events	Abatacept (Orencia)	Adali-(mumab humira)	Anakinra (Kineret)	Certolizumab pegol (Cimzia)	Efalizumab (Raptiva)	Etanercept (Enbrel)	Natali-zumab (Tysabri)	Infliximab (Remicade)	Rituximab (Rituxan)
Infusion reactions	✓						✓	✓	✓
Local injection site reactions		✓	✓	✓	✓	✓			
Malignancies	✓	✓	✓	✓	✓	✓		✓	✓
Progressive multi-focal leukoen-cephalopathy (PML)							✓		✓
Immunosuppression/infections	✓	✓	✓	✓	✓	✓	✓	✓	✓
Hepatotoxicity		✓				✓	✓	✓	✓
Hematological events		✓	✓	✓	✓	✓		✓	✓
Hepatitis B reactivation		✓		✓		✓		✓	✓
Neurological events		✓		✓		✓		✓	✓
Cardiac events		✓		✓		✓		✓	✓

certain infectious diseases. Although immunoglobulin gamma (IgG) has been used for a variety of conditions, in the United States there are six FDA-approved indications: immune thrombocytopenic purpura (ITP); primary immunodeficiency; chronic lymphocytic leukemia; pediatric HIV infection; Kawasaki disease; or for prevention of graft-versus-host disease (GVHD) and infection in patients undergoing bone marrow transplantation (*IDF Guide for Nurses,* 2007). The dynamic of immunoglobulin use is rapidly changing, and immunoglobulin is being used to treat a growing range of off-label conditions, including a variety of neurological diseases, immunological disorders, and hematological conditions. However, the use of immunoglobulin in these off-label conditions will not be included in this chapter.

Many theories exist as to how immunoglobulin works but the exact mechanism of action is unknown. Inhibition of cytokines, competition with autoantibodies, complement "sponging," interference with the binding of crystallized fragment (Fc) receptors on cells of the reticuloendothelial system, interference with antigen recognition by T cells, and a negative feedback effect on the factories of antibody production are just a few of the theories, although the actual effects are probably multifactorial (Swenson, 2000).

There are various immunoglobulin products licensed in the United States and these are made from carefully screened and tested donors. The production processes of all of the products include dedicated steps such as low-pH treatment, pasteurization, solvent/detergent treatment, and/or nanofication, designed to remove and inactivate bloodborne pathogens. However, potential transmission of bloodborne pathogens or emerging pathogens cannot be absolutely ruled out (*IDF Guide for Nurses,* 2007). The intravenous immunoglobulin (IVIG) preparations are lyophilized or liquid. Stabilizers (such as sorbitol, maltose, or sucrose) are added to several products to stabilize the IgG and keep the molecules from aggregating. All currently available products contain varying concentrations of IgA, and certain patients may be at risk for anaphylaxis if IgE is produced by the patient against the IgA. Table 16-3 is a list of

available immunoglobulin products licensed for use in the United States.

Considerations for which product is appropriate for the patient will depend on factors such as the patient's risk factors, including kidney function; history of diabetes, hypertension, or stroke; history of thromboembolic events; the concentration of the product; the IgA levels present in the product; the product form (such as liquid preparation or lyophilized powder); and the time it takes to prepare the product for administration (Duff, 2006).

When a patient is identified as a candidate for immunoglobulin therapy, the route of administration must be determined. In the United States, patients can receive immunoglobulin either by intravenous infusion or by subcutaneous infusion. The intravenous route is the most common method of administration, generally tolerated by most patients, and larger doses could be given, with resultant improvement in the patient's condition (*IDF Guide for Nurses,* 2007). The subcutaneous route of administration involves giving smaller doses more often, which may eliminate some of the adverse effects associated with intravenous infusions (*IDF Guide for Nurses,* 2007). Considerations for subcutaneous infusion of immunoglobulin include clinical information and factors related to the patient's living circumstances. Box 16-3 summarizes the considerations in selecting the route of administration for immunoglobulin therapy.

A majority of patients receive immunoglobulin infusions in an outpatient setting or in a hospital inpatient setting. About 20% of patients treated with immunoglobulin receive infusions at home (Duff, 2006).

ADVERSE EVENTS OF IMMUNOGLOBULIN THERAPY

It is estimated that up to 30% of patients experience adverse events associated with the use of immunoglobulin therapy (*IDF Guide for Nurses,* 2007). Most adverse events occur during the first 30 to 60 minutes of the infusion, with the severity ranging from mild to severe and self-limiting. The types of adverse

TABLE 16-3 Immune Globulin Products Available in the United States[*]

Brand name	Gammagard S/D 5%, 10%	Gammagard liquid	Carimune NF	Vivaglobin	Flebogamma 5%	Octagam	Gamunex
Manufacturer	Baxter Corp./BioScience Division	Baxter Corp./BioScience Division	CSL Behring	CSL Behring	Grifols	Octapharma	Talecris
Methods of production (including viral inactivation)	Cohn-Oncley fractionation, ultrafiltration, ion-exchange chromatography, solvent/detergent treatment	Cohn-Oncley fractionation, solvent/detergent treatment, ANX chromatography, 35-nm nanofiltration, low pH/elevated temperature incubation	Kistler Nitschmann fractionation, pH 4.0, trace pepsin, nanofiltration	Cold alcohol fractionation, ethanol-fatty alcohol/pH precipitation, pasteurization, diafiltered and ultrafiltered	Cold alcohol fractionation, PEG ion-exchange chromatography, pasteurized at 60° C for 10 hr	Cohn-Oncley cold ethanol fractionation, ultrafiltration, chromatography, solvent/detergent treatment	Cohn-Oncley fractionation, caprylate/chromatography purification, cloth and depth filtration, final container low pH incubation
Form	Lyophilized	Liquid	Lyophilized	Liquid	Liquid	Liquid	Liquid
Shelf life	24 months	36 months	24 months	24 months	24 months	24 months	36 months
Reconstitution time	<5 min at room temperature > 20 min if cold	None (liquid solution)	Several minutes	None (liquid solution)	None (liquid solution)	None (liquid solution)	None (liquid solution)
Available concentrations	5%, 10%	10%	3-12%	16% (160 mg of protein/mL)	5%	5%	10%
Maximum recommended infusion rate	5%: 4 mL/kg/hr 10%: 8 mL/kg/hr	5 mL/kg/hr	>2.5 mL/kg/hr	20 mL/hr	6 mL/kg/hr	<4.2 mL/kg/hr	4.8 mL/kg/hr
Time to infuse 35 g[†]	5%: 2.5 hr 10%: 0.6 hr	1 hr	<3.3 hr (6% solution)	Time will vary[‡]	1.6 hr	2.5 hr	1.0 hr
Sugar content	5%: 20 mg/mL glucose 10%: 40 mg/mL glucose	No added sugars	1.67 g of sucrose/g of protein	None	5% D-sorbitol (polypol)	100 mg/mL maltose	None
Sodium content	5%: 8.5 mg/mL sodium chloride 10%: 17 mg/mL sodium chloride	No added sodium	<20 mg of sodium chloride/g of protein	3 mg/mL	<3.2 mmol/L	≤30 mmol/L	Trace amounts
Osmolarity/osmolality	5%: 636 mOsm/L 10%: 1250 mOsm/L	240-300 mOsm/kg	192-1074 mOsm/kg	445 mOsm/kg	240-350 mOsm/kg	310-380 mOsm/kg	258 mOsm/kg
pH	6.4-7.2	4.6-5.1	6.4-6.8	6.4-7.2	5.0-6.0	5.1-6.0	4.0-4.5
IgA content	<2.2 mcg/mL in 5% solution	37 mcg/mL	720 mcg/mL	<1700 mcg/mL	<50 mcg/mL	<100 mcg/mL	46 mcg/mL
Approved method of administration	Intravenous	Intravenous	Intravenous	Subcutaneous	Intravenous	Intravenous	Intravenous

[*]Check product label for storage temperatures, which vary among immunoglobulin brands. Check package insert for detailed prescribing information. Privigen and Flebogamma 5% DIF also available.
[†]The time to infuse is based on the maximal infusion rate: 0.5 g/kg for a 70-kg adult = 35 g; 5% concentrations: 1 g = 20 mL; 10% concentrations: 1 g = 10 mL.
[‡]Time will vary depending upon volume and tolerability. Using 35 g as monthly dose, calculate weekly dose = 8.75 g = 55 mL infused into 4 sites at a rate up to 20 mL/hr/site, which can range from 45 minutes to 3 hours.
From The Immune Deficiency Foundation website, Immunoglobulin Products page:http://www.primaryimmune.org/patients_families/prod_safe/ivig_chart.pdf. Accessed 3/1/08.

reactions reported with infusions of immunoglobulin are listed in Table 16-4.

Adverse events related to subcutaneous administration of immunoglobulin include a low incidence of systemic effects, but a high incidence of local reactions at the infusion sites. The low incidence of systemic effects is attributed to the slower equilibration of the IgG into the circulation. Rates of local infusion site reactions were reported to be as high as 80% to 90% with the initial infusion, decreasing to less than 30% within 1 to 2 months of continued weekly infusion (Ochs et al, 2006). Local reactions at the infusion site often include swelling, erythema, and a sensation of burning or itching. The swelling and erythema dissipate completely within 24 hours after the infusion is finished (Berger, 2008).

Box 16-3   CONSIDERATIONS FOR SELECTION OF ROUTE OF ADMINISTRATION FOR IMMUNOGLOBULIN THERAPY

Clinical Factors	Lifestyle/Psychological Factors
Ability to establish IV access	Distance from/accessibility of infusion center
Adverse effects during IV infusions or following peak	Availability of transportation
Adverse effects/suboptimal health at trough when IV infusion due	Patient's schedule
History of thromboembolic events	Availability of home nursing services
Risk of thrombosis, renal failure, hyperviscosity	Ability to learn and perform infusions
	Availability of partner/parent/ "infusion buddy"
	Home environment
	Reliability of patient
	Reimbursement issues

From Berger M: Subcutaneous IgG therapy in immune deficiency diseases, *Clin Focus Primary Immune Defic* 13:1-10, 2008.

NURSING CONSIDERATIONS AND PATIENT MANAGEMENT

The advances in drug technology and our increased understanding of the immune basis of many diseases led to the expansion of the clinical application for biologic agents. This advancement can become an ongoing challenge for both experienced and new infusion nurses as they provide care and manage patients receiving parenteral biologic therapies. One of the key points to remember is biologic agents are not like the chemical compounds or drugs we have traditionally administered to our patients. Biologic agents have unique characteristics and features very different from traditional drugs, and therefore may require a different management approach. The following discussion on the nursing considerations in managing patients receiving biologic therapies will include patient assessment; patient education; drug preparation, handling, and administration; monitoring and management of adverse events such as infusion reactions; documentation; and reimbursement.

PATIENT ASSESSMENT

One of the greatest contributions of nurses to patient care is patient assessment. In the patient receiving biologic therapy, patient assessment is performed before initiation of therapy to obtain baseline information and to screen the patient. Information that should be obtained incorporates new facts as well as the patient's past medical history, including any significant illnesses or diseases (e.g., cancer or malignancies, cardiac or pulmonary problems, neurological disorders, hepatic or liver disorders, hematological disorders or blood dyscrasias, diabetes,

hypertension, and serious viral, fungal, or bacteria infections). The patient's past medical history will help the nurse be aware of risk factors that may place the patient at a higher risk for developing adverse events associated with biologic therapy. In patients receiving biologic therapy that suppresses TNFα, the nurse must screen for a history of tuberculosis and other infections such as histoplasmosis and coccidioidomycosis, as well as active infections. A tuberculin skin test and/or a chest x-ray must be administered and results read before the initiation of therapy. TNFα is critical for containing and killing *Mycobacteria* and other intracellular pathogens, and chronically suppressing TNF by anti-TNF agents appears to remove these protections and may reactivate latent tuberculosis (Vizcarra, 2003).

A medication and allergy profile must be obtained, including history of prior treatments and current symptoms related to the prior treatment or the underlying disease process. Always be aware of any allergies the patient may have to drugs or food with special attention to allergic reactions associated with biologic therapy. A detailed review of the patient's medication history is important, looking closely at concurrent medications for possible interactions (Vizcarra and Belcher, 2006). Patients are discouraged from taking medications similar to the parenteral biologic therapy they will be receiving because of the increased risk of potential side effects with no additional medical benefit.

After a detailed past medical history is obtained, the patient's current health status and condition must be assessed. Before each treatment, take note of the patient's current weight, vital signs, hydration status, skin integrity, and appearance. It is important to establish the baseline function and status of the renal, hepatic, hematological, cardiovascular, and pulmonary systems (Vizcarra and Belcher, 2006). Laboratory assessments may be necessary depending on the biologic agent and underlying disease process. Laboratory tests may include a complete blood count with differential, platelet and reticulocyte counts, prothrombin time, partial thromboplastin time, liver and kidney function tests, including electrolytes, and a thyroid panel (Rieger, 2001). There are special considerations to remember with the elderly. They are more likely to have alterations in renal and hepatic functioning, as well as a decrease in cardiac function, which may affect dosing, clearance, and tolerance of the biologic agents. Special attention is required to their medication profile since they are often taking several medications (Rieger, 2001).

On an ongoing basis, the patient's response to treatment should be assessed, paying particular attention to the patient's progress or lack of progress. In certain diseases such as rheumatoid arthritis (RA), a patient self-assessment tool, such as a health assessment questionnaire (HAQ), including a disability index and pain scale, can be valuable in providing a clearer perspective related to the patient's illness. The Health Assessment Questionnaire Disability Index and Pain Scale was developed jointly by Stanford University Arthritis Center and the Arthritis, Rheumatism, and Aging Medical Information System, with funding support from the National Institutes of Health (NIH). A reduction in the HAQ score over time indicates improvement. A similar self-administered health-related quality-of-life assessment tool is available for use in patients with Crohn's disease and other inflammatory bowel diseases. The Inflammatory Bowel Disease Questionnaire (IBDQ) was developed by the School of Nursing, Department of Clinical Epidemiology and Biostatistics, and Department of Medicine, McMaster University, Hamilton, Ontario, Canada. As a result

TABLE 16-4 Adverse Events Related to Immune Globulin Therapy

	Nursing intervention
Anaphylactoid Reactions	
Chills/rigors	Slow rate or stop infusion, administer ibuprofen, aspirin, and/or diphenhydramine hydrochloride.
Headache	Administer acetaminophen, ibuprofen, or NSAIDs. Alternate after infusion every 3-6 hours for 24-48 hours based on physician's recommendations.
Migraine headache	To have better success with resolution of symptoms, administer prescribed antimigraine medications as soon as first signs of migraine occur. Oral or IV steroids may help decrease intensity of headache. This is based on physician's recommendations. Nonpharmacological interventions may include: turn off lights, apply cold compresses, and increase fluid intake before and during infusion.
Malaise/flulike symptoms; Myalgia/arthralgia	Educate patient that resting after IVIG infusion may help minimize muscle aches or pain; patient should avoid excessive fatigue. Some children have opposite effect, with increased amount of energy, but then usually require increased amount of sleep.
Allergic Reactions	
Urticaria	In patients who have not experienced transient urticaria with many of their previous infusions, development of urticaria should trigger immediate stopping of infusion. Contact physician or call 9-1-1. Administer ordered medications such as antihistamines and/or steroids. Observe for signs of true anaphylaxis and give epinephrine if indicated.
Vasomotor symptoms: Hypotension, hypertension, flushing, or tachycardia	Slow or stop infusion, or administer fluid with hypotension, based on physician's order. Administer diuretics on physician's order if fluid overload is likely.
Nausea/vomiting	Stop or slow infusion. Administer antacids as needed. If ordered, administer IV hydration and/or antiemetic medication.
Adverse Reactions	
Back pain/hip pain/arthralgias	Stop or slow infusion, administer ibuprofen to help with discomfort, apply heating pad, and administer other medications per physician's orders.
Anaphylaxis: Hypotension, strong uncomfortable feeling, tightening in or around neck, chest, or abdomen; difficulty swallowing, choking sensation, or difficulty breathing; wheezing, rash or hives, rapid or weak pulse, sweating, or upset stomach with or without vomiting and diarrhea	Immediately turn off infusion. Administer an antihistamine. Notify health care provider. If symptoms do not resolve, patient should lie flat and be given a single dose of adrenaline (EpiPen); arrangements should be made for patient to be evaluated. Call 9-1-1 if adrenaline is used in home care environment. Literature supports that second dose of adrenaline may need to be administered.
Aseptic meningitis: Patients with aseptic meningitis develop symptoms of severe headache with nuchal rigidity, drowsiness, fever, and lethargy; symptoms often begin 24-48 hours or more after infusion has been completed	Patients exhibiting these symptoms should undergo thorough neurological evaluation, including CSF studies, to rule out other causes of meningitis. Symptoms are not relieved by slowing or stopping infusion, and headache does not resolve with acetaminophen or NSAIDs. Using a different IVIG preparation may be helpful in preventing recurrence of aseptic meningitis. Severe cases requiring discontinuation of therapy are rare.
Thrombotic events	Patients with these risk factors should follow a conservative infusion protocol, using a product with a low (5%) concentration, and proceed slowly and cautiously with incremental increases in rate of infusion to maximum of 4 mL/kg of body weight per hour.

From The Immune Deficiency Foundation Nursing Advisory Committee: *IDF guide for nurses on immune globulin therapy for primary immunodeficiency diseases,* ed 2, Bethesda, Md, 2007, Immune Deficiency Foundation. Accessed 3/1/08 at http://www.primaryimmune.org/publications/book_nurse/Nurses_Guide.pdf.

of their assessment and the health care provider's assessment, the patient may need treatment manipulation related to drug dose or schedule.

PATIENT EDUCATION

The purpose of therapy, treatment schedule, potential side effects, cost, and reimbursement concerns are discussed with the patient before the initiation of therapy (Rieger, 2001). Possible adverse events associated with the biologic agents should be discussed along with recommendations to prevent, minimize, or alleviate them. The nurse should assess what the patient has been told by others regarding the disease and possible treatment to avoid misunderstanding and confused expectations. It is important for the nurse and other health care providers to

work together in giving accurate information that can be easily understood by the patient. With all the new and ongoing therapies reported by the media in newspapers, on the Internet, and on national television, patients may have many questions about current and new therapies not yet approved. It is the responsibility of the nurse to be aware and have access to educational material and information in order to answer questions appropriately. Proper patient preparation through patient education and effective communication is instrumental in promoting quality of life and compliance with the prescribed therapy (Vizcarra and Belcher, 2006).

Educational resources for the patient and family support should be provided as needed. The manufacturers of biologic agents and immunoglobulin products often provide up-to-date educational information and financial resources for patients and families. Several other organizations offer many direct services and resources for patients, families, and health care providers, including, but not limited to, the following: Immune Deficiency Foundation (IDF) and Crohn's Colitis Foundation of America (CCFA).

DRUG PREPARATION, HANDLING, AND ADMINISTRATION

Depending on the setting where the therapy will be given, the nurse may also be responsible for drug preparation, handling, disposal, and administration. Follow the institution's policy on preparation of intravenous medications. Biologic agents are generally a protein powder preparation, and must be reconstituted by closely following the procedure recommended by the manufacturer. The nurse must be very cognizant of the drug dosage and the maximum concentration recommended for proper administration. The drug, before and after reconstitution, must be handled properly to avoid destabilization of the protein. Do not shake or use heat since it can destroy some of the sensitive protein components of the drug. This precaution includes delivery of the product through a pneumatic tube system. Throughout the reconstitution and preparation, it is necessary to observe aseptic technique, particularly if the drug is not reconstituted in the pharmacy (Vizcarra and Belcher, 2006). Products used for intravenous immunoglobulin therapy are packaged as lyophi-

lized powders or liquid preparations. Follow the manufacturer's recommendation on the reconstitution of lyophilized products. The average time for the product to go into full solution is 15 to 30 minutes. Avoid vigorous agitation as this can denature the IgG protein (*IDF Guide for Nurses, 2007*).

Currently, there are no OSHA guidelines for the handling and disposal of biologic agents. Biologic agents, such as monoclonal antibodies by themselves, are not mutagenic since they do not alter DNA; thus they are not considered genotoxic substances (Estes, 2002). However, monoclonal antibodies conjugated with chemotherapy drugs or radioactive substances should be handled in the same manner as chemotherapy or radiotherapy. All biologic products and supplies used for reconstitution must be disposed according to the institution's policies and procedures.

Biologic therapies are usually administered either through intravenous infusion or by subcutaneous injection. If given intravenously, venous access must be established and may become a challenge to the nurse. Many patients requiring biologic therapy have been receiving high-dose steroids or other medications, causing skin changes that can make vein assessment and access difficult. A patient with a history of diabetes may have thicker vein walls and may have sensitive or rough skin surfaces. Hyperglycemia in diabetic patients causes vasoconstriction, which makes it more difficult to access a vein. Patients with hypertension may also have thicker vein walls that may not

---

FOCUS ON EVIDENCE

Subcutaneous Administration of Immunoglobulin Therapy

- An original article cited subcutaneous immunoglobulin G (SCIG) infusions as life-long replacement therapy in patients with primary antibody deficiencies (PADs). However, only a few published pharmacokinetic studies that used this route of administration are available. Therefore the pharmacokinetics of a 16% immunoglobulin G (IgG) preparation intended for subcutaneous use were investigated in patients with common variable immunodeficiency and X-linked agammaglobulinemia. SCIG infusions (200 mg/kg body weight) were administered to 12 adult patients every 14 days for 24 weeks (total of 144 infusions). Pharmacokinetic parameters were determined based on serum IgG trough levels and antibody levels against tetanus. The median half-lives of the total serum IgG and the tetanus antibodies were 40.6 and 23.3 days, respectively. Median in vivo recovery levels of serum IgG and tetanus immunoglobulins were 36% and 46%, respectively. Median preinfusion serum IgG trough levels per patient were high without major variations between infusions and ranged from 7.24 to 7.86 g/L. Safety, in terms of adverse events including systemic adverse reactions and local tissue reactions at infusion sites, was monitored throughout the study. Six mild, local tissue reactions were observed during the study in one patient. No systemic adverse reactions related to the study drug were observed and no serious other adverse event occurred during the study. It is concluded that the bi-weekly SCIG therapy was well tolerated in the study and that it results in high and stable serum IgG levels, offering an alternative therapy regimen to patients suffering from PAD (Gustafson et al, 2008).
- A review article highlighted findings from international studies and demonstrated the following results: (i) SCIG therapy is safe, with very few adverse effects; (ii) the therapy can be used for patients

with previous adverse effects to intravenous administration of IgG; (iii) the therapy leads to high serum IgG levels and good protection against infections; (iv) the therapy facilitates home therapy, as the infusion technique is easy for children, adults, and elderly people to learn and there is no need for venous access; (v) SCIG home therapy leads to significantly improved life situations for the patients; (vi) the SCIG home therapy regimen in particular reduces the costs of treatment (Gardulf, 2007).
- A review article described the health-related quality of life and health of patients suffering from primary antibody deficiencies before and after the initiation of life-long IgG replacement therapy, and before and after the introduction of a home therapy regimen program. The importance of including patient-reported or parent-reported outcomes in evaluations of treatment and care of this group of patients is also discussed. Adequate IgG replacement therapy means a dramatically improved life situation. Home therapy programs should be encouraged, as self-infusions at home further improve health-related quality of life and self-perceived health (Gardulf and Nicolay, 2006).
- Case studies described how patients tolerate subcutaneous infusions despite previous adverse reactions to intravenous immunoglobulin. Large overall monthly doses can be spread out over time, and attentive nursing practices can limit infusion site reactions. The impact of experienced nursing management and individualized therapy positively affect the outcome of therapy (Murphy, Burton, and Riley, 2007).
- A review article described the use of subcutaneous infusion of immunoglobulin as an alternative administration method for both children and adults. Subcutaneous infusion of immunoglobulin is well tolerated, safe, and clinically efficacious (Kirmse, 2006).

FOCUS ON EVIDENCE

Infusion Reactions Associated with Infusions of Biologic Agents

- In a retrospective study of 165 consecutive patients with Crohn's disease who received a total of 429 infliximab infusions during the period of July 1, 1998, through January 2001, there were several clinical features that suggest that the infusion reactions may not be IgE-mediated acute hypersensitivity reactions. After managing the initial infusion reaction, patients were successfully retreated with a reduction in the rate of infusion. Despite significant respiratory compromise and dyspnea in some cases, no objective evidence was found of wheezing on pulmonary auscultation, a hallmark of an allergic reaction. In addition, the levels of tryptase, an enzyme elevated after IgE-mediated acute hypersensitivity reactions, were within the normal range. The serum IgE levels were also measured and found to be within the normal range. The study concluded that the acute infusion reactions did not seem to be a true IgE-mediated acute hypersensitivity event and this explains why the majority of the infusion reactions can be managed and prevented by a reduction in the rate of infusion (Cheifetz et al, 2003).

- A review article describing the increasing use of monoclonal antibodies as a treatment modality for a number of immune-mediated and malignant diseases has yielded great promise. However, problems with infusion reactions were encountered. Two forms of reactions have been identified: acute and delayed. The reactions were largely not anaphylactic (IgE mediated), making it possible to retreat patients using specific protocols detailed in the article (Cheifetz and Mayer, 2005).

- Case studies described two rheumatoid arthritis patients with a history of severe acute infusion reactions to infliximab who subsequently underwent successful infusion using a prophylactic treatment with a combination of H_1 and H_2 receptor blockers, hydrocortisone, and diphenhydramine. Although successful, prophylaxis does not always prevent subsequent infusion reactions; thus the risks and benefits of treatment need to be carefully considered (Uthman et al, 2006).

- A review article described the characteristics and management of hypersensitivity reactions to monoclonal antibodies and commonly used chemotherapy agents. Hypersensitivity or infusion reactions to platinum compounds are acquired; reactions to taxanes and monoclonal antibodies are immediate and typically occur during the first few minutes of the first infusion. The different time of onset should be considered when developing strategies for preventing and managing hypersensitivity reactions. The decision to rechallenge or discontinue treatment after a reaction occurs depends on the severity of the reaction and other clinical factors (Lenz, 2007).

- A case study reported on the successful use of a prophylactic regimen including H_1- and H_2-receptor blockade plus prednisone and colchicine in the treatment of infusion reactions associated with the infusion of rituximab (Lin, 2004).

PATIENT OUTCOMES

Expected outcomes for the management of infusion reactions during infusion of biologic agents include:

- Stop the infusion; administer 0.9% sodium chloride solution.
- Assess patient, obtain vital signs.
- Administer medications, such as antihistamines, acetaminophen, and/or corticosteroids or prednisone as ordered by the physician.
- Observe the patient for symptom resolution; notify the physician of patient's progress.
- Follow physician's order to either resume or discontinue infusion.
- Document.

constrict or dilate. During the infusion, follow the manufacturer's recommendations on rate, volume, duration, frequency, and the need for a filter during the infusion, as well as the type of administration set to be used (Vizcarra and Belcher, 2006).

If the biologic agent is to be administered subcutaneously, the injection will be either weekly or bi-weekly, and may be administered by the nurse or self-administered by the patient. For self-administration, the patient must be educated about drug preparation, administration of subcutaneous injections, the importance of site rotation, actions to take when doses are missed, and signs or symptoms that should be monitored or reported during and after the injection. Compliance is extremely important for patients who are self-administering subcutaneous injections as missed doses could lead to worsening of the disease.

The administration of immunoglobulin by subcutaneous infusion allows for the slow and gradual absorption of IgG. With the use of a subcutaneous catheter, immunoglobulin therapy is administered by giving smaller doses more often, once or twice a week; in most cases two or more sites simultaneously deliver therapy over 1 to 3 hours with the use of an infusion pump. Subcutaneous immunoglobulin (SCIG) therapy can be self-administered, or administered by a parent to a child or by a caregiver to a patient. As mentioned previously, compliance and adherence to the SCIG dosing are very important for the success and effectiveness of the therapy (Berger, 2008).

PATIENT MONITORING

During the infusion, many manufacturers recommend that the patient be monitored closely for any problems, including monitoring vital signs before and after infusion or as frequent as every 15 to 30 minutes. As with any infused agents, the potential for infusion reactions can accompany the intravenous administration of many protein-derived drugs and biologic agents. The exact mechanism and cause for the infusion reactions related to biologic agents are unknown and often believed to be non-IgE mediated. According to Cheifetz et al (2003), there are several clinical features that suggest that the infusion reactions associated with biologic infusions may not be IgE-mediated acute hypersensitivity reactions. The types, severity, and manifestations of infusion reactions vary among biologic agents, but have some commonality. These include symptoms such as dizziness, headaches, and chest tightness, or signs such as rash or hypotension. Cheifetz et al (2003) described the severity of infusion reactions as mild, moderate, or severe, and classified the type as acute (occurring within 1 to 2 hours of an infusion) or delayed (occurring up to 14 days after treatment). Treatment protocols were developed based on the commonly reported symptoms associated with mild, moderate, or severe acute infusion reactions and the corresponding treatment and prophylaxis. Infusion reactions were usually controlled by slowing or stopping the infusion and administering acetaminophen, antihistamines, corticosteroids, and epinephrine (Cheifetz et al, 2003; Vizcarra, 2003). The nurse should be prepared to manage acute infusion reactions by having an understanding of how biologic agents work as well as the treatment orders and the equipment needed. Ideally, biologic agents should be infused separately through a side port or low Y site of a primary administration set. This method is used in the event of an acute infusion reaction; the infusion of the biologic agent can be stopped and intravenous solutions can be initiated immediately. Medications for treating infusion reactions can be administered intravenously through an injection port.

Although many infusion reactions occur during the first infusion, infusion reactions can also develop during subsequent exposures (Rieger, 2001). The use of routine prophylaxis protocols, such as the administration of acetaminophen and antihistamines, before the infusion would allow patients to be safely retreated, but prophylaxis does not always prevent subsequent infusion reactions (Cheifetz et al, 2003). While Cheifetz et al (2003) state that most acute infusion reactions are not IgE mediated, the risks and benefits of retreating a patient after a severe infusion reaction should be carefully considered because biologic agents will still be perceived as "foreign" by the patient's immune system. Refer to Focus on Evidence Box: Infusion Reactions Associated with Infusions of Biologic Agents.

Delayed infusion reactions are generally manifested as arthralgia, myalgia, malaise, fever, urticarial rash, fatigue, and gastrointestinal symptoms. Together these clusters of constitutional signs and symptoms are called flulike syndrome. The pathophysiology of flulike syndrome as a result of biologic infusion therapy is unclear and dependent on the type of biologic agent. In patients receiving monoclonal antibodies, recent reports suggest that flulike syndrome is probably related to the elimination of the circulating target antigen (Rieger, 2001). While flulike syndrome is not life threatening, it can contribute substantially to the debilitation already experienced by the patient and can adversely affect the patient's quality of life. Management of flulike syndromes includes the use of hydration and medications such as acetaminophen, antihistamines, and steroids as well as nursing comfort measures to decrease chills and fever (Rieger, 2001).

Because many biologic agents interact with the immune system, several have the potential to increase the risk or severity of infections. While common infections such as upper respiratory tract infections (sinusitis, pharyngitis, and bronchitis) or urinary tract infections do occur, some patients may develop more severe infections. In the patient receiving anti-TNF therapy, the risk of more serious infections (such as tuberculosis, histoplasmosis, coccidioidomycosis, or reactivation of hepatitis) is increased because of the suppression of TNFα, which would normally protect the patient. The patient should be instructed to avoid areas where they can be exposed to these infections, to monitor symptoms, and to immediately report symptoms or see a physician.

A number of adverse events have been associated with the use of immunoglobulin therapy in both children and adults. There are factors that may identify patients at greater risk for having a reaction. Infusion reactions are most likely to occur in patients receiving immunoglobulin for the first time, and whenever a patient is receiving a new product or one the patient has not received in recent months. Severe anaphylactic reactions are rare. Reading the specific prescribing information provided with each of the immunoglobulin products is recommended, as the incidence and types of potential adverse events may vary (*IDF Guide for Nurses*, 2007).

DOCUMENTATION

Documentation serves many different purposes; one important value it serves is the validation of the care performed by the infusion nurse. It provides the details related to the care provided and the patient's response to that care. The *Infusion Nursing Standards of Practice*, published in 2006, outlines the standard and practice criteria for documentation (INS, 2006). The practice guidelines are highly recommended for all care settings where biologic infusions are administered. In addition, the reader is referred to Chapter 28 of this textbook for more documentation considerations.

REIMBURSEMENT

The advent of biologic products represents both a clinical opportunity and a financial challenge for payers and health plans. With the expanded use of biologic products to treat familiar chronic conditions outside of cancer, autoimmune diseases, and HIV/AIDS, few payers have yet determined how to make these treatments available in a cost-effective manner (Herskovitz, 2005). The vast majority of biologic therapies are administered as an outpatient service; thus reimbursement will depend on whether the policy covers prescriptions or self-administered drugs (Rieger, 2001). Reimbursement for biologic therapies is still limited, restricted, or non-existent, and the effect is felt directly by the patient seeking treatment and by the health care providers. For the nurse caring for the patient receiving biologic therapy, it becomes a responsibility to be informed about the reimbursement for a recommended therapy, such as a biologic infusion. Be knowledgeable about the process of working with insurers or payers by developing a working relationship with case managers or medical directors. Assist patients by educating them about financial responsibilities for specific aspects of the therapy, discuss reimbursement issues related to "off-label" use of drugs, and provide patients with pharmaceutical company sponsored reimbursement services or patient assistance programs. Employ cost-effective plans when making clinical decisions for equipment and treatment strategies, balancing cost and quality clinical care.

 SUMMARY

Biologic therapy is the use of agents derived from biological sources or of agents that affect biological responses. These agents differ from most drugs as they are not small chemical compounds; instead, they are proteins structurally similar to autologous proteins and they are not metabolized like drugs. Thus adverse reactions might be different from those elicited by drugs. Having the knowledge of how the immune system functions in health and illness will provide the foundation in understanding how biologic agents work. Biologic therapy is a rapidly growing field in the treatment of disorders of the immune system. There are several biologic agents used for the treatment of autoimmune disorders. Immunoglobulin therapy is a treatment option for patients with select primary immune or secondary immune deficiencies. Several immunoglobulin products are available in the United States, each with its own characteristics and features. While most often immunoglobulin therapy is administered intravenously, the therapy can also be administered by the subcutaneous route.

The area of biologic therapy will continue to grow at a pace that health care providers will find challenging. For the nurse providing care to the patient receiving parenteral biologic therapy, an understanding of the basic principles of these agents, specific administration protocols, monitoring parameters, and the management of potential adverse events is crucial to ensuring good patient outcomes.

■ REFERENCES

Abatacept [Orencia] prescribing information, Bristol Myers Squibb, Princeton, NJ, April 2008.

Adalimumab [Humira] prescribing information, Abbott Laboratories, North Chicago, Ill, Feb 2008.

American Medical Association: *Monoclonal antibodies.* Accessed March 2008 at http://www.ama-assn.org/ama/pub/category/13280.html.

Anakinra [Kineret] prescribing information, Amgen, Thousand Oaks, Calif, Dec 2006.

Berger M: Subcutaneous IgG therapy in immune deficiency diseases, *Clin Focus Primary Immune Defic* 13:1-10, Feb 2008.

Certolizumab pegol [Cimzia] prescribing information, UCB, Smyrna, Ga, April 2008.

Cheifetz A, Mayer L: Monoclonal antibodies, immunogenicity, and associated infusion reactions, *Mt Sinai J Med* 72(4):250-258, 2005.

Cheifetz A, Smedley M, Martin S et al: The incidence and management of infusion reactions to infliximab: a large center experience, *Am J Gastroenterol* 98:1315-1324, 2003.

Chen G, Goeddel DV: TNF-R1 signaling: a beautiful pathway, *Science* 296(5573):1634-1635, 2002.

Copstead-Kirkhorn LE, Banasik JL: *Pathophysiology,* ed 3, St Louis, 2005, Elsevier Saunders.

Duff K: You can make a difference in the administration of intravenous immunoglobulin therapy, *J Infus Nurs* 29(3):S5-14, 2006.

Efalizumab [Raptiva] prescribing information, Genentech, San Francisco, Calif, June 2005.

Estes JM: Handling and disposal of monoclonal antibodies, *Clin J Oncol Nurs* 6(5): 290-291, 2002.

Etanercept [Enbrel] prescribing information, Amgen/Wyeth/Immunex, Thousand Oaks, Calif, June 2008.

Feldmann M, Maini RN: Anti-TNF-therapy of rheumatoid arthritis: what have we learned? *Annu Rev Immunol* 19:163-196, 2001.

Gardulf A: Immunoglobulin treatment for primary antibody deficiencies: advantages of the subcutaneous route, *Biodrugs* 21(2):105-116, 2007.

Gardulf A, Nicolay U: Replacement IgG therapy and self-therapy at home improve the health-related quality of life in patients with primary antibody deficiencies, *Curr Opin Allergy Immunol* 6(6): 434-442, 2006.

Gustafson R, Gardulf A, Hansen S et al: Rapid subcutaneous immunoglobulin administration every second week results in high and stable serum immunoglobulin G levels in patients with primary antibody deficiencies, *Clin Exp Immunol* 152(2):274-279, May 2008.

Herskovitz S: Payers' dilemma: looming costs for chronic conditions, *Biotechnol Healthcare* 29-34, April 2005.

Immune Deficiency Foundation Nursing Advisory Committee: *IDF guide for nurses on immune globulin therapy for primary immunodeficiency diseases,* ed 2, Bethesda, Maryland, 2007, Immune Deficiency Foundation.

Infliximab [Remicade] prescribing information, Centocor, Horsham, Pa, Aug 2008.

Infusion Nurses Society: Infusion nursing standards of practice, *J Infus Nurs* 29:1S, 2006.

Kirmse J: Subcutaneous administration of immunoglobulin, *J Infus Nurs* 29:3(S15-20), May/June 2006.

Lenz HJ: Management and preparedness for infusion and hypersensitivity reactions, *Oncologist* 12:601-609, 2007.

Lin RY: Rituximab infusion reaction prophylaxis using histamine receptor blockade, prednisone, and colchicines, *Internet J Asthma Allergy Immunol* 3:1, 2004.

Mackay IR: Science, medicine, and the future: tolerance and autoimmunity, *Br Med J* 321:93-96, 2000.

Medicinenet.com: *Biologic therapy.* Accessed 3/1/08 at http://www.medicinenet.com/biological_therapy/article.htm.

Murphy E, Burton J, Riley P: Nursing approaches to a novel subcutaneous immunoglobulin therapy, *Infusion* 13:4, July/Aug 2007.

Natalizumab [Tysabri] prescribing information, Biogen Idec, Cambridge, Mass, Jan 2008.

Ochs HD, Gupta S, Kiessling P et al: Safety and efficacy of self-administered subcutaneous immunoglobulin in patients with primary immunodeficiency diseases, *J Clin Immunol* 26:265-273, 2006.

Oldham R: Cancer biotherapy: general principles. In Oldham R, editor: *Principles of cancer biotherapy,* ed 4 (pp 1-17), Dordrecht, The Netherlands, 2003, Kluwer Academic Publishers.

Olsen N, Stein M: New drug therapy for rheumatoid arthritis, *New Engl J Med* 350:2167-2179, 2004.

Papadakis KA, Targan SR: Role of cytokines in the pathogenesis of inflammatory bowel disease, *Annu Rev Med* 51:289-298, 2000.

Pichler WJ: Adverse side effects to biological agents, *Allergy* 61(8): 912-920, 2006.

Rieger PT: *Biotherapy: a comprehensive overview,* ed 2 (pp 3-37), Sudbury, Mass, 2001, Jones & Bartlett.

Rituximab [Rituxan] prescribing information, Biogen Idec/Genentech, San Francisco, Calif, Jan 2008.

Swenson M: Autoimmunity and immunotherapy, *J Infus Nurs* 23(S5):S8-15, Sept/Oct 2000.

Thibodeau GA, Patton KT: *Anatomy & physiology,* ed 6, St Louis, 2007, Mosby.

Understanding autoimmune disease (website). Accessed 3/1/08 at www.http://www.nutritionadvisor.com/autoimmune-diseases.htm.

Uthman I, Touma Z, El-Sayyad J et al: Successful retreatment with infliximab in patients with prior severe infusion reactions, *Clin Rheumatol* 25:540-541, 2006.

Vizcarra C: New perspectives and emerging therapies for immune mediated inflammatory disorders, *J Infus Nurs* 26(5):319-325, 2003.

Vizcarra C, Belcher D: Management of the patient receiving parenteral biologic therapy, *J Infus Nurs* 29(2):63-71, 2006.

17 PARENTERAL NUTRITION

Elizabeth A. Krzywda, MSN, ANP, and Doug Meyer, RPh, MBA*

The administration of specialized nutrients intravenously is termed *parenteral nutrition* (PN). The term *total parenteral nutrition* (TPN) is typically used as a general term for whichever type of parenteral solution is used at a particular institution. The term *parenteral nutrition* is becoming more accepted as the preferred choice of nomenclature for parenteral nutritional therapy, replacing TPN. This unique way of providing nutrition circumvents the usual pathway of nutrient digestion, the gastrointestinal system. Intravenous nutrients are circulated to the portal venous system for metabolic processing by the liver. PN is a source of nutrition for patients who are unable to receive adequate nutrition with oral feedings, supplements, or enteral feeding. The ability to provide patients PN is viewed as a major advance in medical science. The success of PN is due to the efforts of many researchers and clinicians, as well as patients who have been a key component of this therapy.

The purpose of this chapter is threefold. The first is to highlight key concepts of metabolism and nutrition as well as to identify and assess malnutrition. The second goal is to review components of PN therapy including physiology, indications, and potential complications. Lastly, this chapter seeks to promote safe and evidence-based concepts of nutrition support.

HISTORY OF PARENTERAL NUTRITION

Many milestones have lead to the development of PN and its use in the clinical setting. The history of PN can be traced as far back as 1656 when Sir Christopher Wren is credited with the first intravenous (IV) injection (Dudrick, 2006). To fashion an IV administration set he used a goose quill and pig's bladder to infuse wine, ale, and opium into the veins of dogs. Developments over the next 300 years included understanding of microbes and infection, knowledge of IV solutions used in fluid resuscitation, and technology of using plastic cannulae to access the venous system. Over the past half century, PN has become a recognized and valuable means of nutrition support. It is a life-saving therapy supporting metabolism and nutrition in both health and disease.

The achievements that formed the framework for PN are extensive (Vinnars and Wilmore, 2003; Ochoa and Caba, 2006). Key developments include the classic studies of protein metabolism and the understanding of essential amino acids by Rose in the 1930s. In 1952 Aubaniac is credited with the first successful subclavian vein catheterization to provide blood transfusions in wounded French military personnel. In 1961 A. Wretlind introduced a safe IV fat emulsion known as Intralipid®. The ability to administer total nutrition intravenously, as well as the use of central venous access as a safe route to administer these hyperosmolar solutions, laid the groundwork for the landmark studies of successful nutritional support (Dudrick et al, 1969). In 1966, under the guidance of Dr. Jonathan Rhoads, Drs. Dudrick, Wilmore, and Vars provided intravenous nutrition support to beagle puppies, using central access for up to 267 days. In 1967 they applied this therapy to a female infant born with small bowel atresia dying of starvation. Using the same infusion catheters as for the puppies, these researchers inserted a catheter via cutdown into the right external jugular vein and advanced it into the superior vena cava. She was subsequently fed intravenously for 22 months.

NUTRITION AND METABOLISM—BASIC CONCEPTS

A balance between nutrient intake and requirements results in a stable nutritional status. Nutrients are required for the provision of energy, the growth and support of tissues, and the

*The authors and editors wish to acknowledge the contributions made by Jeanne M. Wilson and Nancy L. Jordan as authors of this chapter in the second edition of *Infusion Therapy in Clinical Practice*.

regulation of physiological processes within the body. Malnutrition is present when an imbalance occurs between nutrient intake and requirements. Although malnutrition is often associated with lack of appropriate nutrient intake, the definition also encompasses states of excessive nutrient intake.

Malnutrition can result from both acute and chronic diseases related to decreased nutrient intake, abnormal digestion, altered nutrient absorption, or increased metabolic needs. Often malnutrition is more specifically referred to as protein-calorie malnutrition. Marasmus and kwashiorkor are two forms of severe malnutrition initially identified in children of developing countries (Hill, 1997). Marasmus is related to both protein and calorie deficiencies leading to wasting of fat and muscle tissue, while kwashiorkor is characterized by generalized edema and primarily protein malnutrition. These categories of malnutrition have been applied in the clinical setting. Marasmus is malnutrition in a patient who has more than 10% weight loss and has clinical signs of reduced stores of fat and protein. Kwashiorkor can be seen in the hypermetabolic patient after major trauma or stress with resultant decreased serum albumin levels and generalized edema. A third category that describes malnourished or depleted patients who then experience an episode of stress such as sepsis is marasmus kwashiorkor.

The work of the human body is centered on tasks essential for life. Energy is needed to support these tasks, and the fuels to provide the needed energy include protein, carbohydrates, and lipids. Energy stored within the chemical bonds of these fuels is converted to support key life-sustaining functions. Calories are the measurement of energy. When referring to body metabolism a kilocalorie or 1000 calories is the standard measurement used (Smith, Frankenfield and Souba, 2005). Conceptually, the total body mass can be divided into the following categories: fat, extracellular mass, and body cell mass. The body cell mass is the metabolic engine while the extracellular mass forms the structure of support.

Glucose is the preferred energy fuel for the body while fat is stored for future oxidation (Wooley and Frankenfield, 2007). Protein is primarily needed to support the structure and functions of the body and is not used primarily as a source of energy, although during protein turnover energy is provided (Young, Kearns, and Schopfel, 2007). Total body protein in a 70-kg person averages 10 to 11 kg and is predominantly in the skeletal muscle. Protein turnover is the measurement of the rate of protein synthesis and breakdown.

Anabolism is a state of positive energy balance, allowing primarily for protein synthesis. Catabolism occurs when energy is not available and the body cannibalizes or breaks down its own tissues and substrates to provide a source of energy. A sustained lack of exogenous fuel leads to a depletion of carbohydrates and lipids as a source of energy, leading to protein breakdown or catabolism for energy. One gram (g) of protein will provide 4 kcal (kilocalories) of energy (Smith et al, 2005).

MACRONUTRIENTS: PROTEIN, CARBOHYDRATES, AND LIPIDS

PROTEIN

The word protein is derived from the Greek "protos," translated as "first"; protein is considered the premiere macronutrient (Young et al, 2007). Proteins are essential to cell function and structure. Key roles of protein include acting as building blocks for muscles, tendons, enzymes, hormones, and antibodies; maintaining plasma oncotic pressure; and serving as transport molecules, such as hemoglobin transport of oxygen.

The daily protein requirement in healthy adults is 0.8 g/kg of body weight. Amino acids form the building blocks of proteins. There are 20 amino acids classified as either essential or nonessential. Essential amino acids cannot be physiologically manufactured within the body and therefore must be supplied by exogenous sources such as diet. Peptides are amino acids linked together by peptide bonds. Proteins are composed of peptides. The human body contains an estimated 10,000 to 50,000 different types of proteins, each with a specific function (Young et al, 2007).

Protein digestion occurs within the gastrointestinal (GI) tract. As proteins enter the GI tract they are digested into peptides and amino acids through a series of enzymes and feedback mechanisms (Colaizzo-Anas, 2007). This process begins in the stomach where hydrochloric acid is released by the parietal cells to denature proteins and increase susceptibility to enzyme activity. Within the small intestine, enzymes released from both the pancreas and the brush borders of the small intestine break down proteins into amino acids and peptides that are absorbed across the membrane of the small intestine and often transported to the liver. The liver plays a key role in the regulation of amino acids as well as the synthesis of certain amino acids, including albumin.

CARBOHYDRATES

Carbohydrates serve as the prime energy source and provide 45% to 65% of daily energy needs (Ling and McCowen, 2007). The hematopoietic and central nervous systems preferentially utilize glucose as an energy source. Carbohydrates are classified as either simple or complex. Classification is based on the number of sugar units, with monosaccharides having one sugar unit and disaccharides consisting of two units. Glucose, galactose, and fructose are common monosaccharides. Simple carbohydrates include both monosaccharides and disaccharides. The basic unit of carbohydrate metabolism in humans is glucose. Nearly all dietary carbohydrates are broken down into glucose and oxidized for energy (Smith et al, 2005).

Multiple units of monosaccharides joined together form polysaccharides or complex carbohydrates, often composed of hundreds to thousands of monosaccharides (Ling and McCowen, 2007). Examples of complex carbohydrates include starch and glycogen. Typically food will contain varied carbohydrate content, usually containing 60% complex carbohydrates.

The process of digestion begins in the mouth where food is broken down and mixed with saliva and salivary amylase (Colaizzo-Anas, 2007). Salivary amylase is an enzyme that initially breaks down some of the polysaccharide bonds. In the intestine, pancreatic amylase and brush border enzymes break down carbohydrates into monosaccharides for absorption. Once in the bloodstream, most nutrients pass through the liver, where a significant amount of glucose is removed. Insulin production is stimulated by the increase in blood glucose level and promotes blood glucose uptake by the cells. Each gram of carbohydrate provides 4 kcal of energy.

In the body, limited amounts of glucose can be stored as glycogen (Smith et al, 2005). Through glycogenesis, glycogen is formed and stored in the liver and skeletal muscles. In addition during times of fasting or carbohydrate deprivation, proteins can be used to form glucose via gluconeogenesis.

LIPIDS

Lipids serve as important sources of energy and also provide metabolic and structural functions (Hise and Brown, 2007). Lipids are the most calorically dense nutrient and provide 9 kcal of energy per gram. Additional functions of lipids include insulation and support of organs; precursors for steroid hormones, prostaglandin, and thromboxane; and carriers of essential nutrients such as fat-soluble vitamins. Lipids are composed of triglycerides, sterols, and phospholipids. Fats or fatty acids are hydrocarbon chains ranging up to 24 carbons. While the majority of fatty acids can be synthesized by the body, two fatty acids are essential. These essential fatty acids are linoleic and linolenic acids.

NUTRIENT METABOLISM: STARVATION AND STRESS

Starvation is an adaptive response to the lack of nutrients (Smith et al, 2005). The breakdown of glucose stores in the liver (glycogenolysis) provides glucose for approximately 24 hours. The brain then relies on a supply of glucose from protein breakdown, which is termed gluconeogenesis. After 2 days of starvation the brain begins to adapt to ketone bodies from the conversion of lipids (Young et al, 2007). As an adaptive measure, a reduction in energy expenditure and a hypometabolic state are noted. Weight loss is gradual in an attempt to preserve protein and body stores.

The metabolic response to stress, sepsis, and trauma is termed the systemic inflammatory response (Hasenboehler et al, 2006). As a result of neuroendocrine and cytokine activation, a hypermetabolic response occurs (Todd, Kozar and Moore, 2006). This hypermetabolic response is characterized by increased energy expenditure, hyperglycemia, and insulin resistance. This catabolic response leads to a decrease in protein, glycogen, and fat stores. In view of the insulin resistance, appropriate utilization of nutrient stores is blunted. As the systemic response continues, protein catabolism increases with key protein losses. Prolonged catabolism of skeletal muscle leads to respiratory compromise, impaired wound healing, immunosuppression, and significant decrease in strength. In comparison to pure starvation, the development of malnutrition in the stressed host is rapid (Cresci et al, 2007; Martindale, Sawai, and Wareen, 2007).

In both settings, starvation and stress, a continued loss of protein will lead not only to decreased function but also eventually to death. In ill patients the interplay between nutrition and disease is not always definable. Providing safe and efficacious nutrition support involves identification of patients at risk as well as providing appropriate nutrition.

NUTRITIONAL ASSESSMENT

Nutrition assessment is defined by the American Society for Parenteral and Enteral Nutrition (ASPEN) as a comprehensive approach to defining nutritional status that uses medical, nutrition, and medication histories; physical examination and anthropometric measurements; and laboratory data (ASPEN, 2005c). A key word in this statement is the term *comprehensive,* as there is no one single nutrition assessment parameter that is without limitations in assessing nutritional status.

The following are goals of nutritional assessment:
- To establish baseline subjective and objective nutrition measurements
- To identify specific nutritional deficits
- To determine nutrition risk factors
- To establish nutritional needs
- To identify medical and psychosocial factors that may influence nutrition support

Nutritional assessment is best performed by members of a multidisciplinary team in consultation with a nutritional support team. Understanding the components of a nutritional assessment and their relevance enables the nurse to provide optimal nursing care and seek appropriate consultation with all disciplines involved in nutritional support.

Nutrition screening is a process to determine if a nutritional assessment is required to identify those at risk for malnutrition. According to The Joint Commission (TJC; formerly the Joint Commission on Accreditation of Healthcare Organizations [JCAHO]), nutrition screening is mandated within 24 hours of hospital admission (JCAHO, 2005).

WEIGHT HISTORY

Height and body weight are the most used, noninvasive, and easily attainable anthropometric measurements. In assessing the importance of weight loss, current body weight is compared with the usual and ideal body weights. Usual weight is the patient's preillness weight. Weight loss is a good marker of nutritional status. Unintentional weight loss of more than 5% in 1 month or 10% in 6 months is clinically significant (DeLegge and Drake, 2007). Comparison of a patient's current weight to the patient's usual weight is more useful than comparison to the ideal body weight (Russell and Mueller, 2007). Excess fluid and fluid shifts can affect weight and need to be assessed. Body mass index (BMI) accounts for differences in body composition. This measurement is used as an index of both obesity and malnutrition.

BMI is calculated by dividing the weight in kilograms by the height in meters squared (kg/m^2) (ASPEN, 2002). A BMI of 14 to 15 is associated with significant mortality. The following are guidelines used to interpret BMI: 29.2 to 25, overweight; 25 to 18.5, normal weight; 18.4 to 17, malnutrition.

Specific anthropometrics to measure body components to assess protein and fat stores are limb circumference and skinfold thickness. The measurement of the triceps skinfold with a caliper is an indirect marker of body fat. The measurement of the circumference of the midupper arm is an indirect measurement of body protein stores. Measurements are then compared to established tables. Limitations to anthropometric measurements include observer variability, standards developed from nonhospitalized patients, and difficulty accessing the arm in seriously ill patients (DeLegge and Drake, 2007; Russell and Mueller, 2007).

Bioelectrical impedance analysis (BIA) is an alternative tool for studying body composition by measuring electrical conductivity (Earthman et al, 2007). BIA is formulated on the simple concept that tissue rich in water and electrolytes offers less resistance to passage of an electrical current than does lipid-rich adipose tissue. A plethysmograph is used to pass an undetectable, painless electrical current (50 kHz). In healthy individuals, the measurements can be used to calculate body composition. Interpretations are based on the patient's own baseline and evaluated through serial measurements. A decrease from baseline indicates a gain in total body water and/or extracellular body water. Although BIA can be done at the bedside, specific conditions such as ascites, anasarca, severe peripheral edema, and massive overhydration may limit its accuracy as a method of assessing body composition, especially in critical illness.

LABORATORY TESTING

Routine laboratory tests may be helpful in detecting nutritional status from a biochemical standpoint. Several laboratory tests reveal certain aspects of nutritional deficiencies. Determinations of levels of serum total protein, albumin, and transferrin were the first biochemical tests included in nutritional assessment. Serum total protein level is of little value as a nutritional index because it is not specific and is affected by the state of hydration, clinical condition, and hypermetabolism.

SERUM PROTEIN ASSESSMENT

Easily measured serum proteins have been used as nutritional markers to reflect protein stores, synthesis, and catabolism. The most referenced serum protein used for assessment has been serum albumin (DeLegge and Drake, 2007). Albumin is the major protein synthesized by the liver and has a half-life of approximately 20 days. This important visceral protein maintains plasma oncotic pressure, and functions as a carrier for substances such as metabolites, enzymes, drugs, hormones, and metals in the circulation. Measurement of serum albumin has been used as a single nutritional test to predict outcome in multiple studies. In the stressed patient serum albumin level is often decreased in response to fluid shifts, liver function, and renal losses. The inflammatory response associated with stress exerts a significant influence on all serum proteins but especially albumin. These factors make this particular marker a poor choice for nutritional assessment of the acutely ill patient.

Other measurable proteins in the blood with shorter half-lives have been proposed as markers of both nutritional status and nutritional repletion. These proteins include transferrin (half-life 8 days), prealbumin (half-life 2 to 3 days), and retinol-binding protein (half-life 2 days) (Fuhrman, Charney, and Mueller, 2004). Serum transferrin is a β-globulin synthesized predominantly in the liver that transports iron in the plasma. Because of its shorter half-life and smaller body pool, serum transferrin levels are believed to more accurately reflect protein malnutrition in its initial stages and during refeeding. Transferrin is present in the serum at a concentration of 250 to 300 mg/dL. Prealbumin functions to transport thyroxine and as a carrier for retinol-binding protein. Retinol-binding protein transports retinol in the plasma.

Many researchers have demonstrated that in general, serum proteins more accurately reflect overall health as opposed to specific nutritional status (Fuhrman et al, 2004). Serum markers have been shown to correlate well with the morbidity associated with disease. Low serum values indicate the severity of disease and the heightened risk of malnutrition.

NITROGEN BALANCE

A calculation of nitrogen balance is used to determine the adequacy of protein intake. This calculation studies the total protein provided in a 24-hour period. For the purpose of calculation,

protein is converted into nitrogen by dividing grams of protein by 6.25 (Russell and Mueller, 2007). A 24-hour urine is collected and tested for nitrogen. Since other body fluids contain nitrogen, a factor to account for nonurinary nitrogen loss is added:

Calculation of conversion of protein to nitrogen:

$$6.25\,g \text{ of protein} = 1g \text{ of nitrogen}$$

Nitrogen balance calculation:

$$24\text{-hr nitrogen intake} - (\text{Total nitrogen measured in } 24\text{-hr urine collection} + \text{factor for nonurinary nitrogen losses from } 2\text{--}4g) = \text{Nitrogen balance}$$

For example:

$$\text{Nitrogen intake} - 12\,g\,(75\,g \text{ of protein}) - (\text{Urinary nitrogen of } 8\,g \text{ plus } 3\,g \text{ for total of } 11\,g) = \text{Positive } 1\,g \text{ nitrogen balance}$$

A positive nitrogen balance reflects an anabolic state or one of protein synthesis (DeLegge and Drake 2007). A negative nitrogen balance reflects protein breakdown with protein losses exceeding protein intake. Increased nitrogen losses are characteristic of the stress response. Anabolic states are common in such settings as pediatric growth and pregnancy, while a catabolic state occurs during starvation.

IMMUNE FUNCTION

Since a loss of protein function results in decreased immune function, measurements to look at that parameter have been proposed in the past (Russell and Mueller, 2007). Delayed cutaneous hypersensitivity testing involves the use of an intradermal injection of an antigen that would normally result in an antibody response. A healthy individual exhibits a response with induration, similar to the concept of tuberculosis (TB) skin testing. The second measurement of immune status is determination of the total lymphocyte count. Total lymphocyte count is calculated by multiplying the white blood cell count by the percentage of lymphocytes. Unfortunately both measures of immune competence can be affected by pharmacological agents, disease, infection, and stress.

PHYSICAL EXAMINATION

Physical assessment is an essential part of a standard nutritional assessment. Special emphasis is placed on signs and symptoms relating to nutritional deficiencies. Signs of nutritional deficiencies are observed most commonly in the skin, hair, eyes, and mouth. Less commonly affected are the glands and nervous system. It is important to relate the findings of the physical examination to the patient's diet and medical history. Knowledge of specific nutrient functions is also helpful in recognizing nutritional deficiencies. Physical signs of nutritional deficiencies may not appear until there has been significant nutritional depletion. Detection of these signs should prompt further evaluation and consultation with the nutritional support team.

DIETARY HISTORY

To identify any possible dietary deficiencies, a thorough dietary history can delineate eating patterns (e.g., dietary intake, frequency, quantity, and types of foods); identify possible food allergies, preferences, and intolerances; and consider socioeconomic, ethnic, and religious influences. Actual observation of the patient's eating patterns at mealtimes can be helpful in illuminating improper nutrition habits, including overconsumption and underconsumption. The patient's usual and current intake should be assessed by a 24-hour intake report, food records, or food frequency questionnaire (Russell and Mueller, 2007). The 24-hour intake report is a simple documentation of what the patient recalls eating for the past 24 hours, and is a rough estimation of the patient's usual eating patterns. For patients suspected of having poor oral consumption, a dietary intake record for 3 to 7 days is valuable. Questionnaires are also available to analyze dietary intake. From data collected, the dietitian can evaluate nutrient intake to define specific nutrient deficiencies and develop a plan of care.

DIRECT MEASUREMENTS OF FUNCTION

Functional impairment secondary to protein loss is thought to be one of the most important assessments of nutritional status (Hill, 1997). Function can be observed by assessing physical activities and abilities as well as wound healing and respiratory status. Handgrip strength has been used as an assessment tool with the use of a handgrip dynamometer (DeLegge and Drake 2007).

CLINICAL SCORING SYSTEMS

Recognizing the limitations of individual nutrition assessment parameters, scoring systems that combine various factors have been developed to provide a comprehensive approach to nutrition assessment. The Subjective Global Assessment (SGA) is one example of a clinical scoring system. This tool reviews changes associated with weight, dietary intake, functional capacity, gastrointestinal symptoms, and disease. Five physical findings are assessed: loss of subcutaneous fat, muscle wasting, ankle edema, sacral edema, and ascites. Based on these findings, nutritional status is categorized as either well nourished, moderately malnourished, or severely malnourished. The assessment tool was initially validated in hospitalized patients admitted for elective surgery (Detsky et al, 1987). The SGA has since been used and validated in a variety of patients including long-term geriatric residents and patients with digestive diseases, and has been modified for oncology patients (Sacks et al, 2001; Baccaro et al, 2007).

ENERGY REQUIREMENTS

Providing adequate energy preserves metabolic functions and sustains life. Careful attention to calorie requirements will prevent overfeeding and underfeeding, both of which may have deleterious effects on recovery. Despite the availability of more than 200 calculation methods, the accurate estimation of energy needs of a critically ill patient remains challenging (Wooley and Frankenfield, 2007).

Total energy expenditure in a healthy individual is divided into three major components:
1. Basal, or resting, metabolic rate, which is the measurement of metabolic rate immediately upon awakening in a fasting individual
2. Thermogenic effect of digestion, which is the increase in the metabolic rate following consumption of a meal
3. Energy associated with physical activity

Illness and metabolic stress, a fourth component of energy expenditure, can result in hormonal changes and initiate a hypermetabolic response. As a result of this response, an increase in energy expenditure of 10% to 20% in general surgery and medical patients and up to 50% to 70% in septic patients has been documented (Smith et al, 2005; Stapleton, Jones, and Heyland, 2007). Methods of measuring energy expenditure include both direct and indirect calorimetry (Wooley and Frankenfield, 2007). Direct calorimetry is a measurement of heat released and usually requires the individual to be in an enclosed chamber. This is based on the principle that energy derived from macronutrient oxidation is released as heat, and therefore this method directly measures energy expenditure.

Because of the constraints of this method, indirect calorimetry using a metabolic cart has been implemented for use in many intensive care units. These calorimeters measure respiratory gas exchange to calculate resting energy expenditure and respiratory quotient. Respiratory quotient (RQ) is defined as the ratio of CO_2 produced to O_2 consumption (DeLegge and Drake 2007). This measurement indirectly reflects substrate metabolism. A respiratory quotient greater than 1.0 indicates lipogenesis or overfeeding. A respiratory quotient less than 0.82 suggests underfeeding or lipid catabolism.

Methods using mathematical equations have been developed and are commonly used in many clinical settings to estimate energy expenditure and calories as part of the specialized nutrition support. One of the classic equations used is the Harris-Benedict equation, which was developed in 1919 by using indirect calorimetry on a healthy group of men and women (Wooley and Frankenfield, 2007). This limitation of the formula has been criticized for not accurately reflecting both critically ill and overweight patients. Despite this, the Harris-Benedict equation is still commonly used. The Harris-Benedict equation and stress factors added to correct for the disease process are given in Table 17-1.

A calculation to estimate calories per kilogram of body weight (kcal/kg) is a simple and clinically useful calculation when other methods are not available. ASPEN recommends a range of 20 to 35 kcal/kg for daily energy needs (ASPEN, 2002). This method allows clinicians to estimate energy expenditure in a variety of settings without requiring additional technology.

TABLE 17-1 Harris-Benedict Equation and Stress Factors Used to Correct for the Disease Process

Harris-Benedict Equation:[*]

$$\text{BMR (male)} = 66.5 + (13.75 \times W) + (5.0 \times H) - (6.8 \times A)$$

$$\text{BMR (female)} = 665 + (9.56 \times W) + (1.7 \times H) - (4.68 \times A)$$

Condition	Stress factor
Mild starvation	0.85-1.00
Postoperative recovery	1.00-1.05
Cancer	1.10-1.45
Peritonitis	1.05-1.25
Severe infection or multiple trauma	1.30-1.55

[*]W, Weight in kilograms; H, height in centimeters; A, age in years.

INDICATIONS FOR PARENTERAL NUTRITION

Since the 1970s, a wealth of research into the usage of PN and outcomes has occurred. While significant advances in patient care have been accomplished with the use of PN, it has also been associated with complications, expense, and lack of demonstrated outcomes in certain settings (Mirtallo, 2007). Defining the benefits of PN is linked to identifying the appropriate clinical indications for its use. Specialized nutrition support defines both enteral and parenteral forms of nutrition support (ASPEN, 2002). Enteral nutrition is the preferred form of nutritional support for several reasons. Enteral nutrition is more physiological as it uses the gastrointestinal tract for nutrient absorption, is less costly than PN, promotes the health of gastrointestinal tract immune function, and prevents villous atrophy.

The American Society for Parenteral and Enteral Nutrition has published guidelines to promote safe and effective patient care by nutrition support practitioners. The initial set of guidelines addressing the use of parenteral and enteral nutrition was published in 1999. In 2002 the guidelines were updated and provide the most current recommendations addressing the use of parenteral and enteral nutrition in both adult and pediatric

patients (ASPEN, 2002). Information in this section is based on the recommendations of the ASPEN guidelines. Universal principles that define the indications for nutrition support include the following:

- When specialized nutrition support is required, enteral nutrition should generally be used in preference to PN.
- PN should be used when the gastrointestinal tract is not functional or cannot be accessed and in patients who cannot be adequately nourished by oral diets or enteral nutrition.
- Specialized nutrition support should be initiated in patients with inadequate oral intake for 7 to 10 days, or in those patients in whom inadequate oral intake is expected over a 7- to 14-day period (Figure 17-1).

DISEASE STATES AND NUTRITION SUPPORT

Specific disease states have implications for both maintaining nutritional status and delivering nutritional support. The pathophysiology associated with a specific disease will often place patients at risk for malnutrition. In general, any disease

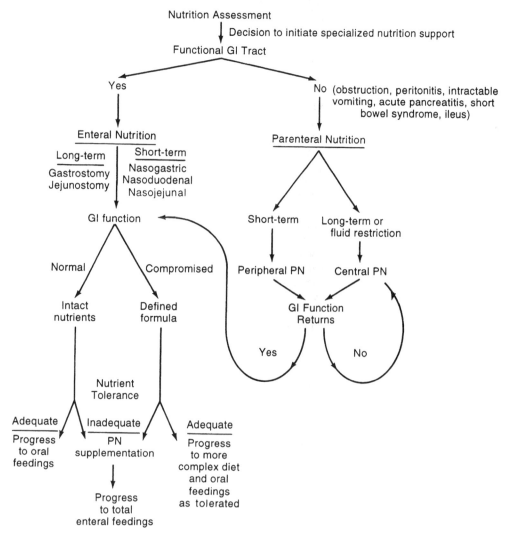

FIGURE 17-1 Clinical decision algorithm: route of nutrition support. (Reprinted from ASPEN Board of Directors: Guidelines for the use of parenteral and enteral nutrition in adult and pediatric patients, *J Parenter Enter Nutr* 17[suppl]:7SA, 1993.)

affecting the gastrointestinal tract can affect nutrient intake and absorption (Parrish et al, 2007). Gastrointestinal diseases can include diseases of the esophagus, such as esophageal dysmotility and carcinomas that may prevent nutrients from passing from the oral cavity into the stomach. Gastric dysfunction such as gastroparesis may delay nutrient emptying from the stomach into the intestine. Small bowel diseases and significant surgical resections can alter the amount of absorptive surface into the small bowel, leading to decreased nutrient absorption. Finally, loss of the function of the large bowel can lead to significant fluid losses. When these diseases prevent adequate nutrition for a prolonged amount of time, specialized nutrition support including both enteral and PN may be indicated. In most cases, enteral nutrition is the preferred method.

Certain disease states in addition to those directly affecting the gastrointestinal tract have also been demonstrated to affect nutrient metabolism. A review of the key features of specific diseases and their nutritional implications based on published guidelines can be found in Box 17-1 (ASPEN, 2002).

CARDIAC DISEASE

Cardiac cachexia is a syndrome associated with severe malnutrition that leads to depletion of lean body mass including vital organs such as the heart. Although rare, this syndrome has been associated with decreased survival in patients with congestive heart failure. While as a general principle preoperative malnutrition has been associated with increased morbidity, the majority of patients undergoing cardiac surgery are not significantly malnourished. In this particular population, research has shown a link between blood glucose control and infectious complications. Most often nutrition support in patients with cardiac disease includes sodium and fluid restriction. An increase in total body fluid can alter the interpretation of laboratory measurements such as protein status and body weights. The use of PN should be reserved for patients who experience postoperative complications, and nutrition using the GI tract is not a safe option. Decreased cardiac output can be associated with decreased mesenteric blood flow. It is advised not to use the GI tract in patients who are hemodynamically unstable as bowel necrosis has been reported.

PULMONARY DISEASE

A strong association exists between pulmonary disease and malnutrition. In patients with chronic obstructive pulmonary disease (COPD), malnutrition is common. The physiology of COPD includes increased energy expenditure and decreased nutrient intake, both of which promote malnutrition. Decreased pulmonary function is a well-established consequence of prolonged malnutrition and often the cause of death. Overfeeding patients with excessive calories does result in increased carbon dioxide production and worsening of an already altered respiratory function. Close assessment of caloric needs is recommended, and theoretically providing a larger percentage of calories as fat may decrease carbon dioxide production. Phosphate is important for diaphragmatic function and should be closely monitored in patients with pulmonary disease.

LIVER DISEASE

Malnutrition and nutrient deficiencies are common in liver disease. The liver plays a central role in the metabolism and storage of nutrients; thus liver disease has a significant impact on nutritional status. The high rate of malnutrition in liver disease patients has been attributed to anorexia; early satiety secondary to ascites; micronutrient deficiencies including zinc and vitamins A, D, E, and K; and altered nutrient metabolism. In certain liver diseases increased protein catabolism and altered amino acid metabolism have been demonstrated, with low levels of circulating branched chain amino acids. However, the general guideline to limit protein or alter amino acids provided is no longer universally recommended. Protein restriction is reserved for acute management of hepatic encephalopathy. The high incidence of malnutrition associated with liver disease mandates close nutrition screening in these patients.

PANCREATITIS

Pancreatitis is a common disorder that can range from acute pancreatitis that is a mild self-limiting disease, to chronic pancreatitis with fibrosis and lack of pancreatic function, to acute necrotizing pancreatitis with a mortality rate of up to 20%. The pancreas has two main roles in nutrient absorption. First, it supplies pancreatic enzymes delivered by the pancreatic duct into the duodenum for use in the digestion of carbohydrates, fats, and proteins. Second, as an endocrine organ it produces insulin and glucagon to support cellular glucose metabolism. In the past, PN was exclusively chosen as the form of nutrition support in patients with severe and prolonged pancreatitis. PN allowed nutrition support to be provided while the pancreas was allowed "to rest." Research has demonstrated the effectiveness and safety in using enteral nutrition, and therefore enteral nutrition is now the preferred route of nutrition support. The placement of a feeding tube beyond the duodenum into the jejunum and providing a low-fat formula will decrease pancreatic stimulation. PN is reserved for those instances when enteral feeding is not tolerated. Only in patients with triglyceride levels greater than 400 mg/dL should IV lipids be restricted. In patients who have sustained a significant loss of pancreatic tissue either secondary to disease or as a result of surgical resection, steatorrhea and malabsorption of primarily fat, vitamins, calcium,

---

Box 17-1   CONSIDERATIONS FOR PARENTERAL NUTRITION

Patient evaluation for parenteral nutrition is based on various objective measurements:

- Any patient who is unable to ingest sufficient nutrients through the gastrointestinal (GI) tract is a potential candidate for parenteral nutrition.
- The least invasive, least expensive means of supporting a patient's nutritional status must be considered.
- The GI route should always be used, if appropriate. There can be serious adverse effects associated with a totally resting GI tract. Enteral nutrition preserves intestinal mass and structures, as well as hormonal, enzymatic, and immunological function, better than intravenous nutrition.
- Generally, nourished patients unable to eat for as long as 7 to 10 days do not require parenteral nutrition. However, the general rule is that whenever 5 to 7 days have passed with insufficient enteral intake, parenteral nutrition should be considered.
- The indications and disease states for which parenteral nutrition is clearly beneficial are continually being established and reassessed.

magnesium, and zinc can occur. In this setting, supplemental pancreatic enzymes are required for nutrient absorption.

SHORT-BOWEL SYNDROME

Short-bowel syndrome results when a significant amount of small bowel is either surgically resected or diseased, affecting adequate nutrient and fluid absorption. The two leading causes for this symptom are multiple surgical resections for Crohn's disease and mesenteric infarction leading to inadequate blood supply of the small bowel. Short-bowel syndrome often requires PN for an extended time, including the need for long-term home PN. While short-bowel syndrome is associated with malnutrition and fluid loss, additional nutrient losses lead to several metabolic disorders. These diseases include metabolic bone disease such as osteoporosis and oxalate nephrolithiasis. After surgical resection, the remaining intestine may adapt and increase nutrient absorption for a period up to 2 years. In recent years, select programs aimed at intestinal rehabilitation have been successful in weaning some patients from PN through the use of factors to stimulate intestinal function such as growth hormone and glutamine. Small bowel transplantation has been used in patients who have lost all available vascular access for continued PN because of either multiple infections and/or thrombosis.

RENAL FAILURE

Renal failure can be classified as both chronic and acute renal failure. With both conditions the associated metabolic abnormalities can result in altered nutrition. Malnutrition, increased protein catabolism, and impaired protein synthesis are recognized abnormalities in renal failure. Protein restriction is often recommended for patients with progressive renal failure that are receiving dialysis. In patients receiving dialysis, protein is not restricted, but rather is advantageous to achieve a positive protein balance. Fat-soluble vitamins, especially vitamin A, needs to be monitored closely to avoid elevated levels.

CANCER

Malnutrition often contributes to death in cancer patients. Cancer cachexia is a syndrome associated with wasting, anorexia, and weight loss. This syndrome is believed to be secondary to increased host cytokine and hormone response to the malignancy and treatments. This syndrome is common and occurs in approximately half of cancer patients. In spite of the frequency of malnutrition in this patient population, it is often overlooked. Weight loss that occurs before treatment has been identified as a prognostic factor influencing survival. In this population, it has been difficult to assess positive improvement in nutritional parameters with specialized nutrition support, and therefore no recommendation for routine use of PN as an adjunct to chemotherapy, radiation therapy, or surgery has been supported. Palliative use of specialized nutrition support is rarely indicated. In patients undergoing active treatment and unable to ingest adequate nutrients for a prolonged time, specialized nutrition support is appropriate.

BURNS

Patients who sustain a significant burn have been recognized to have pronounced hypermetabolism and protein catabolism. Specialized nutrition support has been shown to positively affect outcome and should be recognized as a priority in these patients. Enteral nutrition that is started early after the injury is the preferred form of nutrition support and PN is rarely indicated.

CRITICAL ILLNESS

Critical illness is often associated with a systemic inflammatory response that is characterized by several metabolic abnormalities. Hypermetabolism and hyperglycemia are prominent factors in this setting. These factors are also accompanied by insulin resistance, increased energy expenditure, accelerated lipolysis, and protein catabolism. This response is fueled by the activation of endogenous mediators, and cannot be totally reversed by nutrition support. Enteral nutrition is often the preferred form of nutrition support in critically ill patients. In patients where enteral nutrition is not possible and they are anticipated to be without nutrient intake for 5 to 10 days, PN is used. The effects of supplementing specialized nutrients have not clearly demonstrated an improvement in overall outcome.

ACQUIRED IMMUNODEFICIENCY SYNDROME (AIDS)

While protein-calorie malnutrition is common in human immunodeficiency virus (HIV) infected patients, new antiretroviral therapy has markedly reduced the incidence of malnutrition. AIDS wasting syndrome has significant nutritional implications and is characterized by involuntary weight loss. The Centers for Disease Control and Prevention (CDC) defines this syndrome as an involuntary weight loss of greater than 10% from baseline, chronic diarrhea, or documented fever greater than 30 days, and associated weakness (Wasserman and Segal-Maurer, 2007). Wasting is associated with high morbidity and mortality. The causes of this wasting syndrome include decreased appetite, nutrient malabsorption perhaps related to enterocyte injury, and metabolic abnormalities, primarily protein catabolism. Anabolic agents, resistance training, testosterone, and appetite stimulants have been used in patients with AIDS wasting syndrome. Specialized nutrient support has a very limited role in this syndrome, and is reserved for patients undergoing active treatment who are unable to meet requirements through oral feeding.

 COMPONENTS OF PARENTERAL NUTRITION

Parenteral nutrition solutions are extremely complex admixtures containing macronutrients (i.e., protein, carbohydrate, fat, and water) and micronutrients (i.e., electrolytes, vitamins, and trace elements), which are all vital for the maintenance of normal metabolism and growth. In general terms, macronutrients (dextrose and fat) are used as an energy source and for structural substrate support (proteins and fats). Micronutrients help support a variety of metabolic activities necessary for cellular function, such as enzymatic reactions, fluid balance, and electrophysiological processes (Mattox and Reiter, 2005). The proportions of these ingredients and the total calories provided must be carefully individualized to meet the patient's needs and clinical condition (Taskforce for the Revision of Safe Practices for Parenteral Nutrition, 2004). In this section, each component of PN will be described in terms of its nutritional importance, as well as considerations for use in PN solutions.

FLUIDS
Nutritional background

The body consists of approximately 50% to 60% water. The average healthy adult requires 2 to 3 L of fluid per day, or approximately 30 to 40 mL/kg/day (Mirtallo et al, 2004). Ideally, fluid balance should be maintained; that is, intake and output should be approximately equal. Individual fluid requirements vary greatly and can fluctuate daily; therefore accurate patient intake and output records and weights are invaluable in determining fluid requirements. Fluids are lost through the kidneys, lungs, bowel, and skin. Insensible losses also occur, but are not measurable and can only be estimated. Insensible fluid losses include losses from perspiration, respiration, third spacing, hemorrhage into soft tissue or the abdominal cavity, ascites, and drainage from burns and wounds. Estimates of fluid maintenance requirements can be obtained from body weight or body surface area (BSA). However, determinations made from body weight may overestimate fluid requirements of obese patients and underestimate requirements of thin patients. This is because adipose, or fat, tissue is the least hydrated in the body, so patients with more body fat have proportionally less total body water content (Rose and Post, 2001). In these instances, BSA in which both height and weight are considered is more accurate.

Component of PN solution

Maintenance fluid requirements for the adult are estimated by using one of two formulas. The first estimate is based on a simple formula: 30 to 35 mL/kg/day. The second formula calculates 1500 mL for the first 20 kg of body weight, adding an additional 20 mL/kg for actual weight beyond the initial 20 kg (Holcombe, 1995). This second formula can also be used for pediatric patients weighing 20 kg or greater.

It is important to consider the patient's cardiac, respiratory, and renal status, as well as the preexisting hydration status. Critically ill patients may become fluid overloaded if calculations used to determine fluid requirements do not incorporate fluids yielded during oxidation of nutrient substances (approximately 500 mL of water daily in typical PN regimens), fluid liberated from muscle catabolism (500 mL daily during severe catabolism), and other exogenous sources such as IV fluids and medications.

Normal fluid losses include renal losses (30 to 120 mL/hour) and insensible losses (800 to 1000 mL/day in the adult). Increased fluid losses occur during fever, diarrhea, vomiting, GI suction or drainage, high respiratory rates, burns, wounds, or osmotic diuresis. These increased losses may indicate the need for additional fluid replacement (Lenssen, 1998).

Care must be taken to continually assess the patient's hydration status during PN therapy. Monitoring hydration includes accurately measuring daily intake and output; assessing for signs of cardiac, respiratory, and renal compromise; observing for rapid weight changes; evaluating peripheral edema; and managing levels of serum electrolytes.

PROTEIN
Nutritional background

Protein is essential for body growth, maintenance, and repair of tissue. When proteins are digested, they are absorbed as amino acids (AAs), the basic structural unit of protein. Approximately 20 different amino acids are commonly found in proteins. Amino acids are classified according to whether the body can produce them endogenously (internally) or if they must be obtained exogenously (from the diet). Nonessential amino acids can be synthesized by the body, and are precursors for the synthesis of carbohydrates, fats, and other amino acids. Amino acids that the body cannot synthesize, called essential amino acids, must be obtained from the diet. Amino acids can also be considered "conditionally essential" in certain situations. These AAs can be manufactured by the body under normal circumstance (nonessential), but in some cases the body's demand exceeds its ability to produce them, so they must also be supplied exogenously. For example, tyrosine is a nonessential AA that is synthesized by the essential AA phenylalanine. However, if inadequate phenylalanine is produced, then tyrosine becomes conditionally essential. Histidine is essential in infants but not necessarily in healthy children or adults. Cysteine and glutamine are other examples of AAs that can at times be conditionally essential (Young et al, 2007). Thus essentiality can be the result of a total inability to make the amino acid or the inability to make an adequate amount. In either case, the body does not store excess amino acids. Available amino acids are used for energy, and excess nitrogen is excreted in the urine as urea (Krzywda, 1996). In terms of physiological need, all amino acids are ultimately essential, as all are necessary for optimal nutrition.

Amino acids are metabolized primarily in the liver, which monitors amino acid uptake and regulates its release. Specific essential amino acids (e.g., phenylalanine, tryptophan, methionine, threonine, and lysine) and all of the nonessential amino acids are catabolized in the liver. The liver is also the site for urea synthesis, where nitrogenous wastes must be converted to urea before being transported to the kidneys for excretion.

Each amino acid has a distinct metabolic pathway that leads to oxidation and its conversion to carbon dioxide, water, and urea. Urea contains two amino groups, one oxygen, and one carbon. Incomplete oxidation yields only a portion of the energy available from protein. Protein yields approximately 4 kcal/g of available energy when oxidized. In addition, when some amino acids are split, they yield carbon structures that can produce glucose through gluconeogenesis. In gluconeogenesis, the carbon structures fit into the glycolytic pathway and are either metabolized as if they were carbohydrate, producing energy, or resynthesized to form glucose. Other amino acids are ketogenic, in which the carbon structures fit into the lipid metabolic pathways and can form ketone bodies. Ketogenic amino acids cannot contribute to the formation of glucose. Other amino acids have branched chains, meaning that a portion of their carbon structure is glucogenic and a portion is ketogenic. Box 17-2 presents the classifications of amino acids.

Body proteins are constantly undergoing catabolism and anabolism, and approximately 40% of the body's resting energy expenditure is used for these processes. During growth and in pregnancy, the body is making more protein than it is breaking down. Therefore the body is in a state of positive nitrogen balance, as described earlier. Under other conditions, such as restricted food intake, disease, or trauma, the body might be in negative nitrogen balance. Clinically, the balance between protein synthesis and degradation can be estimated by measuring the nitrogen balance.

Component of PN solution

Protein is provided in PN solutions by the addition of crystalline amino acid (CAA) solutions. Commercially available CAA solutions vary widely in their concentration (range 3% to 20%)

Box 17-2 CLASSIFICATIONS OF AMINO ACIDS

Essential amino acids	Nonessential amino acids
Histidine	Alanine
Isoleucine	Arginine*
Leucine	Asparagine
Lysine	Aspartic acid
Methionine	Cysteine*
Phenylalanine	Glutamic acid
Threonine	Glutamine*
Tryptophan	Glycine
Valine	Proline
	Serine
	Tyrosine*

*Conditionally essential.

as well as their content of individual amino acids. Amino acid solutions also differ in their nitrogen content per gram, electrolyte content, osmolarity, and pH. Despite these differences in available products, their effects on markers of protein utilization are not clinically different (Furst and Stehle, 1994). Amino acid solutions with electrolytes included usually contain amounts of the most common electrolytes needed to meet an adult's requirements. Based on the specific amino acid profile, standard or specialized solutions are available. Standard amino acid solutions contain a balanced profile of essential and nonessential amino acids and are used for a majority of PN compounding. Specialized amino acid solutions have a modified amino acid profile to meet age- or disease-specific amino acid requirements. Specialized amino acid preparations have been developed for use in specific disorders such as renal and hepatic failure. Disease-specific amino acids are discussed later in this chapter.

A patient's estimated protein requirement depends on age, level of activity, nutritional status, renal function, hepatic function, and presence or absence of hypermetabolism or stress. Aside from these quantitative differences, there may also be differences in the requirements for specific amino acids. Certain amino acids perform unique physiological functions that may have a therapeutic or damaging effect on a particular patient. Thus the optimal provision of amino acids during PN depends on the total quantity provided *and* the specific amino acid composition.

Normal protein requirements depend on utilization and losses (i.e., protein turnover and catabolism). The recommended dietary allowance for protein is based on the amount of protein needed to maintain nitrogen equilibrium, and the fact that energy needs are met by nonprotein sources. A protein intake of 0.8 g/kg body weight per day is recommended for healthy adults. Conditions that increase protein utilization, such as illness or metabolic stress, will increase the body's protein requirements. During periods of stress, injury, or infection, patients may require protein intake up to 1.5 g/kg body weight per day (Hutchins and Shronts, 1998). Burn patients may require protein intake up to 2.0 g/kg body weight per day (Jacobs et al, 2004). Provision of protein in quantities greater than 2.0 g/kg/day in PN solutions is controversial and rarely required (Mirtallo et al, 2004).

An interaction exists between calorie and nitrogen substrates. Increasing the caloric support reduces the nitrogen required to achieve nitrogen balance, and increasing the nitrogen intake reduces the calories required to achieve nitrogen balance. The optimal calorie/nitrogen ratio in the patient requiring nutritional support remains individualized. The currently used calorie/nitrogen ratio ranges from 100:1 to 200:1. This means that for each gram of nitrogen, 100 to 200 calories must be provided for protein sparing. It is logical that patients under severe stress are likely to have a different optimal ratio than those who are chronically malnourished. A lower calorie/nitrogen ratio results in greater nitrogen retention, increased plasma transferrin, and a lower respiratory quotient when a patient is hypermetabolic (Hutchins and Shronts, 1998).

CARBOHYDRATES
Nutritional background

Carbohydrates are organic compounds composed of carbon, hydrogen, and oxygen and provide approximately 45% to 65% of our daily energy. Carbohydrates in the diet are classified as complex or simple. Simple carbohydrates are monosaccharides, meaning one sugar, and are commonly referred to as simple sugars. Disaccharides, also considered simple carbohydrates, are formed when two monosaccharides join together. The major monosaccharides are glucose and fructose; the others are galactose and mannose. Disaccharides include sucrose (the most abundant disaccharide), maltose, and lactose. Disaccharides and monosaccharides can be joined together to form complex carbohydrates, or polysaccharides.

The metabolism of carbohydrates involves a number of intricate chemical processes that depend on the presence of insulin, glucagon, and, to a lesser extent, hormones such as epinephrine and norepinephrine. Carbohydrate metabolism, like all forms of metabolism, has a constructive phase called *anabolism* and a destructive phase called *catabolism*. Carbohydrate catabolism is the process whereby the body breaks carbohydrates down into smaller molecules and uses the energy that is released in the process. The three major processes involved in carbohydrate catabolism are glycolysis, the Krebs cycle, and glycogenolysis. The initial process in carbohydrate catabolism is glycolysis, which results in a breakdown of the glucose molecule into smaller pyruvate molecules and a release of energy. Adenosine triphosphate (ATP) is formed during glycolysis, which results in the storage and release of energy from the cells. Glycolysis only results in the creation of a small amount of energy from glucose cells. The Krebs cycle (also called the citric acid cycle) completes carbohydrate catabolism much more efficiently, and results in the total breakdown of glucose into carbon dioxide, water, and more net energy (e.g., ATP) than is produced during glycolysis (Berg, Tymoczko and Stryer, 2002). When the blood glucose level is abnormally low, glycogen stores are converted to glucose by *glycogenolysis*.

Carbohydrates are stored in the body in the form of glycogen. Only about 5% of ingested glucose is stored as glycogen; the rest is oxidized into energy. Carbohydrate anabolism is a process whereby catabolic products of carbohydrates, fat, or protein are chemically converted into glycogen and stored, primarily in the liver and skeletal muscle. Unlike catabolism, anabolism does not release energy, but instead uses the body's energy. Two major processes are involved in carbohydrate anabolism: glycogenesis and glyconeogenesis. *Glycogenesis* is the process whereby glucose is converted to glycogen. It is the reverse of glycogenolysis and depends on the release of insulin. *Glyconeogenesis* is the breakdown of fats and proteins into glucose or glycogen for use by cells as fuel. This process occurs when carbohydrates are not available.

Component of PN solution

Carbohydrates are the body's preferred fuel, as well as its immediate source of energy. Dextrose is used almost exclusively in PN solutions as the source of carbohydrate calories and it provides 3.4 kcal/g of energy. The body burns carbohydrates rather than fats or protein, provided the carbohydrate intake is adequate, sufficient insulin is available to allow passage of glucose into the cells, and glycogen is present.

There are no specific minimum requirements for carbohydrates during PN, but they are an important component of most PN regimens. Dextrose has a relatively low caloric density (3.4 kcal/g) and is available in concentrations ranging from 2.5% to 70%. Higher concentrations of dextrose are used in PN solutions to minimize the volume of dextrose in the overall admixture, thus allowing greater volume for amino acids and fats. For example, 1 L of 5% dextrose (found in conventional IV solutions) contains only 170 kcal (50 g of dextrose per liter × 3.4 kcal/g). A liter of 70% dextrose (used for compounding PN solutions) contains 2380 total kcal (700 g of dextrose per liter × 3.4 kcal/g).

Dextrose solutions with concentrations exceeding 5% are increasingly hypertonic. The normal serum osmolarity is approximately 310 mOsm/L. Parenteral solutions with an osmolarity of up to 900 mOsm/L may be administered peripherally. However, tolerance of solutions with 900 mOsm/L or less varies greatly by patient and vein condition and administration guidelines vary (see Focus on Evidence box). In general, parenteral solutions with a final dextrose concentration greater than 10%, or greater than 900 mOsm/L, should be administered through a central vein (Dickerson, Brown and White, 1993; American Society of Parenteral and Enteral Nutrition, 2004).

The optimal dose of dextrose differs for infants, children, and adults. In general, for balanced PN, dextrose is used to provide 40% to 60% of the total caloric intake. In adults, the optimal dose for maximal suppression of gluconeogenesis and glucose oxidation is 2 to 5 mg/kg/min (Dickerson et al, 1993). This represents a PN regimen that contains 150 to 200 g of dextrose per liter administered centrally at a rate of 1.5 to 2.5 L/day. Overfeeding by supplying glucose in excess of this rate does not accentuate nitrogen retention and produces adverse effects such as fatty liver and increased carbon dioxide

FOCUS ON EVIDENCE

Peripheral Infusion of Parenteral Nutrition, Osmolality, and Phlebitis

- Practice guidelines from the American Society of Parenteral and Enteral Nutrition (2004) recommend that intravenous fat emulsions of either 10% or 20%, which are isotonic, can be infused separately via a peripheral vein or as part of a peripheral nutrient admixture not exceeding 900 mOsm/L.
- The *Infusion Nursing Standards of Practice* (INS, 2006) state that infusions not appropriate for peripheral administration include infusates with osmolality of greater than 600 mOsm/L.
- A total of 56 references addressing peripheral parenteral nutrition in adults were obtained from a search for clinical trials in MEDLINE, EMBASE, and Cochrane databases. Early studies (late 1970s) using an amino acid/glucose-based solution noted that osmolarity greater than 600 mOsm/L resulted in phlebitis. However, later studies using amino acid/glucose/lipid-based solutions (1200-1700 mOsm/L) found no difference in the incidence of peripheral vein phlebitis (Anderson, Palmer, and MacFie, 2003).
- In a literature review of 13 selected studies on peripheral parenteral nutrition, there were 5 references addressing thrombophlebitis. Based on the literature, the authors recommend that parenteral nutrition solutions should have an osmolality between 600 and 900 mOsm/L within a pH range of 7.2 to 7.4 (Culebras et al, 2004).
- An experimental study examined the effect of changing osmolality of nutrient infusions on peripheral venous endothelial cells in a rabbit model. Two test solutions (748 and 718 mOsm/kg) were infused into peripheral veins for 12 and 24 hours. After both infusions, the veins were examined histopathologically and graded based on findings of the loss of venous endothelial cells, inflammatory cell infiltration, edema, and thrombus. As a second test, the solutions with the same nutrient composition were diluted (648 and 514 mOsm/kg) and infused, and the veins were examined. This study concluded that dilution of solutions with the same nutrient composition and infusion time resulted in significant decreases in phlebitis (Kuwahara, Asanami, and Tamura, 1998b).
- This experimental research study examined varying infusion rates and osmolality on venous phlebitis. In a rabbit model, test solutions ranging in osmolality from 917 to 539 mOsm/kg were infused for 8, 12, and 24 hours. After infusions were completed, the veins were examined histopathologically and graded based on findings of the loss of venous endothelial cells, inflammatory cell infiltration, edema, and thrombus. In this model, the infusion tolerance of peripheral venous cells was estimated to be 820 mOsm/kg for 8 hours, 690 mOsm/kg for 12 hours, and 550 mOsm/kg for 24 hours. Researchers propose that infusion phlebitis may be decreased by higher rates of infusion (Kuwahara, Asanami, and Kubo, 1998a).
- A randomized study was undertaken to determine if increasing osmolality increases the incidence of thrombophlebitis. Thirty-six patients were randomized to receive either a low osmolality solution (1200 mOsm/L) or a high osmolality solution (1700 mOsm/L). The mean duration of peripheral IV nutrition was between 6 and 7 days in both groups. In this small study, there was no significant difference in the rate of thrombophlebitis between the two groups; the overall phlebitis rate was high, however, at 30% (Kane et al, 1996).
- Phase A of this two-phase study looked specifically at infusing three peripheral nutrition solutions containing heparin (400 mOsm/L, 900 mOsm/L, 900 mOsm/L with cortisol) at 125 mL/hour for 3- to 10-day periods in 15 adult malnourished patients. In each subject, solutions were altered in a random fashion and continued until infiltration or tissue reaction was noted. (Phase B was a metabolic nutrient balance study and is not further discussed here). The 900 mOsm/L solution was stopped on an average of 4 hours while the 900 mOsm/L with cortisol was stopped at 120 hours average. The researchers concluded that peripheral infusions containing 900 mOsm/L, heparin, and cortisol are feasible (Isaacs et al, 1977).

production, which may aggravate preexisting respiratory distress.

Other sources of parenteral carbohydrates include glycerol, fructose, galactose, invert sugar, maltose, sorbitol, and xylitol. Other than glycerol, these carbohydrates are no longer commercially available because of the high potential for adverse effects (Holcombe, 1995). Glycerol, a sugar alcohol also known as glycerin, is available as an IV carbohydrate-like solution used in PN, but is used infrequently. Glycerol is commercially available in premixed PN solutions that are intended for peripheral administration. For example, Procalamine® is ready for infusion after vitamins and trace elements are added. Procalamine® contains 3% amino acids and 3% glycerol premixed in 1-L bottles. It has a caloric density of 250 kcal/L and a solution osmolarity of 735 mOsm/L, and can therefore be administered peripherally. Because it is a partial nutritional solution, Procalamine® is used only for patients whose nutritional requirements can be met by the nutrients and electrolytes present (Dickerson et al, 1993).

FAT
Nutritional background

Fats, organic substances that are insoluble in water, are responsible for a wide range of metabolic and structural functions. Fats are a particularly efficient form of energy because they are calorically dense (9 kcal/g) and are stored in the anhydrous state. Along with carbohydrates, fats are burned for energy in protein sparing. Fats function to support and pad critical organs, such as the kidneys, and to insulate the body against heat loss. Fats are an important component of cell membranes and are precursors of the regulatory compounds, such as the prostaglandins, glucocorticoids, mineralocorticoids, estrogens, androgens, and bile acids. Fat in food serves as a vehicle for fat-soluble vitamins (vitamins A, D, E, and K), which are essential to body metabolism. The major classes of lipids found in plasma include triglycerides, phospholipids, cholesterol, and free fatty acids.

The two essential fatty acids for humans are linoleic and α-linolenic acids. These fatty acids are necessary for cell membrane structure and stability and are precursors of prostaglandins (Krzywda, 1996). The primary fatty acid in the diet is linoleic acid, a precursor to arachidonic acid. Linoleic acid is considered essential because the body cannot synthesize it, and it must therefore be supplied from an exogenous source, such as diet or parenteral feedings. The role of linolenic acid in adults is unclear, and its essentiality is controversial. Arachidonic acid can be synthesized from linoleic acid if there is an adequate supply.

Long-term inadequate intake of long-chain fatty acids or malabsorption can cause essential fatty acid deficiency (EFAD). The clinical signs and symptoms of EFAD are dry, thick, desquamating skin, alopecia, brittle nails, thrombocytopenia, anemia, hepatic dysfunction secondary to fatty liver, and growth retardation in infants (Kumpf and Gervasio, 2007). An increase in the specific laboratory test to measure the lipid triene/tetraene ratio (greater than 0.2) will confirm the diagnosis (Sax, 1993; Hise and Brown, 2007).

Patients receiving a seemingly appropriate amount of essential fats in the diet or from IV lipid emulsion who continue to demonstrate clinical signs and symptoms of EFAD may have a carnitine deficiency. Carnitine is a naturally occurring substance that transports long-chain fats into the mitochondria, where they are converted into energy. Serum carnitine levels are used to determine carnitine deficiency. If serum levels are normal and carnitine deficiency is still strongly suspected, a

muscle biopsy may be indicated. Carnitine is a commercially available intravenous product and can be added to PN for patients with a suspected or documented deficiency (Barber, Rollins, and Sacks, 2007).

Component of PN solution

Intravenous fat emulsion (IVFE) serves two purposes in PN. It is a source of calories and of essential fatty acids needed to prevent essential fatty acid deficiency. Fat is the most calorically dense substrate available (approximately 9 kcal/g), providing more than twice the caloric density of carbohydrate and protein. Fat emulsions provide varying amounts of linoleic and linolenic acids sufficient to prevent or treat essential fatty acid deficiency.

In PN lipid emulsions should at least be provided in quantities sufficient to prevent essential fatty acid deficiency. Depending on the baseline nutritional status and co-morbid disease states, EFAD can occur in as little as 4 weeks, if the patient is given a fat-free PN (Mirtallo et al, 2004). The minimum requirement needed to prevent essential fatty acid deficiency is 2% to 4% of the total caloric intake, or at least 2.4 g of linoleic acid per 2000 kcal of nutrient intake. Fats also provide calories for meeting energy requirements to optimize protein utilization and, when needed, to decrease the carbohydrate load. The optimal dose of lipid for the provision of calories is unknown. However, the maximum safe dose is no more than 60% (most patients receive 15% to 30%) of the daily caloric intake, and should not exceed 2.5 g/kg for adults or 3 g/kg for pediatric patients (Dickerson et al, 1993).

The parenteral lipid emulsions currently in use are emulsions of soybean oil or a combination of soybean and safflower oils. Other components of fat emulsions include egg phospholipids, which act as an emulsifier, and glycerol, which adjusts the osmolarity to make the emulsion isotonic. Isolated reports of patients with an allergy to one parenteral lipid emulsion have yielded other formulations of lipid emulsions. Lipid emulsions are available in concentrations of 10%, 20%, and 30%. Ten percent lipid emulsion provides 1.1 kcal/mL, 20% lipid emulsion provides 2.0 kcal/mL, and 30% provides 2.9 kcal/mL. The content of glycerol is constant in all three formulations, resulting in caloric contents that are not proportional. Lipid concentrations of 10% and 20% could be infused alone, either centrally or peripherally. Thirty percent lipids are for PN solution compounding only and should not be infused independently (Mattox and Reiter, 2005).

Adverse reactions to fat emulsions are rare (<1%) but it is prudent to monitor patients the first time they receive lipids for dyspnea, chest tightness, palpitations, and chills. If fat emulsions are administered too quickly, headache, fever, and nausea may also be seen (Mattox and Reiter, 2005).

ELECTROLYTES
Nutritional background

Electrolytes play a critical role in almost all of the body's physiological functions. Disorders of electrolyte homeostasis are associated with many disease states. In the patient requiring nutritional support, abnormal electrolyte concentrations reflect the primary disease, its complications, or its treatment. Electrolytes commonly used in a PN formula include sodium, potassium, calcium, magnesium, chloride, and phosphorus. Electrolytes are included in the formula to meet daily requirements and to correct deficits. The management of electrolytes for these patients can be one of the most time-consuming aspects of monitoring and managing nutritional support. The important points for minimizing electrolyte complications associated with nutritional support are close monitoring, awareness of preexisting deficits and factors that predispose a patient to electrolyte imbalance, and the recognition of signs and symptoms of deficiency.

Sodium (Na)

Together with chloride and bicarbonate, sodium is the major osmotic force in the extracellular fluid. Sodium is actively involved in the absorption of sugars and amino acids. It is the most abundant cation and contributes to the osmolarity of the extracellular fluid.

- Hyponatremia (serum sodium concentration <135 mEq/L) is common in hospitalized patients. Headache, nausea, vomiting, muscle cramps, lethargy, disorientation, and depressed reflexes may be seen when concentrations reach <125 mEq/L. The etiology of hyponatremia may or may not represent a deficiency of total body sodium levels. Correction of hyponatremia should be done carefully to avoid osmotic demyelination.
- Hypernatremia (serum sodium concentration >145 mEq/L) is many times caused by other interventions or therapies. Hypernatremia can occur with low, normal, or (rarely) high total body sodium stores. The majority of cases result from net body loss of water.

Potassium (K)

Potassium is the main intracellular cation. It plays a role in cell metabolism, participating in such processes as protein and glycogen synthesis. Potassium absorption in the ileum is a passive process and depends on the concentration gradient. Potassium loss may be increased by diarrhea and the chronic use of laxatives.

- Hypokalemia (serum potassium concentration <3.6 mEq/L) is found in over 20% of hospitalized patients (Paice et al, 1986). Hypokalemia is frequently the result of potassium depletion secondary to losses in the urine or stool. Symptoms of hypokalemia are nonspecific and include generalized weakness, lethargy, and constipation. Hypokalemia is often symptom free unless concentrations fall below 3.0 mEq/L.
- Hyperkalemia (serum potassium concentration >5.0 mEq/L) is uncommon in healthy individuals because of the body's regulatory mechanisms. Hyperkalemia most frequently occurs in the presence of renal failure. Symptoms of elevated potassium concentrations present as changes in neuromuscular and cardiac function, including muscle twitching, cramping, weakness, ascending paralysis, and electrocardiogram (ECG) changes including widening QRS complex and shortened QT interval.

Calcium (Ca)

Calcium is one of the most abundant ions in the body and constitutes 1% to 2% of total adult body weight, primarily in bones and teeth (Langley, 2007). Calcium is present in the body as complexed, protein bound, or ionized. Ionized calcium is the metabolically active form and not influenced by serum proteins, such as albumin. In malnourished patients, serum calcium levels may be low because of decreased levels of albumin, to which half of calcium is bound. For each 1 g/dL decrease in serum albumin level below 4.0 g/dL, total calcium level decreases by approximately 0.8 mg/dL (Singer et al, 1977). Total calcium level may be estimated with a correction formula:

$$\text{Corrected total calcium (mg/dL)} = \text{Measured total calcium (mg/dL)} + 0.8 \, [4 - \text{albumin concentration(g/dL)}]$$

However, accurate assessment of metabolically active calcium in the body is best accomplished by the measurement of a serum ionized calcium concentration (Popovtzer, 2003). Calcium is responsible for the preservation and function of cell membranes, propagation of neuromuscular activity, regulation of endocrine and exocrine secretory functions, blood coagulation cascade, platelet adhesion process, bone metabolism, muscle cell excitation-contraction coupling, and mediation of the electrophysiological slow-channel response in cardiac and smooth muscle tissue.

- Hypocalcemia (serum calcium concentration <8.6 mg/dL) frequently occurs as a result of hypoalbuminemia and may not be clinically significant if the ionized calcium level is normal. Low calcium level is common in critically ill patients with sepsis, rhabdomyolysis, and blood transfusions. Symptoms include decreased blood pressure, muscle cramps, distal paresthesias, tetany, and seizures.
- Hypercalcemia (serum calcium concentration >10.2 mg/dL or ionized calcium >1.5 mmol/L) most commonly occurs secondary to hyperparathyroidism and cancer with bone metastases. Nonspecific symptoms include fatigue, nausea, vomiting, constipation, and confusion. Bradycardia may present in severe cases.

Magnesium (Mg)

Sixty percent of magnesium is bound to bone and unavailable for metabolism. The remaining magnesium is largely intracellular. Serum magnesium concentrations do not accurately reflect total body magnesium level. Magnesium is necessary for the control of neuromuscular irritability. Most of the absorption of magnesium takes place in the ileum. Resected ileum and excessive diarrhea can cause magnesium deficiency.

- Hypomagnesemia (serum magnesium <2.8 mg/dL) occurs frequently in hospitalized patients (Whang and Ryder, 1990). Neuromuscular hyperexcitability, latent tetany, and generalized seizures may occur in severe cases. Hypokalemia and hypocalcemia are commonly present when hypomagnesemia exists. In these scenarios, the magnesium concentration should be corrected first, followed by potassium or calcium levels (Langley, 2007). Intravenous supplementation is often preferred because of the slow onset of effect and GI intolerance frequently seen with oral magnesium supplementation. The kidneys have a threshold for magnesium, so supplementation rates greater than 1.0 g/hour should be avoided in asymptomatic patients (Oster and Epstein, 1988).
- Hypermagnesemia (serum magnesium >2.3 mg/dL) is seen primarily in renal insufficiency or with increased intake, such as with magnesium-containing antacids or aggressive replacement in patients with renal disease. Symptoms include nausea, vomiting, diaphoresis, flushing, and drowsiness.

Chloride (Cl)

Chloride is the principle anion of the extracellular fluid. It is essential for the diagnosis and maintenance of appropriate acid-base balance. Along with sodium, chloride contributes to the total osmolarity in blood and urine, and plays a major role in water balance and extracellular fluid volume control. Chloride is generally excreted with sodium.

Phosphorus (P)

Phosphorus is the major intracellular anion. It is the essential element in phospholipid cell membranes, nucleic acids, and phosphoproteins required for mitochondrial function. It regulates the intermediary metabolism of carbohydrates, fats, and proteins and regulates enzymatic reactions, including glycolysis. Phosphorus is a source of high-energy bonds of adenosine triphosphate, and is therefore important in muscle contractility, electrolyte transport, and neurological function.

- Hypophosphatemia (serum phosphorus concentration <2.7 mg/dL) may be seen with chronic alcoholism, critical illness, respiratory or metabolic alkalosis, and as an unwanted effect of patients receiving aluminum-containing antacids or sucralfate (Peppers, Geheb, and Desai, 1991). The refeeding syndrome may present if malnourished patients receive large carbohydrate loads without adequate phosphate supplementation. This can cause the serum phosphate level to drop significantly and quickly (Brooks and Melnik, 1995).
- Hyperphosphatemia (serum phosphorus concentration > 4.5 mg/dL) most often occurs in the presence of renal insufficiency. Metastatic and vascular calcification of nonskeletal tissue is the most serious concern with this electrolyte disorder (Block and Port, 2000).

Component of PN solution

Because electrolytes play a critical role in almost all of the body's physiological functions, they are included in the administration of PN to meet daily requirements and to prevent or correct preexisting deficits. Although general guidelines for electrolyte requirements during PN exist for adults and pediatric patients, these recommendations are based on normal requirements in healthy individuals, so patient-specific needs must be considered when making electrolyte decisions for the PN formulation. Patients with preexisting conditions, such as long-term diuretic use or ongoing losses of electrolytes such as with fistulas or diarrhea, can be anticipated to have increased electrolyte requirements. It may be necessary to restrict electrolyte intake in patients with severe renal dysfunction, edema, or congestive heart failure.

Electrolytes may be added to parenteral solutions individually or in combination; electrolyte mixtures are available in concentrations designed to meet the standard adult electrolyte requirement. Several amino acid products contain electrolytes in amounts designed to meet adult requirements if 2 L/day are given. The use of these products in PN is usually limited to stable adult patients whose electrolyte balance can be achieved by the contents of these products. The patient's acid-base status will determine which salt should be used when calculating electrolytes in parenteral solutions. For example, sodium and potassium can be administered as the chloride, acetate, or phosphate salts, based on the patient's clinical status. Table 17-2 shows standard electrolyte ranges for PN solutions based on normal organ function and losses.

VITAMINS
Nutritional background

Vitamins are diverse organic compounds essential to normal tissue growth, maintenance, and function. They are involved in enzymatic processes that are important to energy and macronutrient (protein, carbohydrate, and fat) metabolism. Vitamins function primarily as co-enzymes of energy-yielding nutrients, and as co-factors in the storage and utilization of energy.

Thirteen vitamins are considered essential for humans. Based on their physical solubility, vitamins are classified as fat- or water-soluble. Fat-soluble vitamins are stored in fatty tissues, but water-soluble vitamins have limited storage options. Because they can be stored, fat-soluble vitamins possess the potential for serious toxicity. Box 17-3 lists the fat- and water-soluble vitamins.

Because the body cannot synthesize vitamins, they must be obtained from dietary sources. Vitamin deficiencies can occur as a result of inappropriate or decreased food intake, diminished absorption, or increased requirements. Deficiencies may occur as a result of fad diets, from anorexia nervosa, and in conditions such as malabsorption, malignancy, immunosuppression, alcoholism, and infectious disease treated with prolonged broad-spectrum antibiotics; deficiencies may also be seen in the elderly. Table 17-3 presents the clinical signs of malnutrition.

Vitamins are essential during nutrition support. Their key role in numerous metabolic processes makes their inclusion critical to the appropriate and efficient use of other nutrients. Standard parenteral maintenance doses of all vitamins should be provided as additives to the total parenteral solution, unless the patient's condition necessitates the limitation or exclusion of selected vitamins.

Fat-soluble vitamins
Vitamin A

Vitamin A (retinol) is required for many body functions, most prominently the visual process. Retinol is found in the visual pigments of the eye for dim light vision and color vision. In

TABLE 17-2   Daily Electrolyte Additions to Adult PN Formulations*

Electrolyte	Standard requirement
Sodium	1-2 mEq/kg
Potassium	1-2 mEq/kg
Phosphorus	20-40 mmol
Magnesium	8-20 mEq
Calcium	10-15 mEq
Chloride	As needed to maintain acid-base balance
Acetate	As needed to maintain acid-base balance

*Standard intake ranges based on healthy individuals with normal losses. Adapted from Mirtallo J, Canada T, Johnson D et al: Safe practices for parenteral nutrition, *J Parenter Enter Nutr*, 28:S39-S70, 2004.

Box 17-3   FAT- AND WATER-SOLUBLE VITAMINS

Fat-soluble vitamins	Water-soluble vitamins
Vitamin A (retinol)	Vitamin B_1 (thiamine)
Vitamin D	Vitamin B_2 (riboflavin)
Vitamin E (tocopherol)	Pantothenic acid
Vitamin K	Vitamin B_6 (pyridoxine)
	Vitamin B_{12} (cyanocobalamin)
	Biotin
	Vitamin C (ascorbic acid)
	Folic acid
	Niacin

TABLE 17-3 Clinical Signs of Malnutrition

Area of examination	Signs associated with malnutrition	Nutrient deficiency
Hair	Dull, dry, sparse, lackluster, easily plucked (inspect comb, pillow, bed for hair), changes in pigmentation	Protein, calorie, zinc, linoleic acid
Eyes	Pale, red conjunctiva	Vitamin A
	Bitot's spots—dry, grayish, yellow or white foamy spots on whites of eyes	
	Xerophthalmia:	
	Conjunctival—dull, roughened, pigmented whites and inner lids	
	Corneal—dull, milky, hazy, or opaque	
	Keratomalacia:	
	Cornea becomes soft	
	Eyes become gelatinous mass	
	Pale conjunctiva	Iron
	Red conjunctiva	Riboflavin
	Angular blepharitis—red, cracked, inflamed corners of eyes	Riboflavin, niacin
Lips	Cheilosis—vertical cracks of lips usually at center	Riboflavin, niacin
	Angular stomatitis—cracks, redness at corners of mouth; may result in scars when healed	Riboflavin, iron, niacin, pyridoxine
Tongue	Magenta (purplish red)	Riboflavin
	Glossitis—beefy red	Folate, niacin
	May be painful, hypertensive, burn with fissures	
	Atrophic papillae—may appear smooth, pale	Riboflavin, iron, B_{12}
Teeth	Mottled enamel—white or brownish patches	Fluorine excess
Gums	Spongy, bleeding	Vitamin C
Glands	Enlarged thyroid	Iodine
	Enlarged parotid	Protein
Skin	Xerosis—dryness, flakiness	Vitamin A
	Follicular hyperkeratosis—looks like "goose flesh" that does not disappear with rubbing or warming	Essential fatty acid
	Petechiae—hemorrhagic spots on skin at pressure points	Vitamin C
	Pellagrous dermatosis—hyperpigmentation on body parts exposed to sun	Niacin
	Casal's necklace—hyperpigmentation along neck where exposed to sun	
Nails	Spoon-shaped, thin, concave	Iron
Musculoskeletal	Osteoporosis—loss of bone mass; bones become brittle and sparse	Vitamins C, D
	Distance between long trabeculae increases with decrease in transverse trabeculae	
	Fractures and deformities result, most often crush fractures of spine	
	May be non-nutritional (postmenopausal, congenital defects, endocrine disorders)	
	Osteomalacia—adult form of rickets	
	Mineral deficiencies lead to soft, brittle bones that bend rather than fracture	
	Usually results from malabsorption from gastrointestinal losses such as in sprue, pancreatic insufficiency, inflammatory bowel disease	
	Rachitic rosary—small lumps (beading) on ribs	
	Pigeon chest	
	Epiphyseal enlargement—enlargement of ends of long bones	
Organ	Hepatomegaly	Protein
	Splenomegaly	
	Tachycardia	Iron, thiamine
Neurological	Confusion, listlessness	Protein
	Sensory-motor, vibratory	Thiamine, B_{12}

From Curtas S: Nutrition assessment of the adult. In Hennessy KA, Orr ME, editors: *Nutrition support nursing,* ed 3, Silver Springs, Md, 1996, ASPEN.

addition, vitamin A is required for the synthesis of certain polysaccharides and is essential in the formation of many membranes. Vitamin A is also necessary for proper immune function, particularly antigen recognition, and is essential for the integrity of epithelial surfaces.

Vitamin D

Vitamin D includes both ergocalciferol (vitamin D_2) and cholecalciferol (vitamin D_3). Vitamin D is converted to hormones that are directly involved in the regulation of calcium and phosphorus levels. This regulation includes the absorption of calcium, the deposition and release of calcium from the bones and teeth, and the entrance of calcium into certain cells or cell nuclei. Deficiency has been documented in the elderly, extended care facility residents, dark-skinned individuals, individuals who have minimal sun exposure, and infants fed exclusively breast milk (Clark, 2007).

Vitamin E

Vitamin E (tocopherol) is an important antioxidant that protects other organic compounds from being oxidized, thus protecting cell membrane integrity during normal metabolic processes. In particular, it protects unsaturated phospholipid cell membranes from oxidation (i.e., degradation) by "donating" a hydrogen ion to oxygen species and other free radicals. This converts the free radicals into nonoxidative metabolites and is known as free radical scavenging (Gallager, 2004). Because oxidation products from unsaturated lipids may be carcinogenic, vitamin E may play a role in inhibiting the development of neoplasms by decreasing the oxidation of unsaturated fatty acids. Epidemiological evidence suggests that low serum vitamin E concentrations are related to increased incidence of certain types of cancer (Sitren, 1997; Gottschlich and Mayes, 1998). Individuals at risk of vitamin E deficiency include those having prolonged steatorrhea (that is, fat malabsorption from, e.g., resection of ileum or small intestine) or requiring prolonged delivery of high oxygen concentrations via mechanical ventilation (Ross, 2004).

Vitamin K (phytonadione)

Vitamin K is involved in blood clotting and the formation of certain dicarboxylic amino acids that bind calcium. True deficiency of this vitamin is rare, but may be manifested by a prolonged prothrombin time or International Normalized Ratio (INR) and possibly bleeding. In patients receiving the anticoagulant warfarin (Coumadin), it is important to remember that vitamin K was added as an option to commercial multiple vitamin formulations in 2000. Small amounts are also present in intravenous fat emulsions (Camilo et al, 1998). While typically not clinically significant, these sources should be considered if reaching or maintaining a therapeutic INR in these patients is difficult.

Water-soluble vitamins
B vitamins

Vitamin B_1 (thiamine) is an important vitamin in the oxidation conversion of pyruvic acid and therefore in the Krebs cycle. Thiamine is also part of certain nerve cells and is required for the proper transmission of nerve impulses. The disease that is historically linked to thiamine deficiency is beriberi. Today, the most common cause of thiamine deficiency is alcoholism, due to impaired absorption and decreased dietary intake (Clark, 2007).

Vitamin B_2 (riboflavin) is necessary for cellular growth and repair. It is also an integral part of several oxidative enzyme systems necessary for electron transport, and thus for the efficient production of cellular energy.

Pantothenic acid is a constituent of co-enzyme A and is the prosthetic group on an acyl carrier protein. It is necessary for the metabolism of glucose, protein, and fat.

Vitamin B_6 (pyridoxine) is a co-factor for more than 100 enzymatic processes affecting the metabolism of protein, amino acids, lipids, gluconeogenesis, central nervous system development, heme synthesis, and many other reactions (Clark, 2007).

Vitamin B_{12} (cyanocobalamin) is a co-enzyme involved in the synthesis of DNA nucleotides and in lipid and amino acid metabolism. Biotin is required for the normal activity of the numerous enzyme systems involved in carbohydrate, fat, and protein metabolism.

Folate (folic acid) is transformed to numerous compounds (folates) that serve as co-enzymes in a variety of one-carbon transfer reactions involved in purine biosynthesis and amino acid metabolism.

Niacin (consisting of two active forms: nicotinic acid and nicotinamide) functions in the metabolism of amino acids, fatty acids, and carbohydrates. The classic disease associated with niacin deficiency is pellagra, which presents as three Ds: dermatitis, diarrhea, and dementia (Clark, 2007).

Vitamin C

Vitamin C (ascorbic acid) is required for normal amino acid metabolism and for the synthesis of collagen, adrenal hormones, vasoactive amines, and carnitine. It is important in cholesterol and folic acid metabolism and leukocyte function. Scurvy is the classic vitamin C deficiency disease that is characterized by connective tissue defects (Boosalis, 2003).

Component of PN solution

Vitamins play an essential role in metabolism and cellular function; therefore a multiple-vitamin preparation should be added to the PN solution each day. Adult vitamin mixtures containing fat- and water-soluble vitamins are commercially available and typically contain 12 or 13 vitamins (with or without vitamin K). If vitamin K is not included in the commercial multiple vitamin infusion (MVI) product, 5 to 10 mg may be given weekly either by the intramuscular (IM) or by the subcutaneous (subQ) route. If patients are receiving warfarin anticoagulant therapy, they should be monitored closely if receiving vitamin K either via MVI or weekly injections.

Parenteral vitamin requirements generally are significantly lower than dietary vitamin requirements because the parenteral route bypasses the digestive and absorptive functions of the GI tract. Guidelines for parenteral vitamin intake have recently been revised following collaboration between the Food and Drug Administration (FDA) and the American Medical Association (AMA). This group recommended that the dosage of some vitamins be increased and that vitamin K be added to parenteral formulation for adults and children older than 11 years of age (U.S. Department of Health and Human Services, 2000). Specific disease states and certain drugs may alter vitamin requirements, but typical needs can be met by adding standard MVI formulations to the PN solution.

TRACE ELEMENTS
Nutritional background

Trace elements (TE) are inorganic compounds that are present in the body in only "trace" amounts, that is, less than 0.005% of total body weight (DeBiasse-Fortin, 2003). Not all trace elements have been confirmed as essential nutrients. A trace element is considered essential if there is evidence for its physiological role in metabolism; if it is present in healthy tissue in constant concentration; if its absence causes physical, structural, or biochemical abnormalities; and if its provision prevents or corrects the abnormality. The trace elements that have been identified as essential in humans perform many biological functions, including a role in carbohydrate, lipid, and protein metabolism, immune function, cell membrane integrity, oxygen transport, and hormonal activity.

Trace element requirements vary by age, gender, and clinical and metabolic status. Deficiencies result from decreased intake, increased losses, excessive metabolic requirements, or impaired GI absorption. Excessive intake of certain trace elements will cause toxicity. Careful monitoring and serum testing will help determine deficiency and replenishment status. Table 17-4 presents the clinical signs of trace element deficiency and toxicity.

Copper (Cu)

Body stores of copper are regulated primarily by biliary excretion rather than absorption (Clark, 2007). Copper is a component of proenzymes that participate in oxygen utilization. Copper deficiency and copper toxicity are uncommon (Clark, 2007). Symptoms related to copper deficiency include hypochromic and microcytic anemia, leukopenia, and neutropenia. Patients at greatest risk of copper deficiency are those with chronic diarrhea, those consuming a milk-based diet, those recovering from intestinal surgery, and dialysis patients (Andris, 1996; Misra and Kirby, 2000).

Chromium (Cr)

Chromium is required for glucose and lipid metabolism and also potentiates the action of insulin. Increased urinary excretion of chromium may be seen in type 2 diabetes and pregnancy, so supplementation may be necessary in those patients. Deficiency, while uncommon, may present as hyperglycemia not controlled by insulin and could develop in long-term PN patients who do not receive trace element supplementation (Andris, 1996; Clark, 2007).

Iodine (I)

Iodine is an important component of the thyroid hormones—thyroxine (T_4) and triiodothyronine (T_3). Iodine deficiency may manifest as goiter, reduced metabolic rate, increased cholesterol level, and impaired fertility (Andris, 1996; Clark, 2007).

Iron (Fe)

The principal function of iron is the transport, storage, and utilization of oxygen. Iron deficiency is the most common nutritional deficiency in the United States, largely because of the needs of women and children. Iron deficiency presents as anemia, with physical symptoms that may include tachycardia, poor capillary refilling, fatigue, and pallor (Andris, 1996). Those at highest risk of iron deficiency include women of childbearing age, hospitalized patients with blood loss or multiple blood

TABLE 17-4 Clinical Signs of Mineral and Trace Element Deficiency and Toxicity

Element	Deficiency symptoms	Toxicity symptoms	Parenteral supplement
Iron	Microcytic hypochromic anemia: dyspnea on exertion, fatigue, pallor, low serum iron and ferritin levels, high TIBC	Hyperpigmentation of skin, cirrhosis, diabetes, sterility, cardiac arrhythmias, arthropathy	Not supported
Zinc	Diarrhea, hair loss, delayed growth and wound healing, impaired taste	Copper deficiency, microcytic anemia, reduced immune response, renal failure	2-4 mg/day*
Copper	Microcytic hypochromic anemia, neutropenia	Vomiting, hepatic necrosis, ataxia, cirrhosis	0.5-1.5 mg/day
Manganese	Dermatitis, hypocholesterol, neuromuscular dysfunction	Weakness, anorexia, somnolence, muscular rigidity, staggered gait, fine tremor	≤100 mcg/day
Selenium	Cardiomyopathy, muscle pain, weakness	Hair loss, peripheral neuropathy, fatigue, nail and teeth changes	≤100 mcg/day
Chromium	Glucose intolerance, elevated cholesterol and triglyceride levels, reduced HDL cholesterol levels	None reported from dietary intake	10-20 mcg/day
Iodine	Hyperthyroid goiter, hypothyroidism, decreased basal metabolic rate, mental sluggishness	Acnelike lesions, "iodine goiter" or "toxic goiter" caused by inhibition of thyroid hormone synthesis	Not recommended
Molybdenum	Mouth and gum disorders, hypouricemia, mental disturbance	Anorexia, listlessness, diarrhea, anemia, slow growth	None specified
Aluminum	None	Vitamin D resistant osteomalacic bone disease, dementia, microcytic hypochromic anemia	Not recommended

*Amount to supplement in addition to the standard maintenance trace element preparation.
HDL, high-density lipoprotein; *TIBC*, total iron-binding capacity.
Modified from DeBiasse-Fortin MA: Minerals and trace elements. In Matarese LE, Gottschlich MM, editors: *Contemporary nutrition support practice: a clinical guide*, St Louis, 2003, Saunders.

samples for lab testing, and individuals with malabsorption states (e.g., celiac disease), Crohn's disease, and gastric or intestinal surgeries (Clark, 2007).

Manganese (Mn)

Manganese functions in energy metabolism and antioxidant protection and is necessary for the action of vitamin K, which is responsible for clotting. It is a soluble co-factor in a number of enzymatic reactions. The mechanism of manganese absorption is not clear, but it may be similar to iron absorption. Manganese toxicity is rare, but populations most at risk include long-term PN patients who develop biliary duct obstruction, as almost 100% of manganese is excreted via the bile into the feces. Deficiency is rare unless the mineral is completely absent from the diet (Clark, 2007).

Molybdenum (Mo)

Molybdenum is required as a co-factor in oxidation-reduction reactions for several enzymes (xanthine oxidase, sulfite oxidase, and aldehyde oxidase). Molybdenum deficiency is rare and occurs predominantly in patients with short-bowel syndrome and those receiving unsupplemented long-term PN. Signs of deficiency include mouth and gum disorders, hypouricemia, and mental and visual alterations (DeBiasse-Fortin, 2003).

Selenium (Se)

Selenium plays an important role in the protection of cell membrane integrity and the immune system. Deficiency of selenium is not common, although may be seen in critically ill patients and in those receiving long-term PN solutions. Muscle weakness and pain are the most common manifestations of deficiency. Signs of toxicity are also nonspecific and include nausea, hair loss, peripheral neuropathy, fatigue, and changes in nails and teeth (DeBiasse-Fortin, 2003).

Zinc (Zn)

Zinc is the most abundant of all the trace elements, second only to iron in body content. It functions in numerous important biochemical processes including cellular respiration, bone metabolism, wound healing, cellular membrane stability, antioxidant function, appetite regulation, and protein synthesis (DeBiasse-Fortin, 2003). Zinc is important for normal functioning of the immune and reproductive systems and the development and functioning of the nervous system (Misra and Kirby, 2000). It also functions as a co-factor in more than 200 enzyme systems (DeBaisse-Fortin, 2003). Clinical situations and diseases that predispose to zinc deficiency include malabsorptive syndromes (e.g., celiac disease, Crohn's disease, short-bowel syndrome, jejunoileal bypass), burn patients, elderly patients, pancreatic insufficiency, alcoholism, and pregnancy. Increased GI losses (diarrhea, fistula, and nasogastric suction) may also predispose patients to zinc deficiency. Clinically, zinc deficiency presents nonspecifically as inadequate growth, skin lesions, impaired night vision, anorexia, alterations in taste and smell, and poor wound healing (Clark, 2007).

Component of PN solution

The efficient use of substrates for energy production and protein synthesis depends on the availability of trace elements. To ensure adequate amounts and prevent deficiency states, trace elements are routinely added to PN solutions. While 17 trace elements have been shown to have biological importance,

deficiencies in humans have only been reported for iron, iodine, cobalt (as vitamin B_{12}), zinc, and copper (Greene et al, 1988; Misra and Kirby, 2000). The trace elements that the American Medical Association (AMA) considers essential for PN are zinc, copper, and chromium (AMA, 1979). It is particularly important to assess individual trace mineral requirements in malnourished patients who may have preexisting micronutrient deficiencies, and in neonates who have limited body stores of trace elements and whose needs are critical for growth. Monitoring trace element status is based on regular clinical assessment for the presence of the signs and symptoms of deficiency.

Trace elements are inefficiently absorbed through the GI tract from dietary sources, so there are substantial differences between amounts required when nutrition is delivered enterally rather than parenterally. Intravenous trace elements are commercially available either as the single component or as multimineral combinations. Most provide the recommended daily requirements for the essential trace elements recommended by the AMA (Mattox and Reiter, 2005). Individual trace elements may be added in higher amounts if the patient's clinical condition warrants increased supplementation. For example, higher doses of zinc may be indicated in patients with high-output ostomies or diarrhea because of increased zinc losses in these conditions. There are no formal recommendations for selenium and molybdenum for adults, but clinical practice suggests inclusion of these trace elements during the PN of select patient groups, including long-term PN patients and those with preexisting deficiencies.

 ## PARENTERAL NUTRITION ADMINISTRATION ISSUES

DRUG COMPATIBILITY

The compatibility of drugs in PN solutions is often in question and is difficult to answer because of the many factors that affect compatibility, such as the solubility, stability, and pharmacokinetics of drugs. However, a number of drugs have been added to PN solutions without any apparent incompatibility complications.

The complex composition of PN solutions renders them highly susceptible to compatibility and stability concerns. Adding drugs to PN admixtures or piggybacking them into the PN access line poses an increased risk of physical and chemical incompatibility and solution contamination. Comprehensive reference sources exist that specifically address compatibility and stability questions related to PN, including *Trissel's Handbook of Injectable Drugs* and *King Guide to Parenteral Admixtures* (Mattox and Reiter, 2005). In many cases, the specific compatibility question is not studied in available references, which then requires the use of other published primary literature, clinical judgment, principles of chemistry, and experience. The pharmacist may be used as a resource to assist in determining the answer to these sometimes complicated questions.

MEDICATION ADMINISTRATION

Using PN solutions to deliver drugs has some advantages, such as efficient utilization of limited IV access, conservation of fluids in volume-restricted patients, decreasing the number of times the registered nurse (RN) must manipulate the vascular access device for drug administration, and the potential economic benefits of reduced personnel time and material savings. However, this practice is not recommended for the routine administration of medications because of the complexity of the PN solutions and the risk of physical and chemical compatibility concerns (Mirtallo et al, 2004). In some cases, there may be limited alternatives. In these situations, only medications that should be considered for inclusion in a PN admixture are those with distinct dosage regimens, documented stability and compatibility with the PN, and evidence to support the efficacy of the agent given in this manner (i.e., as a continuous infusion). Medications that may be added to PN solutions and are commonly used include regular insulin, heparin, and H₂-receptor antagonists (e.g., cimetidine, famotidine, ranitidine).

Insulin

Diabetes is a common metabolic disorder that is characterized by a relative or absolute lack of insulin. Diabetic patients on PN typically will have a blood glucose goal in the 100 to 200 mg/dL range, but the high glucose loads provided by PN can cause blood glucose control challenges for diabetic and nondiabetic patients. In the intensive care unit (ICU), insulin requirements are typically the highest, and most variable, during the first day in the ICU (Mirtallo et al, 2004). Regular insulin may be added to the PN solution; however, it should be added gradually and cautiously. Initial blood glucose management should be provided with subcutaneous dosing or a continuous insulin infusion, which can be more easily adjusted. When the patient's 24-hour insulin needs are stable, a portion of that dose may be added to the PN. Caution should be taken not to add too much insulin too quickly, as a hypoglycemic event would require that the entire PN solution be discontinued and wasted. It is also important to recognize that insulin will adsorb to polyvinyl chloride (PVC) tubing and PN bags, so a certain percentage of the dose added will be lost if PVC products are used. If the blood glucose concentration cannot be controlled by exogenous insulin, the amount of dextrose may need to be reduced and additional calories provided from lipids.

Heparin

Subtherapeutic doses of heparin (0.5 to 1 unit/mL) are sometimes added to peripheral PN solutions to prevent venous thrombus formation (Anderson et al, 2003). However, concerns related to the possibility of heparin-induced thrombocytopenia (HIT) and long-term heparin administration causing osteoporosis have decreased this practice.

H₂-receptor antagonists

H₂-receptor antagonists inhibit gastric acid secretion and are used during PN to prevent stress ulceration. They are effective in counteracting metabolic alkalosis induced by nasogastric suctioning or use of crystalline amino acid solutions that contain large amounts of acetate (Krzywda, 1996).

PIGGYBACKING MEDICATIONS

Ideally, the central venous access device lumen used for the administration of PN should be dedicated to the PN infusion and not used for other purposes. Frequently, the lack of IV access necessitates considering use of the PN line for administering other medications concurrently, or "piggybacking" medications with the PN. Antibiotics, pain medications, and sedatives are examples of medications that often need to be piggybacked. Antibiotic compatibility information is limited for 3-in-1 solutions. Each PN solution is an individualized product, with unique substrate concentrations, pH, and final volume, for example, so compatibility generalizations are difficult to make. Available compatibility references and the pharmacist should be consulted any time a medication is being considered for piggybacking directly with the PN solution. If a medication is compatible and will be infused with the PN solution, it should be administered via a piggyback infusion at the catheter hub to minimize direct mixing with the PN solution.

STANDARD PN SOLUTIONS

The two most commonly used types of PN solutions are "2-in-1," which consists of amino acids and dextrose with or without intravenous lipid emulsions (IVLE) piggybacked into the infusion line, and "3-in-1," or total nutrient admixtures (TNA). TNA contain dextrose, amino acids, fat emulsion, electrolytes, trace elements, and multivitamins in one container. The addition of fat emulsion is the unique part of these admixtures. The components are mixed in a single bag, providing a 24-hour nutritional supply for the patient. Final volumes of TNA bags may be as much as 3 L. Total nutrient admixture solutions offer advantages compared to PN regimens that infuse IVLE separately, including reduced costs (fewer infusion pumps, less tubing and other supplies), less time to prepare and administer, fewer manipulations of the venous access device, and ease of delivery and storage for patients receiving home PN (Campos, Paluzzi and Meguid, 1990). Disadvantages of 3-in-1 solutions include increased infectious risk, because of the addition of the lipid solution, solution stability concerns, and increased risk for undetected incompatibilities (Mattox and Reiter, 2005). PN formulations vary considerably as each is usually tailored to the individual patient's nutritional needs.

ADMINISTRATION CONSIDERATIONS

The administration and preparation of PN solutions have many considerations for the infusion nurse specialist. These pertain to both "2-in-1" and "3-in-1" formulations and will be reviewed briefly here.

Filtering

The addition of an in-line filter to PN solutions helps to prevent both bacterial and particulate contamination. Studies have shown that the following bacteria are effectively removed by a 0.22-micron filter: *Staphylococcus epidermidis*, *Escherichia coli*, and *Candida albicans* (Mershon et al, 1986). However, a filter this small will not allow the fat particles in the intravenous fat emulsion to pass. Current FDA recommendations for filtering call for the use of a 1.2-micron filter for any PN solution containing IVFE. While this filter will not remove the *E. coli* and *S. epidermidis* that a 0.22-micron filter will, *C. albicans* will be prevented from entering the bloodstream. Particles 5.0 microns or larger in size are capable of obstructing blood flow and potentially leading to pulmonary embolus (ASPEN, 2002). Of note, in-line filters will also increase the incidence of occlusion alarms, warning of possible blockage. These alarms should be investigated and if they cannot be resolved, the infusion of the

PN solution should be halted. The in-line filter should never be removed if the PN solution is continuing (Barber et al, 2007). If a PN "2-in-1" solution is used, a 0.22-micron filter is recommended; it is also acceptable to use a 1.2-micron filter for both types of PN solutions (ASPEN, 2002).

Hang time of IVFE and PN-containing IVFE

Intravenous fat emulsions (10% and 20%) are isotonic, so they may be administered peripherally. Fat emulsions may be administered through a separate site or given through a lower Y connector in the existing PN administration set. Fat emulsions may or may not require filtration depending on manufacturer's directions and individual institutional policy. In cases in which filtration is required, a 1.2-micron filter may be used. Guidelines for the amount of time that lipid emulsions can remain hanging depend on if they are infused alone, or as part of a PN solution. Concern about the potential for a contaminated IVFE solution to support bacterial or fungal growth resulted in the recommendation that IVFE given alone as a piggyback be limited to a hang time of 12 hours (CDC, 2002). If lipids are included in a "3-in-1" formulation, the hang time of the bag is extended to 24 hours (Mirtallo et al, 2004).

Calcium and phosphate precipitation

The Food and Drug Administration (FDA) issued a safety alert in 1994 based on the reports of two deaths and two cases of respiratory distress in PN patients. The sentinel events were ultimately confirmed to be the result of pulmonary embolism secondary to calcium phosphate particulates developing from PN solutions (Knowles et al, 1989; FDA, 1994). These unfortunate incidents heightened awareness of the risk of calcium and phosphorus compatibility in PN solutions. Evaluation of the risk of this precipitation is not as straightforward as determining the amount of calcium and phosphate in the solution. Factors that can affect this risk include amino acid concentration, pH of the final PN solution, dextrose concentration, temperature of formulation, order of mixing, and others (Barber et al, 2007). It is important that the ordering practitioner be aware of the potential risks, utilize the clinical pharmacist, and adhere to institutional recommendations and limits when ordering calcium and phosphate in the PN formulation.

Propofol and IVFE

Propofol is an anesthetic agent commonly used as a sedative in the intensive care unit, particularly in mechanically ventilated patients. It is desirable for ICU sedation because it is easily titrated to effect and is rapidly cleared from the body when discontinued (Hise and Brown, 2007). It is formulated in a 10% fat emulsion and its caloric content is the same as that of standard 10% IVLE. Long-term use of propofol infusions need to be considered as part of the patient's caloric and fat intake, as propofol provides 1.1 kcal/mL. Possible effects on triglycerides should also be considered.

Peripheral parenteral nutrition (PPN)

Parenteral nutrition solutions that are intended for peripheral infusion contain the same components as central PN, but in lower concentrations. The solution is more dilute than a central solution (600 to 900 mOsm/L), requiring larger volumes of fluid to provide nutritional therapy that still may fall short of the patient's energy and protein requirements. The inclusion of calorie-rich IV fat emulsion will increase the energy content of the PPN, but it remains difficult to achieve therapy goals. The use of PPN is controversial as the risk versus benefit can be argued. PPN is challenging because of frequent episodes of phlebitis in superficial veins potentially requiring the peripheral access site to be changed every 2 to 3 days. PPN is often used in patients with mild to moderate malnutrition for short periods of time, or as a temporary therapy until central access can be placed. Contraindications to PPN highlight the limited role of this therapy. Those contraindications include: (1) significant malnutrition, (2) severe metabolic stress, (3) large nutrient or electrolyte needs (e.g., high concentrations of potassium cannot be infused peripherally), (4) fluid restriction, (5) need for prolonged PN (more than 2 weeks), and (6) renal or hepatic compromise (Stokes and Hill, 1993).

A typical standard PPN solution will contain final concentrations ranging from 1.75% to 3.0% amino acids and from 5% to 10% dextrose plus 10% to 20% IVFE. Electrolytes, trace elements, and vitamins are also included in similar amounts as used with central PN. To avoid vein phlebitis and injury, the final concentration of dextrose should not exceed 10% in a peripheral PN and the final osmolarity should be less than 900 mOsm/L (Mirtallo, 2007).

DISEASE-SPECIFIC PRODUCTS

Specialized amino acid solutions are available to support specific medical conditions, such as renal or hepatic disease, fluid restriction, and metabolic stress. These products offer some advantages in certain situations, but their use should be under the guidance of providers familiar with their advantages, including cost versus benefit considerations. Best practice guidelines addressing the use of these products are available (ASPEN, 2002). These solutions are briefly discussed here.

Renal failure

The rationale behind amino acid solutions for renal failure is that nonessential amino acids will be recycled from urea in patients with renal disease, so these products provide primarily essential components (Barber et al, 2007). Ironically, these "essential amino acid" formulations are usually more dilute (e.g., 5.2% to 6.5%) compared to standard AA solutions (10% to 15%). This will result in the fluid-restricted patient receiving more fluid when these products are used. These products offer no significant clinical advantage in patients with renal disease (Melnick, 1996). Using smaller doses of standard amino acid solutions is often the approach used in patients affected by renal disease (Barber et al, 2007).

Hepatic failure

Patients with hepatic failure have abnormal plasma amino acid profiles, characterized by high levels of aromatic amino acids (AAAs) and low levels of branched-chain amino acids (BCAAs). It has been theorized that this abnormal profile contributes to "false neurotransmitter" synthesis and the development of encephalopathy. Hepatic failure formulas contain little or no AAAs and high concentrations of BCAAs. These formulations are sometimes called "modified" amino acids and also have limited clinically significant value (O'Keefe, 1993).

Fluid restriction

These are highly concentrated formulations (15% to 20%) that are otherwise similar in content to standard formulations (typically 10% concentration). Some electrolytes may be present in different amounts (e.g., chloride, acetate), so acid-base balances should be monitored (Barber et al, 2007).

Other modified amino acid solutions

Other products are available that also contain higher amounts of BCAAs with the theory that these amino acids are beneficial during metabolic stress because of skeletal muscle breakdown (Barber et al, 2007). Altered protein metabolism is considered a hallmark of the stressed patient. These products have been marketed for use in such conditions as trauma, burn injuries, and hypercatabolic states. Nitrogen balance has been improved in some patients receiving these products, but outcomes have not been shown to be significantly improved (Klein et al, 1997; ASPEN, 2002).

Respiratory insufficiency

Because of its large carbohydrate load, the standard PN formula administered to a critically ill patient can adversely affect the respiratory quotient (RQ). Fat emulsions can be used as an alternative source of calories, allowing for a reduction of the carbohydrate load. The production of CO_2 increases as the amount of infused glucose increases. In a patient with normal respiratory function, the effect of the infusion on the RQ is not a major consideration. However, in the patient with compromised ventilation, increasing CO_2 production may precipitate respiratory failure or may delay or prevent weaning from a ventilator. Therefore, in patients with respiratory insufficiency, maintenance caloric requirements must be defined more precisely. When a patient is being weaned from a ventilator, the caloric intake is stabilized at maintenance levels. If weaning is hindered by CO_2 retention, the carbohydrate load is reduced to provide about 60% to 70% of the maintenance caloric requirements as glucose, and 30% to 40% of requirements as lipid emulsion (Wilmore and Van Woert, 1992).

PARENTERAL NUTRITION INFUSION

Parenteral nutrition solutions should be compounded in a pharmacy using a laminar flow hood to ensure sterility. The solutions should be used immediately after preparation or refrigerated and removed 60 minutes before administration to minimize patient discomfort from infusion of the chilled solution. To reduce the risk of bacterial contamination, PN solutions must be infused or discarded within 24 hours after hanging.

Maintenance of administration sets and tubing

To assure product sterility and minimize the risk of infectious-related complications, guidelines exist for proper care of administration sets and tubing products used for PN (Mirtallo et al, 2004; INS, 2006). Those recommendations are summarized here:

- "3-in-1" (TNA) administration sets are changed every 24 hours or immediately if contamination is suspected.
- Any associated extension tubing, filters, or needleless devices should be changed along with the extension set every 24 hours. The purpose is to maintain the PN administration in a closed system.

- Administration sets used for IVFE being infused independently (not with PN solution) and periodically, such as three times a week, are discarded after each bag or bottle is infused.
- Sets used with separate IVFE units that are administered continuously shall be changed every 24 hours.
- PN formulations containing only dextrose and amino acids ("2-in-1") shall be changed every 72 hours.

Initiation and discontinuation of PN

The catheter tip location must be confirmed before initiating central PN. Before PPN is started, the peripheral site must be assessed carefully. The solution and container should be checked for leaks, cracks, clarity, discoloration, and expiration date. This visual inspection is more complex in TNA (lipid-containing) solutions because the opaque mixture makes particulates difficult, if not impossible, to see.

Parenteral nutrition solutions may be initiated and gradually increased as the patient's fluid and glucose tolerance allows, over 12 to 24 hours, until the final goal rate is reached. Similarly, when the PN solution is discontinued, it may be weaned over the same amount of time. The rationale for tapering up and down is to minimize the risk for development of hyperglycemia and rebound hypoglycemia. Changes in the rate of administration should be gradual because fluctuations in glucose levels can occur if the infusion is interrupted or irregular in rate. Initial glucose infusions should not exceed 250 g over 24 hours to allow for adequate endogenous insulin secretion. Solution administration may then be advanced to the required nutritional level, increasing by 1000 kcal/day. This approach has been recommended for patients receiving intermittent subcutaneous insulin; patients with severe liver or hepatic disease, diabetes, or pancreatic cancer; or patients taking medications that may mask the signs of hypoglycemia, such as beta-blockers (Mattox and Reiter, 2005). It has been shown that patients with normal renal function and stable baseline glucose levels are able to tolerate both abrupt initiation and abrupt discontinuation of PN (Dickerson, 1985; Kryzwda et al, 1993).

PPN solutions containing less than 10% dextrose concentration usually can be discontinued safely without a tapering regimen because of the decreased risk of rebound hypoglycemia. There are a variety of approaches to tapering a PN solution (Leupold-DeCicco and Monturo, 1996).

- *Transition feeding:* Initiate oral or enteral feeding while tapering PN concomitantly. Oral or enteral intake should provide two thirds to three fourths of the daily nutritional requirements before PN is discontinued (Krzywda, 1996).
- *Replacement with a peripheral IV:* This approach is used when a central catheter must be removed suddenly. Dextrose 5% or 10% may be initiated at the same rate of infusion.
- *Tapering technique:* Tapering the rate over 2 to 3 days may be required to reduce the incidence of rebound hypoglycemia if the patient is receiving more than 1000 kcal/day. The diagnosis, patient's condition, and length of therapy must be considered to evaluate whether tapering is necessary. The appropriate protocol for discontinuing PN has been controversial, and practice patterns vary among institutions (Dickerson, 1985; Speerhas et al, 2003). The patient may have complicating conditions that predispose him or her to hypoglycemia

following the rapid tapering of PN, such as concurrent insulin administration or existing renal or hepatic disease. In the unstressed patient, rapid tapering can be accomplished by reducing the rate by 50% during the first hour and by 50% during the second hour (Speerhas et al, 2003).

Cyclic regimens

Cyclic administration regimens involve the infusion of PN intermittently over 8 to 16 hours rather than the standard continuous infusion over a 24-hour period. Indications and benefits of cyclic infusions are presented in Box 17-4. PN can be transitioned to cyclic administration once tolerance to 24-hour continuous infusion has been obtained. The switch to cyclic infusion is accomplished by a gradual reduction in the hours of infusion, usually 1 to 4 hours a day. The hourly rate is determined by dividing the total required volume of PN by the number of hours the PN is to be infused. Cyclic PN is usually administered at a rate no higher than 200 mL/hour. The ability to tolerate the glucose and fluid volume determines how rapidly the solution can be infused. With the average patient receiving 2 to 3 L, this usually requires 12 to 16 hours to complete. Patients receiving 2 L of fluid may tolerate 8-hour infusions to maximize freedom. Cyclic infusions are generally infused at night and turned off during daytime hours.

VASCULAR ACCESS

PN solutions require access into a central vein, allowing rapid dilution of the solution to prevent phlebitis, pain, and thrombosis. Central venous access systems include subcutaneous venous ports, tunneled catheters, nontunneled catheters, and peripherally inserted central catheters. Central access generally involves insertion into one of the major veins of the upper neck or chest, with the tip located in the superior vena cava. Generally speaking, subcutaneous venous ports and tunneled catheters are used for long-term IV therapy. Nontunneled catheters and peripherally inserted central catheters are used for short-term therapy.

Guidelines for vascular access and catheter care are basically the same for PN as for any other infusion. However, it is generally recommended that access devices be dedicated solely to the use of PN to decrease potential contamination. As discussed earlier, peripheral venous access for PPN, a lower osmolar solution, should be limited to short-term or supplemental therapy especially if PPN does not provide the patient's nutrient requirements.

 ## COMPLICATIONS

Perhaps the most important complication of nutritional support is the failure to achieve the desired goals of therapy because of inadequate monitoring. The general goals of nutritional intervention are to support the lean body mass; support the structure and function of the organs to prevent nutrient deficiencies; and, perhaps most importantly, to do no harm. The nurse plays an important role in monitoring patients receiving nutritional support therapy. Measuring vital signs, recording intake and output, monitoring laboratory values, understanding the PN prescription, and observing, interpreting, and accurately reporting changes in the patient's condition and physiological responses are vital for the successful management and care of the patient.

The complications of PN may be divided into three areas: metabolic, technical, and septic. The causes, treatment, prevention, and monitoring of these types of complications are summarized in Table 17-5.

 ## PARENTERAL NUTRITION IN THE PEDIATRIC PATIENT

Nutritional support in children presents many differences from adults, including nutritional requirements and monitoring, special administration sets and access devices, different administration techniques, and unique nutritional solutions used to prepare the parenteral formulation (Testerman, 1989). This chapter will primarily focus on PN in full-term and pediatric populations. Parenteral nutrition therapy specific to high-risk, preterm neonatal infants is beyond the scope of this section, but recent reviews can provide the reader with up-to-date information related to this special patient population (Valentine and Puthoff, 2007).

Box 17-4   CYCLIC PARENTERAL NUTRITION: BENEFITS AND INDICATIONS

BENEFITS

1. Improved quality of life through resumption of normal daily activities; allows the patient freedom from pumps during daytime hours, increased psychological well-being
2. Allows for increased mobility, which maintains somatic muscle mass
3. Allows for more physiological hormonal responses and stimulation of appetite
4. Prevention or treatment of hepatotoxicities induced by continuous PN; reversal of fatty liver and enzyme level elevations and faster albumin level recovery
5. Prevention or treatment of essential fatty acid deficiency in patients receiving fat-free PN; reduced insulin levels during PN-free periods allow for lipolysis and release of essential linoleic acid

6. In hospitalized patient with limited venous access, allows uninterrupted and complete PN while freeing up IV lines for other uses during the day

INDICATIONS

1. Patients who have been stable on continuous PN and require long-term parenteral nutrition
2. Patients who are receiving home PN
3. Patients who can handle the total infusion volume in a shortened time period
4. Patients who require PN for only a portion of their nutritional needs
5. Patients who have hepatic steatosis or for its prevention

PN, Parenteral nutrition.

TABLE 17-5   Complications of Parenteral Nutrition

Cause	Symptoms/Signs*	Treatment	Prevention	Monitoring
I. METABOLIC				
A. Fluid and Electrolyte Imbalance				
1. Overhydration				
Excess fluid administration, particularly for renal insufficiency or immediately after trauma		Reduce fluid administration, provide diuretics	Initiate parenteral nutrition (PN) only after fluid balance is stable, careful intake and output (I/O) monitoring with calculation of fluid needs and intake from other sources	I/O, daily weights, blood urea nitrogen (BUN) levels, serum sodium (Na) levels, and hematocrit
2. Dehydration				
Inadequate fluid administration, overdiuresis, excessive unreplaced fluid loss		Increase fluid administration	Same as overhydration	Same as overhydration
3. Hyperkalemia				
Renal insufficiency or excessive potassium (K) administration		Reduce K or K binders provided	Careful laboratory monitoring and calculation of K levels	Serum K levels
4. Hypokalemia				
Inadequate amounts provided; increased loss from diarrhea, fistulas, and burns; increased needs related to anabolism		Adjust amount of supplement provided	Same as hyperkalemia	Same as hyperkalemia
5. Hypernatremia				
Excessive water loss		Reduce Na in infusion and fluid replacement	Avoid excessive intake and careful fluid replacement	Serum and urinary Na levels, I/O
6. Hyponatremia				
Depletion of fluid through sweating or excessive gastrointestinal (GI) losses, excessive diuretic therapy, dilutional states, including congestive heart failure (CHF) and syndrome of inappropriate antidiuretic hormone (SIADH)		Adjust fluid and Na intake as condition indicates	Provide Na replacement unless contraindicated by cardiac, renal, or fluid status	Same as hypernatremia
B. Glucose Metabolism				
1. Hyperglycemia				
Rapid infusion of concentrated dextrose solution; high-risk conditions include diabetes, sepsis, and steroid medication		Provide insulin and/or part of nonprotein calories as lipid	Slow initial administration of dextrose, reduce dextrose provided, provide insulin as needed	Frequent blood and urine determinations
2. Hypoglycemia				
Rapid discontinuation (DC) of PN		Administer dextrose	Taper PN solution; if abrupt DC occurs, hang 10% dextrose to prevent rebound hypoglycemia	Frequent blood or urine determinations especially during DC

TABLE 17-5 Complications of Parenteral Nutrition—cont'd

Cause	Symptoms/Signs*	Treatment	Prevention	Monitoring
C. Mineral Imbalance *1. Hyperphosphatemia* Seen in long-term PN with phosphorus-containing solutions; also seen in decreased renal excretion	Paresthesia of extremities, flaccid paralysis, listlessness, mental confusion, weakness, hypertension, cardiac arrhythmias, prolonged elevated phosphorus levels, which may result in tissue calcification	DC phosphorus (P); provide serum calcium (Ca) repletion	Reduce P as indicated by serum levels	Serum levels 1-2 × weekly
2. Hypophosphatemia Often seen in malnutrition; predisposing factors include alcohol abuse, diabetes mellitus, antacid ingestion, and increased phosphorus requirements of anabolism	May include respiratory distress	Administer intravenous phosphate (PO_4) or add PO_4 to solution	Use P in PN, 13.6 mmol/day; has been shown to prevent PO_4 depletion in most patients	Serum level 1-2 × weekly; more frequently with replacement
3. Hypermagnesemia Excess magnesium (Mg) administration; inability to excrete Mg because of renal insufficiency	Sharp drop in blood pressure and respiratory paralysis; cardiac toxicity progressing from increased conduction time, hypotension, and premature ventricular contractions to cardiac arrest	Remove or decrease Mg in PN; severe cases may require mechanical ventilation, dialysis, correction of fluid deficit, and administration of calcium gluconate	Restrict as appropriate	Plasma levels 1-2 × weekly; or more frequently as indicated
4. Hypomagnesemia Risk factors include diuretic use, diabetic ketoacidosis, GI disease, aminoglycoside use, alcoholism, and chemotherapy	Nonspecific symptoms; GI and neuromuscular hyperactivity, convulsions, and cardiac arrhythmia	Administer peripheral magnesium; add Mg to solution	Provide Mg in PN solution	Serum levels 1-2 × weekly during initiation of PN and weekly thereafter; more frequent monitoring may be necessary during hypomagnesium, repletion, and chemotherapy
5. Hypercalcemia Neoplasia, excess vitamin D administration, prolonged immobilization, and stress	Thirst, polyuria, muscle weakness, loss of appetite; nausea, vomiting, constipation, itching	Administer isotonic saline, provide inorganic PO_4 supplement, mithramycin, corticosteroids	Restrict as appropriate	Plasma Ca levels 1-2 × weekly
6. Hypocalcemia Decreased vitamin D intake; hypoparathyroidism; reduced Ca intake, increased GI losses, decreased PO_4 intake	Paresthesia; tetany	Provide additional amounts of Ca	Administer approximately 15 mEq daily to achieve Ca balance	Plasma Ca levels 1-2 × weekly; if serum albumin level is depressed, obtain ionized Ca level
D. Nutritional *1. Carbohydrate Overfeeding* Rapid increase of feedings above requirements, particularly in patients with compromised pulmonary or cardiac function	CO_2 retention, cardiac tamponade	Decrease infusion to acceptable level	Carefully calculate nutrient requirements; ensure appropriate distribution of energy substrate	Respiratory quotients may help determine proper energy substrate mix

(Continued)

TABLE 17-5 Complications of Parenteral Nutrition—cont'd

Cause	Symptoms/Signs*	Treatment	Prevention	Monitoring
2. Protein Overfeeding				
Continued infusion of protein in excess of requirements	Elevated BUN levels; excess nitrogen excretion	Reduce amino acid content	Carefully calculate protein requirements; provide adequate calories from carbohydrate and/or fat	Serum BUN levels 1-2× weekly; nitrogen balance weekly
3. Essential Fatty Acid Deficiency				
Inadequate fat intake; biochemical signs appear 1-2 weeks on fat-free regimen	Dermatitis; alopecia; changes in pulmonary, neurological, and red cell membranes	Provide lipid emulsion at least 2× weekly	Provide 2%-4% of caloric needs as linoleic acid, or 8%-10% of calories from fat; fat intake achieved by 500 mL of 10% fat emulsion 2-3× weekly	Physical examination for symptoms
4. Thiamine Deficiency				
Concentrated glucose infusion without adequate thiamine	Elevated blood and urine lactate and pyruvate levels, abnormal ECG, cardiomegaly, and dyspnea	Adequate thiamine intake per intravenous RDA	Provide thiamine daily in PN	Blood and urine lactate and pyruvate levels 2× weekly in patients at risk
E. Hepatic				
1. Fatty Liver				
Presumed to be infusion of carbohydrate in excess of hepatic oxidative capacity; overfeeding of calories and/or fat	Moderate elevation shown in liver function tests	Reduce amount of carbohydrate administration; cycling of PN has been tried, but results are inconclusive; rule out (R/O) other causes	Balanced nutrient solutions containing energy from carbohydrate and fat; avoid overfeeding	Liver function tests at least 1× weekly
2. Cholestasis				
Unknown	Progressive increases in total serum bilirubin level; elevated serum alkaline phosphatase level	Prevent overfeeding; known to resolve at DC of PN and return to normal diet; R/O other cause	Use GI tract if possible	Liver function tests at least 1× weekly
F. Refeeding Syndrome				
Initiation of PN, especially in severely malnourished patients	Acute fluxes: fluid-dependent edema, CHF, pulmonary edema Electrolytes—decreased serum K, P, Mg, as result of intracellular shift; water-soluble vitamin deficiency, glucose intolerance as lethargy, weakness, and confusion	Adjust electrolytes, minerals, and vitamins as needed Administer diuretics as needed	Careful initiation and slow advancement of PN Careful monitoring during first 24-48 hr of PN therapy	Serum electrolyte monitoring daily and more frequently as indicated during PN initiation
II. TECHNICAL **A. Pneumothorax**				
Venous anomalies; inexperience with catheter placement technique		Small pneumothorax may resolve untreated Larger pneumothorax may require chest tube placement	Experience with catheter placement is necessary; some institutions ensure this by restricting privileges for central line insertion	Chest x-ray is performed and line placement is confirmed before line is used
B. Air Embolism				
Central line interrupted and patient inspires air while line is open	Dyspnea, cyanosis, chest pain, tachycardia, elevated central venous pressure, disorientation, shock, coma, cardiac arrest	High death rate if immediate action not taken Place patient in reverse Trendelenburg's position on left side immediately	Proper dressing and catheter care techniques; proper training of patient and caregivers	Observe for signs and symptoms

TABLE 17-5 Complications of Parenteral Nutrition—cont'd

Cause	Symptoms/Signs*	Treatment	Prevention	Monitoring
C. Catheter Embolization				
Pulling catheter back through needle used for insertion		Catheter snare technique or surgical removal of catheter tip	Remove needle and catheter at same time	Ensure catheter is intact when removed; if not obtain chest x-ray
D. Venous Thrombosis				
Mechanical trauma to vein; hypotension; infection; solution osmolality or precipitates		Urokinase, streptokinase, catheter change	Proper selection of catheter material; addition of heparin to PN	Observe corresponding arm for swelling
E. Catheter Occlusion				
Failure to flush catheter with heparin; fibrin sheath formation; precipitate formation	Inability to aspirate blood Resistance to flushing; sluggish infusion Tissue plasminogen activator (TPA)	Urokinase, streptokinase, catheter change	Proper catheter care	Observe for inability to infuse
III. SEPTIC **A. Catheter-Related Sepsis**				
Improper technique in catheter insertion; infusion of contaminated solution; multiple-line violation and manipulation; skin colonization adjacent to catheter site; hematogenous seeding of catheter by bloodborne organisms from other distant infections	Unexplained fever; chills; red, indurated area or purulent discharge around catheter site; positive catheter tip culture and positive blood culture to confirm infection	Removal of catheter and replacement at another site and concurrent antibiotic therapy	Strict adherence to aseptic technique during line insertion, line manipulation, and catheter care	Monitor for signs and symptoms; assess for glucose intolerance as possible early warning sign of impending sepsis

*For the symptoms/signs of Fluid and Electrolyte Imbalance and Glucose Metabolism, refer to Chapter 11: Fluids and Electrolytes.

Malnutrition is a problem in hospitalized pediatric patients and has been estimated to be as high as 25% (Hendricks et al, 1995; Wessel et al, 2005). Parenteral nutritional therapy must be modified in pediatric patients to meet the special demands of growth and development. These increased needs often result in greater nutritional requirements on a per-kilogram basis when compared to adults, attributable to a higher basal metabolic rate per unit of body weight, increased evaporative fluid losses, and immature kidneys with decreased clearance (Taylor and O'Neill, 1991). Additionally, pediatric patients have lower nutrient reserves compared to adults. Thus the tolerance period of starvation for a neonate ranges from 1 to 5 days, compared with 7 to 10 days in the older child or adult.

A complete nutritional assessment of the pediatric patient is indicated in cases of recent weight loss greater than 10% (excluding dehydration), weight/height ratio below the 5th percentile, serum albumin level less than 3.5 g/dL, and a diagnosis associated with the development of protein-calorie malnutrition (Hennies et al, 1996). Similar to the adult, nutritional assessment of the pediatric patient includes medical and dietary history, physical examination, and review of clinical growth charts. The Centers for Disease Control and Prevention (CDC) most recently updated these curves and these are representative standards for American children (CDC, 2008). The charts include expected growth curves based on age, gender, weight-for-age, weight-for-height, length-for-age, head circumference, and others (Davis and Stanko-Kline, 2003). Each of these measurements has a potentially important and distinct role in the

nutritional assessment. For example, excessive weight-for-age indicates the child is overweight, underweight-for-age is seen with acute malnutrition, and weight-to-height ratio evaluates body weight in proportion to height and is used to differentiate wasting from dwarfism (WHO Working Group, 1986). Head circumference is used to assess brain growth and screen for specific developmental and neurological disorders. Serious malnutrition during critical stages of brain development may affect this measurement (Hennies et al, 1996). However, head circumference is the last anthropometric marker to be affected by nutritional status (Davis and Stanko-Kline, 2003). Visceral protein stores are evaluated by determining serum albumin, serum transferrin, prealbumin, and retinol-binding protein levels (Taylor and O'Neill, 1991). Finally, a complete nutritional assessment of the pediatric patient may also include other biochemical measurements such as vitamin levels, phosphorus, trace elements, and iron deficiency anemia screening. It is important to remember that normal values for these tests differ between adults and pediatrics and also vary depending on the age of the child. Also, some tests may be utilized differently in children, such as alkaline phosphatase level, which may be decreased if a child is zinc deficient (Davis and Stanko-Kline, 2003).

INDICATIONS

When the GI tract can absolutely not be used, PN is indicated. Most pediatric patients requiring PN fall into two major categories: (1) patients with congenital or acquired anomalies

Box 17-5   INDICATIONS FOR PEDIATRIC PARENTERAL NUTRITION

- Paralytic ileus
- Necrotizing enterocolitis
- Severe acute pancreatitis
- Gastroschisis
- Malrotation/volvulus
- Severe inflammatory bowel disease
- Omphalocele
- Short-gut syndrome
- Congenital malformation
- Intestinal atresia
- Chronic idiopathic intestinal pseudo-obstruction
- Severe Hirschsprung's disease
- Microvillus inclusion disease
- Small bowel ischemia
- Severe motility/absorptive/secretory disorders
- Gardner's syndrome
- Hypermetabolism with limited enteral tolerance and/or access:
  - Sepsis
  - Multisystem organ failure
  - Multiple or major trauma
  - Malignancy, bone marrow transplantation
  - Severe burns

From Matarese LE, Gottschlich MM, editors: *Contemporary nutrition support practice: a clinical guide*, ed 2, St Louis, 2003, Saunders.

TABLE 17-6   Nutrient Requirements

Category	Age or weight	Amount per 24 hours
Fluid	0-10 kg	100 mL/kg
	11-20 kg	1000 mL + 50 mL/kg over 10 kg
	>20 kg	1500 mL + 20 mL/kg over 20 kg
	High-risk neonate	120-150 kcal/kg
Calories	Infants (birth-1 yr)	90-120 kcal/kg
	Children (1-7 yr)	75-90 kcal/kg
	Children (7-12 yr)	60-75 kcal/kg
	Adolescents (12-18 yr)	30-60 kcal/kg
	Adults (>18 yr)	25-30 kcal/kg
Fats	Infants	0.5-3.0 g/kg
	Children	0.5-3.0 g/kg
Protein	Low birth weight	3.0-4.0 g/kg
	Infants, full term	2.0-3.0 g/kg
	1-10 yr	1.0-1.2 g/kg
	Adolescence (boys/girls)	0.9/0.8 g/kg
	Children	2.0-3.0 g/kg
	Critically ill child/ adolescent	1.5 g/kg

Adapted from ASPEN Board of Directors and the Clinical Task Force: Guidelines for the use of parenteral and enteral nutrition in adult and pediatric patients, *J Parenter Enter Nutr* 26(suppl):1SA-138SA, 2002; Hazinski MF: *Nursing care of the critically ill child*, ed 2, St. Louis, 1992, Mosby.

of the GI tract, and (2) patients with intractable diarrhea syndromes. A list of conditions that may require PN is provided in Box 17-5.

NUTRITIONAL REQUIREMENTS

A thorough assessment of the pediatric patient's nutritional needs should be done before initiating any nutritional plan, including PN (ASPEN, 2005b). Multiple tables and methods of calculating nutritional requirements of protein, carbohydrates, and total calories exist. Tables 17-6 and 17-7 are representative of customary recommendations for these nutrients. Nutritional needs can vary based on multiple variables in pediatric patients and these tables provide guidelines and should be used in conjunction with clinical judgment. Objective measurements, such as indirect calorimetry and urinary nitrogen assays, should be considered when available to decrease the risk of overfeeding (Thomson et al, 1995). The Harris-Benedict equation, often used in adults to predict energy needs, should only be used in postpubescent adolescents, as it does not include a validated growth factor for younger patients (Davis and Stanko-Kline, 2003).

Fluid requirement estimations are important to prevent both over- and underhydration. Many factors can affect requirements in pediatrics, such as heat shields, thermal blankets, phototherapy, and radiant warmers. Fluid and hydration status should be evaluated each day (Davis and Stanko-Kline, 2003). Calculations used to determine fluid requirements in pediatric patients are as follows: 100 mL/kg for children weighing 3 to 10 kg; 1000 mL + 50 mL/kg for each kilogram over 10 kg for children weighing 11 to 20 kg; and 1500 mL + 20 mL/kg for each kilogram over 20 kg for children weighing 20 kg (Hennies et al, 1996).

Current recommendations for the caloric components in pediatric nutritional supplementation are that carbohydrates make up 40% to 50% of total calories, protein 15%, and fat 35% (Taylor and O'Neill, 1991). Peripheral PN uses 10% to 12.5% glucose and 2.5% protein. Central PN may use up to 30% glucose and 3.5% protein (Hennies et al, 1996).

Protein requirements in pediatrics vary according to age. Neonate and infant requirements range from 2.0 to 4.0 g/kg body weight parenterally per day. Infant protein requirements gradually decrease to 1.0 to 1.2 g/kg body weight per day by 12 months of age until about 10 years of age, and then decline again slightly in adolescence (Warner, 1991; ASPEN, 2002). Clinically, to accommodate for metabolic stress, it is common to provide hospitalized children 1.5 g/kg/day of protein (Shew and Jaksic, 1999). When protein requirements for pediatrics are compared to adults on a weight basis, the recommendations are higher for neonates and children. Also, amino acids such as histidine, tyrosine, and cysteine, which are nonessential in adults, may be essential for infants and young children because of a limited ability to synthesize them in the body. This explains why some of these protein sources (e.g., cysteine) are found in high concentrations in breast milk (ASPEN, 2002). Special amino acid formulations for pediatric PN formulations contain both essential and nonessential components to meet these needs. A positive nitrogen balance usually requires 200 kcal/g of nitrogen in children.

Fats are necessary to prevent essential fatty acid deficiency (EFAD). Children require approximately 1% to 2% essential fatty acids in their diet. EFAD develops more rapidly in children than in adults, in as little as 1 week using fat-free solutions. The use of lipids may be harmful in the infant with jaundice. Fatty acids displace bilirubin from albumin and produce unbound bilirubin, which increases the risk of kernicterus (Warner,

TABLE 17-7	Nutritional Requirements for the Pediatric Patient

Requirements	Term infants and children (Dose/Day)
Vitamins (Lipid Soluble)	
Vitamin A	700 mcg (retinol equivalent)
Vitamin E	7 mg
Vitamin K	200 mcg
Vitamin D	10 mcg (400 IU)
Vitamins (Water Soluble)	
Ascorbic acid (Vitamin C)	80 mg
Thiamin (Vitamin B_1)	1.2 mg
Riboflavin	1.4 mg
Pyridoxine (Vitamin B_6)	1.0 mg
Niacin	17 mg
Pantothenic acid	5 mg
Biotin	20 mcg
Folic Acid	140 mcg
Cyanocobalamin (Vitamin B_{12})	1.0 mcg
Trace Elements	
Chromium	0.2 mcg/kg
Copper	20 mcg/kg
Iodine	1 mcg/kg
Iron	Maintenance dose not established
Electrolytes and Minerals	
Sodium	2-4 mEq/kg
Potassium	2-4 mEq/kg
Chloride	2-4 mEq/kg
Magnesium	0.25-1.0 mEq/kg
Calcium	0.45-3.15 mEq/kg
Phosphorus	0.5-2.0 mmol/kg

Adapted from ASPEN Board of Directors and the Clinical Task Force: Guidelines for the use of parenteral and enteral nutrition in adult and pediatric patients, *J Parenter Enter Nutr* 26(suppl):1SA-138SA, 2002; Davis AM, Stanko-Kline R: Pediatrics. In Matarese LE, Gottschlich MM, editors: *Contemporary nutrition support practice: a clinical guide,* St Louis, 2003, Saunders.

1991). To prevent ketonemia, no more than 60% of nonprotein calories should be from fats.

Vitamins and trace elements for infants and young children

Vitamins are essential in the pediatric PN formula. Separate recommendations for adult and pediatric formulations were updated in 1988 by the AMA's Nutrition Advisory Group and the American Society of Clinical Nutrition (Greene et al, 1988). Commercially available products for pediatric MVI injections differ for children less than 11 years of age. After the age of 11, the addition of vitamin K (phytonadione) is recommended (ASPEN, 2002). Requirements for electrolytes and minerals depend on such factors as diuretic administration, electrolyte losses, hydration, and renal function. As stated earlier, a greater need for these minerals exists in early infancy. Trace elements (zinc, copper, selenium, chromium, and

manganese) should routinely be added to pediatric PN solutions (Leung, 1995; ASPEN, 2002). Molybdenum is another trace element that affects protein synthesis, metabolism, and growth. While not routinely supplemented in PN, it may be necessary to include in long-term PN in pediatrics (Friel et al, 1999).

ADMINISTRATION
Vascular access

The basic principles of vascular access and catheter care for adults also apply to pediatric patients. A major responsibility is maintaining asepsis and preventing technical problems with the catheter, which is the most common complication requiring interruption of therapy in children (Warner, 1991). Signs of sepsis in the neonate include lethargy, fluctuating temperature, increased serum bilirubin level, and increased metabolic complications, such as hyperglycemia while on the same formulation that has been tolerated in the past (Davis and Stanko-Kline, 2003).

Monitoring

Initial management of pediatric patients receiving PN includes strict measurement of intake and output and measurements of daily weights, temperature, stool frequency and consistency, and daily electrolytes. In addition to urine glucose measurements, serum glucose measurements may be done every 8 to 12 hours initially. Serum triglyceride and free fatty acid levels are measured weekly. Liver function tests are performed biweekly. Growth determinations include routine measurements of weight, height, head circumference, and anthropometric measurements for the duration of therapy. It is not uncommon for substrate adjustments to be necessary during long-term PN in pediatrics to support normal growth cycles.

Many children require long-term (greater than 4 weeks) PN support at home. The potential accumulation of aluminum must be considered in these patients as some PN components contain high levels of aluminum, such as intravenous calcium, phosphorus, and albumin solutions. Accumulation of aluminum in bone, which can occur as early as 3 weeks, can result in metabolic bone disease, encephalopathy, and cholestasis (Popinska et al, 1999). The FDA requires that the aluminum content in amino acid solutions, concentrated dextrose solutions, and sterile water for injection be less than 25 mcg/L (Kumpf and Gervasio, 2007).

Metabolic complications

As in the adult patient, metabolic complications in the pediatric patient are generally related to disorders of glucose metabolism or to deficiencies of specific components in the solution. Additionally, fluid status is important to monitor in a pediatric patient, as this patient population is vulnerable to both overhydration and underhydration (Davis and Stanko-Kline, 2003). Hepatobiliary dysfunction is one of the more common complications, second only to technical complications of the catheter. A pattern of cholestasis is seen with conjugated hyperbilirubinemia and an early elevation of serum glutamyltransferase (GGT) level (Warner, 1991). This cholestasis can appear in pediatric patients after 2 weeks of PN (Davis and Stanko-Kline, 2003). Management includes decreasing protein intake, cycling the infusion, and providing minimal amounts of enteral feeding if possible.

HOME PARENTERAL NUTRITION

Home parenteral nutrition (HPN) therapy was first attempted in 1967 and although the patient survived only a few months, a new conceptual advance was established, extending hospital care into the home setting (Shils et al, 1970). While HPN is a complex component of modern home health care, compared to patients receiving similar therapy in a hospitalized setting, it has been shown to be cost-effective (Marshall et al, 2005). Today, approximately 40,000 patients are receiving PN at home (Ireton-Jones et al, 2003).

CANDIDATE IDENTIFICATION

In a majority of cases, home PN patients are transitioned from a hospital to home on nutritional therapy. Because of the complexity of HPN, planning for continuation of PN at home begins very early in the patient's hospitalization. It is increasingly important to recognize candidates for HPN early as hospital length of stays continue to shorten, not only as a result of improved ambulatory and home care services but also because of diminished reimbursement from third-party payers. Patients who are candidates for HPN are otherwise medically stable and do not require frequent or drastic changes in their PN formulation.

In addition to a suitable home situation from an environmental standpoint (Box 17-6), four major factors in successful HPN have been identified (Lin, 1991). The first factor is patient acceptance of this therapy in the home environment. Patients must be motivated and committed to being an active participant in their home health care. Without the desire and dedication to make the necessary changes in lifestyle required by HPN, patient compliance and the therapy outcome will suffer. Attention to possible mental health consequences (depression, alteration in body image, anxiety, fear) should be included in the ongoing emotional assessment of the home PN patient. Short- or long-term HPN will potentially affect quality of life, and acceptance of therapy varies by patient (Smith, 1993). Psychological counseling should be considered if indicated.

Second, the financial impact must be considered. Although less expensive than hospitalization, the cost is considerable and the patient's available insurance coverage must be investigated before initiation of therapy. It is not prudent to assume that HPN will be covered by the patient's insurance or government agencies (DeLegge and Ireton-Jones, 2007). Guidelines vary among regional providers and are changing with the current concerns over health care costs and reforms. Declaration of disability or application for medical assistance may be necessary. Case management strategies may be implemented to help the patient and family meet the financial burden.

Third, the patient and/or caregiver must have the capability to understand and be willing to participate in the program at home. Physically, they must possess adequate eyesight and dexterity to manipulate the equipment and maintain catheter care.

Fourth, there must be adequate long-term central IV access for infusion of the solution. Peripheral venous access is only appropriate in home PN as a short-term solution until central access is available (ASPEN, 2005a).

INDICATIONS

Depending on the reason for HPN, patients may receive either short- or long-term therapy. While most HPN patients receive therapy for less than 6 months for short-term bowel rest, some may receive therapy for the rest of their lives (DeLegge and Ireton-Jones, 2007). In general, indications for HPN mimic those for hospitalized patients, but home care patients differ in that overall they are stable enough to be managed at home. Disease states in which HPN may be indicated include the following:

- Short-bowel syndrome
- Functional, mechanical, or pseudo-obstruction
- Fistulas
- Chronic radiation enteritis
- Inflammatory bowel disease
- Congenital bowel defects
- Carefully selected malignancy patients
- Disorders of malabsorption, including sprue, pancreatitis, and cystic fibrosis

---

Box 17-6   HOME ASSESSMENT CRITERIA FOR PARENTERAL NUTRITION

Electricity	Is electricity available in the home and is it compatible with the use of an infusion pump (i.e., three-pronged outlet)? Is there frequent interruption of the electrical service that would warrant the use of a backup pump? Does the infusion pump have sufficient battery backup? Has the electric company been notified about the presence of medical equipment in the house?
Refrigeration	Is a refrigerator available for storage of the PN solutions and, if so, can it accommodate 1 to 2 weeks of PN and related supplies?
Telephone	Is a telephone available for emergency calls to the nursing/home infusion agency or ambulance service?
Water	Is water available for cleaning preparation areas and for handwashing?
General cleanliness	Is the home free of insects and rodents? Is there an area that can be used for supply storage that is secure from children and pets?
Safety issues	How difficult is it for the patient to get from the bedroom to the bathroom? Can an intravenous pole and pump be maneuvered into the bathroom or does the patient need a bedside commode?
	Are there stairs that need to be negotiated during the infusion period? Do area rugs pose a safety threat?
	Is there an area for sharps disposal that can be placed out of reach of small children?

From Ireton-Jones C, DeLegge M, Epperson L et al: Management of the home parenteral nutrition patient, *Nutr Clin Pract* 18:310-317, 2003.

- Acquired immunodeficiency syndrome
- Dysmotility disorders

ADMINISTRATION CONSIDERATIONS

Infusion devices used for HPN range from the larger devices commonly seen in the hospital setting to small, compact, battery-operated devices suitable for the more ambulatory patient. Devices for the home patient should be user-friendly and should have various safety features, including sophisticated alarm systems, variable pressure settings, and tapering features that allow programmed rate changes during the infusion. Tapering programmability allows patients receiving cyclic therapy to taper infusion rates automatically within a given time and volume at the beginning and end of their daily infusion. Tapering at the beginning and end of infusions allows for gradual increase and decrease in insulin production to prevent hyperglycemia and hypoglycemia.

HPN solutions are individualized according to the patient's specific needs. The solutions have a stability that typically allows 1 week's supply to be delivered and stored in the patient's home refrigerator and are usually supplied by a home infusion pharmacy. Parenteral nutrition solutions that do not contain lipids may have a longer shelf life.

Dual-chamber PN bags provide the lipid component in a separate chamber from the protein and carbohydrate solutions. A rigid divider between the two chambers is disengaged just before administration, allowing the solutions to mix. Keeping the solutions separate increases shelf life and may make the solution viable for up to 2 weeks (Figure 17-2).

Parenteral nutrition solutions should be taken out of refrigeration and left at room temperature 1 to 2 hours before administration to decrease hypothermic infusion effects. Because of short stability, multivitamins (MVI) is added daily by the patient or caregiver to the rest of the solution just before infusion. Once the MVI has been added, the infusion should be used within 24 hours.

Continuous infusions are the least desirable in the home care setting but may be required because of caloric need, glucose fluctuations, fluid intolerance, or underlying diseases, such as diabetes mellitus, renal disease, or cardiac dysfunction (Ireton-Jones et al, 2003). Cyclic infusions given over a period of 8 to 16 hours allow the patient flexibility and an improved quality of life (Speerhas et al, 2003). When possible, cyclic PN infusions are infused overnight while the patient sleeps.

PATIENT AND FAMILY EDUCATION

The most critical factor in the success of HPN may be the adequate education of the patient and caregiver by the clinician. Reduced complications and improved clinical outcomes have both been shown when repeated education of the patient in the home setting is emphasized (Weston-Eborn and Sitzman, 2005). Teaching is initiated using an individualized plan before discharge from the hospital and is a collaborative effort among all members of the health care team, including staff from the home care agency. Teaching methods may involve audiovisuals, mannequins, and written procedures. The patient and/or caregiver should be able to verbalize and/or demonstrate the care of a central venous access device, simple IV troubleshooting, infection control practices (handwashing, sterile technique), and emergent procedures. In the first phase of education, the patient and caregiver observe the procedure being performed by the nurse. In the second phase, the patient or caregiver performs the procedure under nursing supervision. The goal is for the learner to demonstrate proficiency in

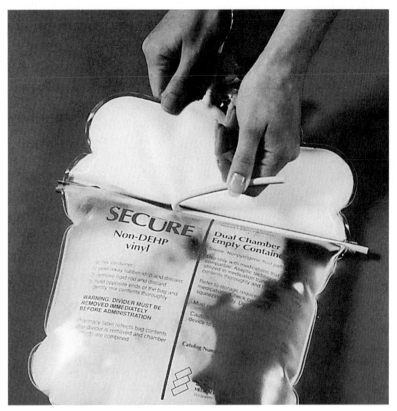

FIGURE 17-2 Dual chamber bag. (Photo courtesy Metrix Company.)

each phase of the procedure. Each training session should be adequately documented.

PATIENT MONITORING

Monitoring of patients receiving home PN requires expertise and experience in recognizing potential issues specific to this patient population. Issues to consider when monitoring home PN patients include status of the venous access device, changes in long-term nutritional goals, psychosocial considerations, caregiver reliability, and changes in medications or co-morbid disease states. As in institutional settings, a multidisciplinary approach involving physicians, nurses, pharmacists, and dietitians is desirable.

While the concept of a home nutritional support team (HNST) mimics the model used in hospitals, the approach and focus are different, as the home patient is faced with issues not apparent in the hospitalized patient. For example, a detailed physical assessment may be a more critical monitoring tool in the home setting because of the relative infrequency of laboratory testing, which often is available daily in the hospital (DeLegge and Ireton-Jones, 2007). The home care nurse should be in attendance for initially starting the infusion, assessing the home environment, evaluating the storage and work areas, and assessing the patient's and caregiver's response to discharge. Reiteration of the procedures is often necessary during the first week at home and may require frequent visits by the home care staff. Clinical self-monitoring is documented in a diary, including weight, temperature, urine or glucometer testing for glucose levels, and changes in urinary volume. Frequency of laboratory monitoring in HPN patients is controversial and also is affected by the existing comorbid disease states. There is no single, accepted standard for how often to utilize laboratory monitoring. As with the PN formulation, the monitoring plan should be individualized according to the patient's clinical condition (DeLegge and Ireton-Jones, 2007). An example plan could include laboratory monitoring of various blood levels performed once or twice weekly at first, and then less frequently as the patient becomes stable. In all cases, patients and caregivers should have 24-hour access to resources (nursing, pharmacy, dietary) to handle unexpected problems.

COMPLICATIONS

Catheter-related sepsis is the most prevalent and serious complication of home PN, as it is in patients receiving PN in the hospital. The organisms most commonly responsible for these infections include *Staphylococcus epidermidis, S. aureus,* and *Candida* species (Buchman et al, 1994). Appropriate care of the catheter site and hub and aseptic techniques are critical to minimize the risk of infections. Adequate teaching of all individuals involved with the home PN, which reinforces proper technique and the ability to recognize early signs of infection, is key. Although some catheter infections can be treated successfully with antibiotics, catheter sepsis remains the main reason for catheter removal or hospitalization (Ireton-Jones et al, 2003).

Vascular access device (VAD) occlusion may be caused by a variety of reasons, including mechanical malfunction and precipitate formation secondary to recent infusions of medications, lipids, or electrolytes. Thrombolytic agents, such as tissue plasminogen activator (tPA), have been successful in restoring patency to the occluded catheter when the obstruction or dysfunction is related to a thrombus. Catheter occlusion may also occur as a result of medication precipitates, calcium phosphate crystal precipitate, or lipid residue. Medication precipitates with a low pH can be cleared with 0.1 N hydrochloric (HCl) acid or 0.1 N sodium hydroxide. High-pH drug precipitates can be cleared using sodium bicarbonate, while ethanol 70% can be used to clear lipid residue. Routine flushing of vascular access devices is equally effective using either 0.9% sodium chloride or heparinized solutions (Breaux et al, 1987; Steiger, 2006). Depending on the location of damage, broken catheters can sometimes be repaired.

The use of long-term PN at home has been observed to produce biochemical and morphological evidence of hepatic insult. Elevations in liver function tests and occasionally bilirubin level occur. The changes are typically transient and are decreased by cyclic HPN administration, which has been shown to reduce serum hepatic enzyme and bilirubin concentrations when compared to continuous PN (Hwang, Jue and Chen, 2000).

Metabolic complications that are similar to those seen in hospitalized PN patients include disorders of glucose metabolism and fluid or volume intolerance. Complications that may be more common in long-term HPN patients include vitamin, trace element, and essential fatty acid deficiencies. These can be avoided by laboratory monitoring and adequate supplementation in the PN solution. Metabolic bone disease has been reported in long-term HPN patients, and is characterized by increased serum calcium levels, excessive losses of calcium and phosphorus in the urine, low plasma levels of vitamin D, and low-normal plasma levels of parathyroid hormone. Metabolic bone disease results in osteopenia, mild to moderate bone pain, and fractures. The etiology is unclear and likely has several contributing factors, including: (1) excess infusions of aluminum, calcium, protein or glucose; (2) cyclic versus continuous PN administration; and (3) the patient's previous nutritional state (McCullough and Hsu, 1987; Seidner and Licata, 2000). The treatment of metabolic bone disease is unclear. Some have reported a reversal of bone disease with the cessation of PN or withdrawal of vitamin D supplementation. Further research continues in this area.

Home parenteral nutrition provides a viable option for medically stable patients who require prolonged nutritional therapy. While not without risks and potential complications, it can be a safe mode of therapy that can significantly improve the quality of life for these patients. The desire to shorten hospital length of stay will likely increase the utilization of this practice in the future.

NURSING ASSESSMENT AND DIAGNOSIS

ASSESSMENT

Using the nursing process, the nurse's care of the patient receiving nutritional support begins with assessment. As noted earlier a nutritional assessment will include adequacy of nutrients provided and any potential complications related to administration of nutritional support, as well as a general physical assessment. Higher risk patients for metabolic complications during PN can include the very young and elderly; those with glucose intolerance, renal dysfunction, neurological damage, or excessive fluid loss such as fistula output or secretions; and patients who are intubated or receiving steroids or diuretics.

The nurse should also assess other factors that indicate fluid balance, such as intake and output, weight, vital signs, peripheral or dependent edema, lung sounds, appearance of mucous membranes, skin turgor, and jugular vein distention. Baseline laboratory values are obtained early in the patient's course of therapy. Daily determinations are necessary to guide the concentration and formulation of the PN solution until the patient is stable.

The nurse collaborates with the physician to ensure that tests are ordered and evaluated regularly to assess the objective status of nutrition and endocrine function. Laboratory tests measure total proteins, albumin, blood urea nitrogen, electrolytes, minerals, and vitamins. Additional laboratory tests include the serum magnesium level, complete blood count, prothrombin time, and liver function tests. All patients receiving nutrition support should have frequent assessments of blood glucose levels, as hyperglycemia is a common complication and can precipitate osmotic diuresis and hyperosmolar dehydration, and be an early symptom of sepsis.

Patients receiving PN for long periods may need a great deal of emotional support. Nutrition is normally associated with food and eating; not eating can have a major psychological effect on some people. Patients initially may have hunger pains and food cravings, even though their physiological requirements are being met. Eventually, however, appetites are suppressed by PN, and the patient needs to be assured that appetite and bowel activity gradually return to normal when the parenteral feedings are discontinued.

DIAGNOSIS

Establishing a nursing diagnosis provides an important framework for identifying problems, setting goals, initiating interventions, and evaluating outcomes. Individual patient circumstances require additional diagnoses to be formulated. The North American Nursing Diagnosis Association's (NANDA International) nursing diagnosis list is helpful in identifying an acceptable nursing diagnosis. Box 17-7 is an example of a nursing care plan for a patient receiving nutritional support.

Documentation remains an important nursing function. Documentation of information regarding the patient's status and response is critical to the success of nutrition therapy. Standardized forms may be used to record information pertinent to the patient's clinical progress, nutrition support regimen, fluid intake and output, and laboratory data, facilitating communication and documenting patient progress. Thorough documentation and evaluation of the plan of care also are important

in substantiating the appropriateness of services provided and securing proper reimbursement.

 ## ETHICAL CONSIDERATIONS

PN may be a factor in supporting and sustaining life, sometimes for long periods. As with other life-sustaining therapies, decisions to provide, withhold, or withdraw nutritional support can also provide dilemmas. The dilemma of withholding versus withdrawing therapy has been a topic of much debate and many publications. The distinction between withholding and withdrawing may lead to undertreatment if treatment is withheld to avoid having to withdraw it later. Patients may also be overtreated because physicians believe that they cannot withdraw treatment that has been started. However, there is no ethical requirement that a treatment must be continued once started, especially if the treatment is against the patient's wishes. It is admittedly more difficult to withdraw a treatment once started, especially if that action results in the patient's death. Establishing goals at the beginning of therapy and repeatedly evaluating the goals and outcomes throughout the course of therapy have been proposed as a means of guiding decision makers.

Questions about ethics continue to loom large in the health care arena, as the paradigm of physician-driven health care shifts to health care team–driven and patient-driven care. Since December of 1991, health care institutions that participate in Medicare and Medicaid have been required to provide patients with educational materials about the patient's right to terminate treatment. Today, patients are encouraged to choose a "health care proxy" or "health care agent" to act in their stead regarding health care should they become incapable of making their own decisions. Advance directives help guide the health care team and health care proxy or surrogate in determining the patient's wishes, goals, and values in the decision-making process. Because of the emotional nature of these decisions, many institutions have created ethics committees and multidisciplinary teams that consult with and assist the health care team.

The most widely accepted principles of medical ethics can be applied to these difficult situations:
- *Beneficence:* acting to benefit the patient
- *Nonmaleficence:* to do no harm
- *Autonomy:* respecting the privacy of the patient's or surrogate's rights

---

Box 17-7   EXAMPLE OF A NURSING CARE PLAN

NURSING DIAGNOSIS

Alteration in nutrition, less than body requirements

GOAL

Stabilize weight and gradually increase to 10% of ideal

INTERVENTIONS

1. Work with patient to establish a scale of weight outcomes from most desirable to least desirable.
2. Weigh patient daily and record until the desired weight is reached.

3. Administer nutrition solution as prescribed. Monitor and record intake and output.
4. Collaborate with nutrition support team to monitor and evaluate patient's nutritional status.

EXPECTED OUTCOMES

1. Weight is stabilized (immediate outcome).
2. Weight gain is 1 pound every 3 weeks, increasing to 1 pound every 2 weeks (most desirable outcome).

- *Disclosure:* providing adequate, intelligible, and truthful information for making medical decisions
- *Social justice:* allocating medical resources justly and equitably according to medical need, exercising reasonable economic stewardship, and with social sensitivity.

In 1992 the American Nurses Association (ANA) *Code of Ethics* recognized anorexia and reduced appetite as a normal component of the dying process (ANA, 1992). In addition, a distinction was made between oral food and water and artificial hydration and nutrition. These ANA statements note no obligation to use extraordinary measures such as specialized nutrition support in the dying patient. ASPEN encourages providers to be familiar with the benefits and burdens of specialized nutrition support (Andrews and Geppert, 2007). It is recommended that patients be encouraged to develop advance directives, recognizing their right to decline artificial fluids and nutrition in certain circumstances.

As with all ongoing debates regarding end-of-life issues, the ideal scenario is decisions be made by the patient or proxy and health care team, with the assistance of the ethics committee. With nutritional support experts armed with research demonstrating clear clinical efficacy, knowledgeable patients and surrogates, a health care team comfortable with their own end-of-life issues, and a supportive ethics committee all working in unison, decisions can be made in a respectful, peaceful, and dignified atmosphere.

SUMMARY

Quality nutrition support is enhanced by specialized training in nutrition, vascular access, and disease management. Infusion therapy nurses are knowledgeable in these areas and often are involved in providing PN. In addition, specialized certification in nutrition support nursing is available from the National Board of Nutrition Support Certification (DiMaria-Ghalili et al, 2007). PN is also a core content area assessed in the CRNI® (Certified Registered Nurse Infusion) exam. While credentialing has elevated the recognition of the nutrition support nurse as a skilled health care professional, it has also provided a framework for professional growth within the field of nursing and competent patient care.

The role of nursing for patient advocacy in nutrition support can be traced back to 1859 and Florence Nightingale, who is credited with noting the relationship between nourishment and its effect on sustaining life (Guenter et al, 2003). This understanding of the role of nutrition as a mitigating factor in disease has evolved over the past 150 years into the modern science of nutrition support. Today, the field of nutrition support is an interdisciplinary science that involves the collegiality of physicians, dietitians, pharmacists, research scientists, and nurses. Throughout time, nursing has been a pioneer in nutrition support and remains a key member of the nutrition support team.

REFERENCES

American Medical Association: Guidelines for essential trace element preparations for parenteral use: a statement by the nutrition advisory group, *J Parenter Enter Nutr* 3:263-267, 1979.

American Nurses Association: *American Nursing Association code of ethics*, 1992. Accessed 3/12/08 at http://nursingworld.org/ethics/code/protected_nwcoe813.htm.

American Society of Parenteral and Enteral Nutrition: Safe practices for parenteral nutrition, *J Parenter Enter Nutr* 28:S39-S70, 2004.

Anderson AG, Palmer D, MacFie J: Peripheral parenteral nutrition, *Br J Surg* 90:1048-1054, 2003.

Andrews MR, Geppert CM: Ethics. In Gottschlich MM, editor: *The ASPEN nutrition support core curriculum* (pp 740-760), Silver Spring, Md, 2007, ASPEN.

Andris DA: Substrate metabolism—micronutrients. In Hennessy KA, Orr ME, editors: *Nutrition support nursing*, ed 3, Silver Spring, Md, 1996, ASPEN.

ASPEN Board of Directors: Guidelines for the use of parenteral and enteral nutrition in adult and pediatric patients, *J Parenter Enter Nutr* 17 (suppl):7SA, 1993.

ASPEN Board of Directors and the Clinical Task Force: Guidelines for the use of parenteral and enteral nutrition in adult and pediatric patients, *J Parenter Enter Nutr* 26 (suppl):1SA-138SA, 2002.

ASPEN Board of Directors and the Standards for Specialized Nutrition Support Task Force: Standards for specialized nutrition support: home care patients, *Nutr Clin Pract* 20:579-590, 2005a.

ASPEN Board of Directors and the Standards for Specialized Nutrition Support Task Force: Standards for specialized nutrition support: hospitalized pediatric patients, *Nutr Clin Pract* 20:103-116, 2005b.

ASPEN Board of Directors and the Standards Committee: Definition of terms, style, and conventions used in ASPEN guidelines and standards, *Nutr Clin Pract* 20:281-285, 2005c.

Baccaro F, Moreno JB, Borlenghi C et al: Subjective global assessment in the clinical setting, *J Parenter Enter Nutr* 31:406-409, 2007.

Barber JR, Rollins CJ, Sacks GS: Parenteral nutrition formulations. In Gottschlich MM, editor: *The ASPEN nutrition support core curriculum* (pp 277-299), Silver Spring, Md, 2007, ASPEN.

Berg JM, Tymoczko JL, Stryer L, editors: *Biochemistry*, New York, 2002, WH Freeman.

Block GA, Port FK: Re-evaluation of risks associated with hyperphosphatemia and hyperparathyroidism in dialysis patients: recommendations for a change in management, *Am J Kidney Dis* 35:1226-1237, 2000.

Boosalis MG: Vitamins. In Matarese LE, Gottschlich MM, editors: *Contemporary nutrition support practice: a clinical guide* (pp 145-163), St Louis, 2003, Saunders.

Breaux CW et al: Calcium phosphate crystal occlusion of central venous catheters used for total parenteral nutrition in infants and children: prevention and treatment, *J Pediatr Surg* 22:829, 1987.

Brooks MJ, Melnik G: The refeeding syndrome: an approach to understanding its complications and preventing its occurrence, *Pharmacotherapy* 15:713-726, 1995.

Buchman AL, Moukarzel A, Goodson B et al: Catheter-related infections associated with home parenteral nutrition and predictive factors for the need for catheter removal in their treatment, *J Parenter Enter Nutr* 18:297-302, 1994.

Camilo ME, Jatio A, O'Brien M et al: Bioavailability of phylloquinone from an intravenous lipid emulsion, *Am J Clin Nutr* 67:716-721, 1998.

Campos ACL, Paluzzi M, Meguid MM: Clinical use of total nutrient admixtures, *Nutrition* 6:347-356, 1990.

Centers for Disease Control and Prevention: Guidelines for the prevention of intravascular catheter-related infections, *MMWR* 51 (RR-10):1-28, 2002 [erratum 51:711, 2002].

Centers for Disease Control and Prevention: *National Center for Health Statistics (NCHS). 2000 CDC growth charts: United States*. Accessed 3/8/08 at http://www.cdc.gov/growthcharts.

Clark SF: Vitamins and trace elements. In Gottschlich MM, editor: *The ASPEN nutrition support core curriculum* (pp 129-159), Silver Spring, Md, 2007, ASPEN.

Colaizzo-Anas T: Nutrient intake, digestion, absorption, and excretion, In Gottschlich MM, editor: *The ASPEN nutrition support core curriculum* (pp 3-18), Silver Spring, Md, 2007, ASPEN.

Cresci GA, Gottschlich MM, Mayes T et al: Trauma, surgery, and burns, In Gottschlich MM, editor: *The ASPEN nutrition support core curriculum* (pp 129-159), Silver Spring, Md, 2007, ASPEN.

Culebras JM, Martin-Pena G, Garcia-de-Lorenzo A et al: Practical aspects of peripheral parenteral nutrition, *Curr Opin Nutr Metab Care* 7:303-307, 2004.

Curtas S: Nutrition assessment of the adult. In Hennessy KA, Orr ME, editors: *Nutrition support nursing*, ed 3, Silver Springs, Md, 1996, ASPEN.

Davis AM, Stanko-Kline R: Pediatrics. In Matarese LE, Gottschlich MM, editors: *Contemporary nutrition support practice: a clinical guide* (pp 357-375), St Louis, 2003, Saunders.

DeBiasse-Fortin MA: Minerals and trace elements. In Matarese LE, Gottschlich MM, editors: *Contemporary nutrition support practice: a clinical guide* (pp 164-172), St Louis, 2003, Saunders.

DeLegge MH, Drake LM: Nutritional assessment, *Gastroenterol Clin North Am* 36:1-22, 2007.

DeLegge MH, Ireton-Jones C: Home care. In Gottschlich MM, editor: *The ASPEN nutrition support core curriculum* (pp 725-739), Silver Spring, Md, 2007, ASPEN.

Detsky AS, McLaughlin JR, Baker JP et al: What is subjective global assessment of nutritional status? *J Parenter Enter Nutr* 11:8-13, 1987.

Dickerson RN: How fast can I taper a TPN in a hospitalized patient? *Hosp Pharm* 20:620-621, 1985.

Dickerson RN, Brown RO, White KG: Parenteral nutrition solutions. In Rombeau JL, Caldwell MD, editors: *Clinical nutrition: parenteral nutrition*, ed 2, Philadelphia, 1993, WB Saunders.

DiMaria-Ghalili RA, Bankhead R, Fisher AA et al: Standards of practice for nutrition support nurses, *Nutr Clin Pract* 22:458-465, 2007.

Dudrick SJ: History of vascular access, *J Parenter Enter Nutr* 30:S47-S56, 2006.

Dudrick SJ, Wilmore DW, Vars HM et al: Can intravenous feeding as the sole means of nutrition support growth in the child and restore weight loss in an adult? An affirmative answer, *Ann Surg* 169:974-984, 1969.

Earthman C, Traughber D, Dobratz J et al: Bioimpedance spectroscopy for clinical assessment of fluid distribution and body cell mass, *Nutr Clin Pract* 22:(4)389-405, 2007.

Food and Drug Administration: Safety alert: hazards of precipitation associated with parenteral nutrition, *Am J Hosp Pharm* 51:1427-1428, 1994.

Friel JK, MacDonald AC, Mercer CN et al: Molybdenum requirements in low-birth-weight infants receiving parenteral and enteral nutrition, *J Parenter Enter Nutr* 23(3):155-159, 1999.

Fuhrman MP, Charney P, Mueller CM: Hepatic proteins and nutrition assessment, *J Am Diet Assoc* 104:1258-1264, 2004.

Furst P, Stehle P: Are intravenous amino acid solutions unbalanced? *New Horizons* 2:215-223, 1994.

Gallager ML: Vitamins. In Mahan LK, Escott-Stump S, editors: *Food, nutrition, and diet therapy* (pp 75-119), ed 11, Philadelphia, 2004, Saunders.

Gottschlich MM, Mayes T: Micronutrients. In Skipper A, editor: *Dietitian's handbook of enteral and parenteral nutrition*, ed 2, Gaithersburg, Md, 1998, Aspen.

Greene HL, Hambidge KM, Schanler R et al: Guidelines for the use of vitamins, trace elements, calcium, manganese, and phosphorus in infants and children receiving total parenteral nutrition. Report of the Subcommittee on Pediatric Parenteral Nutrient Requirements from the Committee on Clinical Practice Issues of the American Society for Clinical Nutrition, *Am J Clin Nutr* 48:1324-1342, 1988.

Guenter P, Curtas S, Murphy L et al: The impact of nursing practice on the history and effectiveness of total parenteral nutrition, *J Parenter Enter Nutr* 28(1):54-59, 2003.

Hasenboehler E, Williams A, Leinhase I et al: Metabolic changes after polytrauma: an imperative for early nutritional support, *World J Emerg Surg* 1:29, 2006.

Hendricks KM, Duggan C, Gallagher I et al: Malnutrition in hospitalized pediatric patients: current prevalence, *Arch Pediatr Adolesc Med* 149:1118, 1995.

Hennies GA et al: Pediatrics. In Hennessy KA, Orr ME, editors: *Nutrition support nursing*, ed 3, Silver Spring, Md, 1996, ASPEN.

Hill GJ: Nutrition assessment and intravenous nutritional support. In Nyhus LM, Baker RJ, Fischer JE, editors: *Masters of surgery* (pp 50-67), ed 3, Boston, 1997, Little Brown and Co.

Hise ME, Brown JC: Lipids. In Gottschlich MM, editor: *The ASPEN nutrition support core curriculum* (pp 48-70), Silver Spring, Md, 2007, ASPEN.

Holcombe BJ: Adult parenteral nutrition. In Young LY, Koda-Kimble MA, editors: *Applied therapeutics: the clinical use of drugs*, ed 6, Vancouver, Wash, 1995, Applied Therapeutics.

Hutchins AM, Shronts EP: Metabolic stress and immune function. In Skipper A, editor: *Dietitian's handbook of enteral and parenteral nutrition*, Gaithersburg, Md, 1998, ASPEN.

Hwang TL, Jue MC, Chen LL: Early use of cyclic TPN prevents further deterioration of liver functions for the PTN patients with impaired liver function, *Hepatogastroenterology* 47:1347-1350, 2000.

Infusion Nurses Society: Infusion nursing, standards of practice, *J Infus Nurs* 29(1 suppl): S1-S92, 2006.

Ireton-Jones C, DeLegge M, Epperson L et al: Management of the home parenteral nutrition patient, *Nutr Clin Pract* 18:310-317, 2003.

Isaacs JW, Millikan WJ, Stackhouse M et al: Parenteral nutrition of adults with a 900 milliosmolar solution via peripheral veins, *Am J Clin Nutr* 30:552-559, 1977.

Jacobs DG, Jacobs DO, Kudsk KA et al: Practice management guidelines for nutrition support of the trauma patient, *J Trauma* 57:660-679, 2004.

Joint Commission on Accreditation of Healthcare Organizations: *2005 Comprehensive accreditation manual for hospitals*, Oakbrook Terrace, III, 2005, Author.

Kane KF, Cologiovanni L, Mckiernan J et al: High osmolality feedings do not increase the incidence of thrombophlebitis during peripheral IV nutrition, *J Parenter Enter Nutr* 20(3):194-197, 1996.

Klein S, Kinney J, Jeejeebohy K et al: Nutrition support in clinical practice: review of published data and recommendations for future research directions, *J Parenter Enter Nutr* 21:133-156, 1997.

Knowles JB, Cusson G, Smith M et al: Pulmonary decomposition of calcium phosphate crystals as a complication of home parenteral nutrition, *J Parenter Enter Nutr* 13:209-213, 1989.

Krzywda EA: Substrate metabolism—carbohydrate, lipid, and protein. In Hennessy KA, Orr ME, editors: *Nutrition support nursing*, ed 3, Silver Spring, Md, 1996, ASPEN.

Krzywda EA, Andris DA, Whipple JK et al: Glucose response to abrupt initiation and discontinuation of total parenteral nutrition, *J Parenter Enter Nutr* 17:64-67, 1993.

Kuwahara T, Asanami S, Kubo S: Experimental infusion phlebitis: tolerant osmolality of peripheral venous endothelial cells, *Nutrition* 14:496-501, 1998a.

Kuwahara T, Asanami S, Takumi T et al: Dilution is effective in reducing infusion phlebitis in peripheral parenteral nutrition: an experimental study in rabbits, *Nutrition* 14:186-190, 1998b.

Kumpf VJ, Gervasio J: Complications of parenteral nutrition. In Gottschlich MM, editor: *The ASPEN nutrition support core curriculum* (pp 323-339), Silver Spring, Md, 2007, ASPEN.

Langley G: Fluid, electrolytes, and acid-base disorders. In Gottschlich MM, editor: *The ASPEN nutrition support core curriculum* (pp 104-128), Silver Spring, Md, 2007, ASPEN.

Lenssen P: Management of total parenteral nutrition. In Skipper A, editor: *Dietitian's handbook of enteral and parenteral nutrition*, ed 2, Gaithersburg, Md, 1998, Aspen.

Leung FY: Trace elements in parenteral micronutrition, *Clin Biochem* 28(6):561-566, 1995.

Leupold-DeCicco C, Monturo CA: Stress states: trauma, burns and sepsis. In Hennessy KA, Orr ME, editors: *Nutrition support nursing*, ed 3, Silver Spring, Md, 1996, ASPEN.

Lin EM: Nutrition support: making the difficult decisions, *Cancer Nurs* 14:261, 1991.

Ling P, McCowen KC: Carbohydrates. In Gottschlich MM, editor: *The ASPEN nutrition support core curriculum* (pp 129-159), Silver Spring, Md, 2007, ASPEN.

Marshall JK, Gadowsky SL, Childs A et al: Economic analysis of home vs hospital based parenteral nutrition in Ontario, Canada, *J Parenter Enter Nutr* 29:266-269, 2005.

Martindale RG, Sawai R, Wareen M: Sepsis and infection, In Gottschlich MM, editor: *The ASPEN nutrition support core curriculum* (pp 129-159), Silver Spring, Md, 2007, ASPEN.

Matarese LE, Gottschlich MM, editors: *Contemporary nutrition support practice: a clinical guide*, ed 2, St Louis, 2003, Saunders.

Mattox TW, Reiter PD: Parenteral nutrition. In DiPiro JT, Talbert RL, Yee GC, editors: *Pharmacotherapy: a pathophysiologic approach* (pp 2591-2613), New York, 2005, McGraw-Hill.

McCullough ML, Hsu N: Metabolic bone disease in home total parenteral nutrition, *J Am Diet Assoc* 87(7):915, 1987.

Melnick G: Value of specialty intravenous amino acids solutions, *Am J Health-Syst Pharm* 53:671-674, 1996.

Mershon J, Nogami W, Williams JM et al: Bacterial/fungal growth in a combined parenteral nutrient solution, *J Parenter Enter Nutr* 10: 498-502, 1986.

Mirtallo J: Overview of parenteral nutrition. In Gottschlich MM, editor: *The ASPEN nutrition support core curriculum* (pp 264-276), Silver Spring, Md, 2007, ASPEN.

Mirtallo J, Canada T, Johnson D et al: Safe practices for parenteral nutrition, *J Parenter Enter Nutr* 28:S39-S70, 2004.

Misra S, Kirby DF: Micronutrient and trace element monitoring in adult nutrition support, *Nutr Clin Pract* 15:120, 2000.

Ochoa JB, Caba D: Advances in surgical nutrition, *Surg Clin North Am* 86:1483-1493, 2006.

O'Keefe SJD: Parenteral nutrition and liver disease. In Rombeau JL, Caldwell MD, editors: *Clinical nutrition, vol II, total parenteral nutrition*, Philadelphia, 1993, WB Saunders.

Oster JR, Epstein M: Management of magnesium depletion, *Am J Nephrol* 8:349-354, 1988.

Paice BJ, Paterson KR, Onyanga-Omara F et al: Record linkage study of hypokalemia in hospitalized patients, *Postgrad Med J* 62:187-191, 1986.

Parrish CR, Krenisky J, Willcutts K et al: Gastrointestinal disease. In Gottschlich MM, editor: *The ASPEN nutrition support core curriculum* (pp 508-539), Silver Spring, Md, 2007, ASPEN.

Peppers MP, Geheb M, Desai T: Endocrine crises: hypophosphatemia and hyperphosphatemia, *Crit Care Clin* 7:201-214, 1991.

Popinska K, Kierkus J, Lyszkowska M et al: Aluminum contamination of parenteral additives, amino acid solutions and lipid emulsions, *Nutrition* 15:683-686, 1999.

Popovtzer MM: Disorders of calcium, phosphorus, vitamin D and parathyroid hormone activity. In Schrier RW, editor: *Renal and electrolyte disorders* (pp 216-277), ed 6, Philadelphia, 2003, Lippincott Williams & Wilkins.

Rose BD, Post TW: *Clinical physiology of acid-base and electrolyte disorders*, ed 5, New York, 2001, McGraw-Hill.

Ross V: Micronutrient recommendations for wound healing, *Support Line* 24:3-9, 2004.

Russell MK, Mueller C: Nutrition screening and assessment. In Gottschlich MM, editor: *The ASPEN nutrition support core curriculum* (pp 163-186), Silver Spring, Md, 2007, ASPEN.

Sacks GS, Dearman K, Replogle WH et al: Use of subjective global assessment to identify nutrition-associated complications and death in geriatric long-term care facility residents, *J Am Coll Nutr* 19:570-577, 2001.

Sax H: Complications of total parenteral nutrition and their prevention. In Rombeau JL, Caldwell MD, editors: *Clinical nutrition, total parenteral nutrition*, vol 2, Philadelphia, 1993, Saunders.

Seidner DL, Licata A: Parenteral nutrition-associated metabolic bone disease: pathophysiology, evaluation, and treatment, *Nutr Clin Pract* 15:163, 2000.

Shew SB, Jaksic T: The metabolic needs of critically ill children and neonates, *Semin Pediatr Surg* 8:131-139, 1999.

Shils ME et al: Long term parenteral nutrition through external arteriovenous shunt, *New Engl J Med* 283:341, 1970.

Singer FR, Bethune JE, Massry SG: Hypercalcemia and hypocalcemia, *Clin Neph* 7:154-162, 1977.

Sitren SS: Vitamin E. In Baumgartner TG, editor: *Clinical guide to parenteral micronutrition*, ed 3, Melrose Park, Ill, 1997, Fujisawa USA.

Smith CE: Quality of life in long-term parenteral nutrition patients and their family caregivers, *J Parenter Enter Nutr* 17(6):501-506, 1993.

Smith JS, Frankenfield DC, Souba WW: Nutrition and metabolism. In Mulholland MW, Maier RV, Lillemoe KD et al, editors: *Greenfield's surgery: scientific principles and practice* (pp 53-75), ed 4, Philadelphia, 2005, Lippincott Williams & Wilkins.

Speerhas R, Wang J, Seidner D et al: Maintaining normal blood glucose concentrations with total parenteral nutrition: is it necessary to taper total parenteral nutrition? *Nutr Clin Pract* 18:414-416, 2003.

Stapleton RD, Jones N, Heyland DK: Feeding critically ill patients: what is the optimal amount of energy? *Crit Care Med* 35:S535-S540, 2007.

Steiger E: HPEN Working Group: Consensus statements regarding optimal management of home parenteral nutrition (HPN) access, *J Parenter Enter Nutr* 30:S94-S95, 2006.

Stokes MA, Hill GL: Peripheral parenteral nutrition. A preliminary report on its efficacy and safety, *J Parenter Enter Nutr* 17:145-147, 1993.

Taskforce for the Revision of Safe Practices for Parenteral Nutrition, *J Parenter Enter Nutr* 28:539-570, 2004.

Taylor L, O'Neill JA: Total parenteral nutrition in the pediatric patient, *Surg Clin North Am* 71:477, 1991.

Testerman EJ: Current trends in pediatric total parenteral nutrition, *J Intraven Nurs* 12:152, 1989.

Thomson MA, Bucol S, Quirk P et al: Measured versus predicted resting energy expenditure in infants: a need for reappraisal, *J Pediatr* 126:21-27, 1995.

Todd SR, Kozar RA, Moore FA: Nutrition support in adult trauma patients, *Nutr Clin Pract* 21:421-429, 2006.

U.S. Department of Health and Human Services (HHS): Parenteral multivitamin products, *Fed Regist* 65:21200-21201, 2000.

Valentine CJ, Puthoff TD: Enhancing parenteral nutrition therapy for the neonate, *Nutr Clin Pract* 22:183-193, 2007.

Vinnars E, Wilmore D: History of parenteral nutrition, *J Parenter Enter Nutr* 27:225-231, 2003.

Warner B: Parenteral nutrition in the pediatric patient. In Fischer JE, editor: *Total parenteral nutrition*, ed 2, Boston, 1991, Little, Brown.

Wasserman PJ, Segal-Maurer S: Human immunodeficiency virus (HIV) infection. In Gottschlich MM, editor: *The ASPEN nutrition support core curriculum* (pp 619-648), Silver Spring, Md, 2007, ASPEN.

Wessel J, Balint J, Crill C et al: Standards for specialized nutrition support: hospitalized pediatric patients, *Nutr Clin Pract* 20:103-116, 2005.

Weston-Eborn R, Sitzman K: Selecting effective instructional resources, *Home Health Nurse* 23:402-403, 2005.

Whang R, Ryder KW: Frequency of hypomagnesemia and hypermagnesemia. Requested vs. routine, *JAMA* 263:3063-3064, 1990.

WHO Working Group: Use and interpretation of anthropometric indicators of nutritional status, *Bull World Health Org* 64:924-941, 1986.

Wilmore DW, Van Woert JH: Enteral and parenteral nutrition in hospital patients. In Rubenstein E, Federman DD, editors: *Scientific American medicine*, vol 4, New York, 1992, Scientific American.

Wooley JA, Frankenfield D: Energy. In Gottschlich MM, editor: *The ASPEN nutrition support core curriculum* (pp 19-47), Silver Spring, Md, 2007, ASPEN.

Young LS, Kearns LR, Schopfel SL: Protein. In Gottschlich MM, editor: *The ASPEN nutrition support core curriculum* (pp 71-87), Silver Spring, Md, 2007, ASPEN.

18 ANTINEOPLASTIC THERAPY

Lisa Schulmeister, MN, RN, APRN-BC, OCN®, FAAN*

Cancer is a chronic condition that consists of a large group of diseases characterized by abnormal cells. An estimated 1,444,920 new cases of cancer were diagnosed in the United States in 2007 and 559,650 deaths were caused by cancer. Cancer is the second most common cause of death in the United States, exceeded only by heart disease. Because of advances in cancer treatment, more than 10.5 million Americans with a history of cancer are alive and considered cancer survivors (American Cancer Society, 2007).

The term antineoplastic therapy refers to treatment intended to prevent, halt, or eradicate cancer. Antineoplastic therapies include surgery, radiotherapy, hyperthermia, cancer vaccines, gene therapy, immunotherapy, biotherapy, molecularly targeted therapies, hormonal therapy, and chemotherapy (Polovich, White, and Kelleher, 2005). Because chemotherapy is often administered as an infusion therapy, it is the focus of this chapter.

Chemotherapy may be given as the primary cancer treatment or administered adjuvantly, in conjunction with other treatments such as radiotherapy. Neoadjuvant chemotherapy is administered before another cancer treatment; for example, chemotherapy is sometimes given before surgery to reduce the size of a large cancer so it may be more easily removed. Induction chemotherapy, initial treatment with high doses of chemotherapy, is used to treat aggressive types of cancer, such as acute leukemia, with the goal of inducing remission of the disease. Postremission chemotherapy may consist of standard dose consolidation chemotherapy, intensification chemotherapy, or ablative chemotherapy (high-dose chemotherapy followed by stem cell transplantation). The goal of postremission chemotherapy is to prevent disease recurrence (Polovich et al, 2005).

For some types of cancer, chemotherapy is curative. In the 1950s only 10% of children responded to cancer treatment. Today, nearly 80% are cured (Singh, 2006). Similarly, the overall survival for all stages of testicular cancer, including metastatic disease, is 80%, and 99% of patients with early-stage testicular cancer are cured (Kopp et al, 2006). Chemotherapy also may be administered

with the goal of controlling disease progression and extending survival. In some cases, such as patients with large tumors obstructing organs or causing pain, chemotherapy is given for palliation.

Although chemotherapy has historically been considered a cancer treatment, chemotherapy also has efficacy in treating noncancerous conditions, such as rheumatoid arthritis (Donahue et al, 2008), and has become an accepted alternative to surgical options for treatment of ectopic tubal pregnancy (Lipscomb, 2007).

Chemotherapy may be administered by the oral, subcutaneous, intravenous (IV), intraarterial, intrathecal, intraperitoneal, intrapleural, intravesicular, and intralesional routes. Some treatment protocols include chemotherapy administered via multiple routes; for instance, two chemotherapy agents are administered intravenously while a third is given intrathecally. Whenever the route of chemotherapy administration is unclear or not specified, clarification of the order should be sought in order to prevent a medication error (wrong route) from occurring (Polovich et al, 2005).

CELL CYCLE

Normal cells and cancer cells go through the same division cycle (or cell cycle) (Figure 18-1). The DNA in a parent cell replicates and divides, and two "daughter" cells are produced. The initial phase of the cell cycle is the resting phase, designated as G_0. A cell in this phase performs its designated function during this stage of the cell cycle; for example, renal cells filter the blood and gastric cells digest food. Enzymes needed for DNA synthesis are produced in this phase. Although G_0 is commonly referred to as the resting phase of the cell, it is sometimes called the postmitotic or presynthetic phase (Park and Lee, 2003; Vermeulen et al, 2003).

When a cell is ready to divide, it enters into the next phase, called gap 1 and designated as G_1. Synthesis of the proteins for RNA occurs during the G_1 phase. Enzymes necessary for synthesis of DNA are activated in the S or synthesis phase. The length of time that the cancer cell is in this phase usually differs from that of normal cells. The second gap phase is designated

---

*The author and editors wish to acknowledge the contributions made by Katherine V. Vandegrift as author of this chapter in the second edition of *Infusion Therapy in Clinical Practice*.

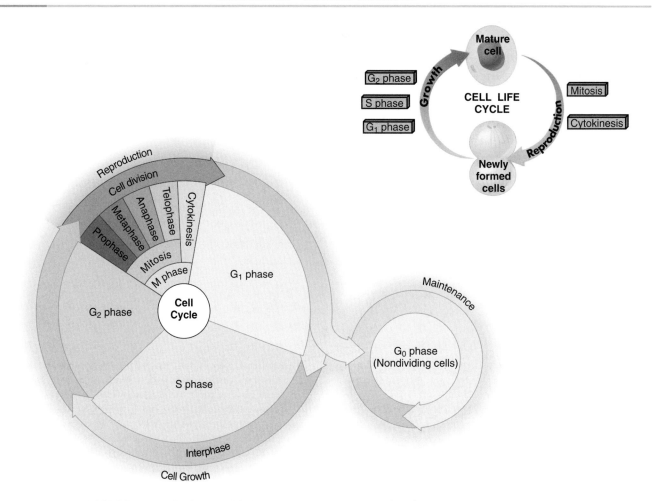

FIGURE 18-1 Cell cycle. (From Thibodeau GA, Patton KT: *Anatomy & physiology,* ed 6, St Louis, 2007, Mosby.)

as G_2. At this time, DNA synthesis stops and RNA synthesis and protein synthesis continue while the cell prepares for mitosis (Park and Lee, 2003; Vermeulen et al, 2003).

Mitosis occurs during the final stage of the cell cycle, the M phase, and usually lasts 30 to 90 minutes. This phase is subdivided into four steps. In *prophase* the nuclear membrane is broken down and the chromosomes clump. In *metaphase* the chromosomes line up in the middle of the cell. During *anaphase* the chromosomes segregate into centrioles. In *telophase,* the final step, there is chromosome replication and cell division, which produces two daughter cells. These cells then go into the resting phase, G_0 (Park and Lee, 2003; Vermeulen et al, 2003).

Although a few chemotherapy agents are given alone as single agents, most are administered in combination with other chemotherapy agents. Combining agents that act in different phases of the cell cycle increases the number of cells exposed to their cytotoxic effects and enhances cytotoxicity.

CHEMOTHERAPY CLASSIFICATIONS AND NOMENCLATURE

Chemotherapy agents can be classified by their effect on the cell cycle, pharmacological action or chemical structure, potential to cause tissue necrosis if extravasated, or emetogenic potential.

Cell cycle–specific chemotherapy kills cells that are in a specific phase and actively dividing. For example, a type of chemotherapy derived from vinca rosea plants and classified as plant alkaloids is cell cycle specific in the M phase. These chemotherapy agents kill only those cells in the M phase of the cell cycle. Cell cycle–nonspecific chemotherapy kills cells in any phase of the cell cycle, including G_0, the resting phase. An example of this type of chemotherapy is the anthracyclines, which are classified by their action as antitumor antibiotics. Vesicant chemotherapy has the potential to cause tissue necrosis when extravasated while nonvesicant chemotherapy does not alter tissue integrity when it infiltrates (Polovich et al, 2005). Chemotherapy agents have varying risks of causing nausea and vomiting, from minimal risk (<10% without antiemetics) to high risk (>90% without antiemetics), and may be classified by their emetogenic potential (Feeney et al, 2007). Each of these chemotherapy classifications is discussed in more detail in the following sections.

Chemotherapy treatment protocols often are assigned an acronym or protocol name and/or number. For instance, the breast cancer treatment acronym "CMF" refers to the multidrug combination of *c*yclophosphamide, *m*ethotrexate, and *f*luorouracil. Southwest Oncology Group (a national clinical research group) protocol SWOG-50337 is a clinical trial evaluating gemcitabine treatment for patients with recurrent bladder cancer. Most cancer clinical trials are funded and coordinated by the National Cancer Institute (NCI), and its website contains a database of trials that are open to patient enrollment (NCI, 2008). Some of the trials involve chemotherapy agents that are commercially available but are being studied in a new way while others are trials of investigational agents to determine their efficacy and toxicity.

CHEMOTHERAPEUTIC AGENTS

Chemotherapy agents have a very narrow therapeutic window; under- and overdosing of these agents can negatively impact the patient's treatment outcome. Similarly, other errors in administration—such as wrong drug, wrong dose, wrong time, wrong route, or wrong patient—may cause patient harm. Chemotherapy orders must be reviewed and verified before administration by a trained clinician in chemotherapy administration to ensure that the correct chemotherapy drug and correct dose are administered to the right patient at the right time. Nurses and other health care providers should always compare a patient's chemotherapy orders with the patient's prescribed plan of care, treatment protocol, and other resources to ensure that the orders do not inadvertently contain errors or omissions (Schulmeister, 2006). Because chemotherapy doses are individualized and vary with the disease being treated, usual dosages are not stated in this chapter and the reader is referred to the manufacturer's package insert for full prescribing information.

ANTIMETABOLITES

Antimetabolites are cell cycle–specific agents that act in the S phase and interfere with DNA and RNA synthesis by acting as "false" metabolites, which block the production of essential enzymes and prevent cell division. Their major toxicities are hematopoietic and gastrointestinal. Other common side effects are elevated liver function tests, photosensitivity, and alopecia (Wilkes and Barton-Burke, 2008).

Gemcitabine HCl

Gemcitabine (Gemzar), an antimetabolite, inhibits DNA synthesis and is cell cycle specific in the S phase. It is indicated for first-line treatment of pancreatic cancer (in combination with paclitaxel), unresectable non–small cell lung cancers (in combination with cisplatin), and women with metastatic breast cancer (in combination with paclitaxel) who have not responded to prior anthracycline chemotherapy. Gemcitabine (in combination with carboplatin) also is indicated for the treatment of patients with advanced ovarian cancer that has relapsed at least 6 months after completion of platinum-based therapy. Myelosuppression is the dose-limiting toxicity, with a nadir of 7 to 14 days. Gemcitabine has a low (10% to 30% risk) emetic risk. Diarrhea, stomatitis, and constipation also occur. Other common side effects are fever, flulike symptoms, and mild to moderate rashes involving the trunk and extremities. Alopecia is minimal, involving about 15% of patients, and is reversible. Flulike symptoms occur in 20% of patients with the first treatment dose, and transient febrile episodes occur in 41% of patients (Thigpen, 2006; Eli Lilly, 2007a).

Methotrexate

Methotrexate (amethopterin, Mexate, Folex) is a folic acid antagonist that interferes with the synthesis of purine and thymidylate. It is cell cycle specific in the S phase, and it is used as a single agent or in combination with other drugs. Methotrexate is active against acute lymphocytic leukemia, lymphomas, sarcomas, mycosis fungoides, gestational trophoblastic carcinomas, and cancers of the breast, lung, head, and neck. Methotrexate can crystallize and precipitate in acidic solution and can cause renal damage in the presence of urine with a low pH. When high doses of methotrexate are given, the patient's urine should be alkalinized both before and after methotrexate administration. Sodium bicarbonate is given orally or intravenously to neutralize the urine and keep the urinary pH greater than 7. Following high doses, leucovorin (folinic acid) is usually given as a rescue agent within 24 to 36 hours. The blood urea nitrogen (BUN), creatinine, and serum methotrexate levels determine the dosage and frequency of leucovorin. The purpose of the leucovorin is to reduce bone marrow toxicity. Methotrexate has a low (10% to 30%) emetic risk. Antiemetics should be given beforehand to control the dose-related nausea associated with this drug. Hydrating fluid is usually given before and after methotrexate dosing. The patient needs to be encouraged to increase oral fluids, and the fluid balance should be monitored. Stomatitis and esophagitis, which can impair eating and swallowing, can range from mild irritation and tenderness with sensitivity to spicy or acidic foods to full-blown, painful sores. With prolonged use of methotrexate, an elevation in liver function tests, hepatic fibrosis, and occasionally cirrhosis can occur. Pneumonitis may develop and is not always reversible. Methotrexate can cause photosensitivity, with the patient's skin having an increased tendency to burn if exposed to bright, intense sunlight. It is recommended that the patient cover the exposed skin or use a sunscreen with a sun protection factor (SPF) of 15 or more. Radiation recall has been seen with this drug. Methotrexate interacts with many drugs, including 5-fluorouracil, asparaginase, and vincristine. The patient should be instructed to avoid the use of aspirin, nonsteroidal anti-inflammatory drugs, folic acid preparations, sulfa vaccines, and alcohol during treatment with methotrexate (Bedford Labs, 2005a; Wilkes and Barton-Burke, 2008).

5-Fluorouracil

Another antimetabolite, 5-fluorouracil (fluorouracil, Adrucil, 5-FU), inhibits the synthesis of DNA and RNA and is cell cycle specific for the S phase. It is indicated in the treatment of gastrointestinal (GI) malignancies, especially colorectal, pancreas, head, neck, breast, prostate, skin (administered topically), and liver (administered intraarterially) cancers. The dose-limiting toxicities are stomatitis and diarrhea. Toxicity may be delayed 1 to 3 weeks. 5-Fluorouracil has a low (10% to 30%) emetic risk. Rarely, GI ulceration can lead to hemorrhage. Myelosuppression is usually moderate, with a nadir of 7 to 14 days. Other side effects are anorexia, fatigue, alopecia, and photosensitivity. 5-Fluorouracil is an irritant, and a central venous access device is recommended for continuous infusions. The patient should be instructed to avoid exposure to direct sunlight, to wear long sleeves and pants outdoors, and to use a sunscreen with an SPF of 15 or higher. Hyperpigmentation of the nail beds and peripheral veins is common. Hand-foot syndrome may occur, involving painful, erythematous desquamation of palms and soles (Wilkes and Barton-Burke, 2008).

Floxuridine

Floxuridine (FUDR) interferes with cell replication and inhibits DNA synthesis. It is cell cycle specific for the S phase and is indicated in the treatment of liver, biliary, pancreatic, oral cavity, and breast cancers. Floxuridine is administered intraarterially into the hepatic artery, usually via continuous infusion for 14 to 21 days. When given intravenously, floxuridine is transformed to 5-fluorouracil; IV administration is being investigated.

Dose-limiting toxicities are stomatitis and diarrhea. Myelosuppression is mild. Alopecia and dermatitis are common. Plantarpalmar syndrome may occur and is characterized by painful swelling and peeling of the hands and feet. Hyperpigmentation of the veins occurs with peripheral infusions (Bedford Labs, 2000).

Fludarabine

Fludarabine (Fludara, fludarabine phosphate) interferes with and inhibits DNA function. It is used to treat mycosis fungoides, low-grade lymphomas, and chronic B-cell lymphocytic leukemia that have not responded to standard treatment. Fludarabine has a minimal (<10%) emetic risk. Common side effects are anorexia, diarrhea, fever, chills, rash, myalgia, fatigue, weakness, GI bleeding, visual disturbances, and urinary tract infections. Cardiac problems such as arrhythmias, congestive heart failure, and myocardial infarction have occurred. Respiratory side effects include cough, dyspnea, pneumonia, and upper respiratory tract infections. The concurrent use of pentostatin is not recommended because of severe risk of pulmonary toxicity. Because myelosuppression can be severe, with a nadir of 7 to 14 days, fludarabine should not be administered with other severe myelosuppressants such as 5-fluorouracil or methotrexate. Confusion, coma, and death have been reported with very high dosages. Tumor lysis syndrome is common and usually begins with flank pain and hematuria. Most toxic effects are dose dependent and increase with advanced age, bone marrow impairment, and renal insufficiency (Bayer Pharmaceuticals, 2007).

Cytarabine

Cytarabine (ara-C, Cytosar-U, cytosine arabinoside) is a cell cycle–specific (S phase) antimetabolite that inhibits DNA synthesis. It is indicated in the treatment of acute nonlymphocytic leukemia, acute lymphocytic leukemia, acute myelogenous leukemia, chronic myelocytic leukemia, and meningeal leukemia (administered intrathecally). Myelosuppression is the dose-limiting toxicity, with a nadir of 7 to 14 days. Anemia with megaloblastic changes in the bone marrow is common. Cytarabine has a low (10% to 30%) emetic risk. Anorexia, diarrhea, and anal ulceration may occur. Alopecia is common, as are rashes, especially hand-foot syndrome (i.e., a rash on the palms and soles followed by blisters and desquamation). Tumor lysis syndrome, which is caused by rapid lysis of tumor cells, may occur when a patient with acute leukemia undergoes induction therapy or has a large tumor burden. Corticosteroid eyedrops are usually started before cytarabine administration to prevent conjunctivitis, which is often seen. Cytarabine is incompatible with 5-fluorouracil and heparin when given through the same administration set (Upjohn Pharmaceuticals, 2002).

Pentostatin

Pentostatin (Nipent) is an antimetabolite that interferes with DNA replication and disrupts RNA processing. It is cell cycle nonspecific and is indicated primarily in the treatment of refractory hairy cell leukemia and other leukemias unresponsive to therapy. Anorexia, nausea, vomiting, stomatitis, abdominal pain, diarrhea, headache, fatigue, rashes, chills, fever, pain, depression, and nervousness are common. Leukopenia and thrombocytopenia are severe with a granulocyte nadir of 15 days. Pulmonary complications such as pulmonary edema can be life-threatening. Infections and hypersensitivity reactions are common and severe. Myocardial infarctions, arrhythmias, heart failure, and death have occurred. Coma has been reported in more than half of patients (SuperGen, 1998).

Pemetrexed

Pemetrexed (Alimta) is an antimetabolite that inhibits key metabolic enzymatic steps that are needed for pyrimidine and purine synthesis. It is indicated in the treatment of malignant pleural mesothelioma (in combination with cisplatin) and non–small cell lung cancer. Bone marrow depression is the dose-limiting toxicity. Pemetrexed has a low (10% to 30%) emetic risk. Common side effects include anorexia, stomatitis, and diarrhea. A rash occurs in 22% of patients; oral dexamethasone is usually prescribed on the day before, day of, and day following pemetrexed treatment. The antitumor effect of pemetrexed is dependent upon the size of the cellular folate pools, so oral folic acid must be concurrently administered to increase the efficacy of pemetrexed and minimize its toxicity. Patients also receive vitamin B_{12} injections every three treatment cycles, beginning 1 week before treatment and continuing throughout treatment every three treatment cycles thereafter (Eli Lilly, 2007b; Wilkes and Barton-Burke, 2008).

PLANT ALKALOIDS

The plant alkaloids consist of two groups: the vinca alkaloids, derived from the vinca rosea plant; and other plant alkaloids, such as etoposide, which is a derivative of mandrake (may apple plant). The plant alkaloids inhibit mitosis and are cell cycle specific for the M phase. Major toxicities of these agents affect the hematopoietic, integumentary, neurological, and reproductive systems. All of the vinca alkaloids have a minimal (<10%) emetic risk. The vinca alkaloids are for IV administration only and are usually fatal when inadvertently given intrathecally. All of the vinca alkaloids are vesicants (Feeney et al, 2007; Wilkes and Barton-Burke, 2008).

Vinblastine

Vinblastine (Velban) is cell cycle specific for the M phase and blocks cellular division. It is used to treat Hodgkin's disease (stages 3 and 4); lymphoma; acquired immunodeficiency syndrome (AIDS)-related Kaposi's sarcoma; mycosis fungoides; histocytosis; testicular, bladder, renal cell, and non–small cell lung cancers; and choriocarcinoma. The major toxicity of this drug is dose-related bone marrow depression. Neurotoxicity may occur after several courses of treatment; symptoms include jaw pain, paresthesias, loss of deep tendon reflexes, and peripheral neuropathy. The patient should be monitored for footdrop and difficulty performing fine motor movements (e.g., fastening buttons). Acute bronchospasm and shortness of breath may occur, especially if the patient is also receiving mitomycin. Constipation is common, and the prophylactic use of stool softeners is recommended. Nausea, vomiting, and alopecia are mild (Bedford Labs, 2001).

Vincristine

Vincristine sulfate (Oncovin) is cell cycle specific for the M and S phases and blocks cell division during metaphase. It is indicated in the treatment of acute leukemia, Hodgkin's disease, non-Hodgkin's lymphoma, rhabdomyosarcomas, neuroblastoma, Wilms' tumor, multiple myeloma, and breast carcinoma.

Vincristine has the same neurotoxicities as vinblastine, but those for vincristine are usually more severe and may be permanent. Fine motor movements, such as the ability to pick up and handle small objects, should be monitored. The patient's gait should also be monitored for difficulty in walking, especially for a slapping gait, which indicates footdrop. Other side effects of vincristine are much the same as those for vinblastine, except myelosuppression is milder (Mayne Pharma USA, 2004; Schulmeister, 2004).

Vinorelbine

Vinorelbine tartrate (Navelbine) is a semisynthetic vinca alkaloid that inhibits mitosis. It is used to treat Hodgkin's disease and metastatic breast and ovarian cancers. It is also indicated in the treatment of nonresectable advanced non–small cell lung cancer as a single agent or in combination with cisplatin, and it is used in combination with cisplatin for stage III non–small cell lung cancer. Granulocytopenia is the dose-limiting toxicity and the risk of bone marrow suppression is increased when used in combination with cisplatin. Acute shortness of breath and severe bronchospasm have been noted to occur, especially when vinorelbine is administered with mitomycin. Mild to moderate nausea and vomiting, stomatitis, anorexia, and diarrhea are common. As with other vinca alkaloids, constipation is common, as is peripheral neuropathy. Transient elevations in liver enzymes, alopecia, and fatigue are common (Bedford Labs, 2005b).

Etoposide

Etoposide (VP-16, VePesid), another plant alkaloid, is indicated in the treatment of small cell lung, testicular, and ovarian cancers; relapsed Hodgkin's and non-Hodgkin's lymphoma; gestational trophoblastic tumors; and Ewing's sarcoma. Etoposide is cell cycle specific, with activity in the G_2 and S phases and inhibition of DNA synthesis. Etoposide also inhibits topoisomerase II, an enzyme necessary for cell division. Myelosuppression is dose limiting. Patients experience mild to moderate nausea and vomiting, anorexia, and diarrhea. Alopecia is seen in about 66% of patients, with thinning of the hair in the remainder. Etoposide should be administered over 30 to 60 minutes to minimize the risk of hypotension and bronchospasm (wheezing). Anaphylactic reactions have been reported and are more common during the initial infusion. A metallic aftertaste may occur throughout the infusion of the drug and can sometimes be relieved by having the patient suck on hard candy. Radiation recall has also been reported. Etoposide is considered an irritant if it infiltrates from the vein (Bedford Labs, 2006).

ALKYLATING AGENTS

Most alkylating agents are cell cycle nonspecific. They interfere with DNA replication by crosslinking DNA strands, breaking DNA strands, and abnormally pairing base proteins. Major toxicities are hematopoietic, gastrointestinal, and reproductive (Wilkes and Barton-Burke, 2008).

Mechlorethamine HCl

The first nonhormonal chemotherapeutic agent, introduced in 1946, was mechlorethamine hydrochloride (nitrogen mustard, Mustargen). It is a cell cycle–specific alkylating drug. Its multiple mechanisms of action result in DNA miscoding, breakage, and failure of the cell to replicate. Although it was widely used in the treatment of Hodgkin's disease, non-Hodgkin's lymphoma, chronic lymphocytic leukemia, bronchogenic carcinoma, and polycythemia vera, its use has diminished in the past decade, largely because of the introduction of newer, more effective, and less toxic chemotherapy agents. Nitrogen mustard has a very short stability when reconstituted and rapidly undergoes chemical transformation and decomposition. Therefore nitrogen mustard is given by IV bolus within 15 minutes of preparation. If inadvertent contact with skin occurs, the area should be washed with copious amounts of water, followed by a rinse of 2.5% sodium thiosulfate solution. Nitrogen mustard is a vesicant and can cause severe tissue necrosis and sloughing in the event of an extravasation. Nitrogen mustard has a high (90%) emetic risk. Nausea and vomiting, which usually start within 30 minutes of administration, may last up to 36 hours. Anorexia and diarrhea are also common. The patient may note a metallic taste immediately after administration. Bone marrow suppression can be profound when nitrogen mustard is given with radiation therapy. Patients receiving this form of chemotherapy not uncommonly develop menstrual irregularities or impaired spermatogenesis (Merck and Co., 1999).

Dacarbazine

Dacarbazine (DTIC-Dome, imidazole, carboxamide) is cell cycle nonspecific and inhibits DNA, RNA, and protein synthesis. It possesses limited ability to cross the blood-brain barrier. Dacarbazine is active against Hodgkin's disease, malignant melanoma, neuroblastoma, and soft tissue sarcomas. Patients may experience discomfort at the infusion site. Adequately diluting the drug and slowing the infusion may decrease the burning sensation and vasospasm. Slowing the infusion and applying ice above the injection site can also be helpful. Dacarbazine has a high (>90%) emetic risk. Myelosuppression, with a nadir of 7 to 14 days, and flulike symptoms are the most common side effects. The flulike syndrome can last for several days, with primary symptoms of fever and myalgias. Many patients complain of a metallic taste, which may interfere with nutritional intake. Skin reactions of pruritus, erythema, and photosensitivity have occurred. Exposure to the sun during the first 48 hours can cause facial flushing, paresthesia, and dizziness. Patients should avoid taking dong quai and St John's wort while receiving dacarbazine treatment (these herbs increase photosensitization) (Merck Manuals Online Medical Library, 2008; Wilkes and Barton-Burke, 2008).

Cyclophosphamide

Cyclophosphamide (Cytoxan, Neosar) is one of the most widely used alkylating agents. It is cell cycle nonspecific and causes cell death by crosslinking with DNA and interfering with RNA transcription. It is active in the treatment of lymphomas, leukemias, multiple myeloma, mycosis fungoides, neuroblastoma, retinoblastoma, sarcomas, and cancers of the breast, ovary, testes, lung, and bladder. Hemorrhagic cystitis is the most serious side effect; it can be severe and fatal. Vigorous hydration with 2 to 3 L of fluid a day is necessary before and after administration. The patient should be encouraged to void every 2 hours to lessen the time the drug dwells in the bladder. Mesna, a drug that prevents the formation of cyclophosphamide metabolites, is given with high-dose cyclophosphamide to lessen the incidence and severity of cystitis. Long-term administration of cyclophosphamide may cause fibrosis of the bladder. Leukopenia is the dose-limiting toxicity, with a nadir of 7 to 14 days. Thrombocytopenia and pulmonary fibrosis may occur with high dosages. Cardiotoxicity can occur with high dosages and in combination with doxorubicin. High-dose cyclophosphamide has a high (>90%) emetic risk while the risk is moderate (30% to 90%) with lower doses (Wilkes and Barton-Burke, 2008).

Ifosfamide

Ifosfamide (Ifex) is cell cycle nonspecific and inhibits DNA synthesis. It is indicated in the treatment of third-line germ-cell testicular cancer and is used to treat soft tissue sarcomas, non-Hodgkin's lymphoma, and lung cancer. Myelosuppression is dose related and common side effects are alopecia, somnolence, and dose-dependent nausea and vomiting. Ifosfamide has a moderate (30% to 90%) emetic risk. Confusion has occurred, and coma and seizures have been reported. The most serious and dose-limiting side effect is hemorrhagic cystitis. Vigorous hydration is recommended before, during, and after administration. The patient should be instructed to void every 2 hours. Scheduled doses of mesna should always be administered with ifosfamide to prevent or lessen the severity of bladder toxicity (Wilkes and Barton-Burke, 2008).

Cisplatin

Cisplatin (cis-diamminedichloroplatinum, platinum, Platinol) is a heavy metal that is cell cycle nonspecific and inhibits DNA synthesis. It is indicated in the treatment of testicular, ovarian, bladder, head, neck, non–small cell lung, small cell lung, esophageal, cervical, breast, gastric, thyroid, and neurological cancers, as well as in Hodgkin's and non-Hodgkin's lymphoma, sarcomas, melanoma, and advanced prostate carcinoma. Cisplatin has a high emetic risk (>90%). Antiemetics should be administered before the infusion because nausea and vomiting are usually severe, starting 1 to 4 hours after the infusion and lasting up to 5 days. Persistent anorexia and taste alterations often occur. Myelosuppression is dose dependent. Ototoxicity occurs in 31% of patients and is usually manifested by tinnitus and high-frequency hearing loss. Peripheral neuropathy occurs and has a cumulative effect. Although rare, anaphylactic reactions have occurred within minutes of the start of the infusion. Renal toxicity is common, severe, and dose dependent. Vigorous hydration is administered before and after treatment, along with mannitol or furosemide, to maintain urinary output. Renal function should be monitored during treatment. Amifostine (Ethyol) reduces the toxic effects of cisplatin and protects the renal cells without interfering with the action of cisplatin. The most common adverse effects of this cytoprotectant are transient hypertension, nausea, and vomiting, which can be severe. The patient should be well hydrated before administration, and should not be hypotensive or receiving antihypertensive therapy within 24 hours of administration. A baseline blood pressure should be taken, with blood pressure monitoring every 5 minutes. Amifostine is given rapidly (less than 15 minutes) with the patient in a supine position. Potassium and magnesium are usually added to the prehydration fluids to prevent hypokalemia and hypomagnesemia. Cisplatin reacts chemically with aluminum and forms a precipitate, so only stainless-steel needles should be used in preparation and administration (Hussain et al, 2003; Kostova, 2006; Rybak, 2007; Yao et al, 2007).

Carboplatin

Carboplatin (Paraplatin), an analog of cisplatin, is cell cycle nonspecific. Its method of action is thought to be crosslinking of DNA strands. Carboplatin is indicated in the treatment of advanced ovarian cancer, endometrial carcinoma, non–small cell lung cancer, metastatic seminoma, recurrent brain tumors in children, relapsed and refractory acute leukemia, and head and neck cancers. Carboplatin has a moderate (30% to 90%) emetic risk. Mild anorexia and taste changes may occur. Myelosuppression is severe and dose related, with a nadir of 7 to 14 days. Hypersensitivity reactions are common after several courses of the drug have been administered (they are acquired rather than immediate reactions), and are characterized by flushing, rashes, dyspnea, hypotension, and tachycardia. Premedication with histamine-1 (H_1) and histamine-2 (H_2) blockers decreases the risk of developing carboplatin hypersensitivity. Epinephrine, corticosteroids, and antihistamines must be available. Cardiac failure, embolism, and cerebrovascular accident have been reported. Alopecia occurs in about 50% of patients. Needles or IV administration sets containing aluminum should not be used because aluminum reacts with carboplatin, causing precipitate formation and loss of potency. Carboplatin is contraindicated in patients with a history of allergies to cisplatin, platinum-containing compounds, or mannitol, as well as in those with severe bone marrow depression or bleeding. The patient should be instructed to avoid using products containing aspirin (Navo et al, 2006; Winkeljohn and Polovich, 2006; Lenz, 2007).

Oxaliplatin

Oxaliplatin (Eloxatin) is a third-generation platinum analog. It blocks DNA replication and transcription and is indicated for the adjuvant treatment of patients with stage III colon cancer and for first-line treatment of metastatic colon and rectal cancers (in combination with 5-fluorouracil and leucovorin). Oxaliplatin has a moderate (30% to 90%) emetic risk. Peripheral neuropathy is a dose-limiting toxicity. Two distinct neurotoxicity syndromes may occur: an acute syndrome that persists for less than 14 days and chronic persistent peripheral neuropathy. Acute neurotoxicity, caused by irritation of ion channels in the nerves, occurs in 56% of patients. It is often precipitated by exposure to cold and is characterized by decreased sensation, particularly in the hands and feet. Peripheral neuropathy affects 48% of patients and most often occurs when a cumulative dose of 800 mg/m² of oxaliplatin has been administered. Symptoms include decreased sensation (often in a stocking and glove distribution) and impairment of proprioception. Delayed hypersensitivity may occur after 10 to 12 courses of treatment. Symptoms range from rash to anaphylaxis. Common symptoms include dyspnea, hypotension, and urticaria. Desensitization protocols have been developed to reduce the risk of hypersensitivity (Sanofi-Aventis, 2006; Kim and Erlichman, 2007; Stordal et al, 2007; Wilkes, 2007; Wilkes and Barton-Burke, 2008).

Thiotepa

Thiotepa (triethylenethiophosphoramide, TSPA, Thioplex) is cell cycle nonspecific and causes crosslinking of DNA. Thiotepa is indicated in the treatment of breast and ovarian cancer, Hodgkin's disease, chronic granulocytic and lymphocytic leukemia, bronchogenic carcinoma, and superficial bladder cancer. Nausea and vomiting are dose dependent. Myelosuppression is the dose-limiting toxic effect. The patient should be instructed to avoid use of aspirin-containing products. Allergic reactions with hives, rash, and bronchospasm have been reported. The patient may experience pain at the infusion site, which may be relieved by diluting the drug, slowing the infusion, or placing an ice pack above the site (Wilkes and Barton-Burke, 2008).

Nitrosoureas

The nitrosoureas are lipid-soluble alkylating agents, most of which can cross the blood-brain barrier because of their lipid solubility. They interfere with DNA replication and repair and are cell cycle nonspecific. Their major toxicities are hematopoietic, gastrointestinal, and reproductive (Wilkes and Barton-Burke, 2008).

Carmustine

Carmustine (BiCNU, BCNU) is a nitrosourea that acts as an alkylating agent by interfering with DNA and RNA synthesis through alkylation. It is cell cycle nonspecific and is indicated in the treatment of brain tumors, Hodgkin's disease, non-Hodgkin's lymphoma, and malignant melanoma. Carmustine has a high emetic risk (>90%). Severe nausea and vomiting may occur 1 to 2 hours after infusion and last 6 to 8 hours. Stomatitis is common. Cumulative bone marrow suppression, which is delayed 4 to 6 weeks, is the major dose-limiting toxicity. Concomitant use of cimetidine is avoided because it may increase bone marrow toxicity. Pulmonary fibrosis has been reported with cumulative doses and may be progressive and fatal. Delayed onset has occurred from 9 days to 15 years after treatment. Nephrotoxicity progressing to renal failure and reversible hepatotoxicity have been reported. Carmustine is an irritant, causing intense pain at the infusion site. To decrease pain, the infusion can be slowed and ice placed above the infusion site. Contact of the drug with skin causes brown staining (Wilkes and Barton-Burke, 2008).

Streptozocin

Streptozocin (Zanosar, streptozotocin) is a cell cycle–nonspecific drug that inhibits DNA synthesis through crosslinking. It is indicated in the treatment of insulinomas, carcinoid tumors, non–small cell lung and colon cancers, hepatoma, and squamous cell carcinoma of the oral cavity. Renal toxicity, which is severe and often fatal, is dose related and cumulative. Proteinuria is an early sign of nephrotoxicity. Renal function should be evaluated before and after treatment. In patients with preexisting renal disease, the potential benefit of streptozocin must be weighed against the risk of further renal damage. The use of other nephrotoxic drugs, such as the aminoglycosides, should be avoided. Liver dysfunction and hypoglycemia caused by sudden insulin release have been reported. Myelosuppression is mild, with a nadir of 1 to 2 weeks. Severe nausea and vomiting is common, particularly with daily treatments. Streptozocin is an irritant and commonly causes pain and burning at the infusion site. Slowing the infusion, diluting the concentration of the drug, and applying ice above the site may decrease the symptoms (Wilkes and Barton-Burke, 2008).

ANTITUMOR ANTIBIOTICS

Although the antitumor antibiotics have some anti-infective qualities, their major action is cytotoxic. They interfere with nucleic acid synthesis and inhibit RNA synthesis by intercalation.

They react with or bind to DNA and therefore inhibit DNA synthesis. Most are cell cycle nonspecific. Their major toxicities are cardiac, hematopoietic, gastrointestinal, and reproductive. All of the antibiotics except bleomycin are vesicants. The largest category of the antibiotics is the anthracyclines, including doxorubicin, daunorubicin, epirubicin, and idarubicin. In addition to myelosuppression, the anthracyclines can cause alopecia, nausea, vomiting, and stomatitis (Wilkes and Barton-Burke, 2008).

Doxorubicin HCl

Doxorubicin hydrochloride (Adriamycin, Rubex) inhibits DNA and RNA synthesis and is cell cycle nonspecific. It is indicated in the treatment of acute lymphoblastic and myeloblastic leukemia, soft tissue and bone sarcomas, neuroblastoma, Wilms' tumor, Hodgkin's and non-Hodgkin's lymphoma, and breast, bladder, thyroid, lung, gastric, and ovarian cancers. Cardiotoxicity is the major dose-limiting toxicity, presenting as arrhythmias (which can be life-threatening), left ventricular heart failure, and irreversible cardiomyopathy. An electrocardiogram and cardiac ejection fraction (MUGA scan) should be obtained as a baseline before administering doxorubicin, and cardiac function is monitored periodically throughout the course of treatments. The recommended lifetime cumulative dose is 550 mg/m². Dexrazoxane is often given to those patients who have received a cumulative dose of 300 mg/m² and are continuing treatment. Dexrazoxane is specifically indicated for women with metastatic breast cancer who have reached the 300 mg/m² dose level and need to continue doxorubicin treatment. Myelosuppression is severe, with a nadir of 7 to 14 days. Doxorubicin has a moderate (30% to 90%) emetic risk; however, emetic risk increases when doxorubicin is given in conjunction with cyclophosphamide. Common side effects are stomatitis, photosensitivity, radiation recall, hyperpigmentation, and flare reaction. Complete alopecia occurs in 3 to 4 weeks. The patient should be informed that the urine turns red-orange for 1 to 2 days. Doxorubicin is physically incompatible with 5-fluorouracil and heparin when given through the same administration set. This drug causes very severe tissue damage and necrosis if extravasated (Cortes-Funes and Coronado, 2007; Hideg and Kalei, 2007; Schulmeister, 2007a).

Daunorubicin HCl

Daunorubicin hydrochloride (daunomycin hydrochloride, Cerubidine) interferes with DNA synthesis and is cell cycle nonspecific. It is indicated for remission induction in acute nonlymphocytic and lymphocytic leukemia. Chronic cardiotoxicity is dose related and presents as congestive heart failure, with a mortality rate of 50%. A MUGA scan is indicated before treatment. Acute cardiotoxicity may occur within minutes of administration and presents as supraventricular arrhythmias. Preexisting cardiac disease or exposure to other anthracyclines or cardiotoxic drugs increases the risk for cardiotoxicity. The recommended cumulative lifetime dose is 500 to 600 mg/m². Bone marrow suppression occurs, with a nadir of 7 to 14 days. Daunorubicin has a moderate (30% to 90%) emetic risk. Common side effects are diarrhea, mucositis, hepatotoxicity, complete alopecia (3 to 4 weeks), radiation recall, flare reaction, and photosensitivity. Extravasation will cause severe soft tissue necrosis. Mixing daunorubicin hydrochloride with dexamethasone or heparin in the same administration set causes precipitation (Wilkes and Barton-Burke, 2008).

Epirubicin

Epirubicin (Ellence) is an anthracycline antitumor antibiotic analog. It inhibits nucleic acid and protein synthesis and causes cleavage of DNA by topoisomerase II. It is indicated in the treatment of breast cancer. Epirubicin has a moderate (30% to 90%) emetic risk. Common side effects are diarrhea, mucositis, and complete alopecia. Concurrent administration of cardiovascular drugs, such as calcium channel blockers, increases the risk of congestive heart failure. A MUGA scan is indicated before treatment, and cimetidine should not be given to patients receiving epirubicin; renal toxicity is increased. Tissue sensitization to radiotherapy may occur (radiation recall reaction). Soft tissue necrosis occurs if epirubicin extravasates. Secondary acute myelogenous leukemia (AML) has been reported in patients with breast cancer treated with anthracyclines, including epirubicin (Gluck, 2005; Pfizer, 2007; Wilkes and Barton-Burke, 2008).

Idarubicin HCl

Idarubicin hydrochloride (Idamycin) is a synthetic anthracycline. It is cell cycle specific for the S phase and acts by inhibiting DNA synthesis. It is indicated in the treatment of acute myeloid leukemia, chronic myelogenous leukemia, and acute lymphocytic leukemia. Cardiotoxicity is the dose-limiting toxicity and can be fatal. Baseline cardiac function should be determined before the initial treatment and monitored throughout the course of treatment. Congestive heart failure, myocardial infarction, arrhythmias, electrocardiogram changes, and cardiomyopathy may occur. The maximum safe dose is unknown. Risk increases with preexisting cardiac conditions, radiation to the mediastinal area, and prior treatment with anthracyclines. Myelosuppression is severe and dose related, with a nadir of 7 to 14 days. Idarubicin has a moderate (30% to 90%) emetic risk. Other common side effects are cramps, diarrhea, and mucositis. Although rare, severe enterocolitis with perforation has occurred. Alopecia, generalized rash, urticaria, and bulbous erythrodermatous rash on the palms and soles are common. Radiation recall and flare reaction may occur. The patient should be informed that the urine may be red for 2 to 3 days. Idarubicin is a vesicant capable of severe tissue necrosis if extravasated. Idarubicin should not be mixed with heparin in an administration set or central venous access device as the drug will precipitate (Wilkes and Barton-Burke, 2008).

Dactinomycin

Dactinomycin (actinomycin D, Cosmegen) is cell cycle nonspecific and inhibits DNA replication and RNA synthesis. It is indicated in the treatment of Wilms' tumor, rhabdomyosarcoma, carcinoma of the testes and uterus, Ewing's sarcoma, gestational choriocarcinoma, and melanoma. Nausea and vomiting are severe and usually occur within the first 1 to 2 hours after the start of treatment. Other common adverse reactions are anorexia, diarrhea, erythema, alopecia, and radiation recall. Myelosuppression may be severe, with a nadir of 7 to 14 days. Hepatotoxicity and anaphylaxis may occur. Dactinomycin is contraindicated in patients with existing or recent exposure to chicken pox or herpes zoster; life-threatening reactions may occur. Dactinomycin is a vesicant that can cause severe tissue necrosis if extravasated (Wilkes and Barton-Burke, 2008).

Mitoxantrone

Mitoxantrone (Novantrone) is cell cycle nonspecific and exerts its antitumor effect by interfering with DNA and RNA synthesis. It is indicated in combination therapy in acute and chronic leukemias, advanced or recurrent breast cancer, ovarian cancer, and advanced hormone-refractory prostate cancer pain. Myelosuppression is the dose-limiting toxicity, with a nadir of 7 to 14 days. Mitoxantrone has a low (10% to 30%) emetic risk. Common adverse effects are mucositis, diarrhea, abdominal pain, headache, fever, rash, dyspnea, and alopecia. Seizures, heart failure, arrhythmias, and a decrease in left ventricular ejection fraction have been reported. Cardiac toxicity may be more common in patients with a history of heart disease, radiation to the mediastinum, or prior anthracycline therapy. Hydration before and after administration is necessary to prevent uric acid nephropathy. Mitoxantrone turns the urine a blue-green color within 24 hours and may cause a bluish discoloration of the sclera. Mitoxantrone is an irritant with vesicant potential. If extravasation occurs, ulceration is rare unless a concentrated dose infiltrates. The skin in the involved area will turn blue. Mitoxantrone is incompatible in the same administration set with heparin (Wilkes and Barton-Burke, 2008).

Mitomycin

Mitomycin (mitomycin-C, Mutamycin) inhibits DNA and RNA synthesis and is cell cycle nonspecific. It is indicated in the treatment of adenocarcinoma of the stomach, pancreas, and colon and in advanced breast, non–small cell lung, ovarian, uterine, cervical, head, and neck cancers. Myelosuppression is delayed 4 to 8 weeks and is cumulative. Mitomycin has a low (10% to 30%) emetic risk. Anorexia, diarrhea, alopecia, purple bands on the nails, and pain at the infusion site are common. Interstitial pneumonitis may occur, with a nonproductive cough and fever as the presenting symptoms. When administered with vinca alkaloids, mitomycin may cause acute respiratory distress. Mitomycin is a vesicant, and extravasation should be avoided (Wilkes and Barton-Burke, 2008).

Bleomycin sulfate

Bleomycin sulfate (Blenoxane) is cell cycle specific in the G_2 phase and inhibits DNA synthesis. It is indicated in the treatment of testicular carcinoma, lymphoma, malignant pleural effusions, and squamous cell carcinoma of the head, neck, skin, cervix, vulva, and penis. Bleomycin has a minimal (<10%) emetic risk. The most significant toxicity of bleomycin is pulmonary. The earliest symptoms are dyspnea and rales, followed by pneumonitis and progressing to pulmonary fibrosis. This occurs in about 10% of patients and is fatal in 1%. Increased risk includes age older than 70 years, total cumulative dosage greater than 400 units, previous lung disease, history of radiation to the thoracic area, and concomitant use with other antineoplastics, especially methotrexate. Respiratory effort and lung sounds should be monitored frequently. Anorexia and stomatitis are common but mild. Myelosuppression, if it occurs, is mild, with a nadir of 10 days. Febrile reactions, which may be delayed for 3 to 6 hours, are very common, especially in patients with lymphoma. Premedicating with diphenhydramine and acetaminophen may lessen the fever and chills. Hyperpigmentation, photosensitivity, nail changes, erythema, rash, skin tenderness, and alopecia occur in nearly half the patients.

A test dose of 1 to 2 units is recommended because anaphylaxis may occur, especially in patients with lymphoma. Bleomycin is the only antitumor antibiotic that is not a vesicant (Wilkes and Barton-Burke, 2008).

LIPOSOMAL ANTHRACYCLINES

Daunorubicin citrate liposome (DaunoXome) and doxorubicin hydrochloride liposome (Doxil) are two traditional drugs encapsulated with a polyethylene coating that allows the drug to evade detection by the immune system, thereby increasing the amount of drug reaching the tumor cell. The benefits of liposomal encapsulation are increased circulation time, decreased side effects, and the ability to penetrate altered vasculature. Toxicities are similar to those for daunorubicin and doxorubicin but are less severe. Liposomal anthracyclines do not discolor the urine, and alopecia, nausea, and vomiting are rare. Their most common side effects are myelosuppression, cardiac events, stomatitis, skin reactions (e.g., hand-foot syndrome), and hypersensitivity reactions. Mild to moderate cardiac events may occur, presenting as chest pain, palpitations, and tachycardia. Allergic reactions have been reported (7%) in the first 5 minutes, with presenting symptoms of back pain, facial flushing, chest tightness, headache, chills, or hypotension. Doxil and DaunoXome are approved for use in the treatment of advanced human immunodeficiency virus (HIV)-related Kaposi's sarcoma. Doxil is also approved for the treatment of ovarian carcinoma and multiple myeloma. Doxil and DaunoXome should never be administered through an in-line filter because this will rupture the encapsulating coating. Liposomal anthracyclines are classed as irritants, not vesicants. Extravasations should be treated by applying ice. Although maximum lifetime dosage does not appear to be a factor, a baseline cardiac assessment including MUGA scan should be done before treatment. Neither Doxil nor DaunoXome should be mixed with 0.9% sodium chloride, bacteriostatic agents (benzyl alcohol), or any other solution (Batist, 2007; Ortho Biotech, 2007; Petre and Dittmer, 2007; Rahman et al, 2007; Samad et al, 2007; Udhrain et al, 2007; Wilkes and Barton-Burke, 2008).

TAXANES
Docetaxel

Docetaxel (Taxotere) inhibits cancer cell growth by preventing cellular mitosis or division. It is indicated in the treatment of locally advanced or metastatic breast cancer, non–small cell lung cancer, prostate cancer, gastric adenocarcinoma, and head and neck cancer. Bone marrow suppression is the most common and dose-limiting toxicity. Docetaxel has a low (10% to 30%) emetic risk. Other common adverse reactions are stomatitis, diarrhea, weakness, fluid retention, alopecia (80%), and severe hypersensitivity reactions. All patients should be premedicated with corticosteroids before and during administration of docetaxel to reduce the incidence and severity of fluid retention and hypersensitivity reactions. Docetaxel is contraindicated in patients with a known allergy to polysorbate 80, a sorbitol ester used in drug manufacturing (Sanofi-Aventis, 2007; Wilkes and Barton-Burke, 2008).

Paclitaxel

Paclitaxel (Taxol) is a natural product obtained by a semisynthetic process from the needles and bark of the Western yew tree. Paclitaxel is an antimicrotubule agent and induces abnormal arrays or "bundles" of microtubules throughout the cell cycle (Jordan and Kamath, 2007). It is indicated as first-line and subsequent therapy for the treatment of advanced ovarian carcinoma, as adjuvant treatment of node-positive breast cancer, and as treatment for breast cancer after failure of combination chemotherapy for metastatic disease or relapse within 6 months of adjuvant chemotherapy. In combination with cisplatin, it is indicated for the first-line treatment of non–small cell lung cancer in patients who are not candidates for potentially curative surgery and/or radiation therapy. Paclitaxel is also indicated for the second-line treatment of AIDS-related Kaposi's sarcoma. Bone marrow suppression, especially neutropenia (90%), is dose related and is the major dose-limiting toxicity. If paclitaxel and cisplatin or carboplatin are being administered in the same treatment, paclitaxel should be given first; studies have shown that myelosuppression is profound if it is given after cisplatin. Paclitaxel has a low (10% to 30%) emetic risk. Mucositis and diarrhea are common and occur more often with 24-hour infusions versus 3-hour infusions. Alopecia is very common, occurring in about 82% of patients. Hypersensitivity occurs in 10% of patients, and anaphylaxis characterized by dyspnea and hypotension requiring treatment, angioedema, and generalized urticaria has occurred in 2% to 4% of patients receiving paclitaxel. Fatal reactions have occurred in patients despite premedication. All patients should be pretreated with corticosteroids, diphenhydramine, and H_2 antagonists, and the paclitaxel should be infused over 3 hours via an infusion pump or controller. Patients who experience severe hypersensitivity reactions to paclitaxel should not be rechallenged with the drug. Peripheral neuropathy has been observed in 62% of patients, and the occurrence increases with cumulative doses. This is usually manifested by numbness, tingling, and pain in the hands and feet. There may be loss of deep tendon reflexes and fine motor skills. A baseline electrocardiogram with cardiac assessment should be performed before administering the first dose because of the potential cardiac side effects of the drug. Severe conduction abnormalities have been documented. If this occurs, the patient should receive cardiac monitoring with subsequent doses. Paclitaxel must be mixed in a glass or polyolefin container and infused via a paclitaxel-compatible administration set to prevent leaching of DEHP (diethylhexylphthalate) found in most polyvinylchloride IV administration sets. An in-line 0.2-micron filter must be used to remove particulate matter that forms in the solution. Paclitaxel is contraindicated in patients with a hypersensitivity to polyoxyethylated castor oil, which is a vehicle often used to transport drugs in solution (Bristol-Myers Squibb, 2007; Kingston and Newman, 2007; Marupudi et al, 2007).

Although paclitaxel is not classified as a vesicant, there have been reports of cellulitis, induration, skin exfoliation, necrosis, and fibrosis following paclitaxel infiltration. In a review of these published reports, Stanford and Hardwicke (2003) concluded that paclitaxel may be a "mild vesicant" because tissue necrosis can occur but it is not severe.

TOPOISOMERASE I INHIBITORS

Topoisomerase I inhibitors are a class of semisynthetic antineoplastic agents extracted from the Chinese tree *Camptotheca acuminator*. They specifically target topoisomerase I, an essential human enzyme, and are combined with other antineoplastic agents with activity dependent on DNA disruption, such as cisplatin and etoposide (O'Brien et al, 2007).

Irinotecan HCl

Irinotecan hydrochloride (Camptosar) is a topoisomerase I inhibitor that prevents the production of the enzyme topoisomerase I, which is necessary to DNA replication. It is indicated in the treatment of metastatic carcinoma of the colon or rectum that has reoccurred or progressed after 5-fluorouracil therapy. Irinotecan hydrochloride can cause severe diarrhea that is either acute (within 24 hours) or late onset (3 to 11 days after treatment). Severe sweating and orthostatic hypotension may occur. The patient's fluid status and serum electrolyte levels must be monitored to prevent dehydration and electrolyte imbalances, which can be life-threatening. The patient should be informed about the potential for severe diarrhea and instructed to avoid use of laxatives. Myelosuppression is severe. Irinotecan has a moderate (30% to 90%) emetic risk. Other common side effects are anorexia, abdominal enlargement, flatulence, constipation, flushing, shortness of breath, and alopecia. Insomnia, dizziness, headache, back pain, and muscular weakness are common central nervous system (CNS) side effects. Irinotecan hydrochloride is an irritant and should not be allowed to contact the skin. If contact does occur, the skin should be washed thoroughly with soap and water. If extravasation occurs, the infusion should be stopped immediately, ice applied, and the physician notified (Seiter, 2005; Wilkes and Barton-Burke, 2008).

Topotecan HCl

Topotecan hydrochloride (Hycamtin) is a topoisomerase I inhibitor that prevents the production of the enzyme topoisomerase I, which is essential to DNA replication. It is indicated in the treatment of metastatic carcinoma of the ovary after failure of initial or subsequent chemotherapy and in the treatment of small cell lung cancer after failure of first-line chemotherapy. Bone marrow suppression, primarily neutropenia, is the dose-limiting toxicity, with a nadir of 11 to 15 days. The severity of myelosuppression may be increased if topotecan is administered in combination with cisplatin. Topotecan has a low (10% to 30%) emetic risk. Common adverse reactions are stomatitis, anorexia, abdominal pain, diarrhea, constipation, dyspnea, fever, and fatigue. Headache is the most commonly reported CNS toxicity. Most patients will experience at least some alopecia, with about 30% having total alopecia (Pommier, 2006; Wilkes and Barton-Burke, 2008).

MISCELLANEOUS DRUGS
Asparaginase

Asparaginase (L-asparaginase, Elspar) is an enzyme that destroys asparagine, an amino acid necessary for protein synthesis. It is indicated in the treatment of acute lymphocytic leukemia and acute and chronic myelocytic leukemia. Nausea and vomiting are mild but common. Mild bone marrow suppression occurs. Prolongation of clotting factors may occur, and disseminated intravascular coagulation may develop. Renal failure, hepatotoxicity, hemorrhagic pancreatitis, fatal hyperthermia, depression, fatigue, coma, confusion, and death have been reported. Hypersensitivity reactions are common. Intradermal skin testing with 2 international units of asparaginase is recommended before the first dose, and should be repeated if doses are 7 days or more apart. The chance of a reaction increases with repeated doses and is more likely to occur in adults than in children. The

site should be observed for at least 1 hour. A wheal indicates a positive response and is a contraindication to therapy (Wilkes and Barton-Burke, 2008).

CHEMOTHERAPY DOSING

Optimal chemotherapy doses are based on clinical trial data. Doses are individualized and calculated using the patient's body surface area (BSA) for adults, the area under the curve (AUC) for carboplatin dosing in adults, or the patient's weight (on a milligram per kilogram basis, usually for pediatric doses). A patient's BSA, expressed in meters squared (m^2), is determined by entering the patient's measured height and weight into a BSA calculator or computerized program. BSA should be verified by two independent checks of the calculation. If a chemotherapy dose is 50 mg/m^2, for example, and the patient's BSA is determined to be 2 m^2, the patient's chemotherapy dose would be 100 mg (Kaestner and Sewell, 2007).

The current practice of using BSA to calculate chemotherapy doses recently has been criticized. There is variation among patients in how chemotherapy is metabolized, and therapeutic drug monitoring with dose adjustment may be of more clinical value. Flat-fixed chemotherapy dosing regimens also have been suggested to avoid potential dose calculation errors, which in some cases may be fatal. A dosing strategy based on a genetic variant involved in a chemotherapy agent's metabolic pathway has also been suggested (and is under investigation) as a patient-tailored dosing strategy in cases where a genetic variant is known to affect the pharmacokinetics of the chemotherapy agent. For an increasing number of new chemotherapy agents in development, the use of BSA is no longer included in dose calculation in the early phases of drug development. Although the patient's BSA has been the basis of chemotherapy dose calculation for over 50 years, alternative strategies are likely to be developed and adopted in the near future (Mathijssen et al, 2007).

Because renal function (especially glomerular filtration rate [GFR], which can be estimated using the Cockcroft-Gault formula) affects the efficacy and toxicities of carboplatin, the AUC is used to determine carboplatin dosing. The AUC is the area under the curve when the concentration of a drug in plasma is plotted against time. The target AUC is ordered by the prescriber of the chemotherapy and usually is 5 to 7 mg/mL/minute. The Calvert formula is used to calculate a carboplatin dose:

Dose of carboplatin in milligrams = (Target AUC) × (GFR ± 25)

Dosing based on milligrams per kilogram is commonly used to calculate chemotherapy doses for young children and infants. Measured weights should be obtained at the time the chemotherapy is prescribed to help ensure accurate dosing.

Dose adjustments may be needed because of the patient's clinical status or manufacturers' recommendations. Patients' weights must be measured before each chemotherapy treatment cycle, and doses adjusted for weight gain or loss. Dose adjustment may be needed for obese patients, patients with ascites, or those with amputated limbs. A dose reduction may be indicated when organ impairment or toxicity from previous chemotherapy is present. The manufacturers of a few chemotherapy agents specify a maximum dose. For instance, although a typical dose of vincristine is 1.4 mg/m^2, a maximum dose of 2 mg is recommended.

Higher chemotherapy dose intensity has been studied as a way of improving clinical outcomes. Dose intensity or dose-dense therapy is a function of dose and frequency of administration. Chemotherapy dose intensity correlates strongly with clinical response, median survival, and median progression–free survival. However, in clinical practice in the United States, more than half of patients being treated with curative intent frequently have doses reduced or treatment delayed. Consequently, chemotherapy dose intensity is significantly reduced (Lyman, 2006).

A cumulative chemotherapy dose refers to the total amount of a chemotherapy agent that a patient has received. Doxorubicin is an example of a chemotherapy agent that is cardiotoxic, so its dose limit (the maximum amount a patient should receive in his/her lifetime) is 550 mg/m^2. When a patient is receiving doxorubicin, the cumulative chemotherapy dose is monitored and the drug is discontinued once the maximum lifetime dose is reached.

CHEMOTHERAPY ADMINISTRATION

Before administering chemotherapy, the nurse should prepare the patient for chemotherapy and teach the patient about the prescribed chemotherapy agents, their side effects, and symptom management. The planned treatment schedule, including plans for monitoring the patient's complete blood count, needs to be reviewed. Information given to patients should be easy to read and in appropriate language, and include pertinent phone numbers and contact information. If the patient is receiving multiple medications, especially for a co-morbid condition, a pharmacy consultation may be indicated. The nurse reviews the chemotherapy orders against the patient's treatment plan or protocol, verifies chemotherapy dose calculations, obtains equipment as needed (e.g., infusion pump, monitoring devices), and ensures that a chemotherapy spill kit and emergency drugs and equipment are available. Additional actions, such as obtaining the patient's written consent for chemotherapy, should be performed in accordance with organizational policies and procedures (Box 18-1) (Polovich et al, 2005).

VESICANT CHEMOTHERAPY ADMINISTRATION

Vesicant chemotherapy agents can cause tissue necrosis if they leak from the vein or are inadvertently administered into the tissue (e.g., accidentally injected into the muscle or infused into the tissue when a noncoring needle dislodges from an implanted port). Vesicant agents include the anthracyclines (doxorubicin, daunorubicin, epirubicin, and idarubicin), plant alkaloids (vincristine, vinblastine, vinorelbine), nitrogen mustard, and paclitaxel, which is classified as a mild vesicant (Box 18-2).

 ## SYMPTOM MANAGEMENT

NAUSEA AND VOMITING

Nausea and vomiting are two of the most common side effects of chemotherapy. Vomiting is a reflex controlled in the emetic center of the brain stem. The emetic center releases signals via various neurotransmitters and receptors to end organs, such as the stomach. Most of the activity occurs at the dopamine, serotonin, and neurokinin-1 receptors. Uncontrolled nausea and vomiting can lead to fluid and electrolyte imbalances, impaired nutrition, nonadherence to chemotherapy treatment, and a reduced quality of life. When antiemetics are optimally used, nausea and vomiting can be prevented in 70% to 80% of patients (Jordan and Kamath, 2007; Warr, 2008).

Three distinct patterns of emesis are associated with chemotherapy administration. Acute emesis occurs in the first 24 hours and is the most severe. Delayed emesis begins 18 to 24 hours after treatment and may continue for several days. Anticipatory emesis is a conditioned response that is triggered by chemotherapy-associated sights, smells, visual cues, thoughts, and anxiety (Aapro et al, 2005; Feeney et al, 2007).

Antiemesis guidelines have been developed by the American Society of Clinical Oncology (ASCO), the Multinational Association of Supportive Care in Cancer (MASCC), and the National Comprehensive Cancer Network (NCCN). Acute chemotherapy-induced nausea and vomiting are prevented and treated with serotonin receptor antagonists, dexamethasone, and aprepitant. Dexamethasone and aprepitant are used to treat delayed nausea

---

Box 18-1   PRINCIPLES OF CHEMOTHERAPY ADMINISTRATION

- Insert a new venous access device before administering peripheral chemotherapy.
- Use a flexible IV catheter for chemotherapy administration. Avoid use of rigid, steel-winged needles.
- Preferably, choose an infusion site in the patient's forearm. Avoid the dorsum of the hand, wrist, and antecubital fossa areas.
- Secure the venous access device and place a transparent dressing over the site to allow visualization of the site.
- Establish a blood return and ensure patency of the device.
- Use appropriate personal protective equipment to administer the chemotherapy in accordance with organizational guidelines.
- Teach patients about the chemotherapy agents they are receiving, side effects, and signs and symptoms to report.

Box 18-2   VESICANT EXTRAVASATION PREVENTION

- All peripherally administered vesicants should be given via a newly placed venous access device, ideally in the forearm.
- Noncoring needles of adequate length should be securely inserted into implanted ports before vesicant administration.
- Instruct the patient to refrain from movement during vesicant administration and report any change in sensation at or around the administration site.
- Ensure that a blood return is obtained before, during (every 3 to 5 seconds), and following vesicant administration. Vesicant administration should only proceed when there is a blood return or other evidence of correct placement or patency (e.g., dye study for implanted ports).
- Monitor closely for swelling, redness, lack of a blood return, and an IV flow rate that slows or stops.
- When in doubt, err on the side of caution, and restart a peripheral IV or insert a new noncoring needle.

and vomiting. Cognitive therapy and benzodiazapines are used to prevent and treat anticipatory nausea and vomiting (Kris et al, 2006; Feeney et al, 2007; NCCN, 2006; MASCC, 2007).

Serotonin receptor antagonists

Serotonin receptor antagonists are the most effective agents to prevent acute nausea and vomiting. Serotonin receptors are major neuroreceptors in the initiation of nausea and vomiting, particularly in the acute phase. There are a number of agents available (dolasetron [Anzemet], granisetron [Kytril], ondansetron [Zofran], and palonesetron [Aloxi]) that are all highly effective at recommended doses. Serotonin receptor antagonists are administered immediately before emetogenic chemotherapy and continued for a few days. The major side effects of these antiemetics are headache, diarrhea, fatigue, fever, and drowsiness (Feeney et al, 2007; Vrabel, 2007).

Neurokinin-1-receptor antagonists

Neurokinin-1-receptor antagonists block the neurokinin-1 (NK-1) receptor, which is found in the vomiting and vestibular centers of the brain. Aprepitant (oral Emend) and fosaprepitant dimeglumine (Emend for injection) are the only drugs in this class that are currently available. When combined with a serotonin receptor antagonist and dexamethasone therapy, they have added efficacy in treating both acute and delayed nausea and vomiting (Dando and Perry, 2004; Olver et al, 2007; Merck and Co., 2008a, 2008b).

Corticosteroids

Dexamethasone is the most commonly used antiemetic corticosteroid. Corticosteroids are synergistic with other agents and are particularly important in the prevention of delayed nausea and vomiting. The most common side effects with short-term use include insomnia, gastric irritation, and transient hyperglycemia (Feeney et al, 2007).

Dopamine receptor antagonists

Dopamine receptor antagonists include metoclopramide, prochlorperazine, promethazine, and haloperidol. Although the overall efficacy of these agents when used alone is low, they are sometimes used in conjunction with other antiemetics for breakthrough emesis. Prochlorperazine is particularly useful as an additional or rescue antiemetic because it is available as a suppository and can be given via the rectum when a patient is vomiting and cannot take oral antiemetics (Feeney et al, 2007).

Benzodiazepines

Benzodiazepines can reduce anxiety that some patients anticipate and experience before and during chemotherapy. They are not antiemetics but are used in conjunction with antiemetics. The benzodiazepine lorazepam can be given sublingually, which may be preferable to oral administration for patients who have severe anticipatory nausea and vomiting (Feeney et al, 2007).

Nonpharmacological measures

In addition to antiemetic administration, there are several nursing care measures that may help reduce nausea and vomiting. It is helpful to obtain a nausea history and institute any intervention that may have been helpful in the past. Patients should avoid eating or drinking 1 to 2 hours after chemotherapy treatments. Many patients find that cold food or foods served at room temperature taste better and do not have as strong an odor as hot foods. Dry toast or crackers may help settle the patient's stomach, especially first thing in the morning. Bland foods rather than spicy or strongly flavored foods are better tolerated. Clear liquids such as gelatin, juice, ginger ale or other carbonated beverages, and herbal tea provide fluids to prevent dehydration. Sport drinks also furnish limited amounts of electrolytes. Liquids should be sipped slowly. Tart foods such as sour hard candy, dill pickles, or lemons may be helpful to some patients. Foods that are known to increase nausea, such as fried fatty foods or foods with a strong odor, should be avoided. Soft, relaxing music; low lights; and a quiet atmosphere can be helpful. Some patients respond well to diversions such as card games, movies, or crafts. Acupressure, acupuncture, behavior modification, progressive muscle relaxation, yoga, hypnosis, massage therapy, and guided imagery also may be helpful (Molassiotis et al, 2002; Yoo et al, 2005; Raghavendra et al, 2007; Tipton et al, 2007).

MYELOSUPPRESSION
Neutropenia

Myelosuppression is the most common dose-limiting factor in chemotherapy administration. Leukopenia and, more specifically neutropenia, predispose the patient to infection. Patients are at a moderate risk for infection when their absolute granulocyte count (AGC) is 1500 to 2000/mm^3 and are at high risk for infection when their AGC is lower than 500/mm^3. Neutropenia may require chemotherapy treatment delays or dose reductions that may impact patients' treatment outcomes (Cairo, 2000).

Infection prevention measures—such as handwashing and evidence-based practice with respect to skin preparation before venipuncture, catheter site care, and changing of intravenous administration sets—reduce the risk of infection in patients with cancer (Friese, 2007).

Colony-stimulating factors (CSFs) enhance granulocyte production and shorten the nadir, or lowest point, between chemotherapy treatments. The 2008 National Comprehensive Cancer Network's (NCCN's) *Myeloid Growth Factor Guidelines* incorporate the most recent evidence in supporting the use of CSFs for the management of chemotherapy-induced neutropenia. All adult patients with solid tumors and nonmyeloid malignancies should be assessed for the risk of neutropenic complications before each chemotherapy cycle. Risk factors include older age, female gender, poor performance status, poor nutritional status, decreased immune function, co-morbidities, bone marrow disease, advanced stage of cancer, and high-dose chemotherapy treatment. CSFs (filgrastim or pegfilgrastim) are recommended for prophylaxis of febrile neutropenia and maintenance of scheduled dose delivery. An algorithm and guidelines for identifying patients at risk for febrile neutropenia, along with CSF dosing guidelines, are available at the NCCN website: www.nccn.org (National Comprehensive Cancer Network, 2008).

Thrombocytopenia

A normal platelet count ranges between 150,000 and 400,000/mm^3. The risk of bleeding increases when the count is below 100,000/mm^3. Signs and symptoms of thrombocytopenia include bleeding gums, petechiae, nosebleeds, and multiple bruises. Spontaneous, frank bleeding usually does not occur until the platelet count is below 20,000/mm^3. Thrombocytopenia places the patient at risk for intracranial and gastrointestinal bleeding. The patient is usually transfused with platelets if actively bleeding or if the platelet count is below 20,000/mm^3.

The platelet growth factor recombinant human interleukin-11, also known as oprelvekin (Neumega), can be given by subcutaneous injection to prevent severe thrombocytopenia and to reduce the need for platelet transfusions. The most common side effects are edema (which can be severe), dyspnea, headache, atrial flutter or fibrillation, syncope, nausea, vomiting, and rash (Bhatia et al, 2007).

Pressure should be applied to all venipuncture sites for 3 to 5 minutes after the venous access device is removed. Shaving should be done with an electric razor rather than a blade. Tampons should be avoided to decrease the potential for vaginal bleeding. Hazardous activities that may cause injury, such as contact sports and working with sharp instruments, should be avoided. Patients should be cautioned against using aspirin, ibuprofen, indomethacin, warfarin, quinidine, and other drugs that prolong clotting. Patients should be instructed to report easy bruising, nosebleeds, bleeding gums, and bloody stools.

Anemia

A patient is considered anemic if the hemoglobin level is lower than 8 g/dL. Anemic patients may be asymptomatic or present with headache, dizziness, lightheadedness, shortness of breath, fatigue, pallor, hypothermia, and pale nail beds and conjunctiva. Many physicians do not transfuse if the patient is asymptomatic. One unit of red blood cells (RBCs) can be expected to raise the hemoglobin level by 1 g/dL.

Erythropoiesis-stimulating agents, such as epoetin alfa (Epogen and Procrit) and darbepoetin (Aranesp), can be effective in stimulating RBC production. Erythropoietin mimics the natural hormone produced in the kidneys, stimulating and increasing the rate of RBC production. A Cochrane review of 57 clinical trials involving nearly 10,000 patients concluded that the lowest dose of erythropoietin that will gradually increase the hemoglobin concentration to the lowest level sufficient to avoid red blood cell transfusion should be administered. The review also found that erythropoiesis-stimulating agents increase the risk for death and for serious cardiovascular events if administered when the hemoglobin level is greater than 12 g/dL (Bohlius et al, 2004).

Common side effects of erythropoiesis-stimulating agents are headache, fever, fatigue, nausea and vomiting, diarrhea, shortness of breath, rash, and injection site reactions. Pain in the long bones and pelvis with cold sweats may occur for several hours after the injection. Blood pressure should be monitored often because hypertension resulting from a rapid hematocrit rise may precipitate seizures and vascular accidents (Wilkes and Barton-Burke, 2008).

FATIGUE

Cancer-related fatigue is the most common side effect of cancer and its treatment. It is often under-recognized, under-reported, and under-treated (Schwartz, 2007).

A systematic review and meta-analysis of 41 randomized controlled trials of psychological and activity-based interventions for cancer-related fatigue found that there is limited support for nonpharmacological interventions (e.g., exercise, relaxation, education programs, measures to optimize sleep quality) (Jacobsen et al, 2007). However, while exercise may not completely alleviate fatigue, studies have shown that it reduces the intensity of fatigue and the distress associated with its occurrence. Treatment of anemia and use of psychostimulants also may be helpful (Dimeo, 2001; Sood and Moynihan, 2005; Mitchell et al, 2007).

ANOREXIA AND TASTE ALTERATIONS

Anorexia and taste alterations are common among patients receiving chemotherapy. Lack of interest or an aversion to food can lead to anorexia, inadequate nutritional intake, and significant weight loss, which can affect the patient's overall quality of life.

Dysgeusia, which is also referred to as taste blindness, is a condition in which the gustatory sense is impaired. This results in familiar foods tasting entirely different and in some circumstances unpleasant. Patients receiving cisplatin, cyclophosphamide, vincristine, or 5-fluorouracil often experience dysgeusia. Some patients experience a bitter or metallic taste or no taste at all. Most patients prefer to have their food served on glass dishes, and many use a plastic fork if they have a metallic taste in their mouth. The nurse can do many things to help the patient and family members cope with this distressing symptom (Box 18-3). The patient should be advised that gum and hard candy, especially the sour types, may be beneficial between meals. The patient should also be instructed to brush his or her teeth often to help eliminate unpleasant tastes. Rinsing the mouth with a nonirritating mouthwash is often refreshing. The patient and caregiver should be encouraged to experiment with different spices and flavorings. This is particularly important because the taste buds have changed and need to be stimulated. Most patients find they have an aversion to meats, especially red meats, which usually have a bitter taste. Many foods have an exaggerated sweetness that can increase the patient's nausea. Patients should be made aware that the food is not spoiled; rather their sense of taste has been affected by the chemotherapy. Cold foods or foods served at room temperature are usually better tolerated than hot foods. Cold fruits and cheeses are often a better alternative to a hot meal. Many patients tolerate multiple small meals better than three large meals. Patients should be encouraged to eat. Artificial saliva or water sprayed in the mouth can help moisten the mucous membranes. Hard, dry food can cause discomfort and is difficult to swallow, whereas soft, moist foods are more pleasing to the palate. Commercial mouthwashes, smoking, and alcohol should be avoided because these products can irritate the mucous membranes (Berteretche et al, 2004; Bernhardson et al, 2007).

Box 18-3   NURSING SUGGESTIONS TO HELP THE PATIENT AND FAMILY COPE WITH TASTE ALTERATIONS

- Provide oral hygiene before meals.
- Arrange food attractively.
- Avoid strong cooking odors, such as cabbage or broccoli.
- Eat in a pleasant, relaxed environment.
- Use pleasant odors, such as cloves.
- Avoid noxious odors, such as fish.
- Enhance food flavors with herbs, spices, or marinade.
- Serve cold foods rather than hot foods.
- Eat frequent, small meals.
- Administer antiemetics before meals.
- Drink high-energy shakes.
- Serve food on glass dishes and use plastic silverware.

CONSTIPATION

Constipation is the difficult, and sometimes painful, passage of hard, dry stool. The severity of the problem can vary from mild discomfort to the development of a paralytic ileus. There are many causes of constipation in addition to chemotherapy, including anxiety, depression, opioids, muscle relaxants, hypercalcemia, immobility, dehydration, dietary deficiencies, and tumor involvement resulting in intrinsic or extrinsic bowel compression. Treatment of constipation depends on the underlying cause. Patients at high risk for constipation, such as those taking opioids and patients receiving vinca alkaloids, may require prophylactic stool softeners or stimulants. Patients at risk for constipation should be instructed to increase their dietary intake of fresh fruits, vegetables, and fiber. Unless contraindicated, the patient should have at least 2 to 3 L of fluids daily. Cheese, eggs, refined starches, chocolate, candy, and foods known to be constipating should be avoided. Eating at the same time each day helps regulate bowel movements. Because physical activity and exercise stimulate peristalsis, patients should be encouraged to be as active as possible. Patients also should be instructed to respond to the urge to defecate immediately and not wait (Thomas, 2007).

DIARRHEA

Diarrhea, the abnormal passage of five or more loose or watery stools in a 24-hour period, often is accompanied by abdominal cramping. The GI tract produces up to 8 L of fluid per day, and the colon reabsorbs the fluid and produces formed or semiformed stool. As with constipation, there are many causes of diarrhea. Postoperative intestinal resection, inflammatory bowel syndrome, *Clostridium difficile* and other intestinal infections, malabsorption syndrome, and cancer-related treatments of chemotherapy, radiation, and biologic therapy can cause diarrhea. The epithelial cells lining the GI tract can be destroyed by the antimetabolites (e.g., 5-fluorouracil), which causes inadequate absorption and digestion of nutrients resulting in diarrhea. Patients with six or more diarrhea stools a day are at risk for dehydration and electrolyte imbalance. Nursing management of diarrhea includes instructing the patient on the importance of early intervention to avoid complications. Patients should be instructed to increase their intake of constipating foods such as cheese and eggs. Many patients have a lactose intolerance, which results in diarrhea; consequently, these patients need to use caution with dairy products. Buttermilk and yogurt contain *Lactobacillus* and can usually be tolerated by lactose-intolerant patients. Foods high in pectin, bulk, and fiber help slow peristalsis. Fluid replacement prevents dehydration. Patients should avoid spicy foods, which irritate the GI tract. Fatty or greasy foods stimulate evacuation of the colon. Raw fruits and vegetables, nuts, caffeine, seeds, popcorn, and alcohol should also be avoided. Foods and liquids should be served at room temperature. Nursing interventions also include accurately recording intake and output. The stool should be measured, if possible. The consistency and number of stools should be noted. Three or more stools a day is an indication for intervention. Patients need to have at least 2 L of fluid per day. Because electrolytes are lost through the diarrhea, an electrolyte solution is recommended. Potassium is one of the major electrolytes lost; therefore fluids and foods high in

this element should be used. Pharmacological intervention should be started as soon as possible to avoid complications of fluid and electrolyte loss. Several prescription and over-the-counter medications are designed to control diarrhea. In cases of severe diarrhea, IV fluid replacement and antimotility agents, such as loperamide (Imodium), diphenoxylate (Lomotil), or octreotide (Sandostatin), may be indicated (Schiller, 2007).

ALOPECIA

For most patients, especially women, the fear of alopecia is second only to the fear of chemotherapy-induced nausea and vomiting. Although hair loss is temporary, alopecia may adversely affect self-image. Rapidly dividing cells, including the hair follicles, are affected by chemotherapy. Hair loss may be thinning, partial, or complete, and may involve not only the scalp but also the eyebrows and eyelashes and facial, axillary, pubic, nasal, and body hair. Hair loss may begin in 7 to 10 days after treatment, and is usually complete in 1 to 2 months. Regrowth usually occurs 3 to 6 months after the last chemotherapy treatment, but sometimes begins before treatments are completed. Patients should have an opportunity to obtain a wig, hat, or scarf before hair loss occurs. Purchasing a wig before losing hair allows a closer match of color and style to the natural hair. Care of the scalp should be the same as that for any area of exposed skin (Box 18-4). Patients should be instructed to use a gentle soap. Lotion or a moisturizer helps keep the scalp from becoming dry but should not be used during radiation treatments to the head. The skin on the scalp is tender and burns if exposed to bright sunlight. Scarves, turbans, or hats provide comfort, protect against the sun, and preserve body heat in the winter (Dougherty, 2007; Frith et al, 2007).

STOMATITIS AND MUCOSITIS

The mucous membranes of the GI tract, especially those of the mouth, can become red, irritated, and inflamed. Stomatitis can range from a mild irritation and sensitivity when eating acidic or spicy foods to full-blown sores, with difficulty swallowing. Chemotherapy-related stomatitis usually begins 5 to 7 days after treatment and lasts about 10 days. Good oral hygiene is imperative in reducing the amount of bacteria in the mouth and decreasing the potential for infection (Box 18-5). A soft toothbrush or gauze prevents further irritation to the delicate tissue. When the mouth is particularly tender, it is advisable for patients to remove their dentures or partial plate at night and as much as possible during the day.

Box 18-4   RECOMMENDATIONS FOR THINNING HAIR

- Use mild shampoo and conditioner and avoid excessive shampooing.
- Avoid using such appliances as curling irons, hot combs, and blow dryers.
- Avoid hairstyles that place tension on the hair, such as ponytails and braids.
- Use a wide-tooth comb to groom hair rather than a brush.
- Avoid chemicals, such as permanents, coloring, or hair spray.

Box 18-5   PREDISPOSING FACTORS FOR DEVELOPMENT OF STOMATITIS
• Poor fitting dentures • Poor nutritional status • Head and neck radiation • Concurrent steroid therapy • High-dose chemotherapy • Advanced age • Antimetabolites, especially 5-fluorouracil and methotrexate • Antitumor antibiotics • Continuous infusion of chemotherapy versus short infusions • Hematological malignancies

Box 18-6   RISK FACTORS FOR CARDIOTOXICITY
• Prior radiation to the mediastinum or left chest wall • Hypertension • History of smoking • Advanced age • Cardiac disease • Multiple cardiac drugs • High-dose therapy and doses over recommended lifetime dosage

The patient should be instructed to eat soft foods with a smooth consistency. Usually, cold, wet foods are soothing to the irritated mucous membranes. Special attention should also be given to the lips to prevent cracking and drying. Applying lip balm, aloe vera, or a petroleum-based gel keeps the lips moist and promotes comfort and healing. Care should be taken to provide adequate nutrition and hydration. In cases of severe stomatitis, the patient may need to be hospitalized for fluid support and pain management (Polovich et al, 2005).

A Cochrane review of 277 studies of mucositis (caused by radiation as well as chemotherapy) noted that a variety of drugs and substances to prevent or treat mucositis have been studied. Although there were concerns about the rigor of many of the studies, ice chips were found to effectively prevent or reduce mucositis in patients receiving 5-fluororuracil (Worthington et al, 2000).

CARDIOTOXICITY

Cardiotoxic chemotherapy agents include the anthracyclines, doxorubicin and daunorubicin, mitoxantrone, paclitaxel, and, in high doses, cyclophosphamide (Polovich et al, 2005). Early signs of chemotherapy-induced cardiotoxicity may be difficult to detect. An electrocardiogram may show a decrease in voltage of the QRS complex or nonspecific ST- or T-wave changes. The anthracyclines can damage the myocytes, weakening the cardiac muscle. This results in decreased cardiac output, with progression to congestive heart failure. The patient usually is asymptomatic until signs and symptoms of congestive heart failure appear. Patients complain of shortness of breath, especially on exertion, and a nonproductive cough. The physical examination shows neck vein distention, tachycardia, gallop rhythm, and edema. A drop in the baseline ejection fraction signals a decrease in left ventricular function. In these situations, the risk of cardiac damage and complications must be weighed against a meaningful tumor response. Most physicians obtain a baseline MUGA scan or an echocardiogram with an ejection fraction and repeat these tests at the halfway point of the total accumulated lifetime dose and at the end of therapy. Frequent electrocardiogram monitoring to detect changes in the voltage of the QRS complex helps identify early signs of impending toxicity (Box 18-6). In selected patients, a percutaneous endomyocardial biopsy is indicated to determine the degree of myocyte damage (Jones et al, 2006; Scully and Lipshultz, 2007; Bird and Swain, 2008).

NEUROTOXICITY

Neurotoxicity is a debilitating side effect of chemotherapy. The incidence of this side effect is increasing because more neurotoxic chemotherapy agents are in use and patients are living longer and receiving multidrug chemotherapy regimens (Wickham, 2007). Neurotoxicity may affect the central nervous system (CNS) or peripheral nervous system. CNS toxicity includes encephalopathy, seizures, cerebellar dysfunction, mental status changes, ophthalmic toxicities, and ototoxicities. Peripheral toxicity causes axonal degeneration or demyelination involving sensory and motor dysfunction. Paclitaxel, cisplatin, carboplatin, and the vinca alkaloids are the agents most likely to cause neurotoxicity. Peripheral neuropathy usually does not occur until after five or more treatments. The exception to this is paclitaxel, which can produce paresthesia within 5 days of administration. When cisplatin is used concurrently with paclitaxel, the patient has an increased potential for neurotoxicity. Patients usually complain of numbness and tingling of the hands and feet (Hausheer et al, 2006; Wilkes and Barton-Burke, 2008).

Tools to reliably and accurately measure neuropathy are in development. There is limited evidence that supports the psychometric properties of the Total Neuropathy Score, a composite measurement tool (Smith et al, 2008).

As the toxicity increases, the patient begins to complain of muscle pain, weakness, and disturbances in depth perception, particularly with ambulation. Patients need to be cautioned about loose rugs, steps, and articles lying on the floor that may cause the patient to trip. Because there is a decrease in sensation, the patient needs to exercise caution with temperature changes. Hot water, heating pads, electric blankets, hot stoves, and radiators are more likely to cause burns with decreased perception of temperature. Exposure to cold is also a concern because these patients are less likely to realize the severity of the temperature. Patients should be adequately dressed for the weather, with special protection for the hands and feet. Constipation and paralytic ileus are other concerns in this patient population. Symptoms can be manifested within 2 days, and this is particularly true in patients receiving vinca alkaloids. Vincristine has good tissue-binding capacity, which results in prolonged exposure of the neural tissue. The patient should be observed for abdominal distention and active bowel sounds, and the diet should be regulated according to the patient's needs, adding fresh fruits and vegetables, fiber, and fluids. Constipation can be compounded in the patient who is also receiving concurrent narcotics. Prophylactic stool softeners can assist in maintaining regularity, and suppositories, oral laxatives, or lubricants may be used. Enemas should be used with caution in the neutropenic patient. Depending on the severity, symptoms of neuropathy usually disappear in a few weeks. If treatment continues, deep tendon reflexes may not return, and muscle weakness may be a problem for many months. In severe cases, motor function may never return to normal (Visovsky et al, 2007).

RENAL TOXICITY

The chemotherapeutic agents that may cause renal toxicity are cisplatin, carmustine, streptozocin, methotrexate, mitomycin-C, and, to a lesser degree, carboplatin. Concurrent administration of amphotericin, the aminoglycoside antibiotics, and vitamin C potentiates nephrotoxicity. Baseline laboratory values of the BUN and creatinine levels need to be obtained before administration of these nephrotoxic agents. When patients have preexisting renal impairment, the risk-versus-benefit ratio must be weighed carefully. Chemotherapy doses that could produce a meaningful tumor response may need to be reduced to protect the patient from further renal damage and to compensate for the longer half-life resulting from renal dysfunction. Vigorous hydration is often administered before nephrotoxic chemotherapy agents. Mannitol and furosemide (Lasix) may also be given to promote diuresis. Accurate intake and output with frequent weights need to be monitored and recorded (Wilkes and Barton-Burke, 2008).

Mesna (Mesnex) is a cytoprotectant effective in reducing the incidence of ifosfamide-induced hemorrhagic cystitis. Mesna does not prevent hemorrhagic cystitis in all patients; therefore a morning urine sample should be checked for hematuria after ifosfamide administration. Common side effects are diarrhea, headache, fatigue, nausea, and hypotension (Wilkes and Barton-Burke, 2008).

Methotrexate precipitates in an acid solution, obstructing the renal tubules. Raising the urinary pH can be accomplished by administering an alkalylating agent to the patient before giving high-dose methotrexate in the form of bicarbonate, orally or intravenously. Measurement of the urinary pH is often ordered to ensure that the pH is greater than 7. If the pH drops below 7, additional bicarbonate is given (Wilkes and Barton-Burke, 2008).

PULMONARY TOXICITY

A few chemotherapy agents have the potential to damage the endothelial cells of the lung. Bleomycin at dosages exceeding a lifetime dose of 400 units and carmustine in total doses of 1500 mg/m^2 predispose patients to pneumonitis and interstitial fibrosis. Toxicity appears to be increased with the concurrent use of cyclophosphamide. Other antineoplastics known to cause pulmonary toxicity include mitomycin and methotrexate. Pulmonary toxicity usually develops over weeks to months but can develop within hours. The patient usually presents with dyspnea, a nonproductive cough, fatigue, and fever. Auscultation of the lungs reveals end-inspiratory basilar rales. The chest radiograph is nonspecific or has streaky infiltrates and consolidation. Elderly patients and patients with a smoking history, current or past radiation therapy to the lungs, or a preexisting pulmonary condition appear to be at greater risk for pulmonary toxicity (Wilkes and Barton-Burke, 2008).

SEXUAL AND REPRODUCTIVE DYSFUNCTION

Chemotherapy adversely affects gonadal function. As cancer treatments have become more effective and survival rates continue to improve, there are more cancer survivors for whom parenting is an important consideration and/or goal. Preservation of fertility is an active area of research (Kwon and Case, 2002; Marsden and Hacker, 2003).

In males, chemotherapy reduces the sperm count and temporary or permanent infertility may result. Men often are offered the option of sperm banking before the initiation of chemotherapy. Men receiving chemotherapy report decreased sexual desire, activity, and satisfaction, and ejaculatory difficulty is common (Fegg et al, 2003).

Chemotherapy suppresses ovarian function in women. Within 6 months of starting chemotherapy, women may experience amenorrhea or changes in their menstrual cycle. Many women have symptoms of a medical menopause, including hot flashes, irritability, insomnia, and vaginal dryness. Gametes or embryos may be frozen before chemotherapy and ovarian tissue may be frozen and stored, with several pregnancies documented after subsequent grafting. There is also increasing interest in protecting the ovaries by using gonadotropin-releasing hormone analogs during chemotherapy (Minton and Munster, 2002; Stern et al, 2006).

VESICANT EXTRAVASATION

Vesicant chemotherapy has the potential to cause tissue necrosis if these agents leak (extravasate) from the vein or are inadvertently administered into the tissue. The extent of tissue necrosis is dependent on several factors, such as the type of vesicant (DNA-binding or non–DNA-binding), concentration and amount of vesicant extravasated, extravasation location (e.g., hand, wrist, antecubital area), and patient factors (older age, co-morbidity). DNA-binding agents, such as the anthracyclines (daunorubicin, doxorubicin, epirubicin, and idarubicin), bind to the DNA in healthy cells when they extravasate into the tissue and cause cell death. These agents are retained in the tissue for long periods of time and cause progressive tissue necrosis. Historically, extravasations of DNA-binding agents have usually required wound debridement and skin grafting or flap placement. In September 2007, the FDA approved the first anthracycline extravasation treatment, Totect (dexrazoxane for injection), which has a 98% efficacy in diminishing tissue damage and allows the majority of patients to continue with scheduled chemotherapy (Schulmeister, 2007a, 2007b; TopoTarget USA, 2007).

Non–DNA-binding agents, such as the plant alkaloids (e.g., vincristine, vinblastine, and vindesine), do not bind to the DNA in healthy cells when they extravasate. Because they are metabolized in the tissue, agents that facilitate dispersion into the tissue, such as hyaluronidase, often are effective in minimizing tissue damage induced by these agents (Box 18-7) (Schulmeister, 2007a).

Much of the research in the area of vesicant extravasation management has been conducted on animals (primarily rodents), and differences in animal anatomy and physiology limit the application of these research findings to humans. Anecdotal reports and small studies of clinically diagnosed vesicant extravasations have been reported with mixed results. Because these extravasations were clinically diagnosed, it is uncertain if they were in fact extravasations, or possibly infiltrations of fluid or nonvesicant chemotherapy agents (Schulmeister, 2007a). The only research that has been conducted on patients with biopsy-confirmed vesicant extravasations was clinical studies evaluating Totect.

Box 18-7   VESICANT CHEMOTHERAPY EXTRAVASATION MANAGEMENT

- If a vesicant chemotherapy extravasation occurs or is suspected, stop the infusion immediately and evaluate for swelling and blood return. If there is any doubt about the patency of the vein, restart the peripheral venous access device in a new site.
- Aspirate residual drug from the venous access device or noncoring needle.
- Apply ice to anthracline, nitrogen mustard, and paclitaxel extravasations per organizational policy (usually 15 to 20 minutes 4 to 6 times daily for 24 to 48 hours).
- Apply heat to vinca alkaloid extravasations per organizational policy (usually 15 to 20 minutes 4 to 6 times daily for 24 to 48 hours).
- Elevate the extremity (peripheral extravasations).
- Avoid exposing the extravasation area to sunlight.
- Administer antidotes and treatment as outlined below.

MECHLORETHAMINE (NITROGEN MUSTARD)

Antidote: Sodium thiosulfate
Mechanism of action: Sodium thiosulfate neutralizes mechlorethamine to form nontoxic thioesters that are excreted in urine.
Preparation: To prepare a 1/6th molar solution, mix 4 mL of sodium thiosulfate 10% with 6 mL of sterile water for injection.
Administration: Inject 2 mL of the solution for each milligram of mechlorethamine suspected to have extravasated. Inject the solution into the extravasation site using a 25-gauge or smaller needle (change needle with each injection). Store the solution at room temperature between 15° and 30° C (59° and 86° F).

VINCA ALKALOIDS (VINCRISTINE, VINBLASTINE, VINORELBINE)

Antidote: Hyaluronidase
Mechanism of action: Hyaluronidase is a protein enzyme that degrades hyaluronic acid and promotes drug diffusion.
Preparation: Available hyaluronidase preparations include:
- **Amphadase** [bovine] (hyaluronidase injection, Amphastar Pharmaceuticals, Rancho Cucamonga, Calif)
  - Vial contains 150 units per 1 mL.
  - Do not dilute. Use solution as provided.
  - Store in refrigerator at 2° to 8° C (36° to 46° F).
- **Hylenex** [recombinant] (hyaluronidase human injection, Baxter Healthcare Corp., Deerfield, Ill)
  - Vial contains 150 units per 1 mL.
  - Do not dilute. Use solution as provided.
  - Store in refrigerator at 2° to 8° C (36° to 46° F).

- **Vitrase** [bvine] (hyaluronidase injection, ISTA Pharmaceuticals, Irvine, Calif)
  - Vial contains 200 units in a 2-mL vial.
  - Dilute 0.75 mL of solution with 0.25 mL of 0.9% sodium chloride (final concentration is 150 units per 1 mL).

Administration: Administer 1 mL of the solution as five 0.2-mL injections into the extravasation site using a 25-gauge or smaller needle (change needle with each injection).

ANTHRACYCLINES (DAUNORUBICIN, DOXORUBICIN, EPIRUBICIN, IDARUBICIN)

Treatment: Totect (dexrazoxane)
Mechanism of action: The mechanism by which Totect diminishes tissue damage resulting from the extravasation of anthracycline drugs is unknown. Some evidence suggests that it reversibly inhibits topoisomerase II.
Preparation: The recommended dose of Totect (dexrazoxane for injection, TopoTarget USA, Rockaway, NJ) is as follows:
- Day 1: 1000 mg/m^2
- Day 2: 1000 mg/m^2
- Day 3: 500 mg/m^2

The first infusion should be initiated as soon as possible and within 6 hours of the anthracycline extravasation. The maximum recommended dose is 2000 mg on days 1 and 2 and 1000 mg on day 3. The dose should be reduced 50% in patients with creatinine clearance values <40 mL/minute. Totect is provided in a carton containing 10 vials of Totect (dexrazoxane for injection) 500 mg and 10 vials of 50 mL of diluent. Each vial of Totect must be mixed with 50 mL of diluent. The patient's dose of Totect is then added to a 1000-mL 0.9% sodium chloride infusion bag. The Totect carton should be stored at 25° C (77° F).

Administration: Totect should be infused over 1 to 2 hours in a large vein in an area other than the extravasation area (e.g., opposite arm). Cooling, such as ice packs, should be removed at least 15 minutes before Totect administration. Dimethyl sulfoxide (DMSO) should not be applied to the extravasation area. Instruct the patient about Totect treatment side effects (e.g., nausea/vomiting, diarrhea, stomatitis, bone marrow suppression, elevated liver enzyme levels, and infusion site burning). Monitor the patient's complete blood count and liver enzyme levels.

The assessment and management of a vesicant chemotherapy extravasation should be documented in accordance with organizational procedures. Some organizations create a specific documentation tool or form. Common elements of vesicant chemotherapy extravasation documentation include the date and time the extravasation occurred or was suspected, type and size of peripheral venous access device or type of central venous access device and gauge/length of noncoring needle (implanted ports), location and patency of peripheral or central venous access device, description and quality of a blood return before and during vesicant administration, concentration and estimated amount of extravasated vesicant, signs and symptoms (including measurement of the area), photographs (when indicated), immediate nursing interventions and treatments, and patient instructions (Schulmeister, 2007a).

 SAFE HANDLING

Chemotherapy agents are hazardous substances and require special handling because of potential health risks associated with exposure to these agents. Care in preparing, handling, and administering chemotherapy reduces accidental exposure from spills and sprays. Personal protective equipment should be worn whenever there is a risk of hazardous drugs being

- A double-blinded clinical study compared recombinant human hyaluronidase to a 0.9% sodium chloride control in 100 human volunteers. The volunteers were injected intradermally with hyaluronidase in one forearm and injected with 0.9% sodium chloride in the other forearm. They were evaluated for allergic responses and injection site side effects. Injection site discomfort (e.g., stinging, burning, other discomfort) occurred in 28% of the arms injected with 0.9% sodium chloride and in 3% of the arms injected with hyaluronidase. No allergic reactions occurred. Recombinant human hyaluronidase was successful in reducing local injection site discomfort that has been observed to occur with animal-derived hyaluronidase products (Baxter Laboratories, 2007).

- Two open-label, single-arm, multicenter studies were conducted in Europe to determine if Totect administration could reduce tissue injury following anthracycline extravasation and thereby reduce or avoid surgical intervention. In the two studies, anthracycline extravasation was confirmed by skin biopsies. A total of 80 patients were enrolled in the 2 studies and 57 were evaluated. The anthracyclines most commonly associated with extravasation were epirubicin (56%) and doxorubicin (41%). Sites of extravasation were the forearm (63%), hand (21%), antecubital area (11%), and implanted port (5%). Most patients presented with swelling (83%), redness (78%), and pain (43%). The median baseline extravasation area was 25 cm^2 (range 1-253 cm^2). In study 1, none of the 19 evaluated patients required surgical intervention and none had serious late sequelae. In study 2, 1 of the 38 evaluated patients required surgery. One additional nonevaluated patient required surgery for tissue necrosis. Thirteen patients had late sequelae at the event site such as site pain, fibrosis, atrophy, and local sensory disturbance; all were judged as mild except in the one patient who required surgery. None of the four patients with implanted ports required surgical intervention (Mouridsen et al, 2007).

PATIENT OUTCOMES

Expected outcomes with intravenous chemotherapy administration include:

- The patient will state the names of the chemotherapy agents to be administered, planned frequency of chemotherapy treatment, and schedule for laboratory and follow-up visits.
- The patient will list the chemotherapy side effects that may occur and describe measures to help prevent their occurrence.
- The patient will accurately describe self-care activities that need to be performed before chemotherapy administration (e.g., oral premedications, antiemetics) and will adhere to the planned administration schedule.
- The patient will describe the process for contacting health care providers and list signs and symptoms that need to be reported, such as persistent or severe nausea and vomiting, signs and symptoms of infection, unusual bleeding or excessive bruising, changes in mental status or cognition, and unrelieved diarrhea or constipation.
- The patient will report any changes in sensation at the chemotherapy administration site during chemotherapy administration.
- The patient will not experience acute complications or adverse reactions, such as hypersensitivity or vesicant extravasation.
- The patient will not experience chemotherapy-induced toxicity, such as pulmonary or renal toxicity.
- The patient will receive the correct intravenous chemotherapy agent in the correct dose via the correct route at the correct time.
- The patient will receive chemotherapy treatment without dosage adjustments or treatment delays.
- The patient will achieve the goal of chemotherapy treatment as identified for that patient (e.g., cure, control, palliation).

(OSHA) guidelines recommend that gloves, gowns, and eye/face protection are worn during chemotherapy administration (OSHA, 2008).

A vertical laminar flow hood, class II biologic safety cabinet, is used to prepare chemotherapy to prevent the release of aerosol spray in the air and potential exposure to toxic substances. Bottles and bags should be spiked and administration sets primed in the chemotherapy preparation area before adding the antineoplastic agent. This provides an added safety margin for the nurse when connecting the infusion to the patient. After the infusion has been completed, the administration set should be flushed with 0.9% sodium chloride or a solution compatible with the drug to eliminate the potential for an accidental spill while disconnecting it. If a chemotherapeutic agent comes in contact with the skin, the area must be thoroughly cleansed with mild soap and large amounts of water (OSHA, 2008).

Inadvertent spills should be cleaned up immediately. Most institutions have a chemotherapy spill kit that contains a sawdustlike substance or an absorbent, plastic-backed sheet to soak up the solution. Spills are cleaned starting from the outside edges and working toward the center. Traffic in the spill area needs to be limited to prevent spread of the contamination. Broken glass is gathered with a disposable scoop. The involved area should be washed with copious amounts of soap and water at least three times. Protective clothing, including a low-permeability gown or cover-up and safety glasses, face shield, or goggles, should be worn while cleaning a spill of chemotherapeutic agents and disposed of properly (OSHA, 2008).

All contaminated material, such as gloves, administration sets, and filters, should be discarded in a double-thick, leak-proof, and sealable plastic bag and labeled as a biohazard. Sharp instruments, including needles, syringes, and ampules, should be placed in a leak-proof, puncture-resistant container and disposed in accordance with federal, Environmental Protection Agency, and OSHA regulations. State regulations may vary and have other specific requirements that must be followed.

Many chemotherapy drugs are excreted in the urine and stool. The nurse needs to exercise caution when handling

released into the environment. Gloves should be designed specifically for chemotherapy or double gloving is recommended. Gloves should be changed after each use, after 30 minutes of wear, or if they become torn or exposed to chemotherapy. Occupational Safety and Health Administration sputum, emesis, or excreta from patients receiving chemotherapy. Gloves should always be worn when cleaning an incontinent patient or when emptying a Foley catheter or bedpan. The primary caregiver needs to be aware of and use standard precautions when caring for the patient. Hands should be washed before applying and after removing gloves (Polovich et al, 2005).

FUTURE DIRECTIONS IN ONCOLOGY

Although hundreds of new antineoplastic agents are currently in use and many more are in development, treating more than 200 distinct types of cancer remains a challenge. The three principal modalities of cancer treatment—surgery, radiotherapy, and chemotherapy—have begun to give way to new targeted therapies. Targeted therapies interact with specific molecular targets, altering gene regulation and protein networks. Oral chemotherapy is increasingly replacing intravenous chemotherapy and has comparable efficacy. Several cancer vaccines that prevent cancer are in development and one is currently available (Gardasil [human papillomavirus quadrivalent (types 6, 11, 16 and 18) vaccine, recombinant]. Emerging therapies include microRNA modulators, personalized cancer treatment based on a patient's genetics and biochemistry, and agents that disrupt histone deacetylase (commonly called HDAC inhibitors) (Aisner, 2007; Murdoch and Sager, 2008).

SUMMARY

With the prevalence of antineoplastic therapy, infusion nurses need to be knowledgable of the numerous chemotherapy agents and the potential side effects associated with each drug. Symptom management and patient education are necessary to minimize any risk to the patient and ensure safe delivery of care.

REFERENCES

Aapro MS, Molassiotis A, Olver I: Anticipatory nausea and vomiting, *Support Care Cancer* 13(2):117-121, 2005.

Aisner J: Overview of the changing paradigm in cancer treatment: oral chemotherapy, *Am J Health Syst Pharm* 64(9 suppl 5):S4-S7, 2007.

American Cancer Society: *Cancer facts and figures 2007*, Atlanta, 2007, Author.

Batist G: Cardiac safety of liposomal anthracyclines, *Cardiovasc Toxicol* 7(2):72-74, 2007.

Baxter Laboratories: Hylenex (hyaluronidase human injection, recombinant) [Package insert], Deerfield, Ill, 2007.

Bayer Pharmaceuticals: Fludara (fludarabine phosphate) [Package insert], Wayne, NJ, 2007.

Bedford Labs: Floxuridine [Package insert], Bedford, Ohio, 2000.

Bedford Labs: Vinblastine [Package insert], Bedford Ohio, 2001.

Bedford Labs: Methotrexate injection [Package insert], Bedford, Ohio, 2005a.

Bedford Labs: Vinorelbine [Package insert], Bedford, Ohio, 2005b.

Bedford Labs: Etoposide for injection [Package insert], Bedford, Ohio, 2006.

Bernhardson BM, Tishelman C, Rutqvist LE: Chemosensory changes experienced by patients undergoing chemotherapy: a qualitative interview study, *J Pain Symptom Manag* 34(4):403-412, 2007.

Berteretche MV, Dalix AM, d'Ornano AM et al: Decreased taste sensitivity in cancer patients under chemotherapy, *Support Care Cancer* 12(8):571-576, 2004.

Bhatia M, Davenport V, Cairo MS: The role of interleukin-11 to prevent chemotherapy-induced thrombocytopenia in patients with solid tumors, lymphoma, acute myeloid leukemia and bone marrow failure syndromes, *Leuk Lymphoma* 49(1):9-15, 2007.

Bird BR, Swain SM: Cardiac toxicity in breast cancer survivors: review of potential cardiac problems, *Clin Cancer Res* 14(1):14-24, 2008.

Bohlius J, Wilson J, Seidenfeld J et al: Erythropoietin or darbepoetin for patients with cancer, *Cochrane Database Systematic Rev*, issue 3, article CD003407, DOI: 10.1002/14651858.CD003407.pub4, 2004.

Bristol-Myers Squibb: Taxol (paclitaxel injection) [Package insert], Princeton, NJ, 2007.

Cairo MD: Dose reductions and delays: limitations of myelosuppressive chemotherapy, *Oncology* 14(9 suppl 8):21-31, 2000.

Cortes-Funes H, Coronado C: Role of anthracyclines in the era of targeted therapy, *Cardiovasc Toxicol* 7(2):56-60, 2007.

Dando TM, Perry CM: Aprepitant: a review of its use in the prevention of chemotherapy induced nausea and vomiting, *Drugs* 64(7):777-794, 2004.

Dimeo FC: Effects of exercise on cancer-related fatigue, *Cancer* 92 (6 suppl):1689-1693, 2001.

Donahue KE, Gartlehner G, Jonas DE et al: Systematic review: comparative effectiveness and harms of disease-modifying medications for rheumatoid arthritis, *Ann Intern Med* 148(2):124-134, 2008.

Dougherty L: Using nursing diagnoses in prevention and management of chemotherapy-induced alopecia in the cancer patient, *Int J Nurs Terminol Classif* 18(4):142-149, 2007.

Eli Lilly: Gemzar (gemcitabine for injection) [Package insert], Indianapolis, Ind, 2007a.

Eli Lilly: Alimta (pemetrexed for injection) [Package insert], Indianapolis, Ind, 2007b.

Feeney K, Cain M, Nowak AK: Chemotherapy induced nausea and vomiting—prevention and treatment, *Aust Fam Physician* 36(9): 702-706, 2007.

Fegg MJ, Geri A, Vollmer TC et al: Subjective quality of life and sexual functioning after germ-cell tumour therapy, *Br J Cancer* 89(12):2202-2206, 2003.

Friese CR: Prevention of infection in patients with cancer, *Semin Oncol Nurs* 23(3):174-183, 2007.

Frith H, Harcourt D, Fussell A: Anticipating an altered appearance: women undergoing chemotherapy treatment for breast cancer, *Eur J Oncol Nurs* 11(5):385-391, 2007.

Gluck S: Adjuvant chemotherapy for early breast cancer: optimal use of epirubicin, *Oncologist* 10(10):780-791, 2005.

Hausheer FH, Schilsky RL, Bain S et al: Diagnosis, management, and evaluation of chemotherapy-induced peripheral neuropathy, *Semin Oncol* 33(1):15-49, 2006.

Hideg K, Kalai T: Novel antioxidants in anthracycline cardiotoxicity, *Cardiovasc Toxicol* 7(2):160-164, 2007.

Hussain AE, Blakley BW, Nicolas M et al: Assessment of the protective effects of amifostine against cisplatin-induced toxicity, *J Otolaryngol* 32(5):294-297, 2003.

Jacobsen PB, Donovan KA, Vadaparampil ST et al: Systematic review and meta-analysis of psychological and activity-based interventions for cancer-related fatigue, *Health Psychol* 26(6): 660-667, 2007.

Jones RL, Swanton C, Ewer MS: Anthracycline cardiotoxicity, *Expert Opin Drug Saf* 5(6):791-809, 2006.

Jordan MA, Kamath K: How do microtubule-targeted drugs work? An overview, *Curr Cancer Drug Targets* 7(8):730-742, 2007.

Kaestner SA, Sewell GJ: Chemotherapy dosing part I: scientific basis for current practice and use of body surface area, *Clin Oncol* 19(1):23-37, 2007.

Kim GP, Erlichman C: Oxaliplatin in the treatment of colorectal cancer, *Expert Opin Drug Metab Toxicol* 3(2):281-294, 2007.

Kingston DG, Newman DJ: Taxoids: cancer-fighting compounds from nature, *Curr Opin Drug Discov Devel* 10(2):130-144, 2007.

Kopp HG, Kuczyk M, Classen J et al: Advances in the treatment of testicular cancer, *Drugs* 66(5):641-659, 2006.

Kostova I: Platinum complexes as anticancer agents, *Recent Patents Anticancer Drug Discov* 1(1):1-22, 2006.

Kris MG, Hesketh PJ, Somerfield MR et al: American Society of Clinical Oncology guideline for antiemetics in oncology: update 2006, *J Clin Oncol* 24(33):2932-2947, 2006.

Kwon JS, Case AM: Effects of cancer treatment on reproduction and fertility, *J Obstet Gynaecol Can* 24(8):619-627, 2002.

Lenz JH: Management and preparedness for infusion and hypersensitivity reactions, *Oncologist* 12(5):601-609, 2007.

Lipscomb GGH: Medical therapy for ectopic pregnancy, *Semin Reprod Med* 25(2):93-98, 2007.

Lyman GH: Chemotherapy dose intensity and quality cancer care, *Oncology* 20(14 suppl 9):16-25, 2006.

Marsden DE, Hacker N: Fertility effects of cancer treatment, *Aust Fam Physician* 32(1-2):9-13, 2003.

Marupudi NI, Han JE, Li KW et al: Paclitaxel: a review of adverse toxicities and novel delivery strategies, *Expert Opin Drug Saf* 6(5):609-621, 2007.

Mathijssen RHJ, de Jong FA, Loos WJ et al: Flat-fixed dosing versus body surface area based dosing of anticancer drugs in adults: does it make a difference? *Oncologist* 12(8):913-923, 2007.

Mayne Pharma USA: Vincristine sulfate injection [Package insert], Paramus, NJ, 2004.

Merck and Co.: Mustargen (mechlorethamine HCl) [Package insert], Whitehouse Station, NJ, 1999.

Merck and Co.: Emend (aprepitant capsules) [Package insert], Whitehouse Station, NJ, 2008a.

Merck and Co.: Emend for injection (fosaprepitant dimeglumine) [Package insert], Whitehouse Station, NJ, 2008b. Accessed at http://www.merck.com/product/usa/pi_circulars/e/emend_iv/emend_iv_pi.pdf.

Merck Manuals Online Medical Library: *Dacarbazine* (website). Accessed 2/3/08 at http://www.merck.com/mmpe/print/lexicomp/dacarbazine.html.

Minton SE, Munster PN: Chemotherapy-induced amenorrhea and fertility in women undergoing adjuvant treatment for breast cancer, *Cancer Control* 9(6):466-472, 2002.

Mitchell SA, Beck SL, Hood LE et al: Putting evidence into practice: evidence-based interventions for fatigue during and following cancer and its treatment, *Clin J Oncol Nurs* 11(1):99-113, 2007.

Molassiotis A, Yung HP, Yam BM et al: The effectiveness of progressive muscle relaxation training in managing chemotherapy-induced nausea and vomiting in Chinese breast cancer patients: a randomised controlled trial, *Support Care Cancer* 10(3):237-246, 2002.

Mouridsen HT, Langer SW, Buter J et al: Treatment of anthracycline extravasation with Savene (dexrazoxane): results from two prospective multicentre studies, *Ann Oncol* 18(3):546-550, 2007.

Multinational Association of Supportive Care in Cancer: *Consensus conference on antiemetic therapy*, 2007. Accessed 2/2/08 at http://www.mascc.org/media/Resource_centers/MASCC_Guidelines_Update.pdf.

Murdoch D, Sager J: Will targeted therapy hold its promise? An evidenced-based review, *Curr Opin Oncol* 20(1):104-111, 2008.

National Cancer Institute: *Clinical trials* (website). Accessed 1/28/08 at http://cancertrials.nci.nih.gov/clinicaltrials.

National Comprehensive Cancer Network (NCCN): *Clinical practice guidelines in oncology: antiemesis. Version 2*, 2006. Accessed 1/3/08 at www.nccn.org/professionals/physician_gls/PDF/antiemesis.pdf.

National Comprehensive Cancer Network: *Practice guidelines in oncology v.1.2008: myeloid growth factors*, 2008. Accessed 1/17/08 at http://www.nccn.org/professionals/physician_gls/PDF/myeloid_growth.pdf.

Navo M, Kunthur A, Badell ML et al: Evaluation of the incidence of carboplatin hypersensitivity reactions in cancer patients, *Gynecol Oncol* 103(2):608-613, 2006.

O'Brien M, Eckardt J, Ramlau R: Recent advances with topotecan in the treatment of lung cancer, *Oncologist* 12(10):1194-1204, 2007.

Occupational Safety and Health Administration: *OSHA technical manual. Section VI, section 2. Controlling occupational exposure to hazardous drugs*, 2008. Accessed 2/23/08 at http://www.osha.gov/dts/osta/otm/otm_vi/otm_vi_2.html.

Olver I, Shelukar S, Thompson KC: Nanomedicines in the treatment of emesis during chemotherapy: focus on aprepitant, *Int J Nanomedicine* 2(1):13-18, 2007.

Ortho Biotech: Doxil (doxorubicin HCl liposome injection) [Package insert], Raritan, NJ, 2007.

Park MT, Lee SJ: Cell cycle and cancer, *J Biochem Mol Biol* 36(1):60-65, 2003.

Petre CE, Dittmer DP: Liposomal daunorubicin as treatment for Kaposi's sarcoma, *Int J Nanomedicine* 2:(3)277-278, 2007.

Pfizer: Ellence (epirubicin hydrochloride) [Package insert], New York, NY, 2007.

Polovich M, White JM, Kelleher LO: *Chemotherapy and biotherapy guidelines and recommendations for practice*, ed 2, Pittsburgh, 2005, Oncology Nursing Society.

Pommier Y: Topoisomerase I inhibitors: camptothecins and beyond, *Nat Rev Cancer* 6(10):789-802, 2006.

Rahman AM, Yusuf SW, Ewer MS: Anthracycline-induced cardiotoxicity and the cardiac sparing effect of liposomal formulation, *Int J Nanomedicine* 2(4):567-583, 2007.

Raghavendra RM, Nagarantha R, Nagendra HR et al: Mechanisms of cisplatin ototoxicity and progress in otoprotection, *Curr Opin Otolaryngol Head Neck Surg* 15(5):364-369, 2007.

Samad A, Sultana Y, Aqil M: Liposomal drug delivery systems: an update review, *Curr Drug Deliv* 4(4):297-305, 2007.

Sanofi-Aventis: Eloxatin (oxaliplatin injection) [Package insert], Bridgewater, NJ, 2006.

Sanofi-Aventis: Taxotere (docetaxel) [Package insert], Bridgewater, NJ, 2007.

Schiller LR: Management of diarrhea in clinical practice: strategies for primary care physicians, *Rev Gastroenterol Disord* 7(suppl 3):S27-38, 2007.

Schulmeister L: Preventing vincristine sulfate medication errors, *Oncol Nurs Forum* 31(5):E90-E96, 2004.

Schulmeister L: Preventing chemotherapy errors, *Oncologist* 11(5):463-468, 2006.

Schulmeister L: Extravasation management, *Semin Oncol Nurs* 23(3):184-190, 2007a.

Schulmeister L: Totect: a new agent for treating anthracycline extravasation, *Clin J Oncol Nurs* 11(3):387-397, 2007b.

Schwartz AL: Understanding and treating cancer-related fatigue, *Oncology* 21(11 suppl):30-34, 2007.

Scully RE, Lipshultz SE: Anthracycline cardiotoxicity in long-term survivors of childhood cancer, *Cardiovasc Toxicol* 7(2):122-128, 2007.

Seiter K: Toxicity of the topoisomerase I inhibitors, *Expert Opin Drug Saf* 4(1):45-53, 2005.

Singh TP: Clinical trials of newly developed anti-cancer agents in children with acute leukemia, *Contemp Clin Trials* 27(6):493, 2006.

Smith EM, Beck SL, Cohen J: The total neuropathy score: a tool for measuring chemotherapy induced peripheral neuropathy, *Oncol Nurs Forum* 35(1):96-102, 2008.

Sood A, Moynihan TJ: Cancer-related fatigue: an update, *Curr Oncol Rep* 7(4):277-282, 2005.

Stanford BL, Hardwicke F: A review of clinical experience with paclitaxel extravasations, *Support Care Cancer* 11(5):270-277, 2003.

Stern CJ, Toledo MG, Gook DA et al: Fertility preservation in female oncology patients, *Aust N Z J Obstet Gynaecol* 46(1):15-23, 2006.

Stordal B, Pavlakis N, Davey R: Oxaliplatin for the treatment of cisplatin-resistant cancer: a systematic review, *Cancer Treat Rev* 33(4):347-357, 2007.

SuperGen: Nipent (pentostatin) [Package insert], San Ramon, Calif, 1998.

Thigpen T: The role of gemcitabine in first-line treatment of advanced ovarian carcinoma, *Semin Oncol* 33(2 suppl 6):S26-S32, 2006.

Thomas J: Cancer-related constipation, *Curr Oncol Rep* 9(4):278-284, 2007.

Tipton JM, McDaniel RW, Barbour L et al: Putting evidence into practice: evidenced-based interventions to prevent, manage, and treat chemotherapy-induced nausea and vomiting, *Clin J Oncol Nurs* 11(1):69-78, 2007.

TopoTarget USA: Totect (dexrazoxane for injection) [Package insert], Rockaway, NJ, 2007.

Udhrain A, Skubitz KM, Northfelt DW: Pegylated liposomal doxorubicin in the treatment of AIDS-related Kaposi's sarcoma, *Int J Nanomedicine* 2(3):345-352, 2007.

Upjohn Pharmaceuticals: Cytosar-U (cytarabine) [Package insert], Kalamazoo, Mich, 2002.

Vermeulen K, Van Bockstaele DR, Berneman ZN: The cell cycle: a review of regulation, deregulation and therapeutic targets in cancer, *Cell Prolif* 36(3):131-149, 2003.

Visovsky C, Collins M, Abbott L et al: Putting evidence into practice: evidence-based interventions for chemotherapy-induced peripheral neuropathy, *Clin J Oncol Nurs* 11(6):901-913, 2007.

Vrabel M: Is ondansetron more effective than granisetron for chemotherapy-induced nausea and vomiting? A review of comparative trials, *Clin J Oncol Nurs* 11(6):809-813, 2007.

Warr DG: Chemotherapy- and cancer-related nausea and vomiting, *Curr Oncol* 15(suppl 1):S4-S9, 2008.

Wickham R: Chemotherapy-induced peripheral neuropathy: a review and implications for oncology nursing practice, *Clin J Oncol Nurs* 11(3):361-376, 2007.

Wilkes G: Peripheral neuropathy related to chemotherapy, *Semin Oncol Nurs* 23(3):162-173, 2007.

Wilkes GM, Barton-Burke M: *Oncology nursing drug handbook*, Boston, 2008, Jones and Bartlett.

Winkeljohn D, Polovich M: Carboplatin hypersensitivity reactions, *Clin J Oncol Nurs* 10(5):595-598, 2006.

Worthington HV, Clarkson JE, Eden OPB: Interventions for preventing oral mucositis for patients with cancer receiving treatment, *Cochrane Database Systematic Rev,* issue 1, article CD000978, 2000.

Yao X, Panichpisal K, Kurtzman N et al: Cisplatin nephrotoxicity: a review, *Am J Med Sci* 334(2):115-124, 2007.

Yoo HJ, Ahn SH, Kim SB et al: Efficacy of progressive muscle relaxation training and guided imagery in reducing chemotherapy side effects in patients with breast cancer and in improving their quality of life, *Support Care Cancer* 13(10):826-833, 2005.

19 PAIN MANAGEMENT

Melanie H. Simpson, PhD, RN-BC, OCN®, CHPN*

PAIN MANAGEMENT

Pain is the most common reason patients seek health care and yet most health care professionals have very little current education in assessing, managing, and treating pain. According to the International Association for the Study of Pain (IASP), the definition of pain is "an unpleasant sensory and emotional experience associated with actual or potential tissue damage described in terms of such damage." Patient advocacy is at the forefront of pain management, whether it involves acute pain or chronic pain. Nurses in any setting are obligated to support the patient's right to appropriate pain management (Brennan, Carr, and Cousins, 2007). To accomplish this, nurses must be armed with the knowledge of what is appropriate—of what constitutes undertreatment and overtreatment. When technologies are used, one must be able to assess their appropriateness and whether they fit into the patient's lifestyle, frame of mind, and support system. The Joint Commission now requires that hospitals provide pain management across the continuum of care. This requirement demands that the pain management plan is outlined from admission to discharge and that patients are part of that planning process when possible. Nurses need to ensure that patients and their families are well educated regarding what is available for pain management intervention and what to expect from each intervention, including side effects and complications.

BARRIERS TO EFFECTIVE PAIN CONTROL

Many health care professionals have inadequate knowledge and skills regarding the pharmacology of pain medications, physiology of pain, assessment of pain, and pain management techniques. This lack of knowledge persists despite efforts to set standards of practice and to educate health care providers. The Agency for Health Care Policy and Research (now known as the Agency for Healthcare Research and Quality) developed

and distributed pain management guidelines in the early and mid 1990s, and the American Pain Society (APS) continues to provide guidelines with the most recent publication in 2003 (APS, 2003). Yet pain control for both acute and chronic pain conditions continues to be inadequate.

A landmark study published in the *Annals of Internal Medicine* (Marks and Sacher, 1973) showed that pain is greatly undertreated. This study revealed that authorized prescribers underprescribe analgesic agents, nurses administer fewer analgesics than prescribed, patients request fewer analgesic medications than they need, and the as-needed regimen of administering opioid agents ensures that the patient will experience pain. More recent studies (Furstenberg et al, 1998; Peretti-Watel et al, 2003) show very little has changed over the years in health care providers' attitudes, knowledge, and behaviors in managing pain appropriately.

Studies have shown that we can educate health care professionals extensively and repeatedly about pain management; however, without institutional commitment for pain management implementation, it will not likely be done (Cromley and Banks, 2000; Farber et al, 1998). A pain management champion is needed to start the process. Guidelines, policies, and standards must then be established to facilitate appropriate pain management. Continuous quality improvement must be in place as well to ensure continued assurance to these guidelines.

One of the most difficult barriers in pain management is the use of negative language. For example, the term "narcotic" is now pharmacologically obsolete, because it is more a historical term (Bond and Simpson, 2006), yet both patients and health care providers continue to use this word. The word narcotic carries a negative connotation; it is therefore difficult to educate patients on the benefits of the use of these types of medications in managing pain. The correct word or term is opioid. Opioids are natural, semisynthetic, and synthetic drugs that bind at opioid receptor sites and provide analgesia.

Another frequent misuse of a term is when the health care provider says or writes that a patient "complains of pain." Patients are asked about their pain and then it is reported that the "patient is complaining of pain of eight out of ten," instead of the "patient reports or states a pain level of eight out of ten." Patients, for the most part, want to be "good" patients and not seen as complainers, so it is then difficult to get them to report

*The author and editors wish to acknowledge the contributions made by Barbara St. Marie as author of this chapter in the second edition of *Infusion Therapy in Clinical Practice*.

the information needed for a thorough pain assessment if they feel they are perceived as complaining.

Attitudes and beliefs of health care professionals serve as additional barriers to effective pain control. Some professionals believe that pain is normal or expected so there is no sense of urgency when a patient reports severe pain. The concern for iatrogenic addiction (addiction inadvertently caused from valid medical use of opioids) from families and health care providers alike is completely out of proportion to the true incidence, which in psychologically intact patients is less than 1%. The daily media are filled with information about drug abuse and addiction that feeds the fears of health care providers and the public about potential drug addiction. These concerns can inhibit the use of opioids even when recent articles (Bloodworth, 2006; Kahan et al, 2006; Guarino and Myers, 2007) show they can provide more effective pain control without a significant majority of the patients developing a problem.

Health care providers and lay people alike use the terms addiction, physical dependence, and tolerance interchangeably, yet they are all very different. This led to the publication of a consensus statement from the American Academy of Pain Management, the American Pain Society, and the American Society of Addiction Medicine (Savage et al, 2001) with the following definitions:

- *Addiction* is a primary, chronic, neurobiological disease, with genetic, psychosocial, and environmental factors influencing its development and manifestations. It is characterized by behaviors that include one or more of the following: impaired control over drug use, compulsive use, continued use despite harm, and craving.
- *Physical dependence* is a state of adaptation that is manifested by a drug class–specific withdrawal syndrome following abrupt cessation, rapid dose reduction, decreasing blood level of the drug, and/or administration of an antagonist.
- *Tolerance* is a state of adaptation in which exposure to a drug induces changes that result in a diminution of one or more of the drug's effects over time.

Health care providers are cautioned about using terms in patients' charts or in conversations with patients and other health care providers that are negative or suggestive of misuse of pain medications as well. The use of words or phrases such as drug seeking, clock watcher, or addicted to their pain medications should be avoided. Very often the patient is in no way behaving inappropriately; it is simply that the treatment for the patient's pain is not the right medication, dose, or dosing interval and needs to be addressed.

Laws and regulations were once designed to prohibit the use of opioids except in severely limited circumstances. Current regulations have tried to emphasize using opioids for treating pain in the appropriate patient population. Many organizations that address pain management issues, such as the American Pain Foundation, the American Pain Society, and the American Society of Pain Management Nursing, have been formed to organize efforts to overcome the lack of knowledge and unclear regulations. These organizations provide education for health care providers about pain management practices. Most have government relations' committees that lobby legislators and regulatory authorities regarding current pain management issues.

DISCIPLINES INVOLVED

The discipline of pain management has transformed over the years. This is no longer a subspecialty of anesthesiology alone. Physicians from anesthesiology, physical medicine and rehabilitation,

neurology, psychiatry, oncology, palliative care, internal medicine, and family medicine specialties have chosen to specialize in pain management as well. Some organizations also have nurses, pharmacists, psychologists, and ancillary professionals (e.g., physical and occupational therapists and social workers) who specialize in pain management. Teams of nurses responsible for pain management have been formed in some hospitals, hospices, and home health agencies. The nursing responsibilities of these teams range from actually administering the pain medications to educating nurses and other health care providers about proper dosing, delivery, and side effects. A pain team may also identify and solve problems associated with pain management.

A pain management medical director is usually a physician who specializes in pain management. The medical director serves as a resource to those involved in pain management and also acts as liaison and educator of other physicians. The medical director needs to understand and respect the nursing role in pain management, thereby enhancing the care that nurses give to patients in pain.

The rapidly developing discipline of pain management is in need of professional support and development. To provide this support and development with education and networking, societies and associations have been organized to advance the art of pain management for health care professionals. The American Society for Pain Management Nursing, founded in 1991, recognizes this need and responds by educating nurses and supporting nursing research in pain management. The society has established the role of the nurse in pain management, provides a professional publication, *Pain Management Nursing,* and offers national certification. As more information becomes available about pain pathways, new medications, and new routes of analgesia administration, nurses are invited to help implement advances in pain management. Continuing education regarding advances in pain management warrants high priority.

▌ PHYSIOLOGY OF PAIN

Pain warns the individual that something is wrong, but once it serves that purpose, it should be relieved. Pain is harmful to the body if left untreated (Box 19-1). There are significant endocrine responses to pain—increased heart rate, vasoconstriction, and decreased gastrointestinal (GI) motility. Pain also causes muscle splinting, which can diminish pulmonary function and lead to atelectasis or pneumonia. These findings make it even more evident that health care professionals need to take pain control seriously to reduce morbidity and mortality, reduce the length of the hospital stay, and promote a more rapid general recovery (Bond and Simpson, 2006).

PAIN NOCICEPTION

Matching clinical indicators with the appropriate pain intervention requires at least basic knowledge of the biochemical response to pain, the pain pathway, and opioid receptor sites. Melzak and Wall (1965) proposed the gate control theory of pain modulation. Current theory supports four processes involved to describe how pain becomes conscious or the nociception of pain. Those four basic processes in the nociception of pain are: (1) transduction, (2) transmission, (3) perception, and (4) modulation (McCaffery and Pasero, 1999) (Box 19-2).

Box 19-1   SELECTED HARMFUL EFFECTS OF UNRELIEVED PAIN

Area affected	Response to pain
Cardiovascular	Increased heart rate, increased cardiac output, increased peripheral vascular resistance, hypertension, deep vein thrombosis
Cognitive	Decreased cognitive function, mental confusion
Developmental	Increased behavioral and physiological responses to pain, irritability, higher somatization, addictive behavior, anxiety states
Endocrine	Increased adrenocorticotropic hormone, increased cortisol, increased antidiuretic hormone, increased epinephrine, increased norepinephrine, decreased insulin, decreased testosterone
Future pain	Debilitating chronic pain syndromes, phantom pain, postherpetic neuralgia, postmastectomy pain, post-thoracotomy pain
Gastrointestinal	Decreased gastric and bowel motility
Genitourinary	Decreased urinary output, urinary retention, fluid overload, hypokalemia
Immune	Decreased immune response
Metabolic	Gluconeogenesis, hepatic glycogenolysis, hyperglycemia, glucose intolerance, insulin resistance, muscle protein catabolism
Musculoskeletal	Muscle spasm, impaired muscle function, fatigue, immobility
Quality of life	Sleeplessness, anxiety, fear, hopelessness, increased thoughts of suicide
Respiratory	Decreased flows and volumes, atelectasis, shunting, hypoxemia, decreased cough, sputum retention, infection

Not all of these are body systems (future pain, developmental, quality of life).
Adapted from McCaffery M, Pasero C: *Pain: clinical manual*, ed 2, St Louis, 1999, Mosby.

Box 19-2   PROCESSES INVOLVED IN PAIN NOCICEPTION

1	Transduction	Noxious stimulus causes cell damage → release of sensitizing substances → action potential begins pain signal
2	Transmission	Signal moves through afferent or peripheral nerve fibers to spinal cord → up spino-thalamic tract to thalamus and cortex
3	Perception	Cortex interprets signal and pain becomes conscious
4	Modulation	Neurons from brain stem send signals down descending pathway → release of endogenous opioids, serotonin, and norepinephrine to inhibit or modulate pain signal

The fourth process is modulation; during this process neuronal impulses from the brain stem move down the descending pathway and release substances that inhibit the pain message, such as endogenous opioids, serotonin, and norepinephrine. This is a very basic explanation of how pain occurs. It is important to understand the sequence of these four distinct processes involved to help understand how specific treatments interact within a process.

Many other factors influence the pain response. These factors include past experiences of pain; anxiety and anticipatory pain; emotional, physical, or sexual abuse; history of chemical dependency; and the patient's support structures. This is why a comprehensive assessment is so important and experts agree that the patient's self-report is the gold standard for measuring pain.

PAIN NERVE FIBERS

Specialized nerve endings in the skin and viscera send messages of noxious stimuli, such as mechanical, chemical, or thermal, to the brain. These specialized nerve endings, or receptors, send impulses along specific fiber types, all of which are peripheral nerves. Most fibers that transmit acute nociceptive pain information are identified as A-delta and C fibers (Sorkin, 2005). These fibers differ in their rate of impulse conduction and their diameter. The myelinated A-delta fibers are the largest and most rapid conductors, and they transmit well-localized, sharp pain (McCaffery and Pasero, 1999). Unmyelinated C fibers have the smallest diameter and are the slowest conductors, transmitting poorly localized, dull, and aching pain. A-delta fibers tend to conduct intense pain but are more receptive to local anesthetics and nonsteroidal anti-inflammatory drugs (NSAIDs). C fibers tend to conduct dull pain and are most responsive to opioids by any route.

Dermatomes constitute the segmental distribution of the spinal nerve sensations and are labeled according to their exit point on the spinal cord. Dermatome charts (Figure 19-1) are useful for tracking the nerves innervating the area of pain. With a nerve block or the intraspinal route of analgesia, medications can be delivered directly to those nerves that are the origin of an individual's pain (Bonica, 1990).

By understanding the dermatomal distribution of pain when working with epidural infusions of opioids and local anesthetics, the nurse can collaborate with the anesthesiologist to determine the appropriate dermatomal distribution of

The first process, transduction, begins in the periphery when the skin is cut or damaged. This trauma or pain stimulus causes a number of sensitizing substances to be released at the site of injury, including prostaglandins, bradykinin, serotonin, substance P, and histamine. In order for this pain stimulus to be changed to an impulse, an action potential must be generated. Changes in the neuronal membrane and the processing or abnormal processing of the sensitizing substances establish if the pain will be perceived as nociceptive or neuropathic (see Categories of Pain).

Transmission is the next process, which allows the impulse to be carried through the afferent or peripheral nerve fibers into the spinal cord. The pain impulse continues to be carried through the dorsal horn and ascends the spinothalamic tract to the brain—in particular, the thalamus. The pathway continues as the impulse travels to the cerebral cortex, which interprets the signal as pain at the site of the cut.

The third process is called the perception of pain, during which the cortex interprets the signal of pain and the pain becomes conscious.

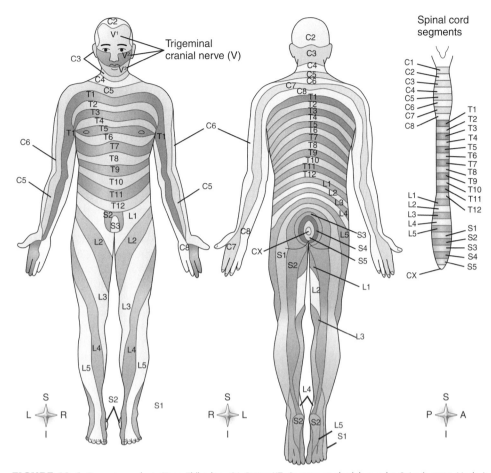

FIGURE 19-1 Dermatome chart. (From Thibodeau GA, Patton KT: *Anatomy & physiology*, ed 6, St Louis, 2007, Mosby.)

opioid and local anesthetic to the painful area. For example, when fentanyl, a lipid-soluble opioid, is used, the rate of infusion may need to be increased to widen the spread of analgesia (see Figure 19-1). The intraspinal route for medication delivery is addressed in Chapter 27.

 PAIN MANAGEMENT BASICS

People are now more aware of pain and the significant problems associated with it than in any time in history. Therefore it is important that nurses and other health care professionals have up-to-date knowledge of pain including pathophysiology, pain assessment, and treatment strategies. Years ago, the International Association for the Study of Pain established three different categories of pain: acute, chronic, and cancer (Bonica, 1990). Current theory supports that the patient's perception of pain is not different simply because the patient has a diagnosis of cancer, and therefore both cancer pain and noncancer pain should be treated equally.

CATEGORIES OF PAIN
Acute pain

Acute pain is caused by such occurrences as traumatic injury, a surgical procedure, or a medical disorder. With acute pain, the patient may show a clinical picture of tachycardia, hypertension, tachypnea, shallow respirations, agitation or restlessness,

facial grimacing, or splinting. The incidence of acute pain in hospitalized patients is astounding. The challenges of acute pain become greater when individuals also suffer from chronic pain and have other co-morbidities, a history of substance abuse, or any communication barriers.

Chronic pain

Chronic pain is persistent, often lasting more than 6 months. However, some practitioners believe that pain that exists for a shorter duration than a 6-month period may qualify as chronic pain. An individual who has chronic pain may show the same clinical picture as the person suffering from acute pain, or the individual may not appear to be in pain at all. It is simply from the patient's self-report that we know the severity of the patient's pain. It is estimated that about 26% of Americans, or 76.5 million Americans, report that they have had a persistent pain problem with a duration of more than 24 hours (of note, this does not include acute pain) (National Center for Health Statistics [NCHS], 2006).

Nociceptive pain

Nociceptive pain is the result of complex interactions between the peripheral nerves and the central nervous system as mentioned earlier. Nociceptive pain is divided into two categories as well: somatic and visceral. Somatic pain is soft tissue or musculoskeletal pain. It is usually well localized and described as achy, throbbing, or tender. Visceral pain is often caused by the abnormal stretching or distention of the smooth muscle wall of the visceral muscles or mucosa (Silver and Mayer, 2007). Visceral pain is not well localized and is described as tight, pressure, cramping, stretching or distention. Nonsteroidal anti-inflammatory drugs (NSAIDs) and opioids are the treatment of choice for these types of pain.

Neuropathic pain

Neuropathic pain is a result of disrupted or injured nerves of the peripheral or central components of the nervous system (Strassman, 2003). This type of pain is often described as numbness, burning, tingling, radiating, shooting, or electric-like. A clue that the patient is describing neuropathic pain is when the pain moves (e.g., wraps around the waist, goes down the back of the leg). Opioids alone are usually not very helpful for neuropathic pain. Antidepressants and anticonvulsants are the treatment of choice.

ASSESSMENT OF PAIN

A comprehensive pain assessment is the key to effectively managing pain. Pain assessment requires an extensive knowledge of pain, its causes, and its management. Taking the time to ask the important questions gives the nurse the information needed to formulate an accurate treatment plan. Yet sometimes in clinical practice we know there are exceptions. A brief assessment of pain is performed when the patient is in absolute distress and delaying pain management would have harmful effects. A brief assessment includes the patient's description and rating of the pain, its timing, and location; any associated symptoms; what lessens the pain or makes it worse; and what medications are being used. The brief assessment is beneficial for postoperative pain, trauma pain, and acute medical disorders. The goal of a brief assessment is to determine what pathways the pain is taking and to intervene with medications that affect those pathways directly.

A comprehensive assessment of pain is used to formulate a long-term plan for pain management. There are many components to a comprehensive pain assessment and many ways to document them (Figure 19-2). Regina Fink (2000) developed one such acronym, WILDA, as a way for health care providers to remember the primary components. WILDA stands for words, intensity, location, duration, and aggravating and alleviating factors.

The words the patient uses to describe the pain give the nurse information about what type of pain the patient may be experiencing. For example, when the patient uses words like numbness, tingling, or burning, the nurse can document that the patient has described a neuropathic pain syndrome. This should also give the nurse an idea of the appropriate intervention for that type of pain (i.e., the use of an antidepressant or anticonvulsant) (Backonja, 2002).

Knowing the intensity or pain rating is very important in selecting the treatment. In 1990 the World Health Organization (WHO) introduced a three-step ladder to use as a framework for the use of analgesics in cancer pain, and those in the field of pain are currently discussing the necessity of revising this concept (Figure 19-3) (IASP, 2005). While a very good guideline, some of the terms are outdated. The original intent for this ladder was to assist the health care provider in choosing which class of analgesic or adjuvant to use in relation to the intensity of the patient's pain.

The WHO analgesic ladder uses a 0 to 10 scale for pain intensity. On that scale, 0 represents no pain, a pain intensity of 1 to 3 represents mild pain, 4 to 6 is moderate pain, and 7 to 10 is severe pain. Each level has suggestions for what class of analgesic or adjuvant medication to use for that patient's level or intensity of pain.

For those patients who are unable to rate their pain with a number, there are many other scales that can be used. For example, with the verbal descriptor scale, patients are asked to describe their pain as mild, moderate, severe, very severe, or worst pain possible. With the faces scale, patients are asked to choose the facial expression that best represents how their pain makes them feel.

Assessing the location of pain is important because very often patients have more than one site of pain. It is essential that each location be fully assessed to determine if the patient has more than one type of pain. The duration of pain is assessed by asking, "Is the pain present more than 50% of the time or does it come and go?" If a patient has constant pain then the use of a long-acting pain medication or a basal or continuous rate of opioid infusion may be warranted. If the patient reports only episodic or transient pain, then the use of "as needed" medications is appropriate.

Aggravating and alleviating factors can be assessed by asking the patient, "What makes the pain better, and what makes the pain worse?" This information can help to determine the etiology of the pain. Most importantly, it can help decide how effective the treatments have been. In addition, other factors that need to be assessed include pain history, medical history, psychosocial issues, and any other accompanying symptoms, such as sleep, appetite, activity, concentration, mood, and relationships. Asking these questions will give the health care provider an indication of how disruptive the pain is for the patient's quality of life, such as level of activity and the ability to sleep and interact with others. When the variables of the pain have been determined, then an appropriate treatment plan can be implemented.

NON-OPIOID, ADJUVANT, OR CO-ANALGESIC AGENTS

Non-opioid, adjuvant, or co-analgesic medications can be useful in pain control, either alone or in combination with opioids. They may have independent analgesic activity, enhance the effects of opioids, or counteract the side effects of opioids (APS, 2003). They are recommended on each level of the WHO analgesic ladder. These drugs include NSAIDs (e.g., ibuprofen, naproxen) and COX-2-selective NSAIDs (e.g., celecoxib), tricyclic antidepressants (e.g., amitriptyline, nortriptyline), anticonvulsants (e.g., gabapentin, pregabalin), alpha$_2$-adrenergic agonists (e.g., clonidine), and many others. For the purposes of this chapter, just a few are listed as examples. These medications need to be considered when evaluating patients with acute and chronic pain.

NSAIDs and COX-2s

NSAIDs and COX-2s target two types of cyclooxygenase (COX) enzymes in the process of relieving pain. Cyclooxygenase type 1 (COX-1) produces prostaglandins that are beneficial to renal and gastric function and are responsible for platelet aggregation. Cyclooxygenase type 2 (COX-2) produces prostaglandins related to the inflammatory process. NSAIDs that are nonselective inhibit both COX-1 and COX-2, which means patients

1. Intensity:

PAIN SCALE

```
        0   1   2   3   4   5   6   7   8   9   10
No
Pain
```

Worst Pain Imaginable

Pain Rating _____ mm

2. Where is your pain located?   (I = Internal)
    Patient or Nurse mark drawing.   (E = External)

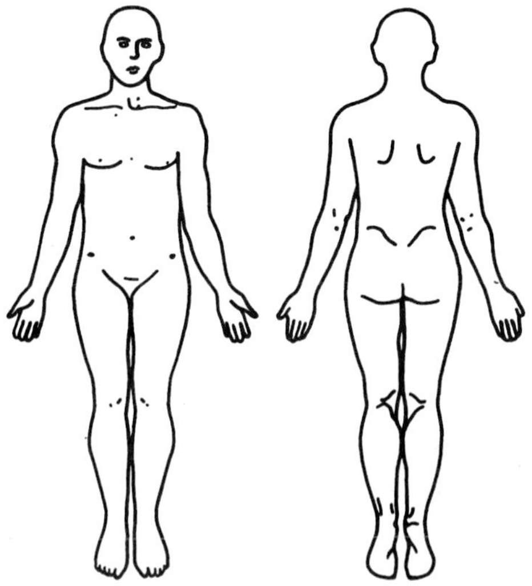

3. How and when did your pain begin?
    Does something trigger your pain?
    _____
    _____

4. How long have you had the pain?
    Is it continuous or intermittent?
    Describe any patterns or changes.
    _____
    _____
    _____

5. Describe in your own words what your pain feels like: _____
    _____
    _____
    _____

6. What makes the pain better? _____
    _____

7. What makes the pain worse? _____
    _____

8. What has helped in the past? _____
    _____

9. What has not helped in the past? _____
    _____

10. What other symptoms accompany your pain? _____
    _____

11. How does your pain affect your: _____
    Sleep? _____
    Appetite? _____
    Physical activity? _____
    Concentration? _____
    Emotions? _____
    Social relationships? _____

12. What do you think is causing your pain now?
    _____

13. Current Analgesic Regimen? _____
    _____

14. Plan/comments _____
    _____
    _____

JPI-DR-019-4A

FIGURE 19-2 Pain assessment form.

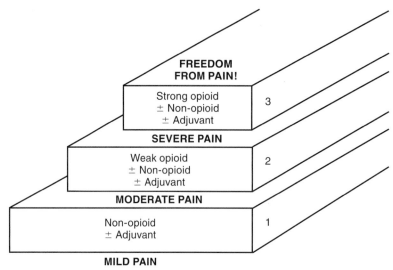

FIGURE 19-3 Analgesic ladder. (1) Assess pain severity. (2) Begin treatment at proper step of ladder. (3) Move up ladder until pain controlled. (Adapted from World Health Organization: *Cancer pain relief*, Geneva, 1990, Author.)

taking these NSAIDs can be at risk for gastrointestinal effects or increased bleeding. COX-2-selective agents selectively inhibit COX-2. When this happens, inflammation is reduced. COX-2-selective agents provide the benefit of analgesia by blocking COX-2, without affecting COX-1, which benefits the kidneys and stomach lining.

NSAIDs and COX-2s, which can be given orally, intravenously, or rectally, inhibit the synthesis of prostaglandin by inhibiting cyclooxygenase. Because of this prostaglandin-inhibiting activity, studies have shown that adjuvant use of NSAIDs (Barden et al, 2004; Mason et al, 2004) and COX-2s (Recart et al, 2003; Reuben and Ekman, 2005) (Celebrex is currently the only one available) is opioid-sparing in controlling pain postoperatively. Careful consideration should be given to the patient before administering NSAIDs or COX-2s, especially in the elderly. The patient's medical history and physical condition should be evaluated, and current medications need to be identified. For instance, if a patient has a history of renal disease or has an elevated creatinine level, the use of NSAIDs and COX-2s may be contraindicated. If the patient has a coagulopathy or is taking anticoagulants, the use of NSAIDs needs to be evaluated carefully. Because certain NSAIDs can be irritating to the stomach, patients with a history of peptic ulcer disease need to be evaluated carefully for this method of pain management because NSAIDs inhibit the production of the very prostaglandins that protect the stomach lining from gastric acids. As a result, the patient may need to receive gastrointestinal (GI) prophylaxis.

Tricyclic antidepressants

Tricyclic antidepressants are important medications for deafferentation of neuropathic pain (Iosifescu et al, 2003) caused by surgical trauma, radiation therapy, chemotherapy, or malignant nerve infiltration and have been used for many years. They are beneficial in pain control because they contribute to an increase in serotonin level in the descending pain pathway, resulting in a release of enkephalins (see Opioids section) in the spinal cord and a decrease in pain. Because of this function, tricyclic antidepressants are physiologically responsible for terminating nerve-transmitting activity. Side effects include hypotension,

sedation, constipation, and dry mouth. A contraindication for tricyclic antidepressant therapy is coronary artery disease in patients with ventricular arrhythmias.

Anticonvulsants

Anticonvulsants are used to relieve lancinating neuropathic pain arising from peripheral nerves. They can be used to treat conditions such as trigeminal neuralgia and postherpetic neuralgia. Gabapentin has been a popular anticonvulsant over the years for the treatment of neuropathic pain (Wiffen et al, 2005) because it has a low side effect profile, has no metabolite, and rarely interferes with other medications. Recent studies (Montazeri, Kashefi, and Honarmand, 2007; Turan et al, 2006) have shown that the use of gabapentin preemptively and throughout the perioperative setting decreases the use of opioids postoperatively and improves patients' satisfaction with their pain management dramatically. However, the gabapentin dose must be reduced in patients with renal insufficiency. Currently there are many other anticonvulsants as well now being used with good pain response (Backonja, 2002).

Alpha₂-adrenergic agonists

Clonidine has been approved by the U.S. Food and Drug Administration for the treatment of pain. Clonidine is effective against tactile allodynia or neuropathic pain (Wallace, 2006). It is available for epidural administration in a 100 mg/mL concentration. Hypotension, bradycardia, and sedation are possible side effects, but these are uncommon at low dosages.

OPIOIDS
Endogenous opioids

The body has its own protection against pain—endogenous opioids. These substances keep us pain-free through normal daily living. Endogenous opioids include endorphins and enkephalins. Endorphins, which are located in the brain, are mimicked by the systemic administration of opioids. Enkephalins, which are located in the spinal cord, are mimicked by the intraspinal administration of opioids. Activities that promote the release of endogenous opiates are physical exercise, deep relaxation, sexual activity, crying, and laughter. Situations that decrease the release of endogenous opioids are stress, chronic pain, chemical dependency, and depression.

Opioid receptors

Understanding opioid receptors helps us understand how opioids work to break the painful impulses. Opioid receptors are parts of cells that link with particular opioids to create analgesia and various side effects. There are three opioid receptors found within the dorsal horn of the spinal cord: mu, kappa, and delta. Of these, mu and kappa receptors are targeted by analgesics. Mu receptors are the most dense (Davis, Glare, and Hardy, 2005) in the spinal cord but are also present in the gut.

The most effective opioid receptor for producing superior analgesia is the mu receptor. Opioids that bind only at mu receptor sites are considered pure mu opioid agonists. Common examples of these include codeine, fentanyl, hydrocodone, hydromorphone, morphine, oxycodone, and oxymorphone. It has been discovered that there are subsets of the mu receptor: mu-1 and mu-2. The mu-1 receptor is responsible for analgesic effects and mu-2 for side effects. Efforts are now being made to find opioids that can combine only with mu-1. The kappa and delta receptors are much weaker than mu and may be less likely to produce physical dependency.

Agonist-antagonist

An agonist-antagonist can also reverse a mu receptor opioid (Goodman, Le Bourdonnec, and Dolle, 2007). Agonist-antagonist opioids combine at the kappa receptor site, thus producing lower quality analgesia than would a mu agonist. A commonly used agonist-antagonist that combines with the kappa opiate receptor site is nalbuphine (Nubain). Working with agonist-antagonist medications requires understanding when this kappa agonist is administered in relation to a mu agonist. When given alone, nalbuphine produces mild analgesia. Nalbuphine is given while a mu agonist is in the patient's system; however, it acts to reverse the mu agonist's analgesia and side effects. For example, a chronic back pain patient who is accustomed to taking sustained-release oral morphine (240 mg/day) is seen in the emergency department of the hospital for sudden severe onset of headache pain. An order is written to administer 10 mg of nalbuphine intravenously now for pain to supplement the oral morphine. The nalbuphine may be ordered because it has fewer side effects, but in this situation it will reverse the effects of the oral morphine, thereby producing severe pain and, most likely, symptoms of withdrawal.

Antagonist

The advantage of administering opioids for pain management is that their effects can always be reversed. Early intervention allows opioid side effects to be reversed before the situation becomes an emergency. Two types of medication can reverse a mu receptor opioid. A commonly used pure antagonist is naloxone (Narcan). This drug competitively inhibits opioids at the opioid receptor sites and thus reverses their side effects. However, naloxone (Narcan) should be given with great caution (see Box 19-3 for naloxone administration).

Box 19-3   GUIDELINES FOR USE OF NALOXONE (NARCAN) FOR RESPIRATORY DEPRESSION

1. Dilute naloxone 0.4 mg in 9 mL of 0.9% sodium chloride.
2. Give 0.5 mL slow IV push every 2 minutes until patient awakens.

   Note: Respiratory depression is rare in patients who have been receiving chronic opioid therapy, but is a significant risk in opioid-naïve patients requiring high doses for acute pain. If naloxone must be used, careful titration is required to avoid the production of acute withdrawal, seizures, and severe pain. The duration of action of naloxone is shorter than that of most opioids, so repeated dosing may be necessary.

PARENTERAL OPIOIDS

Parenteral opioid administration is considered IV (intravenous), IM (intramuscular), and Sub-Q (subcutaneous) (see Chapter 26 for subcutaneous infusion). Parenteral opioids are available in a variety of forms including continuous infusions, intermittent doses, combinations of these, and patient-controlled analgesia. Opioids may be delivered through central or peripheral venous access. Selection of opioid depends on the type of pain reported by the patient and the availability of the nursing staff for administering it appropriately.

Continuous infusion

Continuous opioid infusion provides analgesia at a steady state. For example, if the patient reports constant pain, a continuous infusion of opioids may be indicated. Before the continuous infusion is initiated, it is best to administer small doses of the opioid around the clock for 24 hours or until the pain is controlled. A problem with this system is that accumulation may occur, causing the patient to feel oversedated and possibly develop respiratory depression. To ascertain the appropriate hourly dose, consideration needs to be given to the patient's age, size, disease process, concurrent diseases, and opioid tolerance. Continuous infusions of opioids are appropriately used in trauma, postsurgical, and terminal care settings. The routes of continuous infusion include the intravenous, subcutaneous, and intraspinal (epidural or intrathecal) routes.

Intermittent doses

Patients may receive intermittent doses of opioids when they state that the pain is episodic. In these cases, it may be more desirable to treat pain only when experienced, with fast-acting opioids that are effective for short periods. For example, if the patient has a kidney stone that produces only intermittent yet severe pain, an intermittent dose of immediate-release opioid can be effective. Frequent intermittent doses of opioids can be administered through the oral, sublingual, buccal, rectal, IV, subcutaneous, or intraspinal routes. Administering opioids less frequently in larger doses can create periods of oversedation interrupted by periods of inadequate pain relief. It is more desirable to use small doses of opioid frequently than large doses infrequently. Although the frequent administration of an opioid is often time-consuming for the nurse, it is the safest method for administering opioids. Although this may be feasible for nurses attending to patients in critical care settings and postanesthesia care units (PACUs), it may not be feasible for nurses who work on postsurgical, oncology, or medical-surgical floors, where the patient/nurse ratio is larger. To solve this dilemma, the nurse should consider recommending to the authorized prescriber a patient-controlled analgesia (PCA) delivery system in which the patient can self-administer small, frequent doses of opioids.

Combination

A patient may receive a combination of continuous opioid infusion and intermittent doses of opioids. For example, if a patient is comfortable at rest but has increased pain when turned or during dressing changes, giving an additional bolus before the activity or procedure will help the patient to maintain good pain control.

Patient-controlled analgesia (PCA)

PCA has been used for many years to provide for a more customized analgesic regimen. There has been much controversy regarding the benefits associated with PCA therapy. According to a recent Cochrane Review (Hudcova et al, 2006), PCA provided better pain control and consistently rated higher in patient satisfaction than traditional as-needed dosing of IV opioids.

PCA allows patients to deliver their own opioids for pain control. PCA involves small doses of an opioid administered frequently, with the goal being to provide a steady state of analgesia, thus avoiding the peaks and valleys of analgesia, sedation, and pain (APS, 2003). PCA delivery does not, however, prevent the accumulation of an opioid and its subsequent side effects. Therefore patients need to be assessed regularly for respiratory effects and sedation level changes. A successful PCA program needs to be safe for the patient while providing adequate pain relief. PCA protocol involves the following:
- Defining appropriate candidates for PCA
- Preparing a list of teaching tools
- Selecting the medications and concentrations used

- Establishing consistency of use and dosage
- Defining who can manage the side effects
- Providing an appropriate avenue of communication between the patient and nurse to determine the quality of pain relief experienced by the patient.

The types of patients who are candidates for PCA are listed in Box 19-4.

Specific patient populations require different guidelines for setting the PCA dose and frequency. Most opioids are metabolized in the liver or kidney, so any impairment in these systems may cause accumulation. Precautions such as lowering the drug dose and increasing the time between PCA doses decrease the likelihood of opioid accumulation. Frequent nursing assessment of the patient's sedation level can detect early signs of accumulation so that doses can be adjusted accordingly.

The cooperation of nursing personnel is necessary for a successful PCA program. Infusion devices are sometimes difficult to program and troubleshoot. When patients sense a nurse's frustration in trying to program the infusion device, their faith in the pain management program can waiver. The number one error reported with PCA is programming errors. For this reason, a second nurse should always validate the correct pump settings by performing an independent double-check before initiation of therapy or with any setting changes. Nurses should receive inservice training about the infusion device before implementation and should be tested regularly for competency in operating the device.

The *Infusion Nursing Standards of Practice* (Infusion Nurses Society, 2006) emphasizes the nurse's vital role in educating the patient. The patient should become familiar with the PCA infusion device before surgery because the stress of surgery along with amnesic medications received perioperatively may cause the patient to forget any teaching that occurred in the same-day surgery area, in the PACU, or on the surgical floor postoperatively. Patient education should include discussion of the following:
- How to use patient-controlled analgesia
- When the patient is to push the bolus button
- When to communicate with the nurse (e.g., pain not controlled with PCA, feeling of sedation)
- Fear of administering too much medication
- Fear of addiction to opioids with PCA therapy
- Expected outcomes for the patient

Most patients who use PCA are more comfortable than those treated with intermittent nurse-administered opioid therapy. They have control over their own pain management and can keep their opioid blood level at a steady state, allowing them to participate in activities of recovery such as ambulation and deep breathing. An expansion of the idea of patient-controlled analgesia is Authorized Agent Controlled Analgesia (AACA), in which someone other than the patient activates the dosing, also known as "PCA by proxy." The American Society for Pain

---

FOCUS ON EVIDENCE

Pain Management with PCA

- A Cochrane review included 55 studies with 2023 patients receiving PCA and 1838 patients in the control group. The review demonstrated that PCA provided slightly better pain control and increased patient satisfaction when compared to conventional methods (Hudcova et al, 2006).
- A meta-analysis of 15 randomized controlled trials comparing the outcomes of conventional analgesia (as-needed intramuscular dosing) and patient-controlled analgesia found that patient preference strongly favors PCA over conventional analgesia (Ballantyne et al, 1993).
- A review of current evidence-based postoperative guidelines found a lack of recent IA evidence to support the use of IV PCA over IM or nurse-administered IV medications. The conclusion states that this should not be misconstrued as a lack of support for PCA, but that the absence of recent studies is a testament to its acceptance as a commonly used method of opioid delivery (Rosenquist and Rosenberg, 2003).

Box 19-4   CANDIDATES FOR PCA

- Patients who are anticipating pain that is severe yet intermittent
- Patients who have constant pain that gets worse with activity
- Patients old and young who can comprehend the technique
- Patients who have the ability to manipulate the dose button
- Patients who are motivated to use this system
- Patients who are not already sedated from other medications

PATIENT OUTCOMES

Expected outcomes for the management of the patient using PCA include:

- The patient will be able to use PCA to assist in the management of his/her pain.
- The patient will achieve his/her personal pain goal.
- The patient will verbalize discomfort or if pain intensity increases.
- The patient and family will verbalize understanding of the medication used in the PCA, potential side effects, and management of side effects.

Management Nursing does not support the use of the term PCA by proxy but has recently released a position statement (Wuhrman et al, 2007) that supports the practice of AACA. The position statement describes the criteria for appropriate use of AACA, including guidelines for selection and education of the authorized agent, prescription and monitoring recommendations during therapy, and quality improvement activities to ensure safety and effectiveness. Before an organization decides to initiate this form of analgesia, careful consideration should be given to the quality of education given to the person who will push the button.

Subcutaneous administration

Patients who are intolerant of or unable to take oral or rectal pain medications or patients in whom vascular access is not reliable or desired may want to consider the subcutaneous route of opioid administration. This route is less invasive and less costly than other parenteral opioid routes. Continuous infusions of subcutaneous opioids have all the advantages of IV opioid administration, without the need for vascular access. Subcutaneous and IV opioid infusions produce similar blood levels and provide comparable analgesia and side effects. However, the subcutaneous boluses have a slower onset, longer offset, and lower peak effect than IV bolus dosing (APS, 2003). This needs to be considered in conversion for subcutaneous dosing of opioids as well.

Morphine and hydromorphone are most often used, and no difference has been found between these two opioids in regard to pain control or side effects. Morphine is not recommended in patients with renal failure because of the active metabolite M-6 glucuronide. Methadone is not recommended because of irritation of the infusion site (Coyle, 1996). Hydromorphone has a high analgesic potency per milliliter, which makes it particularly attractive for patients who require a high-dose infusion with a small volume (Glare, 2005). This property minimizes the volume of infusion and is useful in opioid-tolerant patients who require higher hourly dosages for adequate pain relief. The effective elimination half-life of hydromorphone is 2.6 hours (Glare, 2005). Morphine has a slightly longer effective elimination half-life. It has been speculated that higher lipid solubility creates a depot effect and that higher water solubility (such as that of morphine) decreases absorption from the subcutaneous compartment into the systemic circulation, resulting in decreased bioavailability. In their study, Moulin and Kreeft (1991) showed that although plasma concentrations of opioid subcutaneous and IV infusions are similar at 24 hours, at 48 hours the plasma concentration of a subcutaneous infusion drops to 78%

of an IV infusion. Therefore adjustments may need to be made during the second day.

Subcutaneous infusions or boluses of opioids are limited to the absorption of the opioid at the subcutaneous site. The subcutaneous tissue can tolerate opioid infusions with less irritation if the infusion rate is slower than 2 to 3 mL/hour (Coyle, 1996). The preparation of opioid concentrations is therefore important to the success of subcutaneous infusions for pain control. Local toxicity from chemical irritation of the opioid is uncommon but is more likely to occur with the extremes of higher volume infusions and higher concentrations of opioid.

Problems associated with subcutaneous infusions are skin irritation at the insertion site and subcutaneous scarring. Skin irritation can be resolved with more frequent site changes and less concentrated opioids. Subcutaneous scarring interferes with the absorption of the opioid, resulting in unpredictable analgesia. Reducing opioid volume and rotating the site more often prevent scarring.

Special considerations

Although IM (intramuscular) injections are still occasionally used, they are dangerous and not recommended for analgesic administration and should be abandoned. There are many disadvantages, including painful administration, erratic absorption, lag time to peak effect, and rapid falloff of action (APS, 2003). Repeated injections can cause sterile abscesses, fibrosis of muscle and soft tissue, and the possibility of nerve injury. Another consideration is obesity, making it difficult to reach muscle through the large amounts of subcutaneous tissues in many patients.

Regional pain management using continuous infusions of local anesthetics and/or opioids with perineural catheters (PNCs) is quickly gaining favor as postoperative pain control, particularly in orthopedic surgeries (Neuburger et al, 2007). Recent studies demonstrate that continuous perineural techniques provide the benefits of prolonged analgesia with fewer side effects (Liu, 2005). More common block sites include interscalene, infraclavicular, femoral, and popliteal. Anesthesiologists place these catheters either during or after the surgery and then connect the catheters either to a traditional patient-controlled analgesia (PCA) device for inpatients or to an ambulatory disposable pump (e.g., ON-Q) for outpatients to continue at home.

NURSING CARE

Monitoring patients receiving parenteral and intraspinal opioid medications requires that the nurse document consistently. The nurse should have knowledge of the pharmacological implications of the medications along with baseline information about the patient, such as pulse rate, respirations, blood pressure, known drug allergies, history of opioid use, and the patient's pain level before opioids are given. Once the pain management plan is implemented, nurses need to reassess the patient regularly and monitor for therapeutic response, record untoward side effects, and document nursing interventions. If the reassessment warrants that the patient's pain management regimen be altered, the authorized prescriber should be notified immediately.

Nursing management of complications related to the administration of opioids requires knowledge and prompt intervention to remedy the situation. Complications include inadequate pain relief, oversedation that may progress to respiratory depression, and, with epidural administration, infection and catheter migration.

Inadequate pain relief

Nurses often do not know how to respond when patients do not receive adequate pain control from their medications. This frustration may reflect disbelief that the patient has pain or a desire to withhold opioids because of fear of addiction. These conditions often occur after a pain control measure sedates the patient to allow sleep, but when awake, the patient reports pain. The nurse needs to realize that patients in pain often do sleep and that sleep is not a good indicator of effective pain management. It can be reassuring to the nurse whose patient does not have adequate pain control to realize that there is no perfect method of pain control. Breakthrough pain may occur with any pain control method, but constant attempts to control pain should continue. In general, treating breakthrough pain with small, repetitive doses of IV opioid is a safe and effective practice that should be used routinely until the medication can be adjusted or the technique of pain management altered.

Inadequate pain relief for patients receiving epidural analgesia may occur for other reasons such as insufficient dosages of opioids and local anesthetics, an undetermined surgical complication, advancing disease process, site infection, or epidural catheter migration.

Respiratory depression

Monitoring for respiratory depression is routine to most nurses who administer opioids. Alteration of mental status such as confusion or sedation is the first indicator that the patient is receiving too much opioid. Using a level-of-sedation scale may be helpful (Box 19-5). Respiratory depression may occur with any route of opioid administration. If the nurse monitors the patient's sedation level and level of consciousness regularly, such as every 1 to 2 hours, respiratory depression can be identified early. Early identification allows the opioid dose to be reduced or stopped, or IV naloxone to be given before the respiratory depression begins. Respiratory rates should be counted for a full minute. If they drop below a predefined limit, such as 7 to 10 respirations/minute, or become shallow or noisy with poor quality and the patient is difficult to arouse, the opioid is stopped and reversal of the opioid is necessary. An abrupt reversal of all analgesia will cause the sudden onset of severe pain and may produce hypertension, tachycardia, rapid respirations, decreased GI motility, and hypercoagulability. By administering small doses of naloxone slowly (see Box 19-3), the nurse can reverse the side effects without reversing the analgesia. When reversal takes place, the patient should still be monitored for return of decreased level of consciousness and respiratory depression because the duration of some opioids can be longer than the duration of naloxone. Naloxone administration may need to be repeated. A low-dose infusion of naloxone might even be considered.

Other ways to monitor for respiratory depression include technologies such as apnea monitors, pulse oximetry, and capnography. An apnea monitor is a device frequently used that detects movements of the thorax, which it records as a ventilation rate. It varies in reliability from one patient to another and occasionally can emit loud false alarms that disrupt normal sleep in monitored patients. In many people, normal sleep is characterized by intermittent periodic breathing and short periods of apnea. Patients may develop progressive respiratory depression characterized by rapid, shallow breathing, and this is not detected by apnea monitors. Significant respiratory depression with infusions of opioids is consistently accompanied by progressive sedation that may lead to somnolence and obtundation. Therefore the best monitoring involves nursing checks every 1 to 2 hours, with observation of respiratory patterns and assessment of level of consciousness. During nighttime sleep, patients need only be touched to see that they arouse easily, and the respiratory rate can be counted without disturbing sleep. Sleep deprivation related to apnea monitor false alarms may have adverse medical consequences.

Monitoring oxygen saturation (SpO_2) with pulse oximetry is another tool used for patients receiving opioid therapy. There are mixed results about this method detecting hypoventilation in a patient. Fu et al (2004) did a two-part study using pulse oximetry to determine the effect of supplemental oxygen on the detection of hypoventilation. They found that hypoventilation can reliably be detected by pulse oximetry only in patients who breathe room air with spontaneous ventilation. Those patients who received supplemental oxygen often masked the pulse oximetry's ability to detect hypoventilation, making pulse oximetry a useful tool only in the absence of supplemental inspired oxygen.

Capnography is the monitoring of the concentration or partial pressure of exhaled carbon dioxide (CO_2) in the respiratory gases in order to assess physiological status or determine the adequacy of ventilation. This was developed as a monitoring tool for use during anesthesia and conscious sedation, but has recently become much more common with patient-controlled and epidural analgesia. Capnography monitoring has been discussed, and some hospitals are currently exploring its use with opioid administration. Hutchison and Rodriquez (2008) reported in their study of 54 opioid-naïve postoperative orthopedic patients that capnography provided better detection of respiratory depression than pulse oximetry and respiratory assessment. They concluded that capnography may be more appropriate for those patients who are at high risk for obstructive sleep apnea (Box 19-6). Currently there is differing research in this area. The American Society for Pain Management Nursing (ASPMN) has assembled a task force to develop practice guidelines for the monitoring of opioid-related sedation and respiratory depression in the hospitalized adult.

Side effects

Side effects occur with all routes of opioid administration and are often dose related. They include excessive somnolence or confusion, nausea and vomiting, urinary retention, pruritus, and constipation, and with epidural administration, numbness in the lower extremities.

Excessive somnolence or confusion may indicate that significant levels of the opioid are present in the brain, a cause for

Box 19-5	LEVEL OF CONSCIOUSNESS SCALE FOR MONITORING MENTAL STATUS
Level	Patient Response
I	Alert
II	Sleepy
III	Lethargic
IV	Responds only to maximal stimulation; response to painful stimulus still present
V	Coma

concern. Excessive somnolence may herald impending respiratory depression. The opioid infusion should be stopped, the respiration rate counted for 1 full minute while observing the quality of respirations, and the authorized provider notified. The administration of naloxone may be necessary if the level of consciousness is markedly abnormal or if there is poor-quality respiratory status.

Nausea and vomiting may result from a number of causes unrelated to the use of opioids, including postsurgical ileus, certain non-opioid medications, and the effects of general anesthetics. Nausea is often associated with opioids by any route. Glare (2005) reports that 30% to 60% of opioid-naïve patients will have nausea and/or vomiting. Many antiemetics can alleviate nausea, or the opioid may need to be changed in some instances.

Urinary retention is not a common side effect of systemically administered opioids, but may occur 10 to 20 hours after the first injection of intraspinal opioid. Intraspinal opioids may prevent the bladder from emptying and therefore cause it to overdistend. If this occurs and there is no mechanical urinary obstruction, it can be treated with medications that contract the bladder, such as bethanechol. A single bladder catheterization may also reverse the retention problem, but it may expose the patient to the risk of urinary tract infection. For postoperative patients with epidural analgesia, some surgeons or anesthesiologists prefer to maintain the Foley catheter until the epidural catheter is ready to be discontinued.

Pruritus is a side effect that may be related to a sensitivity or allergy to the drug or its vehicle. Administering an antihistamine is often effective, but may result in sedation, or the opioid effects can be reversed with an antagonist. Use of another opioid should be considered. Pruritus from intraspinal opioids is not caused by histamine release but by the opioid interacting with the opioid receptor sites in the dorsal horn. It is best treated with an antagonist rather than with an antihistamine. After an epidural injection, 8.5% of all patients experience pruritus; after an intrathecal injection, 46% experience pruritus.

Opioids can slow bowel function, resulting in constipation. Bowel sounds need to be monitored and elimination patterns to be tracked. Stimulant laxatives in combination with stool softeners are given to prevent opioid-induced constipation when necessary. Managing pain in chronically ill patients needs to be done simultaneously with managing or preventing constipation. In these patients, poorly managed pain, immobility, poor diet, and dehydration, as well as opioids, can reduce GI motility. Elimination patterns must be monitored to facilitate a bowel movement at least every 3 days. A stool softener combined with a peristaltic agent is most likely necessary. If bowel evacuation is delayed for longer than 3 days, the designated provider should be notified immediately and a more aggressive bowel program defined.

Continuity of care

The importance of continuity of care for patients in pain cannot be stressed enough. If one or two nurses caring for the patient are not knowledgeable about the level of care given, the patient is left feeling isolated, helpless, and in pain. Pain management in the home setting or long-term care facility involves the transfer of knowledge to the staff. Documentation of pain level and compliance with the pain treatment plan is important. Nurses in home health care and long-term care need to be familiar with the use of non-opioids, adjuvants, or co-analgesics and opioids for patients suffering from chronic pain. They need to be able to communicate effectively to determine the patient's goals for pain management. The patient needs to be educated regarding the various methods and routes of pain control; only by being educated can the patient be involved in the decision-making process. Given the lack of available resources in the home setting, it is particularly important that home health care nurses be able to recognize side effects and complications and know how to intervene immediately.

Clinical indications for quality improvement

Organizational trends in pain management can be improved through a process of continuous quality improvement. Predetermined clinical indicators related to pain management can be identified, such as assessment of pain, respiratory depression, or documentation of pain, and these can be monitored quarterly. Other measurements can be determined by using patient satisfaction questions and monitoring costs and charges for pain management interventions. It is through these measures that health care professionals can link cause and effect to intervention and outcome.

It is clear that there are valuable benefits to having a well-organized system in place for delivering pain management services. Good communication among health care professionals can empower nurses to provide effective analgesia to their patients, and it is well documented that effective pain management reduces complications, thereby decreasing length of hospital stay. A good system also ensures that up-to-date approaches to pain management are used efficiently.

There have been many recent discoveries in the field of pain management. These discoveries should help improve patient outcomes, but it takes motivated personnel to keep up with the latest information. The quality of pain management depends on the knowledge and expertise of health care professionals. Infusion nurses should seize the opportunity presented by these advancements and accumulate the knowledge needed to facilitate pain control for their patients.

MODERATE SEDATION/ANALGESIA (CONSCIOUS SEDATION)

DEFINITION AND GOALS

Moderate sedation/analgesia (conscious sedation) is produced when the administration of pharmacological agents, by any route, results in a depressed level of consciousness but allows the patient to independently maintain a patent airway and respond appropriately to verbal commands or physical stimulation. Patients should be able to retain their protective reflexes. Moderate analgesia/sedation enables the patient to tolerate unpleasant procedures by relieving anxiety, discomfort, and pain. The difference in analgesia and moderate sedation/analgesia is the *intent*. With moderate sedation/analgesia the *intent* is to produce an altered mental state as opposed to analgesia or pain relief.

An American Society of Anesthesiologists (ASA) task force on sedation and analgesia guidelines for nonanesthesiologists decided that the term sedation/analgesia more accurately defines this therapeutic goal than the term conscious sedation (ASA, 2002). They defined four levels of sedation:

1. *Minimal sedation* (anxiolysis). At this level, the patient is awake or arouses easily but is under the influence of the drug administered. The patient maintains normal respiration, normal eye movements, and intact protective reflexes. Amnesia may or may not be present.
2. *Moderate sedation/analgesia* (conscious sedation). At this level, the patient is in a pharmacologically controlled state of limited or minimally depressed consciousness. The patient independently and continuously maintains protective reflexes and a patent airway. The patient responds appropriately to physical stimulation and verbal commands. This level will be the topic of this chapter.
3. *Deep sedation/analgesia*. This is a controlled state of depressed consciousness during which patients cannot be easily aroused and have partial or complete loss of protective reflexes, including the ability to maintain an airway independently and continuously. Although this level is not the intent of sedation/analgesia, the patient may occasionally achieve this level of sedation. The clinician should be medically prepared to respond to this event.
4. *General anesthesia*. This is a controlled state of unconsciousness, loss of protective reflexes, and inability to respond to physical stimuli or verbal commands.

The primary goal of moderate sedation/analgesia is to reduce the patient's anxiety and discomfort and to facilitate cooperation between the patient and the nurse. The objectives for the patient receiving conscious sedation/analgesia include the alteration of mood, maintenance of consciousness, enhanced cooperation, decreased pain, minimal variation of vital signs, some degree of amnesia, and a rapid, safe return to activities of daily living. Patient selection criteria for receiving sedation/analgesia depend on meeting these objectives.

PATIENT SELECTION AND PREPROCEDURAL ASSESSMENT

A complete and thorough assessment is mandatory before the administration of sedation/analgesia (Waring et al, 2003). The patient should be cooperative and have the ability to follow simple commands. In children and uncooperative adults, moderate sedation/analgesia may expedite procedures that are not particularly uncomfortable but require that the patient remain still. A minimal loss of protective reflexes is recommended. Protective reflexes include the ability to breathe independently, the gag reflex, the ability to cough and swallow, and eye movements.

The nurse whose role is to monitor moderate sedation/ analgesia should be familiar with the relevant aspects of the patient's medical history. The initial assessment should include pertinent medical and anesthetic history, nothing-by-mouth (NPO) status (Box 19-7), baseline vital signs, weight, current medications, allergies, mental status, and a history of tobacco, alcohol, and substance use or abuse. The patient's underlying medical condition should guide preprocedural lab studies. Unsuitable candidates include patients requiring more extensive monitoring and sedation, as in high-risk patients with underlying medical problems, severe cardiovascular problems, or severe respiratory problems, or patients undergoing extremely painful procedures.

A thorough airway assessment is required, because positive-pressure ventilation may be necessary if respiration is compromised. Factors that may influence airway management include a history of stridor, snoring, or sleep apnea; significant obesity; previous problems with anesthesia or sedation; facial abnormalities; and advanced arthritis. Head, jaw, and neck deformities, including such findings as short neck, limited neck extension, neck mass, cervical spine disease, trauma, and tracheal deviation, may also create potential airway problems. An examination of the mouth may reveal a nonvisible uvula, tonsillar hypertrophy, small mouth opening, edentulism, protruding incisors, loose or capped teeth, or a high, arched palate. All of the aforementioned abnormalities may increase the likelihood of airway obstruction during sedation/analgesia.

MONITORING AND EQUIPMENT

Monitoring equipment required for sedation/analgesia must be in the patient's room or procedure room before the administration of any medication. This equipment should include oxygen and oxygen delivery devices, suction apparatus, noninvasive blood pressure device, electrocardiograph, and pulse oximeter.

Along with the respiratory rate and oxygen saturation, monitoring criteria should include blood pressure, cardiac rate and rhythm, level of consciousness, and skin condition. Monitoring the patient's level of consciousness (see Box 19-5) reduces the risk of complications by allowing for early detection of adverse drug responses (ASA, 2002). Undesirable changes in the patient's condition should be brought to the designated provider's attention immediately.

Box 19-7 NPO RECOMMENDATION FOR SEDATION/ ANALGESIA*

Ingested material	Minimum fasting time (Hours)
Clear liquids†	2
Breast milk	4
Infant formula	6
Nonhuman milk	6
Light meal‡	6

*Recommendations apply to healthy patients who are undergoing elective procedures. *NPO*, nothing by mouth.

†Examples of clear liquids include water, fruit juices without pulp, carbonated beverages, clear tea, and black coffee.

‡Light meal is typically toast and clear liquids. Meals that include fried or fatty foods may prolong gastric emptying.

From the American Society of Anesthesiologist (ASA) Task Force: Practice guidelines for sedation and analgesia by non-anesthesiologists, *Anesthesiology* 96(4):1004-1017, 2002.

Continuous intravenous access should be determined on a case-by-case basis. The facility's policy and procedures and the designated provider's preferences determine the type of IV access. If the patient is receiving sedation intravenously, IV access should be continuously maintained throughout the procedure. An individual with the skills to establish IV access should be immediately available in all instances.

Not all facilities require continuous electrocardiographic (ECG) monitoring throughout the procedure. According to the *Practice Guidelines for Sedation and Analgesia by Non-Anesthesiologists* (ASA, 2002), patients with a history of cardiac problems or other underlying diseases that may cause problems, such as hypertension or diabetes, should be monitored continuously. The need to continuously monitor the ECG must be determined by the preprocedural assessment.

Because diminished reflexes, depressed respiratory function, and impaired cardiovascular function may occur within seconds or minutes after the administration of medications, an emergency cart must be immediately available whenever sedation/analgesia is administered. The cart should include resuscitative medications, including opioid and sedative reversal medications, and equipment such as a defibrillator. The nurse must maintain a current certification in cardiopulmonary resuscitation (CPR) and maintain knowledge in the use of the emergency cart and the medications and equipment on that cart. The *Practice Guidelines for Sedation and Analgesia by Non-Anesthesiologists* (ASA, 2002) recommends that a clinician with certification in advanced cardiac life support (ACLS) be immediately available (within 5 minutes).

The nurse monitoring the patient should have no other responsibilities. The patient should never be left unattended. The nurse must be clinically competent to immediately identify complications and respond to adverse reactions during the procedure. The nurse should understand the pharmacology of the administered agents, and the role of pharmacological antagonists for opioids and benzodiazepines. The nurse must also have the skills necessary to assess, diagnose, and treat any complications that may arise during the course of care.

PHARMACOLOGY

Agents used for sedation/analgesia depend on the type, duration, and intensity of the procedure. The patient's health status should be considered when selecting and administering medications. Although the designated provider orders the type and amount of medication for administration, it is the nurse's responsibility to validate the order, obtain the medication, and ensure proper administration. This section discusses the most commonly used medications: benzodiazepines, opioids, and their respective reversal agents (Table 19-1).

Benzodiazepines

Benzodiazepines can be administered as preprocedure medication, during the procedure for sedation/analgesia, and during postprocedure care. They have anticonvulsant, antianxiety, sedative, muscle relaxant, and amnesic properties. Three benzodiazepines are used in sedation/analgesia. Midazolam (Versed) is the most commonly used benzodiazepine for sedation/analgesia because it has a fast onset of action, is short acting, and produces a high degree of retrograde amnesia (Waring et al,

2003). Diazepam and lorazepam are longer acting and are not as well suited for shorter procedures.

Midazolam

Midazolam (Versed), a short-acting benzodiazepine, is a central nervous system (CNS) depressant and a sedative-hypnotic. It may be administered intravenously, orally, rectally, or nasally. The most common route is IV. The starting IV dose is 0.5 to 2 mg and may be repeated every 2 to 3 minutes if needed, titrating to effect. The usual total dose is 2.5 to 5 mg. Slurred speech is an excellent indicator of an adequate dose. Midazolam must be given slowly intravenously and never administered by rapid or single-dose bolus. Rapid or excessive IV doses may result in respiratory depression or arrest.

Doses of midazolam should be individualized, and patients must be monitored carefully. Premedicated patients usually need 30% less midazolam than nonmedicated patients. If used with other CNS depressants, half the usual dosage should be given. Lower dosages should be given to patients who are older than 60 years of age, debilitated, or chronically ill, or who are receiving opioids. The best rule for administration of midazolam is to start with small doses and administer slowly. By following this simple rule, serious complications can be avoided.

Midazolam is contraindicated in patients with known benzodiazepine hypersensitivity or acute narrow-angle glaucoma. Adverse reactions from IV administration include hiccups, nausea, vomiting, oversedation, headache, coughing, and pain at the injection site.

Diazepam

Diazepam (Valium), a benzodiazepine used as an anticonvulsant, is a CNS depressant. It may be administered via the IV, rectal, or oral routes. The initial IV dose is 2.5 to 5.0 mg and may be repeated every 5 to 10 minutes. The maximum dose should not exceed 30 mg in 2 hours. When given intravenously, diazepam needs to be administered slowly over 1 minute for each 5 mg. As with midazolam, slurred speech is an excellent indicator of an adequate dose. Lower dosages should be used in the elderly or in debilitated patients. This drug cannot be mixed with other medications or diluted because of the risk of precipitate formation. It must be injected as close to the IV injection site as possible because of the risk of thrombophlebitis.

Lorazepam

Lorazepam (Ativan), a benzodiazepine used as an anxiolytic, is a CNS depressant and sedative-hypnotic. It is occasionally administered for its sedative effects during procedures that last more than 2 hours and is not appropriate for short-term procedures. The dosage is 1 to 2 mg intravenously 15 to 20 minutes before the procedure or orally 2 hours before the procedure. Half the original dose may be repeated every 10 to 15 minutes. The maximum adult dosage by all routes is 10 mg unless the patient's airway is controlled.

Flumazenil

Flumazenil (Romazicon) is a benzodiazepine antagonist. The dosage is 0.2 mg intravenously every 45 to 60 seconds until the desired effect is achieved or until 1 mg is given. This dose can be repeated at 20-minute intervals. No more than 3 mg should be given in a 1-hour period. The duration of this medication is influenced by the dose administered and the dose of

TABLE 19-1 Moderate Sedation/Analgesia: Adult Medications

Drug	Age	Route	Dose/titration	Onset	Duration	Side effects/ precautions
Opioids—For pain control only. Not appropriate for sedation, amnesia, or relief of anxiety.						
Morphine (Various brands)	Adults	PO PR IV	10-30 mg 10-20 mg 2.5 mg given slowly initially 5-20 mg total dose	PO: 60 minutes IV: 5-10 minutes	PO/IV: 7 hours $T_{1/2}$ = 2-4 hours	Dose dependent— Respiratory depression, orthostatic hypotension, nausea, itching, painful injection Decrease dosages in hepatic and renal insufficiency, and elderly, debilitated patients
Fentanyl (Various brands)	Adults	IV	1-2 mcg/kg in 25-mcg increments, slowly titrated over 1-2 minutes	PO: <20 minutes IV: 1-3 minutes	PO/IV: <60 minutes $T_{1/2}$ = 2-4 hours	Respiratory depression, apnea, hypotension, bradycardia, dizziness, nausea Decrease dosages in hepatic and renal insufficiency and elderly, debilitated patients
Opioid Reversal Agent						
Naloxone (Narcan)	Adults	IV	Dilute in 10 mL, 0.9% sodium chloride and titrate to effect; maximum of 2 mg in adults	1-2 minutes	1-4 hours $T_{1/2}$ = 1.5 hours	Pulmonary edema, nausea, sweating, tachycardia
Benzodiazepines—For sedation, amnesia, and relief of anxiety only. Not for pain control.						
Midazolam (Versed)	Adults	IV	1-5 mg, given in 1-mg increments over 2 minutes; titrated to effect	PO: 30-60 minutes IV: 1-5 minutes	PO/IV: 2-6 hours $T_{1/2}$ = 1-4 hours	Respiratory depression, hypotension, bradycardia, hiccups, apnea Decrease dosages in hepatic and renal insufficiency, and elderly, debilitated patients
Benzodiazepine Reversal Agent						
Flumazenil (Romazicon)	Adults	IV	0.2 mg/min in incremental doses up to 1 mg	IV: 1-3 minutes	45-90 minutes $T_{1/2}$ = 30-90 minutes	Hypoventilation, may precipitate seizure
Other Agents						
Chloral hydrate (Various brands)	Adults	PO	500-1000 mg 30 min before procedure; maximum dose 2 g/24 hours	PO: 0.5-1 hours	4-8 hours $T_{1/2}$ = 8-11 hours	GI irritation, nausea, vomiting, diarrhea, disorientation, drowsiness Decrease doses in patients with renal insufficiency and avoid in hepatic impairment

From The University of Kansas Hospital: Policy: moderate sedation/analgesia (conscious sedation)— management of patient undergoing procedures, *Corporate policy manual 2, section: care of patients*, 2005.

the agonist. This medication does not reverse hypoventilation or cardiac depression.

Flumazenil should be used with extreme caution in patients with a history of seizure disorders. Patients chronically receiving benzodiazepines are at risk of grand mal seizures with the use of flumazenil. It should not be used routinely and should be administered slowly with careful, continuous patient monitoring.

Opioids

Opioids provide analgesia and sedation and are effective in elevating the pain threshold. They may be administered as a premedication or along with another medication during a procedure. Generally, an opioid and a benzodiazepine are administered along with local or regional anesthesia. Opioids are broken down by hepatic metabolism. Only the most common opioids are covered in this chapter.

Fentanyl citrate

Fentanyl citrate is a synthetic opioid indicated for short-term analgesic action. It has a rapid onset of action. The dosage must be decreased by one fourth to one third if used with another CNS depressant. Rapid administration can lead to a rigid chest wall and difficulty breathing, which can be reversed with naloxone (Narcan). However, a depolarizing muscle relaxant and intubation may be required. Fentanyl can be stored in fat and muscle tissue and consequently returned to the circulation, resulting in a delayed-onset respiratory depression.

Morphine

Morphine may be given intravenously or orally. If administered with another CNS depressant, the dosage is decreased by 30%. Morphine is contraindicated in patients with known hypersensitivity to morphine or codeine.

Naloxone

Naloxone (Narcan) is an opioid antagonist; it works by competing for the receptor site, thereby reversing the effect of the opioid. This means that naloxone reverses not only sedation and respiratory depression, but also analgesia. This sudden unmasking of pain may result in significant sympathetic and cardiovascular stimulation, resulting in hypertension, stroke, tachycardia, arrhythmia, pulmonary edema, congestive heart failure, or cardiac arrest.

DOCUMENTATION, POSTPROCEDURAL CARE, AND DISCHARGE

Documentation of nursing interventions ensures the continuity of patient care, improves communication among health care team members, and provides a mechanism for comparing actual versus expected patient outcomes. The frequency of vital sign monitoring is determined by the medication, route of administration, and patient condition.

The most common complications in the administration of sedation/analgesia are respiratory depression and respiratory arrest. The most common treatment for these complications is the administration of oxygen. The patient should be stimulated by verbal or noxious stimuli and instructed to take a deep breath if the respiratory status becomes compromised. If spontaneous respiration does not occur, a head tilt-jaw lift maneuver should be initiated. Positive-pressure ventilation may be required if respiratory status does not improve. If the patient cannot maintain his or her own airway, an artificial airway is indicated. Although either a nasal or an oral airway may be used, a nasal airway may be more tolerable for a conscious patient. Continuous observation of the patient's respiratory rate and monitoring of pulse oximetry may ward off the need for emergency measures.

Notify the designated provider immediately of the following:
- Rise or fall in systolic blood pressure (BP) of 20 to 30 mm Hg from baseline
- Tachycardia (>150 beats/min) or bradycardia (<50 beats/min)
- *Excessive* rise or fall in respiratory rate
- Oxygen saturation (SaO_2) less than 90% or significantly below presedation level
- Marked decrease in patient responsiveness to verbal or painful stimulation
- Signs or symptoms of medication intolerance or allergy
- Patient not meeting discharge parameters

Postprocedural care

After the procedure, the patient is usually transferred to his or her room in an inpatient setting or to a recovery area until determined ready for discharge. This usually occurs once the patient's vital signs (e.g., blood pressure, pulse, respirations, SpO_2) have returned to and been maintained at presedation levels for at least 30 minutes since the last sedating medications were administered. The designated provider should remain immediately available to participate in the patient's postprocedural care until the risk of respiratory compromise is resolved.

Several scoring systems are available to standardize documentation and the patient's readiness for discharge back to his or her room or to home. Figure 19-4 is one example of a discharge scoring system. A postsedation scoring system is not mandatory as long as prudent guidelines for discharge are met. These include stable vital signs, mental status, and activity; relative freedom from pain, nausea, and vomiting; and the ability to void or take fluids. A physician must evaluate any patient who is unable to meet the discharge criteria.

SUMMARY

As more and more procedures are performed with moderate sedation/analgesia, the need for trained and competent staff to administer and monitor these patients will increase. Every practice setting should have policies and procedures in place. Each facility using sedation/analgesia needs to specify in their policy and procedures the competencies determined necessary for their staff members. An education/competency validation system should be designed to evaluate and document the demonstration of the knowledge, skills, and abilities related to managing the patient receiving sedation/analgesia. A positive patient outcome is the primary goal. This can be accomplished only through education and safe practice by the entire health care team.

Pain management is an aspect of patient care in which patient advocacy is exceedingly important. It is the responsibility of each nurse caring for a patient to ensure quality pain management. Nurses who work at the patient's bedside talk with their patients and know when they are experiencing pain. Nurses must communicate pertinent information to other members of the health care team, and need to teach patients how to help manage their pain effectively.

Infusion nurses can be valuable members of the health care team concerned with pain management. Knowledge gained through infection prevention and control and advances in intravenous (IV) technology have provided the infusion nurse with a background that can make it easy to gain proficiency in pain management. Pain management includes such procedures as piggybacking opioid infusions and supplying patient-controlled doses of opioids into maintenance administration sets. It also involves the delivery of opioids and local anesthetics into regional, epidural, and intrathecal spaces. Infusion nurses have knowledge and expertise that can help resolve the problems that occur with pain management. For example, infusion nurses are familiar with the equipment used to deliver pain-relief medications and can serve as a resource for its operation. As patients become more aware of new technology for providing pain relief, they will demand it in every care setting. The infusion nurse is

Vital signs	Time							
	Temperature							
	Blood pressure							
	Pulse							
	Respiratory rate							
	Oxygen saturation							

Respirations*							
2 = Adult: Regular rhythm; rate between 12 and 28	2	2	2	2	2	2	2
Child: Regular rhythm; lungs sound clear							
1 = Adult: Shallow/on oxygen; rate <12 or >28	1	1	1	1	1	1	1
Child: Abnormal rhythm; lung sounds							
0 = Adult: Dyspnea; rate <10 or >40	0	0	0	0	0	0	0
Child: Stridor with difficulty in breathing							

Circulation							
2 = Post-procedure systolic BP ±20 mm admission BP	2	2	2	2	2	2	2
1 = Post-procedure systolic BP ±20-50 mm admission BP	1	1	1	1	1	1	1
0 = Post-procedure systolic BP ±50 mm admission BP	0	0	0	0	0	0	0

Activity							
2 = Adult: Moves all extremities/able to ambulate on own	2	2	2	2	2	2	2
Child: Normal activity prior to procedure							
1 = Adult: Moves 2 extremities/ambulates with assistance	1	1	1	1	1	1	1
Child: Able to sit up, arousable							
0 = Adult: Moves no extremities/unable to ambulate	0	0	0	0	0	0	0
Child: Asleep							

Pain							
2 = States relief or free from pain	2	2	2	2	2	2	2
1 = Medicated for pain PO/moderate pain	1	1	1	1	1	1	1
0 = Medicated for pain IV or IM/severe pain	0	0	0	0	0	0	0

Bleeding*							
2 = No significant procedural bleeding	2	2	2	2	2	2	2
1 = Moderate procedural bleeding	1	1	1	1	1	1	1
0 = Large amount procedural bleeding	0	0	0	0	0	0	0

Consciousness*							
2 = Awake and alert	2	2	2	2	2	2	2
1 = Arousable to verbal stimulus	1	1	1	1	1	1	1
0 = Unresponsive/responds to pain	0	0	0	0	0	0	0

Nausea and vomiting							
2 = No nausea and vomiting	2	2	2	2	2	2	2
1 = Nausea only	1	1	1	1	1	1	1
0 = Intractable vomiting	0	0	0	0	0	0	0

| Nurse's initials   Score: | | | | | | | |

*Outpatients MUST have a score of 2 to be considered for discharge or a return to baseline.

All patients should attain a minimum score of 12 of 14 or must return to baseline to be discharged from recovery.

FIGURE 19-4 Moderate sedation/analgesia: discharge scoring system. (From The University of Kansas Hospital: Policy: moderate sedation/analgesia [conscious sedation]–management of patient undergoing procedures, *Corporate policy manual 2, section: care of patients*, 2005.)

positioned to provide pain relief with present technological skills supplemented by additional education and training.

 REFERENCES

Agency for Health Care Policy and Research: *Clinical practice guidelines, acute pain management: operative or medical procedures and trauma,* Rockville, Md, 1992, U.S. Department of Health and Human Services.

American Pain Society (APS): *Principles of analgesic use in the treatment of acute pain and cancer pain,* ed 5, Glenview, Ill, 2003, Author.

American Society of Anesthesiologist (ASA) Task Force: Practice guidelines for sedation and analgesia by non-anesthesiologists, *Anesthesiology* 96(4):1004-1017, 2002.

Backonja MM: Use of anticonvulsants for treatment of neuropathic pain, *Neurology* 59(suppl 2):S14-S17, 2002.

Ballantyne JC, Carr DB, Chalmers TC et al: Postoperative patient controlled analgesia: meta-analyses of initial randomized control trials, *J Clin Anesth,* 5(3):182-193, 1993.

Barden J, Edwards J, Moore RA et al: Single dose oral diclofenac for postoperative pain, *Cochrane Database Systematic Rev,* issue 2, article CD004768, DOI: 10.1002/14651858, CD004768, 2004.

Bloodworth D: Opioids in the treatment of chronic pain: legal framework and therapeutic indications and limitations, *Phys Med Rehabil Clin North Am* 17(2):355-379, 2006.

Bond MR, Simpson KH: *Pain: its nature and treatment,* Edinburgh, 2006, Churchill Livingstone Elsevier.

Bonica J: *The management of pain,* ed 2, Vol 1, Philadelphia, 1990, Lea & Febiger.

Brennan E, Carr DB, Cousins M: Pain management: a fundamental human right, *Anesth Analg* 105(1):205-221, 2007.

Coyle N: Cancer patients and subcutaneous infusion, *Am J Nurs* 96(3):61, 1996.

Cromley A, Banks C: Pain management: clinician survey and institutional needs assessment, *BUMC* 13(3):230-235, 2000.

Davis M, Glare P, Hardy J, editors: *Opioids in cancer pain,* New York, 2005, Oxford University Press.

Farber S, Andersen W, Branden C et al: Improving cancer pain management through a system wide commitment, *J Pall Med* 1(4):377-385, 1998.

Fink R: Pain assessment: the cornerstone to optimal pain management, *BUMC* 13:236-239, 2000.

Fu ES, Downs JB, Schweiger JW et al: Supplemental oxygen impairs detection of hypoventilation by pulse oximetry, *Chest* 126:(5)1552-1558, 2004.

Furstenberg CT, Ahles TA, Whedon MB et al: Knowledge and attitudes of health-care providers toward cancer pain management: a comparison of physicians, nurses, and pharmacists in the state of New Hampshire, *J Pain Symptom Manag* 15:335-349, 1998.

Gilfor JM, Viscusi ER: Epidural analgesia. In Wallace MS, Staats PS, editors: *Pain medicine & management: just the facts,* New York, 2005, McGraw-Hill.

Glare P: Hydromorphone. In Davis M, Glare P, Hardy J, editors: *Opioids for cancer pain,* New York, 2005, Oxford.

Goodman AJ, Le Bourdonnec B, Dolle RE: Mu opioid receptor antagonists: recent developments, *Chem Med Che* 2(11):1552-1570, 2007.

Grabinsky A, Boswell MV: Analgesic use in acute pain management. In Smith HS, editor: *Drugs for pain,* Philadelphia, 2003, Hanley & Belfus.

Guarino AH, Myers JC: An assessment protocol to guide opioid prescriptions for patients with chronic pain, *Mo Med* 104(6):513-516, 2007.

Hudcova J, McNicol E, Quah C, et al: Patient-controlled opioid analgesia versus conventional opioid analgesia for postoperative pain, *Cochrane Database Systematic Rev,* issue 4, article CD003348, DOI: 1002/14651858, CD003348.pub2, 2006.

Hutchison R, Rodriguez L: Capnography and respiratory depression, *Am J Nurs* 108(2):35-39, 2008.

Infusion Nurses Society (INS): Infusion nursing standards of practice, *J Infus Nurs* 29(suppl 1S):S1-S92, 2006.

International Association for the Study of Pain (IASP): Time to modify the WHO analgesic ladder? *Pain Clin Updates* 13(5):1-4, 2005.

Iosifescu DV, Alpert JE, Fava M: Antidepressants: Basic mechanisms and pharmacology. In Smith HS, editor: *Drugs for pain,* Philadelphia, 2003, Hanley & Belfus.

Kahan M, Srivastava A, Wilson L et al: Opioids for managing chronic non-malignant pain: safe and effective prescribing, *Can Fam Physician* 52(9):1091-1096, 2006.

Liu SS: Continuous perineural catheters for postoperative analgesia: an update, *IARS 2005 Rev Course Lect,* 48-52, 2005.

Marks RM, Sacher EJ: Undertreatment of medical inpatients with opioid analgesic, *Ann Intern Med* 78(2):173, 1973.

Mason L, Edwards JE, Moore RA et al: Single dose oral naproxen and naproxen sodium for acute postoperative pain, *Cochrane Database Systematic Rev,* issue 4, article CD004234, DOI: 1002/14651858, CD004234.pub2, 2004.

McCaffery M, Pasero C: *Pain: clinical manual,* ed 2, St Louis, 1999, Mosby.

Melzak P, Wall PD: Pain mechanisms: a new theory, *Science* 150(699):971-979, 1965.

Montazeri K, Kashefi P, Honarmand A: Pre-emptive gabapentin significantly reduces postoperative pain and morphine demand following lower extremity orthopedic surgery, *Singpore Med J* 48(8):748-751, 2007.

Moulin E, Kreeft J, Murray-Parson N, Bouquillon AL: Comparison of continuous subcutaneous and intravenous hydromorphone infusions for management of cancer pain, *Lancet* 337:465, 1991.

National Center for Health Statistics (NCHS): *United States chartbook on trends in the health of Americans* (pp 68–71), Hyattsville, 2006.

Neuburger M, Buttner J, Blumenthal S et al: Inflammation and infection complications of 2285 perineural catheters: a prospective study, *Acta Anaesthesiol Scand* 51:108-114, 2007.

Peretti-Watel P, Bendiane MK, Obadia Y et al: The South-Eastern France Palliative Care Group. The prescription of opioid analgesics to terminal cancer patients: impact of physician's general attitudes and contextual factors, *Pall Support Care* 1:345-352, 2003.

Recart A, Issioui T, White PF et al: The efficacy of Celicoxib premedication on postoperative pain and recovery times after ambulatory surgery: a dose-ranging study, *Anesth Analg* 96:1631-1635, 2003.

Reuben SS, Ekman EF: The effect of cyclooxygenase-2 inhibition on analgesia and spinal fusion, *J Bone Joint Surg* 87A(3):536-543, 2005.

Rosenquist RW, Rosenberg J: Postoperative pain guidelines, *Reg Anesth Pain Med* 28(4):279-288, 2003.

Savage S, Covington E, Heit H et al: *Definitions related to the use of opioids for the treatment of pain: a consensus document from the American Academy of Pain Medicine, the American Pain Society, and the American Society of Addiction Medicine,* Glenview, Ill, 2001, American Pain Society.

Silver J, Mayer RS: Barriers to pain management in the rehabilitation of the surgical oncology patient, *J Surg Oncol* 95(5):427-435, 2007.

Sorkin LS: Basic physiology. In Wallace MS, Staats PS, editors: *Pain medicine & management: just the facts,* New York, 2005, McGraw-Hill.

Strassman A: Pathophysiology of pain. In Smith HS, editor: *Drugs for pain,* Philadelphia, 2003, Hanley & Belfus.

The University of Kansas Hospital: Policy: moderate sedation/analgesia (conscious sedation)—management of patient undergoing procedures, *Corporate policy manual 2, section: care of patients,* 2005.

Thibodeau GA, Patton KT: *Anatomy & physiology,* ed 6, St Louis, 2007, Mosby.

Turan A, White PF, Karamanlioglu B et al: Gabapentin: an alternative to the cyclooxygenase-2 inhibitors for perioperative pain management, *Anesth Analg* 102(1):175-181, 2006.

Wallace MS: Chronic spinal drug administration. In Abram SE, editor: *Pain medicine: the requisites in anesthesiology*, Philadelphia, 2006, Saunders.

Waring JP, Baron TH, Hirota WK et al: Guidelines for conscious sedation and monitoring during gastrointestinal endoscopy, *Gastrointest Endosc* 58(3):317-322, 2003.

World Health Organization: *Cancer pain relief*, Geneva, 1990, Author.

Wiffen PJ, McQuay HJ, Edwards JE et al: Gabapentin for acute and chronic pain, *Cochrane Database Systematic Rev*, issue 3, article CD005452, DOI: 10.1002/14651858, CD005452, 2005.

Wuhrman E, Cooney MF, Dunwoody CJ et al: Authorized and unauthorized ("PCA by proxy") dosing of analgesic infusion pumps: position statement with clinical practice recommendations, *Pain Manag Nurs* 8(1):4-11, 2007.

20 INFUSION THERAPY EQUIPMENT

Lynn C. Hadaway, MEd, RN, BC, CRNI®*

The equipment used in health care rapidly changes to meet the demands of all consumers, including health care professionals and our clients and patients. Both groups demand products that are safe and effective. Device manufacturers strive to meet those changing needs while being governed and guided by the regulations of the Food and Drug Administration (FDA).

The patient's role in choices about devices to be used is also changing. While hospitalized, patients are not involved in the decision-making process of equipment acquisition and act more as a passive recipient of device choices made for them. This role changes, however, as the need for long-term therapy becomes apparent and the patient becomes responsible for self-administration of his or her infusion therapy.

Nurses in all health care settings have an active role in making product decisions by serving as the gatekeeper for device decisions, monitoring quality improvement processes to identify the need for device changes or additions, monitoring device implementation processes, and providing staff development on new devices. All these activities serve to enhance patient safety and improve financial outcomes for the organization.

The device manufacturing industry should be considered an active partner in this process and a rich resource for information. The manufacturer employs design engineers, researchers, and regulatory, reimbursement, clinical, sales, and marketing professionals to assist and support the health care professional. Information from the manufacturer can be plentiful and critical to proper application of each device, including but not limited to instructions for use, patient information, laboratory and clinical research, and a variety of professional educational materials. However, it remains the nurse's responsibility to consider all brands of a specific product so that actual product performance can be delineated from salesmanship, thus ensuring the most appropriate choice is made.

Safety for the patient and caregiver is of paramount importance in the development, use, maintenance, and disposal of infusion products and equipment. Device users must be aware of all aspects of the device's purpose, design, and instructions for use. Electrical equipment requires active surveillance to ascertain hazards and mechanical malfunctions, and any equipment known to be malfunctioning must be removed from use until it is repaired. All personnel operating equipment must be properly trained in its safe and effective use. The care provider must also protect patients from infectious hazards resulting from inadequately cleaned equipment, reuse of disposable products, or procedures performed with poor aseptic technique.

Infusion therapy has always posed a high level of infectious risk to nurses; moreover, protecting against these hazards has a new urgency because of our increasing knowledge of bloodborne diseases. A thorough understanding of the risk factors and the products and procedures used can reduce the risk.

Financial accountability and cost containment are necessities in health care. This information is essential for the formulation of plans to evaluate and procure equipment in a cost-effective manner.

The intended outcome of these extensive efforts is the safe use of medical devices and equipment and, ultimately, the protection of the public. The relationship among health care professionals, health care organizations, manufacturers, and clients/patients is one of mutual dependence. The role of each exists because of the presence of the others. The public holds all accountable for the safe and effective delivery of health care.

FROM INVENTION TO THE PATIENT

All equipment used in the process of delivering infusion therapy is regulated by the Center for Devices and Radiologic Health (CDRH) at the Food and Drug Administration (FDA). This organization: (1) reviews requests to research or market medical devices; (2) collects, analyzes, and acts on information about

*The author and editors wish to acknowledge the contributions made by Roxanne Perucca and Krisha S. Scharnweber as authors in the second edition of *Infusion Therapy in Clinical Practice*.

injuries and other experiences in the use of medical devices and radiation-emitting electronic products; (3) sets and enforces good manufacturing practice regulations and performance standards for radiation-emitting electronic products and medical devices; (4) monitors compliance and surveillance programs for medical devices and radiation-emitting electronic products; and (5) provides technical and other nonfinancial assistance to small manufacturers of medical devices (FDA, 2002b).

A medical device is defined as "an instrument, apparatus, implement, machine, contrivance, implant, in vitro reagent, or other similar or related article, including a component part, or accessory which is: (1) recognized in the official *National Formulary*, or the *United States Pharmacopoeia*, or any supplement to them; (2) intended for use in the diagnosis of disease or other conditions, or in the cure, mitigation, treatment, or prevention of disease, in man or other animals; or (3) intended to affect the structure or any function of the body of man or other animals, and which does not achieve any of its primary intended purposes through chemical action within or on the body of man or other animals and which is not dependent upon being metabolized for the achievement of any of its primary intended purposes" (FDA, 2002a). This definition distinguishes a medical device from a drug; however, recent advances have allowed the creation of drug and device combinations.

DEVICE DEVELOPMENT

Typically, device creation begins when a health care professional or design engineer develops an idea to address an unmet clinical need. The owners of the idea then proceed through the process of applying for a patent, giving the inventors exclusive rights to their invention for a limited period of time. While this process provides financial incentive to the owners, it also increases the general knowledge in the industry because it requires the inventors to disclose their idea to the public (Elliott, 2007).

After patent application begins, device prototypes are built followed by laboratory and possibly animal testing. The design engineers seek the advice of nurses, physicians, and other health care professionals during the evolving processes of designing, building, testing, and redesigning. This is very similar to the quality improvement processes nurses employ to improve patient care.

Small manufacturers produce the greatest number of new products, although a few ideas for medical devices originate within academic medical centers. The medical center may develop a prototype and then license the legal rights to the device to a manufacturer. To encourage ideas from academic centers, federal law assigns the legal rights to the academic center if it was created within a federally funded program (Kaplan et al, 2004).

Small manufacturers obtain funding from investors such as venture capitalists to support the cost of bringing a product to market, which may take several years and millions of dollars. Large device manufacturers will improve or refine existing devices to enhance their clinical usefulness using financial resources derived from their business operation.

The type of testing for each device is determined by factors in the regulatory process administered by the CDRH and this may or may not involve clinical research on the device. When clinical research is required, the majority of this clinical research is conducted outside of the United States (Kaplan et al, 2004).

GOVERNMENTAL REGULATION OF DEVICES

Before any device can be sold within the United States, it must complete designated processes with the CDRH at the FDA. Devices are classified based on their risk. Class I devices have the lowest risk with a minimal possibility of harm. Infusion-related devices in this group include manufactured catheter stabilization devices, adhesive tape, pressure infusors for an IV bag, and IV poles. Class II devices have a moderate amount of risk with a greater possibility of harm. IV solution containers, catheters, vessel dilators, introducers, guidewires, and stylet wires fall into this category. Performance standards have been established and all devices must meet or exceed these standards. Class III devices are more invasive and carry the greatest amount of risk. This group includes cardiac pacemakers, replacement heart valves, and other surgical devices.

The class of the device determines the process used by the CDRH for the internal review. For class I devices, the manufacturer must show they have met "general controls" such as proper labeling, adherence to good manufacturing practices, and adequate packaging and storage. The locations of manufacturer and importers involved are then registered with the FDA and the FDA lists the specific product.

Other devices come to the U.S. market by either the premarket notification (PMN) process or the premarket approval (PMA) process. Premarket notification, commonly known as the "510(K) application," is a common process for class II devices. This process documents that the product is "substantially equivalent" to other products legally sold in the United States. This is known as the "predicate" device and the new device will have similar uses and characteristics. New devices with updated characteristics may still fall into this category if there are no new questions of safety and effectiveness. This method usually does not require submission of data from any clinical studies or clinical outcomes with the product. Thus these devices are "cleared" for market rather than receiving a more detailed investigation (Maisel, 2004).

The premarket approval (PMA) process is used for most class III devices. Laboratory, animal, and clinical studies are usually required to demonstrate that the product is safe and effective when used according to the labeled indications. Clinical use of the product before approval requires an Investigational Device Exemption (IDE). The FDA issues this to the manufacturer for use only at the institution(s) conducting the clinical trials. The number of devices entering the market through the PMN or 510(K) process is about 10 times greater than those entering the market through the PMA process (Feldman et al, 2008).

POSTMARKET SURVEILLANCE

When a device is introduced and clinical practice begins, the postmarket surveillance system also begins, working toward the goal of reducing adverse events associated with devices. This system, known as medical device reporting (MDR), involves the manufacturers, health care facilities, and professionals, albeit with vastly different requirements.

All manufacturers are mandated to notify the FDA of reported complaints of device malfunctions, serious injuries, or deaths associated with a device. The manufacturer has strict time limitations within which this reporting must be accomplished. User facilities—defined as hospitals, nursing homes, and outpatient treatment, surgical, and diagnostic facilities—are also required by law to report death or serious injury caused by a device within 10 days to be followed by an annual report. These reports are submitted to the manufacturer and the FDA.

Health care professionals are encouraged to submit voluntary reports through the MedWatch system. These reports may include serious adverse events including death, those that create life-threatening or disabling outcomes, and those that require hospitalization or intervention to prevent permanent injury. Additionally, professionals may report product problems such as defective, contaminated, or improperly labeled devices and product-use errors. Forms for submitting these reports can be submitted online at http://www.fda.gov/medwatch/report/hcp.htm or be downloaded and submitted by fax or phone to the FDA (Figure 20-1).

There are searchable databases on the FDA website that will provide information about events reported with products. The Manufacturer and User Facility Device Experience (MAUDE) database contains drop-down lists of problems with devices and includes information submitted over the past 12 to 15 years. For instance, a search using "Intravenous, intermittent" over the past 6 years pulled up five reports containing a written description of the event along with other product information. This database can be accessed at http://www.accessdata.fda.gov/scripts/cdrh/cfdocs/cfMAUDE/Search.cfm.

Recalling a device for problem correction or complete removal of that device from the market is also part of postmarket activity. Most device recalls are voluntary, but federal law gives the FDA the authority to recall devices. Manufacturers are also required to have a program for tracking devices that are likely to cause serious consequences if they fail and also those devices that will be implanted for more than 1 year. This includes devices such as cardiac pacemakers and implantable infusion pumps. The FDA also has the power to require a manufacturer to conduct postmarket surveillance studies on devices where failure would produce a serious adverse event, those intended to be implanted more than 1 year, or those life-supporting devices used outside a user facility. Data must be actively collected and analyzed in a scientific manner.

The role of the CDRH is to regulate the premarket assessment, manufacturing practices, and postmarket surveillance of health care devices. Neither the CDRH nor any other FDA center has the power to regulate what health care professionals do with those devices in clinical practice. Use of devices in a manner or for an indication not included in the product label is considered to be "off-label" use.

A device's label is printed, written, or graphically depicted on the container of the device. It must clearly indicate the intended use, along with directions for how to use the product and the manufacturer's name and address. Labeling, however, extends to all other supportive material such as brochures or pamphlets, instruction books, posters, and booklets that accompany the device or are assembled with the device after it has been shipped to the user. The practice of distributing published articles containing information about off-label uses of a product is the subject of a guidance document for manufacturers. While a manufacturer's representatives cannot actively promote the off-label use of a device, they can provide information from credible sources about the experiences of other professionals providing that they meet the guidelines from the FDA for these activities.

The Medical Product Safety Network (MedSun) is a collaborative partnership between the CDRH and more than 350 health care facilities across the United States. The primary goal of this program is to work with the clinical community to identify, understand, and solve problems with medical devices. Representatives from each facility are identified and trained to use an Internet-based system for reporting device problems that result in serious illness, injury, or death. Voluntary reports for devices with the potential for harm or any other safety concern are encouraged so that serious injury and death may be prevented (FDA, 2008).

NONGOVERNMENTAL AGENCIES

The International Organization for Standardization (ISO) is a worldwide federation of standard-setting organizations from 140 countries. The American National Standards Institute (ANSI) represents the United States at the ISO. Their purpose is to establish product standards to facilitate international commerce of goods and services. Without standard product definitions, measurements, connection mechanisms, and many other product specifications, the exchange of products between countries would be more difficult. In this organization (ISO), "standard" is defined as a documented agreement about technical specifications that are considered as rules or guidelines to ensure that products meet their intended purpose (Scott and Weeks, 2003).

The Association for the Advancement of Medical Instrumentation (AAMI) is another group that creates standards, reports, and position papers. AAMI is accredited through ANSI and work is conducted through numerous technical advisory groups (TAGs) who vote on behalf of the United States on international documents (Scott and Weeks, 2003).

The Emergency Care Research Institute (ECRI), located in Plymouth Meeting, Pennsylvania, is a nonprofit organization rooted in research and evaluation of medical technologies. *Health Devices* is their monthly journal that publishes technology evaluations and hazard reports. Through their Evidence-based Practice Center, they serve as a major resource for the Agency for Healthcare Research and Quality (AHRQ), providing evidence reports, systematic reviews, and technical expert panel meetings. ECRI is also designated as a collaborating center for patient safety, risk management, and health care technology with the World Health Organization. Other services include print and on-line databases to compare and guide purchasing decisions for capital equipment and disposable supplies. Systems for tracking all product alert and recall information along with medical device problem reporting are also available through their member services. More information can be found at their website (www.ecri.org).

The Advanced Medical Technology Association (AdvaMed), formerly the Health Industry Manufacturers Association (HIMA), located in Washington, DC, is a trade association of health care device manufacturers. This association's members include the manufacturers of more than 90% of the health care devices on the market today, including those that infusion nurses use daily. This organization addresses the common concerns of quality, education, marketing, and legislation.

Proper use of devices is remarkably dependent upon individual technique of the professional using that product and is often an extension of the professional's hands. Poor or improper technique dramatically impacts the clinical outcome with the device, driving the need for appropriate education and training from experienced professionals. This differs significantly from drugs, where the prescription is given but the

U.S. Department of Health and Human Services

MEDWATCH

The FDA Safety Information and Adverse Event Reporting Program

For VOLUNTARY reporting of adverse events, product problems and product use errors

Page _____ of _____

Form Approved: OMB No. 0910-0291, Expires:10/31/08
See OMB statement on reverse.

FDA USE ONLY

Triage unit sequence #

PLEASE TYPE OR USE BLACK INK

A. PATIENT INFORMATION

1. Patient Identifier	2. Age at Time of Event, or Date of Birth:	3. Sex	4. Weight
In confidence		☐ Female ☐ Male	_____ lb or _____ kg

B. ADVERSE EVENT, PRODUCT PROBLEM OR ERROR

Check all that apply:

1. ☐ Adverse Event   ☐ Product Problem (e.g., defects/malfunctions)
   ☐ Product Use Error   ☐ Problem with Different Manufacturer of Same Medicine

2. **Outcomes Attributed to Adverse Event**
   (Check all that apply)

   ☐ Death: _____ (mm/dd/yyyy)
   ☐ Life-threatening
   ☐ Hospitalization - initial or prolonged
   ☐ Required Intervention to Prevent Permanent Impairment/Damage (Devices)

   ☐ Disability or Permanent Damage
   ☐ Congenital Anomaly/Birth Defect
   ☐ Other Serious (Important Medical Events)

3. Date of Event (mm/dd/yyyy)	4. Date of this Report (mm/dd/yyyy) 09/14/2007

5. **Describe Event, Problem or Product Use Error**

6. **Relevant Tests/Laboratory Data, Including Dates**

7. **Other Relevant History, Including Preexisting Medical Conditions** (e.g., allergies, race, pregnancy, smoking and alcohol use, liver/kidney problems, etc.)

C. PRODUCT AVAILABILITY

Product Available for Evaluation? (Do not send product to FDA)

☐ Yes   ☐ No   ☐ Returned to Manufacturer on: _____ (mm/dd/yyyy)

D. SUSPECT PRODUCT(S)

1. **Name, Strength, Manufacturer** (from product label)
   #1
   #2

2.	Dose or Amount	Frequency	Route
#1			
#2			

3. Dates of Use (If unknown, give duration) from/to (or best estimate)	5. Event Abated After Use Stopped or Dose Reduced?
#1	#1 ☐ Yes ☐ No ☐ Doesn't Apply
#2	#2 ☐ Yes ☐ No ☐ Doesn't Apply

4. Diagnosis or Reason for Use (Indication)	8. Event Reappeared After Reintroduction?
#1	#1 ☐ Yes ☐ No ☐ Doesn't Apply
#2	

6. Lot #	7. Expiration Date	#2 ☐ Yes ☐ No ☐ Doesn't Apply
#1	#1	9. NDC # or Unique ID
#2	#2	

E. SUSPECT MEDICAL DEVICE

1. **Brand Name**

2. **Common Device Name**

3. **Manufacturer Name, City and State**

4. Model #	Lot #	5. Operator of Device
Catalog #	Expiration Date (mm/dd/yyyy)	☐ Health Professional ☐ Lay User/Patient
Serial #	Other #	☐ Other: _____

6. If Implanted, Give Date (mm/dd/yyyy)	7. If Explanted, Give Date (mm/dd/yyyy)

8. **Is this a Single-use Device that was Reprocessed and Reused on a Patient?**
   ☐ Yes   ☐ No

9. **If Yes to Item No. 8, Enter Name and Address of Reprocessor**

F. OTHER (CONCOMITANT) MEDICAL PRODUCTS

Product names and therapy dates (exclude treatment of event)

G. REPORTER (See confidentiality section on back)

1. **Name and Address**

Phone #	E-mail

2. Health Professional?	3. Occupation	4. Also Reported to:
☐ Yes ☐ No		☐ Manufacturer ☐ User Facility ☐ Distributor/Importer
5. If you do NOT want your identity disclosed to the manufacturer, place an "X" in this box: ☐		

FORM FDA 3500 (10/05)   Submission of a report does not constitute an admission that medical personnel or the product caused or contributed to the event.

FIGURE 20-1   Voluntary reporting form for MedWatch, the FDA Medical Products Reporting Program. For more information, see www.fda.gov/medwatch/safety/FDA-3500_fillable.pdf.

professional has no control over the clinical outcome with the drug. Additionally, professionals using a device can have tremendous influence on the design and development of that device. Because of this, there is significant interaction between the device manufacturer and the professional, creating the potential for unique conflicts of interest (LaViolette, 2007). To clarify this relationship, AdvaMed has a *Code of Ethics on Interactions with Health Care Professionals*. This document outlines the methods for bona fide research, education, and expansion of professional skills; however, these activities must be conducted in an ethical manner. Product training and education, supporting third-party educational conferences, sales and promotional meetings, arrangements with consultants, gifts, reimbursement and other economic information, and grants and charitable donations are addressed (AdvaMed, 2005).

Professional nursing organizations are also influential public safety advocates. Nursing organizations such as the Infusion Nurses Society, the Association of PeriOperative Registered Nurses, the Oncology Nursing Society, and the Association for Professionals in Infection Control and Epidemiology strive to educate their members about the positive and negative outcomes with medical devices. These organizations offer feedback to manufacturers to initiate needed changes.

 ## PRODUCT PROCUREMENT

Infusion devices and equipment represent one of the most important components of patient safety. Proper choices can enhance safety while lack of attention to numerous details may seriously compromise the safety of both patients and caregivers. Product choices should be based on an interdisciplinary, collaborative effort among nurses, pharmacists, physicians, biomedical technologists, and human factors engineers.

TYPES OF EQUIPMENT

There are three types of equipment used in infusion therapy currently: durable medical equipment, single-use devices, and reprocessed single-use devices.

Durable medical equipment is defined as equipment that is used for long periods, is cleaned between uses, and may be considered property or capital equipment. Examples of durable medical equipment are IV poles, infusion pumps, and ultrasound or infrared devices for vascular visualization.

Single-use devices are discarded after being used once on a single patient. Most infusion products are disposable, including solution containers, administration sets, IV catheters, and dressing supplies.

Reprocessed single-use devices are devices labeled for single use but are reprocessed for uses on multiple patients. Examples of devices in this group include angiography and electrophysiology catheters and implanted programmable infusion pumps. This practice is a complex and controversial one, with an entire subindustry of companies providing reprocessing services. While there have been adverse events, including deaths, reported with reprocessed devices, the pattern does not differ from those seen with new devices. Proponents argue that these products cut costs and dramatically reduce medical waste, but the scientific data to support or disprove the safety of this practice are scarce (Nelson, 2006).

PURCHASING DECISIONS

The goal of all purchasing processes is to identify products that meet the needs of patients, professionals, and the facility. Although not a part of nursing curriculum, there are numerous aspects of business management that affect product decisions. Frequently, product decisions are made within the larger context of solving a patient safety issue (Powers, 2002; Keohane et al, 2005) or as a cost-containment initiative (Kokotis, 2005). Regardless of the approach or need identified, the purchase price of infusion supplies and equipment is a major part of direct resource consumption and requires careful analysis (Pierce and Baker, 2004). Traditionally, product decisions are based on the attributes of cost, quality, efficacy and availability; however, there may be the need to identify "trade-offs" in features that will not compromise patient or health care worker safety.

The nurse's limited knowledge of complex technology is a frequent cause of errors in studies about IV medication errors. While studies have found a very low rate of severe errors, moderate and minor errors delay the desired response to therapy or extend hospital stay (Taxis and Barber, 2003a,b; Husch et al, 2005). New concepts such as human factors engineering (HFE), mistake proofing, failure mode effects analysis (FMEA), and life-cycle thinking are now involved with product purchasing decisions.

Human factors are defined by the FDA as "the study of how people use technology. It involves the interaction of human abilities, expectations, and limitations, with work environments and systems design" (FDA, 2006). The use of human factor principles in the design of devices and systems is known as human factors engineering and is synonymous with usability engineering and ergonomics. Through the use of these principles, human performance is improved, reducing the risk of user error. Additional benefits include safer connections between devices, more effective alarms, easier repair and maintenance, more intuitive devices, and a reduction in the need for training. The most important aspect of this process is to reveal how a human interacts with the device (Gosbee, 2002). In the case of infusion therapy, this is especially applicable to infusion pumps and administration sets.

Heuristic evaluation and usability testing for an infusion pump help to enhance user interface and reduce the risk of adverse events. A list of principles or heuristics for an infusion pump includes consistency of words or symbols, appropriate display of information, elimination of extraneous information, prompt and beneficial feedback to the user, good error messages, and clear indication that each step has begun or ended. Usability testing involves direct observation of nurses using the infusion pump. This may also include videotaping for further examination, asking the nurses to verbalize thoughts about using the pump and to provide comments on their experience (Ladak et al, 2007).

Originating from the Japanese automobile industry, mistake proofing is frequently used in infusion therapy devices and processes. Using design features to prevent errors or the negative outcomes of those errors constitutes mistake proofing. Detection of mistakes and processes that allow for "safe" failure is also part of mistake proofing (Grout, 2007). Examples can easily be found in sharps injury prevention devices and infusion pumps. Short peripheral IV catheters have multiple types of engineered features to prevent the sharp needle from causing a needlestick injury, including spring-loaded, self-blunting, self-sheathing, and other retractable housing mechanisms. Chlorhexidine is now recognized as the most effective skin antiseptic; however, the clear solution cannot show the areas of skin that have been missed during the application. Adding color to provide a tint to the solution delineates the skin area where the solution has been applied. Infusion pumps may have a control switch on the rear panel behind a plastic cover. When activated, this switch prevents tampering with the pump settings, yet the cover does cause some inconvenience for those who need to have access to the settings. This small inconvenience is offset by the added safety of tamper-resistant settings (Grout, 2007). Color-coding is an example of a weak mistake proofing method. Color-coding of wires and their connection sites is frequently used for computer equipment; however, it has not been shown to be effective with preventing medication errors. The limitation of color-coding is that it cannot stop the process if the human ignores the colors. A system of color-coding syringe labels for anesthetics has been shown to produce medication errors (Fasting and Gisvold, 2000; Haslam et al, 2006).

Failure mode effects analysis is the process of analyzing product design to learn how it can fail. This process, typically applied to product development by engineers, is now being applied to hospital processes as a result of requirements from The Joint Commission. A multidisciplinary team uses a multistep process to identify vulnerable aspects of a product or process before harm can reach a patient. The process for using a specific product is listed in step-by-step detail. All possible or potential hazards, faults, or failures are identified and analyzed to determine the causes and the severity or criticality of each failure. Actions and proper interventions can then be determined to prevent the identified failures (Krouwer, 2004). Use of this process identified a 59% reduction in failure modes between the old and new processes for production of pediatric parenteral nutrition solution (Bonnabry et al, 2005).

One positive example of this technique is the selection of infusion pump technology with an integral drug library. Analysis of IV medication administration with the old processes and the new pump technology disclosed many ways to improve the process. The most success with this process was seen by end-users correctly and consistently using the pump features and not choosing to bypass these features or creating ways to "work around" the device (Apkon et al, 2004; Wetterneck et al, 2006).

Life-cycle thinking is the inclusion of all aspects of the product's life to the environment. This includes manufacture, distribution, clinical use, and disposal of the product. Mercury and dioxin are examples of two substances found in significant amounts from medical waste incinerators. During the product decision-making process, the disposal of products must be considered, yet most professionals involved do not have knowledge of environmental sciences. The stream of waste coming from health care facilities includes solid, infectious, hazardous, radioactive, recyclable, compostable, control-substance, confidential paper, and construction and demolition waste.

Infusion therapy products can produce dioxin during incineration. A common example is IV solution containers made of polyvinyl chloride (PVC). Bags made of polyolefin do not produce dioxin upon incineration and perform equally as well as those made of PVC (Kaiser et al, 2001). These processes rely upon involvement of professionals from all disciplines. Nurses, pharmacists, physicians, engineers, information technologists, and materials managers may be involved with each decision. Multiple departments within the organization need to be represented, such as radiology, anesthesia, laboratory, infection control and prevention, and risk management. It is also imperative that frontline caregivers be closely involved with decisions about products they will be expected to use. Infusion therapy is delivered throughout the entire health care spectrum and to all ages. While it is never easy, all needs must be considered in any product decision.

 ## PRODUCT USE

Products involved in the delivery of infusion therapy have the potential to produce electrical, chemical, sharps, and other infectious hazards to patients and health care workers alike. Products must be made available when and where they are needed, yet be properly stored and maintained when not in use.

PRODUCT INTEGRITY

Product integrity begins with an intact package to prevent contamination of the product components inside. Packaging may produce a sterile product on all surfaces, such as a central venous catheter and the components required for the insertion procedure. However, packaging may be designed to act as a dust cover. Most administration sets and prefilled flush syringes are packaged in a clear plastic overwrap or cardboard box. The labeling indicates that the sterile parts are the fluid pathway and the ends covered by protective caps. These products must be inspected to ensure that the end caps remain intact and that the package has not been compromised. Additionally, these products cannot be added to a sterile field because the outer surfaces of the product are considered to be clean and not sterile. Products such as extension sets or prefilled syringes that are completely sterile will indicate this on the package label, and that packaging is made of stronger materials to prevent accidental puncture and contamination.

Sterilization uses steam, heat, gas, or other chemicals to destroy or eliminate all forms of microbial life. Disinfection refers to liquid chemicals or wet pasteurization to eliminate many or all pathogenic microorganisms on inanimate objects except for bacterial spores. For more than 30 years, infection control professionals have used a standardized approach to disinfection and sterilization of patient care equipment. This approach divides all items into three categories—critical, semicritical, and noncritical. Critical items include those that enter sterile tissue or the vascular system or those items in which blood will flow. For obvious reasons, all IV catheters would fall into this group and must be sterile before insertion. Semicritical items come into contact with mucous membranes or nonintact skin and include respiratory and anesthesia equipment. Noncritical items contact intact skin but not mucous membranes. Blood pressure cuffs, crutches, and other environmental surfaces fall into this category (Rutala, 2007).

The growing body of knowledge about biofilm, increasing concern about catheter-associated bloodstream infections, burgeoning technology used with vascular catheters, and elimination of reimbursement for hospital-acquired infections are causing many questions about this popular approach to disinfection of equipment. Needleless connectors are commonly used on most venous catheters. They are exposed to a multitude of microorganisms from the patient's environment such as skin, bed linens, clothing, and body fluids; therefore these devices require disinfection before each use. According to the categories described previously, needleless connectors would be a critical item, yet once attached to a catheter hub there is no method for adequately sterilizing these devices before each use. The other option for sterilization would be high-level disinfection with chemicals such as glutaraldehyde, hydrogen peroxide, or peracetic acid; however, none of these solutions can be used while the device remains connected to the patient. Moreover, these agents require contact for up to 30 minutes. Intermediate- and low-level disinfectants such as ethyl alcohol or isopropyl alcohol are used for semicritical and noncritical items. High-level disinfection with either type of alcohol is not recommended. They may be used for "surface disinfection," although there is no further explanation of what surfaces are being discussed; bacteria are killed in 10 seconds with both alcohols in concentrations of 60% to 95% (Rutala, 2007).

The nurse is responsible for confirming that equipment is cleaned and checked for safety before it is used. Although others perform these functions, the nurse must ensure the usability of equipment. All infusion equipment must be inspected for product integrity before, during, and after use. If the product's integrity is compromised, that product is not to be used. If inspection reveals any defects during or after use, appropriate intervention is initiated and the defective product retained and reported (INS, 2006).

An organization's policies and procedures establish the requirements for disinfection of durable medical equipment, which includes IV poles, infusion pumps, vascular visualization devices, and teaching models. The agent used to disinfect durable equipment should effectively prevent cross-contamination, which is defined as the movement of pathogens from one source to another.

Infusion equipment is usually disinfected by being wiped down or immersed in a germicidal solution. Chemicals used for either of these processes should always be considered hazardous. Once a product is disinfected, it should be allowed to thoroughly dry, and fumes should be avoided. Manufacturers of some chemical disinfection products suggest that the product be aerated for a certain time before reusing.

Policies regarding the use of chemical disinfectants should include guidelines that protect employees from exposure and harm. Use of gloves to protect the hands, ventilation of the work area, and device aeration should be addressed before the product is reused, wrapped, or packaged. Although proper aeration is seemingly a minor point, nurses have reported ill effects from fumes emitted by disinfected products in closed areas, even from face masks removed from sterile packs.

Durable equipment should be disinfected between each patient use. This means that an infusion pump cannot be moved from one patient to another without validating that it has been thoroughly disinfected. In the absence of a centralized equipment pool, knowledgeable personnel on the nursing unit are responsible for such validation; the task should be assigned to a specific person to ensure its completion.

Disinfection should also be performed intermittently during patient use, weekly in the hospital or monthly in the home. The organization should set the precise interval, and this task should also be delegated to a specific department or person.

HEALTH CARE WORKER RISK

Employee protection is the responsibility of the health care facility and each worker. Proper grounding of electronic devices and routine safety checks help to avoid electrical hazards. Mechanical hazards can be avoided by proper inspection of equipment and thorough, up-to-date education regarding the use and upkeep of equipment.

Infusion therapy involves the risk of chemical hazards for the health care worker, and product choices must include consideration of this risk. Many antineoplastic and biological agents require special protection to compound, deliver, administer, and dispose of these medications and related supplies. The products used for protection include ventilated biological safety cabinets for compounding; personal protective equipment, including face shield, chemotherapy gloves, nonabsorbent gowns, and a certified respirator); closed system drug transfer devices; needleless connectors; and proper disposal receptacles. Risk comes from touch contamination, the air, or spills (NIOSH, 2004; Trossman, 2006).

Infusion therapy has always posed a high level of infectious risk to nurses. Sharps pose the risk of percutaneous injury, and blood splashing into broken skin or mucous membranes creates a risk of exposure to numerous bloodborne pathogens. Knowledge of the risks and use of proper products and procedures help prevent these risks.

The risk of legal liability for improper use of infusion equipment is another hazard that is often overlooked. All nurses with responsibility for administering any type of infusion therapy must have documented competency in the use of the equipment and application of policies and procedures. Issues that could be raised in the legal process incorporate deviation from the product instructions for use, failure to have documented competency, and failure to know and conform to the organization's policies and procedures.

ROLE OF BIOMEDICAL ENGINEERING

The profession of biomedical engineering has grown to match the dependence and amount of technology used in health care. The complexity of equipment drives the need for an engineering background to assist with purchase decisions, performance standards, regular maintenance, and repair. This profession is segmented by specialties. Bioinstrumentation involves the use of electronics, including imaging equipment and infusion controlling devices. Biomaterials, or the materials used to manufacture implantable devices, focuses on the mechanical, chemical, and toxic properties of numerous metals, ceramics, polymers, and composite substances. Clinical engineers use their skills to apply the technology in hospitals and other health care facilities.

No single authority exists to set standards for equipment validation by biomedical engineering departments within a health care facility. Manufacturers set instructions for periodic checks of equipment function using standardized tests. The Joint Commission requires that periodic safety and function tests be performed on all electronic equipment. Several other agencies give input into what constitutes acceptable levels of equipment monitoring by biomedical departments.

Organizational policy establishes the process for equipment safety checks and the frequency with which they are performed. When new equipment is introduced to an institution, all aspects of its performance should be checked. After the initial inspection, further performance checks may not be necessary unless a situation arises that indicates a need for testing.

The biomedical department might perform diagnostic tests on any equipment that is considered to have been under undue stress as a result of prolonged use (e.g., an ambulatory pump that is used continuously for many months on the same patient).

The age and service history of a product should be considered when scheduling maintenance checks. Older devices may have impeccable service histories but should be watched with care because all devices have a predictable life span. However, many infusion pumps from past generations still infuse with the accuracy and reliability of new devices. Older equipment, or equipment that malfunctions often, should be logged and tracked to validate poor performance and the extra expense resulting from repairs, supplies, and personnel time.

In the case of rented infusion equipment, some agencies prefer to monitor performance between each patient use. Because infusion equipment supplied for home care may be located far from the provider or support systems, equipment malfunction or failure is inconvenient, at best, and can be dangerous. To minimize these situations, care of equipment is a full-time effort that requires many more hours and tests than are mandated by regulatory agencies.

All tests and uses of equipment are clearly logged and kept as permanent records, as mandated by The Joint Commission; this regimen should also be a part of organizational policy. The maintenance of equipment reduces the associated risk in all health care settings for the safety of the public, the institution, and the employee.

The nurse facilitates problem solving by clearly noting suspected and actual occurrences of malfunction, including questionable product performance. Without clear observation and communication, equipment malfunction may continue undetected. If equipment users and engineers do not work closely together, the assumptions each make about the other can lead to serious compromises in safety.

When equipment is found to be functioning erroneously or is suspected of operating outside normal parameters, its use should be discontinued immediately. The exact problem should be documented, and a detailed description should be attached to the device. If the problem is poorly stated, it may not be found in routine examination. For example, if an infusion pump is not delivering at the prescribed rate, a nonspecific complaint of malfunction to the biomedical engineering department will result in diagnostic tests that do not include long-term infusion-accuracy tests. The scope of routine diagnostic procedures may have to be expanded to isolate a problem that has already been identified by the nurse but not clearly stated.

PRODUCT STORAGE AND ALLOCATION

Stored electrical equipment should be plugged into continuous electric current to prevent depletion of internal batteries, especially under very cold storage situations. Equipment powered only by batteries can be rendered useless by cold, leaving the equipment unusable until returned to room temperature. Equipment powered by any type of commercial battery should be stored without the batteries in place, because batteries corrode and can leak into the internal mechanisms of equipment.

Cleanliness is critical for storage of medical products. The storage area should be free of dust, lint, rodents, and insects. Mechanical equipment should be covered and protected, and products should be stored to prevent damage from stacking or crowding.

Equipment and supplies that are stored off-site, requiring movement and transport, are especially vulnerable to damage. Persons responsible for moving equipment should be educated about the nature of the products entrusted to their care as well as the hazards of damage. If equipment must be transported to the patient care area, proper function and safety should be verified on delivery. In home health care, the verification may be performed by the nurse or by a driver trained in equipment set-up. Contracted services for peripherally inserted central catheter (PICC) insertion drive the need for the nurse to be able to verify performance of ultrasound machines transported between facilities.

Allocation of equipment refers to the method of distribution or sharing throughout the entire organization. This primarily applies to durable equipment such as infusion pumps or vascular visualization devices such as ultrasound machines.

Infusion pump distribution is frequently delegated to a central resource responsible for tracking, transporting, retrieving, cleaning, and documenting the associated charges for equipment use. In many cases, this distribution function is largely taken for granted and undervalued. In hospitals with a decentralized approach, the pumps are kept in the nursing areas and moved from patient to patient as needed. Critical elements for equipment upkeep and accountability, such as knowing the equipment's location and how it is being used, are often unattended.

Ultrasound and infrared equipment for vascular visualization is limited to only those professionals with documented competency in their use. This restriction could make equipment upkeep and accountability easier; however, it could limit the expanded use of these devices to other patient care areas.

There must be physical accountability of equipment at all times, even if the equipment is not returned to a central pool at the end of each use. Tracking equipment is an important record-keeping obligation. If a recall were to occur, a system must be in place to locate the equipment. Logs must be maintained to track safety and calibration checks and to validate that equipment is cleaned between uses. Any equipment leaving the system must be fully checked by the biomedical engineering department before it is returned to use. Any interruption in accountability necessitates that the equipment's function and safety be confirmed.

On discontinuation of therapy, the nurse is responsible for notifying the central equipment pool or, in the case of home health care, the billing office. This action ensures that the patient is not charged needlessly and that the equipment can be retrieved, cleaned, and reallocated as soon as it is needed.

EDUCATION AND TRAINING

The basis for protecting patients and health care workers begins with education. This process involves four components—continuing professional education, orientation, inservice training, and patient education.

Continuing professional education is designed to meet the needs of the professional. It is required when the professional expands the scope of practice to incorporate a new service such as PICC insertion. A PICC insertion course incorporates identifying appropriate patient candidates, indications and contraindications, infection control and prevention, technology characteristics and uses, routine nursing interventions, and complication prevention and management. Continuing education is used for numerous aspects of infusion therapy, such as types of therapy or complication management, and is the responsibility of the individual professional. The instructor or faculty for continuing education must be a qualified professional with experience in what is being taught.

A certificate of completion or attendance is issued at the end of the program.

Orientation is the responsibility of each health care organization upon beginning work at that facility. It encompasses the mandatory training programs such as infection control and prevention, appropriate use and location of the specific products and equipment used by that facility, and policies and procedures for that organization. Orientation is also required when a nurse is temporarily reassigned to a nursing unit outside of their routine place of work. Many types of equipment and supplies vary across hospitals and even between nursing units within the same facility; therefore this orientation serves to acquaint the individual with the critical information needed to successfully perform his or her job responsibilities.

Inservice training is educational programs designed for the benefit of the organization, such as a new policy or a new brand of equipment. One example is an infusion nurse learning the differences about a new brand of PICC and its accompanying kit components. The hospital has chosen to change brands, driving the need to learn the new product. This differs from a continuing education process used for a nurse learning the complete PICC insertion process. The instructor for an inservice training program may be a nurse or educator from the hospital or various product manufacturer's representatives. These programs are usually short sessions and attendance is documented within the facility's personnel records. Inservice training usually does not qualify for awarding continuing education contact hours.

Patient education involves written and verbal communication to educate the patient and family about their specific care, and is critical for positive outcomes in home care. Patients should be involved in making choices about the type of venous access device they prefer for long-term infusion needs. They must master the techniques for administration of medications, catheter maintenance, use of sophisticated equipment, and infection prevention techniques.

Many resources are available to support all of these processes. Each product comes with written instructions for use contained within or on the package. It is the nurses' responsibility to know those instructions before using each device. Many devices such as long-term venous access devices also have patient information booklets and product information cards to enhance the care when patients are transferred to other facilities or other providers see the patient. Other important written information regarding equipment use includes policies, procedures, and handling of nonroutine or emergency situations.

Proper product use requires training of all users, which is a challenge for weekend-only or shift employees. Training should occur when the product is introduced and as often as necessary during sustained use of the product to ensure continued safe practice. Validation of training is mandated by The Joint Commission and should appear in the employee record or a central education database.

Technology is affecting the delivery of all of these processes. Continuing education is available in traditional classrooms, via the Internet, or through other computer- or paper-based self-study processes. Orientation and inservice training programs are organized and delivered through the staff development department in each facility. This could involve traditional classes, required reading with documentation, email messages, an organization's Intranet, or other computer-based processes. Patient education is delivered by one-to-one instruction, videotapes of procedures, or written pamphlets; however, these should be followed by adequate time for the patient and family to ask and receive answers to their questions.

OFF-LABEL USES

Before products are purchased, their intended use should be clearly defined. As a general rule, products should not be used for indications or in a manner other than that specified by the manufacturer. However, products could be used in a manner that is outside the manufacturer's written instructions, also called off-label uses. One common example is the use of a regular PICC for injection of a high-pressure injection for a CT scan. Only catheters labeled for high-pressure injection should be used. Also, infusion of low-dose alteplase (Cathflo, Genentech) over several hours to treat a fibrin sheath on the external catheter surfaces is another off-label use. The only indication is instillation of a 2-mg dose into the catheter lumen, followed by aspiration after 30 to 120 minutes.

Manufacturers cannot actively promote the use of their products outside of their labeling and are governed by FDA guidance on how they provide information about off-label uses. The FDA has no governance over the practice of health care professionals; thus off-label use does occur. Generally, manufacturers are not held legally liable for problems resulting from misuse of their products; however, all off-label use would not be considered misuse. Examples of misuse would include cutting a guidewire or advancing a catheter over a stylet wire not designed for that use.

PRODUCT ERROR

Statistically, the equipment provided for use in health care is very safe. There is no acceptable level of tolerance for critical errors and there is increasing emphasis on creating a culture of safety for all people within the system—workers and patients alike. However, critical events do happen. A recent analysis of the MAUDE database disclosed problems with the use of insulin and patient-controlled analgesia (PCA) pumps in an adolescent population. The report included 13 deaths and several reports involving hypoglycemic and hyperglycemic events that were device-related; however, the prevalent causes were related to compliance, education, or sports-related activities. This report highlighted the special needs of this age group with these devices (Cope, Morrison, and Samuels-Reid, 2008).

Malfunction indicators are built into devices to protect the patient and caregiver. Alarms on infusion devices should never be circumvented. Devices that allow alarms to be silenced invite certain hazards. All alarms have a specific purpose and the proper way to silence the alarm is to discover and correct the cause of that alarm.

Some device problems are not detected by alarms but are discovered by alert caregivers. At times, caregivers confirm that the equipment is functioning without double-checking its performance. An example of this type of performance problem is an infusion device set to infuse at a given rate. The nurse monitors the patient, notes that the pump is infusing, reads the amount infused, and charts the data provided by the pump on the amount infused. Eventually, an observant nurse notices that the solution should have totally infused hours earlier if the pump had actually delivered the amount calculated. In this case, the device is not operating according to its programming, but no alarm has sounded. The infusion device must be used as an adjunct to providing safe care, not as a substitution for careful nursing. From legal, professional, and clinical perspectives, competency is vital to infusion specialists, nurses, nursing staff, non-RN staff, and family members. It is paramount to patients who depend on the health care team to deliver the best care possible.

Negative clinical outcomes should trigger the necessary investigation. Any devices being used must be included in that investigation; however, care must be taken to avoid assumptions that the device is always the cause of the outcome. Complications, unexpected deterioration of the patient, or development of a patient crisis should always cue the caregiver to check the equipment. If a device or product is even remotely involved in a negative patient outcome, the device should be removed, not altered in any way, and taken to the appropriate department such as biomedical engineering or risk management; a full written report should be made. If the equipment appears to be functioning appropriately but cannot be ruled out as a potential problem, it should be removed as soon as safely possible and checked completely.

The nurse must never allow equipment to substitute for nursing assessment and judgment. If the equipment indicates that the patient is doing well but nursing assessment does not confirm it, the nurse's professional skills should supersede the equipment (INS, 2006). It is not necessary to calculate drop factors for infusion pumps, but monitoring the pump's performance is mandatory. If the patient is using a patient-controlled analgesia device, is pain controlled? If not, is the device functioning? If the patient is somnolent, is the pump delivering medication as programmed? These questions should be answered before changing the infusion settings to attain improved patient response.

User-induced malfunctions are numerous, unfortunately (Table 20-1). These problems are the most dangerous, most challenging to identify, and the most difficult to correct. All professionals using infusion equipment must know the proper operation of the device and follow the instructions for use, including indications, contraindications, precautions, warnings, and the specific procedure for use.

Education, product training, and competency documentation, along with performance improvement processes, will help to identify and correct these errors. Identification of the situation that precipitated the problem can aid in the discovery of the actual cause. User errors can result from unfamiliarity with the operational controls of a device or from fundamental misconceptions about functions and capabilities.

Documentation of these errors through incident reports or some other form of communication to a centralized location will increase the early recognition of any trends. Records may be maintained in the departments of infusion therapy, biomedical engineering, purchasing, materials management, or nursing education. Problems with devices should always be considered for inclusion in the medical device reporting program discussed earlier in this chapter. The actual device involved in an incident should be collected and maintained in an unadulterated manner. Manufacturers may request the return of devices to allow investigation by their engineers. Also, the outcome of any malpractice lawsuit could hinge on having the device in question available. For instance, fracture and embolization of a central venous catheter could be related to the insertion procedure, to the care of the device during the dwell time, or to its design or manufacture. Without the actual catheter in question, many questions and subsequent liability could be undetermined or incorrectly placed on the wrong professional. The product's brand name, lot number, and any other identifying numbers or markings should be provided to the manufacturer and kept in the organization's records. All details of the negative occurrence should be documented immediately.

Medical devices suspected of malfunction should be reported as soon as the product defect can be defined and user error can

TABLE 20-1 Types of User-Induced Product Malfunctions and Failures

Device	Error	Potential outcome
Flow control devices	Bypassing a function of device (e.g., air-in-line alarm or lockout function)	Venous air embolus Overdose of narcotics Medication errors
	Incorrect choice of administration set	Over- or underinfusion of fluids or medications
	Ignorance or disregard for proper device operation	Over- or underinfusion of fluids or medications Medication errors
Venous access devices	Forceful injection from any size syringe	Catheter rupture or breakage
	Use of clamps with sharp ridges or teeth	Catheter rupture or breakage Cracking catheter hub
	Alteration of device by bending or cutting	Unraveling of safety design on guidewire, leading to wire embolization
	Incorrect attachment of catheter to port body	Catheter separation from port body with embolization
Administration sets and other add-on devices	Connection of infusion sets to another Luer-locking tubing system	Administration of solutions and medications intended for another route into vein
	Connection of another Luer-locking tubing system to an infusion catheter	Administration of intravenous solutions or medications into another anatomical location (e.g., epidural) Air emboli if misconnected to an automatic blood pressure device or other air-based system
	Lack of sterile cap following intermittent use	Contamination and subsequent bloodstream infection
	Failure to use Luer-Lok™ connection	Air emboli if set and catheter became disconnected Fluid leakage from a loose connection resulting in an incorrect amount of fluid or medication going to patient

be ruled out. Significant trends in user errors could indicate an unrecognized flaw in product design and should be brought to the attention of the manufacturer. Death of a patient or employee known or thought to be associated with any device should be immediately reported to the manufacturer and the FDA. Careful investigation must begin immediately and the role of the device must be clarified.

 ## SOLUTION CONTAINERS

A wide variety of containers for IV solutions are available in all sizes. Glass and plastic containers range from 50 mL to 3 L and syringes range from 1 mL to 60 mL. Each type of container offers advantages and disadvantages to their use.

GLASS CONTAINERS

The first intravenous (IV) infusion container to be mass-produced was made of glass. Glass was and is easy to sterilize, and graduations on glass can be easily and accurately read. However, after 50 years of use, glass remains the container of choice only for infusates that cannot adapt to plastic bags because of incompatibilities with the chemicals or properties of plastic.

Closed system glass bottles are sealed with a thick, hard, rubber disk. The center is designated with a target area, which can be easily perforated with the administration set spike. The hard rubber disk is covered with an easily removable vacuum seal. Once the seal is removed, the bottle should be used immediately to ensure sterility. The seal must be removed before it is spiked with an administration set and cannot be reapplied or resealed. In a sterile compounding program, infusates can be mixed and a second sterile cover applied for delivery to the patient care area.

Because they are noncollapsible, glass bottles must also be vented. For the solution to empty from the bottle, air must replace the solution, which can occur through a venting straw or with a vented administration set. If the bottle is made with a venting straw, it runs the length of the bottle to allow air to be pulled in as the solution infuses. The potential for contamination of the solution is increased with the use of a venting straw because no barrier exists between the external sources of contamination and the interior of the bottle.

The most acceptable method of introducing air into the system is to use a vented administration set designed to allow air to enter the bottle. The administration set spike has a regular channel for the flow of fluid and a very small side channel to introduce air into the bottle. The administration set may be made specifically as a vented set, or may be considered a universal administration set with a capped air channel, requiring the nurse to uncap the air inlet channel when it is used with a glass fluid container (Figure 20-2).

The venting mechanism provided by the manufacturer is intended to allow air to enter without allowing fluid to leak from the venting device. Although this might appear simple, it requires an understanding of droplet formation and the physical composition of the venting outlet. In the absence of a vented administration set, filter needles are available to provide a filtered air source. It is not acceptable to vent a bottle with a regular needle through the rubber disk; this method creates a risk of solution contamination and an open entry for infection. This is also an unsafe use of a needle. When a needle is used inappropriately in this way, solution often leaks from the bottle.

PLASTIC CONTAINERS

Large-scale conversion to plastic IV solution containers came with the need to transport soldiers from the battlefield or field triage areas with treatment already initiated. The same pressure for use of plastic grew from improved emergency care in hospitals. As emergency personnel and treatments evolved and many more treatments were initiated outside the hospital, the need for the safety of plastic became critical for the patient and for the health care provider. Thus flexible polyvinyl chloride (PVC) plastic fluid containers have met requirements for many health care settings. Although it is commonly used for plastic IV solution containers, there are challenges with its use. Polyolefin and ethyl vinyl acetate (EVA) are newer plastics that reduce some of these problems. Some newer plastic containers are made of multiple layers of thermoplastic material to improve safety and eliminate the need for a plastic overwrap.

PVC-based solution containers depend upon the addition of di-2-ethylhexylphthalate (DEHP), a plasticizer added to make them soft and pliable. However, there has been concern for several years regarding leaching of DEHP into the blood and its potential harmful effects. DEHP is commonly found in numerous plastic products such as building products, automobiles, clothing, food packaging, and children's toys. In the United States, it is estimated that an adult is exposed to approximately 1 to 30 micrograms (mcg) per kilogram (kg) of body weight per day. For a person weighing 155 pounds or 70 kg, this would equate to 70 to 2100 mcg daily (Kavlock, 2006).

Exposure to medical procedures with products containing DEHP carries the greatest risk for male fetuses and infants, where the levels of exposure could be as high as 6000 micrograms per kilogram of body weight per day. There is serious concern about the developing male reproductive tract in utero, and up to 1 year of age. This concern is based on studies measuring low testosterone levels in male rodents. Similar concerns cannot be extended to female fetuses or infants nor the general adult population (Kavlock, 2006).

There are many other concerns about DEHP and its possible carcinogenic or hepatotoxic effects. Additionally, there is some evidence that certain drugs cause more leaching of DEHP from the fluid containers and administration sets (de Lemos et al, 2005; Loff et al, 2007; Yang et al, 2007). The possibility of the DEHP molecule size contributing to catheter-related deep vein thrombosis has been reported (Danschutter et al, 2007).

Another issue with plastic fluid containers is the sorption or adherence of certain drugs to the container's surface. As much as 80% of the dose of insulin and nitroglycerin may adsorb or adhere to the PVC-based fluid container, requiring close monitoring and titration to the patient's response (Gahart and Nazazreno, 2008). Testing of several drugs produced evidence that insulin still adsorbs to fluid containers made of polyolefin plastic while other drugs do not (Trissel, Xu, and Baker, 2006).

Research of polyolefin fluid containers has studied multiple drugs known to be associated with the problems of sorption and leaching. For the problem of sorption, amiodarone, carmustine, regular human insulin, lorazepam, nitroglycerin, sufentanil, and thiopental were studied. For the problem of leaching of plasticizers or other polymer products, docetaxel, paclitaxel, tacrolimus, and teniposide were studied. Insulin was the only tested drug to have a problem with sorption to the

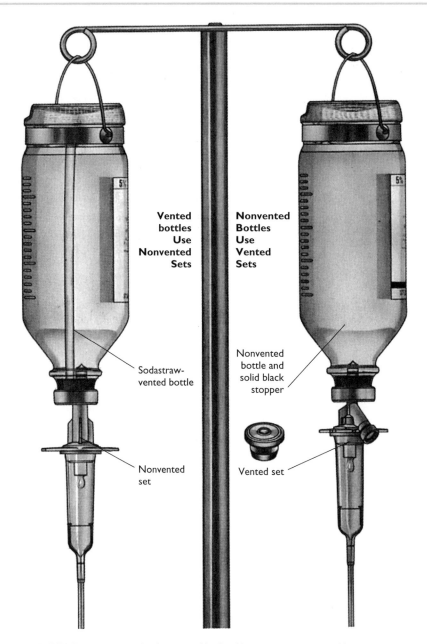

FIGURE 20-2 Vented and nonvented bottle tubing. (Courtesy Baxter Healthcare Corp.)

polyolefin container. Leaching of plastic components was not found with any of the tested drugs (Trissel et al., 2006).

Plastic containers can present mechanical challenges as well. Accuracy of the graduation markings and the volume readings from those markings can be incorrect. The plastic fluid container should be closely inspected before and during use to make sure there are no pinholes or tears. For instance, inserting the spike of the administration set at an angle can easily tear the container, causing solution leakage and the potential for contamination.

Plastic solution containers collapse when they empty, eliminating the need for a venting device either in the bag or on the administration set. Because air is not introduced into the bag, very little air can be accidentally infused.

Because it is relatively light and unbreakable, the plastic container is safer and more practical to store, stack, and move from one place to another. Most plastic containers are not sensitive to fluctuations in temperature or changes in environment.

Because plastic can withstand freezing and thawing, many drugs are provided in prefrozen minibags.

With the trend toward ambulatory and home care infusion, the plastic fluid container has added a significant degree of safety and convenience. The expanding outpatient delivery of infusion therapy is possible because of the development of plastic fluid containers.

OTHER SOLUTION CONTAINERS

Syringes can be correctly identified as solution containers. The syringe, when used in conjunction with a syringe-loaded electronic infusion pump, acts as a fluid container for either intermittent or continuous use. If the syringe contents are withdrawn or aspirated by the pumping mechanism, the administration set must be vented to allow air to displace the solution being extracted. If the pump mechanism only compresses the syringe, any administration set may be used with the syringe.

A syringe is easily and accurately readable for volume given or volume remaining. The syringe is unbreakable, easy to store and transport, and impossible to perforate accidentally. The syringe, in comparison with other solution containers, is inexpensive and available worldwide. The syringe can be prefilled and frozen with an almost unlimited number of solutions and drugs.

The limiting feature of the syringe is the volume it holds. Syringes are seldom seen with volume capabilities greater than 50 to 60 mL because syringes of this size are awkward to handle. This is not a limiting feature in neonatal and pediatric applications. In these areas, syringes can be the primary container for all types of infusions, such as crystalloids, blood products, fat emulsions, medications, and parenteral nutrition. In adults, the syringe is often used for intermittent medications. Continuous infusion via the syringe may be used for small volumes required by such therapies as pain management and titrated concentrated medications.

Solutions for catheter flushing are available in prefilled syringes. These syringes are available in either a clean or a sterile package. If the entire contents of the package are sterile, the syringe can be added to a sterile procedure field; however, the majority are sterile only in the fluid pathway. Aseptically filled syringes use sterile fluid, syringe, and tip cap and are filled in much the same manner as a pharmacy would batch-fill syringes. Terminally sterile syringes have been filled and then processed in an additional sterilization process. Both aseptically filled and terminally sterilized syringes are enclosed in an overwrap that acts as a dust cover (Hadaway, 2008).

Prefilled syringes for catheter flushing do not have the same gradation markings as other syringes and have a fixed label with their contents; 0.9% sodium chloride filled syringes should not be used for diluting other medications because of these wider markings and the fact that there is no way to alter the label to include the drug that has been added. Additionally, the short segment of the syringe barrel beyond the plunger is clean and protected by the dust-cover overwrap. However, complete sterility of the syringe barrel outside of the fill line is not guaranteed. Therefore the plunger should not be retracted into this area of the barrel (Hadaway, 2008).

Infusion pump–specific containers also fall in the category of solution containers. Most of these are reservoirs made specifically for use with a single, unique infusion device. They are not interchangeable. Efforts to use most of these solution containers in devices other than the one for which they were produced may lead to serious and harmful effects. Some are dedicated not only to a specific infusion system but also to a specific therapy, such as chemotherapy or pain control.

The container systems used for specific devices have unique limitations, depending on pump functions and therapies delivered. Limitations include lack of testing for a wider variety of uses and problems arising with commonly used drugs in uncommon concentrations or infusion modes.

USE-ACTIVATED CONTAINERS

Use-activated containers have premeasured drug and diluent in separate compartments. These containers are very helpful for frequently used medications with a relatively short beyond-use date after dilution. Although they are more expensive than the individually supplied products, use-activated containers offer considerable savings of personnel time for drug preparation. These containers play a significant time-saving role in emergency care and are easy to use in acute situations, such as in ambulances, field use, or transport. Ambulatory and home care settings can also benefit from use-activated containers.

To activate the container, the nurse deliberately ruptures the container's seal or diaphragm by compressing opposing parts or by applying pressure to rupture the internal reservoir or remove the barrier between compartments. The primary disadvantage of the system occurs when this step is not completed appropriately. It is not always apparent when the drug has entered the diluent compartment, leaving the diluent infusing without the medication. A more severe concern is the belated rupture of the medication compartment with a potentially harmful concentration of drug being administered.

LIGHT SENSITIVITY

Many drugs require protection from ultraviolet light because they degrade with prolonged light exposure. With regard to plastic versus glass, there is apparently no distinct advantage of one material over another. Efforts have been made to provide a container material that would protect light-sensitive drugs, but such development is not economically practical. A simple solution is to protect the infusate container from light by placing a dark material such as a paper bag over the fluid container. The disadvantage to using paper bags is the inability to see the fluid level and the container labels. There are commercially available plastic bags made of a variety of colors that block the UV light while allowing the fluid level and labels to be seen.

 ## ADMINISTRATION SETS

PURPOSE OF THE SET

Administration sets may have a variety of purposes, although the set design is very similar. The purpose of the set dictates the length of time it may safely be used.

Primary continuous administration sets

A primary set is typically the main administration set used to carry the infusing solution from the container to the patient. It should be a single entity, although adding other components may be required to meet the patient's needs. Primary sets can be a gravity set, an infusion pump set, or even a microbore syringe-pump set if the main solution is being infused with the syringe pump.

The primary set can be selected with varying drop size and length, depending on the intended use, the patient's condition, and the rate of infusion. Administration set length depends on the patient's needs and whether other equipment is used. Administration sets should be long enough to allow patient activity and for appropriate placement of the IV solution container and a flow control device if used. Standard primary sets can range from 60 to 110 inches in length.

The use of add-on devices such as filters or extension sets is discouraged. While these additional devices may be necessary, it is preferable to have a primary set with these devices built on rather than requiring their assembly at the bedside. Each add-on device is a potential source of contamination, misuse, and accidental disconnection.

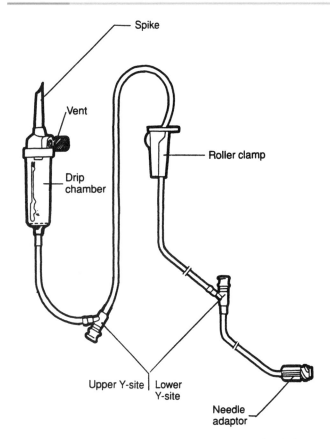

FIGURE 20-3 Primary administration set. (Courtesy MiniMed Technologies.)

Primary administration sets should have Luer-Lok™ connectors to prevent accidental disconnection. The use of needles to access administration set ports is no longer acceptable practice. All set connections require a needleless system. Figure 20-3 depicts a primary administration set. All primary sets should be replaced no more frequently than 72-hour intervals. More frequent replacement has not proven to reduce the risk of infection, although it increases the manipulation of the central venous catheter hub, which is known to increase the risk of contamination and subsequent infection.

Secondary administration sets

A secondary set attaches to the primary administration set for a specific purpose, usually to administer medications. The set may be used for intermittent or continuous infusion; however, compatibility with the primary solution must be assessed. Secondary sets are also known as piggyback sets.

Secondary sets are usually between 18 and 70 inches long, but the most commonly used length is 30 to 36 inches. Secondary sets can be macrodrop or microdrop, depending on the volume and rate of the secondary solution and the patient's condition.

Secondary administration sets can be attached to the primary set by using one of several types of needleless systems. When a secondary set is used, the primary set should contain a back-check valve, which prevents the retrograde flow of fluid from the secondary container into the primary container. The secondary set should remain connected to the primary set, with both being changed simultaneously no more frequently than every 72 hours. If the secondary set is disconnected after each

use and then reconnected, it should be managed as an intermittent set.

Primary intermittent sets

These sets are frequently the same set as the one used for continuous infusion. It extends from the solution container to the catheter hub, or in some cases to another primary continuous set. Primary intermittent sets can be a gravity set, infusion pump set, or even microbore syringe-pump set if the main solution is being infused with the syringe pump. The difference in this set from a primary continuous one is that it is connected and disconnected with each use, thus requiring close attention to proper handling and more frequent change due to the increased manipulation of the set.

After each use, the male Luer end of the intermittent set must be properly covered. If using a needleless system requiring a blunt cannula, the used cannula should be removed and discarded with a new cannula opened and attached. If using a Luer-access needleless system, the male Luer end of the administration set must be protected with a new dead-end cap. The action of inserting the male Luer tip of the administration set into an injection port higher on the same set, referred to as looping, is not considered appropriate. Red blood cells may be present in large quantity without a change in color (Jain et al, 2005), thus providing a growth medium in the entire length of the administration set. Any organisms present on the male Luer end would be spread to the entire administration set as well.

Primary intermittent sets should be changed every 24 hours (INS, 2006). Research on the life of IV administration sets has purposefully excluded sets used intermittently or for medication administration; therefore there are no studies that have examined the length of time that these sets can safely be used (Hadaway, 2007). Guidelines from the Centers for Disease Control and Prevention state that only sterile devices should be used to access injection ports (O'Grady et al, 2002). Extending the use of primary intermittent sets can increase the risk of contamination of the male Luer end. This contaminated set is then reconnected to a needleless connector, consequently increasing the potential for catheter-associated bloodstream infection.

Specialty sets

There are several special uses of administration sets that must be considered. Certain intravenous drugs, parenteral nutrition and fat emulsion, arterial pressure monitoring, and blood and blood components present special requirements for the administration set used for infusion.

Nitroglycerin and insulin adsorb or adhere to the plastic in the administration set and fluid container. The percentage of drug lost to this process depends on the exact nature of the plastic, which varies by manufacturer, the length and type of set, and the length of exposure to the plastic.

This adsorption phenomenon prevents the prescribing physician and the nurse administering the infusion from knowing exactly what percentage of the drug is being delivered. In the clinical setting, the drug is titrated, so the concentration delivered depends on the patient's symptoms, making the actual concentration less critical. Not knowing the actual concentration could be problematic if certain interventions are initiated based on the assumption that a predetermined limit of drug infusion has been reached. The saturation point must be reached with each set change, potentially creating fluctuations in the drug concentrations delivered. Many clinicians are uncomfortable dealing with such an unknown factor in conjunction with such a critical drug.

Nitroglycerin sets can be made with non-PVC material, or the inner lumen can be coated with polyethylene or similarly compatible material. Used with glass containers, both of these alternatives offer a system that does not create an adhering surface for nitroglycerin. Minimal drug loss occurs, making the infusing concentration constant. These nitroglycerin-specific sets are more expensive than standard sets. Safe care could be accomplished with or without nitroglycerin-specific administration sets, as long as the potential risks are understood.

Fat emulsions are provided in glass containers only, although recent research has evaluated the physical stability in plastic syringes for neonatal dosages (Driscoll et al, 2007). Fat emulsion does cause leaching of DEHP from plastic (Loff et al, 2007), making DEHP-free sets necessary (Mirtallo et al, 2004). The glass container also mandates the need for a vented administration set and it should be changed after 24 hours of use (O'Grady et al, 2002; Mirtallo et al, 2004).

Sets used for arterial pressure monitoring have additional components, including a pressure transducer, a continuous flush device, and a three-way stopcock. Manipulations and entries into this system should be kept to a minimum to reduce the risk of introducing microorganisms and air. Disposable transducers are accurate and are preferred. There is a means for attaching the transducer to a cardiac monitor with the capability of measuring arterial pressure; 0.9% sodium chloride with or without heparin is the preferred solution to flow through the system, and dextrose solutions should not be used because they are a growth medium for several microorganisms. The continuous flush segment will usually deliver between 3 and 5 mL of solution and a pressure infuser bag is placed around the solution container. Disinfection of the diaphragm is required before entering the system with a syringe and the stopcock must remain closed. The administration set and all connections must be capable of tolerating the pressures used to keep the system patent. The solution container, administration set, and transducer should all be changed simultaneously at 96-hour intervals (O'Grady et al, 2002).

Blood-specific administration sets are designed to accommodate the viscous properties of blood, allow rapid transfusion (if needed), and provide a dual line for the infusion of 0.9% sodium chloride before and after the blood product is infused. Blood-specific sets can be gravity or pump specific and should be used only for their stated purpose. The large-bore tubing and flow regulation clamp in these sets are not intended for routine infusion of crystalloids or medications.

Blood sets usually contain a large-screen filter to remove coarse fibrin and by-products of stored blood. This filter is usually 170 to 260 microns in size. Add-on filters of smaller pore size, including microaggregate and leukocyte-depletion filters, may be added and are discussed later in this chapter.

Some blood sets incorporate an in-line hand pump to push blood along when rapid infusion is needed. The hand pump should be used with caution. Adverse effects of inappropriate use of a hand pump include damaged vasculature, loss of the venipuncture site, and severe infiltration. Other potential problems can be damage to the infusing red blood cells, pulmonary emboli, and speed shock.

Blood should be given only through blood-specific sets (Figure 20-4). Blood is frequently infused by gravity flow. When strict control of the flow rate is needed, most electronic flow control devices or infusion pumps include blood transfusion

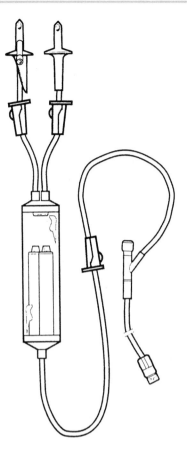

FIGURE 20-4   Sample blood administration set. (Courtesy MiniMed Technologies.)

in their list of indications for use. The administration set must be a blood-specific set that is acceptable with the chosen infusion pump. Infusion pump manufacturers who do not have blood as a labeled indication for use and do not offer these sets should be consulted before blood is infused through one of their devices.

Ideally, one administration set would be used for 1 unit of blood. If more than 1 unit can be transfused within 4 hours, one set could be used for more than 1 unit of blood. Instructions from the manufacturers of the set should be consulted; however, all sets should be changed at 4 hours (INS, 2006; Roback et al, 2008).

Metered-volume chamber sets

A metered set contains a small-volume chamber between the primary fluid container and the administration set. The metered chamber may be purchased as a stand-alone item, which enables its use with various administration sets. It is also available with a large variety of preattached tubing. The increasing use of large-volume infusion pumps and syringe pumps has reduced the use of the metered-chamber set; however, they remain in use in some facilities.

Metered-chamber sets are designed to limit the amount of fluid available to the patient by only filling the chamber with the prescribed fluid volume of 1 or 2 hours of infusion. The chamber usually holds 100 or 150 mL but some neonatal chambers may hold 10 to 50 mL. The graduation marks on a metered chamber are commonly 5 mL but some may be as small as 2 mL. The chamber is semirigid and may have a ball float at the

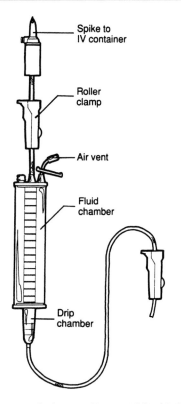

FIGURE 20-5   Metered-volume set. (Courtesy MiniMed Technologies.)

bottom to prevent air from entering the infusion line when the chamber empties.

Another application of the metered chamber is the intermittent infusion of medication. The chamber is filled to a prescribed level to achieve a correct dilution, and the medication is added through an injection port at the top of the chamber. This method is useful when the medication is available in a syringe, the medication is admixed immediately before infusion, or the patient's volume is restricted. The primary infusing solution then becomes the diluent. The drawback to this method is that the medication administration rate could vary greatly from the primary infusion rate, requiring the nurse to return immediately when the medication infuses to reset the infusion rate. There is also a problem when the medication is not compatible with the primary fluid. Figure 20-5 depicts a metered-volume set.

Primary Y sets

Primary Y sets are used for rapid infusion or dual administration, usually in critical care, trauma, or surgery patients, and can be found in gravity as well as in infusion pump configurations. Each leg of the Y set is capable of being the primary set. The Y set has two separate spikes, with a separate drip chamber and a short length of tubing with individual clamps. The junction occurs usually 12 to 20 inches below the spikes and there may be another drip chamber at this level. The fluids mix fully at this point. Primary Y administration sets cannot be used to infuse incompatible fluids.

Because they are meant to infuse large amounts in acute situations, primary Y sets are commonly made with very-large-bore tubing and clamps that lack the rate-controlling capabilities of general-use administration sets. These sets are not intended for general use and pose a risk if used for general-purpose infusion.

The risk of accidental bolus or a runaway infusion is very high because of the design of the set.

Additional precaution is required if a primary Y set is used with a glass bottle. The air vent not only will fill the bottle, but also the air will continue to flow with the infusing solution from the other side into the patient. Primary Y sets are not provided as vented sets, so this caution applies to bottles with venting straws or a venting apparatus added to the bottle. Any air emboli associated with sets of this inner lumen size would be significant.

CHARACTERISTICS OF SETS
Vented and nonvented sets

Vented sets allow air to enter the infusion container to displace the infusing solution. These sets are necessary for glass containers that do not collapse when emptying. A vented set is designed with a small air inlet on the spike portion of the administration set. The fit into the container may be tighter than a nonvented spike, requiring more effort to spike the container. This characteristic is not considered a problem, but the nurse should be aware of it to ensure that the spike is fully inserted into the bottle, preventing accidental dislodgment or impeded flow. Vented sets are available in gravity-infusion administration sets and infusion pump sets.

Some manufacturers prefer to offer a universal set that can be vented or nonvented, depending on need. In these sets, a removable cap exists for the air inlet vent. To create a vented set, the capping device is simply removed.

Nonvented administration sets are designed for plastic fluid containers. No air is admitted into the system; the infusing solution creates a small vacuum that allows the bag to collapse as it empties. This is an important characteristic when a sterile, closed infusion system is the goal. Nonvented sets cannot be used with glass fluid containers. Plastic containers can physically accommodate a vented spike; however, it can create an unnecessary risk of air entering the administration set. If a bag is vented, the infusing solution is displaced by air entering the bag.

Drop factors

The *drop factor* is the number of drops delivered that equal 1 mL and differs by each manufacturer. The drop factor is a specific measurement designed to deliver the calculated number of drops per minute. The user calculates flow rates based on the number of drops allowed to fall each minute. Drop sizes vary from 10 to 60 drops/mL. Drop factors are usually divided into two categories: *macrodrop* and *microdrop*.

Macrodrop is also called *regular drop size*. The 10-, 12-, 15-, and 20-drop/mL sets are macrodrop sets. This common set can be used in any application, although its accuracy decreases as the rate per hour decreases.

Microdrop sets are the most suitable for infusion rates of less than 100 mL/hr. Microdrop sets are usually termed *pediatric*, although it is used as often or even more often in adults in whom high rates are not necessary. Microdrop sizes are usually 50 to 60 drops/mL.

Internal diameter

Internal lumen sizes of solution administration sets are manufacturer-specific and dictate the required priming volume of the set. Industry standards refer to a range of inner lumen sizes, and each manufacturer is allowed to market products that are compatible but not uniform. Administration sets can be categorized into types based on lumen size, but uniformity among manufacturers cannot be assumed. Usually, miniscule differences are acceptable and do not affect performance in situations not calling for such precision. In other instances, these differences can be critical. If performance problems are suspected, the manufacturer of the products should always be consulted to confirm or rule out administration set conflicts. (An administration set tubing conflict means that one piece of tubing interferes with the performance of another.)

Macrobore administration sets are commonly used on blood administration sets or primary Y sets for use in trauma or operating room situations. Macrobore means that the set's inner lumen is larger than standard to facilitate high flow rates. The degree to which the inner lumen is larger depends on the manufacturer. Anesthesia sets and some specialty sets are designed specifically as macrobore sets.

The large inner lumen makes macrobore sets stiffer, which makes it more difficult to accommodate a controlling mechanism such as a roller clamp. The clamp is less reliable for longterm infusion control. Macrobore sets should never be used in electronic infusion pumps that accommodate generic administration sets.

Microbore sets have a smaller than standard inner lumen. Because small administration sets can be extremely flexible, microbore sets often have a smaller inner lumen but a thicker wall, making them resistant to kinking. Many microbore sets are termed *kink resistant* or *noncompliant* (meaning the administration set does not bend or stretch). Again, because administration sets are manufacturer-specific, the qualities of each microbore set should be investigated, not assumed.

Because microbore sets have a narrowed inner lumen, flow is somewhat restricted. Microbore sets can be used as a safeguard against runaway or bolus infusions and offer a very low priming volume, making them suitable for pediatrics, neonatal units, and volume-restricted adult care areas such as cardiology or renal units. Microbore sets are often the sets of choice for syringe pumps, epidural infusion pumps, or ambulatory infusion devices that are designed to deliver small quantities over a long period, such as low-dose chemotherapy or pain-control medications.

Most sets are standard lumen administration sets, and almost all infusions can be accomplished with standard-bore administration sets. All standard-bore sets have a common inner lumen size with very little variation from manufacturer to manufacturer. Again, the standard-bore sets are within a common range but should never be assumed to be exactly the same.

Injection ports

Most primary administration sets are made with one to three injection ports located in strategic places along the tubing, allowing for multiple infusions simultaneously. To eliminate the use of needles for connection of administration sets, most injection ports use a needleless design. Some needleless systems require the use of a blunt plastic cannula, while others will directly accept the male Luer tip of a syringe or administration set.

Injection ports requiring needles are still available, although their use is prohibited by OSHA's bloodborne pathogen standard. They are made of dense latex or a nonlatex rubber and are secured to a portion of the administration set where a hard, molded Y site exits the main infusion tubing. These rubber caps

are tightly secured with a heat-shrunk band to prevent any movement or break in the sterility of the administration set. The port reseals after the needle has been removed.

All needleless injection ports should be able to accommodate numerous uses, although a definitive number does not exist. The port can usually be safely used through the limited life of the administration set. Caution should be taken if an extraordinary number of entries is required, as failure of the port will increase the risk of air and microorganisms entering the system.

The injection port that is found on the upper third of the administration set nearest the fluid container is used for secondary or piggyback administration. The back-check valve in the primary administration set is located in close proximity to this injection port. The injection port that is found nearest the patient is preferred for IV push medications.

Back-check valves

Back-check valves, or one-way valves, are an integral part of many administration sets. These valves allow the solution to flow in one direction only. Back-check valves work much like a float. When the solution is passing through the disk, a small float device holds the passage open. If the flow is reversed, the float device closes off the passageway. Another one-way valve appears similar to a flap valve in the fluid path. When solution is passing correctly, the flap flows open. When the flow is reversed, the flap is forced shut, stopping the flow. Back-check valves have no other purpose than to direct the flow of solution.

The most common use of back-check valves is to administer secondary medications at the injection port on the upper third of the primary administration set. This configuration prevents the secondary piggyback from flowing into the primary infusion container if there is resistance in the infusion system at the patient end. A small air bubble inside the valve could also prevent correct function and can be removed by turning this tubing segment upside down and tapping while the fluid is flowing from the primary container. As long as the secondary solution hangs higher than the primary container, the primary solution stops to allow the secondary solution to flow. When the secondary solution container is empty, the back-check valve reverses its position, allowing the primary fluid to resume flow.

Back-check valves are also found in patient-controlled analgesia (PCA) pump sets. To ensure that the pain medication is flowing from the pump to the patient, the PCA administration set incorporates a back-check valve where the PCA set attaches to the primary set. The valve is on the leg of the Y that infuses the primary solution. This configuration prevents the pain medication from flowing upstream into the primary infusion should the IV access device become occluded (Figure 20-6).

Connections

Manufacturers of administration set connections strive to make them universal, which means that male and female fittings for standard devices should make a correct fit when connected. This standard exists for reasons of safety and efficiency. Recent reports of tubing misconnections have highlighted the fact that this standardization could be a problem. The same fittings appear on tubing used for automatic blood pressure cuffs, enteral feeding tubes, and respiratory equipment. This has lead

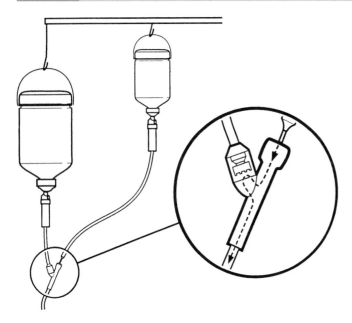

FIGURE 20-6   Back-check valve or one-way valve. (Courtesy MiniMed Technologies.)

to serious error when a variety of tubings are being used, disconnected, and reconnected (ISMP, 2004).

Two basic types of standard connections exist: slip and Luer. Slip connections provide fittings that simply slide into each other and provide a tight connection when twisted. These connections are not absolute in preventing accidental disconnects and should never be used on administration sets connected to central venous catheters. Luer connections screw together two compatible ends. Deliberate twisting motions are required to disconnect a Luer connector, making accidental disconnection almost impossible. Another configuration is a combination of these two types. The male end slips into the female end and a movable locking collar screws around the connection to provide the Luer lock. Most major medical manufacturers offer administration sets and add-on devices with both slip and Luer connections, although slip locking devices are less available.

 NEEDLELESS CONNECTORS

The types of needleless connectors have dramatically increased in recent years, leading to confusion about their use. They have met the original goal of reducing needlestick injuries in health care workers; however, there have been questions about their potential to cause an increased risk of bloodstream infections in patients (Danzig et al, 1995; Kellerman et al, 1996; Do et al, 1999). These connectors can be divided by their design and by how they function.

DESIGN

The original design was a split septum injection cap placed on the catheter hub or built onto the administration set. A blunt plastic cannula is attached to the syringe or IV administration set to pass through the split in the septum. Recent changes to this design include a split septum that will accept the male Luer

end of a syringe tip or administration set directly without using a blunt plastic cannula.

The second device was a mechanical valve. One product is a two-piece system requiring a cap to be replaced after each use. Most others are a one-piece system that is placed on the catheter hub and is accessed directly with a male Luer on a syringe or administration set. There is much variety in size, shape, color, and internal fluid pathways in this group.

Needleless connectors are also available with a pressure-sensitive valve inside the device, and there are two designs available—a split septum accessed with a blunt plastic cannula or a stand-alone valve that can be capped with any needleless connector. Because this device acts by pressure, when the solution flows down the administration set to a certain level, this valve will close. All other devices without this pressure-sensitive valve remain an open conduit until the nurse detaches the IV administration set.

FUNCTION

With early use of these devices, catheter occlusion problems began to increase in frequency. Laboratory demonstration showed the negative fluid displacement that can occur, although these occlusion problems were not published. All split septum devices and some of the mechanical valves fall into the negative displacement category. The withdrawal of the blunt plastic cannula or the movement of the internal valve design encourages blood to move back into the catheter lumen as the syringe or administration set is disconnected.

To address this problem, devices were created that held a small amount of fluid inside an internal reservoir, and became known as positive displacement devices. Upon disconnection of the syringe or IV administration set, this fluid is pushed out to the catheter tip to overcome the blood that has refluxed into the catheter lumen. The quantity of fluid in this reservoir varies among brands of these devices. Based on this quantity, some of these positive displacement devices have instructions allowing for use of 0.9% sodium chloride only as the final flush solution and state that heparin is not required to maintain patency. Another category of these connectors is labeled as neutral displacement devices because they reduce the amount of blood that moves into the catheter upon disconnection. The terms negative, positive, and neutral displacement are used for description purposes but there are no guidelines from the FDA about the amount of fluid displacement required or allowed for a connector to be included in each group.

Additionally, the appropriate flushing technique depends upon the type of device being used. Negative fluid displacement in split septum devices and some mechanical valves is prevented by appropriate flushing techniques. One of two techniques can be chosen. For blunt plastic cannula systems, as the last milliliter of fluid is flushed into the lumen, the plastic cannula is withdrawn. This allows the injected fluid to fill the space left by the large cannula, preventing blood reflux at the catheter tip. The second technique is to flush all fluid in, maintain the pressure on the syringe plunger, close a clamp on the catheter or extension set, and then disconnect the syringe. When using a positive displacement needleless connector, this technique of closing the clamp before disconnection can prohibit the fluid reservoir from pushing fluid out to the catheter tip. These devices must be clamped after disconnection of the syringe. Neutral displacement needleless connectors are not dependent upon flushing technique and can be clamped either before or after syringe disconnection.

There is currently much controversy about these devices and their associated risk of bloodstream infection. The current guidelines from the CDC state, "When the devices are used according to manufacturers' recommendations, they do not substantially affect the incidence of catheter-related bloodstream infection" (O'Grady et al, 2002).

Published studies subsequent to these guidelines have provided more data. Two prospective studies using a sequential group design in a pediatric population have reported that total and partial catheter occlusions were 15.2% and 17.3%, respectively, with the split septum devices using heparin as the final flush. Catheter-associated bloodstream infection rates with the split septum devices were 5.3 and 8.8 infections per 1000 catheter-days. In the cohort with positive displacement Luer-activated connectors using 0.9% sodium chloride only, these same studies reported total and partial catheter occlusions at 11.8% and 8%, respectively, and catheter-associated bloodstream infections at 15.5 and 10.9 infections per 1000 catheter-days (Jacobs et al, 2004; Schilling et al, 2006).

There have been four published reports of serious increases in catheter-associated bloodstream infection rates after hospitals changed from one needleless connector to another type of connector. These studies have involved changing from a negative displacement device to a positive displacement device (Maragakis et al, 2006); from a split septum device to a negative displacement mechanical valve (Salgado et al, 2007); from a split septum to both positive and negative displacement mechanical valves (Field et al, 2007); and from a split septum to a positive displacement mechanical valve (Rupp et al, 2007).

These studies have garnered much attention from ECRI and leading infection prevention professional organizations. An evaluation by ECRI examined the mechanical properties of all connectors including flow rates and human factors such as the ease of connection. This ECRI report assessed the publications about bloodstream infection rates and stated that they did not believe the evidence supported an association between infection rates and a particular design, model, or manufacturer of needleless connectors (ECRI, 2008).

A recent set of recommendations was issued collaboratively from the Society for Healthcare Epidemiology of America (SHEA) and the Infectious Diseases Society of America (IDSA). These guidelines stated that positive-pressure needleless connectors should not be routinely used without a thorough assessment of risks, benefits, and education about their correct use (Marschall et al, 2008). Factors that must be included in this assessment should include both product design and nursing practice. Box 20-1 provides a list of these factors.

The recommendations from these organizations appear to state opposing views. It is imperative that each organization looks carefully at the product design, the current risk factors in its patient population, the presence of adequate policies and procedures to reduce extraluminal and intraluminal sources of catheter contamination, and the adherence of nursing staff to these policies and procedures.

Two approaches are evolving to reduce the infection risk with these devices. Several devices are coated with silver. The device may be coated on internal and external parts or the swabbing surface and fluid pathway. This technology is relatively new and no clinical studies are available to identify the outcomes associated with its use. Another idea is to place a cap

Box 20-1	FACTORS INVOLVED IN THE CHOICE OF NEEDLELESS CONNECTORS
Patient factors	Clinical need to eliminate the use of heparin for catheter locking
	Previous history of catheter-associated bloodstream infection
	Number of catheter lumens required to deliver the prescribed therapy
Facility factors	Policies and procedures about disinfection of all needleless connectors
	Policies and procedures about management of both continuous and intermittent administration sets
	Policies and procedures about the change interval for needleless connectors
	Adequate supply of disinfectants at the patient's bedside and convenience of use
	Adequate supply of blunt plastic cannulae or sterile end caps to protect the male Luer end of intermittent administration sets at the patient's bedside and convenience of use
Nursing practice factors	Compliance with all policies and procedures listed above, especially with disinfection of all needleless connectors before each use
	Ensuring that continuous infusions are not interrupted and disconnected for patient activity
Device factors	Connection surface and the ability to disinfect it
	Gaps between moving parts of the connection surface that may prohibit adequate cleaning
	Tortuous fluid pathways that create more surfaces for growth of biofilm
	Relationship between the device surface and the fluid pathway

loaded with an antiseptic sponge over the needleless connector between uses. Theories supporting this concept include: (1) the prolonged contact between the antiseptic sponge and the connection surface of the needleless connector is much longer than a simple wipe by the nurse, and (2) this process protects the connection surface from contact with microorganisms from many environmental surfaces such as skin, clothing, or linens.

The change interval for needleless connectors should follow the same interval for changing primary continuous administration sets. This may be at 72- or 96-hour intervals. Infusions of fat emulsion or blood transfusions or obtaining blood samples through the needleless connector raises questions about the frequency of change. No studies have specifically addressed these issues; however, the factors that influence these policies should include the design of the fluid pathway of the connector being used, the ability to adequately flush all fat emulsion or blood products from the connector, and the adherence to proper disinfection when using the connector.

 ## OTHER ADD-ON DEVICES

The health care market offers an unlimited number of devices that can be attached to any catheter or administration set. The routine use of add-on devices is discouraged because they add points of connection that could loosen or separate totally. However, there are times when their use is clinically necessary to accomplish a specific purpose. They are used to add length, filtering capabilities, or increased overall function to the infusion system. Limiting their use reduces the incidence of contamination and accidental disconnection, minimizes the manipulation of the sterile fluid pathway, maintains a closed system, and reduces the costs associated with their use. Health care workers should constantly justify the use of add-on devices to ensure they are not used habitually or routinely.

STOPCOCKS

A stopcock is a manually manipulated device used to direct the flow of solution. The stopcock is generally a three-way or four-way device. For example, the stopcock has an inlet from the main administration set and a second portal to direct the solution to the patient. Turning the stopcock to the third portal allows solution to flow from a second container and from the primary container. The fourth portal is an off port, so the first three can be used in any combination of two or three.

Because of its versatility, this device is very useful in critical care, anesthesia, and trauma settings. As useful as it is in these settings, however, the general use of stopcocks is strongly discouraged. Misuse of stopcocks has become a major factor contributing to their unavailability in many health care settings.

The issue of contamination of stopcocks has been addressed in multiple arenas. When the stopcock portals are uncapped, they are vulnerable to touch contamination. The stopcock itself is small and must be handled in such a way that sterility is not compromised. Often, syringes are attached for IV push administration, and the portal is poorly protected after use. Only stopcocks made with Luer-locking connections should be used, reducing the risk of accidental disconnection. If the stopcock is accidentally turned, the infusion may be interrupted or administered incorrectly. The potential for error with stopcocks makes their use worthy of caution.

EXTENSION SETS

Extension sets are used to add length, to provide clamping capability, or to restrict flow. To add length, extension sets can be 20, 30, or 60 inches long. Many specialty sets may be just about any length imaginable. Sets that are made to add clamping capability are usually much shorter, even as short as 2 to 3 inches. Restriction of fluid flow with a microbore extension set is possible but not advisable for a volume-restricted patient.

Extension sets should not be added routinely or for convenience; there must be a clearly defined purpose. The potential for contamination exists with any add-on device, especially if excessive length allows the administration set to lie on the floor or become entangled. To ensure patient safety, only extension sets with Luer-locking connectors should be used. However,

the use of a short extension set on a peripheral catheter will separate the health care workers' hands from the catheter hub and reduce blood contact, and decrease catheter manipulation when converting from a continuous infusion to an intermittent infusion and when giving all intermittent medications.

CATHETER CONNECTION DEVICES

T ports have become common add-on devices. The T port is usually 4 to 6 inches long and is made of standard or microbore tubing with a hard, plastic, T-shaped connector on one end. One side of the T attaches to the catheter hub and the other is an injection port or needleless connector. The long leg of the T attaches to a standard administration set and often has a simple slide or pinch clamp attached.

The T connector has a clamp that allows safe disconnection of the administration set without fear of backflow of blood or air emboli. If the catheter is locked for intermittent use, many patients and practitioners feel more comfortable with the T connector clamped.

Some manufacturers make the slide clamp optional and easy to remove. This feature poses a risk to small children, who find the clamps an irresistible item for small fingers and mouths.

J loops and U connectors have the same intended use as T connectors. Both are rigid and hold their shape when attached to the IV catheter. Their predetermined shape creates a disadvantage if the insertion site is in an awkward location. Their rigid shape does not help prevent catheter movement when the connection is manipulated. Figure 20-7 depicts several types of add-on devices.

MULTIFLOW ADAPTERS AND Y CONNECTORS

Multiflow adapters and Y connectors allow two or three infusions to flow into one catheter lumen. Multiflow adapters and Y connectors require Luer-locking connections. Some have color-coded hubs or clamps attached. The versatility of these devices is enhanced by adding pinch or slide clamps on each leg of the device. It is important to remember, however, that all solutions and medications given through these adapters must be compatible as contact inside the lumen could lead to drug precipitate formation.

Priming each infusion leg of the device before their use is required to prevent small air emboli. The end caps may be air vented for easy priming; however, they cannot be left in place after the system is primed. To adequately close each leg of these adapters, a needleless connector must be attached. If the end cap is not vented, it will need to be removed to accommodate priming and each end should then be attached to an administration set or needleless connector.

BLOOD SAMPLING SYSTEMS

The typical process for obtaining a blood sample from a central venous catheter requires wasting a portion of blood to remove the solution used to lock the catheter or any fluid that has been infused through the catheter. This process can lead to nosocomial blood loss and iatrogenic anemia when frequent blood samples are required. Additionally, collecting blood samples from catheters requires excessive manipulation of the catheter hub, increasing the risk of contamination. Lastly, these procedures require needleless systems designed to collect blood so that all needles and blood exposure are eliminated. To meet

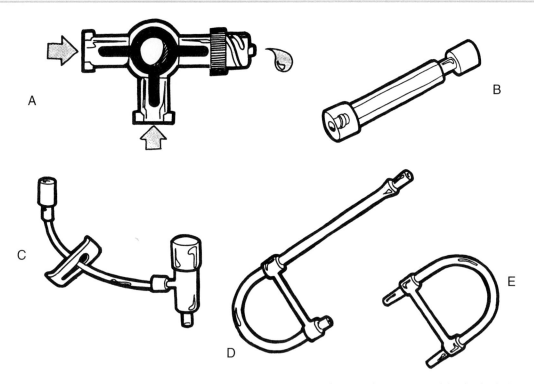

FIGURE 20-7   Add-on devices. **A,** Stopcock. **B,** Injection cap. **C,** T port. **D,** J loop. **E,** U loop. (Courtesy MiniMed Technologies.)

these goals, there are in-line blood sampling systems for both venous and arterial blood samples.

These systems are similar to the system used for measuring arterial pressures and some are designed to be used in conjunction with those monitoring systems. The sampling system consists of a volume-restricted syringe or other form of fluid reservoir mounted near a stopcock, a dense silicone septum built into the tubing, and a Luer-locking connection at the end of the administration set. Fluid and blood are aspirated into the set past the location of the septum and into the reservoir or syringe, and the stopcock is closed to the administration set. A needleless device is inserted into the septum to withdraw the blood sample directly into a vacuum tube or syringe. After collecting the sample, the needleless device is removed, the stopcock is opened, and the line is flushed to reinfuse the solution and blood into the catheter. These systems are available with reservoir volumes suitable for adult, pediatric, and neonatal patients.

CLOSED SYSTEM DRUG TRANSFER DEVICES

Compounding and administration and disposal of hazardous drugs creates substantial risk to all health care workers involved in the process. Hazardous drugs are those chemicals with statistically significant evidence from at least one study that acute or chronic health effects may occur in exposed individuals. This includes carcinogenicity, reproductive toxicity, fetal development toxicity, and other organ or structural toxicity (ASHP, 2006).

Closed system drug transfer devices have been shown to reduce exposure to hazardous drugs. The National Institute for Occupational Safety and Health (NIOSH) defines these as a "drug transfer device that mechanically prohibits the transfer of environmental contaminants into the system and the escape of hazardous drugs or vapor concentrations outside the system"

(NIOSH, 2004). Many available devices are labeled as "chemo adjuncts" but do not meet this definition of a closed system. These usually have a vented spike with a filter to aid in drug reconstitution.

Closed system devices have a needleless injection cannula that is designed to enter the drug vial, a Luer-lock connection, or any connector on an administration set, to lock onto it. There is a membrane system designed to equalize the pressure within the vial, syringe, or administration set. No medication leaks or comes into contact with these connections, eliminating the risk of exposure. While not a substitute for the proper environment of a biological safety cabinet or the use of personnel protective equipment, these devices are included in the guidelines for handling hazardous drugs from the American Society of Health-System Pharmacists (ASHP, 2006).

FLOW CONTROL DEVICES

Controlling the rate of fluid flow is an essential component of all types of infusion therapy. Flow control can be accomplished by a wide spectrum of devices from simple mechanical devices for gravity flow to the most complex electronic volumetric infusion pump. The choice for the most appropriate mechanism depends upon the age and acuity of the patient, the type of therapy being infused, and the health care setting for the infusion therapy. Regardless of the sophistication of the device, flow control devices should be considered an enhancement to patient care and not a replacement for the nurse's responsibility to monitor the infusion of the prescribed therapy (INS, 2006).

Fluid flows by a pressure gradient. The pressure at one end of the system is greater than the pressure at the other end. With the exception of syringe pumps, gravity is used in all types of flow control devices. The gravity could be from the solution container to the catheter or from the solution container to the infusion pump, requiring that the solution container be above the patient or pump. Syringes and the syringe pump can be at the patient's level.

GRAVITY-DEPENDENT FLOW CONTROL

All gravity-dependent systems rely upon pressure generated from the height of the fluid container. A container placed between 3 and 4 feet above the patient will usually produce about 2 pounds per square inch (psi) of pressure. The nurse controls the flow by counting drops passing through the drip chamber on the administration set. Resistance to fluid flow comes from several mechanisms on the IV administration set.

Roller clamps

Roller clamps are found on all standard administration sets and are attached during the manufacturing process. The roller clamp allows the tubing to be incrementally occluded by pinching the tubing as the roller clamp is tightened. Most roller clamps are easily regulated with one hand. The preferred process is to completely close the roller clamp and regulate the rate as you roll the clamp upward to open it. The clamp is designed to hold its place on the tubing, keeping the infusion rate constant between adjustments.

Standard roller clamps on standard-bore administration sets can be as accurate as ±10%. The accuracy of standard roller clamps is directly dependent on the number of variables involved in each administration. Patient movement, patient ambulation, patient transfer, and the height and volume of the solution container are just a few of the things that can affect the accuracy of an adjusted roller clamp. These factors could bring the accuracy rating to ±25%. Safe rate control with roller clamps requires vigilant observation at frequent intervals by the caregiver to confirm the infusion rates.

Roller clamps should be positioned on the upper third of the administration set near the solution container. This placement is convenient for the nurse and, more importantly, is out of the way of the patient, thus preventing accidental manipulation. The clamp should be repositioned along the set at periodic intervals because the tubing develops "memory," making it difficult to regulate. This memory can work in two ways. In the event of "cold creep," the tubing tries to retain its round shape, pushing the clamp open. The other form of memory creates a pinched section of tubing that does not reopen when the clamp is removed. Both of these problems can be avoided by moving the clamp to an unused portion of the administration set when the rate is readjusted.

Slide and pinch clamps are provided on some sets but are not regulating clamps. Both are simple, one-handed clamps whose sole purpose is to provide on-off control; they cannot regulate the flow rate. Both of these clamps are capable of creating a serious crimp or crease in the tubing that can be hazardous.

Manual flow regulators

Manual flow regulators are available as built-on devices or as separate devices to be added onto the administration set. They are used to regulate the flow of fluid instead of using the roller clamp on the administration set. These devices have also been considered to be a modified roller clamp.

These flow regulators may provide a more consistent flow rate than that obtained by preattached roller clamps. They are

accurate within ±10%, which is the same for the roller clamp on standard administration sets. In actual practice, however, some of these clamps have been shown to provide added safety, a benefit that is not easily quantified. With these devices, added protection exists against crimped tubing, cold creep, and drifting of the roller clamp. The add-on controlling devices are not likely to be accidentally reset when bumped or jostled because of patient activity. In addition, they provide added protection from accidental free flow of solutions.

An issue with flow regulators is the accuracy of predetermined settings. On these devices, the nurse sets the dial or indicator to a given number, and the set supposedly delivers at that rate. In actuality, many variables in the patient care setting can alter that rate, such as change in patient position, sharp changes in room temperature, or even decreased volume in the fluid container. The nurse cannot rely on the numbered setting to indicate the actual flow being delivered. Although the numbered dial may have some advantages, the numbers may not be the rate of flow actually being delivered, requiring a count of drops for confirmation.

Careful assessment of the real versus perceived need is required when making a decision about the use of these devices. The proficiency of the nursing staff, the level of illness being treated, the type of patient population, and the care environment need to be considered. For instance, one use could be for patients having a magnetic resonance imaging (MRI) study where an infusion pump made of metal may be prohibited. These devices cannot be considered as a replacement for an electronic infusion pump on a regular basis. Flow regulators add to the cost per administration set in any setting, and they must be changed with the routine administration set changes.

Pressure bags or cuffs

A pressure bag or cuff for the rapid infusion of gravity-drip solutions should be reserved for trauma, anesthesiology, surgery, and critical care needs. The device is placed around the plastic solution container and inflated to maintain consistent pressure on the bag. Most have a warning not to exceed 300 mm Hg or 6 psi.

Pressure bags are frequently used for the maintenance of pressurized arterial lines. The pressure bag maintains consistent pressure on the infusing heparin infusate or 0.9% sodium chloride, which infuses through a restricted access that maintains flow at a very minimal amount (usually 3 mL/hr). The pressure does not allow any backflow of blood, maintaining patency of the arterial catheter.

Mechanical pumps

Mechanical devices have no outside power source; they operate on the physical principle of matter retaining its own shape, such as a balloon or spring or other mechanical restriction on the fluid pathway. These devices are also classified as disposable pumps because all or parts of the device are discarded after a single use.

Flow accuracy in this group is generally ±15% with some being as low as ±20%. Factors that affect flow rates include drug viscosity, temperature, atmospheric pressure, backpressure, partial filling, and the manner in which the devices are stored. Most devices are calibrated to skin temperature although some with higher flow rates are calibrated for room temperature. Changes of 2% to 3% can be expected when the temperature changes by 1° C. Greater fluid viscosity causes slower flow rates. Changes in atmospheric pressure have the greatest impact on negative-pressure devices. The pump's position in relationship to the patient can increase the backpressure. The internal pressure generated by the collapsing balloon or spring pumps is greater when the device is only partially filled. Cold storage can slow the rate of infusion. Devices that have been frozen are stiffer and thus will produce slower flow rates. Cold temperatures also increase the viscosity of fluids, also slowing the flow rate. There are differences with each type and brand of these pumps; therefore careful attention to manufacturers' instructions for use is required (Skryabina and Dunn, 2006).

Elastomeric balloon pumps

Elastomeric balloon pumps are made of a soft rubberized material inside a rigid, transparent housing. The container shape varies by manufacturer. The balloon can be made of rubber, latex, or silicone material. It may also have a single or multiple layers. There is a tamper-proof port for injecting the medication into the balloon.

When filled with fluid, the balloon inflates. There is an outlet port with either a preattached set or an attachable set. The administration set has a low priming volume, an air-eliminating filter, and Luer connections. Resistance to control the rate of fluid delivery is determined by the size of the opening where the tubing joins the balloon. Pressure to cause the delivery of the infusion comes from the collapsing balloon. Multiple-layer balloons exert higher amounts of pressure to overcome the added resistance from large and/or small lumen catheters. There is no additional rate control possible with these devices, but this means there are no additional parts to malfunction or settings to ensure proper infusion. Predetermined rates last from 30 minutes to several days. Infusion pressure ranges from 260 to 520 mm Hg (5.2 to 10.4 psi), and rates of infusion range from 0.5 to 500 mL per hour (Skryabina

and Dunn, 2006). Examples of elastomeric balloons are shown in Figure 20-8.

The elastomeric balloons have been tested extensively for drug compatibility and stability. Types of therapies given with this device include antibiotics, antivirals, chemotherapy, and analgesics.

The PCA elastomeric balloon functions in the same manner, but the controlling mechanism is unique. A restricting orifice exists in the neck of the rigid container. The patient-control option is a push-button regulator on the administration set leading to the patient. The push-button holds a dose of prescribed analgesia in a bolus-dose reservoir, which the patient administers to himself or herself when the need arises. The restricting orifice refills the tiny reservoir slowly over the "lockout period." A patient could push the button more frequently and receive smaller doses of the medication; however, the maximum hourly dose is not exceeded.

Elastomeric balloon pumps can also be attached to catheters that have been placed within the area of a surgical site. These catheters may be open-ended or have a "soaker hose" design at the internal tip. The catheters are usually a 19 gauge in various lengths. The segment designed to allow the medication to infuse or soak the surgical site can be 1, 2.5, 5, 7.5, or 10 inches long. These catheters are also available with a silver coating to provide antimicrobial benefits.

Spring-based pumps

The spring-coil container is a combination of the spring coil and a collapsible, flattened disk. The overextended spring is in an enclosed space between two disks and seeks to collapse, pulling the top and bottom together and forcing the contents out of the restricting orifice. The round, flat shape can accommodate many infusions and volumes and can be carried in a pocket. The external housing is two parts that are screwed together and are reusable. The disposable fluid container is placed

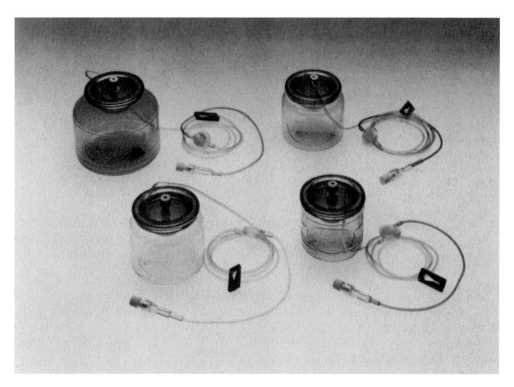

FIGURE 20-8   Elastomeric balloon construction. (Courtesy McGraw, Inc.)

inside this mechanism where the spring produces the pressure to force fluid from the container. Accuracy rating for these devices is usually ±10% (Skryabina and Dunn, 2006).

A spring-coil piston syringe device is equipped with a spring, which powers the syringe plunger in the absence of manual pressure. The syringe piston is withdrawn to overextend the spring. The filled syringe is placed inside the housing that has the rate-controlling administration set attached. As the spring attempts to regain its shape, it forces the piston back down, expelling the contents.

The syringe has no incompatibilities associated with its use, which makes it ideal for the infusion of problematic drugs. Its volumes are easy to read. Syringes can be prefilled and frozen.

Negative pressure pumps

A negative pressure pump has a double-sided chamber with one side being a vacuum or negative pressure and the other being at atmospheric pressure. Filling the drug reservoir causes the creation of a vacuum. Pressure from a moveable wall is exerted against the drug reservoir as a result of the pressure difference between the two chambers. These devices are used to deliver pain medication when connected to a catheter immediately following surgery. The medication is delivered to the surgical site as it flows from the multiple side holes in the catheter.

Electronic infusion pumps

By its name, a pump indicates that pressure is used. The pressure exerted must be sufficient to overcome resistance from many causes along the fluid pathway, including length of the administration set, kinked tubing, and accumulation of particulate matter in the tubing; biofilm, fibrin, thrombus, and/or drug, mineral, or lipid precipitate inside the catheter lumen; and the resistance caused from vascular pressure, the presence of venous valves or fibrin/thrombus near the catheter tip, or the catheter's position against the vein wall. Electronic infusion pumps deliver fluids under positive pressure and fall into two categories—volumetric pumps and syringe pumps. Volumetric pumps can be further divided into pole-mounted and ambulatory varieties. Internal batteries or alternating current, or a combination of both, powers all electronic devices.

Over the past few years, infusion pumps have greatly increased in complexity. Examples of enhanced patient safety range from protection from freely flowing fluid when the administration set is removed to the use of complicated drug libraries. The integration of health information technology and networking capabilities with infusion pumps is in its infancy but is expected to rapidly expand.

The industry standard for accuracy of an electronic IV infusion pump is ±5%, although some may be as accurate as ±2%. Accuracy of pumps with rates of 1 mL/hr or less ranges from ±5.5% to 10%.

Pressure capabilities with pumps can be a confusing issue. The normal pumping pressure is slightly lower than the occlusion pressure. When the pump identifies increasing resistance, it responds by increasing the pumping pressure. This continues until it reaches the preset limit, usually referred to as the occlusion pressure. Some pumps have a fixed occlusion pressure, while others allow the nurse to change the occlusion pressure. Once the pump reaches the set limit, the occlusion alarms sound. Some fixed-pressure pumps can be internally altered by the manufacturer or by biomedical engineering departments. Any fixed-pressure pump that has been altered by increasing

the psi should be clearly marked on the outside to inform all users and should be restricted to certain applications, such as hyperbaric units or dialysis. Variable-pressure pumps allow the user to determine the psi needed to safely deliver therapy and adjust it with a simple programming designation.

Downstream occlusion pressures range from 1.5 to 15 psi. However, in some instances, pressures up to 22 psi are appropriate. Greater-than-normal pressures are needed when infusion pumps are used in conjunction with specialized high-volume, high-pressure treatments, such as hemodialysis, plasmapheresis, cardiothoracic surgeries, and arterial infusion procedures. In each of these cases, which require close medical supervision and specialized nursing personnel, high pressures are used for purposes other than simple fluid infusion.

Another arena for very high pressure is the hyperbaric chamber. Pressures required for the chamber must exceed the greatly exaggerated atmospheric pressure of the therapy. The infusion pump is ideally outside the chamber or room because its pumping function cannot be guaranteed under high pressure. An extension piece allows the pump to reach the patient through a sealed portal. A psi greater than 16 and up to 22 is necessary.

The psi rating for occlusion is a safety factor for the patient. On pumps with variable occlusion pressure, the nurse may increase the psi limit to decrease alarms. This should be done with extreme caution because eliminating a nuisance alarm may actually disable a safety feature.

Electronic infusion pumps do not have any mechanism to detect or prevent escape of the infusion solution from the vein into the surrounding tissue, known as infiltration or extravasation. Many alarms are built into the system to indicate that solution has stopped flowing for some reason. It is the nurse's responsibility to observe the pump, catheter and insertion site, and the patient to identify when solutions are no longer flowing into the vein, artery, or other intended body cavity.

The most important feature of electronic infusion pumps is the internal drug library or the "smart pumps." The computers in these pumps are programmed to contain information on many drugs with upper and lower dosing limits, clinical advisories, drug incompatibilities, and other facility-specific dosing limitations. These libraries have been shown to reduce IV medication errors; however, there are many things that must be considered. Making the technology available will not be sufficient to ensure its successful use.

A culture of safety is necessary to prevent nurses from using techniques to bypass the limits within these drug libraries. Each facility must decide on standardized concentrations of all medications, agree on dosing calculations for milligrams per minute or milligrams per kilogram per minute, consistently use the same name for each medication, and ensure that this information is in agreement with the printed medication administration record.

Types of infusion pumps

Pole-mounted, ambulatory, syringe, and patient-controlled analgesia pumps are the types of electronic flow control devices. All types can be considered volumetric because the pump uses some mechanical method to calibrate the exact volume of fluid being delivered. This could be a peristaltic, piston, or syringe-driven mechanism, which dictates the type of administration sets that can be used with the pump. The administration set or fluid reservoir is manipulated internally by a specific action of the pump. This may require a special set that is dedicated to a specific brand of pump or the pump may be capable of accepting a wide range of administration sets.

Pole-mounted volumetric pumps

These pumps lock onto a stationary or ambulatory IV pole and are used in all practice settings. Configurations of the available pumps appear to be endless with single, dual, and multiple channels, along with modules that deliver patient-controlled analgesia and monitor oxygen and carbon dioxide levels.

Before use, the nurse must ensure his or her knowledge of the chosen pump and its operation. The data entered into each pump may be similar, but the mechanisms for entering those data may be very different. Also ensure that the administration set appropriate for the pump is available. These may be manually primed or placed on the pump for priming and purging all air. There will be a mechanism for preventing free flow of the solution when the set is not on the pump. There could also be a means for allowing gravity infusion by a manual regulator when the pump cannot be used. This may be helpful when transporting the patient from one unit to another or when administering a vesicant medication where the quality of the gravity infusion is needed to assess patency of the vein or catheter.

Interference from other equipment may be possible. Cellular telephones, portable radios, and electrosurgical equipment operate with high-frequency radiowaves that could produce false alarms. When infusing electrolytes on a pump, nonhazardous currents may be created that produce artifacts on electrocardiogram (ECG) tracings. If this is suspected, stopping the pump will cause the artifacts to disappear, indicating that the ECG equipment may not be properly set up.

Multichannel pumps have different configurations. Some are two single-channel devices in one housing. Others have two pump mechanisms with common control and programming panels. Others may be modules attached to the side of the central controlling unit or units stacked laterally up the pole. Programming a multichannel pump can be complex, but offers the benefits of being compact, requiring less space at the patient's bedside.

Intermittent IV piggyback capability may be possible with a single-channel pump by simply programming a secondary infusion rate and volume and placing the secondary solution container higher than the primary container. Medication may also be infused intermittently through a separate channel or module requiring it own administration set and programming.

Ambulatory infusion pumps

Ambulatory infusion pumps are small enough to be easily carried, allowing the patient the freedom to return to work, to school, or to a more normal life pattern. They were developed with the patient's home in mind. Ambulatory devices are capable of delivering most infusion therapies delivered by pole-mounted pumps, including critical care drugs and blood products.

Ambulatory devices range in size and weight; some are small enough to fit into the palm of the hand, whereas others are large enough to necessitate a backpack. Most of these pumps weigh less than 6 pounds. The solution container is often more cumbersome than the actual pump. Ambulatory pumps have pump-specific administration sets made to accommodate only the therapies for which each device is designed.

Ambulatory pumps have the advantage of being small, but they have limitations that prevent the small size from being incorporated into the hospital setting. Reducing the number of programming options is one factor that enables the manufacturer to miniaturize the pump.

Ambulatory pumps use a battery system that necessitates frequent recharging and battery replacement. Most hospital uses are so rigorous that the ambulatory pump's battery is quickly depleted. Ambulatory devices usually infuse at lower rates or intermittently, requiring significantly less power. Hospitals using battery-powered infusion pumps report significant battery replacement costs.

Ambulatory pumps have many features that have improved the quality of life for persons who require infusions outside the hospital. Because one pump cannot perform all of the infusion therapies, pumps have been designed to address a wide range of therapies. Currently, a pump exists that can be synchronized with the patient's biorhythms, giving medications when needed instead of on a schedule. Another pump is able to deliver several different dose ranges at several different intervals to replicate the secretion of hormones. Several medications may be given sequentially by an internal clock, freeing the patient or caregiver from all interventions except reloading of the device. These pumps retain memory of programs, use informational display screens, and have safety alarms that alert the user of potential problems.

Syringe pumps

A traditional syringe is filled with the prescribed solution or medication and then positioned inside a special pump designed to hold it. The withdrawn plunger fits into a housing that controls the rate of force applied and thus the rate of infusion flowing from the syringe tip. Syringe pumps are used to administer a variety of medications and small-volume parenteral infusions. Numerous syringe pumps are specific to anesthesia, oncology, and obstetric applications.

Syringe pump volume is limited to the size and recommended brands of the syringe used in the device. The rate is controlled by the drive speed of the piston attached to the syringe plunger. Syringe pumps are capable of delivering flow rates ranging from 0.01 to 1130 mL per hour. Many are available with complex drug libraries for titration of critical drugs such as vasopressors.

Syringe pumps eliminate the concern for drop size or fluid viscosity, but their alarms and detection of no-flow situations differ from those of other volumetric pumps. They may not be equipped with air sensors or various other safety and convenience alarms. The administration set usually consists of a single, uninterrupted length of kink-resistant tubing without Y injection ports. Syringe pump administration sets can be the primary set or the secondary set, depending on the intended use.

Patient-controlled analgesia pumps

The concept of PCA is not new, but the technology to provide this type of pain control has seen many advances. PCA pumps are available as pole-mounted, ambulatory, and syringe pumps. The programming options are somewhat standardized, although accessory features vary with each pump.

The distinguishing feature of a PCA device is the ability of the pump to deliver doses on demand, which occurs when the patient pushes a button, similar to a nurse call light, on a cord. The pump responds by delivering or denying the dose, recording the request, and perhaps making a small sound to assure the patient that the request was received. Whether the dose is delivered is determined by preset limits set on the pump.

Infusion options of a PCA pump can be categorized into three types: basal, continuous, and demand. All three afford some type of pain control with varying degrees of patient interaction. The nurse and physician must understand the terminology of the therapy offered so that PCA pumps can be used to the maximum potential.

The continuous mode of therapy is designed for the patient who needs maximum pain relief without the option of demand dosing. Continuous infusions of analgesics usually do not fluctuate from hour to hour and should completely relieve pain or achieve a constant affect. This mode is used for epidural narcotic infusions, neonatal infusions, pain-control administration to persons unable to use the demand feature, or any application requiring a constant rate.

The basal mode differs from the continuous mode in that a basal rate can be accompanied by intermittent doses requested by the patient. The basal dose is designed to achieve pain relief with minimal medication, but not necessarily to achieve a pain-free state, allowing the patient to be alert and active without sedation. The demand dose is delivered by intermittent infusion when a button attached to the pump is pushed. The demand dose can be used alone or supplemented by the basal rate.

The PCA pump must be programmed with a lock-out interval to prevent overmedication. A lock-out interval on a PCA device ensures that over a set period the patient can receive only a prescribed dose of medication.

PCA pumps are also capable of dispensing a bolus dose. Practitioners sometimes call the initial bolus dose a *loading dose*. After an initial bolus dose or after a short lapse in medication, the patient may benefit from a one-time dose of medication that is significantly higher than a demand dose to achieve immediate pain relief. After the bolus dose is delivered, the basal or demand doses provide the sustained effect of pain control. The bolus dose is not calculated into the hourly limit of medication and cannot be accidentally delivered.

These features allow for great flexibility with a PCA pump but also require attention to all these details by the prescriber. In addition to the medication, the order must include the continuous or basal rate if needed, the demand dose, the lock-out period between doses, and the maximum hourly dose.

PCA devices frequently contain narcotics so security is required. The solution container and pump controls may be placed inside a locked area requiring a special key for access. Tamper-resistant features require the nurse to repeat a series of simple steps known to any user to change pump settings. In the hospital setting, the PCA device is commonly locked to the IV pole for added security. Narcotic accountability is more defined with the PCA device because the drug is in one reservoir, and all deliveries are automated and recorded on the pump memory.

PCA pumps are built with extensive memory capability, which includes the pump programming, any interventions by the patient or the nurse, and the times of the interventions. The memory is critical for the pump's effective use in pain management. The frequency of patient requests, the tolerated time intervals, and the numbers of bolus injections are a few of the assessments needed to monitor pain tolerance or change in pain intensity. The programming and memory can be viewed on a display screen.

Programming characteristics

Programming the pump to deliver the required infusion, the information displayed on the screens, the alarms, and other safety mechanisms varies with each type and brand of pump.

There are many general aspects that apply to all devices. It is critical that each user have a command of each device being used to ensure patient safety and avoid use of short-cuts or steps to work around the pump's settings. When used properly infusion pumps can enhance safety; however, misuse or wrongful use can result in harmful medication errors.

Standard information programmed into the pump includes rate and volume to be infused, and the pump records volume infused. Other optional programming capabilities are possible.

Rate

Rate is expressed as the volume of fluid that infuses over a unit of time. For example, a 1000-mL volume infusing over 6 hours will be infused at a rate of 2.7 mL/min or 166 mL/hr. Most infusion pumps deliver in increments of milliliters per hour; however, some pumps can be programmed in milligrams per hour. The lowest infusion rate is either 0.1 or 0.5 mL per hour, depending on the brand of device, eliminating the need for different pumps for adults and infants. The highest rate is 999 mL per hour. Some nurses may be uncomfortable using a pump with such a wide range of infusion rates in a neonatal or pediatric population. For example, a nurse may not notice that the decimal is in the wrong place, thereby setting a rate of 440 mL/hr instead of 44.0 mL/hr. Some pumps have a microinfusion capability with limitations on the rate from 0.1 to 99 mL.

Volume to be infused

The volume to be infused is usually the amount of infusate hanging in the fluid container (e.g., 1000 mL). It could be a lesser amount if only part of the fluid is to be administered or some adjustments must be made after a specific volume has infused. When the pump has infused this volume, an alarm will sound. Like the rate, the volume to be infused ranges from 0.1 to 9999.0 mL, measured in 0.1-mL increments.

Volume infused

The volume infused is a common measurement provided by the infusion pump, not a programmable capability. This measurement is the amount the pump has supposedly delivered since it was last set to zero. This could be reset to zero at the end of each solution container, at the end of each shift, or at some other interval required by the patient's situation.

Tapering and ramping

Tapering and *ramping* are terms used to describe the progressive decrease and increase, respectively, of the infusion rate. Some infusates, specifically those with high dextrose concentrations, such as parenteral nutrition, are tapered when they are cycled, discontinued, or initiated. Once the pump is programmed to the patient's needs, it begins infusing at a low rate, usually one quarter to one third of the final rate. Then, at 1- or 2-hour intervals, the rate increases to half and then to three quarters of the final rate, until the full rate is achieved. The hourly increment is individualized, as is the rate increase. Many patients accustomed to the cycle of parenteral nutrition may taper or ramp in a one- or two-step process over 1 to 2 hours. Tapering is also used in reverse for a patient discontinuing parenteral nutrition. The pump may be able to use its internal computer to mathematically calculate the ramping rate once the duration of the infusion and the total volume to be infused are given.

Timed infusion

Timed infusion refers to an infusion governed by a 24-hour clock within the device. With timed infusion, the device must have a sufficient internal back-up battery to maintain the clock accurately at all times. Timed infusions are used for ramping and tapering, automatic piggybacking, and intermittent dosing. Timed-infusion features can greatly simplify many infusion regimens both inside and outside the hospital. A smaller ambulatory pump with this feature must be checked frequently to ensure that the internal power source is sufficient to maintain the accuracy of the internal clock.

Retrievable historical data

Upon request, the device displays how much fluid has infused in a given period (even over days), gives a record of rate changes and alarm situations sensed by the pump, and, for PCA devices, tallies patient requests for pain medications, intermittent doses delivered, and the total amount of medication delivered.

Positive-pressure fill stroke

The positive-pressure fill stroke feature is important in applications in which no tolerance exists for the intermittent loss of positive pressure or for intermittent negative pressure. This feature is very important in arterial pumping, neonatal infusion, or infusion of sensitively maintained, titrated medications. The fill stroke occurs when the pump momentum is temporarily interrupted while the pump reservoir refills. If, during the refill phase, the pressure in the infusion line is reduced or allowed to "backstroke" even a fraction of a milliliter, blood is drawn into the catheter. If the line is a tiny catheter threaded into an umbilical vessel, the catheter and the infusion are compromised. If the fill stroke stops the consistent forward pressure of medication, blood pressure may fluctuate, cardiac indicators may vary, and hemodynamic status may be compromised.

Modular self-diagnosing capabilities

The self-diagnosing feature has made infusion pumps much easier to maintain and repair. It allows the clinical engineering department to perform certain tests on the infusion device to isolate and communicate mechanical or potential infusion problems. The mechanisms within the device are modular, allowing repairs to a specific compartment without affecting the remaining parts. Personnel from bioengineering departments perform repairs quickly and return devices to service readily. In addition, pumps can be upgraded or enhanced by replacing a specific part. With technology changing so rapidly, infusion pumps are able to keep pace with changing needs.

Printer read-out

The ability to obtain a printer read-out of pump activity is available from several manufacturers. The printer may be centrally located and electrically connected to the infusion device, or the printer can be moved from pump to pump with information being passed to the printer wirelessly, much like information is downloaded into a computer. Some pumps have their own printers, which print on self-contained paper much like the narrow strips generated by a cash register.

The printer is able to print all of the pump's activity over a certain time frame. In the case of PCA, this activity might include milligrams and milliliters infused, patient requests, and infusion limits programmed into the pump. Other pumps print out drugs infused, total volumes, alarms experienced, interruptions in use, and, in cases where there are drug libraries having hard and soft limits, reports of overrides and trends for quality assurance purposes.

Nurse call systems

Infusion pumps may have the capability of being integrated with the nurse call system. With these systems, the patient's bedside call light can be activated if the pump sounds an alarm, or the signal can be relayed to a central pump diagnostic station. The pump diagnosis screen may be at the nurses' station, where the nurse can identify the problem without going to the bedside. The screen at the nurses' station is scored, giving each bedside pump a portion of the screen. The section that lights up corresponds to a specific bedside and a specific device. The screen also indicates the type of alarm sounding.

Remote site programming

Remote programming is accomplished by using computer technology, which allows communication with the pump by a wired or wireless network. The pump's activities can be monitored from the base unit, making it possible for the caregiver to monitor the pump without being present. The base unit has the ability to change the pump's infusion settings once an assessment has been made, proving to be cost-effective and efficient. This capability does not circumvent nursing assessment, but rather supports it.

Syringe use for secondary infusion

Syringe use for secondary infusion is a practical alternative to small-volume piggybacks or tedious IV push medications. The syringe is attached directly to the pump administration set and is vented, allowing the solution to flow from the syringe without requiring pressure to be exerted on the syringe piston. This option is available with the primary fluid in the syringe or with the syringe attached to the primary set as a secondary infusion container. Both options offer considerable cost savings if they eliminate the need for syringe pumps in addition to regular pumps. The largest cost savings are realized by using inexpensive syringes in place of more expensive, small-volume plastic bags.

Secondary rate settings

Secondary rate settings are achieved in the same manner as secondary infusions by gravity administration. The secondary container is hung at a higher level than is the primary infusion, so the secondary infusion automatically infuses first. The pump settings are designed to program two separate rates and two separate volumes. After the secondary volume is reached, the pump switches to the primary rate and resumes counting the primary volume. The pump is unable to tell which fluid is infusing because it counts volume infused only. Solution containers must be hung at the correct height to ensure that the pump infuses correctly.

Bar coding

New microtechnology has made it possible for the pharmacist to generate the prescription for infusions into a bar code label. An appropriately equipped infusion device reads the bar code using an attached scanner and programs the pump at the ordered rate. The nurse can check the settings for accuracy by reviewing the display screen. This technology has significantly reduced human error. The pump can be changed immediately to override the system if unplanned interventions become necessary. This device is ideal in home infusion practice because it eliminates any accidental program changes or tampering.

Alarms and safety features

The number and type of alarms that are beneficial must be decided by each health care organization. The nurse should always remember that alarms are for the protection of the patient, not the caregiver. A list of infusion pump alarms is contained in Box 20-2. These alarms are listed generically and may have a different name on the pump being used.

The wide range of safety features is usually taken for granted until they are compromised. An excellent example is the actual pump housing. The housing should be sealed to prevent solutions from entering the internal mechanisms of the pump. Although the housing is not important to most users, biomedical

engineers have witnessed the amazing efforts of infusion devices to function while mired in dextrose solutions. The seal of the housing includes the face, where the indicators and control knobs are located. To achieve a more effective seal, most devices use touch pad technology with liquid crystal display.

The seal cannot be perfect. There must be a vent somewhere on the housing to allow gas to escape from the pump. Gas is a product of battery storage and pump operation, and although minuscule in volume, gaseous build-up can cause the pump housing to rupture. The vent is usually not readily visible, is extremely small, and must be clear to ventilate the device.

Automatic keep-vein-open (KVO) features are not available on all devices but are considered highly desirable. An automatic KVO feature ensures that instead of a device shutting down when an alarm sounds, such as low battery or infusion complete, the pump goes into a KVO rate. The KVO rate is pump specific but usually ranges from 0.1 to 5.0 mL/hr.

Size is considered a safety feature in the current climate of health care delivery. Smaller pumps pose fewer risks to the caregiver and patient in terms of transport and ambulation. Size can cause significant problems in terms of excess weight, bulk, and cumbersome management.

Size should be considered inversely as well. When pumps are miniaturized, certain features, such as the back-up battery, the air-in-line alarm, or the free-flow features, may be affected. Smaller is not always better or safer.

A tamper-proof feature requires that a deliberate series of steps be taken to affect the action of the pump. These steps may not be complex; in fact, they may include nothing more than having to start the pump after it is reprogrammed or started. Tamper-proof features may also include lock-out programs, which require the nurse to enter a sequence of numbers to access the programming capabilities of the pump. For both hospital and alternative care settings, tamper-proof devices are often desirable.

Tamper-proof capabilities are beneficial safety features, but must be tailored to fit the situation. A tamper-proof feature could prove hazardous if it is used in conjunction with life-threatening medications because the time required to override the tamper-proof feature could hinder quick action. All pumps should provide some degree of tamper-proof consideration, especially those used for geriatric and pediatric populations.

Another safety feature is the inability to bypass alarms. Most devices feature an alarm silence button, which is usually self-terminating in less than 5 minutes. This means the alarm can be silenced for only 5 minutes or less. This self-terminating feature prevents the safety features from being overlooked or deliberately ignored. Repeated attempts to fool a safety feature can result in the pump changing to a nonfunctional mode, completely refusing to operate.

Electrical safety is a concern with any equipment connected to an alternating current outlet. Electrical cords should be equipped with grounded plugs and a grounded outlet. Many devices even call attention to their power source if it is in any way inadequate. When any device is used, both the caregiver and the patient must be protected from electrical hazards.

Box 20-2	INFUSION PUMP ALARMS
Alarm	**Purpose**
Air-in-line	An ultrasound-based device near the tubing's exit from the pump detects air inside the line; may include air detection and air removal.
Occlusion	Detects absence of fluid flow in either the upstream (between the pump and the container) or the downstream (between the patient and the pump) location. Upstream alarms are associated with clamped tubing. Downstream alarms are associated with catheter occlusions.
Infusion complete	The preset volume to be infused limit has been reached.
Low battery	Warns the user about the pump's impending inability to function. The device must be connected to an external power source or have the batteries replaced. May trigger switching to a KVO rate instead of the programmed rate.
Low power	Power from an alternating current is not sufficient, causing the pump to draw power from the battery. May occur with power outages, at times of peak power demand, or when emergency generators are inadequate. May trigger switching to a KVO rate instead of the programmed rate.
Nonfunctional or system error	The pump has malfunctioned, cannot be resolved, and requires checking by a biomedical engineer.
Not infusing	Indicates that the pump settings have not been programmed. Most pumps require a start command to begin working.
Parameter	Manufacturer-specific alarms indicate that setting(s) is (are) not complete, such as "set rate" or "set secondary rate."
Tubing	Checks for use of the correct administration set and for the correct loading of the set into the pump.
Door	Indicates that the door to secure the tubing is not closed correctly.
Timing	Indicates that the time allotted for setup or hold has been exceeded.

▌ INFUSION FILTERS

A filter is a device intended to separate solid particles or other unwanted matter from a liquid. The removal of these solid particles, microorganisms, and air is the primary purpose of using filters in infusion therapy. It has long been recognized that unwanted matter appears in all types of solutions and medications, including glass, cotton and synthetic fibers, talc, starch, and insect parts (Lehr et al, 2002). The use of filters to reduce the incidence of catheter-associated bloodstream infection remains very limited, prompting the CDC guidelines to avoid making recommendations for their use as an infection control measure (O'Grady et al, 2002). Air emboli literature has focused on catastrophic events involving large amounts of air; therefore removal of in-line air is not regarded as a distinct need for filters. While the immediate clinical benefit of filters has eluded researchers and clinicians, there is a growing trend in recent literature to support their use.

The United States Pharmacopeia (USP) sets the standards for the amount of particulate matter in each solution container. A solution container meets these standards if it contains no more than 50 particles/mL of 10 microns or larger and 5 particles/mL of 25 microns or larger (O'Grady et al, 2002; Weinstein, 2007). Consequently, solutions are intrinsically filled with particles. Addition of medications and administration sets adds more particulate matter and increases manipulation and the subsequent risk of introducing organisms and air. The average diameter of pulmonary capillaries, the ultimate location of particulates, is about 5 micrometers (μm) (Guyton and Hall, 2006); thus it is likely that even 1 L of IV fluid could introduce enough particles to occlude significant areas of pulmonary circulation. It has been estimated that an adult in a critical care unit could receive more than 10^7 particles greater than 2 micrometers within a 24-hour period of infusion therapy (RA Lingen et al, 2004).

CLINICAL INDICATIONS

Indications for filters include infusions administered via the peripheral and central venous systems and intraspinal and intraosseous routes. Blood filters are used for the routine infusion of blood and blood components. Arterial routes are not filtered because the filter's presence could interfere with successful pressure monitoring, although particulate matter in the arterial system could cause serious injury by occlusion of small arterioles.

Filters are contraindicated for use with certain medications, which are retained on the filter material. Filters made of nylon have been shown to remove 100% of amphotericin B while polyether sulfone filters did not produce the same results (Hirakawa et al, 1999a). Additionally, subsequent re-

FOCUS ON EVIDENCE

Particulate Matter and Filtration

- Significant amounts of particulate matter have been found on autopsy in the lungs of patients following lengthy stays in critical care units. All patients developed irreversible adult respiratory distress syndrome. Lungs of these patients were sampled in 12 locations and assessed by scanning electron microscope and an optical microscope. Microthrombosis was found in the pulmonary capillaries of all patients, along with interstitial and interalveolar edema, interstitial fibrosis, and fat emboli. Further analysis of the particles revealed the majority contained rubber, glass, and latex and a smaller number were composed of metal and silicone. These particles directly caused damage to capillary endothelium, thrombosis, granulomas, and formation of foreign body giant cells (Walpot et al, 1989).
- A study of the number and size of particles in lyophilized antibiotics showed that generic brands had small-particle counts (2 to 10 microns in diameter) 30 times greater than what was contained in the brand name drug. Generic drugs had large particles (25 to 100 microns) at 12 to 28 times the amount in the brand name drug. This study went on to assess the tissue response to infusions of these drugs in animals. In normal tissue, there was no change in functional capillary density; however, tissue that had been ischemic for 4 hours and then reperfused for 2 hours showed a 30% reduction in functional capillary density upon receiving the infusion. This research suggests that the presence of particulate matter can have a detrimental impact on the nutritional blood supply of tissue that has been compromised by trauma, surgery, or disease (Lehr et al, 2002).
- Following aortic valve replacement in a 17-year-old patient requiring numerous medications and continuous fluid infusion, the in-line filter was examined after 72 hours of use. A scanning electron microscope showed numerous particles, mostly with a crystalline look and angular or "spearhead" shape. The authors hypothesized that these particles could have produced endothelial damage leading to respiratory distress syndrome, thrombosis, and inflammatory responses, and possibly even multiple organ failure (Brent, Jack, and Sasse, 2007).
- Injection of contrast medium using high pressure has been documented to contain large and small particles in excess of Japanese and USP recommendations (Hirakawa et al, 1999b).
- A Japanese study assessing the particle counts in multiple drugs found insoluble particles of 5 microns or greater in the bags of normal in-line (mean of 12 ± 3.3 in 5 mL), and in lyophilized drugs (mean of 11 ± 5 per 5 mL to 250 ± 45 per 5 mL) after reconstitution. This study called for the routine use of in-line final filtration for IV drug infusion (Kuramoto, Shoji and Nakagawa, 2006).
- Yorioka and colleagues (2006) found significantly larger numbers of particles for drugs obtained from glass ampules compared to the same drugs derived from prefilled syringes.
- A study in a Singapore hospital found a significant reduction in infusion phlebitis by using final in-line filtration (Chee and Tan, 2002).
- A review of the literature by the Cochrane Neonatal Review Group found only three studies assessing morbidity and mortality in infants from the use of in-line filters. However, they found insufficient data to base a recommendation for or against the use of filtration (Foster, Richards and Showell et al, 2006).
- The introduction of microbubbles of air into infusion systems is reported to be of significant clinical consequences. Small bubbles induce platelet aggregation and cause endothelial damage leading to thrombus generation. While large air embolus can be catastrophic, the infusion of a small air bubbles can be clinically silent. The clinical outcome of repeated exposure to microbubbles is unknown but could be influenced by the patient's co-morbidities (Barak and Katz, 2005).

search produced information about the particle count in amphotericin B exceeding the amount recommended by the USP (Sendo et al, 2001). Filter material differs; therefore no statements can be made about specific drug compatibility. Manufacturers specific recommendations should be followed. Filters are available with tubing that is free of DEHP or other plasticizers. Filters should also be avoided when administering very small volumes of drugs because retention by the filter might seriously decrease the volume of medication received by the patient.

CHARACTERISTICS

Screen and membrane filters are available as infusion filters and there are numerous processes used to manufacture them. Materials include polymers such as polyester, polypropylene, polyvinylidene fluoride, and polyvinyl chloride as well as organic substances such as cellulose and ceramics. The filter "media" is the material responsible for the filtration task.

Screen filters are the simplest type of filter. It is usually made by weaving fine fibers and wrapping them around a core and then placing this in a plastic housing. This process can be locked, creating a relatively constant pore size, while others are not locked, allowing a widening of the pore size. Membrane filters consist of sheets of material with irregular shaped channels. Some manufacturing processes result in a decreasing pore size throughout the material thickness. The surface of the filter material can be treated by applying a variety of chemicals or gases. These processes alter the surface to have features of clinical importance such as hydrophilicity or hydrophobicity or to improve fluid flow rates. Finally, the prepared media is mounted in a housing. It can be flat or pleated sheets in housings with a variety of shapes, all designed to direct the flow of fluid, increase flow rates, or separate the particles from the fluid (Ortolano et al, 2004).

A depth filter consists of multiple layers of material through which fluid must pass. The primary use for this type of filter is in filter needles used to aspirate medication from vials or ampules. Because the pore size of the different layers is not uniform, the filter captures various-sized particles at different layers.

Hollow-fiber filters are used in dialysis filters and the manufacturing processes for medications and vaccines. The hollow-fiber filter housing is cylindrical and consists of many very fine tubes, each of which is porous and allows the passage of fluid through sterilizing membranes. The number of tubes makes high flow rates possible and minimizes clogging over long periods. The hollow-fiber filter achieves good air elimination and primes easily.

Filters are characterized numerically to differentiate filter pore size. The universal scale of measurement is the micron. Common filters are 0.2, 0.45, 1.2, 5.0-micron retentive filters for use with common IV solutions and medications. Larger filters must be used to filter blood products because they capture large particulate matter and allow red blood cells to pass.

The hydrophobic properties of the filter material prevent air passage in the line. The filter housing is designed so that the air is successfully vented out of the system. A surfactant added to the filter material prevents the filter from becoming air-locked, which would prevent the solution from flowing. The air-venting feature works with gravity flow and infusion pumps and is not dependent upon the position of the filter.

Filters should have high-flow capabilities and incorporate hydrophilic and hydrophobic membranes. Hydrophilic filters

are easily wetted and pull the fluid forward, overcoming flow resistance. Most reputable filters can accommodate extremely high flow rates, as much as several liters per hour. The better filters allow high flow rates despite medications being added or being given IV push.

Pressure tolerance is sometimes a misunderstood feature of an IV filter. Filters used in conjunction with a pressure bag or IV pumps may pose a certain risk if the filter membrane ruptures as a result of excessive pressure. Rupture can also occur if an IV push medication is administered upstream or above the filter. If undue pressure causes the filter membrane to rupture, the patient could receive a concentrated infusion of particulate and infectious matter. To prevent this situation from occurring, the filter is made with pounds per square inch (psi) tolerance in the housing. The housing of the filter is designed to rupture, leaving the filter membrane intact and protecting the downstream flow of fluid. When this rupture occurs, the integrity of the infusion system is broken, and the infusate flows from the filter, necessitating a change in the administration set.

Most users associate filter breakage with a malfunctioning filter. However, filter breakage is a patient-protection mechanism intended to warn the user to examine the activity that precipitated the breakage. If the situation calls for extremely high pressure to be used, such as in trauma cases, the filter should not be used. If the filter breaks during routine use, the event precipitating the breakage should be examined carefully. Pressure powerful enough to break the filter could also damage the vasculature or rupture softer infusion catheters.

Infusion filters either are preattached to the primary administration set or are available as a separate add-on piece. The most common micron size is 0.2 for both configurations. Because not all infusates can be filtered, administration sets that do not contain a filter must also be available, which increases inventory and cost.

Filter sets commonly include an injection port after the filter, situated between the filter and the patient. This design allows the nurse to give small-volume IV push medications, avoiding the filter.

BLOOD FILTERS

Routine IV solution and blood filters are not interchangeable. The size of a red blood cell is several hundred times the size of the microorganisms being filtered from routine IV solutions. The American Association of Blood Banks and the *Infusion Nursing Standards of Practice* require the routine use of blood filters for transfusion therapy. Standard, sterile, pyrogen-free transfusion administration sets have a filter pore size ranging from 170 to 260 microns. A filter of this great pore size removes only coagulated products, clots, and debris resulting from blood collection and storage. Microaggregate filters have a pore size of either 20 or 40 microns and remove fibrin and clumps of dead cells; however, their primary use is reinfusion of autologous cells collected during or following a surgical procedure (Roback et al, 2008).

Leukocyte-depletion filters are designed to remove leukocytes and leukocyte-mediated viruses, which greatly increases the safety of transfusions to patients who have received multiple transfusions. These filters have been shown to improve patient response to blood products in patients requiring frequent, repeated transfusions and to prevent febrile reactions in patients who have experienced transfusion reactions. Leukocyte-depletion filters are classified according to efficiency level, not micron size, and can remove up to 99.9% of leukocytes from the blood transfusions and platelets. Prestorage leukocyte depletion is most common, but bedside leukoreduction is possible. Manufacturers' instructions should be followed closely to avoid an air lock, preventing the passage of blood through the filter. Also, patients could experience a serious episode of hypotension with bedside leukodepletion, especially those that are taking an angiotensin-converting enzyme inhibitor. If this occurs, the transfusion should be stopped immediately (Roback et al, 2008).

 VENOUS ACCESS DEVICES (VADs)

Technology has certainly resulted in many advances to the devices used to access the vascular system. We have definitely come a long way from the first crude hollow tubes, with many developments occurring within the past decade. A catheter is defined as a tube for injecting or evacuating fluids. These tubes are made of many types of plastic, metal, or other synthetic material. A venous access device (VAD) is a catheter inserted into any part of the vascular system including veins, arteries, and bone marrow (INS, 2006). Catheters are also used to access other body cavities such as intraperitoneal and intraspinal spaces.

A common way to categorize VADs is by the veins in which the tip resides. This would include veins of the extremities (or peripheral veins) and veins of the thorax (or central veins). Along with these anatomical descriptions there are many types of catheter designs and product characteristics.

The goal of nursing and medical care should be to proactively select the most appropriate device for each patient early in his or her course of infusion therapy. This device should be the one that has the greatest likelihood of reaching end of therapy with the minimal number of devices used. This approach improves clinical outcomes by reducing complications, enhances patient satisfaction by reducing unnecessary pain from excessive venipunctures, and improves the financial considerations by reducing costs. Patients and significant others must be involved in the final device selection as these devices will have a direct impact on their quality of life.

CATHETER CHARACTERISTICS
Catheter material

Over the past century, technology has evolved from stainless steel to rubber and various forms of plastic as the material used to manufacture the tube inserted into a vein. Stainless steel is still used for winged needles; however, their use is limited to blood sampling procedures. The rigidity of the metal prevents its successful use for infusion. Other precursors of current materials included polyvinyl, polyethylene, and nylon (Thomas, 2002).

Most of the materials currently used are polymers, a word derived from the Greek language meaning "many parts." Small molecules are chemically linked together to form a long chain or a large molecule with a spaghetti-like appearance. Adding more molecules changes the properties of the material. Polytetrafluoroethylene (Teflon) is a carbon-based polymer that forms a very stiff material. Fluorinated ethylene propylene (FEP) is another polymer of the same family that offers more flexibility and compatibility with tissue and drugs. These materials are used to make short peripheral catheters and many types of introducers for other longer catheters.

Polyurethane is a urethane-based polymer that can be formulated in many ways. Polyurethane is composed of alternating groups of soft segments and hard segments that provide the flexibility and strength needed for a catheter. The soft segments respond to temperature, resulting in the label of "thermoplastic" for these materials. When a polyurethane catheter is inserted into the human body, the change from room temperature to body temperature increases its softness and flexibility. There is an attraction for moisture, also increasing the flexibility when placed in the bloodstream (Thomas, 2002).

Polyurethanes of many formulations are used to make all types of peripheral and central intravenous catheters. Because of its strength, it can be manufactured with thin walls, allowing for greater fluid flow without the need for a larger diameter of catheter. One challenge with polyurethane is its compatibility with alcohol, which can act as a solvent of some polyurethane catheters. Manufacturer's warning about exposure of polyurethane catheters to alcohol differ because the formulations used by manufacturers also vary. These instructions may be based on testing performed by the original polyurethane manufacturer or by testing conducted on the assembled catheter by the catheter manufacturer. Testing on the polyurethane material may not duplicate the ways that alcohol comes into contact with the catheter in clinical practice. Testing by the catheter manufacturer may be closer to the catheter's exposure to alcohol clinically. Alcohol may be applied to the skin surface at the catheter-skin junction, and there is a growing interest in using ethanol as a locking solution to treat or prevent bloodstream infection associated with catheters.

A recent study examined mechanical properties of catheters made of polyether urethane and silicone after being locked with 70% ethanol inside the lumen. These catheters were compared with a control group of catheters without ethanol exposure. The polyurethane group was exposed to the ethanol for 67 days and the silicone group was exposed for 72 days. There were no significant differences in elongation, strain, or the force required to break the catheters exposed to ethanol in either group (Crnich, Halfmann, Crone et al, 2005). This study examined only one formulation of polyurethane and did not examine the ethanol impact on intraluminal walls and external hubs. Other formulations may have different outcomes; therefore catheter manufacturer's instructions for use must be followed.

Silicone is a polymer material used in a wide variety of industrial and medical applications. It is constructed of inorganic silicone-oxygen with an organic component added, usually methyl groups, to create polydimethylsiloxane (PDMS). This formulation can be created as a liquid, often used as a lubricant for guidewires and catheter tips, or crosslinked with silica filler to form a gel-like or a solid material. The high degree of flexibility allows for the rapid diffusion of water, gases, and some drugs through the silicone matrix. Silicone elastomer materials used for catheters are extremely flexible, requiring they be inserted through an introducer. Some of this flexibility is lost because the catheter wall must be made thicker to achieve the required strength for use as a venous access device (Thomas, 2002). Silicone catheters are not affected by chemicals such as alcohol, as shown in the study of ethanol exposure discussed previously (Crnich et al, 2005).

All catheter material is tested for biocompatibility. These tests include cytotoxicity, sensitization or the risk of allergic reactions, irritation or the potential to cause inflammation, acute and chronic systemic toxicity, genotoxicity, and hemocompatibility (Renner, 1998). All catheter material should be radiopaque to facilitate location of catheter emboli in the event of catheter shearing or fracture. Barium sulfate is a common radiopaque substance added to the polymer and the degree of radiopacity varies between brands.

Catheter geometry

A discussion about catheter geometry includes the catheter sizes, lengths, lumen shapes and sizes, and extension legs. This information usually involves the use of the words "proximal" and "distal;" however, these words have purposefully been avoided because they can lead to confusion. The use of these words requires a reference point. Most nurses regard the center of the patient as their reference point; however, catheter design engineers use themselves as the point of reference. To a nurse the distal end of the catheter would be the external hub; however, to the engineer the distal end would be the internal tip or the end farthest away from them. When using these words, it is always a good practice to clarify the way they are being used.

Size

The diameter of a catheter is measured both inside and outside. The outer diameter (O.D.) is most often, but not always, used to indicate the catheter's size. It is the measurement in millimeters of a straight line from the outside wall through the center of the lumen to the opposite outside wall. The inner diameter (I.D.) is measured from one inside wall through the center to the opposite inside wall. The diameter of the vein's internal lumen must be capable of accommodating the catheter's O.D. without greatly reducing the blood flow around the catheter. The I.D. of a catheter determines the priming volume, the flow rate, and the pressure tolerance of the catheter. Cutting the catheter length to a patient-specific size would alter the priming volume (Lawson and Vertenstein, 1993).

French size is calculated by multiplying the O.D. measurement in millimeters times three. A catheter's O.D. of 2 mm would be labeled as a 6 French (6F) size; consequently, larger numbers would mean larger size catheters. French size is more commonly applied to central venous catheters and ranges from 1.1 French of neonatal catheters to 16-French dialysis catheters.

Gauge size is derived from the industrial wire manufacturers and is best applied to a round catheter, needle, or wire. Smaller numbers indicate larger sizes; thus an 18-gauge catheter is larger than a 22-gauge catheter. Conversion from gauge size to French size is possible but the two systems are not evenly converted. Gauge size is more commonly used for short peripheral catheters and introducers with the sizes ranging from 12-gauge to 26-gauge. Winged metal needles are measured in gauge size also; however, odd numbers are used ranging from 13 gauge to 27 gauge. Gauge size can also be applied to the lumen size of a multiple lumen catheter. When the lumen shape is not round, the surface area is measured and a calculation of the closest equivalent gauge size is used.

Length

Catheter length can be considered in two ways—the total catheter length or the effective catheter length. The effective catheter length is measured from the internal tip to the external junction with the catheter hub or lumen bifurcation.

In other words, this is the length intended for insertion into the vein. The total catheter length would include the effective length along with the length of extension legs and the hubs. A winged needle device may be 3/8 to 1-1/2 inches long and short peripheral catheters are between 5/8 and 2 inches. A midline catheter is usually between 3 and 10 inches effective catheter length, while the length of PICCs can be up to 28 inches.

Central venous catheters may have depth markings to indicate the catheter length; however, there are no requirements for how these markings are applied. These markings could be every centimeter, every 5 cm, or every 10 cm. There could be a series of straight lines or a line with a number. Some brands may have the smaller numbers begin on the catheter's internal tip, but some begin on the external side.

Lumens

Both peripheral and central venous catheters are available with single or multiple lumens. Additional lumens can enhance the ability to infuse complex infusion therapies without fear of mixing incompatible medications, but more lumens means more hubs to manipulate and a potential for a greater risk of catheter-associated bloodstream infection. The patient should be assessed for the appropriate number of lumens based on the complexity of the infusion therapy. Multiple lumen catheters should not automatically be chosen for all patients.

The shape of each lumen depends upon the manufacturing process. A single lumen catheter will have a round shaped lumen. A double lumen catheter may have a wall separating the round lumen into two evenly sized D-shaped lumens. Triple or quadruple lumen catheters could have round, oval, or elliptical-shaped lumens. The size of these lumens depends upon the O.D. of the catheter, the catheter material and wall thickness, and the measured lumen surface area.

Extension legs

Most central venous catheters and a few brands of peripheral catheters have an extension leg on each lumen. The effective catheter length stops at the catheter wing used for stabilization or, in the case of a multiple lumen catheter, at the point where each lumen bifurcates. Each lumen will have a separate extension leg and catheter hub. These legs could be made of a different plastic from the catheter material itself; the composition of the legs varies by catheter brand. Each extension leg could be stamped with the lumen size or other valuable information around the catheter.

The catheter hub is located at the external end of this extension leg and is also made of different types of plastic. All catheter hubs will have Luer-locking threads and are considered to be the female side of the Luer connection. Catheter hubs may have the same or different colors, which could provide information about the preferred uses for each lumen. For instance, the larger lumen could have a red hub, indicating that blood sampling is best through that lumen.

Hubs require careful attention to cleaning at each administration set change to remove any dried blood, drug precipitate, or tape residue, as this could be a major contributor to lumen contamination. Alcohol pads are commonly used to clean the catheter hub and the hub should be allowed to dry thoroughly before a new Luer connection is applied.

Some brands of catheters have a clamp on the extension leg. This could be a removal slide clamp, a permanently attached slide clamp, or a C-clamp. Depending upon the material used for the extension leg, it is recommended that these clamps be applied at different locations on the extension leg to avoid a permanent kink in the tubing. Catheters with removal slide clamps may not be advisable for use on small children as these small objects could be removed and present a choking hazard.

Tip configuration

A few brands of multiple lumen catheters have the lumens exiting at different or staggered locations on the catheter's internal tip. This is especially applicable to hemodialysis catheters where the tip of each lumen is separated by at least 2 cm. The amount of separation between these lumen exit sites on infusion catheters varies between brands but could be less than 1 cm. Many brands of catheters have nonstaggered lumen exit sites, indicating that both lumens exit at the same place on the catheter's internal tip. The significance of staggered versus nonstaggered lumen exit sites has not been firmly established in clinical studies. For central venous catheters, the tip will be located in the superior vena cava where the blood flow is approximately 2000 mL per minute. This could be sufficient to prevent contact between two incompatible fluids or medications; however, drugs that are known to be incompatible with many medications (e.g., phenytoin) could precipitate at the catheter tip when there is contact with fluid infusing from the other nonstaggered lumen. For short peripheral catheters and midline catheters, the tip resides in a peripheral vein with much smaller blood flow. This could easily allow contact between incompatible medications infusing simultaneously.

When there are staggered lumen exit sites, the length of the extension leg may correlate to the position of the exit site. For instance, the shortest extension leg would be attached to the lumen exiting on the internal catheter tip.

Integral valves

Valves are built into various midline and central venous catheters at both the internal tip and the external hub. The original valved catheter has the valve located on the catheter wall near the closed internal tip. During infusion, the valve opens outward; during aspiration, the valve opens inward; and when no pressure is applied, the valve remains in a neutral position. Another design has a valve on the catheter tip that allows fluid to flow inward from the opening on the catheter tip; however, blood is aspirated from an opening on the catheter wall, slightly above the catheter tip.

Valves are also located inside the external catheter hub. One type is a round silicone disk with the valve seated in the catheter hub. On infusion it opens inward; on aspiration it opens outward, and remains closed when no pressure is applied. Another type of valve located in the catheter hub consists of three valves, one for infusion in the center and two for aspiration on the sides.

While these valves have differing designs and function in different ways, the one common aspect is the fact that they can all be flushed and locked with 0.9% sodium chloride. All manufacturers of these catheters state that heparin as the final locking solution is not required.

Anti-infective agents

Some brands of central venous catheters are impregnated with anti-infective agents, which have been shown to decrease the risk of catheter-associated bloodstream infection.

Chlorhexidine and silver sulfadiazine are impregnated into the polyurethane material of nontunneled percutaneously inserted central venous catheters. The antiseptic properties are located on the inner and outer catheter walls, the extension legs, and the hubs.

Minocycline and rifampin are used to impregnate another brand of catheters, available in both polyurethane and silicone catheters. These catheters have the antimicrobial agents on both inner and outer catheter walls and are available in nontunneled central venous catheters and peripherally inserted central catheters (PICCs).

Another brand of nontunneled percutaneously inserted central venous catheters contains silver and platinum in the polymer. Carbon creates an electrically conductive path between the particles, causing the silver to be released while the platinum is retained in the polymer.

High-pressure injection

Several brands of short peripheral catheters, PICCs, and other central venous catheters are designed to tolerate the high pressure required for rapid injection in CT scans. These injections may require pressures in excess of 150 pounds per square inch (psi). The upper pressure limit for most catheters is 40 psi; therefore the high-pressure injection far exceeds the capability of many catheters. Catheters used for high-pressure injection must be labeled for that purpose to avoid serious catheter damage, including catheter fracture and embolization.

Repairability

Most central venous catheters are not repairable, although some brands do provide repair kits. The main criterion for successful catheter repair is to use a brand of repair kit specifically designed for the brand of catheter being repaired. Kits and catheters should not be considered interchangeable because of a variety of catheter measurements. Repairable catheter damage could also lead to sites for microorganisms to enter. If repair must be made, there must be enough external catheter length to allow repair. Usually, tears or ruptures are trimmed and a new connecting hub applied. Catheter repair is a technique requiring advanced skills along with adherence to organizational policy. This policy should address the catheter repair kit and procedure, and answer questions such as the following: "Will this repair be considered permanent or temporary until a new catheter can be inserted?"

Reverse taper

Many brands of central venous catheters are constructed with an enlarged external segment of catheter wall known as a reverse taper. This segment of catheter has an O.D. larger than the remaining catheter length, yet this enlarged segment resides in the smallest vein diameter. The primary purpose of this design is to provide strength to the catheter wall so that kinking will not occur at the transition from the vein to the subcutaneous tissue. Reverse tapers have a variety of lengths. Some brands may allow for a significant amount of large catheter length to reside inside the vein lumen, while others with a shorter reverse taper could have this enlarged segment residing in the subcutaneous tissue. No clinical studies are available to establish the outcome with this design.

TYPES OF VENOUS ACCESS DEVICES
Winged needles

One of the most basic and time-tested devices is the winged needle. The device has flexible plastic wings or flaps extending from either side of the needle hub. The hub is usually plastic and may be color-coded; however, reading the package label is the best method to determine gauge identification. Attached to the plastic hub is a short length of PVC tubing ranging from 3 to 12 inches in length. Syringes or vacuum tube holders attach easily to the connector at the end of the tubing. Safety mechanisms on winged infusion sets allow for the needle to be withdrawn into a protective sheath as it is pulled from the vein.

Winged needles should only be used for obtaining blood samples and not for infusion of solutions or medications. Although easy to insert because of fewer moving parts, winged needles are difficult to stabilize and are associated with higher rates of infiltration.

Short peripheral catheters

A peripheral catheter is one that begins and terminates in an extremity (arm, hand, leg, foot, or neck). The external jugular access is considered a peripheral access if the catheter does not extend into the subclavian vein. Short peripheral catheters are most commonly used when infusion therapy is required for less than 1 week. These catheters are not recommended when the therapy is a vesicant, when the final pH is less than 5 or greater than 9, and when the final osmolarity is more than 600 mOsm/L (INS, 2006).

Short peripheral catheters are available as winged infusion sets or as over-the-needle catheters. Winged infusion sets include a plastic catheter with a needle stylet inside. This stylet has a beveled edge extending beyond the plastic catheter to make the venipuncture. Behind the folding plastic wings, clear plastic tubing is attached with a plastic hub several inches away from the insertion site. The needle stylet is attached to a wire with a plastic tube on the external end that houses the needle after retraction from the vein.

The most widely used infusion device is the over-the-needle catheter (Figure 20-9). This device is a soft plastic catheter with a rigid, plastic hub. A hollow metal stylet (needle) resides inside the catheter and the angled bevel protrudes through the distal tip of the catheter to allow puncture of the skin, subcutaneous tissue, and vessel wall. When the vein is punctured, a flashback of blood appears in a closed chamber behind the catheter hub. The catheter is then threaded off the stylet into the vein, and the stylet is completely removed, leaving the softer, plastic catheter in place.

Several features are designed into the safety mechanism and flashback chamber. The stylet inside the plastic catheter must be held stationary and in a bevel-up position during insertion to prevent vein trauma and to receive early flashback. The hub of the plastic catheter is seated on the safety mechanism/flashback chamber stylet in a preset, clinically correct position with the bevel up. Additionally, there is a silicone seal at the junction of the catheter tip and the bevel of the stylet to maintain the correct position of these pieces. Instructions from some manufacturers may indicate a step to rotate the catheter and break this seal while others may not include this as part of their instructions. Some small gauge catheters have an opening in the stylet near the beveled tip. This allows for blood return to be seen inside the catheter lumen rather than waiting until it has passed into the flashback chamber. This could be beneficial in small infants and/or patients with low blood pressure.

The safety mechanism is located between the catheter hub and the flashback chamber. The metal stylet may be automatically retracted into a plastic housing as the catheter is advanced into the vein, or the stylet may be automatically retracted into the plastic housing by pushing a button. Other mechanisms include a metal clip that closes over the sharp bevel of the stylet as it is retracted from the catheter hub, or a blunting device that is passed through the stylet lumen to render it incapable of causing a puncture.

The flashback chamber is a small space at the hub of the stylet or a continuation of the safety mechanism. When the stylet punctures the vein during catheter insertion, the increased pressure in the vein is immediately relieved into the catheter stylet with a flow of blood in the flashback chamber. Catheters have a closed flashback chamber that allows air to escape and blood to enter but prevents blood from spilling out.

The hubs of short peripheral catheters are completely round or may be flat on the side next to the skin with flexible wings extending from the sides. The flat side and the wings could add to the stability of the catheter when it is secured against the skin.

One challenge with the design of short peripheral catheters is connecting the extension set to the catheter hub with blood flowing from the catheter. This connection site lies very close to the skin, making it easy to contaminate the administration set during this connection. Blood also can flow down the patient's arm or hand if not controlled during the removal of the safety mechanism/flashback chamber and connection of the administration set. A new design for short peripheral catheters addresses this problem. The catheter has wings extending from the sides of the hub along with a permanently attached extension set extending to one side. The blood return is seen inside the catheter lumen as a result of a needle stylet with a notch or hole near the tip. The blood return continues up the catheter lumen and into the extension set. A safety mechanism extends from the back of the catheter hub, where a closed hub is left when the stylet is removed. The extension set has a bifurcated hub with one side having a preattached Luer-activated split septum needleless connector. The other side can be connected to infusing solutions or capped with the same type of needleless connector provided in the package. This closed system allows for a venipuncture technique the same as that used for other short peripheral catheters, while providing the fixed extension set and needleless connector.

Short peripheral catheter hubs are color-coded according to an international standard. Universal color-coding standards allow visual recognition of the catheter gauge size. This standard has not been applied to the gauge sizes of midline or central venous catheters. An inherent danger exists in color-coding

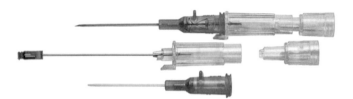

FIGURE 20-9   Over-the-needle catheter. (Used with permission from B. Braun Medical, Inc., Bethlehem, PA.)

of IV catheters, medical products, and other devices because color-coding implies that products can be identified without reading the label. The *Infusion Nursing Standards of Practice* (2006) state that color-coding shall not be used for product or medication identification. However, for ease of sorting, supplying, or reaching for a product, color codes can be useful. After the product is in hand, the label must be read.

Dual lumen peripheral IV catheters may also be used and are available in a range of catheter gauges with corresponding lumen sizes. These catheters have a larger total lumen size, necessitating cannulation of a larger vessel to accommodate both lumens. They have two infusion channels, making it possible to infuse two fluids. Because two infusions may be delivered simultaneously, it is necessary to have as much hemodilution as possible to protect the vessel; thus a very large peripheral vein is necessary. Simultaneous infusions of solutions or medications known to be incompatible are controversial because of the proximity of the lumen exit sites and the limited hemodilution achievable in peripheral vessels.

Midline catheters

The concept of a midline catheter was first introduced in 1989 with a 6-inch-long over-the-needle device; however, midline catheters available now use the same insertion techniques as a PICC. A midline catheter is inserted through the veins of the antecubital fossa or lower portion of the upper arm in adults. The basilic vein is preferred because of its larger diameter; however, the cephalic vein or one of the paired brachial veins could be used if ultrasound guidance is available. The catheter is advanced far enough up the vein to allow the tip to reside in the upper arm, level with the axilla. The tip should always remain below the shoulder joint to reduce the risk of vein irritation from movement of this joint. In infants, other insertion sites include the veins of the head, neck, and lower extremities.

A midline catheter is indicated when the therapy will be longer than 1 week; however, the optimum dwell time has not been established (O'Grady et al, 2002). Midline catheters are not appropriate when the infusion is a vesicant, when the final pH is less than 5 or greater than 9, and when the final osmolarity is greater than 600 mOsm/L. Vein depth at the midline tip location could prohibit the observation of the typical signs and symptoms of complications. Other veins, arteries, and nerves of the upper extremity could be seriously damaged before the complication is detected. A midline catheter can replace the need for multiple peripheral catheter insertions; however, it should not be regarded as a substitute for a central venous catheter.

Midline catheters are made of polyurethane or silicone and are usually 8 inches (20 cm) long. Measurement of the arm from the venipuncture site to the axilla will indicate the length of catheter to insert. Midline catheters may be single or double lumens in sizes from 1.9 to 5 French, although some manufacturers use gauge sizes for midline catheters. Some brands are available with a suture or securement wing and an extension leg. The brands without an extension leg have the effective catheter length ending at the female connection hub.

The midline catheter has a stylet wire inside the catheter to add stiffness so that the soft catheter can easily be advanced into the vein. This stylet wire ends about 1 to 2 cm from the catheter tip. If the catheter length is trimmed, the wire should not be cut but must be withdrawn into a similar position within the catheter lumen. The stylet wire is not intended to be the leading edge moving up the vein. The wire is attached to a flushable extension set seated in the external catheter hub. This allows the catheter to be filled with 0.9% sodium chloride, wetting the stylet wire to facilitate its removal at the end of the procedure.

It is not advisable to use a longer catheter and trim it to a midline length. Most catheters are labeled with the type of catheter on the extension leg or hub. Using a catheter labeled as a PICC, but cut to be a midline catheter will lead to serious infusion errors because the actual tip location is unknown or the primary care nurse is confused by the labeling.

The venipuncture for a midline catheter insertion can be performed with through-the-introducer or modified Seldinger techniques. The traditional introducers are similar to those of peripheral IV catheters with needle safety mechanisms. The venipuncture is made into a visible or palpable vein. The blood return is seen in the flashback chamber. The needle is retracted into the safety mechanism and removed from the introducer catheter. The midline catheter is advanced into the introducer catheter to the desired length, and then the introducer catheter is retracted from the vein. The wings of the introducer catheter are broken and peeled away from the midline catheter. This method requires a large vein because the introducer must be larger than the remaining midline catheter. A small amount of bleeding from the puncture site may be present for a few hours following insertion. The modified Seldinger technique will be discussed with PICCs.

Central venous catheters

A central venous catheter (CVC) or *central line* is any catheter whose tip resides within the superior vena cava near its junction with the right atrium. Before they are used for any infusion, all CVCs must have tip location confirmed by a chest radiograph. CVCs are used when emergency access is required in trauma or surgery situations, when there is a lack of peripheral veins to safely deliver the prescribed therapy, when the prescribed therapy has characteristics that render it inappropriate for infusion through small peripheral veins, and when long-term access to treat a variety of diagnoses is necessary. Nurses, patients, and their caregivers independently manage the delivery of complex infusion regimens through CVCs in all inpatient units, outpatient or ambulatory care, long-term care, and home care.

Device manufacturers have created CVCs with a wide variety of features and insertion methods suitable for insertion into many different anatomical locations. This variety places a great responsibility on the nurse to know the CVC's design, purpose, limitations, warnings, and precautions. Insertion site, insertion techniques, tip location, and nursing care during the dwell time are directly related to the clinical outcomes with these devices. Knowledge of and adherence to national standards of care are critical, along with documented clinical competency.

Peripherally inserted central catheters (PICC)

A PICC is a central line that is inserted percutaneously through the veins of the upper extremity in adults. The catheter is passed through the veins until it resides in the superior vena cava near the junction with the right atrium. In infants, veins of the head, neck, or lower extremities are used for insertion. The tip location will be the same as that in adults except when the lower extremities are used and the tip resides in the thoracic inferior vena cava. The basilic vein is preferred because of its larger diameter; however, the cephalic vein or one of the paired brachial veins could be used if ultrasound guidance is available.

A PICC is indicated for all types of infusion therapy because the tip resides in the central venous circulation. Hemodynamic monitoring is possible through a PICC; however, a PICC that contains an integral valve will prohibit the pressure monitors from working properly.

PICCs are made of polyurethane and silicone. Because of the increasing need for high-pressure injection for CT scans, the use of polyurethane PICCs is increasing. PICC sizes can be as small as 1.1 French for a neonate and as large as 7 French for adults. Single, double, and triple lumens are available in effective catheter lengths up to 70 cm.

Most PICCs have a preloaded stylet wire inside the catheter to add stiffness so that the soft catheter can easily be advanced into the vein. This stylet wire ends about 1 to 2 cm away from the catheter tip. If the catheter length is trimmed, the wire must be withdrawn and repositioned into a similar location within the catheter lumen after cutting. A stylet wire or guidewire should never be cut. The stylet wire is not intended to be the leading edge moving up the vein. The wire is attached to a flushable extension set seated in the external catheter hub. This allows the catheter to be filled with 0.9% sodium chloride, wetting the stylet wire to facilitate its removal at the end of the procedure.

Trimming PICCs to a patient-specific length is at the center of controversy. Manufacturers make catheters with smooth, rounded tips to reduce the trauma to the vein wall. Some brands of catheters have staggered lumen exit sites. Trimming to length removes these features and their subsequent benefits. Studies using neonatal PICCs have highlighted the possible risk associated with this practice (Pettit, 2006; Trotter, 2004). Tools used to trim catheters include scissors, scalpel blades, and a guillotine-type tool sold by one manufacturer. One blinded study trimmed multiple neonatal catheters of polyurethane and silicone using all possible tools. Digital photographs of these catheter tips were taken using high-powered magnification. All catheters trimmed with scissors showed tip irregularities; 75% trimmed with the scalpel blade were irregular; and 17% twimmed with the trimming tool were irregular. Analysis of clinical outcomes of 108 neonatal PICCs showed that 93 were trimmed and 15 were not trimmed. There were three cases of mechanical phlebitis, two of the trimmed catheters and one of the untrimmed catheters. There were no clinically apparent thromboses (Pettit, 2006). This preliminary study highlights the controversy and the need for more well-designed studies. Leaving an excessive length of catheter externally can present additional problems. The best option at this time is to choose a catheter length that is as close to the desired patient length as possible.

The venipuncture for a PICC insertion can be performed with through-the-introducer or modified Seldinger techniques (MSTs). The through-the-introducer procedure was discussed in the section on midline catheters. The modified Seldinger technique is the most prevalent method used for PICC insertion. The venipuncture is made with a 21-gauge metal finder needle that could range from 5 to 10 cm. Some brands of these needles are available with a safety mechanism to house the sharp bevel. Another feature of these needles is the echogenic tip, a special design that makes it more visible when ultrasound is used. Based upon individual preferences, a syringe can be placed on the hub of this needle or it can be used without a syringe. The other option is to use a short peripheral catheter with a safety mechanism. After venipuncture the stylet is removed, leaving the short peripheral catheter in the vein.

A guidewire is advanced into the needle or short peripheral catheter. This guidewire is designed with multiple safety features so that it can be advanced into the vein. It is significantly different from the stylet wire inside the catheter lumen. The guidewire is advanced several inches into the vein to ensure sufficient length for successfully advancing the vessel dilator, also known as "purchasing" the vein. The needle or short peripheral catheter is withdrawn from the vein and off the guidewire. The guidewire should not be advanced beyond the shoulder unless the procedure is being performed under fluoroscopy in the radiology department. Extreme care is required to maintain complete control of this guidewire at all times. Losing control of the wire could mean embolization of the guidewire to the heart or pulmonary vessels.

A scalpel blade is used to slightly enlarge the skin puncture site so that it will accommodate the dilator/peel-away sheath assembly. The dilator/sheath device is threaded over the guidewire and advanced through the skin and into the vein. A twisting motion may be needed to get the dilator/sheath into the vein. The dilator and guidewire are withdrawn from the vein, leaving the peel-away sheath inside the vein. This will leave an open catheter in the vein and bleeding may occur. Digital pressure above the sheath may be helpful to control this bleeding, depending upon the depth of the vein. Another method would be to occlude the sheath lumen with the thumb over the hub. The PICC is advanced through the sheath to the desired length. The sheath is withdrawn, broken, and peeled apart.

Nontunneled, percutaneous centrally inserted catheters

This type of CVC has been the largest group of CVCs but the use of PICCs is rapidly overtaking it. These CVCs are inserted percutaneously into the subclavian, jugular, and femoral veins. For subclavian and jugular insertions, the tip should be located at the superior vena cava and right atrium junction. For those inserted via the femoral vein, the catheter tip should be located in the thoracic inferior vena cava above the level of the diaphragm (INS, 2006).

These CVCs are most commonly made of polyurethane; however, there are silicone devices available. They range in size from 5 to 12 French and from 5 to 25 cm in length. Single, double, triple, and quadruple lumen catheters are available.

These catheters may be inserted using the MST as described previously or by using the Seldinger technique. The Seldinger technique uses the same finder needle and guidewire. The difference is that the catheter is advanced over the guidewire and into the vein. The guidewire is removed from the catheter hub. This procedure requires a longer guidewire and very careful control of the guidewire to prevent its loss into the vein. Guidewires designed for MST and Seldinger techniques are different and are not interchangeable.

Tunneled, cuffed catheters

Tunneling is the technique for placing a segment of the catheter inside a subcutaneous tunnel to separate the vein entry site from the skin exit site. This technique was introduced more than 30 years ago based on the idea that this separation would reduce the risk of bloodstream infections, allow for very long dwell times, and permit self-care. The most common brand names are taken from the physicians that originally created these catheters—Broviac and Hickman. Many companies now make these catheters and these names should be reserved for the specific brands that bear these names.

The catheter can be inserted by the modified Seldinger technique or by a cut-down technique. The venipuncture or *entrance site* is made at a point near the subclavian or internal jugular vein. From this point to a predetermined point lower on the chest where the catheter will exit, a small, pencil-like device called a *tunneler* is passed. The catheter is attached to the tunneler and drawn through the subcutaneous layer as the tunneler is removed. The catheter is then passed through the sheath introducer and positioned at the superior vena cava/right atrial junction. The skin at the vein insertion site may require a few sutures. The tunnel may be 2 to 12 inches long for placement on the chest. If the catheter has a nontraditional entrance and exit site, the tunnel may be even longer. For example, a catheter with a femoral entry site could exit midsternum.

The concept of small-bore tunneled catheters has recently emerged. This was originally thought to reduce the risk of catheter-associated bloodstream infections; however, that has not proven to be successful. The primary use is in renal failure patients. Using the internal jugular vein for insertion bypasses the veins of the upper extremity and subclavian veins, which have a higher risk of thrombosis. Thrombosis in these veins could produce much difficulty in placing a large hemodialysis catheter if required. These catheters may or may not have a cuff. Some brands are capable of high-pressure injection. Therefore the specific brand of catheter and its features must be known.

Catheters unable to be trimmed because of their unique design at the internal tip (e.g., valve-tip or staggered lumen ends) must be inserted in reverse. The catheter is placed in the central vessel, and the external ends (minus the catheter hubs) are pulled through the subcutaneous tunnel from the vein entrance site to the skin exit site. Any trimming to make the catheter shorter occurs at the external end before the catheter hubs are attached. A schematic of tunneling technique is presented in Figure 20-10.

A cuff is a strip of material about 1 cm wide that encircles a catheter. The cuff can be made of various materials, such as nylon or Dacron, although the texture of the cuff before insertion is roughened like Velcro. Approximately 14 days after catheter insertion, the cuff, positioned in the subcutaneous tunnel, becomes firmly attached by the growth of a connective tissue seal. The tissue seal around the cuff stabilizes the catheter. The risk of a catheter-associated bloodstream infection is reduced because of the tunnel and cuff; however, tunnel infections can occur and are very difficult to treat without catheter removal. Because the cuff is firmly adhered to the tissue, the catheter is designed to pull loose from the cuff when sharp tension is applied. This feature prevents tissue tearing if the catheter is accidentally pulled. After the catheter is removed, the cuff can be left behind or surgically removed using local anesthesia.

Another type of cuff is made of silver-impregnated collagen. This cuff is available on one brand of CVC. This cuff is intended to have an antimicrobial effect at the puncture site.

Implanted ports

This long-term VAD is attached to a port body and all components are placed under the surface of the skin inside a surgically created pocket. This pocket is usually created in the upper chest but may also be placed in the upper part of the arm. To use the device, the port body is palpated and accessed with a noncoring needle passed through the skin and into the port septum. Implanted ports are best suited for long-term intermittent needs; however, some patients receiving cyclic parenteral nutrition may learn to access the port for their daily needs.

The implanted port body consists of housing made of titanium, plastic, or stainless steel. Steel interferes with electromagnetic imaging procedures and is quite heavy compared with the other materials. For these reasons, it is no longer used for most port bodies. Titanium has the advantages of steel without the interference problems and is very lightweight. Polymers such as polysulfone are used alone or coated with silicone.

The center of the port body is hollow and covered by a septum made of dense silicone. Port bodies come in a variety of sizes, depths, and shapes. High profile ports are deeper while low profile ports are shallower and have a smaller priming volume. The fluid reservoir may be a rounded configuration or squared. The base of the port body has suture holes around the circumference to enable the port body to remain stable. The outlet stem exits from the base of the port body and provides the attachment for the catheter. Some brands have a preattached catheter while others have catheters that are attached during the insertion procedure. If attachable, there are multiple methods for making this connection. Figure 20-11 depicts a cross section of an implanted port.

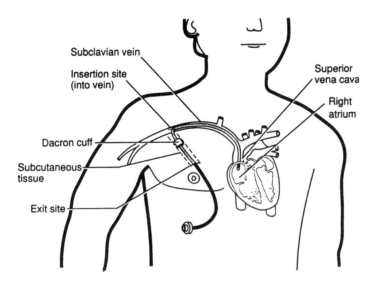

FIGURE 20-10   Schematic of tunneling technique. (Courtesy MiniMed Technologies.)

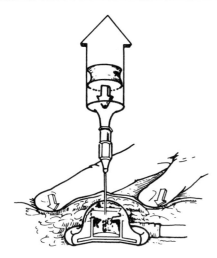
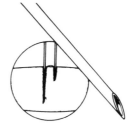

FIGURE 20-11 Cross section of implanted port. (Courtesy Bard Access Systems.)

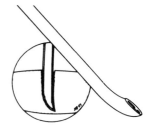

FIGURE 20-12 Comparison of coring versus noncoring needle. (Courtesy Bard Access Systems.)

Interventional radiologists, surgeons, nurse practitioners, and physician assistants insert implanted ports. The catheter is inserted into the subclavian or internal jugular vein and the incision is sutured or suture-taped, leaving no external apparatus. The catheter length is trimmed so it resides at the junction of the superior vena cava and right atrium. This catheter may have a valve at the internal tip or at the end near the port body.

The reservoir septum accommodates a noncoring needle and is critical to the success of the device. It not only allows the needle to enter but also holds the needle tightly. The opposite edges of the septum are palpated through the skin and the needle is advanced into the skin and through the center of the septum. Some implanted ports recess the septum for ease in identification, whereas others have a domed configuration. Regular sized septums are rated to tolerate approximately 2000 punctures, while small port bodies placed in the arm have a smaller septum and are rated to tolerate approximately 750 punctures. The tissue over the septum commonly becomes calloused or scarred, with a loss of sensitivity resulting from the chronic presence of the device and the needlesticks associated with its use. Ports usually have softly molded edges that minimize skin breakdown.

Noncoring needles have a deflected tip designed to slice through the dense septum. If traditional needles are used to penetrate the septum, coring and leakage occur after a few punctures, rendering the device useless. Because the dense septum holds tightly to the needle, there can be a rebound problem when it is removed. This increases the risk of accidental needlestick injuries. Noncoring needles are available with a wide variety of safety mechanisms to house the needle as it is withdrawn. Figure 20-12 compares the construction of coring and noncoring needles.

Implanted ports may be single or dual lumen; a dual lumen has two separate reservoirs inside one port housing. The stem extending from the port body has two channels to accommodate the catheter with two lumens. Implanted ports are also being made that can tolerate the high pressure required for rapid injection in CT scans. In the majority of cases, however, it can be very difficult for the nurse to distinguish by simple palpation whether or not the port is power injectable. The manufacturers generally provide patient information and

identification that should be given to each patient following insertion; the patients should be instructed to carry this information with them at all times.

Hemodynamic monitoring catheters

The lumens of hemodynamic monitoring catheters are function specific, and the device is primarily used in critical care nursing. The lumens will have an inline transducer attached to a data-monitoring device to determine core temperature, cardiac output, and hemodynamic analysis. The catheter itself is longer than 3 feet and is used in fully monitored intensive care units and specialty care areas.

The introducer for these catheters is extremely large to accommodate the catheter passing through it. With these introducers, a rubber seal at the introducer's hub holds tight around the catheter, preventing the introduction of air or bacteria. An added infusion port appears as a side "pigtail" and exits at the internal tip of the catheter. This side port provides an extra infusion lumen, but it is not necessary for the function of the introducer. The side port does not have a separate lumen but allows flow around the catheter inside the introducer.

The introducer should not be regarded as a CVC. The introducer by design is shorter and stiffer than that for a typical CVC and its intended purpose is not that of an infusion device. When the catheter is removed from the introducer, the introducer should be exchanged over a guidewire for a traditional CVC. Allowing these introducers to remain as an infusion catheter poses a risk of air embolism and exsanguination if the administration set connections were to loosen.

Dialysis/pheresis catheters

Dialysis catheters are rarely considered for the routine use of infusions; they are strictly reserved for dialysis, primarily because of the many problems associated with occlusion and the increased risk of a catheter-associated infection. Infusion of medication is often given through these catheters at the end of a dialysis run or they may be used for infusion in an emergent situation when no other vein can be cannulated. Pheresis catheters may be used for the purpose of plasmapheresis and for the routine administration of medications.

Dialysis and pheresis catheters are available in polyurethane for short-term needs and in silicone materials for long-term needs. Dialysis and pheresis catheters have a much larger lumen (usually 13 to 16 gauge) and are shorter and less flexible than those of regular central VADs. They have traditionally been more rigid than other lines to allow high blood volumes and rates.

Dialysis and pheresis catheters are problematic in that they are difficult to secure and maintain because of their rigidity.

Their large size makes them more painful to the patient during movement. The site bleeds easily, making it difficult to keep the dressing clean, dry, and intact.

Silicone dialysis and pheresis catheters may have a cuff located inside a subcutaneous tunnel. The connecting hubs are color-coded to facilitate the identification of lumens for withdrawal and reinfusion.

ALTERNATIVE ACCESS DEVICES
Shunts

Shunts can be placed for many reasons. Only the artificial venous shunt is discussed here as a venous access device. Modern shunts are made of GORE-TEX or silicone material. A shunt bridges two vessels: an artery and a vein. The shunt is usually placed in the forearm between the radial artery and the brachial or cephalic vein. It is accessed with a large-bore dialysis needle and is used for routine hemodialysis.

Newer shunts are able to withstand many needlesticks and are used routinely in some places for infusion purposes other than dialysis. Only knowledgeable persons should access a shunt. If it is inadvertently damaged, surgical replacement is necessary.

Arterial catheters

Catheters that are introduced into the arterial circulation can be used for two purposes: monitoring or administration of organ-specific infusions. When the purpose is monitoring, the arterial catheter, usually at the radial artery located at the wrist, provides an access for blood sampling (including blood gases) and blood pressure monitoring.

The catheter must be able to sustain its shape and be long enough to cannulate the artery, which is normally deeper than a peripheral vein. When properly placed, the arterial catheter may have to bend as it descends to the artery. If the catheter kinks at the bend or collapses on itself with negative pressure, it does not function well as an arterial catheter. For this reason, arterial catheters may have a thicker wall. Arterial catheters are routinely used to monitor blood pressure when they are attached to the appropriate nondistensible tubing and transducer set-up.

Peripherally placed arterial catheters are not used for the infusion of solutions. Medication infused into an artery, even in benign volumes and concentrations, can cause tissue damage because of the close proximity to the capillary bed or terminal point of circulation. Hemodilution is not sufficient to prevent tissue saturation of the drug and resulting cellular hypoxia.

Arterial catheters are placed for organ-specific infusions, with the most common being the hepatic artery catheter. These therapies are for specialized infusions, such as regionalized chemotherapy to a particular diseased organ. Some are attached to an implanted pump or reservoir that is accessible with a special needle.

Intraspinal catheters

Intraspinal means located within the spinal space. Technically speaking, this area can include the epidural and the intrathecal spaces. The intraspinal route has been accessed for many years for many forms of medical treatment, injections, diagnostic tests, and infusions. Advancements in anesthesia have made the intraspinal space more accessible,

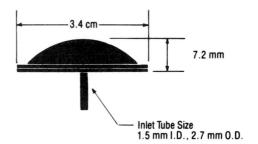

FIGURE 20-13   Ommaya reservoir. (Courtesy American V. Mueller.)

medically functional, and respected as a route for medication administration.

The catheters used for intraspinal infusion are 22 to 26 gauge and are approximately 10 to 30 inches long. They are made of polyurethane or silicone. They can extend several inches into the epidural space, especially if the catheter is intended to be in place long term. Intraspinal catheters can exit directly from the spinal puncture site or can be tunneled subcutaneously to a remote site.

Once successful spinal puncture has been performed, the catheters are threaded through an introducer apparatus. If the catheter is intended for a one-time infusion, it is lightly secured until the procedure is over. The rigid needle is not left in place for any length of time. If the catheter is to be left in place for extended periods, it is threaded farther into the epidural space and taped securely.

Another device that introduces infusate into the spinal fluid is the Ommaya reservoir (Figure 20-13). This is a very specific therapy reservoir that attaches to a catheter and terminates in the cerebral ventricular space. The medication most often infused is concentrated morphine sulfate without preservative. This drug bathes the neurons of the brain and spine directly to achieve maximum pain control. This is also called *intraventricular therapy*.

Subcutaneous access devices

Needles are inserted into the fatty tissue below the skin, providing the name for this procedure, *subcutaneous infusion* or *hypodermoclysis*. The subcutaneous tissue has minimal pain sensors but good absorption rates, making medications and solutions infused into this compartment effective therapy. Needles used to access this space can be regular hypodermic needles less than 1 inch long. The needle is inserted at a 10° to 20° angle, depending on the patient's fatty tissue depth. Specially designed subcutaneous needles built on a flat disk with an adhesive pad at the hub are also available. The needles are ⅜ to ⅞ inch long and are inserted directly into the skin with the disk resting on the skin. These needles are comfortable for the patient and do not dislodge easily.

Intraosseous needles

Intraosseous needles, those inserted into the bone, are categorized with steel needles. The marrow space of the human bone, especially in children, is capable of providing an infusion route for any IV drug or solution.

Several designs of intraosseous needles are available. The tip end of an intraosseous needle is solidly protected by an obturator, is very sharp, and may have circular screwing threads to

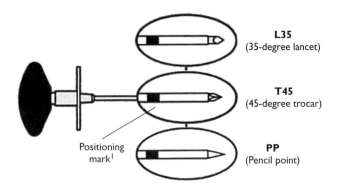

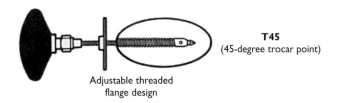

L35
(35-degree lancet)

T45
(45-degree trocar)

Positioning
mark[l]

PP
(Pencil point)

T45
(45-degree trocar point)

Adjustable threaded
flange design

FIGURE 20-14   Intraosseous needle placement. (Courtesy Cook Critical Care.)

help penetrate the bone. The hub end has a large, solid handle that fits into the palm so that pressure can be exerted. Figure 20-14 depicts intraosseous needle design.

The needle size recommended for a child is 18 gauge, and a 15- to 16-gauge needle is used for adults. The long bones of the leg and the iliac crest are usually the point of insertion. Intraosseous administration is thought of as a pediatric procedure, but it can be used in adults. The sternum of adults has been used with mixed opinions. Complications include bone breakage, infiltration, bone infection, and cellulitis.

 ## STABILIZATION DEVICES

When discussing stabilization, there are two areas of concern—the catheter hub and the joint when an IV catheter must be placed near an area of joint flexion. Movement of the catheter and the nearby joint will increase complications. A study from an emergency setting reports that the majority of serious complications occur in the hand or wrist (Kagel and Rayan, 2004).

CATHETER STABILIZATION

The *Infusion Nursing Standards of Practice* focuses on stabilizing a catheter and securing the junctions of administration sets. Dressing any catheter should be considered a two-step process—one to control the catheter movement and one to cover and protect the skin and insertion site. A stabilization device is used for catheter movement; however, there is no evidence that any type of dressing material can adequately stabilize a catheter. Sutures have commonly been an accepted method for stabilizing catheters, although sutures are a common cause of needlestick injuries. Dressing material and sutures are no longer considered to be appropriate methods to stabilize any catheter. No mechanism used to stabilize a catheter should cover the junction of the catheter and skin.

Catheter stabilization devices include devices that are manufactured for that purpose, sterile tape, and surgical wound closure strips; however, a manufactured stabilization device is preferred (INS, 2006). Research has shown significant reduction in complications with short peripheral and central venous catheters when manufactured stabilization devices are used as compared to other stabilization methods (Yamamoto et al, 2002; Schears, 2006). The FDA defines a catheter stabilization device as a device with an adhesive backing that is placed over a needle or catheter and is used to keep the hub of the needle or the catheter flat and securely anchored to the skin. By this definition, a manufactured device must have a means to control the movement of the catheter hub rather than focusing solely on the attached administration set.

A manufactured device can have several mechanisms to control the movement of the catheter hub. All have an adhesive backing that adheres to the patient's skin under the catheter hub. These mechanisms include a plastic cage that is snapped around the hub, posts designed to fit through the suture holes on catheter wings, or elastic bands that crisscross over the hub.

JOINT STABILIZATION

Areas of joint flexion should be avoided when selecting a site for catheter insertion, if at all possible. When this is not possible, an armboard must be used to stabilize the joint (INS, 2006). Peripheral sites in the dorsal aspect of the hand and the cephalic vein of the medial wrist are the most problematic sites demanding the need for joint stabilization. The patient with a catheter in these sites is often expected to use his or her hand for activities of daily living, increasing the movement of the joint and vein damage. There has been concern that armboards used in conjunction with IV catheters should be considered a form of restraint and accordingly prohibited by the regulations on the use of restraints. Federal regulations from the Centers for Medicare & Medicaid Services have a definition of restraints and include an explanation of what is not considered to be a restraint. Basically, a device that is intended to protect the patient from additional risk, such as an armboard, is not considered to be a restraint. Also, The Joint Commission states that a device used for the protection of a surgical or treatment site is not considered to be a restraint (TJC, 2005).

An armboard can be either flat or contoured to fit the extremity. It should be padded for comfort and is intended for use on a single patient and then discarded. The armboard should be placed on the hand in such a way to allow movement of the fingers, yet support the wrist and restrict it from movement. The tape used to secure the board should not obstruct the view of the insertion site, nor should it be so tightly secured that it would compromise the neurocirculatory function of the extremity.

 ## DRESSINGS

Two types of dressings materials are used in infusion therapy—gauze and tape or transparent semipermeable membranes. The choice of dressings for an IV catheter has been the source of much debate over the years; however, there are benefits of each type. Regardless of the type of dressing chosen, the use of skin protectant solutions will allow more adherence of the dressing while preventing the adhesives on the dressing materials from causing skin irritation. Skin integrity at the site of all IV catheters is of paramount importance.

GAUZE

Cotton and cotton blends with synthetics are used to make gauze sponges. Finer-quality sponges have very little lint or are lint free. *Lint free* means that small flecks of cotton do not adhere to tissue. Lint adhering to soft tissue or granulating areas hinders wound healing.

Gauze, which has a higher cotton or all-cotton content, may be more absorbent than synthetic blended gauze. If the intent of the dressing is to cushion or pad an area, blended gauze is an excellent choice because it is very soft. If the intent is to absorb, all-cotton gauze may be superior.

Appealing aspects of gauze are its absorptive quality and clean appearance. A gauze dressing may be less costly than other dressings and readily available in most health care environments. Disadvantages include obscuring the catheter insertion site and preventing easy visual inspection of the site. Once the dressing is lifted to observe the condition of the catheter and the insertion site, a new dressing must be applied. Gauze must be secured with tape across all surfaces to make it an occlusive dressing. If tape is only placed around the outside edges, external moisture can penetrate and carry microorganisms to the catheter insertion site.

Gauze and tape dressings should be changed at least every 48 hours and when the dressing is dirty, wet, or nonadherent to the skin (O'Grady et al, 2002; INS, 2006).

TRANSPARENT DRESSINGS

Transparent dressings are also called *semipermeable membrane dressings*. They are designed to allow moisture to pass through the dressing away from the skin surface. The rate of moisture release varies greatly among products. Even with the best semipermeable membranes, the adhering ability of the dressing is severely tested by wound drainage and perspiration.

Transparent dressings are occlusive, preventing external moisture from contacting the insertion site. They adhere satisfactorily most of the time, minimizing the need for additional tape to secure the dressing.

Transparent dressings are provided in individually wrapped sterile packaging. Each brand has a specific application method. Because transparent dressings remain in place for longer periods, the user must be vigilant to protect against contamination with handling and application. If the dressing is poorly designed or the application technique is complex, there is a greater chance that the dressing will be contaminated.

For a short peripheral catheter, a transparent dressing may remain in place until the catheter is changed. For midline and central venous catheters, a transparent dressing should be changed at least every 7 days or more often if it becomes wet, dirty, or nonadherent to the skin (O'Grady et al, 2002; INS, 2006).

PLASTIC SHIELDS

Devices composed of a plastic molded piece to fit over the catheter and dressing are available as an additional means of site protection. Multiple sizes and shapes are available; however, all are made of clear plastic to visualize the site through the device. Many have soft straps to hold it in place, avoiding the use of additional tape on the patient's skin. These devices are frequently used to prevent small children or any confused or disoriented patient from disturbing the catheter or dressing.

ANTIMICROBIAL BARRIER MATERIALS

Two novel dressing materials are available to add the protection of an antiseptic agent at the insertion site. A circular patch impregnated with chlorhexidine gluconate fits around the catheter at the insertion site under the dressing. This patch releases chlorhexidine gluconate incrementally over several days. Chlorhexidine reduces gram-positive and gram-negative colonization significantly and has been shown to reduce the incidence of catheter-associated infection. Patches are smaller than a regular dressing and have a precut radial slit to allow the catheter to exit at the center. A similar circular patch impregnated with silver is also available. Although silver is an antimicrobial agent frequently used in burn treatment, there are no published clinical studies available showing a reduction in catheter-associated infection when silver is used.

A novel transparent membrane dressing contains a gel pad built into the center of the dressing. This pad is impregnated with aqueous chlorhexidine gluconate that surrounds the catheter-skin junction.

The indications for routine use of these patches are institution specific, but they are especially useful in patients with high infection risks. Children, immunosuppressed patients, or patients with recurring catheter infections may benefit from the use of these forms of antiseptic agents at the insertion site.

VASCULAR VISUALIZATION DEVICES

The need for technology to assist with finding veins and arteries rises as our use of these vessels increases for therapeutic and diagnostic purposes. Traditionally we have relied upon palpation and visualization of peripheral veins and arteries, and for central venous catheterization anatomical landmarks have been used as the only guide. Many reasons now emphasize the serious limitations of these methods. Many chronic diseases cause patients to have a long history of repeated venipuncture, different types of catheters, and lengthy courses of infusion therapy, severely restricting vascular access sites. Diseases such as diabetes and hypertension produce changes in vessel walls making them more difficult to locate and cannulate. Fear of pain from previous bad experiences can produce vasoconstriction in any age. In children, these experiences result in much less cooperation on subsequent attempts. Cardiovascular and respiratory changes occur in infants from cold stress and noxious stimuli. Toddlers and prepubescent children have the highest percentage of body fat, obscuring veins. Finally, the growing number of bariatric patients produces many challenges with locating veins suitable for cannulation.

Ultrasound devices have been successful in finding deep veins for insertion of PICCs and other CVCs. There is also a growing trend to use ultrasound for insertion of short peripheral catheters in patients with difficult or limited venous sites. The insertion success is increased (Brannam, Blaivas, Lyon et al, 2004); however, there are no published data on the clinical outcome of peripheral catheters inserted with ultrasound. The use of ultrasound requires one hand to hold the transducer and one hand to hold the catheter. This alters the traditional method of using one hand to hold skin traction. Because of the vein depth, catheter length may need to be longer than the traditional 1- to 1.25-inch catheters used. The rates of phlebitis and infiltration/extravasation are unknown.

ULTRASOUND DEVICES

Ultrasound devices use sound waves to locate structures in the human body. Sonography, the term used to indicate imaging with ultrasound, can be two or three dimensional for diagnostic purposes. The nurse acts as the sonographer to perform the scan and the sonologist to interpret what is seen.

The system has two major components—the transducer and the imaging instrument. The transducer is held against the patient's skin and generates sounds waves that are passed through the part of the body being examined. These sound waves reflect off of internal structures. Returning echoes pass back to the transducer and the imaging instrument converts these echoes to visible dots on a screen, seen as an image of the veins, arteries, and surrounding tissue. The transducer can be positioned to obtain a transverse or cross-sectional view of the vein or a longitudinal view.

Each pulse or wave of ultrasound produces one scan line on the screen. As multiple pulses are sent, multiple scan lines appear to create the rectangular image. A standard cross-sectional image usually contains between 128 and 256 scan lines. This is known as a linear image. A sector image produces a pie-shaped picture with the pulses originating at the same point but dispersing in slightly different directions (Kremkau, 2002).

Principles of ultrasound

Sound occurs in waves much like the rolling surface of a pond after dropping a rock into it. Sound produces similar mechanical motion in the medium through which it travels. Sound waves involve frequency, speed, length, and intensity. Frequency is the number of complete cycles of a sound wave that occur in 1 second. Frequency is measured in hertz (Hz); 1 Hz is one cycle per second. Infrasound is less than 20 Hz and cannot be heard by humans. Human hearing functions between 20 and 20,000 Hz, but there is wide variation among individuals, especially the elderly. Ultrasound has a frequency greater than 20,000 Hz, or 20 kilohertz, and is too high for human hearing. Medical ultrasound ranges from 2 megahertz to 15 megahertz, or 2 million hertz to 15 million hertz (Kremkau, 2002).

The diagnostic image depends upon the pattern of echoes it produces. Air between the transducer and the skin can reduce the production of echoes. To enhance the sound path, a gel coupling medium is needed. All air must be eliminated as this would reflect the sound and prevent it from entering the body, thus preventing the return echo. As the sound spreads, it weakens in amplitude and intensity, a process known as attenuation. As the path for the sound lengthens, attenuation increases. Although morbidly obese patients or those with extremely muscular arms would have more tissue, this usually does not create a problem for ultrasound machines used for venipuncture. Attenuation occurs primarily by absorption or conversion of sound to heat.

Resolution is a function of the transducer. Increasing the frequency produces a more detailed resolution, or the ability to have small objects appear separated. The price for this improved resolution is the loss of imaging depth because attenuation increases as the frequency increases.

Motion of the sound source, the receiver or reflector, produces the Doppler effect because of a change in frequency and wavelength. Think of an approaching train and the sound you hear. As the train moves closer, the sound has a higher frequency. As it moves away, it has a lower frequency. An ultrasound-imaging instrument may be equipped to record audible sound of fluid flow to evaluate blood flow in the body. Blood, a dense and viscous fluid, flows because of a pressure gradient. As the pressure difference between two points increases, the flow rate also increases. Increases in vessel diameter also increase the flow rate. Increases in vessel length and blood viscosity decrease flow rate. The Doppler effect can record changes in steady (venous) fluid flow and pulsatile (arterial) flow. The narrowing of a vessel because of stenosis produces changes in the flow characteristics that can be detected by Doppler. The presence of flow and its direction, speed, and character can be revealed with Doppler ultrasound. Color-Doppler imaging or color-flow imaging produces real-time illustration of blood flow or tissue motion.

Ultrasound safety

In recent years much attention has been given to the effect of ultrasound on the human body. In vitro and in vivo tests have not disclosed any risks from diagnostic ultrasound. Although there are no known risks, the possibility of risk cannot be overlooked, requiring a conservative approach to the use of medical ultrasound use. Thermal and mechanical means of tissue damage have been and continue to be studied. The principle of ALARA ("as low as reasonably achievable") must prevail in the manufacture and use of all ultrasound equipment. Factors that influence the application of this principle for ultrasound users include the patient's size, attenuation, and ultrasound exposure time. Limiting exposure time and exposure intensity would be the best way to employ the ALARA principle (Kremkau, 2002).

LIGHT DEVICES

Like sound waves, the use of light waves can also be harnessed to produce vascular images for venipuncture. Electromagnetic or light waves are the movement of electric and magnetic energy. These waves are measured on a continuum from longest to shortest. Gamma rays have the shortest length, with x-rays and ultraviolet waves a little bit longer. The next segment in the center of the continuum is the light waves that are visible to humans. This spectrum is represented by colors of the rainbow with violet having the shortest wavelength of about 400 nanometers and red having the longest wavelength of about 700 nanometers. The spectrum continues to the longest waves but outside of what is visible to humans. Infrared, microwaves, and radio waves are included in this section. Near-infrared light is the closest to visible light. It does not produce heat. A common device using infrared light is a remote control for electronic equipment. Far-infrared light is closest to the microwave length and does produce heat.

The wavelength for near-infrared light can be applied to the depth of tissue where veins and arteries are located. The skin ranges in thickness from 1.5 to 4 millimeters, and the thickness of the superficial fascia will vary with the amount of adipose tissue and the location on the extremity. Near-infrared light will have a wavelength between 750 and 800 nanometers, a sufficient amount of light to penetrate the tissue so that veins can be seen.

Two methods are used to illuminate vessels in light-based devices. Transillumination is shining a light through tissue. Reflection is the return of light from a surface with the production of an image like a mirror.

Visible light

Transillumination from flashlights, otoscopes and other fiber-optic devices has been used to locate veins for many years, especially in babies. These devices have produced burns and were the subject of an ECRI *Hazard Report* in 2003. Some neonatal nurses rely heavily on placing a visible light on the opposite side of the infant's extremity to highlight the dark lines that are veins.

Visible light devices designed for finding peripheral veins are small, portable, battery-operated devices. They have a high-intensity light source and moveable arms to widen or narrow the area illuminated. Successful use of these devices requires a darkened room to eliminate competing sources of visible light. The area of illumination depends on the color of the skin, with darker skin tones producing greater difficulty. Some devices have protective covers but they do require adequate cleaning after each use.

Successful use of these devices greatly depends upon personal preference and there are no outcome studies available. There is one study documenting the use of a visible light device to detect IV infiltration in healthy volunteers (Yucha, Russ, and Baker, 1997).

Infrared light

Transillumination and reflection are used in different types of infrared light devices. Transillumination is used when the near-infrared light source is placed against the opposite side of the extremity. Hemoglobin absorbs the light to identify veins and arteries. A viewing scope using the same technology as night vision goggles is used to actually see the vessels.

Transillumination by infrared light produces a good image of veins. Arteries appear larger than veins and have a "fuzzier" appearance, and pulsation can often be seen. The challenges with this system are the use of monovision required by the viewing scope. It also can produce alterations in depth perception, making it difficult to recognize when the catheter tip is in contact with the skin.

Reflection devices use a digital video camera to capture the image reflected from the patient. The image is sent to a processing unit that adds contrast and projects the image to the patient's skin surface. This method produces a good image of veins; however, arteries are not easily identified. The device currently available is very large, making it difficult to move between patients. Smaller portable devices are in developmental stages. Some nurses report depth perception issues of a different nature. The reflected picture shows the vein's location, but not its depth in the tissue, making palpation techniques still necessary. Metals from rings or watches on the nurse's hand may also interfere with the image.

Infrared imaging devices do not require alteration of room lights. Skin tone and body type do not matter when using this device. This is a hands-free device, leaving both hands to perform the venipuncture procedure. This technology is in its infancy but more developments are anticipated.

LOCAL ANESTHETIC DEVICES

Several new devices for the delivery of a local anesthetic agent have taken the practice far beyond simple intradermal injection of lidocaine or topical cream application. These advances coincide with a keen interest in alleviating pain, especially procedure-related pain. The use of these technologies is primarily for insertion of a short peripheral catheter. Because of the vein depth, they have not been used extensively for PICC or other CVC insertions.

IONTOPHORESIS

Iontophoresis is the delivery of many types of drugs through the skin by using an electric current. A drug reservoir or pad soaked with the anesthetic agent is applied to the skin over the planned venipuncture site and secured with an adhesive pad. Another pad is also adhered to the skin beside the drug reservoir pad. Most devices use a combination of lidocaine and epinephrine. One device has both pads constructed together with the electrodes already attached. Another device requires application of separate pads and connection of the electrodes. The positive and negative electrodes attach to a small device that generates a very small electric current. The electric current ionizes the medication, causing it to penetrate the skin and produce anesthesia. The anesthetic effect will last for approximately 10 minutes at the site where the drug reservoir pad was placed.

OTHER FORMS OF ACCELERATED DELIVERY

One system looks like a very large syringe. It is firmly placed against the skin. Pressing downward releases an internal safety lock. Pressing the start button releases helium gas that drives the powder particles of lidocaine into the skin. The effect is felt in 1 to 3 minutes and lasts for about 10 minutes. This device is indicated for children from 3 to 18 years of age.

Another system uses a multiple layer adhesive patch similar to a typical dressing. Holes in the top layer allow oxygen to penetrate the pad and activate a heating element. A mixture of lidocaine and tetracaine is loaded into another layer and is driven into the skin by the effects of the heat. The site is ready for venipuncture in approximately 20 minutes. This system is indicated for adults and children older than 3 years of age (Sethna et al, 2005), although safe use was documented with infants of 4 to 6 months in one study.

Both systems should only be used on intact skin. Check for allergies to any of the medications contained in the chosen system. Local site reactions have been reported with both systems, including redness, blanching, and edema. Since these are common symptoms of local catheter complications, a careful assessment of the catheter and vein patency is required to determine the cause of these adverse reactions.

CATHETER LOCATION SYSTEMS

Systems designed to locate the tip of a CVC immediately after insertion are now available. One group relies on anatomical landmarks while the second group uses changes in ECG tracings to identify tip location.

Several systems have an external device or sensor and a stylet wire containing a magnet. The catheter is inserted after external measurements are taken in a traditional method. When placed over the patient's chest, a visible display or audible alarm indicates the vicinity of the catheter's tip. Some systems are dedicated to a brand of catheters with the stylet wire preloaded in the catheter while another system offers the external device and the stylet wire that can be loaded into any brand of catheter. The external devices must be placed on or near the sterile field, so a sterile clear cover will be needed for it.

These systems may not function correctly when there is interference from other radiofrequency signals such as cellular telephones. Additionally they could interfere with pacemakers or other cardiac rhythm devices.

The use of ECG tracing, specifically a change in the P wave, can also indicate the catheter's tip location. Electrodes are placed on the patient's right and left arms, left leg, and chest in a standard fashion. A metal connection is made between the catheter and the ECG device. The connection can be accomplished by using a stylet wire in the lumen leading to the internal catheter tip or by using a metal needle on a 0.9% sodium chloride filled syringe that is inserted into the injection port on the catheter's hub. As the catheter tip passes the sinoatrial node, the P wave increases in voltage and has an upward spike. This system requires the ability to interpret ECG tracings; however, this method could be the most reliable method to accurately identify the catheter's position.

The standard of practice is to verify a CVC tip location by obtaining a post-procedure chest radiograph. There are not enough studies on the use of these tip-locating systems to alter that standard; however, these devices are helpful to identify that the catheter is close to the correct location before the sterile field is compromised.

SUMMARY

Over the past 10 to 20 years, much technological advancement has radically changed the way we insert catheters and deliver infusion therapy. These changes will continue as many companies work with health care providers to find innovative ways to enhance patient care by providing safer technology. The device is an extension of our hands and the clinical outcome is greatly influenced by our skill with each device. Product changes require outcome tracking to show the positive and potential negative changes resulting from its use. While these devices are beneficial to our patients, none are intended to replace the knowledgeable and skillful health care professional.

REFERENCES

AdvaMed: Code of Ethics on Interaction with Health Care Professionals with FAQs, 2005, Washington, DC, Advanced Medical Technology Association.

Apkon M, Leonard J, Probst L et al: Design of a safer approach to intravenous drug infusions: failure mode effects analysis, *Qual Saf Health Care* (13):265-271, 2004.

ASHP: ASHP Guidelines on handling hazardous drugs, *Am J Health Syst Pharm* (63):1172-1193, 2006.

Barak M, Katz Y: Microbubbles: pathophysiology and clinical implications, *Chest* (128):2918-2932, 2005.

Bonnabry, PL, Cingria F, Sadeghipour H et al: Use of a systematic risk analysis method to improve safety in the production of paediatric parenteral nutrition solutions, *Qual Saf Health Care* (14):93-98, 2005.

Brannam L, Blaivas M, Lyon M et al: Emergency nurses's utilization of ultrasound guidance for placement of peripheral intravenous lines in difficult-access patients, *Acad Emerg Med* (11):1361-1363, 2004.

Brent BE, Jack T, Sasse M: In-line filtration of intravenous fluids retains 'spearhead'-shaped particles from the vascular system after open-heart surgery, *Eur Heart J* (28):1192, 2007.

Chee S, Tan W: Reducing infusion phlebitis in Singapore hospitals using extended life end-line filters, *J Infus Nurs* (25):95-104, 2002.

Cope JU, Morrison AE, Samuels-Reid J: Adolescent use of insulin and patient-controlled analgesia pump technology: a 10-year Food and Drug Administration retrospective study of adverse events, *Pediatrics* (121):e1133-e1138, 2008.

Crnich C, Halfmann, Crone JW, Maki D: The effects of prolonged ethanol exposure on the mechanical properties of polyurethane and silicone catheters used for intravenous access, *Infect Control Hosp Epidemiol* (26):708-714, 2005.

Danschutter D, Braet F, Van Gyseghem E et al: Di-(2-ethylhexyl)-phthalate and deep venous thrombosis in children: a clinical and experimental analysis, *Pediatrics* (119):e742-e753, 2007.

Danzig L, Short L, Collins K et al: Bloodstream infections associated with a needleless intravenous infusion system in patients receiving home infusion therapy, *JAMA* (273):1862-1864, 1995.

de Lemos ML, Hamata L, Vu T: Leaching of diethylhexyl phthalate from polyvinyl chloride materials into etoposide intravenous solutions, *J Oncol Pharm Pract* (11):155-157, 2005.

Do A, Ray B, Banerjee S et al: Bloodstream infection associated with needleless device use and the importance of infection-control practices in the home health care setting, *J Infec Dis* (179):442-448, 1999.

Driscoll DF, Silvestri AP, Bistrian BR et al: Stability of total nutrient admixtures with lipid injectable emulsions in glass versus plastic packaging, *Am J Health Syst Pharm* (64):396-403, 2007.

ECRI: Hazard Report: Common flashlights can cause burns when used for transillumination, *Health Devices* (32)273-274, 2003.

ECRI: Evaluation: needleless connectors, *Health Devices* (37):261-283, 2008.

Elliott G: Basics of U.S. patents and the patent system, *Aaps J* (9):E317-324, 2007.

Fasting S, Gisvold SE: Adverse drug errors in anesthesia, and the impact of coloured syringe labels, *Can J Anaesth* (47):1060-1067, 2000.

FDA: Is the Product a Medical Device?, in *Center for Devices and Radiological Health*, 2002a, Food and Drug Administration.

FDA: Overview of What We Do, in *Center for Devices and Radiological Health*, 2002b, Food and Drug Administration.

FDA: About human factors, in *Center for Devices and Radiological Health*, 2006, Food and Drug Administration.

FDA: *About MedSun, in Center for Devices and Radiological Health*, Rockville, Md, 2008, Food and Drug Administration.

Feldman MD, Petersen AJ, Karliner LS et al: Who is responsible for evaluating the safety and effectiveness of medical devices? The role of independent technology assessment, *J Gen Intern Med* (23)Suppl 1:57-63, 2008.

Field K, McFarlane C, Cheng A et al: Incidence of catheter-related bloodstream infection among patients with a needleless, mechanical valve-based intravenous connector in an Australian hematology-oncology unit, *Infect Control Hosp Epidemiol* (28):610-13, 2007.

Foster J, Richards R, Showell M: Intravenous in-line filters for preventing morbidity and mortality in neonates, *Cochrane Database Syst Rev* CD005248, 2006.

Gahart B, Nazazreno A: *Intravenous medications*, St. Louis, 2008, Mosby.

Gosbee J: Human factors engineering and patient safety, *Qual Saf Health Care* (11):352-354, 2002.

Grout J, Mistake-proofing the design of health care processes, *in* A. f. H. R. a. Quality, Rockville, Md, 2007, AHRG.

Guyton A, Hall J: *Textbook of medical physiology* , Philadelphia, 2006, Saunders.

Hadaway L: Intermittent intravenous administration sets: Survey of current practices, *J Vasc Access* (12):143-147, 2007.

Hadaway L: Misuse of prefilled flush syringes, *Infect Contr Res* (4):2-4, 2008.

Haslam GM, Sims C, McIndoe AK et al: High latent drug administration error rates associated with the introduction of the international colour coding syringe labelling system, *Eur J Anaesthesiol* (23):165-168, 2006.

Hirakawa KM, Makino K et al: Evaluation of the in-line filters for the intravenous infusion of amphotericin B fluid, *J Clin Pharm Ther* (24):387-392, 1999a.

Hirakawa M, Sendo T, Kataoka Y et al: High speed injection of radiographic contrast media induces severe particulate contamination, *Br J Radiol* (72):998-999, 1999b.

Husch M, Sullivan C, Rooney D et al: Insights from the sharp end of intravenous medication errors: implications for infusion pump technology, *Qual Saf Health Care* (14):80-86, 2005.

INS: Infusion Nursing Standards of Practice, *J Infus Nurs* 29(Suppl 1S), 2006.

ISMP, Problems persist with life-threatening tubing misconnections: ISMP Medication Safety Alert, 2004, p. 1.

Jacobs B, Schilling S, Doellman D et al: Central venous catheters occlusion: a prospective, controlled trial examining the impact of a positive-pressure valve device, *J Parenter Enteral Nutr* (28):113-118, 2004.

Jain S, Persaud D, Peri T et al: Nosocomial malaria and saline flush, *Emerging Infectious Disease* (11):1097-1099, 2005.

Kagel E, Rayan G: Intravenous catheter complications in the hand and forearm, *J Trauma* (56):123-127, 2004.

Kaiser B, Eagan PD, Shaner H: Solutions to health care waste: life-cycle thinking and "green" purchasing, *Environ Health Perspect* (109):205-207, 2001.

Kaplan AV, Baim DS, Smith JJ et al: Medical device development: from prototype to regulatory approval, *Circulation* (109):3068-3072, 2004.

Kavlock, R: NTP-CERHR Monograph on the potential human reproductive and development effect of Di(2-Ethylhexyl) Phthalate (DEHP), *in* N.T. Program, U.S. Department of Health and Human Services, 2006.

Kellerman S, Shay D, Howard J et al: Bloodstream infections in home infusion patients: The influence of race and needleless intravascular access devices, *J Pediatr* (129):711-717, 1996.

Keohane CA, Hayes J, Saniuk C et al: Intravenous medication safety and smart infusion systems: lessons learned and future opportunities, *J Infus Nurs* (28):321-328, 2005.

Kokotis K: Cost containment and infusion services, *J Infus Nurs* (28):S22-S32, 2005.

Kremkau F: *Diagnostic ultrasound*, Philadelphia, 2002, Saunders.

Krouwer, JS: An improved failure mode effects analysis for hospitals, *Arch Pathol Lab Med* (128):663-667, 2004.

Kuramoto K, Shoji T, Nakagawa Y: Usefulness of the final filter of the IV infusion set in intravenous administration of drugs—contamination of injection preparations by insoluble microparticles and its causes, *Yakugaku Zasshi* (126):289-295, 2006.

Ladak SS, Chan VW, Easty T et al: Right medication, right dose, right patient, right time, and right route: how do we select the right patient-controlled analgesia (PCA) device? *Pain Manag Nurs* (8)140-145, 2007.

LaViolette P: Medical devices and conflict of interest: Unique issues and industry code to address them, *Cleve Clin J Med* (74)S26-S28, 2007.

Lawson M, Vertenstein MJ: Methods for determining the internal volume of central venous catheters, *J Intraven Nurs* (16)148-155, 1993.

Lehr HA, Brunner J, Rangoonwala R et al: Particulate matter contamination of intravenous antibiotics aggravates loss of functional capillary density in postischemic striated muscle, *Am J Respir Crit Care Med* (165):514-520, 2002.

Loff PD, Subotic U, Oulmi-Kagermann J et al: Diethylhexylphthalate extracted by typical newborn lipid emulsions from polyvinylchloride infusion systems causes significant changes in histology of rabbit liver, *J Parenter Enteral Nutr* (31):188-193, 2007.

Loff S, Hannmann T, Subotic U et al: Extraction of diethylhexylphthalate by home total parenteral nutrition from polyvinyl chloride infusion lines commonly used in the home, *J Pediatr Gastroenterol Nutr* (47):81-86, 2008.

Maisel WH: Medical device regulation: an introduction for the practicing physician, *Ann Intern Med* (140):296-302, 2004.

Maragakis LL, Bradley KL, Song X et al: Increased catheter-related bloodstream infection rates after the introduction of a new mechanical valve intravenous access port, *Infect Control Hosp Epidemiol* (27):67-70, 2006.

Marschall J., Mermel LA, Classen D et al: Strategies to prevent central line-associated bloodstream infections in acute care hospitals, *Infect Contr Hosp Epidemiol* (29):S22-S30, 2008.

Mirtallo J, Canada T, Johnson D et al: Safe practices for parenteral nutrition, *J Parenter Enteral Nutr* (28):S39-70, 2004.

Nelson R: AJN Reports: Reprocessed single-use devices- Safe or Not? *Am J Nurs* (106):25-26, 2006.

NIOSH: Preventing occupational exposures to antineoplastic and other hazardous drugs in health care settings, *in* Health and Human Services, ed., 2004, Cincinnati, OH, NIOSH.

O'Grady, N, Alexander M, Dellinger E et al: Guideline for the prevention of intravascular catheter-related infections, *MMWR*, (51):1-26, 2002.

Ortolano, GA, Russell RL, Angelbeck JA, et al: Contamination control in nursing with filtration. Part 1: filters applied to intravenous fluids and point-of-use hospital water, *J Infus Nurs* (27):89-103, 2004.

Pettit J: Trimming of peripherally inserted central catheter: the end results, *J Vascular Access* (11):209-214, 2006.

Pierce CA, Baker JJ: A nursing process model: quantifying infusion therapy resource consumption, *J Infus Nurs* (27):232-244, 2004.

Powers F: Effectively evaluating and converting your organization to the use of infusion safety products: *J Infus Nurs* (25):S10-S14, 2002.

Renner C: Polyurethane vs. silicone PICC catheters, *J Vasc Access* (3):16-21, 1998.

Roback J, Combs M, Grossman B et al: *Technical manual*, Bethesda, Md, 2008, American Association of Blood Banks.

Rupp M, Sholtz L, Jourdan D et al: Outbreak of bloodstream infection temporally associated with the use of an intravascular needleless valve, *Clin Infect Dis* (44):1408-1414, 2007.

Rutala W, editor: *Disinfection, sterilization and antisepsis: principles, practices, current issues and new research,* Washington, DC, 2007, Association for Professionals in Infection Control and Epidemiology, Inc.

Salgado C, Chinnes L, Paczesny T et al: Increased rate of catheter-related bloodstream infection associated with use of a needleless mechanical valve device at a long-term acute care hospital, *Infect Control Hosp Epidemiol* (28):684-688, 2007.

Schears G: Summary of product trials for 10,164 patients: Comparing an intravenous stabilizing device to tape, *J Infus Nurs* (29):225-231, 2006.

Schilling S, Doellman E, Hutchinson N et al: The impact of needleless connector device design on central venous catheter occlusion in children: a prospective controlled trial, *J Parenter Enteral Nutr* (30):85-90, 2006.

Scott W, Weeks C: Medical device standards, *J Vasc Access* (8):47-48, 2003.

Sendo T, Makino K, Nakashima K et al: Particulate contamination of lyophilized amphotericin B preparation during reconstitution process, *J Clin PharmTher* (26):87-91, 2001.

Skryabina EA, Dunn TS: Disposable infusion pumps, *Am J Health Syst Pharm* (63):1260-1268, 2006.

Sethna NF, Verghese ST, Hannallah RS, Soldink JC et al: A randomized controlled trial to evaluate s-caine patch for redundancy pain associated with vascular access in children, *Anesthesiology* 102:403-408, 2005.

Taxis K, Barber N: Causes of intravenous medication errors: an ethnographic study, *Qual Saf Health Care* (12):343-347, 2003a.

Taxis K, Barber N: Ethnographic study of incidence and severity of intravenous drug errors, *BMJ* (326):684, 2003b.

The Joint Commission: Accreditation Programs: Hospitals-Standards FAQs Behavioral Health Care Restraint and Seclusion , Oakbrook Terrace, IL, 2005, The Joint Commissionwww.jointcommission.org/AccreditationPrograms/Hospitals/Standards/FAQs/Provision+of+Care/Restraint+and+Seclusion/Restraint_Seclusion.htm

Thomas J: The use of polymers in IV catheters, *J Vasc Access* (7):25-33, 2002.

Trissel LA, Xu QA, Baker M: Drug compatibility with new polyolefin infusion solution containers, *Am J Health Syst Pharm* (63):2379-2382, 2006.

Trossman S: Hazardous conditions: the ANA, nurses work to inform colleagues about safer drug handling, *Am J Nurs* (106):75-78, 2006.

Trotter C: Why are we trimming peripherally inserted central venous catheters? *Neonatal Network* (23):82-83, 2004.

van Lingen RA, Baerts W, Marquering AC et al: The use of in-line intravenous filters in sick newborn infants: *Acta Paediatrica* (93):658-662, 2004.

Walpot H, Francke RP, Burchard WG et al: Particulate contamination of intravenous solutions and drug additives during long-term intensive care, *Anaesthesist* (38):544-548, 1989.

Weinstein SM: *Plumer's principles & practices of intravenous therapy*, ed 8, Phildelphia, 2007, Lippincott Williams & Wilkins.

Wetterneck TB, Skibinski KA, Roberts TL et al: Using failure mode and effects analysis to plan implementation of smart i.v. pump technology, *Am J Health Syst Pharm* (63):1528-1538, 2006.

Yamamoto A, Solomon J, Soulen M et al: Sutureless securement device reduces complications of peripherally inserted central venous catheters, *J Vasc Interven Radiol* (13):77-81, 2002.

Yang L, Milutinovic PS, Brosnan RJ et al: The plasticizer di(2-ethylhexyl)phthalate modulates gamma-aminobutyric acid type A and glycine receptor function, *Anesth Analg* (105):393-396, 2007.

Yorioka K, Oie S, Oomaki M et al: Particulate and microbial contamination in in-use admixed intravenous infusions, *Biol Pharm Bull* (29):2321-2323, 2006.

Yucha C, Russ P, Baker S: Detecting IV infiltrations using a Venoscope®, *J Intraven Nurs* (20):50-55, 1997.

21 PRODUCT SELECTION AND EVALUATION

Crystal Miller, BSN, MA, RN, CRNI®*

Product selection and evaluation of infusion therapy equipment are critical to effective infusion nursing practice. With the vast number of products on the market, a methodical approach to product selection and evaluation will help the infusion nurse and health care administrator identify cost-effective, appropriate infusion products for safe, high-quality patient care delivery. A standard process for introducing a new product helps ensure that all patient care areas using a given product will be included. It also helps to prevent duplicate products from entering the system. Standardization simplifies training, procedure development, and the purchasing process, and improves the opportunity to negotiate more cost-effective purchase contracts.

Important steps in the process of selecting a product include recognizing and documenting the need for equipment, scanning the market, and identifying essential features of the device. Once the product has been selected, each member of the product evaluation committee plays a specific role in the comprehensive evaluation process. Verbal and written communication of the process must be conveyed to the users of the equipment to ensure proper evaluation. Finally, the financial aspects of purchasing or leasing new products must be considered. Product pricing must not be the primary factor in product selection because poor-quality products may lead to increased use, patient trauma, or liability issues. Cost analysis and justification will enable efficient and appropriate decisions to be made in choosing a new product or in demonstrating the need to continue using an existing product.

This chapter discusses the related processes of product selection and evaluation. This chapter is intended to help the infusion nurse make educated and informed selections of infusion products, ensuring safe delivery of infusion therapy without compromising quality patient care.

THE ROLE OF NURSES IN PRODUCT SELECTION AND EVALUATION

As the most likely end-users of infusion products, nurses possess the expertise, knowledge, and experience to participate in product evaluation. The nurse's awareness of the cost-effectiveness

FOCUS ON EVIDENCE

Impact of Product Evaluation

- A prospective product trial was conducted to examine the rate of restarts and complications associated with the use of tape versus the catheter stabilization device (StatLock) to secure peripheral IVs (PIVs). Data were obtained from 10,164 patients in 83 hospitals who had 15,004 PIVs. Infusion teams were present in 16 of the hospitals (19%). A 67% reduction ($p <.001$) of complications with a 76% reduction in unscheduled restarts was observed in patients with the StatLock device. Cost savings of \$18,000 per hospital for PIV materials as well as \$277,000 for overall reduction in cost associations with complications were estimated (Schears, 2006).

- A prospective, sequential clinical trial compared three securement methods of peripheral IV catheters (PIVs) to extend dwell times for implementation of a 96-hour scheduled change protocol. Nonsterile tape, StatLock™ and HubGuard™ were evaluated. Results of the trial indicated a 52% survival time for StatLock versus 9% for HubGuard and 8% for nonsterile tape. Despite its descriptive nature, this study does provide evidence supporting the use of mechanical securement devices for a 96-hour PIV change protocol (Smith, 2006).

of current products and new technology is critical to the evaluation process (INS, 1997). Because the nurse provides direct patient care, he or she is cognizant of the benefits and complications associated with infusion products.

The nurse's education and experience should be considered before a product is replaced or a new product is introduced. Depending on the organization's policies and procedures, the practitioner's professional status may determine who uses the equipment. For instance, a licensed practical nurse may not be permitted to regulate IV infusions via an infusion pump but

*The author and editors wish to acknowledge the contributions made by Mary C. Alexander as author of this chapter in the second edition of *Infusion Therapy in Clinical Practice*.

may operate an infusion controller. If the organization's nursing population is largely made up of licensed practical nurses, the most appropriate choice for that institution would be to purchase controllers.

Health care professionals must be educated in the use and operation of the product. The practitioner must know how to operate the equipment to ensure that safe infusion therapy is delivered to the patient and operator error is minimized. Reading the product literature, familiarizing oneself with the product, and observing precautions are necessary measures to guarantee safe, efficient operation. References should be available and supervision provided if the nurse requires additional assistance.

Educational programs should include the reasons for the change in products because staff cooperation and understanding can greatly enhance the effectiveness of the evaluation. During the evaluation, the nurse should be aware of the importance of reporting a product defect or malfunction. Documenting the problem, using another product, returning to the formerly used product until the problem is corrected, and contacting the company representative are appropriate responses to a defect or malfunction. Actively involving the nurse in the evaluation process fosters professional accountability and growth for both the individual and the organization.

PRODUCT SELECTION PROCESS

IDENTIFYING THE NEED FOR A PRODUCT CHANGE

To begin the product selection process, the organization must determine a need for changing equipment or purchasing a new product. Patient care requirements drive this process. The rationale for change should fall into one of the following categories: cost considerations, safety considerations, or product effectiveness.

Because cost containment and fiscal constraints are critical issues, product prices must be carefully compared. Lower prices may not be equated with cost-efficiency. Therefore purchasing a less costly item may not be cost-effective if poor product performance leads to increased product use. If custom-made products are desired, the associated high cost may preclude their use in the organization.

Some products require associated equipment. An electronic infusion device may require a dedicated administration set, whereas extension sets and injection caps may be necessary to complete a catheter insertion component. In the case of IV start kits, buying each item individually may be less expensive than purchasing an assembled kit. When calculating the cost of a device, organizational policies, nursing time, and also the extra expense of the added equipment must be included to reflect the true cost of the product. Other considerations include storage space, the time needed to process the order, and the additional time required for the user to assemble the necessary supplies.

Operating costs must be taken into account in addition to acquisition costs. One product may cost less than another, but if priming the device or training the patient is very time-consuming, any cost advantage may be outweighed by the additional labor involved (Schleis and Tice, 1996).

In addition to the price of the product, the manufacturer's product support capabilities need to be considered. Historically, the length of time the company has been in business is important. Additionally, educational needs must be considered.

Manufacturers' proposals and competitive bidding should be compared to ensure an appropriate and cost-effective arrangement for the organization.

Safety must be considered when initiating the product selection process. As stated in *Infusion Nursing Standards of Practice*, "the infusion nurse...should interact with other members of the health care team to provide safe, quality infusion therapy" (INS, 2006). Technological advancement has resulted in product innovation, evident in the more-concentrated and potent forms of medications being administered. Therefore when products are selected and evaluated, specific product safety features should be considered. For instance, infusion control devices should have features that reduce the risk of accidental free flow and alarms that detect air, malfunctions, or occlusions (INS, 2006). A lock-out mechanism may be necessary to make the device tamper proof. When evaluating venous access devices, needlestick protection features should be assessed. Safety components that capture or resheath needles or those that make it difficult to accidentally or intentionally negate a safety mechanism need to be considered. Inserting catheters with safety features can reduce the risk of accidental needlesticks to the patient and the practitioner. Safer products, although sometimes more expensive, may actually save money by reducing the organization's exposure to liability claims.

The consistency of the product's effectiveness also needs to be assessed. A review of maintenance records and product features will help determine how consistently the product produces the desired results. An on-line search of product complaints and recalls should be conducted. Technological advances and the product's ease and range of use should be examined.

Technological changes have resulted in improved quality and technique. Infusion control devices have become more sophisticated to accommodate the administration of potent medications and therefore are more valuable in acute care settings. Conversely, some infusion control devices have been designed simply enough that the patient can be taught to use them; these devices have become assets in home care settings.

Improved technique can be demonstrated by the use of transparent semipermeable membrane dressings. If these dressings, instead of gauze dressings, are applied on an IV insertion site, the area can be seen and inspected without removal of the dressing.

The ease of product use should be investigated. The education and experience of the end-user may affect the success of a product's introduction. If an organization has a high staff turnover rate, less complicated equipment may facilitate orientation and decrease errors. For home care patients, the complexity of a product may be an issue because the patient and caregiver will need to be taught how to use it competently and be prepared for troubleshooting when necessary.

A product's range of use depends on several factors, including the needs of the patient, the anticipated uses for the product, the patient population using the product, and the clinical settings in which the product will be used.

Patient needs are considered when assessing new products. Particular patient populations have varying needs. For example, home care patients whose homes are not equipped with electricity require battery-powered infusion devices to administer their therapy. The size and weight of ambulatory pumps are concerns for patients who wish to maintain their normal activities.

Anticipated product uses must be defined. For instance, when evaluating infusion control devices, the types of solutions and medications to be administered are considered. Specific features may be required to infuse such therapies as narcotics, chemotherapy, and parenteral nutrition. IV catheters, whether being used for short- or long-term therapy, vary in terms of product design and materials. Many types of peripheral, central, and peripherally inserted central catheters are available.

The patient population using the product is another consideration. An infusion pump used in the hospital may be a more sophisticated device than one used in the home. For instance, in the acute care setting, medications may need to be titrated to one tenth of a milliliter. Patients requiring the administration of epidural anesthesia, vasoconstrictors, or chemotherapy may need specific equipment to closely monitor drug delivery. In the case of the home care patient requiring cyclic parenteral nutrition during the night, the infusion device would need a specialized titrating feature. Therefore the nurse should be aware of the patient's clinical conditions that warrant specific products to deliver the appropriate treatments.

The clinical setting in which the product will be used should be considered. If an infusion pump is used primarily in an intensive care unit, the size of the device (i.e., whether one IV pole can have several pumps safely attached to it) and its ability to titrate medications are major considerations. The size of a pump is also a concern for the home care patient who wishes to maintain normal activities; a compact, portable device is preferred. In the case of the patient receiving long-term antibiotic therapy at home, a peripherally inserted central catheter instead of a short peripheral catheter is usually the appropriate device for medication delivery. The peripherally inserted central catheter may remain in place indefinitely, whereas a peripheral catheter has to be changed every 72 hours or sooner if complications such as phlebitis or infiltration occur (INS, 2006).

TIMING A PRODUCT CHANGE

Incident occurrences may indicate the need for product change. Evolving patterns that demonstrate product errors or defects can threaten safe infusion therapy and patient outcomes, warranting a product change.

It is important to review the patient care areas that will be affected by a product change to ensure that the product selected is representative of the patient's needs. The organization should then determine whether the proposed product is a necessity or a luxury. For example, an infusion control device should have alarms that detect air, occlusion, and malfunction, but a feature for titration may not be necessary if that mode is seldom used.

EXPLORING POTENTIAL PRODUCTS

Once the need for a product has been established, the next step is to document that need, draft a proposal of intention, and explore the market. Reviewing current literature, attending trade shows, and interviewing organizations currently using the product are effective ways to obtain product information.

Conducting a literature review provides material about current products. Marketing brochures and articles in nursing and pharmacy journals about infusion therapy provide useful information on infusion equipment. Scientific, health, and cost-outcomes research that objectively identifies the qualities of patients who will benefit from various types of infusion technology should be requested from manufacturers (McConnell, 1998). Information from the Emergency Care Research Institute (www.ecri.org) may be beneficial. This independent

organization evaluates medical equipment, publishes journals featuring comparative evaluations and ratings of products, and reports hazards and problems of medical devices.

Attending trade shows is another way to obtain product information. Trade shows offer the opportunity to see and use devices and to speak with company representatives. Manufacturing representatives demonstrate their products, enabling cursory evaluations. Trade show reviews help narrow the field of available products early in the selection process by eliminating equipment inappropriate for the organization.

In addition, interviewing other organizations regarding their experiences with products can provide useful information about equipment, including advantages and disadvantages. Site visits also provide an opportunity to visualize use of the product for a given population or a variety of patient populations.

IDENTIFYING NECESSARY PRODUCT FEATURES

Before a product is changed or a new product selected, written criteria should be developed that include the product's necessary features. To ensure that all aspects of a product are considered, the most important as well as the least important features should be included in the criteria (DiGirolamo, 1995). Input from all departments using the product should be considered when developing the guidelines because each practitioner's perspective is valuable. This material will be used to narrow the field for the final hands-on evaluation. In addition, this information will be incorporated into a preliminary evaluation form for product selection. Table 21-1 identifies characteristics worth assessing in four products: catheters, transparent semipermeable membrane dressings, administration sets, and needleless systems.

PRELIMINARY EVALUATION FORM FOR PRODUCT SELECTION

Once product guidelines are established, a product evaluation form is created. The evaluation form may be designed by the infusion team, the product evaluation committee, or a task force addressing a particular product. This evaluation form is helpful in preliminary product selection. The form encourages objective ratings and product comparisons. This process also encourages price bidding and may result in lower costs.

As many products as possible should be reviewed during this initial phase, which helps narrow the field for the actual hands-on evaluations. It is not feasible to evaluate all the devices on the market; the cost of doing so, in time and money, is prohibitive.

To facilitate product selection, the entries on the form should coincide with the product guidelines. Spaces for the product name, manufacturer, person evaluating the product, dates of evaluation, and comments should be included. Figure 21-1 illustrates the information to be included on a preliminary product evaluation form, and Table 21-2 and Box 21-1 provide guidelines for its use.

 CONDUCTING A PRODUCT EVALUATION

PRODUCT EVALUATION COMMITTEE

A product evaluation committee facilitates product selection and evaluation with decision-making. This group should be broad based and multidisciplinary; it should include representatives from departments affected directly or indirectly by the use of

TABLE 21-1 Product Guidelines

Features	Considerations
Catheters	
Packaging	Is the package easy to open? Is sterility easily maintained after the package is opened? Can the package be easily stored or discarded?
Handling	Is the catheter easy to hold? Do features make it awkward to handle?
Length	What lengths are available?
Sizes	What gauge sizes are available? What French sizes are available for PICCs?
Lumens	Is it available with multiple lumens?
Radiopacity	Is it radiopaque?
Ease of insertion	Does the needle penetrate the skin easily or with resistance? Does the needle appear dull?
Catheter advancement	Does the catheter advance easily? Is sterility maintained while it is advanced?
Catheter flexibility	Does the catheter retain its shape? Does it have power injectable capabilities?
Blood return	Is blood return quickly visible?
Needleless feature	Does the needleless feature capture or resheath the stylet after insertion? Is user activation necessary? Can it be determined whether the safety feature is activated? Can the safety feature be deactivated? Does the safety feature remain protective through disposal? Are features available to prevent blood contamination?
Catheter stabilization	Can the catheter be easily secured to prevent movement? Can a dressing be applied that does not interfere with assessment of the insertion site?
Transparent Semipermeable Membrane Dressings	
Ease of application	Is the dressing easy to apply? Is sterility maintained when applying? Is a one- or two-handed method needed for application?
Adhesive quality	Does the dressing adhere adequately to the skin? Is it difficult to remove?
Water resistance	Is it water resistant?
Air permeability	Is it air permeable?
Administration Sets	
Injection ports	How many injection/access ports are available? Are the ports an integral part of the administration set or do they have to be added?
Clamps	How many clamps are available? What types of clamps are on the administration set?
Drop size	What drop sizes are available?
Filters	Is an in-line filter available on the administration set? Can a filter be added to the administration set?
Length	What lengths are available?
Luer-Lok™ design	Is a Luer-Lok™ feature available?
Compatibility with infusates	Does the composition of the infusate make it incompatible for use with certain administration sets?
Compatibility with existing equipment	Can the administration set be used with existing products or devices?
Needleless Systems	
Packaging	Is the packaging easy to open? Is sterility maintained after opening? Will storage and disposal be a problem?
Number of components	Are separate components needed to complete the system?
Ease of use	Is the system easy to handle? Are there features that make it awkward to handle?
Compatibility with existing equipment	Can it be used with existing equipment?
Injection/access port	Does it allow for use of needles? Is it valve activated or a split septum?
Compatibility of infusates	Can all types of infusates be delivered via this system?
Infection prevention	Does the device increase the risk of infection? How easy is it to clean before accessing? To obtain access, does the system have to be opened to the air?

the product. This committee participates in the preliminary selection process and ongoing product evaluations, and acts as an end-reviewer for product decisions. The product evaluation committee considers the product's merits and assesses its range of use within the organization before deciding to either endorse or deny support for the purchase (DiGirolamo, 1995; Hinson and Blough, 1996; Hostutler, 1996; Evans, Riccardi, and Hart, 2007; Valenti and Herwaldt, 1997). The committee should include representatives from infusion therapy, nursing, medical staff, infection control, pharmacy, materials management, and purchasing. Representatives from information technology and biomedical engineering are also included as needed. Each person will have specific concerns relative to his or her discipline. In some situations, one committee member may represent more than one discipline. For instance, in a small home care company, the pharmacist may also be the purchasing agent and the materials management director. Subcommittees or task force groups may be convened to evaluate a specific infusion product.

Product _____   Evaluation Date _____

Evaluator _____

RATING: 4 = highly satisfactory; 3 = more than satisfactory;
2 = satisfactory; 1 = less than satisfactory;
0 = not acceptable

Guidelines	Manufacturer					
Alarms						
Battery life						
Rate range						
Accuracy						
PSI						
Size of machine						
Titration						
Types of infusates						
Easy to read						
Directions on machine						
Free-flow protection						
Tamper proof						
Piggyback mode						
Associated equipment needs						
Total						

Comments: _____

FIGURE 21-1   Example of a preliminary product evaluation form.

The organization may choose to evaluate a product within the facility or do a thorough review of products followed by a site visit to see the product in action. If the product selection includes an evaluation process, a committee should be selected.

Infusion therapy department representatives are integral members of the evaluation committee and infusion nurses are a good choice for committee leadership. Their clinical expertise is beneficial to the process, and they can identify favorable and unfavorable features of a product. In addition, they review products for appropriate and safe clinical use. They should be used as resources during the evaluation process, and their comments are valuable at the point of final product selection. If infusion nurses are not available in an institution, the Infusion Nurses Society or other professional networks may provide useful product information or clinical insight.

The committee should include members of the nursing department. Depending on the product to be tested, staff nurses may participate in the hands-on evaluation of the devices. The evaluators must be aware of the importance of completing the evaluation forms and conveying any comments about the product to the designated person on the committee.

Suggestions from physicians are beneficial because they may identify advantages and disadvantages of the product from a different perspective. Physicians may be involved in the hands-on evaluation. For example, the interventional radiologist and the neonatologist may be asked to evaluate a new brand of peripherally inserted central catheters for pediatric patients.

Pharmacists should also be represented on the evaluation committee. Their knowledge of medication administration and infusion capabilities, including guidelines to safeguard the patient, can be valuable. They can advise the committee on the appropriate distribution of products, particularly infusion control devices, within the organization.

Input regarding the efficacy and safety of a product from the infection prevention department may be important to the evaluation. For instance, when evaluating needleless systems, infection control professionals may assist infusion nurses in monitoring sharps injuries or nosocomial infection rates related to a specific product. The infection prevention department may also be helpful when interpreting data from a manufacturer's clinical trials and scientific studies.

A representative from the biomedical engineering department (also referred to as the medical or clinical engineering department) should be included on the committee, especially when electronic devices are being considered. Representatives from this department perform accuracy and pressure tests and disassemble devices to evaluate the quality of design and workmanship. They also provide information on a product's approximate repair and replacement time and cost. Engineering professionals can warn of any design flaws, possible power inadequacies, or incompatibilities with equipment already in use. They may have information on future upgrade capability and vendor histories (Hostutler, 1996).

Materials management representatives on the committee provide valuable information regarding a product's storage requirements. The overall size of product packaging determines the amount that can be put on the infusion nurses' carts and in department storage units. The materials management department is responsible for storing products in easily accessible, sterile places. They address issues that may limit product distribution, consider duplication of products, and raise awareness of similar products in stock that may be confused with the product in question as well as usage information.

Input from the purchasing and/or contracts management department is imperative. These departments manage information on product prices, shipping costs, and buying groups and contract negotiations that encourage competitive bidding. Their goal is to purchase products at low cost without sacrificing quality. With many organizations facing increasing economic pressures, the price of a product may dictate purchasing decisions. Elaborating on patient safety issues may demonstrate the need to buy a more costly product. In addition, the purchasing department performs cost comparisons. For example, the cost of an infusion pump may be low, but the price of the dedicated administration set required for its operation may be higher than a regular administration set. If a custom-designed product is desired, comparisons with other products need to be performed. This department also has insight into equipment and product reimbursement issues.

With computer-driven infusion pump technology, information technology representation on the committee is essential. Information technologists can evaluate features of a pump and determine the feasibility of its software to communicate with the organization's other computer systems. In addition, the capability of the organization's wireless system needs to be assessed in relation to the incoming technology needs.

TABLE 21-2 Infusion Pump Evaluation Guidelines*

Features	Considerations
Alarms	What alarms are included: air, occlusion, door open, malfunction, low battery, infusion complete? Can alarms be silenced? Can volume be adjusted?
Battery life	How long will the pump operate on battery power?
Rate range	What is the rate range? Are tenths-of-milliliter increments available?
Accuracy	What is the percentage of margin of error?
psi	What is the maximum psi exerted? Is the pressure level adjustable?
Size of machine	Can the pump fit easily on an IV pole? Can several fit safely on one IV pole? Are the size and weight of the ambulatory pump conducive to the patient's normal daily activities?
Titration	Can the pump titrate solutions?
Compatibility of infusates	Can all types of infusates, including opaque parenteral nutrition solutions, be infused?
Easy to read	Are commands and buttons easy to read? Are panel lights available to illuminate in a dark room? Can the lettering on the LED screen be seen from a distance?
Directions on machine	Are there permanent directions on the pump for quick reference? Are they easy to understand?
Free-flow protection	Does the device have an anti–free-flow mechanism? Can it be deactivated or circumvented?
Tamper-proof characteristics	Is there a lock-out mechanism to prevent unauthorized tampering?
Piggyback mode	Is this mode available?
Drug library	What drug classifications are included? Can the library be updated easily? How many clinical care areas can be programmed?
Reports	What reports can be generated and how easy are they to get? How much information can be stored and for how long?
Associated equipment needs	Does the pump need dedicated infusion sets?

*Use these guidelines when completing the preliminary product evaluation form seen in Figure 21-1.
IV, intravenous; *psi*, pounds per square inch.

Box 21-1   COMPLETING THE EVALUATION FORM (See Also Figure 21-1)

1. Identify the type of product to be evaluated (e.g., peripheral catheter or infusion device).
2. Document the evaluation date and evaluator's name.
3. Insert product name and model number.
4. Rate each product feature according to a given scale.
5. Add the ratings for each product to determine the total score.
6. Add comments as necessary.

Compile ratings from the evaluation forms: Once a total rating is determined for each product, the committee can narrow the field to a few products for the final hands-on evaluation. The products with the highest scores are chosen to be evaluated. The "Comments" section must be taken into consideration because negative comments may override a high score.

Box 21-2   PRODUCT SELECTION PROCESS

1. Identify and document the need to purchase or change to a new product. Is the product being considered to improve cost-effectiveness, safety, or efficiency?
2. Research competing products by conducting a literature review, attending trade shows, and interviewing facilities using the product.
3. Develop product guidelines by including the most and least important features desired.
4. Complete the preliminary product evaluation form by rating the product using the corresponding guidelines.
5. Narrow the field for hands-on evaluations or a site visit; compile the results from the evaluation forms and select the product.

Other departments, including radiology, anesthesiology, and emergency and operating rooms, may be affected by a product change as well. Inquiries should be made to determine the impact the change may have on different units, and representatives included as needed.

With all committee members working as a team, an informed product choice can be made. Each representative contributes valuable information (Box 21-2). The product evaluation committee's goal is to choose safe, cost-efficient products that are appropriate for the patient and organization; product selections should never compromise quality patient care.

EVALUATION PROCESS

Once the preliminary selection process has been completed, the final evaluation procedure can begin (Box 21-3). The infusion team or the product evaluation committee rates products using established guidelines. When the field is narrowed, the products chosen should be those that are appropriate for the institution based on established criteria. Once all the products have been rated, the committee determines the number to be evaluated by the staff. Usually, no more than two or three products are selected for hands-on evaluation.

Once the committee establishes the number of products to be evaluated, the group delineates the actual evaluation process. The committee then considers such factors as the timeline, the

Box 21-3 FINAL EVALUATION PROCESS

1. Determine the length of time for the evaluation.
2. Identify the location for the evaluation (i.e., several departments or facility-wide testing).
3. Convey to the evaluators the importance of completing the product evaluation forms.
4. Schedule inservice sessions for proper product operation as near to the evaluation start date as possible.
5. Compile evaluation results and make the final decision for product selection.
6. Communicate throughout the facility which product was chosen.
7. Continuously evaluate new products, as well as the ones in use, to ensure that the appropriate product is being used in patient care.

location (e.g., which patient care units), and the staff involved with the hands-on process.

The timeline for the evaluation varies depending on the product. Weeks or months may be needed to complete an effective evaluation. When evaluating electronic infusion devices, it is important to allow sufficient time. Educating the staff in the correct use of the product could take 1 or 2 weeks; therefore 2 to 4 weeks per product may be necessary for all evaluators to have the opportunity to evaluate the products. Some evaluators may like a product because it is new and others will dislike it for the same reason. The length of the evaluation should be sufficient to diminish the novelty effect. When a product is used many times each day, staff will make the transition more quickly than with a product that is used once a day or once a week.

The number of items that will be rated must also be determined. For example, when catheters are tested, the committee will determine how many catheters must be inserted to allow a thorough evaluation. Another way to rate products may be to have a predetermined time frame, such as 3 to 4 weeks. A sufficiently long trial period helps overcome the learning curve required by some products.

The committee must establish the location of the evaluation. In a large organization, the committee may select several patient care units to participate in the study, whereas in a small organization, the evaluation may be conducted throughout the hospital. One of the advantages of selecting certain units within a facility is that by limiting the number of staff involved, the organization can reduce the number of hours dedicated to training. Another advantage is the ability to select hospital units that use the product often and represent diverse patient populations. Units in which there is a high prevalence of central and peripheral catheter insertion, where multiple types of IV medications are administered, and where blood components are transfused can improve the evaluation process because of the varied delivery methods. Data are generated quickly if the selected department uses the product often.

There are also disadvantages to limiting the evaluation to a small number of departments. When a patient is transferred to a unit that is not evaluating the product, the likelihood of incorrect use and errors in operation increases because the staff may not be familiar with the device. When the entire facility is not represented in the evaluation, it may be difficult for staff in nonparticipating units to obtain comprehensive product information.

It is important that guidelines for product evaluations are also established in home care and alternative care settings. Select nurses may test the product or all staff members may participate.

The next step is communicating the evaluation procedure to those involved. An explanation of the importance of the process is essential. When the evaluators understand the purpose of the evaluation, they are more likely to cooperate with the process.

USER EDUCATION

The next step in preparing for the hands-on evaluation is the education of all evaluators. Inservice sessions should be scheduled with the product manufacturer's representative once the product's availability, evaluation start date, and completion date are established. Infusion nurses and all other evaluators need to know how to use the product correctly, so time must be allowed for hands-on practice. To lessen the chance of forgotten details about product operation, the inservice sessions should be conducted as near to the evaluation start date as possible. Written instructions, operating manuals, computer-based learning modules, and videos should be available as resource materials.

EVALUATION FORM

The evaluation form is essential to product evaluation. Data can be obtained in various ways. One method is to have the evaluators rank product performance on a scale ranging from 0 to 5, from "highly satisfactory" to "not acceptable," or from "strongly agree" to strongly disagree." Another way is to ask closed-ended or open-ended questions. Closed-ended questions require only "yes" or "no" answers and may ask evaluators to compare products. Conversely, open-ended questions allow the evaluators to respond with subjective comments. An effective evaluation combines both types of questions on the evaluation form.

The evaluation form can be generic or specific to the product. Either type should be clear and concise. Figure 21-2 is an example of a generic evaluation form that can be used for any product. If a particular product requires a detailed evaluation, the committee should solicit specific information. Figure 21-3 is an evaluation form specific to infusion pumps.

Evaluators must understand the importance of returning their completed forms after they have taken sufficient time to evaluate the device. The frequency of responses should be determined; the evaluators may respond each time they use a product or after using the product for a specified period. A designated area may be assigned where the forms can be placed, or a specific person may have the responsibility of collecting them. Oral comments, both positive and negative, need to be documented to ensure that all information received about a product is compiled for comparison. Evaluators must report equipment problems and complaints. An evaluation may be terminated before the completion date if extensive difficulties are encountered.

MANUFACTURER SUPPORT

Manufacturer support is an important component of product evaluation. The manufacturer's availability and responsiveness when problems occur during the evaluation should be assessed.

Department conducting evaluation _____

Evaluation period to last _____ Days from _____ to _____

	Existing Product	Proposed Product
Description		
Manufacturer		
Model		

Your comments are important to help conduct a thorough product evaluation; please complete this questionnaire and forward to your supervisor.

	YES	NO
1. Have you been in-serviced on the proper use of the product?	____	____
2. Does the product open from its packaging with ease?	____	____
3. If the product is sterile, does it permit sterile transfer from packaging to use site?	____	____
4. Does this product contain all the components necessary for the procedure to be performed?	____	____
If no, which additional items are required?	____	____

_____

5. Does this product contain unnecessary components (resulting in excessive costs) for the procedure to be performed?   ____ ____

If yes, which ones? _____

6. Which characteristics of this product are inferior to those of the existing product?_____

_____

Which characteristics of this product are superior to those of the existing product?_____

_____

7. Do you recommend this product for use in the hospital?   ____ ____

_____ _____ _____
(Name)   (Date)   (Ext.)

Comments: _____

FIGURE 21-2 Example of a generic product evaluation form.

During the trial, the accessibility and receptiveness of the company representative should be observed. Brochures and teaching materials should be available as references. The quality of the representative's inservice training to the staff is assessed. In addition, the manufacturer's follow-up efforts when responding to requests from staff or resolving product difficulties should be observed. When serious problems occur, it is important to note the representative's response as well as that of the company's management. These characteristics indicate the company's quality of service.

COST CONSIDERATIONS

The *Infusion Nursing Standards of Practice* states that the nurse should be actively involved in and accountable for establishing and maintaining the budgetary process that encompasses staffing, education, and products used in infusion nursing (INS, 2006). Responsible financial decisions regarding new products can be made when the infusion nurse specialist takes an active role in product selection.

The cost of the product needs to be justified, and consideration must be given to associated equipment needs. The cost of custom-made items needs to be assessed because they may prove to be exceedingly high. With custom-made products, the prototype should be retained until the actual item is obtained. If problems arise, a comparison of the item with the prototype is warranted. Written evaluations may substantiate product quality.

When the committee narrows the field to a few products, a cost analysis should be conducted. The costs of the different products, including associated equipment requirements, must be compared. In addition to the price of the product, labor

Product _____   Evaluation date _____

Manufacturer _____   Evaluator _____

Complete this form by rating each statement and adding any comments. Return to the Product Evaluation Committee representative.

RATING: 4 = highly satisfactory; 3 = more than satisfactory; 2 = satisfactory;
1 = less than satisfactory; 0 = not acceptable

1. The alarms were easy to identify and troubleshoot.   _____

2. The pump was accurate and reliable.   _____

3. The pump could be easily positioned at the bedside or on an IV pole. The weight of the
    machine did not hinder patient ambulation or transport.   _____

4. The command panel was easy to read.   _____

5. The pump was easy to prime and load.   _____

6. The pump was easy to operate.   _____

7. The directions on the pump were easy to understand.   _____

8. The lock-out mechanism provided additional patient safety.   _____

9. The featured safeguards prevent accidental free-flow of infusates.   _____

10. The in-service education for operation was adequate.   _____

11. Approximately how many times did you use the pump?   _____

Comments: _____

FIGURE 21-3   Example of a product evaluation form for infusion pumps.

costs need to be included. Nurses' time can be calculated relative to the frequency of product use and the time necessary to educate a patient or caregiver on the product's use (DiGirolamo, 1995). In a home care agency, reducing the time and number of home visits required for nurses to teach patients often justifies use of a more expensive product. In a facility where nursing and pharmacy costs are fixed and staffing is not expected to be reduced, the advantage of shorter training times may not be sufficient to warrant a product change (Schleis and Tice, 1996).

To encourage competitive bidding, the organization's negotiators should carefully compare manufacturers' proposals. The evaluation's cost also needs to be considered; the evaluation price can be reduced by having the manufacturer provide the products, as opposed to the organization having to purchase them.

At this stage of the evaluation, the purchasing department takes a more active role. New equipment can be obtained in many ways: the organization may purchase, rent, or lease the products. Renting or leasing may be more advantageous than purchasing because when the lease agreement expires, an updated version of the product may be obtained. Purchase options may include volume discounts, selected option programs, and maintenance contracts.

Group purchasing arrangements may be available to reduce costs. Depending on the product, bidding may be structured in such a way that allows several manufacturers to bid on an individual item rather than a group of products. With the rapid development of new technology, it may be advantageous to limit the duration of a contract, thus allowing the facility to replace outdated equipment more quickly.

PRODUCT SELECTION

When the product trials are completed, a final selection can be made. The product evaluation committee or specific task force tallies the results of the completed evaluation forms and compiles the evaluators' comments. The committee compares product advantages and disadvantages. At this point, if the products are comparable, an enhanced feature may be the determining factor in the final decision. The organization's plan to standardize the product throughout may influence the selection; some products may not be suited to universal use. The manufacturer may offer a product mix to satisfy the organization's varied needs.

Final product selection involves several factors, including product performance, cost, overall evaluation results, and the manufacturer's performance. Product performance must be acceptable and meet the committee's criteria. From a financial standpoint, the least expensive product may not be a high-quality or efficient device; therefore cost should not be the only consideration. To justify purchasing an expensive or superior product, features that reduce user time or eliminate complications may be favorable. Comments from the overall evaluation may illuminate product or service problems. Finally, the company representative's responsiveness must be assessed with regard to the effectiveness of the inservice training, the frequency of follow-up calls, and the response to problems.

COMMUNICATION OF PRODUCT SELECTION

Once the product evaluation committee selects the final product, it must be communicated throughout the organization. Memoranda should be distributed to all units stating which product will be used and when implementation will begin. Policies and procedures will need to be developed for use of the product. Infusion nurses should be involved in establishing the new product's procedures and guidelines for use. Nursing procedure committees, staff education departments, and nursing management may also participate in this process.

The new product may be introduced immediately or gradually, depending on the size of the organization. Smaller organizations may immediately implement the product throughout, whereas large hospitals may find it more effective to have a phase-in plan.

Inservice sessions must be scheduled, with duration dependent on the complexity and sophistication of the product and staff members' skills and training. Because the sessions may be time-consuming, staffing levels may have to be increased during the evaluation and implementation processes. Around-the-clock inservice sessions with the manufacturer may be necessary for one product, whereas viewing of a video may be sufficient instruction for another. For example, operation of an electronic infusion device will probably require in-depth instruction, whereas application of a transparent semipermeable membrane dressing may be demonstrated adequately on a video.

 ## POSTEVALUATION EDUCATION

Once a product has been selected, postevaluation education and problem solving are necessary. Written procedures, training manuals, or posters describing proper operation should be available. Resource materials and personnel should be readily accessible to the staff using the product. Infusion nurses' knowledge and clinical expertise make them excellent resources. Staff members should be allowed sufficient time to learn how to operate the product and should be supported until a comfort level is attained. If staff members appear to have difficulty using the product, additional inservice programs conducted by the company representative may be needed to ensure proper use of the device.

When a product malfunctions or a defect in the device is identified, the serial and lot numbers of the item should be documented. This information helps the vendor locate a problem that may have developed during the manufacturing process. Incident occurrences should be filed. Accumulated information on the product's performance may demonstrate a need for immediate intervention by the manufacturer. According to the Safe Medical Devices Act of 1990, health care organizations are required to report to the Food and Drug Administration the malfunction of a device that causes serious illness, injury, or death (Deacon, 2004).

To ensure quality infusion care, product evaluation must be ongoing. Practitioners may like the product initially, but over time they may cease using it. Reasons for this failure need to be identified. Additional inservice education may be needed, the device may be faulty, or there may be an inadequate supply to meet the organization's needs.

 ## SUMMARY

Health care organizations must have processes in place to select and evaluate new products to ensure that the most appropriate products are used for patient care. The infusion nurse plays an important role in the product selection and evaluation processes. Educated product selection choices enable safe, efficient delivery of infusion therapy to the patient. A methodical approach facilitates this process. Written evaluations help demonstrate objective rationales for selecting particular products. The evaluation process may demonstrate that a product improves technique or patient safety and is cost-efficient, or it may conclude that the product in use is appropriate for the patient and the organization. Ongoing evaluation of products in use is important in the delivery of high-quality patient care. The infusion nurse's participation with his or her colleagues from other departments enhances commitment to the specialty and to the health care organization and provides personal satisfaction. Assuming an active role in product selection and evaluation contributes to the infusion nurse's sense of professional accomplishment as his or her suggestions and recommendations are applied to clinical practice.

 ## REFERENCES

Deacon VL: The safe medical device act and its impact on clinical practice, *J Infus Nurs* 27(1):31, 2004.

DiGirolamo D: Professional product evaluation, *J Infus Nurs* 18(2):79, 1995.

Evans G, Riccardi C, Hart B: Replacing medical equipment, *24X7*, March 2007.

Hinson EK, Blough LD: Skilled IV therapy clinicians' product evaluation of open-ended versus closed-ended valve PICC lines, *J Infus Nurs* 19(4):198, 1996.

Hostutler JJ: A better way to select medical equipment, *Nurs Manag* 27(9):32, 1996.

Infusion Nurses Society: Infusion nursing standards of practice, *J Infus Nurs* 29(Suppl 1), 2006.

Intravenous Nurses Society: Position paper: the registered nurse's role in product purchase, *J Infus Nurs* 20(2):69, 1997.

McConnell, EA: Infusion devices require educated users, *Nurs Manag* 29(11):55, 1998.

Schears GJ: Summary of product trials for 10,164 patients: comparing an intravenous stabilizing device to tape, *J Infus Nurs* 29(4):225, 2006.

Schleis TG, Tice AD: Selecting infusion devices for use in ambulatory care, *Am J Health Syst Pharm* 53(8):868, 1996.

Smith, B: Peripheral intravenous catheter dwell times: a comparison of 3 securement methods for implementation of a 96-hour scheduled change protocol, *J Infus Nurs* 29(1):14, 2006.

Valenti WM, Herwaldt LA: Product evaluation, *Infect Control Hosp Epidemiol* 18(10):722, 1997.

CHAPTER

22 PATIENT ASSESSMENT AS RELATED TO FLUID AND ELECTROLYTE BALANCE

Rose Anne Lonsway, BSN, MA, RN, CRNI®

Knowledge and recognition of potential problems associated with a fluid or electrolyte imbalance are critical to patient care. This chapter describes basic patient assessment as it relates to fluid volume and electrolyte dynamics. Patient history, clinical assessment, and correct interpretation of laboratory data are valuable components of this process.

ASSESSMENT TECHNIQUES

The physical assessment of a patient is one of the most important functions that a nurse performs. The results of the initial assessment develop the baseline for the patient's care and treatment. Ongoing assessment charts the patient's response to treatment and provides data to measure outcomes. The nurse uses many skills during the assessment and builds a relational database by synthesizing bits of information into a total picture of the patient.

The skills used in assessment include inspection, auscultation, palpation, and percussion, as well as observation, inquiry, and listening. One of the critical skills for the clinician is to provide a safe environment in which to conduct the assessment, enabling the patient to speak freely about personal and private matters. The safe environment allows trust and a level

of comfort to develop between the clinician and the patient, resulting in more accurate data collection. The clinician should also provide information about findings; this helps the patient gain an understanding of his or her state of health and allows mutual goal and outcome development to begin. These skills are used in combination, system by system, as the assessment progresses. This chapter focuses on those aspects of physical assessment related to alterations in fluid and electrolyte balance.

PATIENT HISTORY

To understand how the body responds to its internal environment, a description of the patient's fluid and electrolyte status must be obtained from the patient. It is difficult to determine the absolute amount of total body water and the relationship between that amount and other mechanisms within the body. The more accurate the history obtained from the patient, the more sensitive the monitoring process will be for specific alterations.

Information obtained from the patient should include medical and family history. For example, although the patient may not exhibit signs or symptoms of diabetes, there may be a family history of diabetes. As the course of the patient's treatment unfolds, latent diabetes may manifest itself. When this information is obtained from a comprehensive patient history, the nurse is attentive to signs and symptoms of alterations in levels of blood glucose or electrolytes and to laboratory findings.

The patient's medical history should establish the baseline status or "normal" for the patient, as well as indicate whether there is a risk for or a history of fluid and electrolyte alterations and how the alteration and course of treatment were tolerated. Although the information may not currently be clinically significant, it may be applied to future treatment.

CURRENT STATUS

When reviewing body systems in conjunction with a physical assessment, the nurse should listen carefully to the patient's description of the chief complaint. Many fluid and electrolyte

TABLE 22-1 Fluid and Electrolyte Imbalances Associated with Selected Diseases or Conditions

Disease or condition	Potential imbalance
Crushing injuries	Potassium excess
	Plasma to interstitial fluid shift
Head injury	Sodium deficit
SIADH	Sodium deficit
Renal failure	Sodium deficit
	Phosphorus excess
	Magnesium excess
Gastrointestinal losses	Potassium deficit
	Magnesium deficit
Congestive heart failure	Fluid volume excess
Acute pancreatitis	Calcium deficit
	Magnesium deficit
	Hypovolemia
Dehydration	Calcium excess
Selected tumors	Calcium excess
Diabetes mellitus	Metabolic acidosis
	Fluid volume deficit
Diabetes insipidus	Sodium excess
Emphysema	Respiratory acidosis
Diuretic therapy	Potassium excess
	Potassium deficit
Prolonged immobilization	Calcium excess
Cirrhosis (hepatic)	Fluid volume excess
	Sodium deficit

SIADH, Syndrome of inappropriate antidiuretic hormone.

imbalances are insidious and require careful history taking and monitoring to prevent further problems. If the patient has suffered an injury, the type and degree of injury should be ascertained because injury may affect the patient's fluid and electrolyte balance (Table 22-1).

Patients should be questioned to determine whether they suffer from any illness or condition that affects fluid and electrolyte balance. For example, in heart failure the patient is at risk for fluid volume excess. Metabolic aberrations, such as diabetes mellitus, can put the patient at risk for metabolic acidosis and fluid volume deficits. Episodes of acute pancreatitis can result in calcium deficits. Conditions such as emphysema cause a respiratory acidosis that results from the patient's inability to exchange carbon dioxide. Some tumors interfere with the use or uptake of calcium, leading to calcium excess. Prolonged immobilization of a patient may cause calcium excess caused by loss of calcium from the bone into the extracellular fluid. A patient who drinks excessive amounts of plain water may wash out electrolytes, causing potassium or sodium deficits or metabolic alkalosis if the condition is not corrected (Table 22-2).

MEDICATIONS

A thorough medication history should be obtained because any medications or therapeutic regimens, such as steroids or parenteral nutrition, can disrupt fluid or electrolyte balance. For example, potassium-depleting diuretics may cause potassium deficit. Conversely, potassium-sparing diuretics may cause

potassium excess, the opposite of problems anticipated with diuretics. Overuse of laxatives may also result in potassium deficits.

INTAKE AND OUTPUT

The nurse must ascertain whether the patient has experienced a large loss of body fluids from vomiting, diarrhea, or lack of intake. An assessment of dietary alterations or medically imposed dietary restrictions should be made. Questions are asked of the patient to try to elicit any discrepancies in intake and output. Is the patient producing copious amounts of urine, or is the patient drinking large amounts of plain water? Has the patient experienced any draining wounds or high-output fistulas that would cause a discrepancy between intake and output? The answers to these questions must be examined carefully when the history is analyzed and must be kept in mind as the clinical assessment is begun.

 CLINICAL ASSESSMENT

The clinical assessment of a patient includes the initial intake assessment as well as ongoing assessment to monitor a patient's progress and response to therapy. A systems approach is recommended to assess for fluid and electrolyte balances related to infusion therapy.

BODY WEIGHT

An accurate body weight is one of the initial clinical assessment parameters. Changes in body weight accurately reflect fluid loss or gain. An accurate determination of change in weight provides important information and is sometimes easier to obtain than an accurate intake and output record. Rapid changes in the patient's body weight can reflect problems with the fluid balance status. One way to approximate the amount of fluid gain or loss is to compare the equivalent between kilograms and liters of fluid. One kilogram, or 2.2 pounds of body weight, is approximately equivalent to the gain or loss of 1 L of fluid. Expressed in pounds, a gain or loss of 1 pound is equivalent to 500 mL of fluid.

This gain or loss is usually rapid. It is typically compared with what is called the *dry weight* of an individual. Even under conditions of starvation, a person will lose no more than one third to one half of a pound of dry weight a day. When monitoring for rapid weight gain or loss (and therefore fluid gain or loss), it is important to assess weight daily. Fluid gains or losses are categorized as mild, moderate, or severe, as described in Table 22-3.

The phenomenon of third spacing may complicate the fluid balance picture. Third spacing occurs when a patient has a fluid volume deficit of the extracellular space. Body weight is basically unchanged because the fluid loss is from the extracellular space to other body compartments.

To ensure that accurate weights are obtained, the patient should be weighed at the same time every day, preferably in the morning before breakfast and after voiding. The same scale should be used for each weighing, and the patient should wear the same or similar-weight clothing. It is also important to ensure that the scale is accurate. This requires verifying the scale reading at regular intervals as recommended by the manufacturer.

INTAKE AND OUTPUT

Intake and output is a clinical measurement that is used daily; unfortunately, the accuracy of this measurement may not always be dependable. Intake and output can be recorded as a result of nursing judgment and may be initiated by a nursing order. A physician's order is not necessary. The intake and output should approximate one another, maintaining a balance between all sources in and all sources out in any 24-hour period.

Box 22-1 provides a series of questions the nurse can ask to develop a complete picture of intake and output.

There are many ways to ensure accurate recording of intake and output. First, the importance of the patient's record should be stressed to the clinical staff and to the patient and family so that all may assist in recording intake and output. If the patient is undergoing parenteral fluid replacement, it is important to remember that IV solution containers may be overfilled by up to 10%. This means that a 1-L container may actually contain 1100 mL of fluid rather than the 1000 mL printed on the container. When possible, intake and output amounts should be measured rather than guessed. In addition, *all* input, such as ice chips (a 200-mL glass of ice chips could equal approximately 100 mL of water), must be recorded.

Output is often referred to as either *sensible* or *insensible* loss. Sensible loss is measurable output, whereas insensible loss is difficult to measure, such as perspiration. Water loss by perspiration should be estimated with labels such as excessive, moderate, or mild. The amount of insensible loss is estimated at approximately 300 to 600 mL/day and varies with ambient

TABLE 22-2 Select Assessment Parameters and Application to Conditions Affecting Fluids and Electrolytes

System and assessment points	Assessment technique	Application to fluids and electrolytes
Cardiovascular		
Chest pain	Interview	
Numbness		Hyperkalemia, hypokalemia
Syncope		Hypercalcemia, hypocalcemia
Arrhythmia		Hypotension: potential for decreased cardiac
Palpitations		output
Blood pressure	Auscultation	Decreased total blood volume
Murmur		Hypervolemia
Arrhythmia		Hypovolemia
Palpitations		
Pulses:	Palpation	
Apical		
Radial		
Pedal		
Edema:		Congestive heart failure
Pitting (1+ to 4+)	Inspection	Right-sided congestive heart failure
Jugular vein distention		Congestive heart failure
Dyspnea		
Orthopnea		
Cyanosis		
Respiratory		
Dyspnea	Interview	Fluid volume excess
Shortness of breath:		Excessive fluid intake
with exertion, at rest		Excessive sodium intake
Orthopnea		Infection (e.g., pneumonia)
Cough:		
Productive, nonproductive		
Color		
Amount		
Hemoptosis		
Pain	Palpation	
Respiratory rate		
Breath sounds	Percussion	
Breath sounds diminished	Auscultation	
Crackles		
Rhonchi		
Wheezes		
Cyanosis	Inspection	Fluid volume excess
Mental status		Acute respiratory failure
Anxiety		Pleural effusion
Speech patterns		Pneumothorax
Stridor		Pulmonary embolism
Retractions		
Dyspnea		Fluid volume excess
Shortness of breath:		Excessive fluid intake
with exertion, at rest		Excessive sodium intake

(Continued)

TABLE 22-2 Select Assessment Parameters and Application to Conditions Affecting Fluids and Electrolytes—cont'd

System and assessment points	Assessment technique	Application to fluids and electrolytes
Renal	Interview	Hypervolemia
Incontinence		Hypovolemia
Retention		Edema
Frequency		Diabetes mellitus
Urgency		Hypertension
Polyuria		Acute tubular nephrosis
Dysuria		Acute nephritis
Nocturia		Acute renal failure
Hematuria		Chronic renal disease
Catheter		
Ostomy		
Discharge		
Urine odor, color, volume		
Change in weight	Palpation	
Swelling	Percussion	
Pain	Inspection	
Flank pain		
Skin turgor		
Mucous membranes and tongue		
Chvostek's sign		Tetany
Trousseau's sign		
Hematuria		
Edema		
Odor, color		
Laboratory Results		
Blood chemistry (hemoglobin, hematocrit, sodium, potassium, chloride, calcium, phosphorus, magnesium, blood gasses)		Alterations in electrolyte values, blood chemistries, acid-base balance, and fluid volume and distribution
Urine studies (urinalysis, volume, pH, protein, glucose, ketones, sediment, osmolality, specific gravity, BUN, creatinine, creatinine clearance, sodium)		
Gastrointestinal	Interview	Fluid volume deficit
Pain		Fluid volume excess
Indigestion		Hypokalemia
Dysphagia		
Appetite change		
Weight loss or gain		
Nausea/vomiting		
Hemoptosis		GI bleed
Constipation		
Diarrhea		
Stool incontinence		
Abnormal bowel sounds	Auscultation (always precedes percussion and palpation)	Obstruction
Rigid abdomen		Ileus
Distention	Percussion	Cirrhosis
Ostomy	Palpation	Hepatitis
Feeding tube	Inspection	Pancreatitis
Rigid abdomen		Tumors
Distention		
Girth measurement		

TABLE 22-3 Rapid Fluid Gain or Loss in the Adult

Category	Fluid volume excess (%)	Fluid volume deficit (%)
Mild	2	5
Moderate	5	5
Severe	≥8	≥8

temperature, body surface area, and level of activity (Metheny, 2000; LeFever Kee et al, 2004; Weinstein, 2007). Estimates of fluid from incontinence of stool or urine, wound exudate, and irrigating solutions for bladder or wounds are important parts of intake and output records. Insensible loss increases if respirations increase (Alexander and Corrigan, 2004). For a patient who is in a delicate state of fluid balance or imbalance, it is important to review 8-hour intake and output totals in addition to the 24-hour totals.

(see Chapter 29)

Box 22-1   QUESTIONS USED TO ASSESS INTAKE AND OUTPUT

- How much is the patient drinking? If the patient is allowed oral fluids, is at least 1500 mL of fluid per day ingested?
- How much is the patient urinating?
- What does the urine look like? Is it dilute without odor, or is it very concentrated and highly odoriferous?
- What is the texture of the skin? Is it dry? Is it loose? Is it overly moist or firm?
- Does the patient have a fever?
- Is the patient perspiring excessively?
- Is the patient experiencing excessive drainage anywhere, including nasogastric tubes, fistulas, or any portal from which the patient could lose fluids? It is important to include those amounts in the daily intake and output record.

URINE VOLUME AND CONCENTRATION

During clinical assessment, a nurse needs to synthesize several pieces of information to understand and evaluate urine volume and concentration. Naturally, an accurate intake and output record is extremely important.

Normal urine output averages about 1 mL/kg of body weight per hour, or approximately 1500 mL in a 24-hour period in a healthy adult. The urine output can be as small as 1000 mL or as great as 2000 mL in 24 hours, which is an average of approximately 40 to 80 mL/hour in a healthy adult. Children have lesser amounts of urine volume, based on their age and weight (see Chapter 29). When the body is under stress, urine output may be less than normal because of increased secretion of aldosterone and antidiuretic hormone. In periods of stress, this may lead to an average output of 30 to 50 mL/hour.

Low or high urine volumes may indicate a fluid imbalance. Urine osmolality and specific gravity provide further information on this issue. Urine osmolality is the measure of the number of particles per unit of water. The average normal value is 500 to 800 mOsm/kg H_2O but may range from 50 to 1400 mOsm/kg H_2O (Metheny, 2000; Corbett, 2008).

Urine osmolality depends on the amount of antidiuretic hormone that is in the bloodstream and the rate that solutes are excreted through the kidneys. It more accurately reflects changes in urine content and the ability of the kidneys to concentrate urine than it reflects specific gravity. Urine osmolality depends on the state of hydration; measuring serum and urine osmolality at the same time yields a more accurate reflection of renal concentrating ability than does urine specific gravity (Alexander and Corrigan, 2004).

Urine specific gravity, which ranges from 1.001 to 1.040 (random samples range from 1.015 to 1.025) (Corbett, 2008), measures the amount of solutes in the urine, gives a picture of the patient's state of hydration, and reflects the kidneys' ability to regulate fluid balance. Urine specific gravity increases with any condition that causes hypoperfusion in the kidneys. Hypoperfusion may lead to oliguria, shock, or severe dehydration. The urine specific gravity decreases when the renal tubules are no longer able to reabsorb water and concentrate urine. This phenomenon would occur, for example, during the early stages of pyelonephritis.

It is also wise to look at urine pH, which may range from 4.6 to 8.0, with an average of 6.0. Urine pH increases in metabolic and respiratory alkalosis and decreases in the presence of uric acid stones or metabolic and respiratory acidosis.

It is important to understand and discriminate between the differences in water diuresis and solute diuresis. A low urinary specific gravity, a low urinary osmolality, and a normal or elevated serum sodium level can indicate either a lack of antidiuretic hormone or the inability of the renal tubules to respond properly. These findings indicate water diuresis.

Solute diuresis occurs when tubular absorption of a solute is impaired. Symptoms of solute diuresis are high urinary specific gravity, high urinary osmolality, and normal or low serum sodium level. Solute diuresis may occur in patients with diabetes mellitus or those who have had bladder obstructions corrected.

Water diuresis and solute diuresis usually occur in conjunction with polyuria. The interplay and responsiveness to feedback systems between filtration, reabsorption, and secretion determine the volume and composition of urine released from the body. Diluting and concentrating mechanisms of the nephrons maintain fluid volume in the presence of normal renal blood flow. Dilution results when the kidneys reabsorb solute but not the accompanying water. Concentration of urine is the result of reabsorption of water without solute.

Based on this information, it is apparent that the amount of solute and the amount of waste product in the urine can influence volume. In other words, urine volume would be increased in conditions that cause high levels of solute in the urine. The amount of circulating volume in the extracellular space also affects urine volume. Hypovolemia can result in decreased urinary output. Hypervolemia can cause increased urinary output in the presence of normal renal function.

The color of urine normally ranges from pale yellow to deep amber, depending on the degree of urine concentration. Some color changes can occur because of medications or foods ingested.

VITAL SIGNS

The measurement of vital signs provides important information regarding the patient's fluid and electrolyte status.

Blood pressure

Changes in blood pressure may be associated with fluid volume status. Postural hypotension may indicate a fluid volume deficit. Electrolyte alterations may cause fluctuations in blood pressure as well. For example, magnesium deficits or excess extracellular fluid volume may cause hypertension. Potassium level alterations may cause hypotension. Accurate baseline blood pressure measurements and blood pressure monitoring assist in early recognition and monitoring of fluid and electrolyte status. It is critical that the equipment used to measure blood pressure be calibrated for accuracy regularly and that the cuff of the sphygmomanometer is the proper size for the patient's arm circumference.

Respirations

Respirations should be assessed for their depth, rate, and effectiveness. Respiration is affected by various changes in fluid and electrolyte levels. Potassium level alterations may cause weakness or possible paralysis of respiratory muscles. Fluid volume excess affects respirations because of the increased effort required to move air in and out of the lungs. Respiration is also altered, as a compensatory mechanism, in the presence of acid-base balance deficiencies.

Pulse

The quality, amplitude, rhythm, and rate of the pulse yield information about cardiac status and how the patient is tolerating excesses or deficits of extracellular fluid. Major pulse points should be examined regularly to determine circulatory status and vascular integrity. Areas to assess include the carotid, brachial, radial, ulnar, femoral, popliteal, posterior tibial, and dorsalis pedis arteries. Tachycardia, pulsus alternans, and irregular rhythms may indicate left ventricular failure. A rapid, weak, thready pulse may signal hyponatremia. Hyponatremia accompanied by fluid volume excess may result in a rapid pulse rate with a full quality.

Temperature

Body temperature may increase or decrease in response to fluid and electrolyte imbalances. The skin and core body temperature should be noted when the fluid and electrolyte status is assessed. Changes in skin temperature are discussed later in this chapter.

Core body temperature may be decreased in the presence of fluid deficit, or it may become elevated in response to electrolyte imbalances. For example, hypernatremia may cause an elevation of body temperature.

Temperature elevations increase the fluid requirements of the body. A temperature between 101° F and 103° F increases the 24-hour fluid requirement by at least 500 mL. A temperature greater than 103° F increases it by a minimum of 1000 mL. Because of increased fluid requirements with fever or temperature elevation, additional fluid and electrolyte imbalances may occur if extra fluid requirements are not met.

HEMODYNAMIC MONITORING

Fluid volume alterations may be detected through various hemodynamic monitoring techniques. Central venous pressure (CVP) gives information on the status of intravascular volume. The CVP may be measured with a water manometer or with an electronic transducer. Normal CVP values are 8 to 10 cm H_2O.

The CVP measurement reflects right atrial pressure or the filling of the right side of the heart, known as *preload;* this measurement can be used to guide volume replacement. When fluid challenges are performed, the response of right atrial pressure provides important information regarding the patient's fluid and cardiovascular status.

The CVP can be estimated during the physical examination. With the patient in the supine position, the jugular veins are visually examined for distention. The jugular vein should be distended in this position because it is then at the same level as the right atrium. The patient can then be slowly raised to a sitting position. As the patient rises to the sitting position, the upper portion of the jugular vein will collapse, and a bulge may be seen where blood vessel distention is still occurring within the vessel.

The distance between the bulge, or point of distention, and the right atrium is then a measure of CVP. When a person is fully upright, the sternal notch is approximately 5 cm above the right atrium. The distention of the jugular vein above the sternal notch is then measured in centimeters and added to 5 cm: the resulting value is the CVP. If the jugular veins are not visible above the clavicle, it is assumed that the CVP is less than 5 cm H_2O. CVP adequately reflects right atrial pressure only in

a person with a normal cardiac status. When myocardial dysfunction exists, especially in the presence of right-sided heart failure, the jugular venous pressure is elevated regardless of the patient's extracellular volume.

Various pressures within the cardiac and pulmonary systems can be measured by use of a pulmonary artery catheter. Single pressure measurements may be useful, but an advantage of IV pressure monitoring is the ability to evaluate pressures over time. The CVP or the pulmonary artery catheter can provide a means to monitor a patient's response to therapy for the correction of volume depletion and help determine volume status (Weinstein, 2007).

TISSUE TURGOR

Assessing tissue turgor helps the nurse evaluate the amount of fluid available to the tissues. Tissue turgor is tested by grasping the skin between the fingers in a pinching action and then releasing the tissue and observing the "tented" skin. If a person has fluid volume deficit, the skin remains in the pinched or tented position for an extended time, usually longer than 3 seconds.

Tissue turgor describes the elasticity available to the skin, which depends in part on the presence of interstitial fluid. Tissue turgor is an age-related phenomenon; the geriatric patient commonly has poor skin turgor because the skin loses elasticity with age. Turgor may also be tested over the sternum, the forehead, or the inner aspect of the thighs. Using the skin over the sternum gives the best indication of skin turgor.

The tongue can also give information on fluid balance. A person with normal hydration status has one longitudinal furrow. In a dehydrated patient, additional furrows are present, and the tongue may actually appear smaller. Tongue turgor is generally not affected by age, as is skin turgor.

THIRST

The sensation of thirst is a normal function of the body that encourages the person to ingest sufficient amounts of water for metabolism. If a person has suffered water losses, the thirst mechanism encourages the intake of more water. If the thirst mechanism fails for some reason, a patient may be at risk for developing hypernatremia as a result of decreased circulating fluid.

The thirst mechanism is affected by a rise in plasma osmolarity or a decrease in fluid volume. Cells of the thirst center respond to the movement of water from the cells to the extracellular fluid by shrinking, thus causing the urge to consume fluid (Weinstein, 2007). Psychogenic alterations can also encourage the patient to drink copious amounts of water, thereby leading to water intoxication and placing the patient in danger of fluid volume overload. People expressing a sense of thirst may often complain of a dry mouth; however, a dry mouth may also result from excessive mouth breathing. Oral dryness resulting from mouth breathing can be differentiated from dryness resulting from fluid volume deficit by an examination of the membrane inside the cheek and gum. When the membrane is dry, the dry mouth results from fluid volume deficit. In the older adult, the sensation of thirst diminishes with age.

APPEARANCE OF THE SKIN

Assessing the skin may provide clues to the patient's fluid status because skin changes are related to the amount of fluid in the interstitium. For example, with extracellular fluid volume

Pitting edema is generally not seen until there is a weight gain of 10 to 15 pounds related to retention of excess fluid (Alexander and Corrigan, 2004). Pitting edema is identified by pressing the tissue with the fingers; if an indentation remains, pitting edema is present. It is best to test the ankles or feet of an ambulatory person or the sacral area of a bed-ridden person. A more accurate means of determining edema is by daily measurement with a measuring tape. Pitting is classified from +1 to +4, with +4 being the most severe.

Dependent edema is generally related to gravity. Fluid accumulates in any portion of the body that is dependent. If a person is ambulatory, dependent edema may be seen mostly in the feet and ankles, or possibly in the buttocks if the patient has been sitting for a long period. The sacral area of the patient confined to bed rest should be evaluated for dependent edema.

Some edema is refractory, meaning that it persists after appropriate therapy, such as diuretics or salt-restricted diets, has been implemented. Persons with refractory edema may have persistent weight gain and are usually hypertensive. Edema usually results from an increase in the total body sodium content. Circulatory overload may cause edema and is generally associated with either heart failure or renal failure caused by sodium and water retention.

Edema may be associated with overly aggressive infusion of hypertonic IV solutions. The cause of this edema is generally thought to be an increase in plasma hydrostatic pressure, which forces fluid into the interstitial spaces. Edema may occur when plasma protein level is low, resulting in decreased plasma oncotic pressure. A decrease in plasma protein level occurs in kidney disease, when there is a loss of protein, cirrhosis, serous drainage, or hemorrhage. Edema may also be associated with interference in venous return or obstruction of the lymphatic system.

It is important to remember that edema may manifest itself in various ways, not just in dependent areas of the body. The patient's history may reveal such symptoms as swollen feet, the feeling of tightness in the lower legs, or puffiness of the face or fingers. Rings may fit too tightly. A patient may complain of a rapid weight gain. If the lungs or heart are involved, a patient may speak of dyspnea on exertion or at night. Obtaining daily weights can be beneficial in identifying and monitoring the edematous state and its treatment.

deficits, the skin and mucous membranes are dry. Skin appears cold and clammy and possibly cyanotic if the patient is progressing to shock. Conversely, with intracellular fluid volume deficit, the skin may be warm and flushed. The skin may feel cool and clammy in acute pancreatitis, whereas in respiratory acidosis it may appear warm and flushed.

EDEMA

Edema is the retention of excessive fluid in the interstitial space. Edema may be classified as *pitting* or *dependent*. Systemic symptoms seen in edema are weight gain, high blood pressure, and dyspnea. Inspection of hand veins is a means for evaluating plasma volume. When the hand is elevated, the veins will empty in 3 to 5 seconds; when it is lowered, they will fill in the same amount of time. Filling that takes longer than 3 to 5 seconds may indicate compromised circulation. Hand veins that remain engorged when held higher than the heart for 10 seconds signify overhydration and excessive blood volume (LeFever Kee, 2004).

TEARING AND SALIVATION

Tearing and salivation are most useful in assessing fluid balance in an infant or child. A child suffering from a fluid volume deficit of moderate proportions will not produce tears or salivate.

BEHAVIORAL AND SENSORY CHANGES

Behavioral changes may occur in relation to fluid and electrolyte imbalance. A patient suffering from a fluid deficit may be apprehensive and restless. Coma may occur in severe cases. Fluid volume excess may cause hyperirritability, disorientation, and mental disturbances. Metabolic acidosis may cause apathy, disorientation, delirium, or stupor. Metabolic alkalosis may cause belligerence, irritability, disorientation, or lethargy. Potassium deficit may cause changes in speech, lethargy, apathy, irritability, and mental confusion. Calcium excess may cause lethargy, exhaustion, mental confusion, a loss of interest in surroundings, and irritability. Magnesium deficiency may cause hallucinations, illusions, extreme confusion, or aggressive

TABLE 22-4 Selected Laboratory Values

Laboratory test	Normal values	Laboratory test	Normal values
Blood Chemistry/Electrolytes		Magnesium	1.6-16 mg/dL
Blood urea nitrogen (BUN)	6-20 mg/dL	Chloride	98-107 mEq/L
Serum creatinine	Male: 0.6-1.1 mg/dL	Carbon dioxide	22-28 mEq/L
	Female: 0.7-1.3 mg/dL	Phosphorus	2.3-4.1 mg/dL
Creatinine clearance	Male: 94-140 mL/min	Zinc	70-120 mcg/dL
	Female: 72-110 mL/min	Lithium	Therapeutic: 0.5-1.4 mEq/L
Hematocrit	Male: 39%-49%	Serum proteins	Total: 6.4-8.3 g/dL
	Female: 35%-45%	Albumin	3.5-5.2 g/dL
Hemoglobin	Male: 13.2-17.3 g/dL	Lactic acid	Venous: 8.1-15.3 mg/dL
	Female: 11.7-15.5 g/dL		Arterial: <11.3 mg/dL
Red blood cells	Male: (4.5-5.9) × 10^{12}/L	Serum salicylates	Therapeutic range:
	Female:		Analgesia: <100 mcg/mL
Mean corpuscular volume (MCV)	80-96 fL		Anti-inflammatory: 150-300 mcg/mL
Mean corpuscular hemoglobin (MCH)	27.5-33.2 pg		Toxic range: >500 mcg/mL
Mean corpuscular hemoglobin concentration (MCHC)	33.4%-35.5%	Anion gap	10-20 mEq/L
		Aspartate aminotransferase (AST) (SGOT)	8-20 units/L
Complete Blood Count		Alanine aminotransferase (ALT) (SGPT)	Male: 10-40 units/L
Total leukocytes	(4.5-11.0) × 10^3/μL		Female: 7-35 units/L
Segmented neutrophils	(1.8-7.8) × 10^9/L	Alkaline phosphatase	4.5-13 units/L
Lymphocytes	(1.0-4.8) × 10^9/L		
Monocytes	(0.0-0.8) × 10^9/L	**Serum Bilirubin**	
Eosinophils	(0.0-0.45) × 10^9/L	Total	0.3-1.2 mg/dL
Basophils	(0.0-0.2) × 10^9/L	Direct (conjugated)	<0.2 mg/dL
Platelets	(150-400) × 10^9/L	Indirect (unconjugated)	<1.1 mg/dL
Reticulocytes	(25-75) × 10^9/L	Lactate dehydrogenase (LDH)	100-190 units/L
Prothrombin time	10-15 sec		
	Standard therapeutic: 2.0-3.0 INR	**Urine Chemistry/Electrolytes**	
	High-dose therapeutic: 3.0-4.5 INR	Sodium	75-200 mEq/day (varies with Na+ intake)
Iron	Male: 65-175 mcg/dL	Potassium	40-80 mEq/day (varies with dietary intake)
	Female: 50-170 mcg/dL	Chloride	140-250 mEq/day
Ferritin	Male: 20-250 ng/mL	Calcium	100-240 mg/day (varies with dietary intake)
	Female: 10-120 ng/mL		
Total iron-binding capacity (TIBC)	250-425 mcg/mL	Osmolality	300-900 mOsm/kg H_2O (usually about 1.0-3.0 times greater than serum osmolality)
Transferrin	215-380 mg/dL		
Partial thromboplastin time	Activated: <35 sec		
Fibrinogen	200-400 mg/dL	Specific gravity (SG)	Random samples have an SG of 1.016-1.022
Serum osmolality	275-295 mOsm/kg		
Serum amylase	27-131 units/L	pH	4.6-8.0
Serum glucose	74-106 mg/dL		
		Arterial Blood Gases	
Serum Electrolytes*		pH	7.35-7.45
Sodium	136-145 mEq/L	Pao_2	83-108 mm Hg
Potassium	3.5-5.0 mEq/L	$Paco_2$	32-48 mm Hg
Calcium (total)	8.6-10.0 mg/dL	Bicarbonate	19.8-24.8 mEq/L
Calcium (ionized)	4.6-5.3 mg/dL	Base excess	−2 to +3

*Measurement of electrolytes may be of limited value because of recent administration of diuretics or lack of knowledge of dietary intake.
Adapted from Corbett J: *Laboratory tests and diagnostic procedures* with nursing diagnoses, ed 7, Upper Saddle River, New Jersey, 2008, Pearson; LeFever Kee J, Paulanka BJ, Purnell LD: *Fluids and electrolytes with clinical applications: a programmed approach,* ed 7, Clifton Park, NY, 2004, Delmar; Metheny NM: *Fluid and electrolyte balance: nursing considerations,* ed 4, Philadelphia, 2000, Lippincott; Weinstein S: *Plumer's principles and practice of intravenous therapy,* ed 8, Philadelphia, 2007, Lippincott.

behavior. As seen by these examples, it is important to have a baseline understanding of a patient's normal behavior and reaction to surroundings so that subtle changes in behavior can be recognized.

LABORATORY DATA

Obtaining and evaluating a patient's laboratory data are important adjuncts to the physical and clinical assessment. Laboratory data most useful in evaluating fluid and electrolyte status are the blood urea nitrogen (BUN) level, serum creatinine level, hematocrit, hemoglobin level, serum osmolality, serum electrolyte values (sodium, potassium, chloride, calcium, magnesium, phosphate, and bicarbonate), and arterial blood gases (pH, Pao_2, $Paco_2$, bicarbonate, and base excess). Table 22-4 (Metheny, 2000; LeFever Kee et al, 2004; Weinstein, 2007; Corbett, 2008) provides normal values for these and other tests that are useful in evaluating patients with problems related to infusion therapy. (These values may vary among facilities. "Normal" values must be referenced with the laboratory performing the tests.)

SUMMARY

By using the systems approach for clinical assessment and obtaining information from the patient's medical history, one can more accurately determine a patient's current fluid and electrolyte status. Accurate and timely assessment allows astute observation of subtle changes in the patient's condition. Rapid recognition of these nuances leads to improved outcomes for patients experiencing fluid and electrolyte alterations.

REFERENCES

Ackley BJ, Ladwig GB, Swan BA et al: *Evidenced based nursing care guidelines*, St Louis, 2008, Mosby.

Alexander M, Corrigan A: *Core curriculum for intravenous nursing*, ed 3, Philadelphia, 2004, Lippincott Williams & Wilkins.

Corbett J: *Laboratory tests and diagnostics procedures with nursing diagnoses*, ed 7, Upper Saddle River, NJ, 2008, Pearson.

Faes MC, Spigt MG, Olde Rikkert MGM: Dehydration in geriatrics, *Geriatr Aging*, 2007. Accessed 6/5/08 from www.medscape.com/viewarticle/567678.

Heo S, Doering LV, Widener J et al: Predictors and effect of physical symptom status on health-related quality of life in patients with heart failure, *Am J Crit Care* 17(2):124-132, 2008.

LeFever Kee J, Paulanka BJ, Purnell LD: *Fluids and electrolytes with clinical applications: a programmed approach*, ed 7, Clifton Park, NY, 2004, Delmar.

Leibovitz A, Baumoehl Y, Lubart E et al: Dehydration among long-term care elderly with oropharyngeal dysphagia, *Gerontology* 53(4):179-183, 2007.

Luckey AE, Parsa CJ: Fluid and electrolytes in the aged, *Arch Surg* 138(10):1055-1060, 2003.

Metheny NM: *Fluid and electrolyte balance: nursing considerations*, ed 4, Philadelphia, 2000, Lippincott Williams & Wilkins.

Weinstein S: *Plumer's principles and practice of intravenous therapy*, ed 8, Philadelphia, 2007, Lippincott Williams & Wilkins.

23 PERIPHERAL VENOUS ACCESS DEVICES

Roxanne Perucca, MSN, CRNI®*

When nurses first began to administer infusion therapy, the sole requisite was the ability to perform a venipuncture skillfully. Today, with the technological development of venous access devices, the use of multiple delivery systems, and the administration of highly specialized treatment modalities, the nurse must be knowledgeable and clinically competent to ensure the safe delivery of infusion therapy. The nurse must be committed to the delivery of safe, cost-effective, quality infusion care.

PREPARATION OF PATIENT AND EQUIPMENT

VERIFICATION OF PRESCRIBED THERAPY

The initiation of infusion therapy requires an order by the physician or other authorized prescriber, in the patient's medical record. The order must be complete and consist of the name of the solution or medication to be used; the dosage; the volume to be infused; and the rate, frequency, and route of administration. The nurse must assess and ensure that the order is appropriate for the patient. If the order is incomplete, unclear, or inappropriate, the prescriber should be contacted for clarification.

COMPATIBILITY CHECK

After the order has been verified, the nurse assesses the order and its implications for the patient. Particular attention is given to identifying allergies to medications, iodine, latex, and tape. The patient's status is evaluated, and the outcome goal is reviewed.

When multiple solutions or medications are to be infused, consideration must be given to compatibility. More than one infusion site may be required if the medications to be infused are incompatible. A pharmacist or pharmaceutical compatibility reference guide should be consulted to determine compatibilities.

If the compatibility of the solution or medications is not known, the IV system must be flushed with a compatible solution. The IV administration set or device can be flushed by using a syringe filled with 0.9% sodium chloride or by establishing a 0.9% sodium chloride or 5% dextrose and water administration system that is used before and after the administration of incompatible medications. Some facilities have established flushing policies that take into consideration the number of medications to be administered per day. For example, if two or fewer medications are administered per day, the sodium chloride syringe method can be used to flush the IV line. If more than two medications are to be administered per day, a separate administration system to flush the IV line must be established.

EQUIPMENT CHECK

After the orders have been verified and the type of infusion system has been determined, the nurse gathers the equipment. The solution container is examined to verify that the type and volume of parenteral solution match the order, taking note of any medications that are to be added. The container is checked for leaks, and the expiration date is verified. The solution is observed for clarity and particulate matter. If there are any doubts regarding the suitability of the parenteral fluid, it must be returned to the dispensing department.

INITIATING THE INTRAVENOUS SETUP

If the venous access device (VAD) is to be inserted for intermittent therapy, a syringe of 0.9% sodium chloride and an injection cap/needleless device must be collected. The remaining venipuncture equipment is gathered. IV start kits are advantageous because they can contain all the necessary insertion equipment except the catheter. When equipment is gathered separately, an item may be forgotten and therefore unavailable when needed. Many start kits are available that provide any combination of the following venipuncture equipment: 70% isopropyl alcohol, antimicrobial solution, sterile gauze, transparent dressing, tape, tourniquet, and label. The organization's policies and procedures for IV catheter insertion determine the required venipuncture equipment for use.

*The author and editors wish to acknowledge the contributions made by Maxine Perdue in the second edition of *Infusion Therapy in Clinical Practice.*

PROCEDURE FOR PREPARING A SOLUTION CONTAINER AND ADMINISTRATION SET

1. Verify order.
2. Gather administration set, electronic infusion device if needed, and labels.
3. Perform hand hygiene.
4. Remove container outer wrap.
5. Examine container and solution, checking for particulate matter, cloudiness, and leaks.
6. Close roller clamp on administration set.
7. Remove protective cap from the solution container.
8. Remove protective cap from spike of administration set. Caution must be taken to avoid touch contamination of the spike. If it is accidentally contaminated, a new administration set must be obtained.
9. Insert administration set spike into container.
10. Hang container on IV pole.
11. Squeeze chamber to at least ⅓ to ½ full.
12. Open clamp slightly and allow administration set to fill slowly.
13. If electronic infusion device is used, purge air from administration set according to manufacturer's recommendations.
14. Close roller clamp.
15. Write date and time initiated on a time strip, and tape it to solution container.

Adapted from Infusion Nurses Society: *Policies and procedures for infusion nursing,* ed 3, Norwood, Mass, 2006b, Author.

PATIENT IDENTIFICATION AND ORIENTATION

Before the venous access device is inserted, the patient's identity must be confirmed using at least two identifiers. The patient should be asked to state his or her name. The nurse should verbally repeat the patient's name to ensure accuracy and confirm patient identification. A patient's identity can be verified by comparing information on the identification bracelet (patient name, medical record number, or date of birth) with the physician's order, request form, or patient label.

After verifying the patient's identification, the nurse identifies himself or herself to the patient. Next, the nurse assesses the patient's psychological preparedness while explaining the following: the purpose of therapy, possible duration of therapy, method of administration, insertion procedure, expected side effects, care and maintenance of the device, and any limitations or restrictions on mobility.

It is essential for the nurse to establish trust. The patient should be approached in a calm and reassuring manner. Encouraging the patient to ask questions provides information that helps alleviate fear and anxiety. When answering a patient's questions, the nurse must be honest and forthright. The nurse should always convey self-assurance and appear confident. The nurse can reduce the patient's anxiety by encouraging him or her to be an active participant in the placement process; active participation communicates that the patient's concerns are important and that the nurse is interested in the whole person and not just in performing the technical procedure. The patient

should also be encouraged to report any discomfort experienced during or after the insertion procedure.

Occasionally, despite appropriate patient teaching and reassurance, the patient may remain uncooperative. These situations require careful nursing assessment and judgment. The patient has the right to refuse treatment. When the patient refuses to cooperate with the ordered medical intervention, the rationale for therapy should be explained again and the patient's physician notified. Possible alternative routes of medication administration should be assessed with the physician and the patient. The nurse's actions and the physician's orders are recorded in the patient's medical record.

VASCULAR ASSESSMENT

PATIENT PREPARATION

After the patient has been properly identified, the nurse must provide privacy by pulling the curtain around the patient's bed, asking visitors to step outside the room, and closing the door to the patient's room. In addition, adequate lighting of the environment is essential for performing accurate venous assessment and catheter insertion. If the lighting in the patient's room is inadequate, the patient may be transported to a treatment room that has adequate lighting.

The nurse should ensure that the patient is comfortable. The patient should be able to extend and stabilize his or her arm on a firm, flat surface. Sometimes, it is helpful to place a pillow or roll a blanket or towel under the extended arm. Attention must also be given to the comfort of the nurse. The height of the bed can be adjusted, if necessary, to prevent unnecessary bending.

In alternative care settings, particularly the home, the nurse may have to adapt to poor lighting, not having an adjustable bed, and lack of privacy. In the home setting, the kitchen table is often a good setting for catheter placement because usually there is good lighting above the table. Creative thinking and forethought will often allow the nurse to change a given situation to provide patient comfort, privacy, and safety. For example, if a patient lives in a one-room apartment with another individual, the caregiver may want to take a walk or run an errand while care is being given. The patient is provided privacy and the caregiver has the opportunity to complete an errand. A large flashlight can provide better visibility when lighting is poor. Regardless of the circumstances, the nurse should be creative and manipulate the environment as needed to provide quality infusion care.

After ensuring privacy and comfort, the nurse performs hand hygiene before proceeding with an overall assessment of the patient's upper extremities. As venous access of the patient is evaluated, the nurse needs to consider the following questions regarding the prescribed therapy: What is the anticipated duration of the prescribed therapy? What clinical procedures are to be performed? What extremity or location does the patient prefer? Which arm is dominant? Prior consideration of these factors often determines the success of the infusion, which ultimately results in preserving the patient's veins. To determine which arm should be selected, the nurse performs an overall assessment of the patient's upper extremities taking into consideration the purpose of the insertion and, if possible, the patient's dominant side. Any injury or absence of sensation to the arm restricts the use of the extremity for venipuncture.

An extremity with an arteriovenous (AV) fistula or graft is never used for routine peripheral catheter insertion. An AV fistula or graft is inserted usually for dialysis only and requires special consideration for catheter placement. The cannulation of grafts and AV fistulas should be established within organizational policies and procedures.

The nurse should avoid placing a catheter into the affected extremity of a patient who has undergone a cerebrovascular accident because of the extremity's decreased or absent neurological sensation. If the infusion device infiltrates or develops phlebitis, the patient might be unable to detect these problems. Often, because of decreased mobility, the affected extremity has limited venous access potential.

Catheter placement in the arm of a patient who has undergone a mastectomy or axillary node removal is contraindicated. In some cases (e.g., bilateral mastectomy, chest wall issues), a peripheral VAD may need to be placed. This should be a careful decision based on collaboration between the infusion nurse, the physician, and the patient.

Cannulation of the lower extremities in adults should be avoided because of the increased risk of phlebitis (INS, 2006a). The cannulation of lower extremity veins is acceptable in children until they are of walking age. If a catheter is inserted in the lower extremity of an adult patient, it should be changed as soon as a central venous access device or an appropriate site in an upper extremity can be established. Institutional policy should define the authorization and approval process for cannulation of a lower extremity. Another area contraindicated for venipuncture includes the palm side of the wrist because the radial nerve is located near the vein, causing excessive pain during insertion and potentially resulting in nerve damage. See Table 10-5 for advantages and disadvantages of the various peripheral IV sites.

Applying a tourniquet promotes venous distention. The tourniquet should be applied snugly enough to impede the venous, but not the arterial, flow. To prevent the spread of health care–associated infection, tourniquets are for single-patient use. The tourniquet is applied 5 to 6 inches above the intended insertion site to promote the dilation of the veins. A blood pressure cuff may also be used to distend veins. The cuff should be inflated and the pressure released to just below the diastolic pressure. When a patient has extremely fragile veins, the tourniquet must be applied very loosely. Sometimes, nurses elect not to apply a tourniquet if a patient bruises easily.

After the tourniquet has been applied, the veins must be given time to fill. Another method for promoting venous distention is lowering the extremity below the level of the heart and having the patient open and close his or her fist. Lightly tapping the vein promotes venous distention; however, caution must be taken when using this method. If a vein is tapped too hard, pain may occur and cause vasoconstriction, or the vein may rupture, creating a hematoma. When these methods fail to promote venous distention, warm, moist compresses may be applied to the extremity for 10 to 15 minutes before insertion. The compresses increase blood flow to the area, which promotes venous filling.

With an edematous patient or an individual who has extremely limited venous access, the nurse may be able to locate a vein by its anatomic location. For example, the cephalic vein is located on the lateral wrist extending along the radial forearm and the lateral aspect of the antecubital fossa and biceps; the nurse, by assessment and palpation, may be able to find it. Several commercial products (e.g., ultrasound or hand-held vein finder devices) may also help identify the location of veins.

Veins that are tender, phlebitic, sclerotic, or located in a previously infiltrated area are unacceptable for venipuncture. If damaged veins are used for venipuncture, greater injury to the skin tissue and vascular system will occur. Also, if previous phlebitic or infiltrated areas are used for cannulation, accurate site assessments cannot be performed.

Palpation of the vein is an important assessment technique used to evaluate the condition of a vessel. By always using the same finger to palpate veins, one develops the sensitivity required for accurate assessment. Usually, the index finger and the third forefinger of the nondominant hand have the most sensitivity for palpating veins. A hard, cordlike feeling can identify a sclerosed vein. Successful venipuncture requires a healthy vein that feels soft and bouncy as one palpates over and across the vessel. Valves can be detected by a hard lump or knotlike feeling. Resilient veins, which are easily depressed, are required for venipuncture. Palpation helps determine whether the vein is located in the superficial fascia or deep tissues. Stroking the vessel downward and observing the venous refill is helpful in determining the condition of the vein. Performing venipuncture in areas where valves are palpated or where two veins bifurcate should be avoided. The insertion site should be proximal to a valve or a bifurcation.

Palpation also helps differentiate arteries and veins. The selected vein must not pulsate; aberrant arteries pulsate and are located superficially in an unusual location. Often, aberrant arteries occur bilaterally on the hand or wrist, usually on a thin, emaciated person. An aberrant artery should not be used for peripheral catheter insertion.

 ## PERIPHERAL INTRAVENOUS ADMINISTRATION

SHORT PERIPHERAL CATHETERS
Site selection

The most distal site on the extremity should be selected for peripheral catheter insertion. Peripheral infusion therapy can be maintained longer by starting at the lowest point on the arm and working upward with future catheter insertions. Sites located below previous insertion sites, as well as phlebitic, infiltrated, or bruised areas, should be avoided as medications or solutions infused through the potentially damaged site can result in further infiltration. Areas of flexion, such as the wrist or antecubital fossa, are also not recommended. The antecubital veins should be preserved for as long as possible and are not used for routine IV therapy. A short peripheral catheter inserted into an antecubital fossa vein is at greater risk for the occurrence of mechanical phlebitis and infiltration. The metacarpal, cephalic, basilic, and median veins are recommended for venipuncture because of their size and location.

Site preparation

Health care personnel must perform hand hygiene before and immediately after all clinical procedures and before donning and after the removal of gloves. The Centers for Disease Control and Prevention (CDC) guidelines for hand hygiene (2002a) recommend the use of an alcohol-based hand rub or antibacterial agent to decontaminate hands before the insertion of a peripheral catheter.

Standard precautions are used for catheter placement. Nonsterile gloves are worn to prevent contact with blood and to provide protection for the patient and the health care worker. When splashing of blood is likely to occur, protective eyewear must be used.

If the patient is unusually dirty, the selected extremity should be washed with soap and water before the insertion site is prepared. If hair removal is necessary, it should be clipped with scissors; surgical clippers with disposable clipper heads are also acceptable (INS, 2006a). To prevent cross-contamination, the clipper heads should be changed after each patient use. Shaving can be harmful to the skin because it can cause microabrasions, which can harbor bacteria. Depilatories or hair removal agents are not recommended because of allergic reactions, which can cause skin eruptions.

The CDC's *Guidelines for the Prevention of Intravascular Catheter-Related Infections* (2002b) state that a 2% chlorhexidine-based preparation is preferred; 1% to 2% tincture of iodine, iodophor (povidone-iodine), and 70% alcohol can also be used. A meta-analysis, which included 8 studies involving 1361 peripheral IV catheters, found that chlorhexidine gluconate, as compared to povidone-iodine solution, was associated with a significant reduction in bloodstream infections (Chaiyakunapruk, Veenstra, Lipsky et al, 2002).

Chlorhexidine-based solutions should be applied with friction using repeated back-and-forth strokes for a minimum of 30 seconds. The prepped area should be 2 to 3 inches in diameter. Applicators are intended for single-patient, one-time use only. For the antimicrobial solution to be effective, it should be allowed to air-dry for a minimum of 30 seconds. Fanning, blowing, or blotting the prepared area is contraindicated.

Pain management during IV insertion

For every patient, an assessment of pain, feelings and fear about IV-related procedures, and preferences for pain control is essential and should be incorporated into the care plan. *Infusion Nursing Standards of Practice* (INS, 2006a) recommends consideration and use of anesthetic agents in general and encourage their use with children. The importance of nursing competency and knowledge about their use are also emphasized. Research studies have demonstrated that a variety of anesthetic methods, both topical and injectable drugs, reduce pain. Patients who have experienced an anesthetic before venipuncture prefer it for future IV insertions.

A physician's order should be obtained if local anesthesia is utilized; some organizations include this in standardized order sets or allow it as a nursing order. Note that there are a variety of interventions (topical, injection) that can be used. The infusion nurse must act as a patient advocate to manage pain and use the most appropriate intervention to manage pain associated with peripheral IV insertion (Gorski, 2008).

Catheter selection

The overall goal of infusion therapy is to obtain a positive patient outcome. Selecting the venous access device that best meets the patient's needs is essential in achieving this goal. The increased availability of different catheter designs and configurations adds complexity to the selection process. The duration and composition of the infusion, clinical condition and age of the patient, and size and condition of the vein are some of the factors to consider when selecting the best device for the patient.

FOCUS ON EVIDENCE

Pain Management for Peripheral IV Insertion—Adults

- A meta-analysis of 20 studies analyzing the effectiveness of a topical anesthetic (2.5% lidocaine and prilocaine mixture, EMLA cream) concluded that the use of EMLA significantly decreases venipuncture and IV insertion pain in 85% of the population (Fetzer, 2002).
- A randomized, double-blinded study involving surgical adult patients (N = 47) compared use of intradermal injection either of lidocaine hydrochloride 1% with sodium bicarbonate or of sodium chloride 0.9% with benzyl alcohol. The researcher found no significant difference between the anesthetic effects; both were effective in reducing pain and were safe (Brown, 2004).
- A randomized, double-blinded study involving adult inpatients on medical units (N = 33) compared use of subcutaneous injection of buffered lidocaine 1%, subcutaneous injection of sodium chloride 0.9% with benzyl alcohol, or no injection. The researchers found a significantly improved pain rating associated with use of lidocaine hydrochloride 1% and no significant difference between patients receiving no treatment and those injected with sodium chloride with benzyl alcohol (Hattula, McGovern, and Neumann, 2002).
- A quasi-experimental study involving surgical adult patients (N = 30) compared use of intradermal injection of lidocaine or topical application of EMLA cream with delivery of the Numby Stuff system (i.e., local anesthetic Iontocaine with use of mild electrical current to deliver the medication through the skin). The study found the Numby Stuff® superior to the other methods in decreasing IV insertion pain (Miller, 2001).
- A descriptive study involving adult medical-surgical patients (N = 180) was designed to determine patient preferences regarding the use of intradermal lidocaine before peripheral insertions; significant findings included that subjects who had any type of experience with lidocaine would prefer to have it used for future IV insertions and that the pain associated with lidocaine injection was less than the pain associated with IV insertion (Brown, 2003).

Over-the-needle catheter-type devices are the most commonly used peripheral venous access devices. Dual-lumen peripheral catheter devices are available for multiple infusions. Catheter composition has evolved from polyvinyl chloride and polytetrafluoroethylene (Teflon®) to various polyurethane materials, and there is still controversy over the advantages and disadvantages of the available catheter materials. Ongoing research in polymer technology seeks to develop a catheter material that further decreases thrombogenicity. To promote patient safety, IV catheters are radiopaque. Safety-enhancing designs of over-the-needle catheters prevent accidental needlesticks and exposure to blood and body fluids, and promote the safety of health care workers.

The smallest gauge and the shortest length of catheter that will accommodate the prescribed therapy should be selected (Table 23-1) (INS, 2006a). A small-gauge catheter results in less trauma to the vessel, promotes proper hemodilution of the infusate, and allows adequate blood flow around the catheter wall. All of these factors promote increased catheter dwell time and improve patient outcomes. The diameter of the vein and the ordered therapy to be delivered determine the size of the catheter inserted. Small veins should not be used for vesicants

TABLE 23-1 Recommendations for Catheter Selection

Catheter size (Gauge)	Clinical applications
14, 16, 18	Trauma, surgery, blood transfusion
20	Continuous or intermittent infusions, blood transfusion
22	Intermittent general infusions, children and elderly patients
24	Fragile veins for intermittent or continuous infusions

or irritants. If a large-gauge catheter is required, a larger vein should be selected. Increased osmolality of the solution increases venous irritation. Hyperosmotic solutions must be administered through veins with large blood volume to dilute the IV solution and to reduce vein wall irritation. Fluids with a greater viscosity, such as packed red cells, require a larger catheter. An 18- or 20-gauge catheter has a larger inner lumen, which permits the flow of viscous components. A smaller-gauge catheter may be used in children.

In emergency situations, larger catheters are necessary to accommodate the rapid infusion of solutions. Catheters inserted in emergency situations should be removed and replaced as soon as the patient has stabilized, but within 24 hours of the emergency. This is because one cannot ensure that the site was adequately prepared or that aseptic technique was maintained during an emergency catheter insertion.

Catheter placement

Before the venipuncture is performed, the patient is educated about the need for a peripheral IV catheter and what to expect from the procedure. The bevel of the catheter is inspected for product integrity. Skin stabilization is an important element of successful venipuncture. Veins are stabilized by applying traction to the side of the insertion site with the nondominant hand to prevent the vein from rolling. Traction may be applied to the forearm by the palm of the nondominant hand, which is holding the whole forearm while the index finger and the thumb pull the skin away from the insertion site.

With the bevel up, the catheter is held at a 10- to 30-degree angle as it penetrates the skin (Figure 23-1). The angle used to enter the skin varies slightly with catheters from different manufacturers. The depth of the vein in the subcutaneous tissue also determines the angle used to enter the skin. A vein located superficially requires a small angle (10 to 20 degrees). However, a vein located deeper in the subcutaneous tissue requires a greater angle (20 to 30 degrees). A direct or an indirect approach can be used to insert a catheter into a vein. Using the direct method, the catheter enters the skin directly into the vein. An advantage of the direct method is that the vein is entered immediately. The disadvantage of this method is that with small, fragile veins, direct insertion can cause the vein to bruise more easily or can pierce the opposite side of the vein wall. With the indirect method, the catheter is inserted through the skin, the vein is relocated, and the catheter is then advanced into the vein. An advantage of this method is that a small tunnel space exists between the area of entry through the skin and the vein. When small, fragile veins are cannulated by the indirect method, bruising is less likely to occur because the catheter is inserted with a gentle entry into the vein.

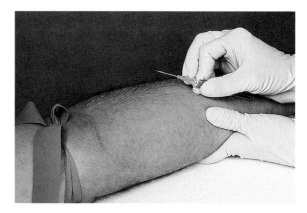

FIGURE 23-1   Peripheral IV catheter insertion, bevel up. (From Elkin MK, Perry AG, Potter PA: *Nursing interventions & clinical skills,* ed 4, St Louis, 2007, Mosby.)

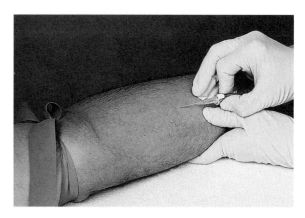

FIGURE 23-2   After the skin has been penetrated, the angle of the needle is decreased as the catheter is advanced into the vein. (From Elkin MK, Perry AG, Potter PA: *Nursing interventions & clinical skills,* ed 4, St Louis, 2007, Mosby.)

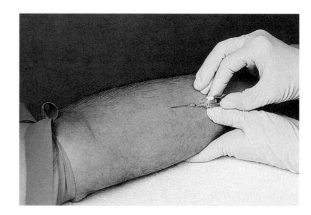

FIGURE 23-3   Blood return in flashback chamber. (From Elkin MK, Perry AG, Potter PA: *Nursing interventions & clinical skills,* ed 4, St Louis, 2007, Mosby.)

After the skin has been penetrated, the angle of the needle is decreased to prevent puncturing the posterior wall of the vein (Figure 23-2). Obtaining a blood return in the flashback chamber confirms the catheter has entered the vein (Figure 23-3). With small-gauge catheters or hypotensive patients, a slow or minimal blood return may be obtained. If a blood return is obtained, the catheter should be advanced an additional $\frac{1}{16}$ inch before the stylet is withdrawn. The catheter is advanced gently into the vein. The catheter can be threaded into the vein by use of a one-handed or a two-handed technique. With the one-handed technique, the same hand that performs the venipuncture also withdraws the stylet while advancing the catheter into the vein. This technique allows skin traction to be maintained while the catheter is advanced. It is also an advantage with the uncooperative patient because the skin traction and the hold on the patient are maintained. In the two-handed technique, one hand performs the venipuncture and the opposite hand grasps the catheter hub while the hand performing the venipuncture withdraws the stylet and advances the catheter with the dominant hand. This method requires the release of skin traction to activate the safety mechanism of the needle, and potentially increases the possibility of contamination from the hand grasping the catheter hub.

Once the catheter is totally advanced into the vein, the tourniquet is removed. If any bruising occurs while the venipuncture is performed, the tourniquet is removed immediately to prevent a hematoma from forming. A stylet is never reinserted into a catheter; doing so can puncture or sever the catheter wall, possibly resulting in catheter fragmentation and catheter embolism. Sometimes, the stylet is removed from the catheter and the solution in a syringe or administration set is used to advance the catheter into the vein. If any difficulty is encountered advancing the catheter or if it cannot be advanced in its entirety, the insertion should be discontinued and a new attempt should be made.

To reduce the risk of infection and phlebitis, it is important to maintain aseptic technique during the insertion of the catheter. Sterility of the catheter should not be violated by laying the catheter on the skin during insertion or by touching the catheter with the fingers. Only one catheter is used for each venipuncture attempt because catheters that have penetrated the skin are contaminated. Once a catheter has been used, it is contaminated. As the catheter enters the skin, it acquires any microorganisms that are on the skin. Also, once a catheter has been used to puncture the skin, fraying of the catheter tip is likely to occur. No more than two attempts at catheter insertion are recommended by any one nurse (INS, 2006a). If a nurse has made two unsuccessful insertion attempts, the nurse with the most advanced IV skills should evaluate the patient's venous access. Further insertion attempts should be made only if the venous access is deemed adequate. Multiple unsuccessful attempts limit future vascular access and cause unnecessary trauma to the patient. If the patient has limited venous access and the veins cannot be cannulated successfully, the patient's physician should be notified; another type of vascular access device should be established or alternative routes for medication administration need to be evaluated.

Catheter securement and dressing

Peripheral catheters may be secured using securement devices or taping methods. Research is supporting the importance of catheter securement in reducing peripheral IV-related complications. Stabilization of the catheter may reduce the risk of phlebitis, infiltration, infection, and catheter migration. By minimizing movement of the catheter, there is less mechanical irritation to the lining of the vein, reducing phlebitis risk. In a systematic review of three prospective studies comparing tape plus a transparent dressing to a manufactured catheter securement device with peripheral IV catheters, there was a reduction in overall complications up to 69%, reduction in catheter

---

PROCEDURE FOR INSERTION OF A PERIPHERAL IV CATHETER

1. Obtain and review order.
2. Ascertain allergies.
3. Gather equipment.
4. Verify patient's identity using two patient identifiers.
5. Explain procedure, benefits, care management, and potential complications to patient.
6. Perform hand hygiene.
7. Assemble equipment.
8. Apply tourniquet.
9. Assess veins, keeping in mind the rationale for therapy and duration of therapy.
10. Apply nonsterile gloves.
11. Wash intended insertion site with antiseptic soap and water (as needed).
12. Remove excess hair from insertion site with clippers or scissors (as needed).
13. Clean intended insertion site with antiseptic solution, working outward using back-and-forth motion.
14. Allow site to air-dry.
15. Perform venipuncture while stabilizing skin with the nondominant hand.
16. Enter skin at a 10- to 30-degree angle. Decrease angle when the skin has been penetrated. When blood is obtained in the flashback chamber, advance catheter $\frac{1}{16}$ inch, and then slightly pull stylet back, advancing catheter gently into vessel. Continue to advance catheter into vein until the catheter hub is against the skin.
17. Release tourniquet.
18. Occlude tip of catheter by pressing finger of nondominant hand over vein to prevent blood spillage.
19. Activate needle safety device before removing stylet. Connect IV administration set or injection cap/needleless device. Begin infusing solutions slowly. Observe insertion site for any signs of swelling. If catheter is for intermittent therapy, flush slowly with 3 mL of 0.9% sodium chloride solution.
20. Stabilize catheter with securement device and/or apply transparent dressing.
21. Label dressing with date, time, gauge and length of catheter, and name of nurse inserting catheter.
22. Discard stylet in sharps container.
23. Remove gloves. Perform hand hygiene.
24. Document procedure in the patient's medical record.

Adapted from Infusion Nurses Society: *Policies and procedures for infusion nursing,* ed 3, Norwood, Mass, 2006b, Author.

---

dislodgement up to 95%, and dwell time prolonged up to 61% (Frey and Schears, 2006). In a prospective, quasi-experimental study that included 659 subjects, 3 peripheral IV catheter securement methods (nonsterile tape, HubGuard™, and StatLock™) were studied; there were significantly longer peripheral catheter dwell times with the StatLock (Smith, 2006).

The use of catheter stabilization devices represents a significant change in practice. There are a growing number of commercially available manufactured stabilization devices. When evaluating potential products, desired qualities for securement devices as well as IV dressings include ease of application, viewing capacity, proper adhesion, appropriate size, moisture-proof characteristics, permeability, durability, patient comfort, ability to immobilize the catheter, ease of removal, and cost-effectiveness.

If the chevron tape method is used instead of a securement device to anchor a catheter, the sterility of the tape must be maintained. Care should be taken to avoid tearing the tape and sticking it to contaminated overbed tables and side rails before insertion. Any microorganisms present on an inanimate object will be transmitted on the tape. When the contaminated tape is placed on the skin-catheter junction site, it may be a potential source of infection. Anchor tape should be applied only to the wings-catheter hub so that the insertion site remains visible and assessment and monitoring of the skin-catheter junction site are not interrupted. Tape should never be placed over the insertion site.

A sterile dressing is applied over the catheter insertion site to prevent the introduction of microorganisms into the intravascular system. The *Infusion Nursing Standards of Practice* (2006a) recommends that sterile gauze or a transparent semipermeable membrane (TSM) dressing be aseptically applied over the insertion site. The most commonly used dressing materials are gauze or a transparent semipermeable membrane. Because it is nonocclusive, a Band-Aid dressing is not recommended unless all four edges are sealed. If gauze is used, the entire surface and all edges must be secured with tape to ensure that the dressing is closed and intact.

Transparent dressings are popular because they allow direct observation of the insertion site. Using only a transparent dressing allows the nurse to visualize and assess the insertion site. The transparent dressing is applied over the insertion site and hub to prevent the catheter from moving (Figure 23-4). If a gauze dressing is used, all the edges must be taped to occlude air flow. The dressing is labeled with the date, time, and gauge and length of the catheter inserted.

After the catheter stylet is disposed in the sharps container, the nurse removes gloves and performs hand hygiene. The nurse should document in the patient's medical record the anatomical location of the insertion site, the gauge and length of the catheter, the number of attempts, evaluation of the

placement (e.g., blood return obtained, flushes easily), and the patient's response to the procedure.

Postinsertion verification

The insertion of venous access devices requires verification that the placement is correct. The presence of a blood return does not always provide absolute verification. If the tip of the IV catheter punctures the posterior wall of the vein, leaving the greater part of the catheter in the vessel, a blood return may be obtained, but at the same time, the fluid could be infiltrating into the tissue. It is important to assess the insertion site for swelling, hardness, coolness, and any patient discomfort. Comparing the infusion site with the same area on the opposite extremity helps determine whether any swelling is present. To ascertain whether an infiltration has occurred, a tourniquet can be applied proximally to the insertion site. When a tourniquet is applied, the venous flow is restricted. However, if the infusion continues regardless of the applied venous obstruction, infiltration of the fluid is confirmed. Arterial placement can be verified by observing the pulsation of bright red blood into the administration set or syringe without applying any traction on the syringe. If there are any questions regarding the patency or placement of the device, the site should be discontinued immediately and a new catheter restarted.

MIDLINE CATHETER

A midline catheter is indicated for patients who require frequent restarts of their peripheral IV catheters, depending on the type of therapy they are receiving. Consideration should be given to the composition of the infusate to be administered. Midline catheters may be appropriate for the infusion of IV solutions, electrolytes, and osmotic or near-osmotic medications that are appropriate for infusion into a peripheral vein. Midline catheters should be inserted by persons who have clinical expertise in IV insertion or their insertion should be supervised by someone who is skilled in such insertion.

Site selection

When the therapy is anticipated to be a few weeks, the placement of a midline catheter may be indicated. The insertion of a midline catheter for the administration of vesicants, long-term antibiotic therapy, solutions with a final glucose concentration greater than 10%, and solutions with a protein concentration greater than 5% is contraindicated.

The basilic and cephalic antecubital veins are the preferred sites for the insertion of a midline catheter. The basilic vein is the largest and recommended as the preferred vein. The cephalic vein is smaller in diameter and more superficial. Because of the risk of additional injury to the vessel and surrounding tissue, previously damaged, sclerotic veins should not be used for the insertion of a midline catheter; an increase in the occurrence of complications, such as phlebitis and infection, could result. An extremity affected by a mastectomy or axillary node removal, an AV graft, or a fistula is also not recommended for the insertion of a midline catheter.

Site preparation

The insertion of a midline catheter is a sterile procedure requiring the use of a mask, sterile gloves and gown, a surgical scrub, and sterile drapes.

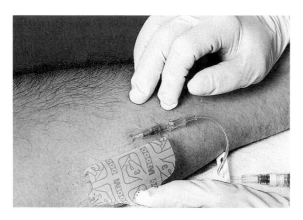

FIGURE 23-4 Apply transparent dressing over insertion site. (From Elkin MK, Perry AG, Potter PA: *Nursing interventions & clinical skills*, ed 4, St Louis, 2007, Mosby.)

Catheter insertion

Only nurses who have validated competency and clinical proficiency in the insertion of short peripheral catheters should insert midline catheters. There is some controversy regarding the necessity of obtaining informed consent signed by the patient or the legally authorized representative for this procedure. Some agencies require a physician's order because of the increased dwell time of the catheter; other agencies do not require a physician's order because the catheter is not entering the central venous system. Each organization should have a written policy regarding the necessity of obtaining documentation of informed consent before the insertion of a midline device.

The insertion procedure varies slightly depending on the midline catheter used. The midline catheter may be inserted through an introducer catheter. With this design, an over-the-needle plastic catheter is used as the introducer for the catheter. After a blood return is obtained and the catheter enters the vein, the needle is removed, leaving the introducer catheter in place. The midline catheter is advanced through the plastic catheter into the vein.

Catheter securement and dressing

Sterile tape and a securement device may be used to secure a midline catheter. Several catheters are available with wings, which snap and lock to a securement device that adheres to the patient's skin. After the catheter is secured, it is covered with a sterile transparent dressing. Junctions on the IV administration set must be secured, preferably with Luer-Lok™ connections, clasping devices, or tape. Accidental tubing separations can cause air embolism, hemorrhage, and contamination of the infusion system.

EXTERNAL JUGULAR PERIPHERAL INTRAVENOUS CATHETER (EJ PIV)

In emergent situations or when no other veins can be accessed, the external jugular vein may be used for the insertion of a peripheral IV catheter (Bernatene, Mason, Rudnick et al, 2007). Only a registered nurse who has validated competency and clinical proficiency in the insertion of short peripheral catheters should insert external jugular catheters (INS, 2008). Qualifications for the insertion of peripheral external jugular catheters must be consistent with federal and state laws as well as organizational policies. It is recommended that the insertion of an external jugular peripheral IV catheter be limited to the acute care setting.

Although the external jugular vein is easy to visualize and locate, it is difficult to cannulate because of its tortuous path and valves and tendency to roll. The insertion, care, maintenance, and monitoring of an EJ PIV are the same as those for a peripheral IV catheter. Peripheral EJs can be secured with a manufactured securement device and transparent tape. The dwell time of a peripheral EJ PIV is limited to 72 to 96 hours. If long-term venous access is required, consideration should be given to the insertion of a central venous access device.

■ MONITORING

The following aspects of the IV administration system should be monitored: solution container, administration set and flow rate, electronic infusion device, IV site dressing, vascular access device,

and insertion site. The frequency for monitoring a peripheral IV site is determined by the prescribed therapy, the condition and age of the patient, and the practice setting. IV insertion sites in acute care settings are often monitored at 4-hour intervals. The pediatric, geriatric, or critically ill patient requires more frequent site assessments. A thorough assessment of the insertion site should be performed when the dressing is changed. The patient receiving care in the home should be taught how to assess his or her venous access device and insertion site several times daily. If administering any medications, the patient should be taught to assess the insertion site before the catheter is flushed or any medication is administered. The home care nurse must provide frequent follow-up and supervision.

A systematic and organized assessment of the IV administration system begins with the solution container and progresses down the tubing to the venous access device and insertion site. The type of solution and medications added are verified against the physician's or other authorized prescriber's order, as is the information printed on the solution container label. The container must be labeled with the date and time that it was hung. Several types of flow strips are available that can be used to identify the time the container was hung and have

PROCEDURE FOR INSERTION OF A MIDLINE CATHETER

1. Obtain and review order.
2. Ascertain allergies.
3. Gather supplies and equipment.
4. Verify patient's identity using two patient identifiers.
5. Explain procedure, benefits, care management, and potential complications to patient.
6. Perform hand hygiene.
7. Assemble equipment; prepare work area.
8. Fully extend patient's arm; abduct the arm at a 45-degree angle.
9. Position protective covering under the patient's arm.
10. Place tourniquet on the mid-upper arm for final vein assessment. Insertion site should be 1 to 1½ inches above or below the antecubital fossa.
11. Remove excess hair from insertion site with clippers or scissors (as needed).
12. Don sterile gloves.
13. Flush catheter with 0.9% sodium chloride solution.
14. Cleanse intended insertion site with antiseptic solution. Apply in a back-and-forth motion, working outward to an area 4 to 5 inches in diameter.
15. Allow to air-dry.
16. Remove and discard gloves.
17. Apply tourniquet.
18. Don second pair of sterile gloves.
19. Drape arm with a fenestrated drape, leaving an opening for the venipuncture. The venipuncture should be two to three fingerbreadths above the bend of the arm or one fingerbreadth below the bend of the arm.

(Continued)

PROCEDURE FOR INSERTION OF A MIDLINE CATHETER—CONT'D

20. Perform venipuncture with the introducer, using the technique recommended by the manufacturer.

21. Withdraw stylet.

22. Slowly continue to advance the catheter via the introducer to the desired insertion length. Intermittently flush with 0.9% sodium chloride, alternating with aspiration for a blood return.
    Caution: If resistance is met during advancement, stop immediately. Techniques that can be used if resistance is met include changing the angle of the arm, rotating the wrist, or having the patient open and close his or her fist. Catheter may be slightly withdrawn, until blood return is aspirated, and slowly advanced while continuing to flush with 0.9% sodium chloride. If resistance continues to be met, catheter insertion must be discontinued.

23. Release tourniquet.

24. Remove guidewire slowly.

25. Remove peel-away introducer.

26. Attach injection cap and/or needleless device.

27. Flush with a 3 syringe of 0.9% sodium chloride.

28. Stabilize catheter with securement device.

29. Cover with sterile transparent dressing.

30. Label dressing with date, time, catheter gauge and length, and inserter's initials.

31. Discard stylet in sharps container.

32. Remove gloves and perform hand hygiene.

33. Document procedure in patient's medical record.

Adapted from Infusion Nurses Society: *Policies and procedures for infusion nursing,* ed 3, Norwood, Mass, 2006b, Author.

interval markings indicating the fluid level at specified times. Sometimes, a tape strip is placed on the container that indicates the time when the container was hung and the fluid level. No matter how the hang time of the container is labeled, the label should not be placed over important information printed on the solution container, such as the name of the solution or the "medication added" label. The solution container should not be labeled by writing with a pen or a felt tip marker on the plastic surface because the ink can penetrate the plastic and leak into the infusate.

The next monitoring criterion to note is the amount of solution remaining in the container. The nurse determines how much solution should remain in the solution container based on the prescribed flow rate and the indicated time. The appearance of the solution remaining in the container is noted: the solution should be clear—free from cloudiness and particulate matter.

The correct type of administration set should be hanging with the solution container and the electronic infusion device. Infusates contained in glass bottles require vented administration sets. Most electronic infusion devices require the use of a dedicated administration set as specified by the specific manufacturer. If an infusion is being administered by gravity at a very slow infusion rate, a microdrop administration set should be used.

Arm boards may be used when an insertion site is located near an area of flexion. Care must be taken when an extremity is placed on an arm board to ensure that it remains in a functional position. Contractures, unnecessary discomfort, skin tears, and neural injuries to the extremity can occur if an arm board is applied incorrectly. Tape or gauze may secure the arm board. If tape is used, it should be back-strapped (tape placed back-to-back) to avoid placing tape directly on the patient's skin. Tape should never encircle an extremity because such practice impairs circulation. If gauze is used to secure an arm board, a window should be left to allow easy observation of the insertion site.

The viscosity of solutions affects the flow rate. Solutions that are thick, including blood, lipid emulsions, or colloidal solutions (e.g., albumin, dextran), can alter flow rates. It may be necessary to administer viscous solutions through a larger-gauge catheter. The temperature of an infusate also affects the flow rate. Refrigerated solution should be removed and allowed to reach room temperature before infusing. Cool fluids can induce venous spasm, which further slows the flow rate. Infusates cannot be submerged in warm water to hasten warming.

The administration set can alter the flow rate if it is crimped or dangling below the bed, a filter is occluded, or the air vent is occluded (with vented administration sets). When assessing the administration set, it is usually helpful to start the evaluation at the drip chamber and work down the length of the set, assessing tubing and access ports, then continuing down to the catheter-tubing junction site. If the filter or an air vent becomes occluded, a new administration set must be used.

The flow rate can be altered, if the position of an IV catheter changes. The catheter tip may become occluded if it lies against the vessel wall or next to a bifurcation in the vein. This condition can sometimes be corrected by pulling the catheter back ⅛ inch or less. When the catheter is pulled back, care must be taken to avoid withdrawing it from the vessel, or an infiltration will occur. In addition, the IV catheter can become occluded if venous pressure increases. An increase in venous pressure occurs when a blood pressure reading is taken on an extremity that has an IV site or when a wrist restraint is placed on or above the IV catheter. Blood pressure readings should be taken on an extremity that does not have a venous access device. Wrist restraints must be applied loosely and should never be placed directly over a venipuncture site.

The flow rate changes if an undetected infiltration, phlebitis, or thrombus is present. As the infiltration progresses, the infusion rate decreases, and the electronic infusion device might sound an alarm. If the electronic infusion device infuses solution using positive pressure, it may not detect an infiltration, in which case it continues to infuse the solution into the subcutaneous tissues. The insertion site must be assessed when any alteration in the flow rate occurs or when the electronic control device sounds an alarm.

The monitoring of the IV infusion system continues with assessment of the electronic infusion device. The electronic infusion device is evaluated to determine whether it is infusing at the prescribed flow rate. When a gravity administration set is being used, the drops of solution per minute are counted to determine the flow rate. The flow rate is altered if the solution container is placed higher or lower than the optimal height, which is 30 to 36 inches above the patient. Raising the height of the container increases the flow rate. The flow rate can also be altered by any change in the patient's position. If the venipuncture site is located on an extremity near a point of flexion, bending of the patient's arm or wrist will alter the flow rate. Sporadic flow rates should be avoided because they result in an inaccurate delivery of solutions and medications.

Many electronic infusion devices are available, and health care professionals must be familiar with the IV equipment being used for each patient. The nurse oversees the overall mechanical operation and troubleshooting when an alarm sounds. Equipment should be monitored to ensure that the prescribed therapy is delivered with minimal deviation. To ensure accurate flow rates, the solution container should be labeled with the date and time it was hung. Some electronic infusion devices decrease the flow rate when the programmed amount of solution has been administered. Other electronic control devices decrease the flow rate if the battery is low. When the electronic infusion device is assessed, it is helpful to read the display panel to note the amount of solution infused and compare this reading with the volume remaining in the container to ensure that the machine is operating properly.

If the catheter-tubing junction site has already been assessed, the nurse can proceed to the IV site dressing. The dressing is monitored to ensure that it remains dry, closed, and intact. An intact dressing is one in which all edges of the dressing are sealed to the skin. If the dressing is damp or its integrity compromised, it must be changed immediately.

The monitoring of the IV system proceeds to the assessment of the insertion site. To thoroughly assess the venous access device, the nurse must know the type and length of the venous access device. Peripheral IV catheters may be as short as 0.7 mm or as long as 20 cm. The length of the IV device determines the area of the patient's arm that requires assessment. If the catheter length is 20 cm, the area of the patient's arm to be assessed begins at the insertion site and follows the catheter tract up the arm to the distal tip. For this reason, the length of the venous access device should be documented on the insertion site dressing and in the patient's medical record.

The venipuncture site must be assessed for pain and tenderness. If a patient experiences pain or discomfort from a peripheral catheter, the site should be discontinued and a new catheter should be inserted because pain can be a precursor to phlebitis. Another cause of discomfort is infusing solutions that are cool. The tunica media, or the middle layer of the vein, contains nerve fibers. When cool solutions are administered, the veins constrict, and venospasm can occur. Therefore refrigerated infusates should be allowed to reach room temperature before they are infused. Solutions can be warmed to room temperature by removing them from the refrigerator 1 hour before they are to be administered. If the infusate cannot be warmed in this way, such as when blood is administered, the infusion should be started slowly and the solution fluid allowed time to warm before the infusion rate is increased. Application of warm, moist packs to the vein promotes vasodilation, relieves venospasm, increases blood flow, and relieves pain.

The peripheral IV site must be assessed for any signs of swelling at or above the venipuncture site. If the tip of the IV catheter punctures the posterior wall of the vein, leaving the greater part of the catheter in the vessel, a blood return may be obtained, but the solution could be leaking into the tissues. The size of the arm with the inserted IV device should be compared with that of the opposite extremity. If the arm with the IV device is larger or if swelling is observed above the insertion site, the catheter must be removed.

Blanching is a white, shiny appearance at or above the insertion site. It is an indicator of an infiltration or a solution leak into the tissue. If any solution leakage is noted at or above the insertion site, the VAD should be changed. Solution leaking at or above the insertion site compromises the integrity of the skin tissue. Any venipuncture site from which solution leaks should be evaluated for signs of cellulitis, which manifests as edema, redness, pain, and irritation that are usually accompanied by weeping skin. *Cellulitis* is an inflammatory response within the subcutaneous tissue that can be caused by the infiltration or extravasation of irritating medications, the lack of aseptic technique during site preparation, or the use of contaminated equipment or solution. Any indications of cellulitis should be reported promptly to the patient's physician.

Redness at the insertion site indicates phlebitis, which is an inflammation of the vein. The VAD should be discontinued and a new venipuncture site established when the first signs of erythema (redness) are observed. Some of the other clinical indicators of phlebitis are swelling, induration, tenderness, and palpation of a venous cord. The degree of phlebitis should be measured according to a uniform phlebitis scale, which provides a consistent standard for measuring the degree of phlebitis. A recommended phlebitis scale is available in the *Infusion Nursing Standards of Practice* (2006a). The accepted phlebitis rate is 5% or less in any given patient population. The degree of phlebitis should be documented in the patient's medical record. The presence of phlebitis may require the application of warm, moist compresses or a medical intervention, such as changing medications, doses, dilution, method of delivery, or venous access devices.

Septic (suppurative) thrombophlebitis can occur when purulent drainage is present at the insertion site. The occurrence of septic thrombophlebitis is related to the presence of an intravascular abscess, which discharges a myriad of microorganisms into the bloodstream. A swab culture of the drainage is obtained, blood cultures are drawn, and the hub and catheter tip are cultured. Removing the catheter does not make the infection disappear. In fact, if any of the infecting organisms are present in the circulatory system, bacteremia can result. The first signs of a catheter-related infection may appear while the catheter is in use or 2 to 10 days after the catheter is removed.

 ## CATHETER CARE

DRESSING CHANGES

Peripheral catheter care should be performed after an IV catheter is inserted, on a routine basis with catheter site rotation, and when the dressing is soiled or no longer intact. The criteria for peripheral site care is established in the *Infusion Nursing Standards of Practice* (2006a). First, the skin-catheter junction should be cleansed with an acceptable antiseptic solution (2% chlorhexidine, tincture of iodine 2%, 10% povidone-iodine, or alcohol), with attention to minimizing disruption and movement of the catheter.

If a stabilization device is used for catheter securement, it is applied before placement of the transparent semipermeable membrane dressing. The transparent semipermeable membrane is the most commonly used insertion site dressing. It is a water-resistant sterile dressing that is permeable to air; it adheres well to the skin and enables continuous visual inspection and observation of the insertion site.

After the dressing has been aseptically applied on a peripheral venipuncture site, a label should be attached to the dressing identifying the date and time, the gauge and length of the catheter, and the name of the nurse who inserted the catheter. If an administration set is being attached to the peripheral catheter, the administration set should be looped and the loop taped to the p atient's skin. This measure helps stabilize the catheter and keeps the administration set out of the patient's way. A transparent semipermeable dressing is not routinely changed on a short peripheral catheter unless it becomes soiled, becomes damp, or is no longer intact. The dressing should be changed at the time the catheter site is rotated.

Although the tip of a midline catheter is not in a central vein, the dressing is changed using sterile technique. Most agencies administer catheter care for midline catheters by following the same policies and procedures as those used for central vascular access devices (see Procedure for site care and dressing change in Chapter 25). Prepackaged dressing kits ensure the availability of all the required supplies and promote continuity in the delivery of care. A sterile dressing change requires the use of a mask and sterile gloves.

Dressings for external jugular insertion sites are difficult to maintain in a manner that is intact and occlusive to air. The jugular area of catheter insertion and movement of the neck create a challenge in applying a dressing that is comfortable to the patient and that remains occlusive. If the jugular insertion site is located near a tracheotomy, moisture repellency is a requirement. With diaphoretic patients, adhesion can be enhanced by applying a skin sealant around the outer perimeter before and after applying the dressing. Numerous skin protectants are available in sterile, single-application packages. If the upper layer of the skin is broken or denuded, the application of a skin sealant is contraindicated because of the alcohol content in these preparations. The application of tincture of benzoin is not recommended because of its drying effect on the skin, which can cause skin irritation.

The optimal time frequency for changing midline and external jugular dressings has not been established. The *Infusion Nursing Standards of Practice* (2006a) recommends that gauze dressings on midline catheters be routinely changed every 48 hours and that TSM dressings are changed at least every 3 to 7 days, sooner if the integrity of the dressing is compromised.

Transparent dressings are preferred because they promote stabilization of the catheter and allow observation of the insertion site. If sterile wound-closure strips and a catheter securement device are used to secure the catheter, they should be replaced with each dressing change. The dressing should be changed immediately when it becomes damp or soiled or if the integrity is compromised.

INJECTION/ACCESS CAPS AND NEEDLELESS SYSTEMS

Peripheral IV catheters are often used for intermittent infusions and injections. Injection/access caps and needleless devices are placed on catheters that are used intermittently. The CDC guidelines (2002b) do not provide recommendations for the use, maintenance, or frequency for changing needleless infusion devices. Much controversy exists regarding the risks of infection associated with needleless devices.

FLUSHES

Many organizations flush intermittent peripheral catheters with 0.9% sodium chloride solution only. Since two meta-analyses published in 1991 concluded that there was no difference in catheter patency when flushed with 0.9% sodium chloride only (as compared to 0.9% sodium chloride plus heparin) (Goode et al, 1991; Peterson and Kirchoff, 1991), practice has changed to eliminate the use of heparin to flush peripheral catheters. Policies and procedures should be established for the flushing of catheters used as intermittent devices.

Manufacturers' guidelines should be used when flushing catheters. If heparin is the flush solution of choice, the lowest possible concentration of heparin should be used. The amount and the frequency of the flush should not alter the patient's clotting factors. When medications are administered that are incompatible with heparin, the VAD is flushed with 0.9% sodium chloride before and after the administration of the medication.

All catheters used as intermittent devices are flushed as follows:

- After each administration of a medication
- After the administration of blood or blood products
- After withdrawal of blood
- When converting a continuous infusion to an intermittent device
- Every 8 to 12 hours when the catheter is not in use

The volume of flushing solution needed to maintain patency is equal to at least twice the volume capacity of the catheter and add-on devices.

A variety of needleless/access devices are available that incorporate positive pressure or antireflux mechanisms to prevent blood from retrograding into the catheter lumen. If resistance is met during flushing, no further attempts to flush should be made. Pressure should not be exerted on the catheter in an attempt to restore patency; applying pressure to an occluded catheter can dislodge the clot into the vascular system or can rupture the catheter.

One way of maintaining positive pressure is to exert a continual push on the syringe plunger while withdrawing the syringe during the administration of the last 0.2 mL of flush solution. Withdrawing the syringe while continuing to push on the plunger replaces the space occupied by the needle during the flush, thereby preventing the reflux of blood within the catheter tip. Some injection ports on administration sets and 0.9% sodium chloride/heparin lock systems (extension set with injection port) have a valve that prevents blood reflux, and the syringe is not withdrawn until all the flush solution has been given.

CHANGING THERAPY

A physician's order is necessary to change the solutions or medications being administered. The nurse uses the nursing process to evaluate the rationale for changing the therapy and intervenes appropriately. Before changing or administering IV solution or medication, the nurse should assess the appropriateness of the prescribed order by evaluating the patient's age and condition and the dosage, route, and rate of the IV solution or medication to be administered. The nurse must be knowledgeable about the indications, actions, dosage, side effects, and adverse reactions associated with each solution and medication administered.

The nurse is accountable for administering medications and solutions safely and for making appropriate nursing interventions. For example, if the nurse questions the prescribed dosage or determines that the patient's condition does not warrant the prescribed medication or solution, the order should not be carried out until it is clarified. If there are any questions regarding the prescribed therapy, the physician should be contacted to clarify the plan of care and to verify the medication order.

The nurse closely monitors the infusion system and the patient's response to the solution or medication being administered. The type and degree of change in the patient's status determine how promptly the nurse must intervene. It may be necessary to discontinue therapy before notifying the physician. For example, if a patient develops hives, hypotension, diaphoresis, or respiratory distress, the nurse must intervene immediately by stopping the medication. These signs and symptoms are indicators of an anaphylactic reaction, and appropriate therapy must be initiated immediately to reverse the complications of the reaction.

SOLUTION CONTAINERS

IV solution containers may be changed to add a sequential container, to avoid exceeding "hang time" restrictions, or in response to a change in the prescribed therapy. Before a new IV solution container is used, the solution in the container should be inspected for clarity and the presence of particulate matter. The infusate container should be inspected for cracks, leaks, or punctures and the expiration date should be verified. If the appearance of the solution is questionable or if the integrity of the container is compromised, the container should be returned to the pharmacy or dispensing department and should be clearly labeled with the reason for the return. If the expiration date has passed or will pass during the infusion, the container should be returned to the originating department or disposed of according to organizational policy.

After a medication has been added to the solution container or when an administration set has been attached, the solution container must be used or discarded within 24 hours. Once the solution container has been accessed, the potential for bacterial growth is increased; therefore CDC guidelines (2002b) recommend that IV solution containers must not hang longer than 24 hours. The solution container should be labeled with the date and time that it was initiated.

ADMINISTRATION SETS

Changing the primary administration set should coincide with the hanging of a new IV solution container or with the changing of the peripheral IV catheter. Each entry into the IV delivery system increases the risk of inadvertent contamination. The *Infusion Nursing Standards of Practice* (2006a) has established that continuous peripheral and central primary sets and secondary administration sets should be changed every 72 hours. However, failure to maintain an ongoing phlebitis rate of 5% or less, or any increased rate of catheter-related bacteremia, requires a return to 48-hour administration set changes.

Primary intermittent sets deliver medication through latex injection caps or needleless system devices. Intermittent devices have a greater risk of touch contamination than continuous devices because of the interruption involved in initiating and discontinuing infusate.

Guidelines from the Centers for Disease Control and Prevention (2002b) recommend that administration sets that include intermittent tubing not be changed any more frequently than every 72 hours. Administration sets used to administer blood, blood products, or lipid emulsions should be changed within 24 hours. The administration set should be labeled with the date and time that it was initiated and should be documented according to organizational policy. The administration set should be labeled to communicate to subsequent shifts, home care nurses, or caregivers when it must be changed.

SITE ROTATION

The *Infusion Nursing Standards of Practice* (2006a) recommends that short peripheral catheters be removed every 72 hours and immediately upon suspected contamination, complication, or when therapy has been discontinued. The CDC guidelines (2002b) recommend that peripheral IV catheters should be rotated every 72 to 96 hours.

When a peripheral rotation policy is strictly followed, venous access may be prolonged, and complications of phlebitis and infiltration are reduced. For routine peripheral site rotation, the extremities should be alternated whenever possible. Using the opposite extremity allows previous insertion sites time to rest and phlebitic or infiltrated areas time to resolve. If a subsequent insertion site is restarted in the same extremity, it must be located proximal to the previously cannulated site. Inserting a catheter proximal to a previously infiltrated or phlebitic site prevents further damage to the tissues.

Some organizations have policies that allow catheter dwell time to be extended in patients who have limited venous access. In these situations, an order must be obtained from the physician to continue the present site, and the physician's order must be documented in the patient's medical record. Peripheral venous sites that are extended beyond the 72- to 96-hour catheter dwell time must be monitored very closely and discontinued at the first indication of tenderness, infiltration, or phlebitis. Documentation by the nurse should include the location and appearance of the insertion site; site care, if administered; and any nursing actions taken to resolve problems associated with the catheter.

Catheters that have been placed in emergency situations should be replaced as soon as possible because aseptic technique or skin preparation may have been compromised. Peripheral catheters must be removed immediately if phlebitis, infiltration, or catheter occlusion occurs. If the peripheral catheter site appears to be infected, the catheter and insertion site should be cultured when the catheter is removed. Culturing will identify microorganisms that are the source of the infection and will determine the medical interventions that follow.

The CDC guidelines (2002b) do not have any recommendations regarding the routine frequency change of a midline catheter.

COMPLICATIONS

Although infusion therapy is usually administered without problems, complications do occur and range from minor to very serious. Some of the more serious complications can result in death if immediate medical intervention is not provided.

The potential for complications is always present in the patient receiving infusion therapy. Complications increase hospital stay, length of therapy, and nursing responsibilities, and can put the patient at risk for other medical problems. Furthermore, the patient experiences additional discomfort, and overall expenses are increased.

For this reason, patient monitoring and catheter care are critical components of IV administration; early detection can prevent many of these complications. Monitoring provides information regarding the patient's response to therapy, confirms the accurate delivery of solution and medications, and detects imminent complications. Catheter care is essential in preventing, detecting, and decreasing the occurrence of complications.

The nurse is responsible for observing and assessing the patient's response and providing appropriate nursing interventions. For example, after beginning the infusion of a newly ordered antibiotic, if a nurse observes that the patient is extremely anxious, is short of breath, and has hives on the face and chest, the nurse should intervene immediately. Interventions for this situation include stopping the remaining antibiotic infusion, notifying the patient's physician, and assessing the patient's vital signs. The patient's response to the administration of IV solutions or medications must be documented in the patient's medical record and communicated to the other members of the health care team.

Fortunately, most of these complications are preventable. A thorough knowledge and understanding of the risks involved with infusion therapy and measures to prevent their occurrence can eliminate many of the hazards associated with this treatment. Patient education in recognizing the signs and symptoms of complications and frequent monitoring by the nurse result in early detection and treatment. These measures may prevent further complications and promote prompt healing.

LOCAL VERSUS SYSTEMIC COMPLICATIONS

The administration of infusion therapy subjects the patient to numerous risks, such as local or systemic complications. Complications associated with infusion therapy are classified according to their location. Local complications, such as phlebitis, infiltration, and catheter occlusion, occur more often than systemic complications. However, systemic complications, such as septicemia, circulatory overload, and embolism, can be life-threatening. Local complications are usually seen at or near the insertion site or occur as a result of mechanical failure. These complications are more common than systemic complications and are not usually serious. Immediate recognition of associated signs and symptoms coupled with nursing intervention can prevent more serious complications from occurring.

Systemic complications are those occurring within the vascular system, usually remote from the infusion site. Although these complications are uncommon, they are usually very serious and can be life-threatening without appropriate medical intervention. Some local complications can lead to more serious systemic complications. For example, thrombophlebitis can develop into a pulmonary embolism if the thrombus becomes detached and floats free in the vascular system. Systemic complications are more difficult to treat than local complications; preventing systemic complications is far easier than treating them.

Local complications

Local complications result from mechanical problems associated with the infusion system or result from trauma to the intima of the vein (Box 23-1). Mechanical problems can result in depriving the patient of needed solutions or medications if vein access is lost. Trauma to the endothelial lining of the vein can lead to extensive edema, depriving the patient of needed solutions and medications, and to necrosis of surrounding tissue; thrombophlebitis, with the subsequent danger of embolism; and sepsis, if an infection at the site is not detected early or remains untreated. Individuals performing infusion therapy procedures must use techniques to prevent trauma to the vein intima and must monitor the system often to detect mechanical difficulties and signs of potential complications. The frequency of monitoring should be stated in established policies and procedures, and compliance should be monitored under the organization's clinical performance improvement program.

Mechanical complications

Mechanical complications relate to a failure of the infusion system to adequately deliver therapy at the prescribed rate. They are usually resolved by correction of the identified problem. If a mechanical problem is suspected, six major areas should be evaluated (Box 23-2).

Tourniquet

Clinicians have been known to fail to release the tourniquet once catheter placement is complete. Solution does not flow, or blood may back up in the administration set. Potential circulatory problems can occur if the tourniquet is not released.

Box 23-1　LOCAL COMPLICATIONS OF INTRAVENOUS THERAPY

- Mechanical failure
- Infiltration
- Extravasation
- Phlebitis
- Postinfusion phlebitis
- Thrombosis
- Thrombophlebitis
- Ecchymosis or hematoma
- Site infection
- Venous or arterial spasm

Box 23-2　STEPS IN THE EVALUATION OF MECHANICAL COMPLICATIONS

1. Check the tourniquet.
2. Check the venipuncture site.
3. Check the catheter.
4. Check the solution container.
5. Check the administration set.
6. Check the involved extremity.

Venipuncture site

The venipuncture site should be checked for swelling at, above, and below the insertion of the catheter. By observing for potential problems associated with the site, one can immediately rule out site-related problems.

Catheter

Proper placement of the catheter should be verified. A catheter tip that lies against a bifurcation or valve, or a catheter that is kinked or bent can slow or stop the infusion. Pulling back slightly on the catheter can often eliminate this problem. Bent catheters should be discontinued and replaced to prevent possible catheter breakage and subsequent catheter emboli.

Placement of a catheter in an area of flexion can also affect the infusion rate. If not obvious, one can easily check for a positional rate by having the patient flex and extend the extremity. If the flow rate slows or increases, the catheter is *positional*. If venous access is limited and the catheter cannot be changed, the application of an arm board should be considered. Arm boards must be used according to agency policies and procedures. Sites in an area of flexion should be avoided, if possible, because they can lead to further complications.

Occasionally, a catheter may leak at the point where it attaches to the hub, or the catheter may be obstructed as a result of the manufacturing process. If either of these situations occurs, the catheter should be removed.

Partially or completely obstructed catheters, regardless of cause, should be removed. They should not be flushed because a clot may be dislodged; the resulting embolus could cause a more serious complication.

Solution container

The solution container should be assessed. An empty container or a lack of adequate gravity flow can lead to an inaccurate flow rate or no flow rate at all. This problem is easily corrected by hanging another bag or by adjusting the height of the IV pole.

The solution container should be checked for a patent air vent. IV solution containers do not need to be vented; however, nonvented bottles require a vented adapter or vented tubing. A vacuum cannot be created within a bottle, and solution will not flow from a bottle unless it is replaced with air. Using a needle to vent a bottle is inappropriate because it opens the system for the entry of bacteria.

Another concern is the bag entry port; if it is obstructed, solution cannot pass. The outlet port seal must be completely penetrated by the administration spike for fluids to flow freely.

Administration set

An administration set that is pinched, crimped, or kinked prevents the delivery of an accurate flow rate. Administration sets may need to be taped to the patient's arm to prevent this problem. Filters can become blocked by particulates and can slow the infusion rate, particularly with the administration of certain medications, such as tetracycline. The filter should be changed when this problem occurs.

Patient

The involved extremity should be checked for constrictive clothing, identification bracelets, jewelry, and restraints. Anything placed above the venipuncture site that constricts the arm may act as a tourniquet and slow or stop the infusion.

Ecchymosis and hematoma

Ecchymosis is a term used to denote the infiltration of blood into the tissues, whereas *hematoma* usually refers to uncontrolled bleeding at a venipuncture site, usually creating a hard, painful lump. Ecchymosis and hematomas are commonly associated with venipunctures that are performed by unskilled professionals or on patients who have a tendency to bruise easily. Patients receiving anticoagulants and long-term steroid therapy are particularly susceptible to bleeding from vein trauma. Ecchymosis and hematomas often occur when multiple entries are made into a vein, or when attempts are made into veins that are difficult to visualize or that cannot be palpated.

The presence of ecchymosis and hematomas limits veins for future use and damages tissues. If a hematoma is severe, it may limit the use of an extremity.

Patient assessment

The venipuncture site and surrounding area should be observed for swelling during cannulation. Ecchymosis may not be noted immediately because of tissue turgor and the amount of blood escaping into the tissues. Ecchymosis occurs first, and if bleeding is allowed to continue a hematoma is formed. If sufficient bleeding is present, it is visible at the moment the catheter pierces the vein as blood escapes into the tissues. Discoloration may be immediate or slow, depending on the amount of subcutaneous tissue between the vein and the skin exterior.

Nursing interventions

If ecchymosis occurs during venipuncture, the catheter should be removed and light pressure should be applied. If heavy pressure is applied, fragile veins within the area may rupture and increase bleeding. These areas usually feel sore, are unsightly, and take 1 to 2 weeks to return to normal.

If a hematoma is noted during a venipuncture attempt, the catheter is removed immediately, direct pressure is applied to the area, catheter integrity is assessed, and the extremity is elevated until the bleeding has stopped. A dry, sterile dressing is applied to the site and the area is monitored for signs of breakthrough bleeding. Ice may be applied to the area to prevent further enlargement of the hematoma. The extremity is monitored for circulatory, neurological, and motor functions.

Preventive measures

Ecchymosis cannot always be prevented. The best prevention for hematomas is to ensure that venipunctures are performed by highly skilled professionals. Inexperienced individuals should never perform venipunctures on patients with fragile veins or veins that are not visible or easily palpable.

Hematomas can also result from excessive pressure being applied to a venipuncture site when a catheter is removed. Direct pressure with a dry, sterile dressing should be applied when catheters are removed. Elevating the extremity while continuing to apply pressure for 1 or 2 minutes helps stop bleeding and prevents hematoma formation. Because alcohol pads inhibit clotting, they should not be used.

Occlusion

Peripheral catheters can become occluded if monitoring or proper maintenance and care are not carried out. Catheters can become occluded with blood when solution containers become empty and when flush solutions are not administered appropriately. The administration of incompatible solutions or medications can also lead to precipitate formation within the catheter with subsequent occlusion.

Patient assessment

Usually, the first sign of a partially occluded catheter is the inability to maintain an accurate flow rate. The infusion rate slows, and readjusting the rate has no effect. When the occlusion intensifies, the infusion stops. Resistance is met when attempts are made to flush an occluded catheter. Prescribed therapy cannot be administered if the catheter is occluded; in addition, a danger exists of thrombophlebitis or pulmonary embolism.

Nursing interventions

Catheters should never be flushed to clear an occlusion. Clearing a catheter occlusion by force releases the occluding substance directly into the vascular system, creating a potential for an embolus. The peripheral catheter should be removed, the integrity of the catheter should be examined, and a dry, sterile dressing should be applied to the site. If therapy is to continue, a new catheter should be placed in another vein.

Preventive measures

Solution containers should be changed when less than 100 mL of solution remains. The use of a time tape to designate the time the solution will reach certain levels is very helpful in determining when a container will empty.

Solutions and medications should be evaluated for compatibilities before they are mixed and administered. The pharmacist should be consulted with questions about compatibilities to prevent the potential for crystallization from the mixing of incompatible solutions.

Infection

An infection can occur at the venipuncture site in the absence of phlebitis. It is usually a local infection at the catheter-skin entry point.

Patient assessment

The venipuncture site should be assessed frequently for signs of local infection while in use and during dressing and site changes. The site should be monitored after the VAD has been discontinued for the possibility of local inflammation at the site. The catheter-skin entry site should be observed for swelling and inflammation, and the surrounding tissue should be observed for discoloration and purulent drainage. An infection at the site may be apparent before or after the catheter has been removed.

Nursing interventions

If the catheter is in place, it should be removed and cultured to determine whether it is the source of the infection. Any drainage from around the site should be cultured, and the skin should be cleansed with alcohol before the catheter is removed for culture. A sterile dressing should be applied, and the physician should be notified. Systemic antibiotic therapy may be necessary, and occasionally surgical intervention is warranted. The site should be monitored until the infection has resolved.

Preventive measures

Usually, the causes of an infection at the site are related to a break in aseptic technique either during catheter insertion, care, or removal. Contaminated equipment or supplies and improper hand hygiene can predispose the site to an infection.

Aseptic technique must be maintained during catheter insertion, therapy delivery, and catheter removal. An infection at the site provides an excellent opportunity for bacteria to enter the venous system unless it is recognized early and appropriate interventions are carried out.

Infiltration

Infiltration is the inadvertent administration of a nonvesicant solution or medication into surrounding tissues. This occurs when the catheter becomes dislodged or the vein ruptures, causing solutions to leak into the surrounding tissue. It is usually recognized by increasing edema at or near the venipuncture site. Infiltration should be rated according to a uniform scale. The scale recommended by *Infusion Nursing Standards of Practice* (2006a) is given in Box 23-3.

Infiltration can result in significant injury. In a retrospective study in a single hospital, researchers reviewed 3 years of peripheral IV complications in patients who were administered IV medications in the emergency department or during hospitalization and found that the most frequent complication was symptomatic IV infiltration (Kagel and Rayan, 2004). The researchers found 26 incidents of minor, self-limited infiltration and 6 incidents of major complications secondary to infiltration. Major complications required surgery or therapy and included skin necrosis, finger stiffness, nerve irritation, neuropathy, and compartment syndrome. Three of the patients experienced scarring, skin depigmentation, and pain/weak hand grip as a result of the infiltration. Infusates included 0.5% and 0.9% sodium chloride, Decadron, Phenergan, cisplatin, and 5-fluorouracil. Most infiltrations occurred in the hand or forearm.

Box 23-3 INFILTRATION SCALE	
Grade	**Clinical Criteria**
0	No symptoms
1	Skin blanched
	Edema <1 inch in any direction
	Cool to touch
	With or without pain
2	Skin blanched
	Edema 1-6 inches in any direction
	Cool to touch
	With or without pain
3	Skin blanched, translucent
	Gross edema >6 inches in any direction
	Cool to touch
	Mild-moderate pain
	Possible numbness
4	Skin blanched, translucent
	Skin tight, leaking
	Skin discolored, bruised, swollen
	Gross edema >6 inches in any direction
	Deep pitting tissue edema
	Circulatory impairment
	Moderate–severe pain
	Infiltration of any amount of blood product, irritant, or vesicant

From Infusion Nurses Society: *Standards of Practice*, Norwood, Mass, 2006a, Author.

Infiltration occurs as a result of mechanical, obstructive, and inflammatory causes (Hadaway, 2007). Examples include catheter dislodgement caused by joint movement when the catheter is placed in an area of flexion, obstruction of solution flow attributable to blood clots from a previously infiltrated venipuncture site distal to the current site, and inflammation resulting from irritating solutions. The first symptom recognized by many patients is the feeling of skin tightness at the venipuncture site that makes flexing or extending the involved extremity difficult. If a large amount of solution is trapped in the subcutaneous tissue, the skin may appear taut or stretched. As more solution gathers in the tissues, blanching and coolness of the skin may occur, the infusion may slow or stop, and the patient may experience tenderness or discomfort at the site. Discomfort experienced by the patient is determined by the type of solution or medication being infused. Isotonic solutions generally do not produce much discomfort when an infiltration occurs. Solutions with an acidic or alkaline pH or those that are slightly more hypertonic are more irritating and usually cause discomfort.

Unless obvious, an infiltration may remain undetected because of dependent edema or the administration of solution at a very slow rate. The venipuncture site must be monitored frequently to prevent this problem.

Patient assessment

A complete assessment of the patient, the venipuncture site, the involved extremity, and the infusion system may be necessary to determine the presence of an infiltration. The site around the tip of the catheter and the extremity should be inspected for swelling, blanching, stretched skin, firm tissues, and coolness. It may be helpful to compare the site with the same area on the opposite extremity. If both extremities appear edematous, the patient's medical status should be evaluated. Patients with hemodynamic problems, such as congestive heart failure, toxic conditions, compromised kidney function, hypothermia, and vascular insufficiency, are particularly prone to vascular edema. The immobilized patient or the patient with muscular weakness or paralysis of an extremity may experience edema of the extremity that is totally unrelated to a problem at the catheter insertion site.

If an assessment of the involved extremity and a review of the patient's medical status are inconclusive, pressure should be applied to the vein with a finger or tourniquet about 2 inches above the insertion site (it must be above the tip of the catheter). If the catheter is in the vein, this pressure will slow or stop the infusion rate. If the infusion continues despite the venous obstruction, an infiltration has occurred.

Checking for a blood return, or backflow of blood, is not a reliable method for determining the absence of an infiltration. A blood return may not be present when small veins are used because they may not permit blood flow around the catheter; one may think the infusion has infiltrated when it has not. In addition, veins that have had previous punctures or that are very fragile may seep fluid at a site above or below the vein catheter entry point; a blood return may be present, yet an infiltration is occurring. The movement of a catheter, such as in-and-out motions, can also cause the skin and the vein entry site to enlarge, allowing fluid to seep at the vein entry site, causing an infiltration.

Nursing interventions

The type of solution being infused should also be considered. If the solution is isotonic and has a normal pH, the patient may not feel much discomfort unless a large amount of solution has infiltrated. In these cases, warm compresses, such as warm, moist towels or chemical packs, may help alleviate the discomfort and help absorb the infiltration by increasing circulation to the affected area. Sloughing can occur from the application of warm compresses to an area infiltrated with certain medications, such as potassium chloride. In these instances, the application of cold compresses is preferred. Established policies and procedures should dictate the use of hot and cold compresses. The involved extremity should be elevated to improve circulation and to help absorb infiltrated solutions.

If weeping of the tissues occurs because of an extensive infiltration or loose, thin tissue, as is often present in the elderly, it may be necessary to apply a sterile dressing to the affected area. It is usually better to leave these areas open because the dressing necessitates the use of gauze and possibly tape, which can increase tissue damage. If a dressing is used, it should be applied loosely. Extreme care should be given to prevent infection. The physician should be notified and measures should be carried out as ordered. If an infusion is needed, a peripheral catheter is placed in the opposite extremity or in a site above and away from the previous site.

Preventive measures

The following strategies can be used to reduce the risk of infiltration:

- Avoiding areas of flexion and lower extremities (exception—infants) when placing peripheral catheters; protecting the site from excessive movement or pressure by use of an arm board
- Placing the smallest gauge and shortest length catheter to accommodate the infusion
- Avoiding subsequent cannulations proximal to previously cannulated sites
- Avoiding infusion of irritating infusates
- Stabilizing the catheter to minimize in-and-out movement
- Monitoring the venipuncture site closely for evidence of infiltration and instructing patients to report any pain, discomfort, or feelings of tightness at the site
- Removing the IV catheter immediately when signs and symptoms occur

Note that if arm boards are used, they should be well padded and applied in a manner that will not cause nerve damage, constrict circulation, or cause pressure areas. They should be removed at frequent intervals and range-of-motion exercises performed. Inadequate or improper use of arm boards or restraints can cause very serious complications.

Patient education is a key factor in the prevention and early recognition of the signs and symptoms of an infiltration. Patient knowledge about the care of the venipuncture site and the infusion system can prevent activities that may cause an infiltration, such as manipulating the catheter, pulling on the administration set or dressing, and using the extremity excessively. A patient who is aware of the signs of infiltration can alert the nurse to the early signs of an infiltration, and immediate care can be initiated, thereby preventing the possibility of more serious complications.

Extravasation

Extravasation is the inadvertent administration of a vesicant solution or medication into the surrounding tissues. A vesicant is a solution or medication that causes the formation of blisters, with subsequent sloughing of tissues occurring from tissue necrosis.

Patient assessment

It is essential that an extravasation be noted early, before an excessive amount of solution is allowed to infiltrate the interstitial tissues. A complete assessment of the patient, the IV site, the involved extremity, and the infusion system should be performed at regular intervals. The flow rate should never be increased to determine the infiltration of a vesicant, nor should a blood return be used as a reliable method to determine an extravasation. Solution can seep into the tissues from a previous puncture site or around the vein insertion site and increase the potential for tissue necrosis (see Infiltration for the assessment process).

Initial indications that tissue sloughing may occur include pain or burning at the site with progression to erythema and edema. Tissue sloughing is usually apparent within 1 to 4 weeks because of tissue necrosis. Necrosis can involve a small or a large area, including underlying connective tissues, muscles, tendons, and bone, necessitating surgical intervention.

The severity of damage is directly related to the type, concentration, and volume of solution infiltrated into the interstitial tissues. The most harmful of the vesicant medications are the antineoplastic agents. Other medications acting as vesicants with the potential for causing tissue necrosis include dopamine hydrochloride (Dopastat, Intropin), norepinephrine (levarterenol bitartrate, Levophed), potassium chloride at high dosages, amphotericin B (Fungizone), calcium, and sodium bicarbonate in high concentrations.

Nursing interventions

When an extravasation is suspected, the infusate is discontinued immediately. Treatment protocols established in written policies and procedures are initiated, and a new site is established, preferably in the opposite extremity or in a site above and away from the extravasated site.

Organizational policies vary as to the treatment of the tissues in which an extravasation has occurred. Usually, the catheter is left in place until any residual medication and blood are aspirated, and an antidote particular to the vesicant is instilled into the tissues. See Chapter 18 for protocols related to the management of extravasation associated with the administration of chemotherapeutic agents. After the catheter is removed, a dry, sterile dressing is applied to the site, and either cold or warm compresses are applied. Cold compresses are usually used for the alkylating and antibiotic vesicants, whereas warm compresses are applied to an extravasation of the vinca alkaloids. The extremity is elevated and observed regularly for erythema, induration, and necrosis. The physician is notified, and tissue damage is evaluated for the possibility of surgical intervention.

Preventive measures

Every effort must be made to prevent an extravasation. Measures to reduce the risk of extravasation are discussed in Box 23-4. Knowledge of the vesicant potential of solutions and medications and identification of associated risk factors are

---

Box 23-4 MEASURES TO REDUCE POTENTIAL FOR EXTRAVASATION

- Only qualified registered nurses who have been trained in venipuncture and drug administration skills and who have knowledge of drugs with vesicant potential should be allowed to administer vesicants. The education program should include the protocols for drug administration, early signs of extravasation, preventive measures, and associated treatment protocols.
- The venous access device should be checked for patency before, during, and after the administration of a vesicant. Infusion of 5 to 10 mL of 0.9% sodium chloride before the administration of a vesicant can help determine vein patency.
- The organization's policies should specify the role of the nurse during the administration of vesicants. Some organizational policies state that a nurse must be in constant attendance during the infusion of a vesicant, whereas others state that the patient and the site should be monitored at specified intervals during the infusion. Others require that two licensed nurses verify vein patency before the administration of a vesicant. The degree to which the patient and site are observed may depend on the location of the patient at the time the vesicant is administered.
- When a vesicant is administered directly into a vein with a syringe, the plunger of the syringe is pulled back every 3 to 4 mL to note blood return. Although a good blood return does not guarantee that an extravasation has not occurred, any change in blood return could indicate the need to investigate the possibility of an extravasation.
- A vesicant should be administered through a side port of a free-flowing infusion because the vesicant is usually concentrated and the severity of tissue damage is related to the amount and concentration of the vesicant. A free-flowing infusion indicates a patent line.
- Catheters should be properly secured to prevent an in-and-out motion, which can enlarge the vein entry site and create an opportunity for the vesicant to seep into interstitial tissues, resulting in an extravasation.
- Vesicants should not be administered in areas of flexion.
- The digits, hands, and wrists should be avoided as intravenous sites for vesicant administration because of the close network of tendons and nerves that would be destroyed if an extravasation occurs.
- Gravity and heat (which maximize vasodilation) should be used to distend small fragile veins, especially those that have been used repeatedly for the administration of chemotherapeutic agents. Venipuncture should be performed without a tourniquet or with a loosely tied tourniquet to decrease the potential for an extravasation in these patients.
- Sites should be protected from excessive movement by using arm boards and restraints when indicated. The use of restraints should be established in written policies and procedures.
- If a catheter has been in place longer than 24 hours, consideration should be given to replacing the venous access device, preferably to the opposite extremity, before a vesicant is administered.
- The use of high-pressure infusion pumps must be avoided when administering vesicant medications.
- Consideration should be given to the placement of a central venous catheter. Some organizations administer vesicants only through central venous catheters, even when viable peripheral veins are available. The use of a central venous catheter should not provide false assurance that an extravasation cannot occur; extravasation has been documented from catheter rupture, catheter leakage, backtracking of an infusate along a fibrin sheath, separation of the port, and dislodgment of the port needle.

essential to the safe administration of these infusates. The nurse must know if the patient has a history of multiple venipunctures, where they were located, and how long ago the sites were used. Vesicants have been known to seep into the tissues at the vein entry site of a previous infusion.

The patient should be educated in the care of the infusion, including the recognition of potential problems, actions to take if a problem occurs, and the dangers associated with extravasation. A well-educated patient can be a vital asset in preventing an extravasation and in minimizing the effects of an existing extravasation.

Phlebitis

Phlebitis, which is the inflammation of the intima of the vein, is a commonly reported complication of infusion therapy. Inflammation occurs as a result of irritation to the endothelial cells of the vein intima, creating a rough cell wall where platelets readily adhere. Phlebitis is characterized by pain and tenderness along the course of the vein, erythema, and inflammatory swelling with a feeling of warmth at the site, streak formation, and/or a palpable cord.

Phlebitis is classified according to its causative factors. The four categories of phlebitis are chemical, mechanical, bacterial, and postinfusion. Phlebitis should be rated according to a uniform scale. The scale recommended by *Infusion Nursing Standards of Practice* (2006a) is given in Box 23-5.

The consequences of phlebitis include pain, discomfort, and limitation of venous access. Phlebitis may result in more serious complications such as purulent thrombophlebitis, sepsis, and thrombosis formation, leading to increased length of hospitalization, need for antibiotics, and possibly surgical intervention. Phlebitis may result from the following:

- Administration of irritating IV solutions or medications
- Injury to the inner lining of the vein by the catheter
- Infection

The following strategies can be followed to reduce the risk of phlebitis:

- Minimizing the risk for phlebitis caused by introduction of bacteria through hand hygiene, site disinfection, and aseptic technique during insertion and while accessing the catheter
- Allowing antiseptic solutions used to prepare the site to completely air-dry before placing the catheter; this avoids tracking the antiseptic into the vein and potentially causing irritation that leads to phlebitis
- Using the smallest gauge and shortest length catheter to accommodate the infusion therapy
- Avoiding areas of flexion and lower extremities (exception—infants) when placing peripheral catheters; use of an arm board

- Stabilizing the catheter to minimize in-and-out movement
- Monitoring the venipuncture site closely for evidence of phlebitis and instructing patients to report any pain or discomfort at the site
- Removing the IV catheter when signs and symptoms such as pain and erythema occur
- Avoiding administration of irritating infusion therapies through a peripheral IV catheter

The *Infusion Nursing Standards of Practice* (2006a) recommend that any incident of phlebitis of grade 2 or greater be reported as an unusual occurrence. In the absence of specialty infusion teams and certified infusion nurses, it is not uncommon for organizations to lack mechanisms for monitoring infusion-related complications. It is important that organizations recognize phlebitis as an adverse outcome and monitor its incidence. The *Infusion Nursing Standards of Practice* state that an acceptable rate for short peripheral IV catheter phlebitis should be 5% or less. When higher rates occur, the data should be analyzed for degree of phlebitis and potential causes in order to develop a performance improvement plan.

Removing and replacing catheters should occur every 72 hours for adults (INS, 2006a) or up to 96 hours (CDC, 2002b) and upon evidence of complications, discontinuation of therapy, or suspected contamination. There is no recommendation for a routine removal and replacement time interval for neonatal and pediatric patients. There is some research (Powell, Tarnow, and Perucca, 2008) that supports longer dwell times in adults but the research primarily involves infusion nurse specialists inserting and maintaining the catheters with ongoing vigorous and cautious assessment. For example, in one study that examined extending peripheral IV catheter dwell time, researchers found that if nonirritating medications were administered and a dedicated team of infusion nurse specialists inserted and evaluated the catheters, catheter dwell time may be extended beyond 72 hours (Catney, Hillis, Wakefield et al, 2001). Clearly there is a need for more well-designed research studies to guide clinical practice in frequency of peripheral catheter replacement.

Box 23-5   PHLEBITIS SCALE

0	No clinical symptoms
1	Erythema at access site with or without pain
2	Pain at access site with erythema and/or edema
3	Pain at access site with erythema, streak formation, and/or palpable venous cord
4	Pain at access site with erythema, streak formation, palpable venous cord >1 inch in length, and/or purulent drainage

From Infusion Nurses Society: *Standards of Practice,* Norwood, Mass, 2006a, Author.

FOCUS ON EVIDENCE

Peripheral IV Catheter Dwell Time

- A correlation descriptive study (N = 413) examining the relationship between extending peripheral IV catheter dwell time from 72 to 144 hours found the following: there was no significant increase in phlebitis or infiltration as the days progressed; drug irritation, catheter size, and personnel inserting the catheter were significant predictors of phlebitis or infiltration; when nonirritating medications were administered and when a dedicated team of IV specialists inserts and evaluates the catheters, catheter dwell time may be extended beyond 72 hours (Catney et al, 2001).

- A prospective descriptive study (N = 2503) found that the rate of phlebitis for peripheral IV catheters at 96 hours was not significantly different from that at 72 hours; peripheral IV catheters were inserted and monitored daily by nurses on the IV team (Lai, 1998).

- A prospective descriptive study (N = 412) found that extended dwell time did not lead to significantly higher rates of phlebitis; catheters were inserted by an IV team whenever possible (Cornely, Bethe, Pauls et al, 2002).

Chemical phlebitis

Chemical phlebitis is associated with a response of the vein intima to chemicals producing inflammation. An inflammatory response can be created by the administration of solutions or medications or as a result of certain catheter materials used for access (Box 23-6).

Normal blood pH is 7.35 to 7.45 and is slightly alkaline. The normal pH for solutions is 7.0, which is neutral. The pH for alkaline, or basic, solutions ranges from 7 to 14; that for acid solutions ranges from 0 to 7. Acidity is necessary to prevent caramelization of the dextrose during sterilization and to maintain the stability of the solution during storage. Some manufacturers also include an additive in the solution to increase the pH. This additive may alter the solution's compatibility status when other medications are added.

Solutions or medications with a pH <5 or >9 or high osmolality predispose the vein intima to irritation. The more acidic an IV solution, the greater the risk of phlebitis. Glucose-containing admixtures (e.g., amino acids, lipid emulsions used in parenteral nutrition), which are acidic, are far more phlebitogenic than 0.9% sodium chloride. Moreover, medications such as potassium chloride, vancomycin hydrochloride (Vancocin, Vancor), amphotericin B, most β-lactam antibiotics, benzodiazepines (diazepam and midazolam), and many chemotherapeutic agents can produce severe venous inflammation.

Also, the addition of certain medications can alter the pH of a solution. For instance, adding vitamin C to IV solutions further decreases the pH, whereas the addition of sodium heparin increases the pH, rarely causing phlebitis.

Osmolality refers to the measure of solute concentration and, depending on the solute present, can irritate the vein intima and predispose the patient to phlebitis. Parenteral solutions are classified according to the tonicity of the solution in relation to normal blood plasma. The osmolality of blood plasma is 290 mOsm/L. Solutions that approximate 280 to 300 mOsm/L are considered *isotonic.* Those with an osmolality higher than 300 mOsm/L are considered *hypertonic,* whereas those with an osmolality lower than 280 mOsm/L are *hypotonic.* The tonicity of infused solutions affects not only the patient's physical status but also the vein intima. The vein intima can be traumatized by the administration of hyperosmolar solutions (having an osmolality greater than 600 mOsm/L), especially if they are administered at a rapid rate or through a small vessel. Isotonic solutions may become hyperosmolar when they are mixed with certain medications, such as electrolytes, antibiotics, and nutrients, and when certain medications are added to 100 mL or less of solutions.

Improper mixture or dilution of medications can result in incompatibilities and the possibility of precipitate formation, thus increasing the risk of phlebitis. When medications are mixed without regard to pH or compatibility, the effect of the drug may be altered. Interactions can occur with no apparent change, but can render one or both of the medications or solutions ineffective or cause a physical change in which crystals are formed and a precipitate is observed.

The infusion rate can be a major factor in the development of phlebitis. A slow rate is thought to cause less venous irritation than a rapid rate. Rapid infusion rates irritate the veins by providing a larger concentration of medications and solutions that come in contact with the vessel walls. Slower rates provide longer absorption times, with hemodilution of smaller amounts of fluids or solutions.

Particulate matter within IV solutions or medications may also contribute to the formation of phlebitis. Particulates are formed when medication particles are not fully dissolved during the mixing process. When infused, they irritate the vein intima, causing inflammation. When IV medications are prepared for administration, using a 1- to 5-micron particulate-matter filter eliminates this problem. A 0.2-micron air-eliminating filter may be used to prevent the infusion of particulates.

Catheters can predispose the patient to phlebitis. Although several different materials are used in the manufacture of catheters, none is absolutely foolproof for the prevention of phlebitis. Catheters made of silicone elastomer and polyurethane have a smoother microsurface, are thermoplastic and more hydrophilic, become more flexible than polytetrafluoroethylene (Teflon) at body temperature, and induce less venous irritation.

The basic principles of aseptic technique and measures to prevent chemical phlebitis must be carried out. Many of the problems associated with chemical phlebitis can be eliminated by implementation of the principles listed in Box 23-7.

The pharmacist should always be consulted for any questions about the mixing of medications or solutions and should be made aware of repeated occurrences of phlebitis associated with certain drugs. Sometimes, the addition of a buffering agent or other additives can help prevent chemical phlebitis.

Mechanical phlebitis

Mechanical phlebitis is associated with the placement of a catheter. Catheters inserted in areas of flexion often result in mechanical phlebitis. As the extremity is moved, the catheter

---

Box 23-6   FACTORS CONTRIBUTING TO CHEMICAL PHLEBITIS

- Irritating medications or solutions
- Medications improperly mixed or diluted
- Medications or solutions administered at a rapid rate
- Particulate matter
- Catheter material
- Extended catheter dwell time

Box 23-7   INTERVENTIONS THAT DECREASE THE POTENTIAL FOR CHEMICAL PHLEBITIS

- Use in-line filters.
- Use recommended solutions or diluents when mixing medications.
- Dilute known irritating medications to the lowest concentration possible.
- Administer intravenous push medications through a port of a compatible free-flowing infusion.
- Administer medications or solutions at the minimal rate recommended.
- Rotate peripheral sites at recommended intervals.
- Use large veins for the administration of hypertonic or acidic/alkaline solutions to provide greater hemodilution.
- Use the smallest gauge catheter that will adequately deliver the ordered therapy.

irritates the vein intima, causing injury that can result in phlebitis. A large catheter placed in a vein that has a smaller lumen than the catheter also irritates the intima of the vein, causing inflammation and phlebitis. Catheters that are poorly secured have a tendency to move in and out of the vein, allowing the catheter tip to irritate the vein intima and resulting in phlebitis. Extensive, unrestrictive movement of an extremity can also result in unwarranted movement of the catheter within the vein.

Several studies have concluded that the use of a specialized infusion team to insert and monitor peripheral IV catheters reduced the risk of complications and cost.

Bacterial phlebitis

Bacterial phlebitis is an inflammation of the vein intima associated with a bacterial infection. It can be very serious and predispose the patient to the systemic complication of septicemia. Contributing factors include those described in Box 23-8.

Hand hygiene is the single most important measure for preventing health care–associated infections. Hand hygiene must be performed before therapy is initiated and after the procedure has been completed. Standard precautions mandate that health care providers must wear gloves when performing venipunctures. Even when gloves are provided in the immediate area, hand hygiene should be performed before gloves are donned; otherwise, contaminants are easily carried into the area and deposited on the gloves.

All equipment and solutions should be checked for expiration date, package integrity, particulate matter, cloudiness, or any signs indicating the presence of contaminants. Containers should be squeezed to reveal punctures, and bottles should be held up to the light and rotated to reveal very fine cracks.

Aseptic technique is essential in the preparation of an insertion site. Appropriate cleansing of the insertion site reduces the potential for infection by minimizing microorganisms on the skin. If the skin is very dirty, it should be washed with soap and water before an antimicrobial solution is applied.

Sterile tape to prevent unwarranted movement of the catheter and a sterile dressing are applied over the catheter site. The catheter is then taped, or a manufactured securement device is used, to prevent in-and-out movement.

Nursing interventions

If an infection is suspected, the catheter should be removed and cultured using established policies and procedures. The surrounding skin should be cleansed with 70% isopropyl alcohol and allowed to air-dry. If purulent drainage is present, a culture of the drainage should be taken before cleansing the skin. The CDC (2002b) recommends a semiquantitative culturing technique. Consideration should be given to obtaining blood cultures to determine proliferation of catheter-related infections. The catheter should be relocated to the opposite extremity, if possible, or to a vein into which the phlebitic vein does not empty. The application of warm, moist compresses promotes healing and patient comfort.

Postinfusion phlebitis

Postinfusion phlebitis, another commonly reported complication of infusion therapy, is associated with inflammation of the vein that usually becomes evident within 48 to 96 hours of catheter removal. The following factors contribute to the development of postinfusion phlebitis:

- Poor catheter insertion technique
- Debilitated patient
- Poor vein condition
- Hypertonic or acidic solutions
- Ineffective filtration
- Large-gauge catheter placed in small vessel
- Failure to change administration sets, dressings, injection access caps, and catheter

Patient assessment. The patient is assessed for postinfusion phlebitis by monitoring the venipuncture site for signs of inflammation after the IV catheter has been removed. The site is observed for erythema, edema, and drainage. The site is palpated for warmth and for vein induration. The degree of postinfusion phlebitis should be measured according to the uniform scale used to measure phlebitis (see Box 23-5).

Nursing interventions. Generally, hot or cold compresses are applied, as described earlier, to the venipuncture site once postinfusion phlebitis is detected. Depending on the degree of postinfusion phlebitis, medical intervention may be required.

Preventive measures. Measures to prevent postinfusion phlebitis are the same as those designed to prevent phlebitis and include those outlined in Box 23-9.

Box 23-8 FACTORS CONTRIBUTING TO BACTERIAL PHLEBITIS

- Poor hand hygiene techniques
- Failure to check equipment for compromised integrity
- Poor aseptic technique in preparation of the venipuncture site or infusion system
- Poor catheter-insertion techniques
- Poorly secured catheter
- Extended catheter dwell time
- Infrequent site observation with failure to notice early signs of phlebitis

---

Box 23-9 MEASURES FOR PREVENTING POSTINFUSION PHLEBITIS

- Ensure that venipuncture is performed by a skilled clinician.
- Use aseptic technique when using or manipulating the infusion system.
- Check compatibility of solutions and medications before mixing and administering.
- Use filters when preparing medications and solutions.
- Use final filtration, when recommended, for administering medications and solutions.
- Add a buffer to known irritating medications and to hypertonic solutions.
- Rotate peripheral infusion sites.
- Change solution container every 24 hours.
- Change injection/access caps and needleless devices on intermittent devices at the time of peripheral catheter change and when the integrity has been compromised.

Thrombosis

A *thrombosis* is the formation of a blood clot within a blood vessel. It is caused by any injury that breaks the integrity of the endothelial cells of the venous wall, and usually occurs at the point at which the catheter touches the intima of the vein. Platelets adhere to the injured wall, and a thrombus is formed. Contributing factors include those listed in Box 23-10.

Patient assessment

When an infusion slows or stops, the causative factors should be assessed. Mechanical and other problems should be ruled out. The possibility of a thrombus should be considered because the formation of a thrombus narrows the lumen of the vein, allowing less fluid to be infused. Usually, a thrombus remains undetected until the infusion stops or the extremity becomes swollen because of circulatory involvement. The area becomes very tender, and redness appears. The degree of circulatory involvement in the affected extremity should be assessed. A thrombosis may impact circulation sufficiently to cause tissue necrosis or result in loss of the involved extremity.

The patient should also be assessed for the possibility of a systemic infection or a pulmonary embolism. Thrombi form an excellent trap for bacteria, whether stationary, carried through the bloodstream from an infectious process located somewhere else in the body, or introduced through a subcutaneous orifice. Although a thrombus is usually well attached, it may in rare circumstances become unattached.

Nursing interventions

If a thrombosis occurs, the infusion should be discontinued immediately and the VAD should be relocated to the opposite extremity. Cold compresses should be applied to the site initially to decrease the flow of blood and increase platelet adherence to the clot that has already formed. The physician should be notified, and the site should be assessed to determine whether surgical intervention is needed; vein ligation may be necessary if the degree of circulatory impairment is sufficient to cause extensive tissue damage. The site should be monitored until symptoms completely resolve.

Preventive measures

To prevent these injuries, venipuncture by skilled professionals is necessary. Cannulation of the lower extremities in adults should be avoided because these veins are very small and allow pooling of blood with subsequent damage to the vein intima and clot formation. The selection of the appropriate venipuncture device is also important; use of the smallest gauge and

shortest device possible to deliver the prescribed therapy decreases the potential of injury to the endothelial lining. Veins over flexion areas should be avoided, and catheters should be anchored securely to avoid in-and-out movements. Consideration should be given to the placement of central venous catheters when venous access is poor.

Thrombophlebitis

Thrombophlebitis denotes a twofold injury: the presence of a thrombus and the occurrence of inflammation. Usually, the first symptom noted is inflammation along the vein that is characterized by erythema. Edema, pain at the site and along the vein pathway, and a feeling of warmth usually follow. The vein becomes hard and tortuous as it thromboses. Marked erythema, increased edema, marked pain along the vein, and aching of the extremity occur.

Any irritation to the intima of the vein can predispose the vein to inflammation and clot formation as platelets adhere to the traumatized wall of the vein. The incidence and severity of inflammation increase with the duration of the infusion.

Patient assessment

The venipuncture site and vein pathway are factors that have been previously discussed under Phlebitis and Thrombosis. The vein should be palpated for induration and tenderness. The patient should be questioned about pain at the site, along the vein pathway, and in the involved extremity. The patient should also be observed for chills and fever, and laboratory values should be evaluated for an elevated white blood cell count.

If the condition remains untreated, the vein becomes sclerosed and is unavailable for future therapy. Although the inherent danger of an embolism always exists when a thrombus forms, these thrombi are generally well attached to the vein wall and do not migrate. Several clinical trials have recommended that patients who have symptomatic infusion thrombophlebitis as a complication of intravenous infusion should be treated with oral diclofenac or nonsteroidal antiinflammatory drugs (NSAIDs), topical diclofenac, or heparin gel for symptom management until resolved or up to 2 weeks (Kearon, Kahn, Agnelli et al, 2008). The risk of septicemia or bacterial endocarditis is greater, particularly if the inflammation is the result of sepsis.

The degree of phlebitis should be measured according to the recommended scale (see Box 23-5). Thrombophlebitis is rated a 3 or 4 on this scale because of the presence of a palpable cord.

Nursing interventions

When thrombophlebitis occurs, the infusion should be discontinued immediately and the physician notified. If an infection is suspected, the catheter should be cultured using a semiquantitative technique. The skin surrounding the catheter should be cleansed with alcohol and allowed to air-dry before the catheter is removed for culture. When purulent drainage is present, a culture of the drainage should be taken before the skin is cleansed.

If infusion therapy is still necessary, a new catheter with a new administration set and solution container should be placed in the opposite extremity, if possible. If using the opposite extremity is impossible, a separate vein that does not form a tributary of the traumatized vein should be used.

Cold compresses should be applied to the site initially to decrease the flow of blood and increase platelet adherence to

---

Box 23-10 FACTORS CONTRIBUTING TO THE FORMATION OF THROMBOSIS

- Venipuncture by an unskilled professional
- Multiple venipuncture attempts
- Use of a catheter that is larger than the vein lumen
- Poor circulation with venous stasis
- Administration of incompatible solutions and medications
- Administration of solutions or medications with high pH or tonicity
- Ineffective filtration
- Use of thrombogenic catheter materials

the clot already formed. Then, warm compresses should be applied. The extremity should be elevated, and the patient should be cautioned that rubbing or massaging the area may cause an embolus. The extremity and the patient are monitored for further complications.

Preventive measures

Thrombophlebitis can lead to serious systemic complications, and measures should be taken to prevent their occurrence. These measures should include those outlined earlier under Phlebitis and Thrombosis.

Venous or arterial spasm

A *spasm* is a sudden, involuntary contraction of a vein or an artery (vasoconstriction) resulting in temporary cessation of blood flow through a vessel. Stimulation by cold infusates or by mechanical or chemical irritation may produce spasms in arteries and veins.

Because arteries supply circulation to large areas of the body, arterial spasms are far more serious than venous spasms. Unlike arteries, many veins supply a particular area, and if one becomes injured, blood is supplied to the area by collateral circulation. In these cases, the supply of blood to the area may be decreased, but not to the extent that it would with injury to an artery.

Patient assessment

It is most important to recognize the signs and symptoms of a spasm. Cramping or pain above an infusion site or a feeling of numbness is usually the first symptom experienced by the patient. Patients experiencing arterial spasms may or may not complain of pain initially; they may not feel pain until tissue damage has occurred. When the patient complains of one of these symptoms, the involved extremity should be observed for localized blanching and the absence of a pulse; these signs would indicate an arterial spasm and a loss of blood flow to the area supplied by the artery.

Nursing interventions

If an arterial spasm occurs, it is usually related to the inadvertent puncture of an artery instead of a vein during venipuncture. If this occurs, the catheter should be removed immediately, pressure should be applied to the site over sufficient time to ensure hemostasis, and a dry, sterile dressing should be applied.

If a venous spasm occurs, discontinuing the infusion is not necessary. The infusion rate should be decreased and, if possible, the medication or solution should be further diluted. If a spasm has occurred as a result of the administration of a cold solution, warm compresses should be applied above the site; the heat provides vasodilation and increases the blood supply, thereby relieving the spasm and the pain.

Preventive measures

Many spasms can be prevented. Ensuring that venipuncture is performed by skilled, experienced nurses can decrease the possibility of an inadvertent arterial puncture. Venous spasms can also be prevented or minimized by infusing medications or solutions known to be irritating at slower rates and by diluting them as much as possible. Blood warmers should be used for rapid transfusions of potent cold agglutinins, exchange transfusions in neonates, and treatment of patients with hypothermia. Fluid warmers may be used to warm IV solutions to prevent or reverse hypothermic conditions. All refrigerated medications and parenteral solutions should be allowed to reach room temperature before they are administered.

Systemic complications

Systemic complications are usually associated with infusion therapy using central venous access devices (see Chapter 25). Systemic complications are usually very serious and require immediate interventions.

Speed shock

Speed shock is a systemic reaction that occurs when a substance foreign to the body is rapidly introduced into circulation. This phenomenon usually results from the administration of a bolus medication or the administration of a medication-containing infusion at a rapid rate. Speed shock should not be confused with pulmonary edema. Pulmonary edema relates to volume, whereas speed shock relates to the rapidity with which a medication is administered; it can occur even when a small volume of medication is given. Rapid injections enter the serum in toxic proportions and flood the heart and the brain with medication.

Patient assessment

When medications are administered, the patient should be observed for dizziness, facial flushing, headache, and medication-specific symptoms. It is vital to note these symptoms early because progression is immediate, with the patient experiencing tightness in the chest, hypotension, irregular pulse rate, and anaphylactic shock.

Nursing interventions

The infusion should be discontinued immediately with recognition of the first symptom, and a patent VAD should be maintained for emergency treatment. The patient should be treated for symptoms of shock, if necessary. The physician should be notified, and the patient should be given additional treatment as needed.

Preventive measures

Speed shock can be prevented. Nurses should know the medication being given and ensure that it is administered at the recommended rate and monitored regularly. Gravity flow administration sets should be checked frequently to make sure that they are infusing at the appropriate rate. Solution containers should be time-taped so that the amount that has infused can be readily observed. Electronic flow control devices or volumetric chambers should be used for patients who are at great risk for developing complications and when critical solutions or medications are administered.

Allergic reaction

An allergic reaction is a response to a medication or solution to which the patient is sensitive. Reactions may also occur from the passive transfer of sensitivity to the patient from a blood donor, or the patient may be sensitive to substances normally present in the blood, as is seen in transfusion reactions. Reactions may be immediate or delayed. The most common reactions are those seen as a result of administering antibiotics and blood products. Reactions to blood and blood products are discussed in Chapter 14.

Patient assessment

Patients receiving infusion therapy should be monitored for symptoms of allergic reactions. The patient may experience chills and fever with or without urticaria, erythema, and itching. Depending on the internal response to the allergen, the patient could experience shortness of breath, with or without wheezing. The patient may also experience angioneurotic edema.

Nursing interventions

The infusion should be stopped immediately, the administration set and solution container changed, and the vein kept open to allow treatment of possible anaphylactic shock. The physician should be notified, and interventions should be carried out as ordered. Antihistamines are usually administered to relieve mild symptoms; epinephrine or steroids are administered for more severe reactions. Sometimes, antihistamines are used prophylactically when an allergic reaction is considered likely.

Preventive measures

Preventive measures include the following:

- An admission assessment should be performed of the patient's previous drug allergies, sensitivities, or idiosyncrasies. The patient's medical record should alert all caregivers of any allergies. In the hospital setting, an allergy alert bracelet may be placed on the patient so that all staff members are aware of any allergies. The pharmacy profile should list all allergies so that all medications can be cross-referenced for allergic reactions.
- Adequate screening of donor and recipient blood can help prevent blood reactions. Policies and procedures should address drawing blood samples for crossmatching, the crossmatching process, the identification process before blood is administered, and interventions to be carried out if a reaction occurs.

 PATIENT OUTCOMES

The desired outcome for all patients receiving infusion therapy is to complete treatment with minimal or no complications. Box 23-11 lists expected outcome criteria for a patient receiving peripheral infusion therapy. When nurses deliver infusion care according to established policies and procedures that are evidence based, the risks associated with a peripheral infusion catheter are significantly reduced. The nurse continuously evaluates patient outcomes to determine whether nursing interventions are appropriate.

 SUMMARY

Although infusion therapy has had great technological advancements—from steel needles to a variety of long-dwelling catheters, from the acute care setting to the home, from continuous to intermittent administration—it is paramount that the nurse provides quality patient care. To ensure the delivery of quality infusion care, potential patient problems must be identified rapidly. Nursing care must be goal directed, and appropriate nursing interventions must be provided. Patient outcomes are evaluated, and appropriate interventions are implemented and communicated to all members of the health care team.

Box 23-11   OUTCOME CRITERIA FOR PERIPHERAL VASCULAR ACCESS DEVICES (PVADs)

OUTCOME CRITERIA: The patient will remain free of complications related to the administration of infusion therapy (PVADS).

1. GOAL

The patient will remain free from infection related to infusion therapy.

Interventions

- IV site will be inspected for signs of infection routinely.
- IV catheter and administration set will be changed every 72 hours.
- IV solution containers will be changed every 24 hours.
- IV catheter will be secured to prevent movement of catheter in and out of the vein.
- IV equipment and solution containers will be inspected for contamination before use.
- Aseptic techniques will be used during IV insertion and administration.

2. GOAL

The patient will remain free of chemical phlebitis associated with the administration of medications.

Interventions

- All medications and fluids will be mixed in the pharmacy under a laminar flow hood. Known irritants will be diluted to the fullest extent possible.
- All fluids and medications will be administered at the recommended rate.
- The venipuncture site will be checked routinely for redness and inflammation associated with chemical phlebitis.
- Infusates should meet *Infusion Nursing Standards of Practice* of pH between 5 and 9 and osmolality <600 mOsm/L.

3. GOAL

The patient will remain free of local complications.

Interventions

- IV sites over areas of flexion will not be used unless absolutely necessary.

4. GOALS

- Patient's level of knowledge for learning will be assessed.
- Patient will be taught care of the venous access device and the associated infusion system.

Interventions

- Patient's level of knowledge for learning will be assessed.
- Patient will be taught care of system.
- Patient will be able to perform routine activities—bathing, movement in bed, and ambulation.
- Patient will be taught emergency measures to follow for complications such as pulling out line, loose or wet dressing, or kinking of tubing.
- Patient will be taught signs and symptoms of complications.

The delivery of safe, quality infusion care requires changing solution containers and administration sets, rotating peripheral IV catheters, changing dressings, and performing site assessments. Careful maintenance of the infusion system, performance of appropriate nursing interventions, and close monitoring minimizes risks to the patient and improve expected patient outcomes. The nurse administering infusion therapy must be knowledgeable about the risks involved and must be able to implement measures to prevent their occurrence.

 REFERENCES

Bernatene K, Mason DL, Rudnick SK et al: Cutting-edge discussions of management policy and program issues in emergency care. External jugular lines: yes or no? *J Emerg Nurs* 33(4):392-393, 2007.

Brown D: Local anesthesia for vein cannulation: a comparison of two solutions, *J Infus Nurs* 27:85-88, 2004.

Brown J: Using Lidocaine for peripheral IV insertions: patient's preferences and pain experiences, *MEDSURG Nurs* 12(12):95-100, 2003.

Catney MR, Hillis S, Wakefield B et al: Relationship between peripheral intravenous catheter dwell time and the development of phlebitis and infiltration, *J Infus Nurs* 24:332-341, 2001.

Centers for Disease Control and Prevention: Guideline for hand hygiene in health-care settings, *MMWR* 51(RR-16):1-44, 2002a.

Centers for Disease Control and Prevention: Guidelines for the prevention of intravascular catheter-related infections, *MMWR* 51(RR-10):1-32, 2002b.

Chaiyakunapruk N, Veenstra DL, Lipsky BA et al: Chlorhexidine compared with povidone iodine solution for vascular site care: a meta-analysis, *Ann Intern Med* 136:792-801, 2002.

Cornely OA, Bethe U, Pauls R et al: Peripheral Teflon catheters: factors determining the incidence of phlebitis and duration of cannulation, *Infect Control Hospital Epidemiol* 23:249-254, 2002.

Elkin MK, Perry AG, Potter PA: *Nursing interventions & clinical skills*, ed 4, St Louis, 2007, Mosby.

Fetzer SJ: Reducing venipuncture and intravenous insertion pain with eutectic mixture of local anesthesia: a meta-analysis, *Nurs Res* 51:119-124, 2002.

Frey AM, Schears GJ: Why are we stuck with tape and suture? A review of catheter securement devices, *J Infus Nurs* 29:34-38, 2006.

Goode C, Titler M, Rakel B et al: A meta-analysis of effects of heparin flush and saline flush: quality and cost implications, *Nurs Res* 40:324-330, 1991.

Gorski L: Standard 40: local anesthesia, *J Infus Nurs* 31:72-73, 2008.

Hadaway L: Infiltration and extravasation, *Am J Nurs* 107(8):64-72, 2007.

Hattula JL, McGovern EK, Neumann TL: Comparison of intravenous cannulation injectable preanesthetics in an adult medical inpatient population, *App Nurs Res* 15:189-193, 2002.

Infusion Nurses Society: Infusion nursing standards of practice, *J Infus Nurs* 29(suppl 1S), 2006a.

From Infusion Nurses Society: *Policies and procedures for infusion nursing*, ed 3, Norwood, Mass, 2006b, Author.

Infusion Nurses Society: *Position paper. The role of the registered nurse in the insertion of external jugular peripherally inserted central catheters (EJ PICC) and external jugular peripheral intravenous catheters (EJ PIV)*, 2008.

Kagel EM, Rayan GM: Intravenous catheter complications in the hand and forearm, *J Trauma* 56(1):123-127, 2004.

Kearon C, Kahn SR, Agnelli G et al: Antithrombotic therapy for venous thromboembolic disease: American College of Chest Physicians evidence-based clinical practice guidelines (ed 8), *Chest* 133(6 suppl):454S-545S, 2008.

Lai KK: Safety of prolonging peripheral cannula and IV tubing use from 72 hours to 96 hours, *Am J Infect Control* 26(1):66-70, 1998.

Miller KA: 1% lidocaine injection, EMLA cream, or "Numby Stuff" for topical analgesia associated with peripheral intravenous cannulation, *AANA J* 69(3):185-187, 2001.

Peterson F, Kirchhoff K: Analysis of the research about heparinized versus nonheparinized intravenous lines, *Heart Lung* 20:631-640, 1991.

Powell J, Tarnow KG, Perucca R: Peripheral intravenous catheter indwell time and phlebitis, *J Infus Nurs* 31:39-45, 2008.

Smith B: Peripheral intravenous catheter dwell times: a comparison of 3 securement methods for implementation of a 96-hour scheduled change protocol, *J Infus Nurs* 29:14-27, 2006.

24 CENTRAL VENOUS ACCESS DEVICES: ACCESS AND INSERTION

Melody Bullock-Corkhill, BSN, BS, MS, CRNI®*

Whether in an acute care setting or in preparation for long-term infusion therapy, decisions regarding venous access device placement are made frequently by nurses on behalf of patients. The need for establishing or maintaining fluid and electrolyte balance; giving bolus infusions for hydration; administering blood products, cardiac drugs, or antibiotics; or attaining hemostasis will direct the decision for intravenous (IV) access. When treatment is delayed because of lack of venous access, patient outcomes are directly affected.

ASSESSMENT FACTORS DETERMINING CATHETER SELECTION

Historically nurses have used peripheral IV access until no further access was possible due to hematomas, phlebitis, and, at times, even necrosis. Peripheral sites were considered less conducive to morbidity and mortality (Galloway, 2002). Evidence-based practice now indicates that an appropriate early assessment will direct the nurse in determination of the type of venous access device (VAD) based on patient needs, expected duration of therapy, medications, and diagnosis. Critically ill patients frequently need immediate venous access for the initiation of life support medications, solutions, antibiotics, and/or steroids. Nurses must be able to rapidly assess the availability of venous access and advocate for the patient. Triage becomes difficult during emergency situations when the patient is at highest risk and multiple attempts for access have been unsuccessful. The ability to administer intravenous medications directly affects the patient's discomfort, morbidity, and mortality, which makes timely decisions even more urgent. The Centers for Disease Control and Prevention (CDC) recommends in the *Guidelines for the Prevention of Intravascular Catheter-Related Infections* that a midline or peripherally inserted central catheter (PICC) should be used if the duration of the therapy is to exceed 6 days (O'Grady et al, 2002).

*The author and editors wish to acknowledge the contributions made by Roxanne Perucca in the second edition of *Infusion Therapy in Clinical Practice*.

The type of intravenous catheter a patient needs depends on several factors. The best time to evaluate venous access is before vascular integrity has been compromised. As soon as a nurse receives a patient for care, venous access availability should be assessed. Vascular damage can be avoided when the appropriate VAD is placed early in the patient's plan of care.

Justification for a particular VAD selection depends on patient needs and the vasculature condition. Drugs known to be acidic, alkaline, hyperosmolar, irritating, or a vesicant require maximum hemodilution. This is accomplished by using venous access that allows the location of the catheter to be in a larger vein, terminating in the central circulatory system (INS, 2006a). When intravenous use will extend for longer periods of time, central venous access devices (CVADs) such as PICCs and tunneled catheters may be ordered. For a more permanent need, an implanted port may be the device of choice.

MEDICATIONS

Central venous access devices should be placed for patients who require medications that are known to cause damage to the inner lumen of the vein. Certain combinations of intravenous medications affect the veins in exponential proportions; damage done over time affects outcomes and may be irreversible (Forauer and Theoharis, 2003). The osmolality, pH, and classification as a vesicant or irritant of the prescribed medications should be considered before inserting a CVAD.

OSMOLALITY

Hyperosmotic describes solutions with a high osmolality—a high concentration of particles in solution—documented to cause trauma to the tunica intima if not diluted when infused (Fletcher and Bodenham, 2000). Many medications and solutions are classified as hyperosmotic including certain contrast media. An order for these medications or solutions should alert the nurse to the need for access that will allow a high rate of blood flow to further dilute the solution.

Solutions being infused should be close to the osmolality of blood serum, which is isotonic (250 to 350 mOsm/L), especially if the medications are infused in the smaller veins of the hands or arms since infusions in these veins may cause cell damage (Florence and Attwood, 2006). Fluids with an osmotic pressure of greater than 400 mOsm/L should also be infused slowly to reduce risk of venous damage. Using central access allows rapid dilution of solutions and medications with an osmolality greater than 500 mOsm/L, and decreases the potential for venous damage.

pH

pH is a significant factor when considering venous access. Device selection early in the course of administration of these drugs with extreme pH ranges will prevent unnecessary injury. Numerous litigious situations have occurred involving the intravenous administration of Phenergan, resulting in damage to veins, arteries, nerves, and tissues, even to the extent of appendage loss that results in significant changes in lifestyle (Shapiro, 2008). Phenergan for injection has a pH of 4.0 to 5.5. Vancomycin, with a pH of 4.0 to 6.0, is another drug that is known to cause vascular damage when mixed for infusion. Medications with a pH of less than 5 or more than 9 should be infused through a CVAD (INS, 2006a).

IRRITANTS/VESICANTS

The classification of a medication as an irritant or vesicant also affects the selection of the venous access device. An irritant is a medication that may cause itching, phlebitis, or reaction along the vessel or at the injection site, whereas a vesicant medication can potentially cause blistering, tissue sloughing, or necrosis when extravasation occurs. Extravasation is "the inadvertent leakage or escape of a vesicant drug or solution from a vein or unintentional injection into surrounding healthy tissues," and may occur in as many as 0.1% to 6% of peripheral infusions, though these incidents are underreported (Wickham et al, 2006). Both cytotoxic and noncytotoxic drugs have the potential for being categorized as irritants and vesicants because of their chemical nature. This may have nothing to do with their pH or osmolality.

LENGTH OF THERAPY

Another factor influencing catheter choice is the prospective length of the prescribed therapy. Short peripheral VADs, midline catheters, and peripherally inserted central catheters are options depending on how long the patient will be needing treatment. While a peripheral site may be appropriate during the acute phase of treatment, a midline or PICC may be considered for a patient going home from the acute setting for extended therapy. Temporary central access is usually reserved for those patients who need immediate access where peripheral IV start attempts have been unsuccessful.

DIAGNOSIS

Because of the nature of certain diseases, many diagnoses will alert the nurse to potential complications and facilitate determining the venous access needs for that patient. Assessing the patient's history and present diagnosis will help the nurse in selecting the appropriate VAD for the patient. Renal disease and diabetes contribute significantly to attaining and maintaining venous access. Common diseases that present infusion problems include cystic fibrosis, scleroderma, certain cancers,

osteomyelitis, Crohn's disease, hypotension, blood dyscrasias, gastrointestinal bleed, pulmonary hypertension, and long-term infections such as methicillin-resistant *Staphylococcus aureus*. These diagnoses can be an indicator for the insertion of a CVAD with a longer dwell time rather than a short-term peripheral device. Rapid assessment and placement of an appropriate VAD and reduction of peripheral venipuncture attempts have also been shown to assist with patient satisfaction (Elliott, 2006).

EXACERBATIONS

Patients with multiple medical conditions who receive numerous medications are prone to complications that may cause extended lengths of stay in acute care facilities and longer courses of intravenous medications, which may affect their lifestyle, their ability to work and continue daily activities, and ultimately their quality of life. A disease process that started out relatively simple can be complicated by secondary effects of the medications. For example, a patient with a respiratory tract illness requiring a relatively simple course of antibiotics and steroids may benefit from early intervention by having a CVAD inserted before the medications cause inner-luminal corrosion and inhibit further peripheral access.

CVAD SELECTION

Once the decision has been made for central rather than peripheral access the most appropriate device can be selected. Central venous access devices are catheters that terminate in the central vasculature, defined as the distal tip dwelling in the lower one third of the superior vena cava to the junction of the superior vena cava and the right atrium (INS, 2006a). There are a variety of soft, flexible CVADs appropriate for placement in patients with short- or long-term needs.

Patients who require multiple medications, such as those in the intensive care unit (ICU), will more likely need a catheter with multiple lumens. Other patients in an acute care facility may need a single- or dual-lumen catheter, depending on the types, amounts, compatibilities, and quantities of medications; the need for blood draws; and the need for the patient to continue using the catheter upon discharge. Placing a single-lumen catheter for patients who require treatment at home may simplify the regimen for home care.

Temporary or short-term devices, such as nontunneled catheters, are those that are removed relatively soon after placement. Most are used for a duration of 5 days to 4 weeks and then removed. In emergent situations where vascular access has been impossible, an intraosseous device may be required until venous access is more feasible. Refer to Chapter 20 for details on the various types of CVADs and their indications for use.

Long-term CVADs, including tunneled catheters such as Broviacs® and Hickman® catheters and implanted ports, can remain in place for years without problems. Implanted ports are indicated for patients with long-term intermittent infusion needs, while a PICC or tunneled catheter is typically used for continuous access. PICCs can remain in place as long as they are functioning properly. The general recommendation is to insert PICCs for therapy anticipated to be less than 1-year duration. CDC recommends central catheters should be replaced only when evidence of catheter-related bloodstream infection (CRBSI) exists (O'Grady et al, 2002). Studies of ICU patients with central venous catheters showed that there was no difference in infection rates between those who had catheters changed as needed and those who had them changed every 7 days (Stephens, 2005).

 ## CVAD INSERTION

Central venous access devices fall under three categories: nontunneled catheters, tunneled catheters, and implanted ports. Tunneled catheters and implanted ports must be inserted and removed using local or general anesthetics. The nurse is responsible for assistance during insertion of the device and for care and maintenance once the catheter is in place. Documentation in the patient's medical record should contain the insertion procedure, including the length of catheter inserted and the location of the catheter tip, skin disinfectant and local anesthetic used, flushing technique and solution used, catheter stabilization method (e.g., manufactured device, sterile tapes, sutures), patient response, and any specific action taken to resolve or prevent adverse reactions.

NONTUNNELED CENTRAL CATHETERS

Nontunneled central catheters are usually inserted at the bedside using a jugular, subclavian, or femoral approach, and are in place less than 14 days (Forauer and Theoharis, 2003). Sometimes these catheters are placed during an emergency or when the patient has no other access, unless the physician or emergency medical technician decides to place an intraosseous device. The *Infusion Nursing Standards of Practice* (INS, 2006a) recommends that catheters inserted during an emergency be replaced no later than 48 hours after placement. Care must be taken to prevent dislodgement, which can easily occur with these catheters.

TUNNELED CENTRAL CATHETERS

Tunneled venous access devices, such as Broviac®, Hickman®, and Hohn catheters, are placed for long-term therapy and are considered permanent since they are meant for use for a much longer time frame. After 10 to 14 days, adhesions form on the Dacron cuff that not only stabilize the catheter but also seal it, which prevents infection from the exit site to the vein. Typically patients with cancer or other chronic illnesses have a tunneled catheter placed for treatments that will be intermittent over a period of time, or for continuous infusions such as parenteral nutrition. After the insertion site is healed, the catheter is more difficult to dislodge and does not require a dressing, making it easier for the patient to maintain the site at home or to receive care in an outpatient setting.

IMPLANTED PORTS

Like tunneled catheters, implanted ports are used for long-term therapies, and are recognized as being beneficial to pediatric patients for their portability. They require no care when the patient does not need access, except for periodic flushing with 0.9% sodium chloride and instillation of heparinized solution. The patient can continue all normal activities when no treatment is being administered. Ports have relatively few mechanical complications compared to their

---

PROCEDURE FOR INSERTION OF A NONTUNNELED CENTRAL VENOUS ACCESS DEVICE

1. Explain procedure to the patient/family. Verify consent has been obtained.
2. Position patient in Trendelenburg or supine position for jugular or subclavian placement.
3. Identify patient using two identifiers. Ascertain patient's allergies.
4. Perform hand hygiene using antiseptic soap for 60 seconds.
5. Prepare sterile field and supplies.
6. Clip hair on and around intended insertion site area.
7. Position drape underneath area to be cannulated.
8. Apply mask, gown, cap, and sterile gloves.
9. Prep site. If using alcohol and povidone-iodine swabsticks, begin with alcohol at the center of the intended site, cleanse using concentric circles, and allow to air-dry. If using chlorhexidine gluconate, use scrubbing motion back and forth for 20 seconds and allow to air-dry.
10. Drape patient using a full-body drape.
11. Change into second pair of sterile gloves.
12. Anesthetize the insertion site with 1% lidocaine.
13. Perform venipuncture into jugular, subclavian, or femoral vein.
14. Remove syringe from needle.
15. Insert spring guidewire through the needle.
16. Remove needle and place dilator.
17. Thread catheter over guidewire, aspirate, and remove guidewire. Flush with 0.9% sodium chloride and place caps on the hubs.
18. Secure catheter in place with a securement device; suture if necessary.
19. Apply sterile transparent membrane dressing over entire insertion site. Date and initial the dressing.
20. Obtain chest radiograph to verify tip placement and to rule out pneumothorax before initiating therapy.
21. Document procedure, patient tolerance during insertion, and monitoring in the patient's medical record.

Adapted from Infusion Nurses Society: *Policies and procedures for infusion nursing,* ed 3, Norwood, Mass, 2006b, Author.

---

length of use and have minimal risk of infection (Dillon and Foglia, 2006). These CVADs are reliable and appropriate for pediatric or adult use for administering parenteral nutrition, antibiotics, and chemotherapy as well as for drawing blood samples.

Obtaining access

Patients with implanted ports can carry on a normal lifestyle when the port is not accessed. An implanted port can be easily accessed for intravenous medications and for flushing to maintain catheter patency. Accessing a port is a sterile procedure requiring sterile gloves, a mask, and sterile supplies. A noncoring needle must be used to prevent openings in the septum from multiple accesses. Most noncoring needles are also 90-angled needles designed for patient comfort. An implanted port can be configured either as a single-lumen or as a dual-lumen device.

An implanted port consists of a small dome-shaped housing with a silicone septum underneath, which is a reservoir that empties into the catheter. A surgeon or interventional radiologist places the implanted port, creating a subcutaneous cavity, usually in the anterior chest wall; the port is attached to the muscle wall and then to a catheter leading into the central venous system. Ports have also been placed in the upper arm, abdomen, back, and side when anterior chest wall placement is not appropriate. In certain pediatric patients, ports have also been placed in the femoral vein with the tip terminating in the inferior vena cava.

To meet the needs of patients requiring repeat computerized axial tomography (CAT) scans with contrast, ports have been developed to withstand the high pressure of power injectors. These ports are recognizable by ridges on the surface or radiographic markings. When using power injectors, noncoring needles that have the tubing attached must also be FDA-approved for power injection to ensure that the tubing and connections will not rupture or separate.

Although the port is sutured into subcutaneous or muscle tissue, it can become unsecured and dislodged, making it difficult to access. If resistance is felt when attempting to access the port, the nurse should attempt again with a new needle. The needle requires only a minimal amount of pressure to access the port completely; and additional pressure may result in the needle bending back on itself, causing damage to the septum when being retracted. Once the needle "taps" the back of the port, a blood return should be visualized. If resistance is unresolved, the port may be partially or completely turned around in the subcutaneous cavity; this will require medical intervention.

When no blood return can be obtained, the nurse may flush the port and then attempt repositioning the patient; patients may be asked to turn their heads in the opposite direction, move their arms, or turn their body to the opposite side. If the port flushes well but no blood is aspirated the physician should be alerted so that an order can be written for an x-ray or dye study to determine the integrity of the catheter, especially if the port will be used to administer vesicants (Rosenthal, 2006).

PERIPHERALLY INSERTED CENTRAL CATHETERS

When assessment indicates the need for prolonged central placement, a PICC can be used for administration of multiple medications and for drawing blood samples. Comparative studies on open-ended PICCs and pulmonary arterial catheters showed correlating hemodynamic measurements, proving them beneficial for this as well (Santolucito, 2007). With almost half of intensive care patients requiring central access, PICC insertions rose from 11% in 1999 to approximately 29% in 2007. Size 6-French PICCs were recently developed, and have proven to be useful when practitioners use upper arm veins of adequate size, ultrasound guidance, and microintroducers for insertion (Nichols and Humphrey, 2008).

PROCEDURE FOR ACCESSING ADD DEACCESSING AN IMPLANTED PORT

1. Verify order for obtaining access. Identify patient using two identifiers, not including the room number.

2. Explain procedure and obtain consent from the patient. Ascertain whether the port is a power port. Apply topical anesthetic if needed.

3. Place patient in recumbent position. Assess the site for signs of inflammation and depth of the port. Clip hair at access site if needed. Determine gauge and length needed for noncoring, access needle. Gather supplies.

4. Wash patient's port site with antiseptic soap and water if needed. Perform hand hygiene. Open supplies. Place noncoring needle, positive-pressure cap, and sterile 0.9% sodium chloride syringe on the field using sterile technique.

5. Place a mask on the patient if needed. Don sterile gloves. Place drapes around site.

6. Prepare noncoring needle by attaching a 10-mL syringe of 0.9% sodium chloride and priming the extension set and needle.

7. Cleanse site with antiseptic. If using alcohol and povidone-iodine swab sticks, start at the center of the skin directly above the port and clean in a concentric circular pattern using alcohol first followed by the iodine solution. If using chlorhexidine, cleanse using a back and forth scrubbing pattern. Allow to dry. Change to new clean sterile gloves.

8. Locate the septum and secure at three points with thumb and two fingers of nondominant hand. Holding the needle with the other hand perpendicular to the site, puncture the skin directly over the center of the septum with the needle, and access the port using one smooth motion until the needle touches the back of the septum.

9. Aspirate for blood return. Flush the port with 10 mL of 0.9% sodium chloride and follow with heparinized solution if the port will not be used for medications or will be deaccessed.

10. If the port will be used for an infusion, fold 2 × 2 gauze in half and place underneath the wings of the needle without obscuring the insertion site for visualization and assessment later; then place a sterile transparent membrane dressing over the site, making sure to cover the entire needle. The insertion site should remain unobscured. Secure the remaining tubing.

11. Document site assessment, procedure, size of needle, and blood return in the patient's medical record.

12. When deaccessing, flush with 10 mL of 0.9% sodium chloride and instill 500 units of heparin in 5 mL of 0.9% sodium chloride or prescribed amount ordered. Remove dressing. Support the port housing with nondominant hand and remove needle without twisting, using a steady perpendicular motion.

13. Apply pressure for hemostasis; then cover with small dressing. Date and initial the dressing.

14. Document procedure, gauge/length of noncoring needle, blood return, instillation of heparin flush, and patient's tolerance to the procedure.

Adapted from Infusion Nurses Society: *Policies and procedures for infusion nursing,* ed 3, Norwood, Mass, 2006b, Author.

Contrast media during computed topography (CT) studies were used for almost half of the exams during a 2006 study consisting of about 35 million cases (Santolucito, 2007). CT scans are ordered for diagnostic information for cancer staging studies, for abdominal pain diagnoses, for trauma, lung disease, and liver or pancreas disorders, to name just a few. Recently new peripherally inserted central catheters have been developed to allow injection of contrast media without rupturing the catheter, making PICCs invaluable to patients with multiple needs and venous access challenges. Many of these patients need CT scans quarterly as well as intravenous medications, and these catheters prevent multiple occasions for painful attempts at access.

Competency

The potential for success in a PICC program is high when certain variables are taken into consideration at the initiation of the program. For that reason, some organizations have requirements that must be met before a nurse is eligible to be taught how to place PICCs. First, they must be a registered nurse with a valid license. Then, many require 2 years experience and demonstrated competency in venipuncture and central line care followed by a program of training (Burns, 2005). Only nurses with documented advanced peripheral venous insertion skills should be considered for training of this advanced skill.

Extensive education and ongoing competency reviews should be the mainstay for nurses that insert PICCs. The learning curve for PICC insertion in adults using ultrasound is extensive, and possibly even more for pediatric placements. Mastery of ultrasound requires practice, usually 30 to 50 attempts (Hunter, 2007). Education should consist of a didactic course of study and testing, followed by hands-on instruction at the bedside. The didactic portion should include an anatomical review of the upper arm and central vasculature, measurement techniques, and placement. Following the PICC education program, a hands-on validation of the procedure with documentation is necessary. Annual competency checks and ongoing data collection regarding individual and team success rates validate the value of the PICC program to the patient and the organization.

Nurses with an understanding of the ultrasound for VAD placement will be at an advantage. Some nurses learn to place peripheral VADs with ultrasound before attempting to place a PICC. PICC education programs using ultrasound include visualization of the entire insertion procedure with incremental advancement of the catheter for proper placement. First the nurse learns to set up the sterile field with the appropriate supplies and how to establish maximum barrier precautions; the nurse then advances to the catheter placement. Most programs require correct placement of three to six PICCs before being "signed off" to practice independently (Burns, 2005). At that point the nurse inserting the PICCs should have someone to call for backup when problems are encountered. This is where a team approach with two nurses placing PICCs is helpful; however, most nurses can practice independently with relatively few problems.

There is debate among PICC teams regarding the length of time needed for a nurse to place a PICC. It is generally agreed that 2 hours is required, which includes the time needed for obtaining informed consent, assembling the supplies and equipment, performing the insertion, and documenting the procedure. A procedure lasting longer than 1.5 to 2 hours is usually not well tolerated by patients. Studies show that insertions requiring

multiple attempts to cannulate the vein may increase the risk of infection or long-term complications (Chapman, Johnson, and Bodenham, 2006), since intraluminal damage may result in thrombosis, leading ultimately to infection. One study concluded that more than two failed punctures were associated with increased complication rates (Maecken and Grau, 2007).

Ongoing competency should be evaluated on a regular basis, and built into organizational policy and procedure. Quality and proficiency data maintained for each nurse will facilitate confidence in the nurse's ability and reduce patient complications. PICC teams could benefit from ongoing data review of each nurse's placement success rate. Some teams place the nurse into training remediation when his or her success rate falls below a certain percentage, and ask the nurse to step down from the team when the rate does not improve or falls a second time. The definition of "success" for an insertion usually refers to a catheter whose tip terminates in the distal superior vena cava. Other quality improvement data to collect that are valuable for improving outcomes would include types and rates of complications, especially infection.

Consent—ABCs

Informed consent has been a topic of importance for many years when it comes to medical procedures. Now, more than ever, it is important for patients to know the ABCs of PICC insertion so they may understand exactly what is happening before making a decision about their care. "A" refers to the alternatives, "B" to the benefits, and "C" to the possible complications. Many organizations have a separate consent for PICC insertion so that all information is readily available for the patient and nurse to discuss the procedure (Figure 24-1).

Alternatives to PICC insertion include continuation of short peripheral devices, sometimes as frequently as every 12 hours when medications are irritating to the vein. The physician may place another type of central catheter that also has to be changed more often, making the PICC more appropriate. Whatever the reason, the patient should know why an alternative VAD is the best solution for the patient's infusion needs.

Benefits of having a PICC placed include the ability to draw blood from the catheter and infuse multiple medications; PICCs also have been shown to have fewer complications (such as pneumothorax or pinch-off syndrome), can be used for cardiac monitoring, provide long-term access, and require relatively simple self-care. The cost is less than that for other types of access requiring insertion by a physician or interventional radiologist, and the insertion does not require general anesthesia.

Full disclosure of complications requires discussions about the following in conversation style and language the patient will understand:
- Bleeding
- Blood clot/thrombus
- Arterial puncture/damage
- Nerve damage
- Irregular heartbeat
- Infection

Supplies

A variety of PICCs are available on the market today, ranging in size from 1.9-French (1.9F) pediatric catheters to 7F triple-lumen catheters for adult patients. Most are made of

INFORMED CONSENT FOR MEDICAL/SURGICAL/DIAGNOSTIC PROCEDURES

I, _____
  (First)   (Middle)   (Last)
give permission to specially trained registered nurses in the **IV Therapy Nursing Department**

(Listing names of nurses, _____) to perform the
following procedure: **Peripherally Inserted Central Catheter Placement.**

_____ has explained to me the purpose of this procedure and the potential
risks and benefits listed below. He/She has also explained medically acceptable alternatives. I understand the results
cannot be guaranteed.

The IV Therapy Nurse has talked with me about the most common **risks** below. I understand that there may be other risks.
  • Bleeding
  • Nerve damage
  • Blood clot (thrombus formation)
  • Irregular heart beat
  • Puncture of an artery
  • Infection

The IV Therapy Nurse has talked with me about the potential **benefits** involved with this procedure including:
  • Fewer needle sticks for lab work, medications, etc.
  • That use of this catheter may substitute for other catheters.
  • I may be discharged home with this catheter.
  • That lab draws may be obtained by this catheter.

The IV Therapy Nurse has talked with me about reasonable **alternatives** to this procedure including:
  • A different type of catheter inserted by your physician
  • Possible multiple IV insertions
  • Possible multiple needle sticks to obtain ordered labs

I understand people may be there during the procedure to watch and consult for professional purposes.

INITIAL (DO NOT CHECK) THE FOLLOWING:
I permit the IV nurse to give me necessary numbing medications:

Yes _____ No _____ Does Not Apply_____

I understand the above and my questions have been answered.

Patient: _____ Date: _____ Time: _____

Patient or person authorized to consent for patient: _____
(Relationship, if other than patient)
(If patient unable to sign, state reason)

Witness_____ Date: _____ Time: _____

FIGURE 24-1   Sample consent form. (Courtesy of Moses Cone Medical Center.)

silastic or polyurethane. PICCs can be open-ended or closed-ended catheters. The Groshong® catheter is closed-ended with a split tip valve to prevent air embolism, blood reflux, and clotting. Reverse-taper PICCs are graduated in size from the catheter to the hub to prevent bleeding at the site after insertion.

Catheter gauge, the measurement of the outer diameter of the catheter, depends on the catheter size. A 3F catheter is 20 gauge and a 4F catheter is 18 gauge, with gauge sizes varying from 18 to 20 gauge, or from 20 to 23 gauge for dual-lumen catheters. Flow rates will vary depending on the catheter gauge. Power-injectable PICCs have been developed to withstand injections of 5 mL of contrast medium per second.

In an effort to stem health care–associated infections, PICCs are being developed with antimicrobial coatings to prevent the formation of biofilm (Roe et al, 2008). The most common antimicrobials used to coat central catheters are chlorhexidine-silver sulfadiazine and minocycline/rifampin. There are chlorhexidene-impregnated foam disks that can be used at the insertion site to prevent infection as well.

Microintroducers are also available both in individual packets and in PICC insertion kits; refer to Chapter 20 for further details. Individual microintroducers are beneficial for cases when a second attempt at insertion is necessary. Any time the vein is to be cannulated more than once, a new needle and guidewire should be used. If only the needle is needed, echogenic needles can be purchased in individual packets as well. Guidewires come in various sizes and materials. To reduce the chance of injury to the vein wall or cardiac structures, flexible tip guidewires, usually 0.018 gauge, are recommended. The guidewire should never be advanced beyond the tip of the catheter.

Use of a PICC insertion kit standardizes the insertion procedure. To maintain sterility the contents of the kit should be checked to see if additional supplies will be needed such as 0.9% sodium chloride, syringes, lidocaine, drapes, gown, surgical cap, and a probe cover. Additional packets of sterile gloves as well as microintroducer kits or sterile echogenic needles should be within reach. With the addition of locator systems, a cover is also needed for the sensor, which is placed on the patient's chest prior to the procedure.

Sterility

PICC insertion is a sterile procedure, requiring implementation of the central line bundle components of maximum sterile barrier precautions. A protective pad placed underneath the patient's arm will shield the bedding. Strict hand hygiene should be performed, and a mask, surgical cap, goggles, sterile gown, and sterile gloves should be worn. The patient should be entirely covered (from head to toe) with a sterile drape, and supplies should be opened using sterile technique and placed on a sterile cover, which is usually provided as a wrap for the PICC insertion kit. A sterile probe cover should be placed on the field for use on the ultrasound machine.

A study addressing catheter-related bloodstream infections (CRBSIs) concluded that maximum sterile barriers proved to be an effective practice, reducing approximately one third of the colonization probability (Carrer et al, 2005). The CDC recommends maximum sterile barrier for central line placement because it substantially reduces CRBSI (McCormick and Rutledge, 2003); and studies are showing dramatic improvements in outcomes since maximum barrier precautions were initiated. One study has shown this practice to be about six times more effective in preventing infection when central catheters are placed (Raad et al, 1994).

Since 90% of catheter-related bloodstream infections occur with central venous catheters, the "central line bundle" (groupings of evidence-based interventions related to a specific procedure or disease process) has been developed to decrease their incidence. When evidence-based interventions are implemented together, patient care outcomes are greatly improved; and when nurses take responsibility for the central line bundle and ensure that maximum barrier precautions are used, the outcomes are even more dramatically improved (IHI, 2007).

After explaining the procedure to the patient, and clearing the room of unnecessary observers, patient comfort should be addressed. Elevating the head of the bed is sometimes easier for the patient, as well as helpful in ensuring the PICC follows the venous path to the superior vena cava rather than the internal jugular vein. A vein is visualized on ultrasound, and the skin marked. Use individual skin markers and discard to avoid cross-contamination between patients. The ultrasound probe should be covered with a disposable cover, such as a small plastic bag, for infection prevention measures.

Measurement

Most PICCs, with the exception of the Groshong®, require premeasuring in order to trim the appropriate length. Many PICCs have graduated markings starting with "0" at the hub end. The nurse trims the PICC according to a predetermined measurement. For PICCs that cannot be trimmed, the catheter length needs to be subtracted from the total length of the PICC. Any extra catheter remaining is left outside the insertion site, coiled, and secured.

Anthropometric measuring (measurement using anatomical landmarks) makes determination of the correct catheter length relatively simple with some practice, unless the patient has anatomical abnormalities or skeletal difficulties that do not allow the patient to lie flat. Measuring from the insertion site to the right sternal notch and then down to the third intercostal space (third intercostal space on the right parasternal line) will closely correlate the distance from insertion to the superior vena cava. This gives the nurse a close estimation for trimming the PICC if it is necessary, or subtracting to find the amount of catheter to leave outside the insertion site.

When the patient is unable to lie flat or the body habitus is prohibitive for accurate measurement by conventional methods, there are ways to mathematically calculate the length of the PICC based on the patient's height (Lum, 2004). When there is no close height available, the nurse should attempt a measurement based on the anatomical landmarks, and adjust as needed to place the tip in the correct position.

Insertion

Until the last few years, PICCs were inserted using visualization, palpation, and a split sheath technique. Since the advent of ultrasound, the placement of PICCs using palpation only is becoming rare. The nurse competent in using ultrasound for PICC placement is at a great advantage in comparison to those inserting PICCs only using palpation. Besides increasing accuracy rates and decreasing complications, ultrasound can detect venous thrombosis and prevent inappropriate placements (Blaivas, 2007).

Modified Seldinger Technique (MST)

The modified Seldinger technique using a microintroducer has greatly improved processes by reducing trauma to the vein and risk of artery or nerve injury (Galloway, 2002). There are MST kits for pediatric catheters as small as 2F and 3F (Wald et al, 2008). The peel-away needle is replaced with a smaller catheter or needle. After accessing the vein with ultrasound, a guidewire is inserted into the vein through the needle. The nurse secures the guidewire to prevent embolism and removes the needle. A small dermatotomy is made, if necessary, and a dilator/introducer is threaded over the guidewire. The guidewire and dilator are then removed. The PICC is threaded into the introducer and vein, where it should follow the blood flow all the way to the vena cava. The introducer is removed by a peel-away method.

The microintroducer technique is advantageous not only because the trauma is minimized but also because it allows the insertion site to be above the antecubital fossa. The peel-away cannula is not as likely to sheer the catheter, decreasing the possibility of catheter embolism.

Another advantage in using this technique is that a small needle is used for cannulation rather than a large-bore metal peel-away needle. A guidewire is placed through the needle when a blood return is noted, and the needle is removed. A dilator is placed over the guidewire, gradually expanding the opening, and the catheter is threaded through the dilator. The insertion is less damaging to the vein wall, and a repeat attempt to access the vein minimizes trauma or development of a hematoma.

Bedside ultrasound

The development of bedside ultrasound has simplified venous selection, and decreased the number of complications related to traumatic placement (Elliott, 2006). Overall mechanical complications occurred up to 21% of the time, and up to 35% of attempts were unsuccessful previous to the use of ultrasound guidance (Feller-Kopman, 2007). One study suggests a reduction in failure rate for PICC placement as much as 60% when using ultrasound (Krstenic et al, 2008). Transverse or cross-sectional views of the vein in "real-time" (Aldrich, 2007) can be obtained when an ultrasound probe is placed on the arm. A small amount of ultrasound gel is required between the probe, the sheath, and the skin. The probe should always be covered with a disposable cover to prevent cross-contamination between patients. An echogenic needle will be seen as a white dot when accessing the vein using a transverse view (Maecken and Grau, 2007). The nurse or physician who uses ultrasound for placement has a much higher success rate after a period of training and experiential self-training (Olivier and Feller-Kopman, 2007). The success rate for image-guided central catheter placement has been reported to be greater than 95% (Lewis et al, 2003). Both physicians and nurses now recognize the improvement in patient outcomes when ultrasound technology is used to access the veins of the upper arms (Maecken and Grau, 2007).

Nurses placing PICCs at the bedside use either a single-operator or a multiple-operator technique. When two nurses are working simultaneously at the bedside, the second nurse can be setting up supplies on the sterile field, providing support for the patient, and assisting when needed to access the vein, insert the guidewire, or thread the catheter.

Veins used most often for PICC placement are the cephalic vein, the median veins, and the basilic vein. An insertion site 2 cm or more above the antecubital fossa, to prevent mechanical irritation or kinking of the catheter when the arm is in movement, has become the site of choice for PICC placement. When visualizing the veins of the upper arm with ultrasound, the basilic vein is the vein of first choice because it is usually the larger vein of the upper arm, and is a direct route with relative lack of obstructions for ease of catheter advancement.

The basilic vein, larger than the cephalic in the majority of patients, extends about 24 cm in the average adult, and runs along the inner aspect of the biceps muscle. It terminates in the axillary vein, which is 11 to 13 cm long. The cephalic vein, 35 to 38 cm long, is along the outer border of the biceps muscle, and also terminates in the axillary vein, with a descending curve just below the clavicle. The subclavian vein is joined by the internal jugular vein and measures approximately 6 cm in length. The superior vena cava adjoins the right atrium and measures about 7 to 9 cm in length.

PROCEDURE FOR PICC PLACEMENT USING ULTRASOUND GUIDANCE AND MODIFIED SELDINGER TECHNIQUE

1. Verify physician or authorized prescriber's order. Determine PICC type based on need (single, dual, or triple lumen; and/or power-injectable PICC). Explain procedure to the patient and obtain consent. Identify the patient using two identifiers. Check patient's allergy status.

2. Place disposable cover on the ultrasound probe. Place tourniquet on patient's upper arm and examine for appropriate veins. Mark expected insertion site. Measure for length of PICC and add 2.5 cm for left-sided placement.

3. Perform hand hygiene for 60 seconds with antimicrobial soap. Don surgical cap, gown, goggles, and mask.

4. Assemble equipment. Prepare sterile field with sterile field drape. Place patient in recumbent position, place nonporous pad underneath the patient's arm, apply locater to chest if appropriate, and adjust the arm to the proper position at a 90-angle from the body.

5. Set up PICC supplies on sterile field. Add any necessary supplies not in the kit (e.g., sterile probe cover, microintroducer kit, echogenic needle, sterile gloves, securement device).

6. Don sterile gloves. Draw up lidocaine and 0.9% sodium chloride in 10-mL syringes using sterile technique, and place on the field in ready-to-use fashion with small-bore needle added to the syringe of lidocaine. Place probe cover on the ultrasound probe.

7. Scrub the intended insertion site with chlorhexidine gluconate swabs. Place full-body drape over patient's entire body, covering everything except the insertion site.

8. Place caps on the hubs of the catheter, and prime each port. Pull the stylet or locater wire back from the catheter and trim the catheter the premeasured length. Advance stylet to the tip of the catheter, being sure to leave entirely covered. Bend the end of the wire at the hub to prevent movement of the guidewire, with resulting trauma upon insertion. Set aside on sterile field.

9. Apply tourniquet. Change to new gloves.

10. Place ultrasound gel on probe, secure position, and anesthetize the area. Cannulate the vein with echogenic needle. Insert guidewire. Make a small nick at the insertion site if necessary.

11. Remove needle. Place introducer/dilator into the vein by threading over the guidewire. Remove the guidewire. Advance introducer the rest of the way into the vein and remove the dilator. Thread the catheter into the vein. Stop about 5 cm past the dilator and activate the locater system. Continue advancing at a slow, steady pace until in position.

12. Break and peel the introducer while pulling away from the insertion. Check for blood return, and flush the catheter. Cleanse site and secure the catheter with securement device.

13. Cover with transparent dressing. Date and initial the dressing.

14. Clean area; dispose of sharps. Provide for patient comfort. Order STAT portable chest x-ray.

15. Document in patient medical record. Note lot number, manufacturer, and type of catheter. Fill out quality improvement (QI) paperwork.

The main artery flanked by median accessory veins will frequently make a "Mickey Mouse" shape on the ultrasound machine, with the two veins making Mickey's ears. The vessels will appear as disks on the screen in the transverse view. When pressing on the vessels with the ultrasound probe, the artery will pulsate and the veins will collapse. Veins that do not collapse may be sclerotic. The integrity of the vein is seen by collapse and rebound when pressing and removing the ultrasound probe. At times the basilic vein will be in the region of the median vessels rather than isolated and more medial to the body. These brachial veins branch into the axillary vein, which gets larger as it nears the central vasculature and connects to the cephalic vein and then to the subclavian vein, which bridges to the superior vena cava. The optimum tip placement is the distal superior vena cava, or the junction of the superior vena cava and the right atrium, called the cavoatrial junction.

Whether placing PICCs independently or with assistance from another nurse, using bedside ultrasound facilitates successful insertion, minimizes unsuccessful venipuncture attempts, and prevents the need to transport the patient to the radiology department, unless the nurse experiences difficulty and interventional radiology is needed. Then the catheter is placed using fluoroscopy. There are patients who are not candidates for placement even by radiology, usually because of stenosis or other vascular issues. Figures 24-2 to 24-10 illustrates the insertion of a PICC using ultrasound guidance and modified Seldinger technique.

Catheter tip verification

Once a PICC is placed, the tip will need to be verified by chest radiograph before it is ready for infusions. There are several states that have added tip verification to their state's nurse practice act, allowing registered nurses who are qualified and competent to confirm tip placement by radiograph. Tip verification

programs are usually in collaboration with a radiologist or the radiology department; these programs educate nurses to identify the correct placement for PICC tips at a point approximately 5 cm below the carina. Initial tip verification allows the PICC to be used or repositioned before the radiologist reads the film. Radiology confirmation of tip placement should occur within 24 hours. When time is of the essence to begin treatment, this can be especially beneficial for the patient.

Catheter tip placement has been an ongoing controversy among physicians, radiologists, and nurses. The "gold standard" among infusion nurses has historically been the distal superior vena cava (SVC). The SVC is referred to as "ideal" placement (Caers et al, 2005; INS, 2006a,b); however, many interventional radiologists and physicians prefer the catheter tip to reside in the right atrium for increased hemodilution and blood flow. These right atrium catheters are placed in an area of greater turbulence to prevent some of the complications of central catheters, namely, thrombosis (Cohn et al, 2001), formation of fibrin sheaths, or tip occlusion (Scott, Kondratovich, and Blum, 2000).

The American Society of Parenteral and Enteral Nutrition guidelines recommend that catheters used for parenteral nutrition are placed with the tip terminating in the superior vena cava "adjacent to the right atrium." A study of 138 catheters used for parenteral nutrition or chemotherapy showed that almost 16% were malpositioned, concluding that all catheters should have tip position verification before initiating parenteral nutrition (DeChicco et al, 2007).

More recent comparison of chest x-rays to CT scans found that an accurate placement identification was possible using the right superior cardiac border as formed by the right atrial appendage (RAA) and the caudal margin of the azygos vein, so that the correct placement for cavoatrial junction was recommended to be 1 to 2 cm below the SVC-RAA junction (Verhey et al, 2008). Measurements from retrospective studies

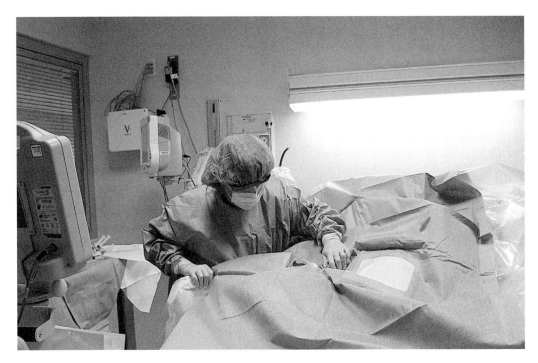

FIGURE 24-2   PICC insertion using maximum barrier protection.

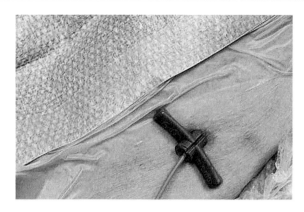

FIGURE 24-3   Image of a vein on ultrasound.

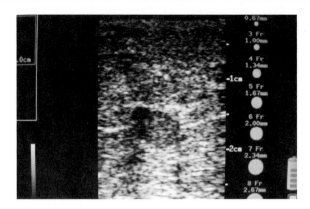

FIGURE 24-7   Advancing PICC through introducer.

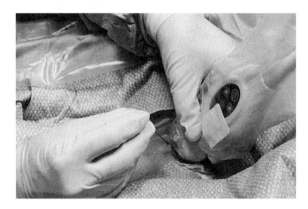

FIGURE 24-4   Accessing a vein with echogenic needle, vascular access probe, and ultrasound.

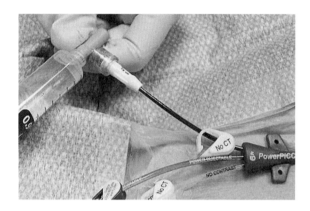

FIGURE 24-8   Aspirating blood return to confirm catheter patency.

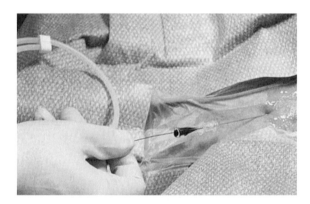

FIGURE 24-5   Inserting guidewire after obtaining venous access.

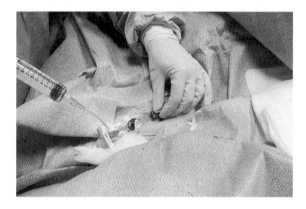

FIGURE 24-9   Flushing catheter with 0.9% sodium chloride in 10-mL syringe.

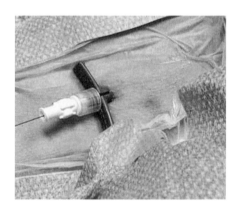

FIGURE 24-6   Removing guidewire from introducer.

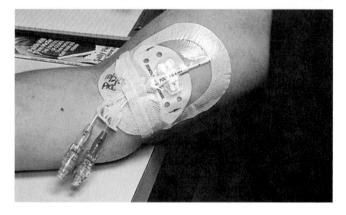

FIGURE 24-10   PICC dressing.

of computed tomographic exams defined a more reliable estimate of the cavoatrial junction as two vertebral bodies below the carina (Baskin et al, 2008).

A review of medical articles shows cardiac and right atrium (RA) placements have been associated with cardiac tamponade (Forauer, 2007), cardiac perforation, arrhythmia, valvular insufficiency, atrial thrombosis, and catheter dysfunction (Baskin et al, 2008). According to a study done by a hospital oncology department (Caers et al, 2005), ports with tips positioned in the right atrium had a higher incidence of thrombosis and dysfunction than those with tips placed in the lower SVC or SVC-RA junction. Arrhythmia has also been directly related to central catheters residing in the right atrium with resulting irritation. When venous or cardiac perforation occurred as a result of central tip placement, the result was frequently fatal, as much as 80% of the time. To avoid cardiac perforation the tip should be placed above the pericardial reflection on radiography, defined as 30 to 50 mm from the carina (Venkatesan et al, 2007). Catheters should also be positioned so that the tip does not make contact with the vein wall.

Evidence indicates heart monitoring can give an accurate picture of the catheter tip position. Central lines placed using electrocardiographic guidance reduced the need for routine chest radiography after central line placement in one study (Davis, 2008). The peak of the P waves during central line placement indicates SVC-RA placement according to another study (Jeon et al, 2006); normally-shaped P waves indicate tip placement in the mid to upper SVC, and biphasic P waves indicate right atrial tip location (Jeon et al, 2006). Nurses placing PICCs in intensive care units or patients being monitored with an electrocardiograph may be able to use electrocardiographic guidance to their advantage.

Midclavicular tip placement has been used in cases where central access was not easily obtained because of anatomical difficulties, but it is not recommended since studies have shown a fourfold increased incidence of thrombosis with midclavicular tip placement (Cook, 2007). Other reasons for placing midclavicular catheters include radiographic cost savings and patient accessibility—some patients cannot be transferred to facilities where central line placement is available. With increased incidents of thrombosis in the midclavicular region, infusion therapy should indicate the need for either a peripheral catheter, a midline catheter, or a central catheter since literature does not support the use of midclavicular catheters.

 ## SPECIAL CONSIDERATIONS

Certain patient populations present unique problem sets related to PICC placement. For the experienced infusion nurse, overcoming these challenges is simply a matter of progressing through the learning curve, but in response to the need, many organizations create specialized teams to handle specific issues. PICC teams specializing in placement in neonates are such an example.

PEDIATRIC

While placing PICCs in older pediatric patients requires the same skills as those for adult placement, younger children and infants can require a different skill-set altogether. Behavioral issues, immaturity, and stranger anxiety are concerns that usually require a two-member team rather than a single nurse in order to address patient comfort and fear. Children require a different approach entirely since younger ones cannot reason or understand the need to remain still and cooperate while undergoing an uncomfortable procedure that may be painful.

Allowing parents or caregivers to remain in the room is beneficial, but requires more confidence from the nurse. Adding another person to the process changes the dynamics even more. Not only is the nurse concerned about the patient, but also the nurse has to be conscious of the observer's fears and reactions. Having a child life therapist in attendance is a valuable resource, especially when a parent will not be able to attend to the child.

Neonatal/infant PICCs are placed in more superficial veins, making ultrasound ineffective. A peel-away device will serve as needle, dilator, and introducer. Warm packs placed underneath the arm and in the axillary region will prevent a certain amount of vasoconstriction. Veins most used in infants under 3 months of age are the temporal vein, lying in front and above the ear, and the posterior auricular vein behind the ear, both of which empty into the external jugular vein. These veins do not have valves. A peel-away catheter is appropriate for the size, depth, and location of the vessels for this patient population, but MST is the most advantageous whenever possible for veins located in the upper arm. Distraction for comfort measures works well in this age group, augmented by swaddling and Sweet-Ease, an oral sucrose solution that helps to soothe and calm distressed babies. Also for infants and older babies, the saphenous vein, which runs along the medial aspect of the foot and threads to the inferior vena cava, is an appropriate choice until they are able to walk. For the toddler and the older child, the median cubital vein and the basilic vein can be accessed if not previously cannulated for blood draws.

A toddler may not be able to tolerate the procedure without general anesthesia or propofol. Many children's hospitals have order sets for Versed and fentanyl. Lidocaine patches or creams can be applied beforehand, and lidocaine infiltrated to the area will help substantially (Mickler, 2008) once it is injected. The *Infusion Nursing Standards of Practice* (INS, 2006a) recommends establishing policies and procedures related to the use of local anesthetic agents as well as adhering to the manufacturer's labeled use(s) and directions. Use of topical anesthetics should be encouraged for children in addition to use of the adjunctive and less invasive anesthetics and anxiolytic therapies. When used, the patient should be monitored because of the potential for allergic reactions or tissue damage.

In addition, pediatric patients present more problems with venous spasm than adults. When accessing the vein, a spasm may prevent the needle from going into the inner layer of the vein, or prevent threading of the guidewire or catheter. The smaller veins are harder to access, and once the nurse attempts and misses, there may not be another chance. Veins and arteries are closer in proximity, and arterial puncture as well as nerve damage is more likely to occur than for adults. This, in combination with uncontrolled movement, can create more tension and less accuracy even for the most skilled and experienced practitioner. Maximum sterile barriers during catheter placement are nonnegotiable to prevent infection (Shah, Smith, and Zaoutis, 2005), even though adhering to the policy is more difficult.

BARIATRIC

The bariatric population presents challenges of its own. According to the National Institutes of Health approximately 34% of Americans are overweight, and of these, 27% are obese. Obesity is determined by body mass index (BMI): a BMI of 25 is considered overweight, 30 is obese, and over 40 is considered morbidly obese (Torpy, Burke, and Glass, 2005).

In 2006 the Centers for Medicare & Medicaid Services (CMS) expanded its coverage for bariatric surgery for morbidly obese patients who also have a secondary diagnosis that would be improved by weight reduction. These conditions include heart disease, stroke, gallbladder disease, sleep apnea, and type 2 diabetes, among others. Patients entering the hospital for any medical reason complicated by obesity have increased problems with venous access.

The research on venous access related to bariatric patients is scant and only mentioned briefly in journal articles or research. Recommendations for VAD placement include the hand, antecubital fossa, and, in instances where access is direly needed and attempts have been unsuccessful, the feet. If the patient has diabetes, a VAD inserted in the foot is not the best option. External jugular placement is often attempted, but even that approach is difficult in some patients, and when access is obtained, it is not effective for a very long period of time because of mechanical complications. If ultrasound guidance is used the external jugular access can be successful more often (Feller-Kopman, 2007).

The best approach for placement in the bariatric patient is using ultrasonography. If peripheral access is difficult, the external jugular placement is exhausted, the VAD will be needed for 5 or more days, and the medications infused will not be irritating or vesicant in nature, a midline is indicated. Adjustments will need to be made to meet special challenges. There are longer echogenic needles available for use in this population. Measurements are more difficult, and harder to be exact when measuring bariatric patient habitus, but using anthropomorphic measurement or calculating by patient height can be done with practice and experience.

RENAL

Long-term use of central catheters has been linked to intraluminal damage, creating problems for patients with renal disease who may need these veins for grafts, fistulas, or hemodialysis catheters later. In a study done postmortem on veins used for central access, all the vessels showed vein wall thickening or intimal hyperplasia and resulting thrombus (Forauer and Theoharis, 2003). Because of the need to use the veins in the upper arm for hemodialysis procedures, patients should be screened for possible renal follow-up before placing a PICC. In one study, the incidence of central vein stenosis and occlusion after PICC and port placements in the upper arm had a 7% chance of developing even though the patients were asymptomatic (Gonsalves et al, 2003).

Many renal physicians request that arm veins be reserved for possible hemodialysis for their patients. Recent data indicate the importance of fistula placement in order to decrease hospitalizations, infection, and mortality in patients with renal disease. CMS has adopted the Fistula First Breakthrough program in an attempt to increase the use of fistulas, instead of catheters, to prevent infection. Dialysis centers that use fistulas more often than catheters have a much lower infection rate, making pre-PICC placement assessment vital (McLennan, 2007). The Kidney Dialysis Outcomes Quality Initiative recommends that glomerular filtration rate (GFR) be checked and education given to patients with a GFR of 30 mL/min/1.73 m^3 or less in preparation for possible renal replacement. They also recommend

forearm venipuncture, PICCs, and subclavian catheters be avoided in patients with end-stage chronic kidney disease; instead intravenous access should be started and maintained in the patient's hands. If alternative access becomes necessary PICC placement should be in the jugular vein (National Kidney Foundation, 2006).

Developing a close working relationship with the renal physicians will prove beneficial to the ongoing care of these patients. Creatinine clearance levels are being used to determine the need for renal clearance on a patient for whom a PICC has been ordered. If the patient has a creatinine clearance level of less than 20 or 30 mL/min/1.73 m^3, depending on the organization, the renal physician will be asked for approval before the device is placed, thereby protecting veins that may someday become the patient's "life-line."

INSERTION-RELATED COMPLICATIONS

Dealing with challenging patient populations is not limited to renal, pediatric, or bariatric patients. Insertion-related complications can occur any time, related to many different disease processes. The patient with severe edema may present an ultrasound of the upper arm as a "cloudy picture." It is often difficult to insert the guidewire through the tunica intima of a patient with diabetes when their blood glucose level is high.

When placing a PICC in a patient with sclerosed veins, there may be difficulty advancing the guidewire. Complications when using a guidewire can be addressed by the following:

- Handle the guidewire gently. Do not force it in or out of the needle to prevent sheering.
- Check for defects in the wire if problems occur. Obtain a new guidewire if any evidence of sheering is noted.
- Place heat packs underneath the arm and in the axillary region underneath the sterile drape when venous spasm is suspected.
- Avoid any veins with diagnosed or suspected sclerosis as seen on ultrasound.
- Reposition the dilator/introducer and reattempt to thread the guidewire.
- Separate the dilator/introducer, attempt with the dilator, and then reassemble the dilator/introducer and attempt reinsertion. Ensure the guidewire is stabilized during separation and reconnection.

When encountering problems advancing the dilator/introducer, and venous spasm is suspected, the nurse should pause, add heat packs, and then reattempt to advance the dilator without the introducer. When successful placement of the dilator is apparent, the introducer can be added and a twisting motion used to place it entirely into the vessel. If the unit will not advance, pull back the dilator/introducer, leaving about 5 cm in the vessel, and when a blood return is noted begin threading the catheter. If the placement is still unsuccessful, check to make sure the dermatotomy is not too small, and the catheter size is not too large.

Patient-related complications include anatomical abnormalities, heart arrhythmias, and behavioral issues, such as those encountered when working with elderly patients with dementia. Mechanical issues such as machine malfunctions, inability to thread either the guidewire or the catheter, and malpositioning into the internal jugular vein or another vein in the upper thorax region may occur.

There is a chance of more serious complications as well. Air embolism can result from air entering the bloodstream from an inadequately primed catheter. Central venous access placement and removal is high on the list of risk for embolism (Mirski et al, 2007). Guidewires can puncture the vasculature, or catheter or wire fragments can embolize, just as with other types of central venous access devices (Surov et al, 2006). Immediate medical intervention is necessary for either of these complications. Guidewire or catheter emboli can cause heart arrhythmias that will usually resolve when the stimulus is removed, or when the catheter is pulled back. Puncture of the artery can occur when

the artery is very close to the veins, and may be avoidable by using ultrasound.

Nerve injury and irritation can be avoided when the patient is alert to signs and symptoms to report to the nurse during placement. Numbness, tingling, or weakness in the hand or arm should alert the patient and nurse that the nerve is being affected. In this case, the needle or catheter should be removed immediately.

The most frustrating complication can be malposition of the catheter into the internal jugular vein, the brachiocephalic vein, or the azygos vein. A PICC can retract on itself or enter

---

Box 24-1   COMPLICATIONS ASSOCIATED WITH IMAGE-GUIDED CVAD INSERTION

- Arterial insertion
- Pneumothorax
- Hemothorax
- Hematoma
- Perforation
- Air embolism
- Wound dehiscence
- Procedure-induced sepsis
- Thrombosis

PATIENT OUTCOMES

The following are expected outcomes related to the insertion of a CVAD:
- The patient will verbalize the alternatives, benefits, and complications before insertion of a CVAD.
- The patient will experience minimal discomfort during the insertion of a CVAD.
- The patient will remain free from infection associated with the insertion of a CVAD.
- The patient will experience no complications associated with the insertion of a CVAD.

FOCUS ON EVIDENCE

Improving Outcomes Related to CVAD Insertion

- A meta-analysis of 8 studies involving 4143 catheters, of which 2782 were CVADs, compared chlorhexidine gluconate with povidone-iodine solution for disinfection of the intended venipuncture site. All studies were randomized, controlled trials conducted in a hospital with patients who had a peripheral or CVA device. Among patients with a central venous catheter, chlorhexidine gluconate reduced the risk for catheter-related bloodstream infection by 49%. The incidence of bloodstream infection is significantly reduced in patients with CVADs who receive chlorhexidine gluconate versus povidone-iodine for insertion site skin disinfection (Chaiyakunapruk et al, 2002).
- In a randomized, controlled, prospective trial, patients received either a PICC or a peripheral IV (PIV) catheter. Outcome measures were patient and parent satisfaction with care, complication of the VADs, number of postoperative venipunctures, and cost-effectiveness. Satisfaction was significantly more frequent in the PICC group (P <0.05), and there were significantly fewer postoperative needle punctures in the PICC group compared with the PIV group. Minor complications were common in the peripheral group; major complications were uncommon in both groups. PICCs should be considered in patients requiring more than 4 days of in-hospital postoperative care, especially if frequent blood sampling or IV access is required (Schwengel et al, 2004).
- In a randomized, controlled trial the safety, efficacy, comfort, and cost-effectiveness of PICCs were compared to peripheral IV catheters. Hospitalized patients requiring IV therapy lasting ≥5 days were randomized 1:1 to PICC or per peripheral catheter (PC). Outcomes were incidence of major complications, minor complications, efficacy, patient satisfaction, and cost-effectiveness. A total of 60 patients were in the study. Major complications were observed in 22.6% of the patients in the PICC group (six deep vein

thrombosis [DVT], one insertion site infection) and 3.4% of the patients in the PC group (one DVT). Superficial venous thrombosis (SVT) occurred in 29% of patients in the PICC group and 37.9% of patients in the PC group. Patients in the PICC group required 1.6 catheters on average, compared with 1.97 catheters in the PC group. Intravenous drug administration was considered very or quite satisfying by 96.8% of the patients in the PICC group, and 79.3% in the PC group. Insertion and maintenance mean cost was $690 (U.S. dollars) for PICC and $237 for PC. PICCs are efficient and satisfying for hospitalized patients requiring IV therapy greater or equal to 5 days. However, the risk of DVT, mostly asymptomatic, appears higher than previously reported, and should be considered before using a PICC (Periard et al, 2008).
- A collaborative cohort study predominantly in the ICUs in Michigan was conducted. A total of 108 ICUs participated in the study and 103 reported data. The analysis included 1981 ICU-months of data and 375,757 catheter days. Over an 18-month period, implementation of the central line bundle resulted in a 66% reduction in catheter-related bloodstream infection (CRBSI) rates (Pronovost et al, 2006).
- A cohort study in an intensive care unit showed that before implementation of the central line bundle physicians were approximately 62% compliant. After implementation of the infection control recommendations in the central line bundle, the CRBSI rate decreased from 11.3/1000 catheter days to 0/1000 catheter days, possibly saving 8 deaths, 43 CRBSIs, and $1,945,922 in additional costs. Conclusions of the study were that multifaceted interventions that helped to ensure adherence with evidence-based infection control guidelines nearly eliminated CRBSIs in the surgical ICU (Berenholtz et al, 2004).

a collateral vessel, which is sometimes impossible to correct when there is an anatomical abnormality or stenosis. Placement of the catheter into the right atrium is easily corrected. The use of location systems during PICC placement has simplified the process, decreased the number of x-rays required after insertion, and resulted in shorter turnaround time for catheter use. Complications associated with image-guided CVAD insertion are listed in Box 24-1.

Frequently, CVADs are inserted in patients who are immunocompromised or critically ill and require hemodynamic monitoring with multiple infusions. Outcomes should be established that provide evidence-based interventions, protecting the nurse and patient from the risks associated with the insertion of CVADs.

Many intensive care units have seen decreased central line infections by initiating the central line bundle. For further details on the central line bundle and the reduction of CRBSIs, refer to Chapters 12 and 25.

SUMMARY

Technological advancements in infusion therapy and the application of evidence-based practice for the insertion of central venous access devices have improved outcomes. Patient satisfaction has greatly improved as a result of fewer venipunctures and the ability to continue treatment at home. Nurses have greater knowledge and expertise in their ability to provide quality care for their patients, with more timely medication administration.

The requirements for reimbursement by CMS have made zero percent infection rates with the use of CVADs and the incorporation of evidence-based interventions into clinical practice even more imperative to health care professionals than ever before. The latest evidence must be incorporated into clinical practice so the focus on improving outcomes related to the insertion of central venous access devices is achieved.

REFERENCES

Aldrich JE: Basic physics of ultrasound imaging, *Crit Care Med* 35(5 suppl):S131-S137, 2007.

Baskin KM, Jimenez RM, Cahill AM et al: Cavoatrial junction and central venous access tip position, *JVIR* 19(3):359-365, 2008.

Berenholtz SM, Provovost PJ, Lipset PA et al: Eliminating catheter-related bloodstream infection in the intensive care unit, *Crit Care Med* 32(10):2014-2020, 2004.

Blaivas M: Ultrasound in the detection of venous thromboembolism, *Crit Care Med* 35(5 suppl):S224-S234, 2007.

Burns D: Clinical investigation: retrospective analysis, the Vanderbilt PICC service: program, procedural and patient outcomes successes, *JAVA* 10(4):1-10, 2005.

Caers J, Fontaine C, Vinh-Hung V et al: Catheter tip position as a risk factor for thrombosis associated with the use of subcutaneous infusion ports, *Support Care Cancer* 13(5):325-331, 2005.

Carrer S et al: Effect of different sterile barrier precautions and central venous catheter dressing on the skin colonization around the insertion site, *Minerva Anestesiol* 71(5):197-206, 2005.

Chaiyakunapruk N, Veenstra DL, Lipsky BA et al: Chlorhexidine compared with povidone-iodine for vascular catheter-site care: a meta-analysis, *Ann Intern Med* 136(11):792-801, 2002.

Chapman GA, Johnson D, Bodenham AR: Visualisation of needle position using ultrasonography, *Anaesthesia* 61:148-158, 2006.

Cohn DE, Mutch DG, Rader JS et al: Factors predicting subcutaneous implanted central venous port function: the relationship between catheter tip location and port failure in patients with gynecologic malignancies, *Gynecol Oncol* 83:533-536, 2001.

Cook LS: Continuing controversy of midclavicular catheters, *J Infus Nurs* 30(5):267-273, 2007.

Davis KA: Assessing procedural and clinical data plus electrocardiographic guidance greatly reduce the need for routine chest radiography after central line placement, *J Trauma* 64(2):542, 2008.

DeChicco R, Seidner DL, Brun C et al: Tip position of long-term central venous access devices used for parenteral nutrition, *JPEN* 31(5):382-387, 2007.

Dillon PA, Foglia RP: Complications associated with an implantable vascular access device, *J Ped Surg* 41:1582-1587, 2006.

Elliott SC: Nurse supported PICC line services, *ACMPE Paper*, p 7, Dec 2006.

Feller-Kopman D: Ultrasound-guided internal jugular access: a proposed standardized approach and implications for training and practice, *Chest* 132:302–309, 2007. Accessed 11/13/08 at www.chestjournal.org/misc/reprints.shtml.

Fletcher SJ, Bodenham AR: Safe placement of central venous catheters: where should the tip of the catheter lie? *Br J Anaesth* 85(2):188-191, 2000.

Florence AT, Attwood D: *Physicochemical principles of pharmacy*, ed 4, pp 70–71, London, 2006, Pharmaceutical Press.

Forauer AR: Pericardial tamponade in patients with central venous catheters, *J Infus Nurs* 30(3):161-167, 2007.

Forauer AR, Theoharis C: Histologic changes in the human vein wall adjacent to indwelling central venous catheters, *J Vasc Interv Radiol* 14:1163-1168, 2003.

Galloway M: Using benchmarking data to determine vascular access device selection, *J Infus Nurs* 25(5):320-325, 2002.

Gonsalves CF, Eschelman DJ, Sullivan KL et al: Incidence of central vein stenosis and occlusion following upper extremity PICC and port placement, *Cardiovasc Interv Radiol* 26(2):123-127, 2003.

Hunter M: Peripherally inserted central catheter placement @ the speed of sound, *Nutr Clin Pract* 22:406-411, 2007.

Infusion Nurses Society: Infusion nursing standards of practice, *J Infus Nurs* 29(1 suppl):S1–S92, 2006a.

Infusion Nurses Society: *Policies and procedures for infusion nursing*, ed 3, Norwood, Mass, 2006b, Author.

IHI org: *Implement the central bundle*, 2007. Accessed 11/5/08 at www.ihi.org/IHI/Topics/CriticalCare/IntensiveCare/Measures/CentralLineBundleComplianceRate.html.

Jeon Y, Ryu H, Yoon S et al: Transesophageal echocardiographic evaluation of ECG-guided central venous catheter placement, *Canada J Anaesth* 53:978-983, 2006.

Krstenic WJ, Brealey S, Gaikwad S et al: The effectiveness of nurse led 2-D ultrasound guided insertion of peripherally inserted central catheters in adult patients: a systematic review, *JAVA* 13(3):120-125, 2008.

Lewis CA, Allen TE, Burke DR et al: Quality improvement guidelines for central venous access, *J Vasc Interv Radiol* 14:S231-S235, 2003.

Lum P: A new formula-based measurement guide for optimal positioning of central venous catheters, *JAVA* 9(2):80-85, 2004.

Maecken T, Grau T: Ultrasound imaging in vascular access, *Crit Care Med* 35(5 suppl):S178-S185, 2007.

McCormick R, Rutledge L: New IV guidelines: what's most critical to know, *Infect Control Today*, 2003. Accessed 11/8/08 at http://www.kchealthcare.com/docs/Guidelines.html.

Mickler P: Neonatal and pediatric perspectives in PICC placement, *JAVA* 31(5):282-285, 2008.

Mirski MA, Lele AV, Fitzsimmons L et al: Diagnosis and treatment of vascular air embolism, *Anesthesiology* 106(1):164-177, 2007.

National Kidney Foundation: *Clinical practice guidelines for vascular access. Update 2006*, 2006 Accessed 12/5/08 at http://www.kidney.org/professionals/KDOQI/.

Nichols I, Humphrey JP: The efficacy of upper arm placement of peripherally inserted central catheters using bedside ultrasound and microintroducer technique, *J Infus Nurs* 31(3):165-176, 2008.

O'Grady NP et al: Guidelines for the prevention of intravascular catheter-related infections, *MMWR* 51(RR10):1-26, 2002.

Olivier AF, Feller-Kopman D: Real-time sonography with central venous access: the role of self-training, *Chest* 132:2061–2062, 2007. Accessed 11/13/08 at www.chestjournal.org/misc/reprints.shtml.

Periard D, Monney P, Waeber G et al: Randomized controlled trial of peripherally inserted central catheters vs. peripheral catheters for middle duration in-hospital intravenous therapy, *J Thromb Haemostasis* 6(8):1281-1288, 2008.

Pronovost P, Needham D, Bereholtz S et al: An intervention to decrease catheter-related bloodstream infection in the ICU, *New Engl J Med* 355(26):2725-2732, 2006 (erratum in *New Engl J Med* 356[25]:2660, 2007).

Raad II, Hohn DC, Gilbreath BJ et al: Prevention of central venous catheter-related infections by using maximal sterile barrier precautions during insertion, *Infect Control Hosp Epidemiol* 15(4 pt 1):231-238, 1994.

Roe D, Karandikar B, Bonn-Savage N et al: Antimicrobial surface functionalization of plastic catheters by silver nanoparticles, *J Antimicrob Chemother* 61:869-876, 2008.

Rosenthal K: What you need to know about ports, *Nursing* 36(1):20-21, 2006.

Santolucito JB: The role of peripherally inserted central catheters in the treatment of the critically-ill, *JAVA* 12(4):208-217, 2007.

Schwengel D, McGready J, Berenholtz SM et al: Peripherally inserted central catheters: a randomized, controlled, prospective trial in pediatric surgical patients. *Anesthes Analg* 99(4):1038-1043, 2004.

Scott WL, Kondratovich M, Blum D: Central venous catheter tip placement and catheter occlusion, Letter to the Editor, *Am J Surg* 180:78-79, 2000.

Shah SS, Smith MJ, Zaoutis TE: Device-related infections in children, *Pediatr Clin N Am* 52:1189-1208, 2005.

Shapiro I: *Cato supreme court review 2007-2008*, p 345, Cato Institute, 2008.

Stephens SS et al: Reduction in central line-associated bloodstream infections among patients in intensive care units—Pennsylvania, April 2001-March 2005, *MMWR* 54(40):1013-1016, 2005.

Surov A, Jordan K, Buerke M et al: Atypical pulmonary symbolism of port catheter fragments in oncology patients, *Support Care Cancer* 14:479-483, 2006.

Torpy JM, Burke A, Glass RM: Bariatric surgery, *JAMA* 294(15):1986, 2005.

Venkatesan T, Sen N, Korula PJ et al: Blind placements of peripherally inserted antecubital central catheters: initial catheter tip position in relation to carina, *Br J Anaesth* 98(1):83-88, 2007.

Verhey PT, Gosselin MV, Primack SL et al: The right mediastinal border and central venous anatomy on frontal chest radiograph-direct CT correlation, *JAVA* 13(1):32-35, 2008.

Wald M, Happel CM, Kirchner L et al: A new modified Seldinger technique for 2- and 3-French peripherally inserted central venous catheters, *Eur J Ped* 167(11):1327-1329, 2008.

Wickham R, Engelking C, Sauerland C et al: Vesicant extravasation part II: evidence-based management and continuing controversies, *ONF* 33(6):1143-1150, 2006.

25 Central Venous Access Devices: Care, Maintenance, and Potential Complications

Lisa Gorski, MS, HHCNS-BC, CRNI®, FAAN, Roxanne Perucca, MS, CRNI®, and Mark R. Hunter, RN, CRNI®*

Central venous access devices (CVADs) are essential to infusion therapy, needed for short-term administration of irritating IV solutions and medications in acute care settings and for short- and long-term infusion therapy in home health and other outpatient settings. Yet, it is important to recognize that all patients with CVADs, commonly called central lines, are at risk for infection, occlusion, and other complications. Outcomes of hospital-associated central line infections include increased length of hospital stay and increased cost, with non–inflation-adjusted costs varying from $3,700 to $29,000 per infection (Marschall, Mermel, Classen et al, 2008). Less is known about the risk of infection as well as other complications in non-ICU acute care units and in alternative care settings, such as outpatient and home care. The risk of all complications is decreased when hand hygiene is practiced and when central lines are appropriately maintained and continually assessed for potential problems, allowing early intervention.

 ## CARE AND MAINTENANCE

Care and maintenance of CVADs includes ongoing assessment of the catheter site and infusion system, site care, dressing changes, catheter stabilization, changing injection caps, and catheter flushing to maintain patency. Implanted venous access ports must be accessed and regularly assessed, and the infusion nurse must also address pain issues during port access. Other CVAD-related care and maintenance activities include blood sampling from the CVAD for laboratory studies, culturing for suspected infection, and removing the catheter as soon as it is no longer needed. For patients living at home with a CVAD, the nurse must educate the patient to check the device and report any signs of complications, and how to manage activities of daily living with a CVAD in place. The goal of care

is safe administration of infusion therapy with the absence of complications and removal of the CVAD when no longer needed.

CVAD ASSESSMENT AND MONITORING

Monitoring of CVADs is encompassed in routine patient assessment and when the CVAD is used for medication or solution administration. The monitoring process includes a review of the patient's medical record. Laboratory results and vital signs are reviewed for indications of infection such as an increase in the number of white blood cells and elevated temperature. The need for the central line is reviewed daily to ensure prompt catheter removal when the device is no longer needed for infusion therapy. Longer duration of central venous catheter (CVC) placement is associated with increased risk of catheter-associated infection. Catheter duration beyond 5 to 7 days significantly increases the cumulative risk of infection (Safdar and Maki, 2005).

A visual inspection is conducted of the entire infusion system from the solution container, progressing down the administration set to the insertion site of the central line. The solution container and administration set should be visually assessed for clarity of the infusate, for integrity of the system (i.e., leakage), and for an expiration date. The solution container and administration sets should be labeled and changed according to organizational policies and procedures.

Assessment of the central line includes the insertion site, catheter tract, and adjacent skin. The infusion nurse must differentiate between the different types and placements of CVADs, whether nontunneled (e.g., subclavian, external/internal jugular, femoral site insertion), peripherally inserted (PICC), tunneled, or implanted port. Regardless of the CVAD type, on a regular basis the insertion site is assessed for integrity of the dressing; for any signs of infection including erythema, drainage, swelling, or induration; and for any other complications such as catheter migration. For patients with tunneled catheters, the tunnel is also assessed for any pain, swelling, drainage, or erythema. The portal pocket for implanted devices is assessed for the same. Beyond the immediate catheter placement site, the adjacent skin, neck area, and extremity on the

*The author and editors wish to acknowledge the contributions made by Maxine B. Perdue in the second edition of *Infusion Therapy in Clinical Practice*.

placement side of the central line are assessed for signs of venous thrombosis. These signs and symptoms may include arm, shoulder, or neck swelling; chest area, limb, jaw, or ear pain; and dilated collateral veins over the arm, neck, or chest. For patients with peripherally inserted central catheters (PICCs), the mid-arm circumference measurement may be regularly assessed (Gorski, 2005); however, the *Infusion Nursing Standards of Practice* do not make specific recommendations for this practice (INS, 2006a). Minimally, a baseline arm circumference may be helpful for later comparison, if deep venous thrombosis (DVT) of the upper arm is suspected. Upper extremity DVT is commonly caused by CVADs (Kearon et al, 2008).

The external length of the catheter should be documented at the time of placement for future comparison in monitoring for potential catheter dislodgment and migration. If leakage of parenteral solutions from the catheter insertion site is noted, catheter integrity should be evaluated immediately. Erythema, drainage, and pain, if noted, should be monitored closely. If drainage is present, the amount, color, and consistency should be noted and reported to the physician. A culture of the drainage is generally ordered.

Frequency of site assessment is dependent upon patient condition and organizational policies (for example, with every shift in an acute care setting). For home care patients, the site should be assessed with every home visit and patients should be taught to inspect their site at least every day (Gorski, 2005). Documentation of central line assessment should be completed in the patient's medical record and should include the parenteral solutions infusing, the location of the device, type of dressing utilized, any complications noted, notification of physicians, and follow-up plans. Patient monitoring in relation to the CVAD is summarized in Box 25-1.

SITE CARE AND DRESSING CHANGES

Site care is performed regularly in conjunction with dressing changes. Aseptic technique is required when providing site care; this includes hand hygiene and use of sterile gloves and mask when dealing with CVADs (INS, 2006a). The CDC *Guidelines for the Prevention of Intravascular Catheter-Related Infections* recommend 2% chlorhexidine as the *preferred* skin disinfectant (O'Grady, Alexander, Dellinger et al, 2002) for patients older than 2 months of age. Chlorhexidine preparations have residual antibacterial activity that persists for hours after application and maintain activity in the presence of organic matter, and they have no or minimal systemic absorption. In a meta-analysis of studies that compared chlorhexidine gluconate with povidone-iodine solutions for catheter site care, the incidence of bloodstream infections was significantly reduced when chlorhexidine gluconate was used (Chaiyakunapruk et al, 2002). Povidone-iodine, tincture of iodine (rarely used), and 70% alcohol are considered acceptable disinfectants by both INS (2006a,b) and the CDC (O'Grady et al, 2002). Povidone-iodine is generally used for infants. An important aspect of site disinfection is to allow the antiseptic solution to fully dry before applying a sterile dressing.

Maintaining a clean, dry, and occlusive dressing is important to protect the catheter insertion site and reduce the risk for infection (Figure 25-1). A dressing is placed at the time of CVAD insertion and is regularly changed in conjunction with site care, which includes site assessment and skin disinfection. The dressing should also be replaced if it is loosened or dislodged or if blood or drainage is present. Implanted ports require a dressing

Box 25-1	MONITORING PATIENT WITH A CVAD

1. Know type and features of the CVAD.
   - Tunneled
   - Nontunneled
   - Peripherally inserted
   - Implanted port
   - Catheter features
     - Valved
     - Nonvalved
     - Number of lumens
2. Review the medical record.
   - Laboratory results
   - Vital signs
   - Continued need for the CVAD
3. Assess the solution container and administration set.
   - Clarity of the infusate (e.g., particles)
   - Solution expiration date
   - Integrity of the system
   - Solution container and administration set are labeled
4. Assess the CVAD.
   - Insertion site dressing
   - Insertion site
     - Drainage
     - Pain or tenderness
     - Erythema or induration
     - Swelling
5. Communicate any problems or evidence of complications to the physician and/or the health care team.
6. Document assessment in patient's record.
   - CVAD location
   - Type of dressing
   - Site assessment
   - Presence of any complications
   - Any actions taken

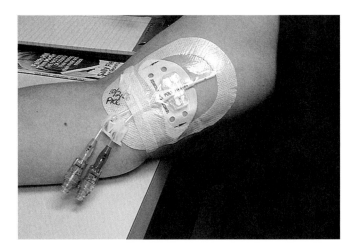

FIGURE 25-1   PICC dressing with StatLock® stabilization.

until the area is healed following the implantation procedure and when accessed with a noncoring needle for intermittent or continuous infusions.

For tunneled catheters in the acute care setting, the dressing regimen is generally the same as that for a nontunneled catheter. In the outpatient setting, if the tunnel is well-healed, no dressing may be required. In a randomized, controlled study of 78 patients with cancer, there were no significant differences in sepsis rates among patients with newly inserted tunneled central venous catheters who were randomized either to a gauze dressing or to no dressing starting at 21 days after catheter insertion (Olson et al, 2004). If the patient is not immunosuppressed and healing at the insertion site is complete, site care may be limited to daily inspection and cleansing with soap and water while bathing.

Dressing choices include the transparent semipermeable membrane (TSM) dressing or a simple gauze dressing. In a systematic review of controlled trials that compared the effects of gauze and tape versus transparent dressings, there was no evidence of difference in the incidence of infectious complications between dressing types (Gillies et al 2003). However, the studies were from small samples and there was a high level of uncertainty regarding risk for infection related to the type of dressing. The authors stressed the need for more research.

Based on limited research and evidence that does not support one choice over another, the type of dressing should be selected based on patient preference and needs. The *Infusion Nursing Standards of Practice* (INS, 2006a) and the CDC guidelines (O'Grady et al, 2002) recommend changing the TSM dressing at least every 7 days and changing gauze dressings every 48 hours. In the event of drainage, site tenderness, other signs of infection, or loss of dressing integrity, the dressing should be changed sooner, allowing the opportunity to closely assess, cleanse, and disinfect the site. Advantages to a TSM dressing include the ability to continually visualize the insertion site without disturbing the dressing as well as cost-effectiveness because of less frequent dressing changes. For example, with home health patients or outpatients, a weekly home or outpatient visit for site care and dressing change is cost-effective and convenient for the patient. However, the patient should be instructed to check the catheter insertion site every day and immediately report any changes, such as redness or drainage or pain at the site.

Gauze dressings are an appropriate choice for the patient who experiences site drainage, perspires excessively, or has a sensitivity reaction to TSM dressings. A gauze dressing is used on a newly placed CVAD when there is bleeding, for at least 24 hours. Often, the transparent dressing is used to secure the gauze dressing. Use of gauze under a TSM dressing is not an uncommon practice, and there is often a misconception, especially among non–infusion nurses, that the dressing is then a TSM dressing and is changed every 7 days. If gauze is used under the TSM dressing, it is considered a gauze dressing and is changed every 48 hours (INS, 2006a).

Antiseptic dressings, such as the chlorhexidine-impregnated foam dressing, are being used more often as research supports their benefits. One such product (BIOPATCH®) is a small, round disk that is placed around the catheter at the exit site, covered with a transparent dressing, and changed every 7 days according to the manufacturer's recommendations. In a meta-analysis, chlorhexidine-impregnated foam dressings were found to be effective in reducing bacterial colonization at both vascular and epidural sites and were identified with a trend toward reduced catheter-associated bloodstream and central nervous system–related infections (Ho and Litton, 2006). The studies included short-term catheters. In a small, randomized trial of adult patients on a hematology unit undergoing chemotherapy, application of chlorhexidine-impregnated foam dressings reduced the incidence of exit site and tunnel infections but there was no

difference in the number of catheter-associated bloodstream infections (CABSIs) (Chambers, Sanders, Patton et al, 2005). There is a lack of research addressing long-term catheters and whether an antiseptic-impregnated dressing has any impact on infection outcome. The CDC did not make recommendations for use of chlorhexidine sponge dressings in 2002 (O'Grady et al, 2002), citing it as an unresolved issue. Evidence-based recommendations from the Infectious Diseases Society of America (IDSA)/Society for Healthcare Epidemiology of America (SHEA) for hospitals recommend their use in the following situations (Marschall et al, 2008):

- The hospital has unacceptably high central line–associated bloodstream infection (CLABSI) rates, despite basic infection prevention measures.
- Patients have limited venous access and a history of CLABSIs.
- There is heightened risk for severe consequences from a CLABSI (e.g., a recently placed prosthetic heart valve).

While the BIOPATCH has been the most commonly used product, there are new and alternative products emerging at the time of publication of this text including the Tegaderm™ CHG. Silver dressings are being promoted as an alternative antiseptic dressing. However, in an in vitro study, researchers found that the chlorhexidine-impregnated foam dressing had larger zones of inhibition than silver dressings and that it was the only dressing effective against *Candida* (Bhende and Rothenburger, 2007). Clearly, this is an area of emerging research.

Before changing a dressing, the patient's medical record should be reviewed for previous history, allergies, condition of the catheter-skin junction site, and dressing material used. The catheter insertion site should be assessed and palpated for redness, tenderness, or drainage. Before proceeding with the dressing change, it is important to teach the patient about the rationale for the dressing change to alleviate concerns and anxiety. Use of a central line dressing kit standardizes the dressing change procedure and improves time efficiency by eliminating the need to gather individual supplies (Figure 25-2). The dressing change procedure begins with removal of the old dressing. This is accomplished by lifting the edge of the dressing beginning at the catheter hub and gently pulling the dressing perpendicular to the skin toward the insertion site. Removing the dressing in this direction will prevent catheter dislodgment should the catheter adhere to the dressing.

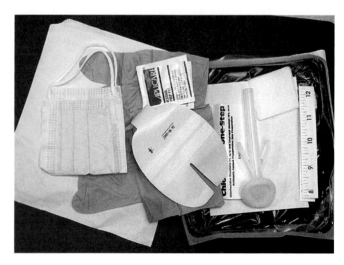

FIGURE 25-2   Central line dressing kit.

PROCEDURE FOR SITE CARE AND DRESSING CHANGE

BEFORE BEGINNING PROCEDURE

1. Wash hands.
2. Assemble equipment.
3. Don sterile gloves and other personal protective equipment (PPE).
4. Use aseptic technique and observe Standard Precautions throughout procedure.

SITE CARE AND DRESSING CHANGE

1. Remove dressing from VAD insertion site.
2. Inspect site and catheter.
3. Disinfect catheter-skin junction using antiseptic solution.
   - Using friction, apply antiseptic solution.
     - If using alcohol, apply friction for a minimum of 30 seconds.
     - If using chlorhexidine gluconate, use friction according to manufacturer's labeled use and directions.
   - Only one application is necessary.
   - Prepared site will be approximately the size of the dressing (i.e., 2- to 4-inches in diameter).
   - Allow antiseptic solution to air-dry (do not blow or blot dry).
   - Repeat twice as necessary depending on antiseptic solution.
4. Dress access site.

POST-DRESSING CHANGE

1. Discard used supplies.
2. Remove gloves.
3. Wash hands.
4. Label new dressing.
5. Document in patient's permanent medical record.

From Infusion Nurses Society: *Policies and procedures for infusion nursing*, ed 3, Norwood, Mass, 2006b, Author.

When completed, the dressing is labeled with the date, time, and initials of the clinician performing the dressing change. Documentation in the patient's medical record should include site assessment, skin disinfectant used, dressing material, catheter stabilization method (e.g., manufactured device, sterile tapes, sutures), patient response, and specific nursing actions taken to resolve or prevent adverse reactions.

CATHETER STABILIZATION

Catheter stabilization, also called catheter securement, is increasingly recognized as an important intervention in reducing the risk for phlebitis, infection, catheter migration, and catheter dislodgment. When the catheter is stabilized, there is less movement of the catheter in and out of the insertion site, and the catheter is less likely to be dislodged. Studies examining catheter stabilization have primarily focused on peripheral IV catheters and peripherally inserted central catheters (PICCs). The *Infusion Nursing Standards of Practice* recommends the use of manufactured catheter stabilization or securement devices as *preferred* over other methods such as sterile tapes and surgical strips. Such devices consist of an adhesive pad and a mechanism to hold the catheter and administration tubing to the pad (e.g., StatLock® [Bard Access Systems, Covington, GA], Grip-Lok [Zefon International, Ocala, FL]).

Promoted by both health care worker safety issues and clinical research, suturing is no longer recommended for catheter securement because of the risk for health care provider needle-stick injuries (OSHA, n.d.). Sutures may also be associated with increased risk for infection. In one prospective randomized study, 170 patients with PICCs were randomized either to sutures or to the placement of a manufactured securement device (Yamamoto, Soloman, Soulen et al, 2002). Significant findings included shorter time to achieve PICC securement (compared to suturing) and fewer PICC-related bloodstream infections in the group using the manufactured securement device; there was one needlestick injury in the suture group.

The use of catheter stabilization devices requires education emphasizing proper use of the product, maintenance of aseptic technique, and catheter stabilization during the placement procedure. There are several commercially available manufactured stabilization devices. Use of the StatLock® stabilization device can be seen in Figure 25-1. It is imperative that the infusion nurse understands the organizational procedures and incorporates specific manufacturer's directions for use and frequency of device replacement.

IMPLANTED PORT ACCESS

A noncoring needle is used to access an implanted port, and the smallest size needle to accommodate the infusion should be used. Smaller needles prolong the life of the port and will also be less painful during access. Standard needles are never used to access the port as they will core a hole in the silicone septum of the port, potentially leading to leakage. If the port is accessed for a continuous infusion, the *Infusion Nursing Standards of Practice* (INS, 2006a) recommends that the noncoring needle is changed at least every 7 days. Aseptic technique, including wearing a mask and attention to skin disinfection, is imperative during the port access procedure. A sterile transparent semipermeable membrane (TSM) dressing is used to cover the accessed needle and administration set. Many nurses place gauze to support the wings of the needle and as long as the gauze does not obscure or cover the catheter-skin insertion site, it is not considered a gauze dressing, and the TSM dressing can be changed at least every 7 days according to the *Infusion Nursing Standards of Practice* (INS, 2006a).

When accessing an implanted port, consideration should be made for use of local anesthesia based upon patient assessment and tolerance to the procedure. While many patients are not concerned about port needle access, some are very anxious and fearful about this procedure. With every patient, assessment of pain, feelings and fear about IV-related procedures, and preferences for pain control are essential and should be incorporated into the care plan. There are an increasing number of effective topical anesthetic creams available. Depending on the product used, the time for effective anesthesia may vary from a few minutes to 1 hour. Other pain management strategies include distraction or relaxation techniques and use of ice over the port site for a few minutes before site preparation and access (Gorski, 2005).

It is critical that patients are educated in daily assessment and monitoring of the site, especially when a noncoring needle is left in place with a continuous infusion. It is not uncommon to deliver infusions of antineoplastic agents, including vesicants, through an implanted port in ambulatory patients at home. Patients should be taught to check the dressing daily, how to dress and undress to avoid pulling at the needle site, and to make sure women's bra straps do not rub over the accessed area. Instruction should also include immediately stopping the infusion pump and calling the nurse to report any signs or symptoms of pain, burning, stinging, or soreness at the site, and calling the agency immediately if there is any wetness, leaking, or swelling noted at the site (Gorski, 2005). See Box 25-2 for an example of a patient education tool.

CATHETER FLUSHING AND LOCKING

The *Infusion Nursing Standards of Practice* (INS, 2006a) state that vascular access devices shall be flushed at established intervals to promote and maintain patency and prevent the mixing of incompatible medications and solutions. Maintaining patency in a CVAD requires either a continuous infusion or periodic flushing. Catheter flushing presents the most controversy, as research has not demonstrated the optimal flushing solution or frequency. Prevention or treatment of catheter-associated infection using antimicrobial solutions is a controversial area of practice and is addressed in the final paragraphs of this section.

Box 25-2   PATIENT EDUCATION TOOL: IMPLANTED PORT BASED INFUSIONS

1. Patient Instructions: Intravenous (IV) Infusion through an Implanted Port

An implanted port is a type of IV that is placed in a large vein in your chest. As you know, your port is placed completely beneath the skin. A special needle is used to enter the port through your skin.

You will be receiving an IV infusion of medication through your port. This means that the needle placed in the port must stay in place until you have received all of your IV medication. Your medication will be infused with a pump.

Name of medication and dose: _____

Duration of infusion: _____

Size of needle in port: _____

Type of IV pump: _____

Your home care nurse will start the infusion. It is important that you help in making sure that your IV medication is safely infused. While your infusion is running, read these instructions and keep them handy in your home as a reminder.

2. If you feel any of the following, turn off your pump and call your nurse **right away:**
   - Pain
   - Stinging
   - Burning
   - Other soreness at port site
3. Look at the dressing over the port every day. If you notice any wetness, swelling, or redness or if the needle seems to be out of place, turn off your pump and call your nurse **right away.**
4. Pick up and carry your IV pump every time you get up to walk.
5. Dress and undress carefully to avoid pulling tubing at the port needle.
6. For women: Make sure bra straps do not rub over port needle area.
7. If you accidentally drop your pump or if the tubing is accidentally pulled at the needle in your port, call your home care nurse **right away** for further instructions.

From Wheaton Franciscan Home Health & Hospice, Milwaukee, Wisc.

There is considerable variance in the types of flushing solution as well as the amounts and frequency used in clinical practice; in addition, there are many unanswered questions about the "optimal" flush to maintain catheter patency. In 2008 INS released *Flushing Protocols,* a user-friendly tool to give recommendations for flushing solution and frequency for all venous access devices based on the type of infusion (INS, 2008). The *Protocols* give direction to both saline flushes and heparin "locking" (Table 25-1). Heparin locking refers to instilling dilute heparin in the unused catheter to prevent blood clotting. The *Protocols* were based on the *Infusion Nursing Standards of Practice* and a review of existing literature. The *Infusion Nursing Standards of Practice* (2006a) recommends the following:

- The flushing volume should be at least twice the internal volume of the central venous access device and injection cap.
- Preservative-free 0.9% sodium chloride flushing solutions should be used to ensure and maintain patency of CVADs at established intervals.
- 0.9% Sodium chloride with preservatives should not be administered to neonates and pediatric patients; if used with adult patients, the volume used should not exceed 30 mL per day.
- Flushing with a heparin solution should occur to ensure and maintain patency of CVADs at established intervals. The heparin concentration should not be in amounts that cause systemic anticoagulation. Concentrations of 1 to 10 units/mL should be used with neonate and pediatric patients.
- Single-use flushing systems are recommended to reduce the risk of contamination and infection.

For central lines, the methods of flushing valved and non-valved CVADs are differentiated in the INS *Flushing Protocols* (INS, 2008). A valved catheter has an intricate valve(s) within the catheter, either at the distal or at the proximal end of the catheter. When the catheter is not in use the valve reduces the backflow of blood into the catheter and reduces the risk of air embolism by remaining closed. Valved catheters can be found in PICCs, nontunneled and tunneled catheters, and implanted ports. Weekly flushing with preservative-free 0.9% sodium chloride is recommended to maintain catheter patency. For the nonvalved, intermittently used CVAD, INS (2008) recommends "locking" the catheter with low-concentration heparin as follows:

- PICC and nontunneled CVAD: Daily heparin lock with 5 mL (10 units/mL)
- Tunneled CVAD: Twice weekly heparin lock with 5 mL (10 units/mL)
- Implanted port: Monthly heparin lock with 3 to 5 mL (100 units/mL)

Catheter locking to maintain patency remains a controversial and underresearched area. Many acute care hospitals and alternative sites (home care, outpatient) use preservative-free 0.9% sodium chloride without heparin to lock catheters and maintain catheter patency. While such organizations cite internal data supporting the maintenance of catheter patency, there is a lack of published data to support this practice. The move to use preservative-free 0.9% sodium chloride results from concern over heparin-induced thrombocytopenia, concern over heparin supporting microbial growth, periodic heparin supply issues, and use of positive/neutral pressure injection caps/valves.

As some drugs are incompatible with preservative-free 0.9% sodium chloride and/or heparin, it is important for the nurse

TABLE 25-1 Flushing Protocols: Saline Flushes/Heparin Locking*

Device	Intermittent	Parenteral nutrition	Blood product administration	Blood draws	Flushing with no therapy	Heparin locking
PIV	Min 2 mL	NA	Preadmin 2 mL Postadmin 10 mL	NA	At least q12 hr	NA
Midline	Min 3 mL	NA	Preadmin 3 mL Postadmin 10 mL	NA	At least q12 hr	3 mL of 10 units/mL heparin
PICC	Min 5 mL	5 mL	Preadmin 5 mL Postadmin 10 mL	Predraw 5 mL Postdraw 10 mL	Nonvalved: at least q24 hr Valved: at least weekly	5 mL of 10 units/mL heparin
Nontunneled	Min 5 mL	5 mL	Preadmin 5 mL Postadmin 10 mL	Predraw 5 mL Postdraw 10 mL	Nonvalved: at least q24 hr Valved: at least weekly	5 mL of 10 units/mL heparin
Tunneled	Min 5 mL	5 mL	Preadmin 5 mL Postadmin 10 mL	Predraw 5 mL Postdraw 10 mL	Nonvalved: at least 1-2 times per week Valve: at least weekly	5 mL of 10 units/mL heparin
Port	Min 5 mL	5 mL	Preadmin 5 mL Postadmin 10 mL	Predraw 5 mL Postdraw 10 mL	Accessed nonvalved: at least 1-2 times per week Valved: at least weekly Deaccessed: at least monthly	3-5 mL of 100 units/mL heparin

From Infusion Nurses Society: *Flushing protocols,* Norwood, Mass, 2008, Author.
*All CVADs require a minimum of a 10-mL syringe for flushing and locking.
Min, minimum; *NA,* not applicable; *PIV,* peripheral IV; *Postadmin,* postadministration; *Preadmin,* preadministration.

to know drug and solution compatibilities. Incompatibility is defined as incapable of being mixed or used simultaneously without undergoing chemical or physical changes or producing undesirable effects (Weinstein, 2007). Signs of incompatibility may include visible precipitation, haze, gas bubbles, and cloudiness. Some precipitates may be microcrystalline, smaller than 50 microns, and not apparent to the unaided eye. Refer to Table 25-2 for a list of drug incompatibilities with NaCl, dextrose, and heparin. The "SASH" method (saline-administration-saline-heparin) is used whenever heparin is used for catheter locking and is outlined in Box 25-3.

If resistance is met or an absent blood aspirate is noted, the nurse should take further steps to assess patency. The catheter should never be forcibly flushed. Pressures in excess of 40 pounds per square inch (psi) may cause catheter rupture with possible embolization (Weinstein, 2007). A wide-barrel syringe (diameter of 10 mL), which exerts less than 10 psi, is recommended for use by many manufacturers of CVADs to avoid excessive pressure and subsequent catheter damage when administering medication and flushing the catheter.

The future will change as ongoing research not only attempts to answer the questions of optimal routine flushing and locking solutions but also discovers novel ways to use flush solutions for eradication of microorganisms within the catheter lumen. Hadaway (2006) proposed an expanded purpose for flushing with antimicrobial solutions (e.g., ethylenediaminetetraacetate [EDTA] and ethanol)—reducing the bacterial biofilm that forms on catheter surfaces. Research is in progress to examine if such novel flush solutions can treat catheter-associated infection and prevent the need for catheter removal and replacement. Some clinicians recommend routine catheter locking with antibiotic or antimicrobial solutions. The 2002 CDC guidelines (O'Grady et al, 2002) state that antibiotic lock solutions should not be routinely used to prevent central line infections but could be used in special circumstances, such as for a patient with repeated infections despite optimal maximal adherence to aseptic technique. The IDSA/SHEA (Marschall et al, 2008) recommends antimicrobial locks for central lines as a preventive strategy in patients with limited venous access and a history of recurrent CLABSIs and in patients with heightened risk for severe consequences from a CLABSI (e.g., recently placed prosthetic heart valve).

INJECTION AND ACCESS CAPS

An injection/access cap is a small molded device with a resealable cap or other configuration designed to accommodate needleless devices for catheter flushing or administration of solutions into the vascular system (INS, 2006a). Types of devices include the following:

- A split-septum injection cap that requires a blunt plastic cannula attached to the syringe or IV administration set to pass through the split in the septum. The male Luer end of a syringe tip or administration set may also be used to access the split septum without using a blunt plastic cannula.
- A mechanical valve, most often a one-piece system, placed on the catheter hub and accessed with the male Luer on a syringe or administration set. There are many types of sizes, shapes, colors, and internal fluid pathways available.

All injection/access caps allow venous access without removing the cap, thereby maintaining a sterile closed infusion system. Injection/access caps can function significantly different from one another even though they look very similar. Some caps can create a negative pressure within the device and

TABLE 25-2 Flushing Protocols: Drug Incompatibilities*

NaCl		DEXTROSE		HEPARIN	
Generic	**Brand**	**Generic**	**Brand**	**Generic**	**Brand**
Aldesleukin	Proleukin	Baclofen	Lioresal	Alteplase	Activase
Amphotericin B cholesteryl sulfate	Amphotec	Bupivacaine	Marcaine	Amikacin	
	Fungizone	Cladribine	Leustatin	Amobarbital	Sodium Amytal
Amphotericin B	Abelcet	Clonidine	Duraclon	Amphotericin B cholesteryl sulfate	Amphotec
Amphotericin B lipid complex	AmBisome	Dantrolene	Dantrium		
Amphotericin B liposomal	Dantrium	Daptomycin	Cubicin	Amphotericin B deoxychoate	Fungizone
Dantrolene sodium	DaunoXome	Dihydroergotamine	D.H.E. 45	Atropine	
Daunorubicin liposomal	D.H.E. 45	Interferon alfa-2	Intron A	Cefmatazole	
Dihydroergotamine mesylate	Procrit, Epogen	Itraconazole	Sporanox	Chlordiazepoxide	Librium
Epoetin alfa	Neupogen	Levothyroxine sodium	Synthroid	Ciprofloxacin	Cipro
Filgrastim	Gammunex		Dolophine	Clarithromycin	Biaxin
Immune globulin	Doxil	Methadone HCl	Dilantin	Codeine	
Liposomal doxorubicin	Vasoxyl	Phenytoin	Streptomycin	Cytarabine	Tarabine
Methoxamine	CellCept	Streptomycin	TNKase	Daunorubicin HCl	Cerubidine
Mycophenolate mofetil HCl	Nitropress	Tenecteplase	Remodulin	Diazepam	Valium
Nitroprusside sodium	Levophed	Treprostinil sodium		Doxorubicin HCl	Adriamycin
Norepinephrine bitartrate	Eloxatin			Doxycycline hyclate	
Oxaliplatin	Rythmol			Droperidol	Inapsine
Propafenone	Diprivan			Drotrecogin alfa	Xigris
Propofol	Synercid			Ergonovine maleate	Methergine
Quinupristin/dalfopristin	Neutrexin			Erythromycin lactobionate	
Trimetrexate glucuronate				Filgrastim	Neupogen
				Gentamicin sulfate	
				Haloperidol decanoate	Haldol decanoate
				Haloperidol lactate	Haldol
				Hyaluronidase	Hydase
				Hydrocortisone sodium phosphate	Solu-Cortef
				Hydroxyzine HCl	
				Idarubicin HCl	
				Kanamycin sulfate	
				Levofloxacin	Levaquin
				Levorphanol tartrate	Levo-Dromoran
				Methylprednisolone	Solu-Medrol
				Mitoxantrone HCl	Novantrone
				Morphine sulfate	
				Nesiritide recombinant	Natrecor
				Norepinephrine bitartrate	Levophed
				Orphenadrine citrate	
				Pentamidine	
				Phenytoin sodium	Dilantin
				Polymyxin B sulfate	
				Prochlorperazine edisylate	Compazine
				Promethazine HCl	Phenergan
				Quinupristin/dalfopristin	Synercid

From Infusion Nurses Society: *Flushing protocols*, Norwood, Mass, 2008, Author.
*Consult with pharmacy for information on drugs not listed in this table.

Box 25-3   SASH METHOD (SALINE-ADMINISTRATION-SALINE-HEPARIN)

- Perform hand hygiene.
- Assemble supplies.
- Disinfect catheter injection cap with 70% alcohol using friction.
- Connect 0.9% sodium chloride filled syringe to injection cap, maintaining asepsis.
- Slowly aspirate until positive blood return is obtained.
  - If resistance is met or there is no blood return, the infusion nurse should take further steps to assess patency. Never forcibly flush the catheter.
- Flush with 0.9% sodium chloride and disconnect syringe.
- Disinfect catheter injection cap with 70% alcohol using friction.
- Connect IV administration set of medication/solution to injection cap.
- Administer medication.
- Disconnect medication from injection cap and cover end of IV administration set with sterile cap.
- Disinfect catheter injection cap with 70% alcohol using friction.
- Connect 0.9% sodium chloride filled syringe to injection cap maintaining asepsis and flush catheter.
- Disinfect catheter injection cap with 70% alcohol using friction.
- Connect heparin syringe to injection cap maintaining asepsis and lock catheter.
- Disconnect syringe from injection cap.
- Discard used supplies in appropriate receptacles.
- Remove gloves; perform hand hygiene.
- Document in medical record.

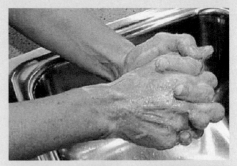
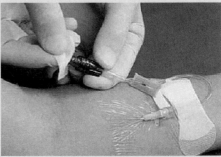
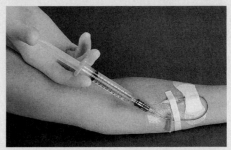
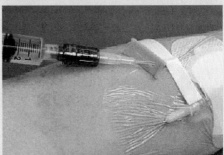
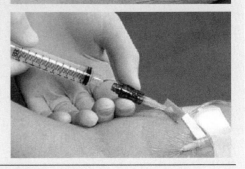

Adapted from Infusion Nurses Society: *Policies and procedures for infusion nursing,* ed 3, Norwood, Mass, 2006b, Author.

catheter when the syringe is removed and create a positive pressure when a syringe is attached. Other caps create a positive pressure within the device and catheter upon removal, and create a negative pressure upon connection.

It is critical that the nurse understand the type of injection/access cap used because the flushing technique will vary based on the type of injection cap. A positive fluid displacement technique is recommended based on the *Infusion Nursing Standards of Practice* (INS, 2006a). For standard injection/access caps (i.e., not positive or negative pressure caps), this means to flush all fluid in, maintain the pressure on the syringe plunger, close the clamp on the catheter or extension set, and then disconnect the syringe. However, if a positive pressure injection valve is used, the technique of closing the clamp before disconnection prevents the fluid reservoir from pushing fluid out to the catheter tip. Positive pressure injection valves must be clamped *after* syringe disconnection. Neutral displacement injection valves are not dependent upon flushing technique and can be clamped either before or after syringe disconnection. Refer to Chapter 20 for more detailed information on injection caps under the heading Needleless Connectors.

The injection/access cap is routinely changed. The *Infusion Nursing Standards of Practice* (INS, 2006a) recommend that injection/access caps be changed with each administration set change, at least every 7 days for catheter maintenance, if residual blood is present in the catheter, and whenever the integrity is compromised. CDC guidelines (O'Grady et al, 2002) recommend changing the valve no more frequently than every 72 hours and at least as frequently as the administration set.

Failure to disinfect the cap when accessing the infusion device or administration set for flushing or medication administration has been recognized as a significant problem. The Institute for Safe Medication Practices (ISMP) (2007) documented infection control problems including failure to disinfect the injection cap/valve when accessing the infusion for flushing or medication administration. This increases the risk for contamination and potential catheter-associated bloodstream infection. INS and ISMP clearly recommend that the injection or access port be aseptically cleansed with an approved antiseptic before use. The 2009 Joint Commission *National Patient Safety Goals* (TJC, 2008) have a specific recommendation to "use a standardized protocol to disinfect catheter hubs and injection ports prior to accessing the port." While there are no specific evidence-based guidelines documenting the optimal disinfectant or duration of cap disinfection, the "scrub the hub" mantra is frequently cited. In an in vitro study, a 15-second scrub using either a 70% alcohol or a 3.15% chlorhexidine/70% alcohol solution was effective in eradicating microbes from four different types of injection access caps that were inoculated with bacteria (Kaler, 2007).

BLOOD SAMPLING

For patients with central lines, blood sampling for laboratory tests is common practice. It is important to recognize that withdrawal of blood can contribute to thrombotic catheter occlusion if the catheter is not adequately flushed. The INS *Flushing Protocols* recommend a 10-mL 0.9% sodium chloride flush after any blood withdrawal from a CVAD. The most common method used to obtain blood is the discard method. The first aspirate of blood is discarded to reduce the risk of drug concentration or a diluted specimen. When the CVAD has more than one lumen, the larger lumen should be used for obtaining specimens.

PROCEDURE FOR BLOOD SPECIMEN COLLECTION FROM A CVAD

FROM CENTRAL VASCULAR ACCESS DEVICE (CVAD)

1. Discontinue administration of all infusates into the CVAD before obtaining blood samples.
2. Check patency of CVAD by flushing with 3 to 5 mL of preservative-free 0.9% sodium chloride (USP).
3. When drawing from multilumen catheters, the distal lumen is the preferred lumen from which to obtain specimen (or the lumen recommended by the manufacturer).
4. Blood samples may be collected from CVAD by syringe method or Vacutainer, as recommended by the manufacturer of the CVAD.
5. Specimens collected from certain CVADs may be adversely affected by catheter composition or material; check with CVAD manufacturer for recommendations on product use.

USING THE VACUTAINER METHOD

1. Clamp catheter.
2. Attach needleless connector to Vacutainer barrel holder.
3. Place blood tube into Vacutainer holder.
4. Disinfect injection or access cap with alcohol.
5. Remove needle cover and insert Vacutainer needleless connector into injection or access cap.
6. Unclamp catheter.
7. Advance blood tube inside Vacutainer holder to activate retrograde blood flow.
8. Hold tube in place until blood flow ceases: this is considered the "discard."
   • The volume should be 1.5 to 2 times the fill volume of the CVAD.
9. Clamp catheter and remove blood tube from Vacutainer holder, leaving needle and holder connected to injection or access cap.
10. Discard blood tube immediately into appropriate container.
11. Insert another blood tube, unclamp catheter, and obtain blood specimens as ordered.
12. After all samples are collected, clamp catheter.
13. Remove Vacutainer holder and needless connector from injection or access cap.
14. Disinfect injection or access cap with alcohol.
15. Flush catheter using 5 to 10 mL of preservative-free 0.9% sodium chloride (USP).
16. Change injection or access cap and extension set, if needed.

USING THE SYRINGE METHOD

1. Clamp catheter.
2. Remove injection or access cap and discard.
3. Disinfect catheter hub with alcohol.
4. Attach empty 5-mL syringe to catheter hub.
5. Unclamp catheter.

(Continued)

PROCEDURE FOR BLOOD SPECIMEN COLLECTION FROM A CVAD—CONT'D

6. Withdraw 1.5 to 2 times fill volume of the CVAD of blood and discard.

7. Reclamp catheter.

8. Remove and discard syringe immediately into appropriate container.

9. Attach second syringe to catheter hub, size to be determined by amount of blood needed.

10. Unclamp catheter.

11. Withdraw blood into syringe.
    - Several syringes may be needed to obtain required amount of blood.

12. Reclamp catheter and remove syringe.

13. Cleanse catheter hub with alcohol.

14. Attach prefilled injection or access cap attached to 10-mL syringe with 5 to 10 mL of preservative-free 0.9% sodium chloride (USP).

15. Unclamp catheter.

16. Flush with preservative-free 0.9% sodium chloride (USP).

17. Transfer blood to collection tubes or vials and rotate vials using appropriate needles or needleless system.

18. If blood does not flow into the blood tube syringe:
    - Have patient change position, cough, move arm above head, or hold a deep breath.
    - Fush catheter with preservative-free 0.9% sodium chloride (USP) and attempt to withdraw blood again.
    - Replace blood tube with a new one.
    - If still unsuccessful, notify physician.
    - Draw the blood specimen peripherally.

From Infusion Nurses Society: *Policies and procedures for infusion nursing,* ed 3, Norwood, Mass, 2006b, Author.

There is limited research guidance on the accuracy of blood specimens drawn from central lines, especially with regard to coagulation studies through a heparinized catheter, and with sampling of drug levels from silicone catheters, if the drug is being administered through that catheter (Pinto, 1994; Mayo et al, 1996; Shulma et al, 1998; Hinds et al, 2002; Frey, 2003; Boodhan et al, 2006).

CATHETER REPAIR

Catheter damage can occur from exerting excessive pressure while flushing, or by accidental cutting from scissors or the catheter clamp. Nurses and patients with a central line must be knowledgeable about immediate actions to take in the event of catheter damage. Patients should be provided instructions on how to clamp or fold the catheter to prevent blood loss or air embolism and to notify the nurse immediately. The infusion nurse must collaborate with the physician regarding the appropriateness of catheter removal versus catheter repair. Factors to consider include risk for infection from the damaged catheter, catheter type and potential for repair, expected duration of catheter need, and patient safety.

Patient benefits from catheter repair include avoidance of the risk, cost, and disruption in life associated with another catheter insertion procedure. The potential risks of catheter repair include the possibility of a catheter-related bloodstream infection attributable either to the catheter or to the catheter repair procedure. The risk of catheter-associated infection is reduced by nursing competence of the repair procedure and use of sterile technique while performing the repair. Catheter repair kits are available and are specific to the manufacturer and size of the catheter. Repair of the external catheter portion of a central venous access device is a sterile procedure. The repairable segment of these catheters is limited to the section of the catheter that is outside of the body.

CATHETER REMOVAL

The *Infusion Nursing Standards of Practice* (2006) state that the catheter should be removed immediately upon discontinuation of infusion therapy, if contamination is suspected, or if a complication is unresolved. Daily review of central line necessity with prompt removal of unnecessary lines is one of the components of the "central line bundle" as originally defined and promoted by the Institute for Healthcare Improvement (IHI, 2008), and this recommendation is also cited by others including the National Quality Forum (NQF) (NQF, 2008) and IDSA/SHEA (Marschall et al, 2008). In The Joint Commission *2009 National Patient Safety Goals* the recommendation for removal of unnecessary central lines applies for all health care settings.

Before removal, a physician's or authorized prescriber's order must be obtained. It is considered a medical act to remove tunneled CVADs and implanted ports. The nurse must be aware of the potential complications of central line catheter removal and be prepared to initiate emergency measures as needed. Air embolism is an underappreciated complication of catheter removal (Peter and Saxman, 2003). Evidence-based interventions to reduce the risk are addressed later in this chapter. Other complications may include, but are not limited to, catheter embolism, pulmonary embolism, and excessive bleeding.

Difficulty with PICC removal has been reported (Marx, 1995; Wall and Kierstead, 1995; Miall et al, 2001). The most common cause for removal difficulty is venospasm. When a PICC is pulled through the vein during removal, an irritation of the lining of the vein causes venospasm. Thrombosis may also result in inability to remove the catheter. Patient anxiety may contribute to the problem. If resistance is encountered, interventions include the following:
- Never pull against resistance as catheter breakage or vein wall damage can occur.
- Stop the procedure and apply a sterile dressing.
- Use a warm compress to dilate the vein proximal to the exit site.
- Consider the use of relaxation techniques.
- Try hand and arm exercises.
- Reattempt removal after a short or intermediate time period.

If all of the above interventions fail, contact the patient's physician. The patient should be sent to interventional radiology for evaluation and catheter removal.

Following catheter removal, inspect the catheter to ensure that the catheter is intact. Documentation of catheter removal should include the catheter length and integrity, site appearance, dressing applied, and patient tolerance. After catheter removal, the dressing should be changed daily to assess the insertion site until the site is epithelialized (INS, 2006a).

PROCEDURE FOR CATHETER REMOVAL

BEFORE BEGINNING PROCEDURE

1. Wash hands.

2. Assemble equipment.

3. Don sterile gloves and other PPE.

4. Use aseptic technique and observe Standard Precautions throughout procedure.

5. Educate patient as to procedure.

6. Place patient in supine position for removal of all CVADs. Patient may assume sitting or reclining position for removal of peripheral-short or midline device.
   - Educate patient in Valsalva's maneuver for all CVAD removal procedures.

CATHETER REMOVAL

1. Discontinue administration of all infusates.

2. Remove dressing from insertion site.

3. Remove stabilization device.

4. Inspect catheter-skin junction.

5. Disinfect catheter-skin junction.

6. Place first two fingers of nondominant hand lightly above catheter-skin junction site with gauze between fingers.

7. Using gentle, even pressure, slowly retract catheter from site with dominant hand while holding site with gauze.
   - Use extreme caution when removing central nontunneled, noncuffed catheters or PICCs to prevent the occurrence of air embolism.
   - Ask patient to perform Valsalva's maneuver.

8. If resistance or complication occurs, discontinue removal and notify physician immediately.

9. Assess integrity of removed catheter. Compare length of catheter to original insertion length to ensure entire catheter is removed.

10. Dress exit site.
    - Apply pressure to site with gauze for a minimum of 30 seconds.
    - Secure gauze to site; cover with occlusive material such as transparent semipermeable membrane (TSM) dressing.

11. For CVAD removal:
    - Apply pressure to site with gauze for a minimum of 30 seconds.
    - Apply new gauze with application of approved antiseptic ointment to exit site.
    - Secure gauze to site; cover with occlusive adhesive material.
    - Change dressing every 24 hours until exit site is healed.
    - Patient should remain in supine position for 30 minutes after CVAD removal.

POST-CATHETER REMOVAL

1. Discard used supplies.

2. Remove gloves.

3. Wash hands.

4. If catheter defect is noted, report to manufacturer and regulatory agencies. Complete Unusual Occurrence Report as established by the organization.

5. Document in patient's permanent medical record.

From Infusion Nurses Society: *Policies and procedures for infusion nursing,* ed 3, Norwood, Mass, 2006b, Author.

CATHETER CULTURES

If catheter-associated infection is suspected, cultures are required. Cultures may be taken from the catheter segment(s), the delivery system, the access site, and/or the infusate. Catheter segments may include the catheter tip or a segment from the subcutaneous area. Two sets of blood cultures are recommended for suspected infection—one obtained via peripheral venipuncture and the other via the catheter.

 ## POSTINSERTION-RELATED COMPLICATIONS

The presence of a central venous access device places the patient at risk for complications during insertion and for as long as the catheter remains within the vascular system. Bloodstream infections, sepsis, venous thrombosis, and air embolism can be life-threatening. The infusion nurse must have a comprehensive understanding and knowledge of signs and symptoms of CVAD-related complications, preventive interventions, and actions to take in the event of their occurrence.

CVAD-ASSOCIATED INFECTION

Health care–associated infections are considered a significant public health issue in the United States. Central line–associated infections are considered preventable with implementation of evidence-based practices such as the "central line bundle" (Institute for Healthcare Improvement, 2008). The bundle includes stringent infection prevention measures at the time of insertion and daily review of central line necessity with prompt removal of unnecessary lines. Research literature has clearly documented sustained success in the reduction of central line–associated bloodstream infections through implementation of the central line bundle in intensive care units (Berenholtz et al, 2004; Berriel-Cass et al, 2006; Pronovost et al, 2006; Venkatram et al, 2007). Refer to Chapter 12 for a detailed discussion about the central line bundle.

It is recognized that all indwelling venous access devices develop a biofilm, a community of microorganisms surrounded by a slime matrix that protects the bacteria from antibiotics; biofilm has also been found on needleless injection access/caps (Donlan, Murga, and Bell, 2001; Hadaway, 2006). Bacteria from the biofilm that detach from the external or internal catheter surface can contribute to catheter-associated bloodstream infection. The patient's

PROCEDURE FOR CULTURING FOR INFUSION-ASSOCIATED INFECTION

PATIENT ASSESSMENT AND EDUCATION

1. Obtain and review physician's or authorized prescriber's order for specific type of culture.
2. Verify patient's identity using two independent identifiers, not including patient's room number.
3. Provide patient with information regarding the procedure.
4. Assess patient.
5. Place patient in recumbent position, as tolerated.

BEFORE BEGINNING PROCEDURE

1. Wash hands.
2. Don gloves.
3. Use aseptic technique and observe Standard Precautions throughout the procedure.

OBTAINING CULTURE SPECIMEN

1. Discontinue administration of all infusates from which culture is to be taken.
2. Remove dressing from access site.
3. For catheter-associated infection, the semiquantitative technique for catheter culture is recommended.
4. Obtain culture specimen using aseptic technique.

Catheter-skin junction

1. If purulent drainage is present, culture of drainage should be taken immediately:
   - Do not cleanse area to be cultured.
   - Swab purulent drainage with sterile swab.
   - Uncap culture tube.
   - Drop swab into culture tube using aseptic technique.
   - Recap culture tube.

Infusion catheter

1. Disinfect venipuncture site with alcohol and allow to air-dry.
2. Place sterile towel in close proximity to catheter-skin junction.
3. Remove catheter, avoiding contact with surrounding skin.
4. Uncap culture tube.
5. Drop catheter into culture tube.
   - For peripheral-short, cut entire length of catheter from hub using sterile scissors.
   - For longer catheters, cut a 2-inch segment from catheter tip with sterile scissors.
6. Recap culture tube.
7. Apply pressure to catheter exit site with sterile gauze and secure with tape.

Infusate

1. Disinfect injection port of infusate container with alcohol.
2. Uncap needle with syringe attached.
3. Insert needle into injection port of infusate bag.
4. Withdraw approximately 5 mL of infusate into syringe.
5. Remove needle from infusate container.
6. Uncap culture tube.
7. Inject syringe's contents into culture tube.
8. Recap culture tube.
9. Discard syringe in appropriate container.

Blood culture from peripheral access site

1. Disinfect intended venipuncture site with antiseptic solution(s), following manufacturer's labeled use and directions.
2. Apply tourniquet proximal to intended venipuncture site.
3. Perform venipuncture.
4. Attach culture tube to Vacutainer holder.
5. Fill culture tube(s).
6. Remove tourniquet promptly.
7. Remove culture tube from Vacutainer holder.
8. Remove access needle; apply digital pressure to achieve hemostasis.
9. Apply sterile gauze dressing to venipuncture site.

Blood culture from VAD

1. Do not discard first draw.
2. Fill culture tube with blood.

POST-CULTURING

1. Discard used supplies.
2. Label culture tube before leaving patient's side with the following:
   - Patient's name
   - Patient's ID number
   - Date and time of specimen collection
   - Contents of culture tube
3. Remove gloves.
4. Wash hands.
5. Send culture tube and infusate with administration set intact to microbiology lab.
   - Place blood specimen in sealed container for transport.
   - Identify container with "BIOHAZARD" label.
6. Document in patient's permanent medical record.
7. Obtain and follow up on lab results.
8. If infusate appears contaminated, notify appropriate regulatory agencies.
9. Complete an Unusual Occurrence Report as established by the organization.
10. Maintain statistical data on incidence of infusion-associated infections.

From Infusion Nurses Society: *Policies and procedures for infusion nursing*, ed 3, Norwood, Mass, 2006b, Author.

skin is the primary source of contamination of the external surface. Attention to skin disinfection before placement is likely the most important intervention in prevention of catheter-associated infection (Ryder, 2006). Microorganisms potentially enter the internal catheter surface anytime the infusion system is manipulated, such as during access and administration set changes. Extraluminal catheter–associated infections typically occur generally within the first week after placement, while intraluminal-associated infections typically occur after 1 week (Ryder, 2006). While attention to central line insertion procedures is reducing the incidence of infection in short-term catheters, optimal care and management of the long-term catheter is less well-researched. Hand hygiene and attention to the catheter hub, including adequacy of disinfection and the optimal type of injection cap to reduce infection risk, are also essential aspects of care as discussed earlier in the Care and Maintenance sections of this chapter.

In an attempt to reduce biofilm within the catheter lumen, antimicrobial solutions (e.g., dilute antibiotic/heparin solutions, ethylenediaminetetraacetate [EDTA], and ethanol) have been used to lock the catheter. Neither the CDC (O'Grady et al, 2002) nor the IDSA/SHEA (Marschall et al, 2008) currently recommends antibiotic lock as a *routine* prevention measure; rather, they recommend this approach only in special circumstances such as high-risk patients with a history of multiple infections despite maximal adherence to aseptic technique. Research related to optimal flushing solutions and their impact on catheter-associated infection is ongoing.

The infusion nurse should also be alert to patient populations who may be at a heightened risk for central line–associated infections (see Focus on Evidence box). The reader is referred again to Chapter 12 in the section titled Prevention of Catheter-Associated Infections for detailed information regarding both general and central venous access device infection prevention strategies including aseptic technique, hand hygiene, CVAD type and insertion site, skin antisepsis at the time of insertion and with ongoing site care, dressing changes, administration set changes, and catheter stabilization.

Patient assessment should include ongoing monitoring of the catheter exit site and implanted port site as well as monitoring for systemic changes indicative of infection including fever. Infections may be local or systemic as outlined in the following CDC definitions (O'Grady et al, 2002):

- *Exit-site infection:* Erythema or induration within 2 cm of the catheter exit site; no evidence of bloodstream infection (BSI) or purulent drainage
- *Clinical exit-site infection:* Tenderness, erythema, or site induration >2 cm from the catheter site along the subcutaneous tract of a tunneled catheter; no evidence of bloodstream infection
- *Pocket infection:* The presence of purulent fluid in the subcutaneous pocket of an implanted port; it may or may not be associated with spontaneous rupture and drainage or necrosis of the overlying skin; no evidence of bloodstream infection
- *Infusate-associated BSI:* Concordant growth of the same organism from the infusate and blood cultures with no other identifiable source of infection
- *Catheter-associated BSI:* Bacteria or fungi in the bloodstream of a patient with an intravascular catheter with at least one positive blood culture obtained from a peripheral vein, signs and symptoms of infection (e.g., fever, chills, hypotension), and no other apparent source for the infection other than the catheter

FOCUS ON EVIDENCE

Risk Factors for CVAD-Associated Infection

- In a descriptive study of 111 catheters that included 1646 catheter days, the incidence of and risk factors for bloodstream infections in patients receiving parenteral nutrition (PN) were studied. The infection rate was 18.8 per 1000 catheter days. Within the patient population, significant risk factors for CABSI included longer duration of catheterization, emergency situation at the time of catheterization, poor patient hygiene, poor hand hygiene, and failure to use maximal sterile barrier precautions (Yilmaz et al, 2007).
- In a prospective cohort study of patients who received PN via nontunneled, non–antimicrobial-coated single- or double-lumen CVCs that were placed in the subclavian or internal jugular vein by physicians, PN was found to be an independent risk factor for CVC-associated infection. Maximal sterile barrier precautions were used during catheter placement and 2% chlorhexidine/alcohol was used for skin antisepsis. Data from 153 patients including 286 catheters were collected. The overall infection rate was 11.7 infections per 1000 days. PN was found to be the only significant risk factor for CVC-associated infections (Beghetto et al, 2005).
- Parenteral nutrition was identified as a risk factor for early catheter-related infection occurring in the first month after catheter placement in a group of patients with cancer. Of 371 patients with a diagnosis of cancer who underwent placement of either an implanted port (*n* = 299) or an external, tunneled catheter (*n* = 72), 14 were followed for 1 month after catheter insertion. In the data analysis, difficulties during the procedure and parenteral nutrition were identified with increased risk for catheter-associated infection (Penel et al, 2007).
- Hosoglu and colleagues (2004) found that renal failure was an independent risk factor in a prospective observational study of 389 catheter insertions in either the subclavian or the jugular site over a 1-year period.
- El-Masri and colleagues (2004) found that the presence of a chest drainage system in patients was associated with a higher risk for catheter-associated infections in a prospective cohort study of 361 critically ill adult trauma patients.
- Being unarousable was a risk factor for CVAD infection in a prospective study of over 4000 patients (Alonso-Echanove et al, 2003).
- Hanna and Raad (2001) performed an analysis of data from a randomized, controlled trial and found that the use of blood products administered through the CVAD was an independent risk factor associated with CABSI.

If the patient develops symptoms of an infection, the physician is notified. Site and/or blood cultures from the central and peripheral lines should be completed. Depending on the clinical condition of the patient, intravenous antibiotics may be initiated and/or the central line may be removed. The CDC (O'Grady et al, 2002) recommends that catheters not be removed on the basis of fever alone as the infection could be related to another location or be attributable to noninfectious causes.

Antibiotic instillation into the lumen of the catheter—the "antibiotic lock" technique—is sometimes used to preserve venous access, especially with long-term catheters. Treatment of an infection with an antibiotic lock is differentiated from regular catheter locking with an antibiotic lock solution as a *preventive* measure for CVAD infection, as discussed previously. This consists of instilling a highly concentrated antibiotic into the catheter lumen for a prescribed duration of time (e.g., 12 hours), and is usually administered in conjunction with systemic antibiotics. Patients who may particularly benefit from the antibiotic lock technique include those who are immunocompromised, patients receiving long-term parenteral nutrition, and patients undergoing hemodialysis through a CVAD (Bagnall-Reeb, 2004).

OCCLUSION

Catheter occlusion is defined as a partial or complete obstruction of the CVAD that limits or prevents the ability to withdraw blood, flush the catheter, and/or administer medications or solutions. It is a significant complication in that infusion therapy may be delayed or interrupted. Catheter occlusion may be due to thrombotic or nonthrombotic causes. The following are signs of occlusion:

- Inability to aspirate blood
- Resistance to flushing
- Sluggish infusion
- Complete inability to flush or infuse
- Increasing occlusion alarm activation with use of electronic infusion devices

Thrombotic catheter occlusion occurs when fibrin or blood within and around the CVAD or within the port reservoir of implanted ports slows down or disrupts catheter flow. The following four categories of thrombotic catheter occlusion are commonly described in the literature:

1. *Fibrin tail or flap:* A layer of fibrin encases the CVAD at the tip. The tail can grow as more cells and blood components are deposited. While solution administration or catheter flushing can be accomplished, if aspiration is attempted the tail acts as a one-way valve as it is pulled over the catheter tip, and blood withdrawal is not possible.
2. *Fibrin sheath or sleeve:* A layer of fibrin forms around the external surface of the catheter, potentially coating the entire exterior wall. Usually there are no symptoms but persistent withdrawal occlusion may occur as a fibrin tail also develops. Administered infusates may travel retrograde along the sheath, potentially causing tissue infiltration or extravasation. In a case report of a pediatric long-term infusion therapy patient with a fibrin sleeve, fibrin was detected after development of severe pain in the infraclavicular region with injection; initially the catheter was easily flushed and blood withdrawn but as symptoms progressed, the catheter became less functional (Ghosh and Griffiths, 2000).
3. *Intraluminal occlusion:* Fibrin accumulates within the internal catheter lumen leading to sluggish flow or complete inability to infuse.
4. *Mural thrombus:* Irritation by the catheter tip against the intima of the vein leads to an accumulation of fibrin, causing the CVAD to adhere to the vessel wall; this may lead to deep vein thrombosis.

Some thrombotic occlusions may be prevented. Intraluminal occlusion may be caused by reflux of blood back into the catheter tip. Proper flushing technique using positive pressure or flushing using the correct method based on the type of injection cap (e.g., positive pressure), as discussed in the preceding section, can reduce the risk of reflux. Changes in catheter and injection access/cap, such as valved catheters and positive and neutral pressure caps, are designed to prevent blood reflux into the catheter lumen. Use of a "push-pause" flushing technique is often recommended to create more turbulence during flushing to better clear the internal catheter; however, there is no clear evidence for this practice.

For suspected thrombotic occlusion, a thrombolytic drug can be used to "declot" the catheter. Low-dose alteplase (recombinant tissue plasminogen activator [t-PA]) is the thrombolytic drug of choice. The efficacy and safety of alteplase in treatment of thrombotic occlusions, defined as inability to withdraw blood, were demonstrated in two major clinical trials (Ponec et al, 2001; Deitcher et al, 2002). Alteplase works by acting on fibrin-bound plasminogen, producing plasmin at the site, which breaks down the thrombus and restores catheter patency. The dose of alteplase is 2 mg in 2 mL (Cathflo Activase), and is the drug of choice for declotting central venous access devices. Some have demonstrated success with lower doses (Davis, Vermeulen, Banton et al, 2000). The alteplase is instilled into the catheter and allowed to dwell from 30 minutes to 2 hours. The dose may be repeated in 2 hours if catheter patency is not restored. While adverse reactions to alteplase are rare, any thrombolytic drug should be used with caution in patients with known or suspected catheter-associated infection, patients with signs or symptoms of catheter-associated deep vein thrombosis, or patients with bleeding disorders or at risk for bleeding (Cathflo Activase, 2005). Alteplase can be used in all settings, including the home setting (Gorski, 2003).

Nonthrombotic causes of CVAD occlusion include drug precipitates, lipid deposits, or mechanical causes such as catheter pinch-off syndrome (see section titled Catheter Pinch-Off Syndrome). Drug precipitates may cause obstruction when incompatible medications or fluids are administered without flushing the catheter. The most common precipitates are calcium, diazepam, and phenytoin. Hydrochloric acid (0.1% N HCl) can be used to dissolve calcium-phosphorous precipitates or precipitates of low-pH drugs such as vancomycin. An amount that approximates the internal lumen of the catheter is used. For high-pH drugs such as phenytoin, sodium bicarbonate is used to neutralize the precipitate. These solutions are instilled into the CVAD for approximately 60 minutes (Hadaway, 1998).

Total nutrient parenteral nutrition (PN) admixtures consisting of dextrose, amino acids, lipids, and other additives in one container can cause a waxy buildup of lipids on the internal catheter lumen, leading to occlusion (Erdman et al, 1994). Instillation of a 70% ethanol solution has been demonstrated to dissolve the buildup (Werlin et al, 1995). Risk factors include long storage periods of PN solutions, common in home care where supplies are often delivered weekly. Use of "split" infusions of lipids and amino acid/dextrose solutions is associated with a decreased risk of occlusion from precipitate or lipids; a plastic bar on the outside of the infusion container is removed, allowing the solutions to mix just before infusion (Erdman et al, 1994). Agents that can be used for catheter clearance are listed in Table 25-3.

Sometimes, malposition of the catheter tip may cause occlusion problems such as the inability to withdraw blood. The catheter tip may abut against the vessel wall, blocking blood withdrawal. This is suspected when difficulty in blood aspiration is resolved with a cough, Valsalva's maneuver, or a body position change such as from lying to sitting. However, persistent inability to obtain a blood return may be an indication of poor catheter tip placement, catheter migration, or fibrin tail formation.

TABLE 25-3 **Agents Used for Catheter Clearance**

Precipitate	Clearing agent	Reason	Concentration	Volume	Caution
Calcium phosphate Low-pH drug (pH 1-5) High-pH drug (pH 9-12) (1 mEq/mL) Fat emulsion residue	Hydrochloric acid (0.1 N) Cysteine hydrochloride Hydrochloric acid (0.1 N) Sodium bicarbonate Ethanol 70% Sodium hydroxide (0.1 N)	To restore catheter's patency when occluded with a precipitate such as calcium phosphate, drugs with high or low pH, fat emulsion residue	See manufacturer's labeled use and directions	Fill-volume capacity of catheter	Should not be used in peripheral-short or midline catheters
Blood	t-PA (1-2 mg/2 mL)	To restore catheter's patency when occluded with blood	See manufacturer's labeled use and directions	Fill-volume capacity of catheter	Should not be used in peripheral-short or midline catheters

From Infusion Nurses Society: *Policies and procedures for infusion nursing,* ed 3, Norwood, Mass, 2006b, Author.

DEEP VEIN THROMBOSIS

While deep vein thrombosis (DVT), or formation of a blood clot in a vein, most often occurs in the lower extremities, DVT may also occur in the veins of the upper extremities or chest, most often associated with the presence of a central venous access device or a diagnosis of cancer (Kearon et al, 2008). Thrombosis may be clinically manifested with the presence of signs and symptoms or, most often, may be a subclinical condition only detected with diagnostic imaging tests or when a complication such as pulmonary emboli occurs (Van Rooden et al, 2005). The subclavian, axillary or brachial veins may be involved and symptoms may include swelling in the neck, supraclavicular area, or arms; dilated collateral veins over the arm, neck, or chest; arm pain; or discoloration (Kearon et al, 2008).

Pulmonary embolism, recurrent DVT, and postthrombotic syndrome are potential consequences of DVT. Postthrombotic syndrome is characterized by venous hypertension leading to extremity swelling and pain, occurring in 15% to 25% of patients who have been treated for upper extremity DVT; treatment includes elastic compression sleeves to reduce symptoms (Kearon et al, 2008).

Virchow's triad remains the time-honored pathophysiological explanation for the formation of venous thrombosis. Three factors are implicated in the development of a thrombus:

1. Vessel wall damage or injury. Causes may include surgery or trauma, the presence of a central venous catheter, or administration of irritating solutions.
2. Alterations in the flow of blood. Causes include venous stasis often associated with immobility, obstruction of the veins, heart failure, and varicosities.
3. Hypercoagulability of the blood. Contributing conditions include a decrease in coagulation inhibitors (e.g., antithrombin III), pregnancy, malignancy, and postoperative states.

Suboptimal internal catheter tip location and left-sided catheter placement are associated with thrombosis in tunneled catheters (Brown-Smith, Stoner, and Barley, 1990). Peripherally inserted central catheters appear to have greater risk in this population than catheters placed via the subclavian or jugular route, and catheter tip position is a factor. When the CVAD tip is in the upper superior vena cava or in a more peripheral location, the risk of DVT is greater than when the tip is at or just above the right atrium (Geerts et al, 2008).

Patients with cancer are particularly predisposed to upper extremity DVT when a central line is in place (Geerts et al, 2008). Use of low-dose warfarin (e.g., 1 mg per day) has often been used to prevent thrombosis in patients with cancer; however, current evidence does not support this practice and the risks of bleeding outweigh any advantages. Currently practice guidelines from the American College of Chest Physicians (ACCP) state that for cancer patients with an indwelling CVAD, clinicians should not use either prophylactic doses of low–molecular-weight heparin or low-dose warfarin therapy as DVT prevention (Geerts et al, 2008). The physician should be notified immediately if vessel thrombosis is suspected. Radiographic studies using dye (venography) are usually performed to verify catheter placement. The ACCP provides evidence-based treatment guidelines for upper extremity–related DVT as follows (Kearon et al, 2008):

- Systemic anticoagulants to prevent extension of the thrombus and pulmonary embolism are recommended.
- Initial treatment with low-molecular-weight heparin, unfractionated heparin, or fondaparinux is recommended.
- Long-term treatment should include at least 3 months with a vitamin K antagonist (e.g., warfarin).
- The CVAD does not need to be removed if it is functioning and necessary.
- If the CVAD is removed, the guidelines do not recommend that long-term anticoagulant therapy be shortened to less than 3 months.

CATHETER PINCH-OFF SYNDROME

Catheter pinch-off syndrome is a significant, yet relatively rare and often unrecognized complication. It occurs when a CVAD inserted percutaneously via the subclavian vein is compressed by the clavicle and first rib. Catheter compression causes intermittent or permanent catheter obstruction and can result in catheter tearing, transection, and catheter embolism, most often to the right side of the heart or pulmonary artery (Masoorli, 2001; Mirza, Vanek, and Kupensky, 2004). The following are signs and symptoms of pinch-off syndrome:

- Intermittent and positional occlusion
- Difficulty with flushing, infusing, or aspirating

- Frequent occlusion alarms
- Occlusion relieved by specific postural changes such as rolling the shoulder back or raising the arm, which opens the angle of the costoclavicular space (Andris and Krzywda, 1997)

An upright chest radiograph should be obtained after placement of a subclavian insertion of a CVAD. Based on a review of the literature, Mirza and colleagues (2004) also recommend chest x-rays at regular intervals for the first 6 months of placement to identify late occurrence of pinch-off syndrome. The interval between CVAD insertion and diagnosis of pinch-off ranged from the day of insertion to 60 months' postinsertion with an average time of about 5 months (Mirza et al, 2004). If pinch-off syndrome is diagnosed, catheter removal is recommended. Should the patient's catheter partially or completely transect, some patients will have no symptoms, while others may experience chest pain, palpitations, swelling in the area of the CVAD, or pain with catheter flushing. The catheter should be removed and the embolized segment should be retrieved. Inserting the catheter lateral to the midclavicular line decreases the risk of catheter pinch-off syndrome (Mirza et al, 2004; Steiger, 2006).

CATHETER DISLODGMENT

Central venous access devices are secured with a catheter securement device or may be sutured. However, devices can still fall out, be pulled out, or become dislodged. Also, ports can become freely movable and migrate from one area to another or flip upside down. The term "twiddler's syndrome" is used in the literature most often to describe patients who nervously touch and potentially dislodge their pacemakers, resulting in dislodged pacer wires. It has also been used to refer to patients who develop a nervous habit of "twiddling" with their ports or catheters, resulting in displacement.

Although it is fairly obvious when a catheter has been pulled out or a port moves when accessed, catheter dislodgment is not always obvious. The CVAD assessment should include measurement of the length of the external part of the catheter at the time of placement. If the external catheter segment extrudes further than at baseline measurement, the catheter tip may no longer be at the correct position. With tunneled catheters, the exit site and tunnel should be palpated for coiling. The exposure of the Dacron cuff of the tunneled catheter is also a sign of catheter dislodgment. Difficulty with aspiration or infusion through the catheter, leaking of solution from the catheter exit site, edema, a burning sensation, or pain when solution is infused can also indicate a displaced catheter.

If displacement is suspected, the physician is notified. Usually, radiographic studies are performed to ascertain catheter tip placement. Depending on findings, the catheter may or may not be repositioned. If the catheter cannot be repositioned, it is removed and a new catheter placed as needed. It is important to note that whenever a catheter is replaced, the administration set and solution container are changed as well.

If a central venous access device is pulled out, an antiseptic ointment and a sterile occlusive pressure dressing should be applied; the rationale for this procedure is to prevent potential air embolism (INS, 2006b). The physician is notified of the dislodgment and the patient prepared for reinsertion of the catheter, if necessary. Preventive measures for central venous access device dislodgment include the following:

- Secure the external catheter with sutures or a manufactured securement device and intact dressing.
- Educate the patient in catheter care, catheter securement, physical activities to avoid, and the danger of pulling the catheter out.

CATHETER MIGRATION

Migration occurs when the tip of a central venous catheter is displaced from a documented, satisfactory position into a neighboring vein. The *Infusion Nursing Standards of Practice* (INS, 2006a) recommend that CVAD tip placement should be in the lower third of the superior vena cava near the junction of the superior vena cava and the right atrium. Tip confirmation is checked immediately following insertion and before using the catheter and periodically reassessed thereafter, although there are no set recommendations for routinely checking tip placement. The catheter tip can spontaneously migrate into the right atrium or into the internal jugular vein after placement. Migrations have also been documented in the axillary veins. Catheter tip migration may result from changes in intrathoracic pressure associated with coughing or sneezing, or from forceful flushing of the catheter as with power injection. In some instances, central venous access device migration has been noted as a result of a disease process. For instance, in patients with congestive heart failure, catheter tip migration has been thought to result from reduced blood flow and the dilated vessels associated with the disease. Migration has also resulted from displacement by invading tissue (tumor) or venous thrombosis. Migration can also be a consequence of suboptimal care, if clinicians accidentally dislodge or advance the catheter into the body.

There may not be obvious signs or symptoms of catheter migration; however, the inability to flush, infuse, or aspirate may mean the catheter tip is no longer at the desired position. Arrhythmias are often indicative of catheter migration into the right atrium or ventricle. The "ear gurgling" or running stream sound is often heard when the catheter is flushed and it has migrated into the internal jugular vein (Figure 25-3). In addition, complaints of headache or pain, swelling, redness, or discomfort in the shoulder, arm, or neck may indicate catheter migration.

When catheter migration is suspected, the physician is notified and venographic studies should be performed to verify catheter tip location. The nurse should prepare the patient for

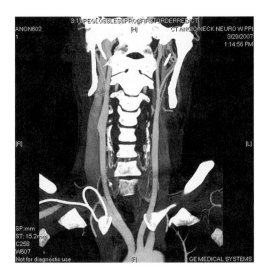

FIGURE 25-3 CT image of contrast being injected through a power PICC and malposition. This is a picture of the neck. The bright white line is the PICC. It has looped up into the jugular during the injection of the dye.

either repositioning the catheter under fluoroscopy or removal and possible reinsertion of another catheter. All infusions should be discontinued.

The following interventions can reduce the risk of catheter migration: preventing trauma to the catheter site, avoiding catheter placement near the site of local disease, and using a catheter securement device.

SUPERIOR VENA CAVA SYNDROME

Superior vena cava syndrome (SVCS) is a rare but serious complication characterized by an obstruction of blood flow through the superior vena cava. It is considered an oncological emergency. It occurs when an internal or external mass, such as a tumor or enlarged lymph nodes, occludes the superior vena cava, impeding venous return of blood to the heart. Venous thrombosis secondary to a CVAD may also be a cause of SVCS. Cancers associated with SVCS include breast, lung, esophageal, and lymphoma (Colen, 2008). The cause of SVCS must be established before assuming the condition results from the CVAD.

Signs and symptoms may be subtle or severe. Early symptoms include nonproductive cough, shortness of breath, dysphagia, hoarseness, chest pain, difficulty buttoning shirt collars, breast swelling, feeling of fullness in the head, jugular vein distention, periorbital edema, ruddy face or cheeks, compensatory tachycardia, and edema of the face, arms, fingers, or neck (Flounders, 2003). A prominent venous pattern usually is present over the chest as a result of dilated thoracic vessels. If the condition remains unnoticed and untreated, the patient may have symptoms including headache (caused by increased intracranial pressure), visual disturbances, and altered mental status. Advanced symptoms include progressive shortness of breath, respiratory distress, irritability, cyanosis of face or upper body, engorged conjunctivae, changes in mentation, tachypnea, orthopnea, stridor, stupor, coma, and seizures (Flounders, 2003).

The physician is notified immediately when the first symptoms of superior vena cava syndrome are observed. The patient should be placed in a semi-Fowler's position and oxygen should be administered to facilitate breathing. Patients with superior vena cava syndrome become very anxious and fearful because of the feeling of suffocation, so it is important to provide emotional support. The patient's fluid volume status should be monitored to minimize further edema, and cardiovascular and neurological status should be monitored. Diagnosis is confirmed by radiographic studies. Treatment is based on the cause. If a tumor is the cause, treatment may include surgery, radiation, chemotherapy or stent placement. If SVCS is due to a CVAD, catheter removal may be necessary or treatment with thrombolytic therapy may be used (Flounders, 2003). The severity of symptoms, the ability to initiate an alternative infusion route, and the type of CVAD in place all contribute to the decision of catheter removal. Anticoagulant therapy is usually prescribed for the patient, and symptoms are treated.

AIR EMBOLISM

Air embolism is caused by the entry of a bolus of air into the vascular system. The air embolus is propelled into the heart, creating an intracardiac air lock at the pulmonic valve that prevents the ejection of blood from the right side of the heart. The right side of the heart overfills with blood and the force of right ventricular contractions increases in an attempt to eject blood past the air lock. Forceful contractions cause small air bubbles to break loose from the air pocket and they are pumped into the pulmonary circulation. This creates an obstruction to forward blood flow resulting in tissue hypoxia. Pulmonary hypoxia results in vasoconstriction of lung tissue, further increasing the workload of the right ventricle. Cardiac output is diminished and shock and death may ensue unless immediate interventions are taken. Conditions or situations that can cause an air embolism include the following:

- Catheter fracture
- Disconnection between catheter connections (e.g., between the injection/access cap and IV administration set)
- Presence of a persistent catheter tract following CVAD removal
- Deep inspiration during CVAD insertion or removal
- Inadvertent infusion of air into the IV administration set (Laskey, Dyer, and Tobias, 2002)

Signs and symptoms of air embolism include palpitations, respiratory distress, hypotension, petechiae, feeling of impending doom, arrhythmias, elevated central venous pressure, loss of consciousness, neurological deficits, and chest, shoulder, or low back pain. A distinctive "mill wheel murmur" is heard over the precordium; this is a continuous churning, drumlike cardiac murmur (Peter and Saxman, 2003). Should an air embolism be suspected, immediate actions are required. The patient should be positioned in the left lateral Trendelenburg position. This moves the air bubble away from the pulmonic valve. The physician is notified; vital signs, oxygen saturation levels, and cardiac rhythm are monitored; and 100% oxygen should be administered. Oxygen causes the nitrogen in the air embolus to dissolve into the blood (Hadaway, 2002). Other potential treatments include hyperbaric treatment or aspiration of the embolus.

Prevention of air embolism is essential. In a review of existing literature including case study reports, Peter and Saxman (2003) identified best practices for preventing air embolism during the CVAD removal procedure as follows:

- Position the patient in a supine position.
- Instruct the patient in Valsalva's maneuver during the catheter removal process; if Valsalva's maneuver is contraindicated, have the patient exhale during the procedure.
- Slowly remove the catheter and place immediate pressure to the exit site until hemostasis is achieved.
- Instruct the patient to perform Valsalva's maneuver again and apply antiseptic ointment, a gauze dressing, and tape to the site (INS, 2006b).
- Have the patient remain in the supine position for 30 minutes following catheter removal.
- Leave dressing in place for 24 hours.

Additional practices to reduce the risk of air embolism include the following:

- Using only Luer-Lok™ add-on devices in the IV system, including injection access/caps (INS, 2006a)
- Frequent checking of administration set junctions, making sure they are secure, especially before patients get out of bed
- Ensuring that the catheter is clamped during IV administration set and injection access/cap changes

Patient education is also important especially with home infusion patients. Though literature is scarce, Laskey and colleagues (2002) reported a case of air embolism in a pediatric patient when the mother inadvertently let an unprimed IV administration set flow by gravity into the patient, resulting in immediate respiratory and neurological symptoms (the patient survived). It is important to teach patients or caregivers to properly prime tubing, to check connections frequently, and to clamp the CVAD at appropriate times. Additionally, should a crack or hole in the catheter occur, clamps should be available to home infusion therapy patients and they should be taught to immediately clamp the catheter close to the skin, above the damaged area of the catheter.

CATHETER DAMAGE

Central venous access devices can be damaged if appropriate measures are not used during insertion, care, and maintenance. Using scissors at or near the catheter during dressing changes can result in the catheter being cut. Catheters are made of non-resealable material; penetration by a needle creates pinholes with subsequent leaking. Catheters can also rupture when excessive force is exerted, such as flushing with a small-volume syringe. Pinch-off syndrome, as discussed earlier, can also result in a transected and potentially embolized catheter segment.

Central venous access devices should be assessed for catheter integrity. Assessment should include observation of the dressing, catheter, and area around the catheter. A wet dressing or leaking at the insertion site during an infusion or flushing may indicate catheter damage. Swelling in the chest area may be indicative of catheter rupture. Tunneled and implanted catheters can usually be palpated to the point at which they enter the vein; if the rupture is in the tunneled segment of the catheter, swelling may be felt at the point of rupture.

If the external catheter segment is damaged, a nonserrated clamp is applied proximal to the damaged part. The damage should be assessed and the appropriate action taken. Damaged catheters must be repaired or removed without delay to prevent serious complications. Any opening in the catheter can serve as a portal of entry for bacteria or air into the vascular system. The entrance of bacteria into the system can predispose a debilitated patient to septicemia. Air may also be drawn into the system because of the negative pressure created within the heart, and the patient can suffer an air embolism. Policies and procedures should be established for the repair of a catheter according to the manufacturer's guidelines. If the catheter cannot be repaired, the physician should be notified immediately and the catheter removed.

Implanted venous access devices can separate at the port-catheter juncture. This phenomenon can result in tissue infiltration or extravasation based on the type of infusate being administered. If either of these conditions is suspected, the infusion should be discontinued immediately, and the physician notified. Radiographic studies should be performed to verify a rupture or a port-catheter separation, and the patient should be prepared for removal of the port and possible replacement of the catheter.

■ NURSING CONSIDERATIONS

Nurses must be able to accurately assess and implement early nursing interventions to achieve positive patient outcomes associated with central venous access devices. By use of the nursing process and a holistic approach, the nurse must implement nursing interventions that provide immediate treatment, promote healing, and prevent further complications. The nurse

must constantly evaluate the care rendered in terms of patient outcomes to promote quality improvement in the delivery of infusion therapy.

The clinical diagnosis of complications is related to the nurse's ability to evaluate the patient's signs and symptoms. Additionally, because many patients with CVADs are at home caring for themselves, with only intermittent care from home health or other alternative settings such as outpatient care, patient education is critical. Patients and their caregivers *must* be instructed in the signs and symptoms of potential complications for which they should be vigilant, the immediate actions they should take if such complications occur, and the importance of calling the nurse or other health care provider immediately. Refer to Table 25-4 for an example of a patient education tool.

Using objective, subjective, and cardinal evaluations, the nurse can make an accurate nursing diagnosis. *Objective symptoms* are visible (e.g., edema, erythema, blanching). *Subjective symptoms* have an internal or mental origin; they relate to the patient's perception of what he or she feels (e.g., pain, tingling sensation, feeling of suffocation). *Cardinal symptoms* relate to the physical body (e.g., pulse, temperature, blood pressure). In addition, signs and symptoms can occur locally or systemically. Local complications usually appear at the site of the invasion of the body and usually produce visible signs and symptoms. Systemic complications occur within the body and usually affect circulation and other body processes.

Other tools often used to evaluate signs and symptoms include differential, exclusion, pathological, and roentgenographic evaluations. *Differential evaluations* can be extremely helpful, such as comparing one arm against another to determine infiltration. *Exclusion evaluations* are often performed when no other reasonable explanation exists for a complication. For example, a patient with a central venous catheter may suddenly develop an elevated temperature, and no other possible explanation exists for the elevated temperature. Sepsis related to the catheter is considered, and interventions for catheter-induced septicemia are initiated.

Pathological evaluations are used to verify the presence of pathological organisms; they are usually performed when drainage from a wound or an elevated temperature occurs, suggesting an infectious process. A good example is the culturing

PATIENT OUTCOMES

Expected outcomes with CVAD include:
- The patient will exhibit no signs or symptoms of CVAD-associated infection.
- The patient will exhibit no signs or symptoms of other CVAD-associated complications.
- The patient will be able to verbalize signs or symptoms of potential complications associated with the CVAD and take appropriate actions including immediate notification of the nurse.
- The home care patient or caregiver will successfully demonstrate care of the CVAD as delegated by the home care nurse. This may include catheter flushing, drug/solution administration, and site care/dressing changes and will include adherence to hand hygiene and aseptic technique.
- The CVAD will be removed when no longer needed for infusion therapy.

TABLE 25-4   **Patient Education Tool: Central Venous Catheter–Associated Problems**

A central venous catheter (CVC) is placed so that the catheter tip is located in a large vein in your chest. It is used to administer intravenous (IV) fluids and medicines. It may also be used to obtain blood samples for lab studies. There are different kinds of CVCs including the PICC (peripherally inserted central catheter), the Hickman (tunneled CVC), and ports. Your home care nurse will see you to check your CVC and to teach you how to care for it. As with any type of treatment, there are certain problems that can occur, which are listed in this table.

Problem	What to do	How to prevent
Redness, pain, warmth, swelling, or pus-like drainage where catheter enters your skin Unexplained fever, chills	These are signs of a possible infection. Call your nurse or doctor immediately.	Check the area around your catheter every day for signs of infection. Wash your hands before doing any IV procedures. Use sterile technique when giving IV fluids or medicines. Perform regular site care of catheter with antiseptic cleansing and a fresh dressing every 7 days (clear dressing) or every 2 days (gauze dressing).
Crack in catheter Leaking of fluid from catheter	Clamp above the crack (nearest to your skin) if a crack or leak occurs. Call your nurse or doctor immediately. Some catheters can be repaired.	Never use scissors or sharp objects near your catheter. Never force flushing solution into your catheter. Carry a spare catheter clamp with you at all times.
Unable to flush catheter	Make sure catheter is not clamped. If clamps are open and catheter still does not flush, call your nurse. Your catheter could have a blood clot; this can be treated.	Flush catheter regularly with heparin or saline as taught by your nurse. Use a "start-stop" technique when flushing.
Shortness of breath, coughing, fast heart rate **(Very rare)**	Call 9-1-1. Lie down on your left side with head flat and feet up.	When changing IV cap, always clamp your catheter (except Groshong-type catheter).
Swelling in your neck, shoulder, face, or arm on the side of the catheter	Stop using your catheter. Call your doctor or nurse immediately.	

From Wheaton Franciscan Home Health & Hospice, Milwaukee, Wis.

of the catheter site, the catheters, or an infusate when a vascular infection is suspected. A pathological evaluation is an effective tool for verifying the disease source. However, it should never be the only tool used because pathological reports usually take time and complications do not wait to be diagnosed—they often progress very rapidly. *Roentgenographic evaluations* can be used to prevent complications (e.g., obtaining a radiograph to verify placement before using a central venous catheter) or to verify a complication (e.g., verifying a pulmonary embolus). The nurse must be alert to all signs and symptoms and must evaluate each one individually. Early recognition of potential complications can prevent further complications and promote quick healing and restoration of health.

SUMMARY

Although observing and evaluating the signs and symptoms of complications is very important, it is far better to prevent complications. The ideal situation is delivering infusion therapy that is free of complications, thereby promoting positive patient outcomes. Outcomes should be established that are based on evidence-based interventions, protecting the patient and nurse from risks associated with infusion therapy. In addition to establishing criteria for patient outcomes, nurses should also monitor the actual patient outcomes. Statistics must be kept regarding the incidence of complications, interventions, and outcomes. They should be reported to staff, the risk management

department, the quality improvement council, and various others involved in the process, and should be used as a tool to recognize areas for improvement.

REFERENCES

Alonso-Echanove J, Edwards JR, Richards et al: Effect of nurse staffing and antimicrobial-impregnated central venous catheters on the risk for bloodstream infections in intensive care units, *Infect Control Hospital Epidemiol* 24(12):916-925, 2003.

Andris DA, Krzywda EA: Catheter pinch-off syndrome: recognition and management, *J Intraven Nurs* 20(5):233-237, 1997.

Bagnall-Reeb H: Evidence for the use of the antibiotic lock technique, *J Infus Nurs* 27(2):118-120, 2004.

Beghetto MG, Victorino J, Teixeira L et al: Parenteral nutrition as a risk factor for central venous catheter-related infection, *JPEN* 29:367-373, 2005.

Berenholtz SM, Pronovost PJ, Lipsett PA et al: Eliminating catheter related bloodstream infections in the intensive care unit, *Crit Care Med* 32:2014-2020, 2004.

Berriel-Cass D, Adkins FW, Jones P et al: Eliminating nosocomial infections at Ascension Health, *J Quality Patient Safety* 32(11): 612-620, 2006.

Bhende S, Rothenburger S: In vitro antimicrobial effectiveness of 5 catheter insertion-site dressings, *JAVA* 12(4):227-231, 2007.

Boodhan S, Maloney AM, Dupuis LL: Extent of agreement in gentamicin concentration between serum that is drawn peripherally and from central venous catheters, *Pediatrics* 118(6):e1650-1656, 2006.

Brown-Smith JK, Stoner MH, Barley ZA: Tunneled catheter thrombosis: factors related to incidence, *Oncol Nurs Forum* 17(4):543-549, 1990.

Cathflo Activase: Prescribing information. Accessed 12/1/08 at http://gene.com/gene/products/information/pdf/cathflo-prescribing.pdf.

Chaiyakunapruk N, Veenstra DL, Lipsky BA et al: Chlorhexidine compared with povidone iodine solution for vascular site care: a meta-analysis, *Ann Intern Med* 136:792-801, 2002.

Chambers ST, Sanders J, Patton WN et al: Reduction of exit-site infections of tunneled intravascular catheters among neutropenic patients by sustained release chlorhexidine dressings: results from a prospective randomized controlled trial, *J Hospital Infect* 61(1):53-61, 2005.

Colen FN: Oncologic emergencies: superior vena cava syndrome, tumor lysis syndrome, and spinal cord compression, *J Emerg Nurs* 34(6):535-537, 2008.

Davis SN, Vermeulen L, Banton J et al: Activity and dosage of alteplase dilution for clearing occlusions of venous access devices, *Am J Health-Syst Pharm* 57(11):1039-1045, 2000.

Deitcher DR, Fesen MR, Kiproff PM et al: Safety and efficacy of alteplase for restoring function in occluded central venous catheters: results of the cardiovascular thrombolytic to open occluded lines trial, *J Clin Oncol* 20:317-324, 2002.

Donlan RM, Murga R, Bell M: Protocol for detection of biofilms on needleless connectors attached to central venous catheters, *J Clin Microbiol* 39(2):750-753, 2001.

El-Masri MM, Hammad TA, McLeskey et al: Predictors of nosocomial bloodstream infections among critically ill adult trauma patients, *Infect Control Hospital Epidemiol* 25(8):656-663, 2004.

Erdman SH, McElwee CL, Kramer JM et al: Central line occlusion with three-in-one nutrition admixtures administered at home, *JPEN* 18:177-181, 1994.

Flounders JA: Superior vena cava syndrome, *Oncol Nurs Forum* 30(4):E84-E90, 2003.

Frey AM: Drawing blood from vascular access devices—evidence-based practice, *J Infus Nurs* 26(5):285-293, 2003.

Geerts WH, Bergqvist D, Pineo GF et al: Antithrombotic and thrombolytic therapy, ed 8: ACCP Guidelines: prevention of venous thromboembolism, *Chest* 133(suppl 6):381S-453S, 2008.

Ghosh A, Griffiths DM: Sleeve thrombus fibrosis causing neck pain, *J Parenteral Enteral Nutr* 24(3):180-182, 2000.

Gillies D, O'Riordan L, Carr D et al: Gauze and tape and transparent polyurethane dressings for central venous catheters, *Cochrane Database Syst Rev* 4:CD003827, 2003.

Gorski LA: Central venous access device occlusions: part 1: thrombotic causes and treatment, *Home Healthcare Nurse* 21(2):115-121, 2003.

Gorski LA: *Pocket guide to home infusion therapy*, Sudbury, Mass, 2005, Jones and Bartlett.

Hadaway LC: Major thrombotic and nonthrombotic complications, *J Intraven Nurs* 21(5 Suppl):S143-S160, 1998.

Hadaway LC: Air embolus, *Nursing* 32(10):104, 2002.

Hadaway LC: Technology of flushing vascular access devices, *J Infus Nurs* 29(3):137-145, 2006.

Hanna HA, Raad I: Blood products: a significant risk factor for long-term catheter-related bloodstream infections in cancer patients, *Infect Control Hospital Epidemiol* 22(3):165-166, 2001.

Hinds PS, Quargnenti A, Gattuso J et al: Comparing the results of coagulation tests on blood drawn by venipuncture and through heparinized tunneled venous access devices in pediatric patients with cancer, *Oncol Nurs Forum* 29(3):1, 2002.

Ho KM, Litton E: Use of chlorhexidine-impregnated dressing to prevent vascular and epidural catheter colonization and infection: a meta-analysis, *J Antimicrob Chemother* 58(2):281-287, 2006.

Hosoglu S, Akalin S, Kidir V et al: Prospective surveillance study for risk factors of central venous catheter-related bloodstream infections, *Am J Infect Control* 32(3):131-134, 2004.

Infusion Nurses Society: Infusion nursing standards of practice, *J Infus Nurs* 29(1 Suppl):S1-S92, 2006a.

Infusion Nurses Society: *Policies and procedures for infusion nursing,* ed 3, Norwood, Mass, 2006b, Author.

Infusion Nurses Society: *Flushing protocols*, Norwood, Mass, 2008, Author.

Institute for Healthcare Improvement: *5 Million lives campaign, getting started kit: prevent central line infections how-to guide*, Cambridge, Mass, n.d., Author. Accessed 6/5/08 at www.ihi.org.

Institute for Safe Medication Practices: *Failure to cap IV tubing and disconnect IV ports place patients at risk for infections,* 2007. Accessed 11/26/08 at www.ismp.org/newsletters/acutecare/articles/20070726.asp.

Kaler W: Successful disinfection of needleless access ports: a matter of time and friction, *J Assoc Vasc Access* 12(3):140-142, 2007.

Kearon C, Kahn SR, Agnelli G et al: Antithrombotic and thrombolytic therapy, ed 8: ACCP guidelines: antithrombotic therapy for venous thromboembolic disease, *Chest* 133(Suppl 6):S454-S545, 2008.

Laskey AL, Dyer C, Tobias JD: Venous air embolism during home infusion therapy, *Pediatrics* 109(1):E15, 2002.

Marschall J, Mermel LA, Classen D et al: Strategies to prevent central line-associated bloodstream infections in acute care hospitals, *Infec Control Hospital Epidemiol* 29(suppl1):S22-S30, 2008.

Marx M: The management of the difficult peripherally inserted central venous catheter line removal, *J Intraven Nurs* 18(5):246-249, 1995.

Masoorli S: A malpractice case history: fracture of an implanted port catheter, *J Vasc Access Devices* 6(4):44-45, 2001.

Mayo DK, Dimond EP, Kramer W et al: Discard volumes necessary for clinically useful coagulation studies from heparinized Hickman catheters, *Oncol Nurs Forum* 23(4):671-675, 1996.

Miall LS, Das A, Brownlee KG et al: Peripherally inserted central catheters in children with cystic fibrosis: eight cases of difficult removal, *J Infus Nurs* 24(5):297-300, 2001.

Mirza B, Vanek VW, Kupensky DT: Pinch-off syndrome: case report and collective review of the literature, *Am Surg* 70(7):635-644, 2004.

National Quality Forum (NQF): *National voluntary consensus standards for the reporting of healthcare-associated infection data*, 2008. Accessed 11/26/08 at www.qualityforum.org/pdf/reports/HAI%20Report.pdf.

Occupational Safety and Health Administration: *Securing medical catheters. OSHA fact sheet*. Accessed 10/28/08 at http://www.osha.gov/SLTC/bloodbornepathogens/factsheet_catheters.pdf.

O'Grady NP, Alexander M, Dellinger EP et al: Guidelines for the prevention of intravascular catheter-related infections, *MMWR Recomm Rep* 51(RR-10):1-29, 2002.

Olson K, Rennie RP, Hanson J et al: Evaluation of a no-dressing intervention for tunneled central venous catheter exit sites, *J Infus Nurs* 27(1):37-44, 2004.

Penel N, New JC, Clisant S et al: Risk factors for early catheter-related infections in cancer patients, *Cancer* 110:1586-1592, 2007.

Peter DA, Saxman C: Preventing air embolism when removing CVCs: an evidence-based approach to changing practice, *Medsurg Nurs* 12(4):223-228, 2003.

Pinto KM: Accuracy of coagulation values obtained from a heparinized central venous catheter, *Oncol Nurs Forum* 21(3):573-575, 1994.

Ponec D, Irwin D, Haire W et al: Recombinant tissue plasminogen activator (alteplase) for restoration of flow in occluded central venous access devices: a double-blind placebo-controlled trial—the cardiovascular thrombolytic to open occluded lines (COOL) efficacy trial, *J Vasc Interv Radiol* 12:951-955, 2001.

Pronovost P, Needham D, Berenholtz et al: An intervention to decrease catheter-related bloodstream infections in the ICU, *New Engl J Med* 355:2725-2732, 2006.

Ryder M: Evidence-based practice in the management of vascular access devices for home parenteral nutrition therapy, *JPEN* 30:S82-S93, 2006.

Safdar N, Maki DG: Risk of catheter-related bloodstream infection with peripherally inserted central venous catheters used in hospitalized patients, *Chest* 128(2):489-495, 2005.

Shulman RJ, Ou C, Reed T et al: Central venous catheters versus peripheral veins for sampling blood levels of commonly used drugs, *JPEN* 22:234-237, 1998.

Steiger E: Dysfunction and thrombotic complications of vascular access devices, *JPEN* 30(1 Suppl):S70-S72, 2006.

The Joint Commission: *2009 National patient safety goals.* Accessed 11/26/08 at www.jointcommission.org/patientsafety/ nationalpatientsafetygoals/.

Van Rooden CJ, Tesselaar MET, Osanto S et al: Deep vein thrombosis associated with central venous catheters—a review, *J Thromb Haemostasis* 3:2409-2419, 2005.

Venkatram S, Murthy S, Loganathan R et al: Reducing central line related bloodstream infections in a university affiliated inner city medical intensive care unit, *Chest* 132(4 Suppl):S493, 2007.

Wall JK, Kierstead VL: Peripherally inserted central catheters— resistance to removal: a rare complication, *J Intraven Nurs* 18(5):251-254, 1995.

Weinstein SM: *Plumer's principles & practice of intravenous therapy,* ed 8 , Philadelphia, 2007, Lippincott Williams & Wilkins.

Werlin SL, Lausten T, Jessen S et al: Treatment of central venous catheter occlusions with ethanol and hydrochloric acid, *JPEN* 19:416-418, 1995.

Yamamoto AJ, Soloman JA, Soulen MC et al: Sutureless securement device reduces complications of peripherally inserted central venous catheters, *J Vasc Interv Radiol* 13(1):77-81, 2002.

Yilmaz G, Caylan R, Aydin K et al: Effect of education on the rate of and the understanding of risk factors for intravascular catheter-related infections, *Infect Control Hospital Epidemiol* 28(6): 689-694, 2007.

26 ALTERNATIVE INFUSION ACCESS DEVICES

Marilyn Parker, MSN, ACHPN, ACNS, BC and
Karin Henderson, MSN, RN, CCRN, CS-GNP

When intravenous (IV) access cannot be obtained because of lack of time, inadequate skills, or patient condition, vascular access by subcutaneous or intraosseous administration are alternative infusion options.

CONTINUOUS SUBCUTANEOUS INFUSION

OVERVIEW

Continuous subcutaneous infusion (CSI) is a useful route for the administration of selected medications. CSI can provide a comfortable, less expensive alternative to traditional IV administration or intramuscular (IM) injections, and can provide patients the added flexibility of receiving prescribed therapies without having to endure venipuncture attempts or painful IM injections. CSI should be considered an option for patients experiencing the following: limited or no venous access, inability to tolerate the burdens of oral therapies (numerous pills), oral therapies not as effective for symptom control or disease management (peak and trough effect), those with a single venous access device (VAD) and incompatible medications, those with medications adaptable to CSI, and patients without a functioning gastrointestinal tract. CSI can be effectively administered in a variety of patient care settings: home care, long-term care, intermediate care, acute care/hospitals, and hospice environments. CSI is used in many settings because it enables patients to manage their illness and/or pain without the risks and expenses involved with IV medication administration (Perry and Potter, 2006).

STRUCTURE OF THE SKIN: A BRIEF REVIEW

As the outermost protective layer, the skin is the largest organ of the body. It plays a major role in homeostasis by serving as a barrier to organisms, regulating body temperature, and maintaining fluid and electrolyte balance. Changes in the skin can also communicate information about a person's health and well-being (Cuzell and Workman, 2006). The thinnest outer layer is the epidermis, less than 1 millimeter (mm) thick; it is able to act effectively as the protective barrier between the body and environment. The epidermis does not have a separate blood supply, but receives nutrients from the dermis by diffusion. The

dermis is the layer of connective tissue between the epidermis and fat layer (also known as the subcutaneous tissue layer). The dermis is an interwoven network of collagen and elastic fibers that give the skin flexibility and strength. The dermis also contains a network of capillaries, lymph vessels, and sensory nerves that promotes oxygen and heat exchange and the transmission of sensation (Cuzell and Workman, 2006). The subcutaneous layer covers muscle and bone, is the site for fat formation and storage, provides heat insulation for the body, and provides protection against injury by absorbing shock and padding internal structures. The thickness of the subcutaneous layer varies with body surface area, age, and gender. Many blood vessels pass through the fatty layer and extend into the dermal layer, forming capillary networks that supply nutrients and remove wastes (Cuzell and Workman, 2006).

Medications and fluids are absorbed into the bloodstream through the network of capillaries and blood vessels. Subcutaneous tissue is less vascular than muscle tissue, so the onset of action is slower than intramuscular or intravenous administration (see Figure 10-1).

CONTINUOUS SUBCUTANEOUS THERAPIES

There are two major categories of continuous subcutaneous therapies: (1) continuous subcutaneous infusion of medication and (2) hypodermoclysis, or "clysis."

Continuous subcutaneous infusion

The goal of giving medication by continuous subcutaneous infusion (CSI) is to attain appropriate blood levels of medications and achieve the desired symptom control or management of disease without the risks, expense, or inconvenience of IV therapies. The most common medications infused via this method are opioids (morphine, hydromorphone, and fentanyl for pain management), insulin (diabetes management), terbutaline (treatment of preterm labor), deferoxamine mesylate (iron chelation), antiemetics, and steroids. Other medications used in palliative care given by CSI include midazolam, haloperidol, and hyoscine (Negro et al, 2002). Recently, clodronate, omeprazole, and methadone have been added to this list; however, methadone is notable for causing a high incidence of tissue irritation (Neasfey, 2005).

Advantages/Disadvantages

The following are advantages of administering medication by CSI: (1) medications are absorbed directly into the bloodstream, avoiding "first pass" effects of liver metabolism; (2) opioids can be titrated rapidly for pain and symptom management; (3) burdens of oral therapy are relieved (e.g., numerous pills, inconsistent medication effects); (4) central nervous system (CNS) side effects associated with intermittent drug therapy (such as nausea, vomiting, and drowsiness) are decreased; (5) a functioning gastrointestinal tract is not required; (6) bioavailability and analgesic efficacy of medications are similar to those from IV administration; (7) therapies are available to patients with limited or nonexistent venous access, or those that have a single VAD with other incompatible medications; (8) it is generally less expensive and less time-consuming than venipuncture, and may be considered less invasive by patients (Neafsey, 2005; Weissman, 2005); (9) clinicians can easily learn the procedure (does not require venipuncture); and (10) it can be safely administered in a variety of patient care settings, including the home (Phillips, 2005).

The major disadvantage of giving medication by CSI is that medications must be concentrated enough to be able to infuse small volumes. Most patients can absorb up to 2 to 3 mL/hour of medication (Pasero, 2002). As the rate of infusion increases, the absorption of medication decreases (Perry and Potter, 2006). Other disadvantages include local discomfort at the infusion site and limited medication choices because of pharmacokinetics and medication properties. Also, the onset of action for medication given by CSI is slower than that when IV administration is used; anticipate about 20 minutes for onset of action as compared to more immediate onset of action when administered by the IV route. Anything affecting local blood flow to the tissues, such as exercise, local application of hot or cold compresses, or altered body temperature, influences the rate of drug absorption (Perry and Potter, 2006). CSI is contraindicated in patients with conditions resulting in decreased local tissue perfusion, such as circulatory shock, hypothermia, and occlusive vascular disease (Perry and Potter, 2006).

Hypodermoclysis

Hypodermoclysis, or "clysis," is the infusion of isotonic fluids into the subcutaneous space for the treatment or prevention of dehydration in the elderly adult (Walsh, 2005).

Because of severe adverse reactions related to the misuse of electrolyte-free or hypertonic solutions in the 1950s, hypodermoclysis was almost completely discontinued. Since the late 1980s, this method has been increasingly rediscovered as an alternative therapy for IV rehydration, especially in the fields of geriatric and palliative medicine (Slesak et al, 2003). In long-term care, the common treatment for patients unable to take adequate fluids by mouth is infusion of IV solutions (Remington and Hultman, 2007), which often necessitates moving the patient to a different level of care, such as the clinic or hospital. With hypodermoclysis, isotonic fluids are infused into the subcutaneous space through a small gauge needle inserted at various sites, including the thighs, back, abdomen, and arms. Fluids can be infused using gravity or a pump at rates of 20 to 125 mL/hr. Over 24 hours, up to 1.5 L can be delivered at one site or 3 L using two sites. Hyaluronidase, an enzyme, may or may not be added to facilitate absorption (Remington and Hultman, 2007).

Advantages/Disadvantages

The following are advantages of hypodermoclysis: (1) it can be administered, after training, in a variety of patient care settings, including the home; (2) it appears to be well accepted by patients and is cost-effective when compared to IV therapy (Slesak et al, 2003); (3) it avoids the need to transfer the patient to another setting; and (4) it does not require venipuncture. The following are disadvantages: (1) local site discomfort or edema, (2) limited application in certain patient conditions, and (3) not effective in emaciated or hypoalbuminemic patients who are edematous. Hypodermoclysis is contraindicated in emergency situations and for patients needing immediate fluid replacement, patients needing large-volume fluid replacement, and patients who require electrolyte-free or hypertonic solutions (Walsh, 2005). Patients with bleeding disorders or skin conditions limiting suitable sites for access device placement are not candidates for hypodermoclysis (Walsh, 2005). Hypodermoclysis is also contraindicated when the patient may be at increased risk for pulmonary congestion or edema, such as severe congestive heart failure (Sasson and Shvartzman, 2001).

ASSESSMENT OF PATIENT BEFORE THERAPY

In addition to other nursing assessments, the patient receiving CSI should have the following assessment parameters evaluated before therapy is initiated:

- Verify physician's order for patient's name, drug name, type of medication, dosage, and route of administration against the medication administration record (MAR).
- Collect drug information necessary to administer drug safely, including action, purpose, side effects, safe dosage range, and nursing implications. Verify that medication can be given through this route.
- Assess the patient's medical history, drug allergies, and medication history.
- Assess for factors that may contraindicate CSI, such as circulatory shock, reduced local tissue perfusion, or pulmonary congestion.
- Assess adequacy of the patient's subcutaneous tissue and skin condition to determine appropriate site.
- Assess patient/family knowledge regarding medication to be received and readiness to learn self-administration.
- Assess the patient's symptoms before initiating the medication therapy. (NOTE: When administering analgesia, assess the patient's level of pain using the appropriate pain scale [Perry and Potter, 2006].) The advanced practice nurse, physician, or pharmacist determines drug dose based on the amount of pain medication the patient used in 24 hours. An equianalgesic chart is used to convert IV, IM, and oral medication doses to CSI doses (Pasero, 2002).
- Check the compatibility of any medications combined in the infusions.

INITIATION OF CONTINUOUS SUBCUTANEOUS INFUSION
Site Selection

Before initiation of therapy, carefully assess the patient's skin condition and the adequacy of subcutaneous tissue stores. Anatomical sites used for subcutaneous injections and the upper chest may be used for CSI (Perry and Potter, 2006). The anterior thigh is more commonly used for subcutaneous injection and the outer thigh area is more commonly used for CSI (Figure 26-1).

Site selection will depend on the patient's activity level, subcutaneous tissue stores, and the type of medication required. For example, pain medications delivered to ambulatory patients are best delivered in the upper chest (infraclavicular area) to allow maximum mobility (Perry and Potter, 2006). In the confused patient, the posterior scapula area may inhibit the patient from pulling at the site (Anderson and Shreve, 2004). Insulin is absorbed most consistently in the abdomen; thus a site in the abdomen away from the belt line is preferred for a continuous insulin infusion (Perry and Potter, 2006). Generally, sites should be located away from the waistline, areas of constriction from clothing, and areas of large underlying muscles or nerves. Avoid bony prominences, irritated or infected sites, and sites around tumors, deep creases, recently radiated areas, and other skin lesions. CSI is not contraindicated for cachectic patients (Pasero, 2002); however, available sites may be limited. The upper abdomen is a recommended site for patients with limited peripheral subcutaneous tissue (Perry and Potter, 2006). Some sources recommend avoiding the chest wall to prevent iatrogenic lung puncture during needle insertion (Weissman, 2005).

Equipment/Supplies

Gather all equipment and supplies before initiating the infusion. An electronic infusion device (EID) is required for all medication infusions. The EID must have a lock-out interval feature, bolus dosing options, and appropriate clinical safety alarms. For subcutaneous infusions of isotonic fluids, an EID or add-on flow regulator may be used to control the fluid infusion rate. Other general supplies include aseptic nonsterile gloves, administration sets, transparent semipermeable membrane (TSM) dressings, tape, gauze pads, alcohol wipes, skin disinfectants, and a subcutaneous access device (e.g., over-the-needle catheter or prepackaged subcutaneous set) (Figure 26-2). Commercially prepared start kits contain the basic supplies; however, a tourniquet is not needed since venipuncture is not required.

Patient preparation

After the orders from an authorized prescriber are verified, the equipment and supplies are assembled, and the patient is properly identified following organizational guidelines. Care is taken to provide privacy and to explain all procedures and rationales to the patient and/or family. Educational materials are provided, if applicable, and time is allowed for questions and answers. Ensure the patient's readiness by assisting the patient to a position of comfort. If initiating an opioid infusion for pain management, assess the patient's pain rating before starting the subcutaneous infusion.

Site preparation

According to the *Infusion Nursing Standards of Practice* "Aseptic technique shall be used and standard precautions shall be observed for subcutaneous access." (INS, 2006a) Hand hygiene is performed before and after all patient care contact. Site preparation for CSI is done in the same manner as for venipuncture. If the skin is visibly soiled, wash the selected site with soap and water before applying skin disinfectants and follow organizational guidelines for site preparation. Excess hair may be clipped with scissors or removed with single-use surgical clippers that have disposable clipper heads.

Device selection

Currently, there are three device options for accessing subcutaneous tissue for infusion of medications or isotonic fluids: (1) stainless steel winged needles, (2) over-the-needle catheters,

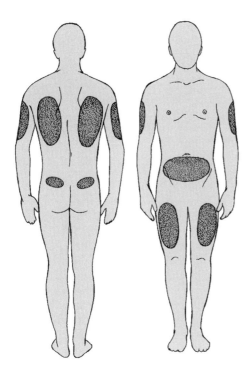

FIGURE 26-1   Common sites for subcutaneous injections. (From Potter PA, Perry AG: *Basic nursing: essentials for practice,* ed 6, St Louis, 2007, Mosby.)

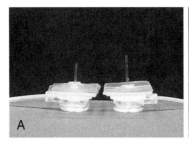 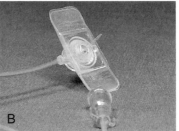

FIGURE 26-2   A, Medtronic standard and micro catheter. **B,** Medtronic Sof-Set. (From Applied Medical Technology, Cambridge, United Kingdom.)

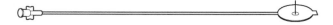

FIGURE 26-3   Sub-Q-Set. (Courtesy Baxter International, Inc., Deerfield, Ill.)

and (3) subcutaneous infusion sets (e.g., Sof-set, Sub-Q-Set). Traditionally, stainless-steel winged needles have been used to obtain subcutaneous access for infusion. However, these devices are intended for short-term duration IV infusions, usually 1 to 4 hours, or a single dose of medication. Over-the-needle catheters (e.g., Vialon™, Teflon®) have been used with reports of increased patient comfort, and decreased risk of tissue damage to the patient or inadvertent needlestick injury to the health care provider. A small gauge over-the-needle catheter (usually 24 gauge) can provide safe and comfortable access into the subcutaneous tissue.

Currently, prepackaged subcutaneous access devices are commercially available with a 90-degree angle needle or a 90-degree angle over-the-needle catheter. These devices are made in a 6- or 9-mm length for optimal access to the subcutaneous tissue (Figure 26-3). A special infusion set is now available exclusively for hypodermoclysis. The Aqua-C Hydration system (Norfolk Medical, Skokie, Ill) combines infusion tubing with an integrated flow regulator spiked into a solution container. The access device is called a "clysis strip" and has two 25- or 27-gauge, 6-mm-long needles placed 1.5 inches apart on an adhesive vinyl strip attached to the end of the tubing (Figure 26-4) (Walsh, 2005).

The needle design allows two sites to be accessed with one device and minimizes the risk of improper needle placement. Using the Aqua-C Hydration system, the maximum infusion rate can be achieved with a single administration setup. The use of a specialized set for hypodermoclysis may also decrease the possibility of mistaking the subcutaneous infusion for an intravenous infusion (Walsh, 2005). According to the *Infusion Nursing Standards of Practice* (2006a), the selected continuous subcutaneous access device should be of the smallest gauge and shortest length necessary to establish subcutaneous access. The National Institute of Occupational Safety and Health (NIOSH, 1999) reports that hollow-bore needles incur the greatest risks of needlestick injuries to health care workers. Of nearly 5000 percutaneous injuries reported by hospitals participating in CDC studies between June 1995 and July 1999, 62% were associated with hollow-bore needles, primarily hypodermic needles attached to syringes (29%) and winged-steel needles (13%). Data from these studies showed that approximately 38% of injuries occur during use and 42% occur after use and before disposal (NIOSH, 1999). Recommendations for avoiding potential needlestick injuries include eliminating unnecessary use of needles, using devices with safety features, and promoting

education and safe work practices for handling needles and related systems (NIOSH, 1999).

Device placement

Insert the subcutaneous device according to the manufacturer's instructions. Over-the-needle catheters are placed into the subcutaneous tissue at approximately a 30- to 45-degree angle depending on the thickness of the subcutaneous tissue. Prepackaged subcutaneous access devices are inserted at a 90-degree angle. These devices are manufactured at specific lengths to optimize access to the subcutaneous tissue, depending on the thickness of the subcutaneous layer.

Device securement and dressing

Subcutaneous access devices are secured with tape and transparent semipermeable membrane (TSM) dressings to allow for site observation and palpation. The administration set and/or pump should be clearly labeled "Subcutaneous Infusion" to prevent the possibility of mistaking the infusion for an intravenous line. Preprinted manufactured labels are available to identify subcutaneous infusions.

SITE ASSESSMENT AND MAINTENANCE
Monitoring

The frequency of monitoring of the subcutaneous infusion site will depend on the patient care setting, the type of medication, whether medications or solutions are being infused, and the overall condition of the patient's skin and subcutaneous tissue. The site may be monitored as frequently as every 2 hours in an acute care setting, to twice daily or daily in the home. Organizational policies should address the frequency of site monitoring.

Site rotation

The subcutaneous infusion site is generally rotated every 3 to 5 days (INS, 2006b) with some sites documented as lasting up to 7 days. Sites should be discontinued when there are signs of complications and restarted in a new location. A decrease in symptom control in the absence of a worsening condition could indicate poor or altered absorption, necessitating changing the site. At present, there appears to be no single protocol for maintaining the subcutaneous site (Anderson and Shreve, 2004).

Discontinuation

Discontinuing a subcutaneous infusion is a simple procedure requiring only a gauze pad and light pressure to the site after the needle or catheter is removed. Needles or subcutaneous access devices with needles must be disposed of in approved sharps containers.

POTENTIAL COMPLICATIONS

Potential complications of CSI or hypodermoclysis are itching or burning at the site, erythema, induration, leaking at the site, bleeding, edema, infection, or tissue slough.

These complications may be treated by providing local site care, rotating infusion sites, and limiting or eliminating irritating medications when possible.

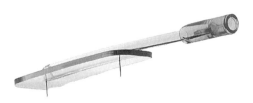

FIGURE 26-4   The Aqua-C Hydration set. (Courtesy Norfolk Medical Products Inc., Skokie, Ill.)

PROCEDURE FOR SUBCUTANEOUS DEVICE PLACEMENT

PATIENT ASSESSMENT AND EDUCATION

1. Obtain and verify physician's order.
2. Verify patient's identity.
3. Provide patient and/or family with educational material/ information regarding procedure.
4. Obtain patient's consent.
5. Assess patient.
6. Place patient in reclining position.

BEFORE BEGINNING PROCEDURE

1. Perform hand hygiene.
2. Apply clean, nonsterile gloves.
3. Use aseptic technique and observe Standard Precautions throughout procedure.

INSERTION SITE AND DEVICE SELECTION

1. Select insertion site with adequate subcutaneous tissue: a fat fold of at least 1 inch (2.5 cm) when thumb and index finger are pinched together. Site selection is also based on patient's anticipated mobility and comfort (and the medication ordered). Sites may include:
   - Supraclavicular area
   - Anterior chest wall (avoid in patients with cachexia)
   - Lower abdomen
   - Outer aspects of the arms and thigh
2. Avoid areas that are:
   - Scarred
   - Infected
   - Irritated
   - Edematous
   - Bony
   - Highly vascular
   - Near the waistline
3. Select access device with smallest gauge and shortest length necessary to establish subcutaneous access.
   - Over-the-needle catheter (22-24 gauge): Insert at 30- to 45-degree angle depending on thickness of subcutaneous tissue.
   - Subcutaneous infusion set (25-27 gauge; specific lengths available to optimize access depending upon thickness of subcutaneous tissue): Insert at 90-degree angle.

INSERTION SITE PREPARATION

1. Wash insertion site with antiseptic soap and water if skin is visibly soiled.
2. Remove excess hair from insertion site, if necessary (do not shave).
3. Disinfect insertion site per organizational guidelines.

DEVICE PLACEMENT AND INITIATION

1. Follow manufacturer's guidelines for access device placement.
2. Inspect access device for defects.

For continuous subcutaneous infusion

1. Prepare equipment and medication to be administered.
2. Inform patient of impending needlestick.
3. Lift skin into small mound between thumb and index finger.
4. Insert primed subcutaneous access device with attached infusion system into the skin (30- to 90-degree angle depending on the type of device and thickness of the subcutaneous tissue).
5. Aspirate to confirm absence of blood return. If blood return is visible, discontinue access device and select another site; repeat insertion procedure.
6. Stabilize access device.
7. Secure connection junctions.
8. Dress access site using transparent semipermeable membrane (TSM) dressing to allow for site observation and palpation.
9. Initiate therapy.
10. Label administration set and/or pump "Subcutaneous Infusion."

SITE CARE AND MAINTENANCE

1. Inspect access site and equipment:
   - Observe site for bleeding, bruising, inflammation, drainage, edema, or cellulitis.
   - Monitor patient for complaints regarding burning or itching at site.
   - Observe previous sites for signs of irritation or infection.
2. Change administration set immediately upon suspected contamination; otherwise, change administration set, including add-on devices and tubing, every 3 to 5 days as long as a closed system is maintained.
3. Change access site dressing immediately upon suspected contamination; otherwise, change TSM dressing every 3 to 5 days during site rotation.
4. Rotate access site every 3 to 5 days. Select a new site at least 1 inch from previous site, preferably dependent on patient comfort.

POST-INSERTION

1. Do not flush subcutaneous access device.
2. Discard used equipment and supplies.
3. Remove gloves.
4. Perform hand hygiene.
5. Document all procedures, patient education, and patient response to procedure in the patient's medical record.

From Infusion Nurses Society: *Policies and procedures for infusion nursing,* ed 3, Norwood, Mass, 2006b, Author.

INTRAOSSEOUS ACCESS

OVERVIEW

It has been over 90 years since infusion of fluids through the bone marrow (intraosseous infusion) was first demonstrated (Drinker et al, 1922). Subsequent research demonstrating the adequacy of the intraosseous (IO) route (Papper, 1942; Tocantins et al, 1941) in the 1930s and 1940s popularized this method of fluid administration. Further studies led to the intraosseous route being routinely adapted by military personnel during World War II to establish vascular access in shock patients with difficult IV access (Morrison, 1946).

However, in the 1950s and 1960s the introduction of disposable medical supplies that allowed the prolonged use of intravenous infusion while reducing the risk of dislodgement quickly overshadowed the benefits of IO methodology and the use of this technique declined sharply. It was not until the 1980s, when numerous studies quantified the ease and reliability of the IO method for pediatric patients, that the procedure regained notoriety for that patient population. With advances in pediatric resuscitation, IO access made a significant reappearance and became a clinical standard of treatment in pediatrics (Turkel, 1983; Orlowski, 1984).

Additional studies in the late 1980s supported the overall reliability of intraosseous access for obtaining most laboratory values and affirmed that they were representative of the general circulation (Grisham and Gastings, 1991). The method was also validated as a viable one for administering virtually all infusates. These later studies opened the door for wider application to the adult population with critical access needs.

Today IO methodology has been recognized by the American Heart Association (AHA) as a standard of alternative vascular access and is cited in the algorithms for American Heart Association Advanced Cardiac Life Support (ACLS) and Pediatric Advanced Life Support (PALS) treatment protocols (AHA, 2006a,b). It is a valuable resource as an alternative method of vascular access when IV cannulation is not feasible or is delayed. A resurgence in use has also been supported by advancements in prehospital resuscitation and emergency medicine (Miller et al, 2005).

INDICATIONS AND CONTRAINDICATIONS FOR USE

The indications for use of the IO route focus on urgent or emergent need for venous access. The treatment and resuscitation of patients experiencing shock, venous collapse, or difficult vascular access have long been noted as a challenge for medical personnel (Fowler et al, 2007). While intravenous access is the preferred administration route, if patient care is compromised because of inability to rapidly establish IV access, then the IO route should be considered. Recently published ACLS guidelines direct IO medication administration as a preferred route over the endotracheal route (AHA, 2006a,b). The new guidelines also support IO as the preferential placement versus that of a central VAD during cardiopulmonary resuscitation (CPR) if peripheral access is unobtainable. Intraosseous routes are temporary solutions to emergent patient situations.

Intraosseous access is an effective route for fluid resuscitation; bolus, drug, and blood and blood product administration; and lab evaluation in all age groups. Any drug or fluid that is appropriate for IV administration can be given via the IO route (AHA Guidelines, 2006a,b). Generally, the volume of fluid given per minute is similar to the rate of fluids infused through a 21-gauge catheter (Miller et al, 2005). Studies by Orlowski (1984) show similar physiological effects and serum drug levels in comparison trials of intravenous and intraosseous routes. Almost any drug, blood product, or resuscitation solution such as 0.9% sodium chloride that can be given intravenously can be given by intraosseous infusion with comparable absorption and effectiveness (Fowler et al, 2007).

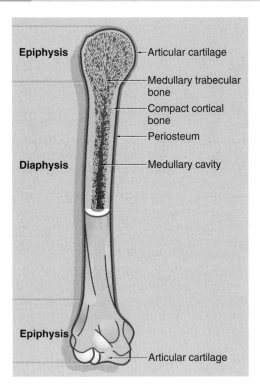

FIGURE 26-5   Intraosseous space. (From Young B et al: *Wheater's functional histology*, ed 5, London, 2006, Churchill Livingstone.)

The most common contraindication for use is bone fracture in the area of IO needle placement. Other contraindications include cellulitis over the insertion site, and diseases such as osteogenesis imperfecta, osteopetrosis, and osteoporosis (Miner et al, 1989; LaRocco and Wang, 2003).

ANATOMY AND PHYSIOLOGY RELATED TO IO THERAPY

The term intraosseous space defines the spongy bone of the epiphysis and the medullary cavity of the diaphysis (Figure 26-5). The intraosseous space is commonly referred to as a noncollapsible vein. Located within the medullary cavity and central to the thin wall of the bone, this space is filled with bone marrow. The marrow consists of blood, a network of blood-producing cells, and connective tissue. This space is directly connected to the central circulation and remains patent, independent of central vasculature collapse or injury (Tocantins et al, 1941).

This space contains thousands of tiny intertwined blood vessels of the yellow and red bone marrow that act like sponges with central circulation for any fluid that comes into the space. Infants and children have only red marrow that changes into yellow marrow in adulthood. While the marrow changes throughout the lifetime in humans, there is no difference in the absorption rates of solutions and medications infused into either type of marrow (VonHoff et al, 2008).

Within the vasculature of the intraosseous space, blood flow remains steady even in shock states. Pressure in the IO space is approximately 35/25 mm Hg or about one third of systemic pressure. Research dating back to the 1940s established that IV and IO infusion had nearly identical effective fluid administration times delivered to the general circulation (Papper, 1942).

TYPES OF IO NEEDLES AND DEVICES

Historically, IO devices have consisted of steel needles with removable trocars. Early practitioners noted the risk of perforating the sternum and puncturing the heart and subsequently developed devices with special trocars and guards to protect against unintentional deep placement (Bailey, 1944). The trocars prevented bone fragments from plugging the insertion site. Special handled and "threaded" shafts of the needles allowed the operator to push the large gauge needle into the bone with a rotating movement. This technique proved optimally successful in pediatric patients with soft bones; however, the thrust pressure necessary for the hard bones in adult patients made it difficult to provide easy and timely IO access. Recently, improved designs and mechanical advances (many using spring-loaded needles) have made IO applications as quick and easy in adults as is in children.

SITE SELECTION

The most common site in the adult patient for IO placement is the sternum; however, other sites may include the proximal tibia, distal femur, radius, ulna, pelvis, clavicle, and calcaneous. In small children and infants the sites available are the tibia, femur, and iliac crest. Site selection should not interfere with treatment interventions such as CPR, spinal immobilization, or treatments (Iserson, 1989; Foex, 2000). Verification of optimal placement is confirmed not by aspiration, but by free flow of fluids into the site. In pediatric patients, optimal placement is the distal femur or proximal tibia.

INSERTION TECHNIQUES

IO insertion uses a range of devices from hand-turned and screwed insertion needles to rapid needle insertion by gun devices. Current IO devices fall into the following three categories: manual, impact-driven, and powered drill. However, any needle can be used, including a steel-winged needle, spinal needle, or bone marrow biopsy needle (a 16- to 18-gauge needle is recommended). Proper placement in the bone marrow is confirmed by assessment of the needle position and flushing with 5 to 10 mL of 0.9% sodium chloride bolus injections that should enter by free-flow or infuse without resistance. The needle should stand up straight as a result of the cortex of the bone holding the needle in position. Aspiration of blood or marrow is not necessary to confirm placement. Because multiple cannulation of a single bone could lead to extravasations, only one IO attempt should be made to each bone. If the cannulation site is to be used less than 24 hours, the needle may be replaced using the same site. Sites of insertion in the adult patient include the iliac crest, femur, proximal and distal tibia, humerus, radius, and clavicle. Preferred insertion sites in the pediatric patient (under 6 years of age) are distal tibia, proximal tibia, and distal femur (Figure 26-6) (INS, 2006b).

CARE AND MAINTENANCE

Once the IO device is inserted, it should be covered with a transparent, occlusive dressing. Assessment of the surrounding tissue for signs and symptoms of infiltration should be performed on a regular basis. Nursing responsibilities may include initiation of access, assessment and maintenance of the site, and termination of access, along with appropriate documentation in the

PROCEDURE FOR INTRAOSSEOUS NEEDLE INSERTION

1. Ensure that none of the following contraindications are present:
   - No bone fractures
   - No previous orthopedic procedures
   - Extremity is not compromised by a preexisting medical condition
   - No infection present over insertion site
   - No cellulitis
2. Perform hand hygiene.
3. Apply nonsterile gloves.
4. Locate appropriate site for IO insertion.
5. Clean skin with antiseptic solution.
6. Disinfect insertion site.
7. Allow site to air-dry.
8. Consider applying a local anesthetic.
9. Insert IO needle using one of the following methods:
   - Hand-turned
   - Pressure
   - Mechanical drill
10. The needle is inserted into the bone until a loss of resistance or a "pop" is felt (indication of entry into the bone).
11. Confirm proper placement:
    - IO catheter stands straight up at a 90-degree angle and is firmly seated in bone.
    - There is a free-flow of fluids without difficulty with no evidence of infiltration at site.
12. Attach the primed administration set with a Luer-Lok™ designed extension and then flush the IO space with 5-10 mL of 0.9% sodium chloride.
13. Initiate the infusion.
14. Secure device and administration set.
15. Apply designated wristband (per organizational policies) noting presence of IO needle.
16. Monitor IO site for 24 hours. After 24 hours, obtain an order for alternative access.
17. Document procedure in patient's permanent record.

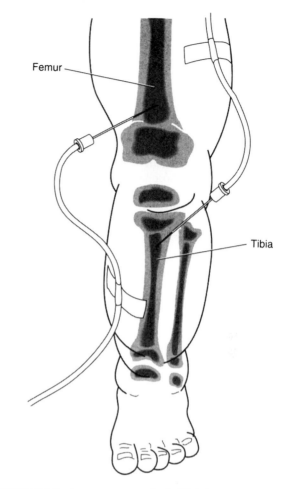

FIGURE 26-6   Intraosseous access sites for IV infusion.

PATIENT OUTCOMES

Expected outcomes with IO or subcutaneous access devices include:
- The patient will experience minimal discomfort during the insertion of an IO or subcutaneous access device.
- The patient will have effective control of symptoms or disease state by fluids and/or medications infused via an IO or subcutaneous access device.
- The patient will have medications effectively delivered via an IO or subcutaneous access device without experiencing local or systemic complications.
- The patient will remain free from infection associated with the insertion of an IO or subcutaneous access device.
- The patient will remain free of complications related to IO or subcutaneous administration.

medical record. Documentation should address the presence of any abnormal findings including redness, warmth, or drainage. The site, after discontinuation of the IO device, should be dressed daily until no drainage is present.

COMPLICATIONS

The risks and complications of the IO route are few. The most common complication is extravasation of fluid. Because IO methodology for infusion therapy is considered a temporary solution, it is necessary to define the optimal dwell time of the IO needle as less than 24 hours. Possible complications of this methodology, though rare, include dislodgments, bone fracture, pain, compartment syndrome, and infection. Complications using this method of access include needle obstruction, osteomyelitis (rare), improper needle placement, or embolization of fat or bony fragments.

SUMMARY

For various reasons there are instances that intravenous access cannot be established in certain patients. Fortunately, there are alternative infusion devices that allow these patients to receive the solutions and medications necessary for treatment. Viable alternatives include medication delivery by continuous subcutaneous infusions and administration of isotonic solutions by hypodermoclysis. Intraosseous access, although reserved for urgent and emergency care, is finding its place in pediatric, emergency, prehospital, and trauma situations to support the access needs of the most fragile patients. Future indications and research opportunities are needed to address possible applications that will benefit patients while enhancing conventional infusion practices.

REFERENCES

Abbas SQ, Yeldham M, Bell M: The use of metal or plastic needles in continuous subcutaneous infusion in a hospice setting, *Am J Hospice Palliative Care* 22:134-138, 2005.

American Heart Association Guidelines for Advanced Cardiovascular Life Support, Dallas, Tex, 2006, Author.

American Heart Association Guidelines: for Pediatric Advanced Life Support, Dallas, Tex, 2006, Author.

Anderson S, Shreve S: Continuous subcutaneous infusion of opiates at end-of-life, *Ann Pharmacother* 38:1015-1023, 2004.

Bailey H: Bone marrow as a site for the reception of infusions, transfusion, and anesthetic agents, *Brit Med J (Clinical Research edition)* 2:181-182, 1944.

Cuzell J, Workman ML: Assessment of the skin, hair, and nails. In Ignatavicius D, Workman ML, editors: *Medical surgical nursing: critical thinking for collaborative care*, ed 5, St Louis, 2006, Saunders.

Dawkins L, Britton D, Johnson I et al: A randomized trial of winged Vialon cannulae and metal butterfly needles, *Int J Palliative Nurs* 6(3):110-116, 2000.

Drinker CK, Drinker KR, Lund CC: The circulation in the mammalian bone marrow, *Am J Physiol* 62:1-92, 1922.

Foex BA: Discovery of the intraosseous route for fluid administration, *JAEM* 17(2):136-137, 2000.

Fowler R, Gallagher JV, Isaacs M et al: The role of intraosseous vascular access in the out-of-hospital environment, *Prehospital Emerg Care* 11(1):63-66, 2007.

Grisham J, Gastings C: Bone marrow aspirates, an accessible and reliable source for critical laboratory studies, *Ann Emerg Med* 20:1221-1224, 1991.

Infusion Nurses Society: Infusion nursing standards of practice, *J Infus Nurs* 29(1 Suppl):S1–S92, 2006a.

Infusion Nurses Society: *Policies and procedures for infusion nursing*, ed 3, Norwood, Mass, 2006b, Author.

Iserson K: Intraosseous infusions in adults, *J Emerg Med* 7(6):587-591, 1989.

LaRocco B, Wang H: Intraosseous infusion, *Prehosp Emerg Care* 7(2):280-285, 2003.

Miller L, Kramer GC, Bolleter S: Rescue access made easy, *JEMS* (Suppl S8–S18), 2005.

Miner WE, Corneli HM, Bolte RG et al: Prehospital use of intraosseous infusion by paramedics, *Pediatric Emerg Care* 5(1):5-7, 1989.

Morrison GM: The initial care of casualties, *Am Practitioner* 1:183-184, 1946.

Neafsey PJ: Efficacy of subcutaneous infusion in patients with cancer pain, *Home Healthcare* 23(7):421-423, 2005.

Negro S, Azuara M, Sanchez Y et al: Physical compatibility and in vivo evaluation of drug mixtures for subcutaneous infusions to cancer patients in palliative care, *Support Care Cancer* 10:65-70, 2002.

NIOSH Alert: *Preventing needlestick injuries in health care settings*, NIOSH Publ. No. 2000-108, Nov 1999.

Orlowski JP: My kingdom for an intravenous line, *Am J Dis Children* 138:803, 1984.

Papper EM: The bone marrow route for injecting fluids and drugs into the general circulation, *Anesthesiology* 3:307-313, 1942.

Pasero C: Subcutaneous opioid infusion, *Am J Nurs* 7(102):61-62, 2002.

Perry AG, Potter PA: *Clinical nursing skills & techniques*, ed 6, St Louis, 2006, Mosby.

Phillips LD: *Manual of IV therapeutics*, ed 4, Philadelphia, 2005, FA Davis.

Potter PA, Perry AG: *Basic nursing: essentials for practice*, ed 6, St Louis, 2007, Mosby.

Remington R, Hultman T: Hypodermoclysis to treat dehydration: a review of the evidence, *J Am Geriatr Soc* 55(12):2051-2055, 2007.

Ross J, Saunders Y, Cochrane M et al: A prospective, within-patient comparison between metal butterfly needles and Teflon cannulae in subcutaneous infusion of drugs to terminally ill hospice patients, *Palliative Med* 16(1):13-16, 2002.

Sasson M, Shvartzman P: Hypodermoclysis: an alternative infusion technique, *Am Family Physician* 9(64), 2001.

Slesak G, Schnurle J, Kinzel E et al: Comparison of subcutaneous and intravenous rehydration in geriatric patients: a randomized trial, *J Am Geriatr Soc* 51(2):155-160, 2003.

Tocantins LM, O'Neill JF, Jones HW: Infusions of blood and other fluids via the bone marrow: application in pediatrics, *JAMA* 117:1229-1234, 1941.

Torre MC: Subcutaneous infusion: non-metal cannulae vs metal butterfly needles, *Brit J Community Nurs* 7(7):365-369, 2002.

Turkel H: Intraosseous infusion, *Am J Dis Children* 137:706, 1983.

VonHoff DD, Kuhn JG, Burris HA et al: Does intraosseous equal intravenous: a pharmacokinetic study, *AJEM* 26(12):31-38, 2008.

Walsh G: Hypodermoclysis—an alternate method for rehydration in long term care, *J Infus Nurs* 28(2):123-129, 2005.

Weissman DE: *Subcutaneous opioid infusions fast fact and concept #28*, ed 2, July 2005, End-of-Life Palliative Education Resource Center. Accessed from www.eperc.mcw.edu.

Young: *Wheater's functional histology*, ed 5, London, 2006, Churchill Livingstone.

27 INTRASPINAL ACCESS AND MEDICATION ADMINISTRATION

Candace K. Stearns, MN, FNP-BC, ONP-C and Jeannine M. Brant, PhD, APRN, AOCN*

Intraspinal access devices are defined as those in the epidural, intrathecal, or ventricular spaces (INS, 2006). The infusion of medications into the intraspinal spaces, a practice employed for decades, involves a multitude of medications, including chemotherapeutic agents, opiates, local anesthetics, alpha$_2$-adrenergic blockers, and N-type calcium channel blockers, as well as others. The infusion of analgesic agents into the intraspinal spaces is sometimes considered the fourth step in the World Health Organization's (WHO) ladder for pain management, that is, the step after other treatment options have been exhausted. Nurses may encounter the intraspinal route of medication administration and access devices in a variety of practice settings from acute care to outpatient and home care (e.g., postoperatively, women in labor, chronic malignant and nonmalignant pain, spasticity control), and as such should demonstrate competency when caring for a patient with this type of device (INS, 2006). The purpose of this chapter is to provide an overview of the intraspinal route of administration. Spinal anatomy, neuropharmacology, assessment of placement and function of the access device, care and maintenance practices, and potential complications shall be addressed. There is a wide array of intraspinal uses; however, this chapter will focus on the infusion of analgesic medications, the most common use of the intraspinal route.

Throughout this chapter, it is important to keep in mind that each state varies in regards to the nursing scope of practice and in the management of intraspinal infusions. Nurses must take responsibility for consulting their individual state board of nursing rules and regulations to ensure actions are within the scope of practice for their individual education level. Some activities are limited to nurses with advanced training, such as Certified Registered Nurse Anesthetists (CRNA), Clinical Nurse Specialists (CNS), or Nurse Practitioners (NP). In addition, the placement of an intraspinal access device is considered a surgical procedure, and placement is dictated by practice laws as well. Additionally, the nurse must follow individual

organizational guidelines and attain and maintain competency for the management of intraspinal infusions and devices (INS, 2006). The following summary describes spinal anatomy and the locations in which intraspinal analgesia and other medications are delivered.

SPINAL ANATOMY

SPINAL STRUCTURE

The spine is divided into four regions—cervical, thoracic, lumbar, and sacral. The spinal column consists of 33 individual vertebrae that are referred to by their location in 1 of 5 regions. The spinal column consists of 7 cervical, 12 thoracic, 5 lumbar, 5 fused sacral, and 4 fused coccygeal vertebrae. Each vertebra consists of an anterior body—the lamina—that protects the lateral spinal cord, and spinous processes that project posteriorly and outwardly from the laminae (Figures 27-1 and 27-2).

The spinal cord itself begins at the base of the skull (foramen magnum) and passes through the vertebral canal of the spinal column. In adults, the spinal cord terminates at the first or second lumbar vertebra. Here, it splits into the cauda equina, which are the lumbar and sacral nerve roots. The spinal cord is located within the bony vertebral column and connective tissues, providing protection from outside injury. The cord consists of a central region of gray matter surrounded by bundles of white matter. The butterfly-shaped gray matter consists of two dorsal (posterior) horns that extend toward the dorsolateral surfaces of the cord and two thicker ventral (anterior) horns that extend toward the ventrolateral surfaces. The right and left regions of gray matter are connected by a gray transverse band of nerve fibers that crosses the middle of the cord. In the middle of the gray band of nerve fibers is the central canal, which is filled with cerebrospinal fluid. The size of the white and gray matter varies according to the function of the spinal segment. White matter is made of approximately 80% lipids. The dorsal horn of the spinal cord is part of the gray matter and is rich in opioid receptors (see Figures 27-3 and 27-4) (Saladin and Porth, 1998; Ghafoor et al, 2007).

*The author and editors wish to acknowledge the contributions made by Barbara St. Marie in the second edition of *Infusion Therapy in Clinical Practice*.

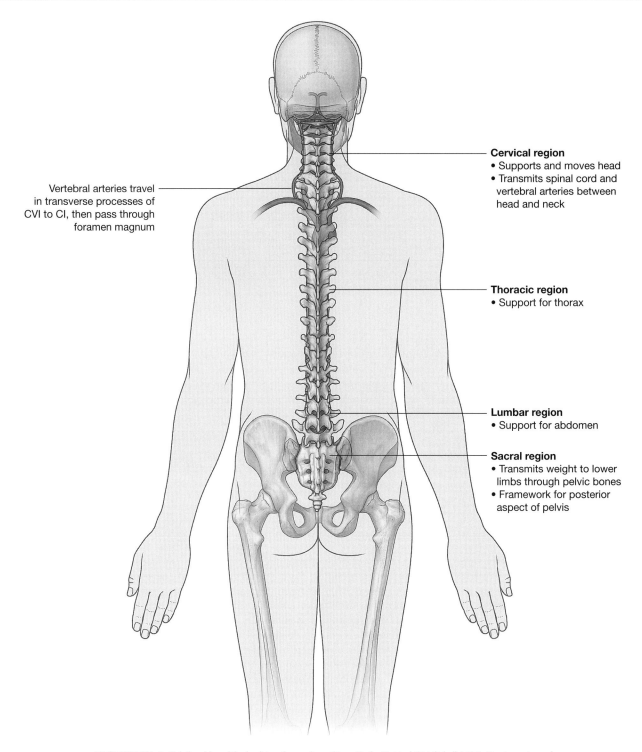

Vertebral arteries travel
in transverse processes of
CVI to CI, then pass through
foramen magnum

Cervical region
• Supports and moves head
• Transmits spinal cord and
  vertebral arteries between
  head and neck

Thoracic region
• Support for thorax

Lumbar region
• Support for abdomen

Sacral region
• Transmits weight to lower
  limbs through pelvic bones
• Framework for posterior
  aspect of pelvis

FIGURE 27-1 Relationships of the back to other regions. (From Drake RL, Vogl W, Mitchell AMW: *Gray's anatomy for students,* London, 2005, Churchill Livingstone.)

SPINAL NERVES

The spinal cord gives rise to 31 pairs of spinal nerves (Figure 27-5). The portion of the spinal cord connected to each pair of nerves is called a segment of the cord. Dermatomes are delineated areas of skin innervated by a spinal cord segment (Figures 27-6 and 27-7). Each spinal nerve except C1 receives sensory input from these specific areas of the skin. This model is used to monitor the level of anesthesia and monitor sensations arising from each level. Dermatomes may overlap at their edges by as much as 50%. Therefore anesthetizing one sensory nerve root does not entirely deaden sensation from a dermatome. It is necessary to anesthetize or deaden three successive spinal nerves to produce a total loss of sensation from a dermatome (Saladin and Porth, 1998; McCaffery and Pasero, 1999). The nurse needs to be familiar with the dermatomes to adequately assess patients who receive intraspinal analgesia.

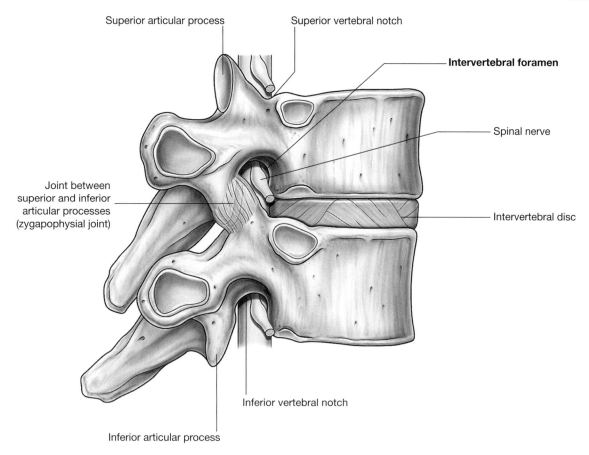

FIGURE 27-2 Intervertebral foramina. (From Drake RL, Vogl W, Mitchell AMW: *Gray's anatomy for students,* London, 2005, Churchill Livingstone.)

SPINAL MENINGES

The connective tissues that provide protection for the spinal cord are also called meninges. The three protective meninges are the dura mater, the arachnoid mater, and the pia mater. The outermost layer is the dura mater, which is the toughest membrane and consists of dense fibrous connective tissue. The arachnoid mater is a thin membrane covering the brain and spinal cord. The arachnoid mater is separated from the dura mater by the extradural or epidural space. The pia mater is the layer closest to the spinal cord and is composed of delicate connective tissue. This tissue clings tightly to the brain and spinal cord (Saladin and Porth, 1998). The epidural space is the area surrounding the spinal cord and its coverings (dura mater, arachnoid, and pia mater). It contains fatty tissue, veins, spinal arteries, and spinal nerves. The space extends from the foramen magnum to the sacrococcygeal membrane. Below the arachnoid space is the subarachnoid or intrathecal space, containing cerebrospinal fluid (CSF) (Saladin and Porth, 1998; McCaffery and Pasero, 1999; Maher et al, 2002). The cerebrospinal fluid that circulates in the intrathecal space is forced down the dorsal surface of the spinal cord and up the ventral side by the pulsatile flow of blood in the central nervous system, and has an important role in distribution of medications (Ghafoor et al, 2007). Drugs are carried upward or rostrally (toward the brain), which may increase the medications' effects away from the targeted area. This concept is referred to as rostral spread (see Figure 27-7) (McCaffery and Pasero, 1999; Ghafoor et al, 2007).

INTRASPINAL ROUTES

EPIDURAL

Epidural opioids are administered adjacent to the spinal cord, and diffuse across the dura mater and into the spine where they bind directly with opioid receptors to block the transmission of pain. Some of the analgesia is lost in the epidural vasculature during the diffusion process, leading to systemic absorption and increased sedation with greater rostral spread (Sloan, 2007). Most typically this type of access is used on a short-term basis (e.g., for postoperative pain management, during labor) (McCaffery and Pasero, 1999). Epidural devices should be aspirated to ascertain the absence of spinal fluid and blood before medication administration (INS, 2006). The doses of medications administered through the epidural route are much lower than systemic doses, approximately one tenth of an intravenous dose and 10 times higher than with the intrathecal route (American Pain Society, 2003).

INTRATHECAL

Intrathecal opioids are administered directly inside the spinal cord, eliminating the need to cross the lipid membrane (dura). This leads to faster action, thereby requiring lower doses of medications when administration is intrathecal rather than epidural (Brant, 1995). Intrathecal administration is often

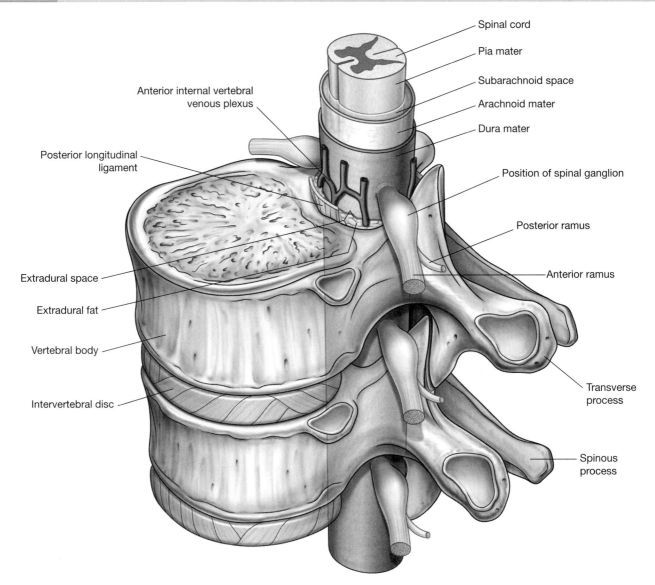

FIGURE 27-3 Vertebral canal. (From Drake RL, Vogl W, Mitchell AMW: *Gray's anatomy for students*, London, 2005, Churchill Livingstone.)

associated with long-term drug administration through catheters that have been surgically implanted. Nurses with advanced training and physicians may inject drugs into these catheters (Potter and Perry, 2007). A drug given intrathecally comes into direct contact with the spinal cord and therefore is effective at a much smaller dose than would be given epidurally. Intrathecal devices should be aspirated to ascertain the presence of spinal fluid and the absence of blood before medication administrations (INS, 2006).

INTRAVENTRICULAR ACCESS

Intraventricular access is usually obtained through a surgically implanted reservoir and provides direct access to ventricular cerebrospinal fluid. This type of access is used primarily to consistently and predictably deliver medications, most often antineoplastic drugs or pain medications, directly into the subarachnoid space and CSF. The majority of chemotherapeutic agents do not cross the blood-brain barrier, so the use

of this type of access device allows more targeted delivery to the source of the cancer. Most typically this type of access is used to target cancers of the head, neck, or spine, or for pain unrelieved by conventional methods (Brant, 1995; Burke et al, 2001). The use of this reservoir also allows samples of the CSF to be extracted for pathological examination and permits the measurement of CSF pressure, which avoids repeated lumbar punctures for the purposes of medication or sampling of CSF (Burke et al, 2001). Usually the volumes of medications administered are small (15 mL or less) and should be injected slowly. Patients receiving medications through this route must be monitored closely for neurotoxicity. Most often physicians will administer the medications through this access. An intraventricular reservoir is rarely removed once implanted unless the device malfunctions or the body develops an infection that cannot be resolved with the device in place. If removal is necessary, the intraventricular reservoir must be removed in surgery (Yarbro et al, 2000; Burke et al, 2001).

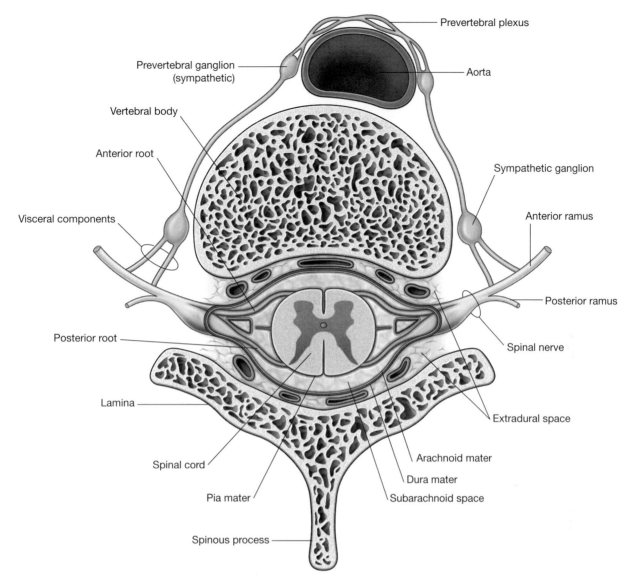

FIGURE 27-4 Spinal nerves (transverse section). (From Drake RL, Vogl W, Mitchell AMW: *Gray's anatomy for students,* London, 2005, Churchill Livingstone.)

EPIDURAL/INTRATHECAL CATHETERS AND ADMINISTRATION SYSTEMS

The choice of short-term or long-term systems for delivery of intraspinal infusion is based on patient needs, contraindications, and cost-benefit evaluations. Externalized systems are typically used for those patients with life expectancy less than 3 months. An implanted system is preferred when life expectancy is greater than 3 months (Krames, 2002; DuPen, 2005; Stearns et al, 2005). Pumps are available in programmable and nonprogrammable forms with reservoir capacities of between 10 mL and 50 mL. Programmable pumps allow immediate adjustments and bolus dosing for patients. Nonprogrammable pumps require dosage adjustments to be made by changing medication concentrations and do not allow rapid medication adjustments for pain control (Krames, 2002; DuPen, 2005). Pumps may be inserted using a local, spinal, or general anesthetic (see Figure 27-8). Additionally, placement is typically aided with the use of fluoroscopic guidance (Krames, 2002; Stearns et al, 2005). Site care of the implanted system is dependent on the individual agency's standards regarding postoperative wound management and the length of time since implantation. It is the nurse's responsibility to ensure familiarity and competency are maintained regarding individual agency pumps, and all users should be aware of factors that may affect the accuracy of medication delivery (Skyryabina and Dunn, 2006).

Intraspinal catheters may be temporary or permanent. Temporary, or "trialing," catheters are typically used for no longer than 7 days, such as in epidural or postoperative analgesia (Figure 27-9). However, they have been used for as long as 11 days for trials before placement of permanent catheters (Figure 27-10) (DuPen, 2005). Permanent catheters may be used for weeks to months. The permanent catheter is tunneled and has a Dacron cuff to aid in the stabilization of the catheter to the tissues. Many have a second Vita cuff impregnated with silver to reduce antimicrobial activity. These catheters are wire guided, which allows for tip advancement and precise positioning.

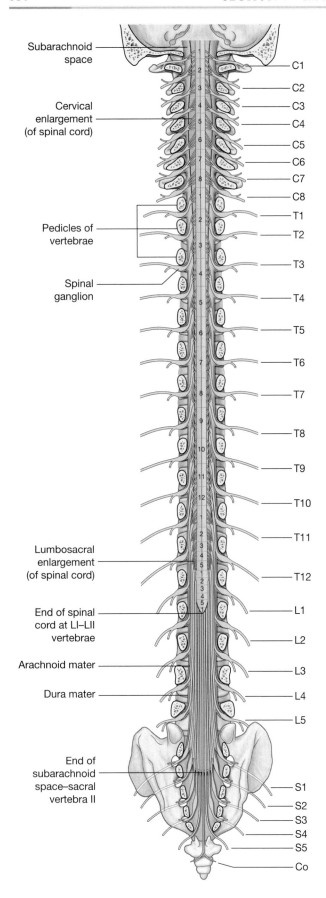

FIGURE 27-5 Vertebral canal, spinal cord, and spinal nerves. (From Drake RL, Vogl W, Mitchell AMW: *Gray's anatomy for students,* London, 2005, Churchill Livingstone.)

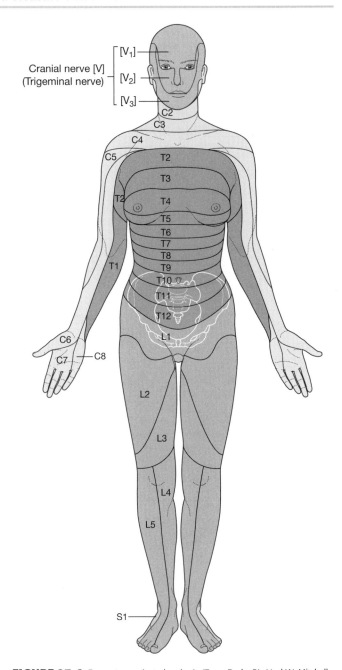

FIGURE 27-6 Dermatomes (anterior view). (From Drake RL, Vogl W, Mitchell AMW: *Gray's anatomy for students,* London, 2005, Churchill Livingstone.)

Catheters that are expected to be used longer than 3 months should be internalized. Catheters may break, disconnect at the site, migrate out of the intrathecal space or epidural space, or disconnect from the pump (Gooch et al, 2003; Albright et al, 2004).

Implanted ports may be used in an effort to decrease infection rates although there are no data to support this. Ports must still be continuously accessed for medication delivery. Care involves weekly transparent dressing change over the firmly secured noncoring needle.

Pump and catheter failures should be reported to allow for improvement in pumps and allow patients to make informed decisions (Gooch et al, 2003; INS, 2006). In children, more complications were found in patients who had implanted pumps with access ports.

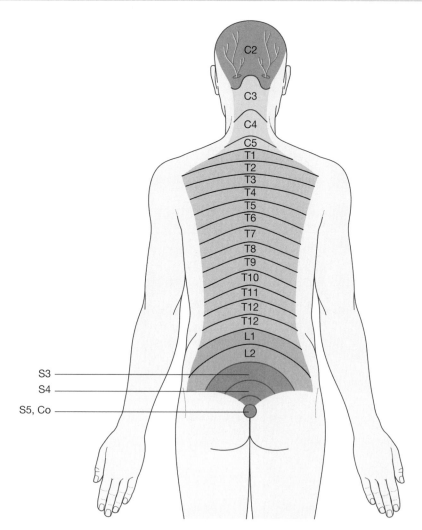

FIGURE 27-7 Dermatomes innervated by posterior rami of spinal nerves. (From Drake RL, Vogl W, Mitchell AMW: *Gray's anatomy for students,* London, 2005, Churchill Livingstone.)

MANAGEMENT OF PUMP DEVICES/ CATHETERS/PORTS

Management of the pump device is entirely dependent on the type of pump device used, and whether the pump device is implanted or external, programmable or nonprogrammable, and the manufacturer's instructions. Regardless of the type of pump used, all pumps should prevent free-flow of medications to avoid overadministration (INS, 2006).

 ## METHODS OF DRUG ADMINISTRATION

Infusion of intraspinal agents may be provided on a short-term or long-term basis. The infusion may be a one-time injection or may be a continuous infusion. Catheters themselves may be internal or external. If long-term intraspinal infusions are used, an implanted device and internal catheter may be warranted to avoid potential complications with infections, malfunctioning of the pump, and/or dislodgement of catheters (Stearns et al, 2005). Patients may receive continuous

or bolus medications, or a combination of both depending on the patient situation. A combination of medications may be provided. Additionally, patients may control the infusion (patient-controlled epidural analgesia [PCEA]). The expected length of time of infusion, method of delivery (intrathecal, intraventricular, or epidural), and patient condition will dictate the prescribed therapy.

Nurses must be aware of relative and absolute contraindications to the use of intraspinal analgesia. Relative contraindications may include spinal column deformities, laminectomy or low back pain, severe headaches or backaches, patients unable to cooperate, and unstable neurological disease. Absolute contraindications include patient refusal, infection at the puncture site, sepsis, allergy to local anesthetics and/or medications to be infused, coagulopathies, uncorrected hypovolemia, and active neurological disease (Brogan, 2006; Sloan, 2007). Contraindications when identified must be communicated by nurses to other members of the health care team. Nurses must also provide patient education, ensure informed consent is completed, and document actions and interventions according to organizational policy and standards of nursing care.

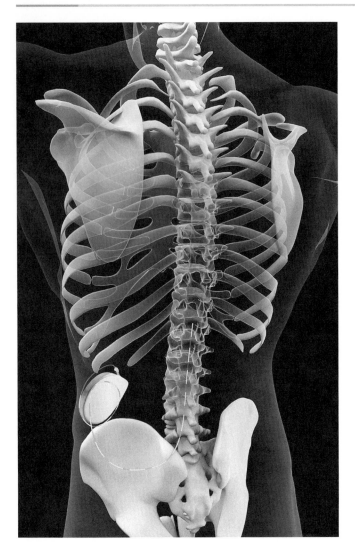

FIGURE 27-8 Spine with implanted pump. (Reprinted with permission from Medtronic, Inc. ©2008.)

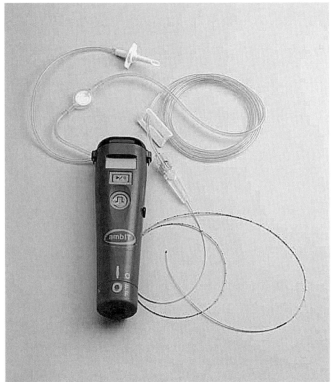

FIGURE 27-9 Trailing pump. (Reprinted with permission from Medtronic, Inc. ©2008.)

 MEDICATIONS

Medications administered may include opioids, alpha$_2$-adrenergics, local anesthetics, and chemotherapeutic agents. Regardless of the medication used, only medications that are preservative-free should be injected into the intraspinal space to avoid neurotoxicity (Prager, 2002; INS, 2006). Any drug packaged in a multidose vial likely has preservatives added and should not be used for intraspinal access (Prager, 2002). Epidural and intrathecal medications must diffuse from the cerebrospinal fluid to the dorsal horn of the spinal cord to produce analgesia (McCaffery & Pasero, 1999; Ghafoor et al, 2007). Doses required to obtain analgesic effects from intraspinal medications are much lower than those required to obtain analgesia from systemic administration, leading to decreased side effects (Kedlaya et al, 2002; Prager, 2002; Farrow-Gillespie and Kaplan, 2006; Cohen and Dragovich, 2007; Ghafoor et al, 2007). Doses are dependent on administration technique (i.e., one-time infusion, continuous), but must be adjusted based on age, weight, patient's opiate tolerance, and condition (American Pain Society, 2003). The onset, peak, and duration of action vary according to the pharmacokinetics of the particular medication.

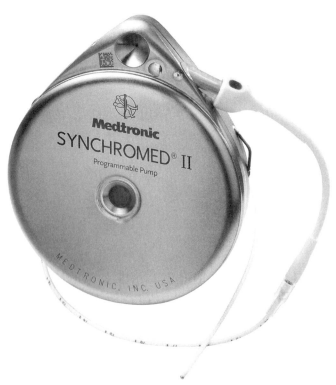

FIGURE 27-10 Programmable pump with catheter. (Reprinted with permission from Medtronic, Inc. ©2008.)

OPIOIDS

Morphine is considered the standard medication for starting spinal opioid therapy and the agent to which all others are compared. Morphine is a hydrophilic-type opiate and has high affinity for mu-receptors in the dorsal horn of the spinal cord. Hydrophilic opioids, like morphine, decline more slowly than lipophilic opioids in cerebrospinal fluid, which accounts for more rostral spread. This may also lead to delayed respiratory depression with initiation of this drug, and increased dermatomal analgesia during long-term administration (Pasero, 2003; Heitz and Viscusi, 2005; Cohen and Dragovich, 2007; Ghafoor et al, 2007; Sloan, 2007). Tolerance can develop when used for extended periods, which may lead to the need for dosage increases (Heitz and Viscusi, 2005). Epidural morphine is 5 to 10 times more potent than intravenous delivery (Kedlaya et al, 2002; American Pain Society, 2003).

Hydromorphone, also hydrophilic, may be used as an alternative to morphine (e.g., intolerability to morphine side effects, titrated doses continue to lack optimal analgesia) (Krames, 2002; Stearns et al, 2005). Hydromorphone has less rostral spread than morphine and an intermediate onset and duration of action (Kedlaya et al, 2002; American Pain Society, 2003). Given epidurally, it is five times more potent than the intravenous formulation (Kedlaya et al, 2002). The use of hydromorphone may produce less pruritus in comparison to morphine (Golembiewski et al, 2005).

Fentanyl and sufentanil are lipophilic in nature; therefore they have more rapid onset of analgesia and less rostral spread (Ghafoor et al, 2007). Fentanyl may have limited access to opiate receptors because of rapid clearing of the drug and more systemic uptake. This issue may lead to little advantage over intravenous infusions. Epidural fentanyl is considered to be equivalent to intravenous administration (Kedlaya et al, 2002; Heitz & Viscusi, 2005).

LOCAL ANESTHETICS

Local anesthetics are sodium channel antagonists and produce analgesia in the epidural space by diffusing across the dura mater to anesthetize nerve roots and the spinal cord (Kedlaya et al, 2002; Heitz and Viscusi, 2005). Many local anesthetics are suitable for epidural infusion, but lidocaine, bupivacaine, and ropivacaine are used most commonly in current practice (Ghafoor et al, 2007). Lidocaine has a fast onset but the shortest duration of action, and is therefore more useful for rescue dosing and catheter testing than for ongoing pain control. Repeated dosing of lidocaine has also been associated with tachyphylaxis (Heitz and Viscusi, 2005). Bupivacaine is often co-administered with morphine and may produce synergistic effects and therefore decrease morphine doses (Ghafoor et al, 2007). Bupivacaine also has the longest duration of action and has been the most extensively used. It does, however, carry a higher risk of cardiotoxicity (Heitz and Viscusi, 2005). Additionally, side effects may include motor blockade, hypotension, diarrhea, and urinary retention (Ghafoor et al, 2007). Ropivacaine, a newer agent, has been shown to have less motor blockade and less potential for cardiotoxicity (Heitz and Vuscusi, 2005).

ALPHA₂-ADRENERGIC AGONISTS

The primary effect of alpha₂-adrenergic drugs is activation of ascending inhibitory pathways on postsynaptic nociceptors in the dorsal horn, thereby blocking pain (Ghafoor et al, 2007).

Clonidine, the most widely used alpha₂-adrenergic agonist, is a centrally acting drug that was initially approved for use as an antihypertensive medication; however, because of sedating side effects, it has been more frequently used as an analgesic. Side effects may include hypotensive effects and dose-limiting toxicity when used as an analgesic. It is most commonly used in conjunction with morphine or bupivacaine (Heitz & Viscusi, 2005; Cohen and Dragovich, 2007). Besides hypotension, other side effects include sedation, nausea, dry mouth, and bradycardia. It is thought to be more effective than opiates in treating neuropathic pain (Kedlaya et al, 2002; Ghafoor et al, 2007).

GABA INHIBITORS

Activation of γ-aminobutyric acid (GABA) receptors results in a decrease in the release of neurotransmitters, and decreased opening of calcium channels to decrease pain. The most commonly used GABA inhibitor is baclofen (Cohen and Dragovich, 2007). Intrathecal administration of baclofen acts directly at the receptor sites in the spinal cord, yielding less systemic toxicity and better therapeutic effect (Zahavi et al, 2004). Baclofen is primarily used in the treatment of spasticity, but may be combined with other medications for pain control. Side effects may include hypotonia, sedation, constipation, erectile dysfunction, loss of sphincter control, and respiratory depression (Cohen and Dragovich, 2007; Ghafoor et al, 2007).

SELECTIVE N-TYPE CALCIUM CHANNEL BLOCKER

Ziconotide is a non-opioid analgesic that blocks pain transmission by binding with selective N-type voltage-sensitive calcium channels (Ghafoor et al, 2007). This drug must be administered intrathecally to maximize effectiveness. It is used to treat refractory pain in patients with cancer, autoimmune deficiency syndrome (AIDS), and/or chronic pain (Staats et al, 2004). Adverse effects include dizziness, nausea, asthenia, somnolence, diarrhea, confusion, and ataxia (Rauck et al, 2006).

COMPLICATIONS OF INTRASPINAL ACCESS DEVICES

Regardless of the method of delivery (epidural, intrathecal, or intraventricular) employed, complications of nonvascular access devices can be categorized as those related to the procedure, medication side effects, or complications related to the device itself. Familiarity with the type of infusions, catheters, and pumps as well as medication side effects is integral to nursing care provided to the patient, and to manage expected effects and complications should they arise.

MEDICATION SIDE EFFECT MANAGEMENT
Pruritus

Pruritus is common with intraspinal analgesia infusions. This side effect may be a result of an allergic-type reaction or may be caused by the stimulation of histamine release secondary to opiate pain medication. The incidence of pruritus has been identified to be higher with epidural analgesia than with systemic, intramuscular, or intravenous routes (Choi et al, 2003; Dolin and Cashman, 2005). Nursing actions for pruritus include providing diversional activities, using cool linens or clothing, or administering medications such as Benadryl, nalbuphine, naloxone, or ondansetron (Slowikowski and Flaherty, 2000; Choi et al, 2003; Rathmell et al, 2005; Kim et al, 2007). Low doses of naloxone, an opioid antagonist, have been shown to reverse pruritus without affecting the analgesic properties of epidural morphine (Choi et al, 2000). Nalbuphine is an opioid agonist-antagonist used for the treatment of pruritus. Titration of both naloxone and nalbuphine must be completed carefully and slowly to avoid reversal of analgesic effects of the opiate pain medications (Choi et al, 2000; Slowikowski and Flaherty, 2000; Kim et al, 2007). If an allergic reaction is suspected, Benadryl can be given to interfere with the histamine release causing the pruritus, leading to cessation of scratching, but Benadryl is rarely effective if the pruritus is not allergic (Slowikowski and Flaherty, 2000; Rathmell et al, 2005). Pruritus is rarely seen with chronic intraspinal opioid administration as tolerance commonly develops.

Nausea and vomiting

Although nausea and vomiting is anticipated to be minimized with the intraspinal route (because of the much smaller doses being administered), it still may occur and may be related to the specific drug being administered (e.g., morphine more than fentanyl) or higher doses of medications (Rathmell et al, 2005). The incidence of nausea and vomiting in patients receiving epidural infusions has been found to be approximately 18.8% for nausea and 16.3% for vomiting. No significant statistical differences have been found in rates of nausea and vomiting between epidural analgesia and systemic analgesia in a recent meta-analysis (Choi et al, 2003). The administration of epidural naloxone has been demonstrated to control nausea and vomiting in epidural infusions, without inhibiting the analgesic effects of the epidural infusion, which may actually be enhanced (Choi et al, 2000; Kim et al, 2007). This side effect may signal overdose caused by catheter migration into the intrathecal space when an epidural infusion has been implemented (McCaffery and Pasero, 1999; Rathmell et al, 2005). The administration of antiemetics (e.g., promethazine, scopolamine) or rotation to another medication may be indicated (Rathmell et al, 2005). The nurse should provide airway management to avoid aspiration if vomiting occurs (Slowikowski and Flaherty, 2000).

Respiratory depression

Respiratory depression occurs less frequently than with systemic analgesia (Choi et al, 2003; Rathmell et al, 2005). Risk factors for respiratory depression include administration of high doses, use of concurrent adjuvant medications, or overdosage in opiate-naive patients. The culprit is not always the opiate, but may actually be the adjuvant medication (e.g., muscle relaxants, additional opiates, sedatives) (Rathmell et al, 2005). The evaluation of all medications being ingested is warranted, and close observation is merited for patients receiving medications. Nurses must be prepared for respiratory emergencies with resuscitation equipment, oxygen, and interventional drugs. Nurses should keep in mind that this side effect may signal overdose attributable to catheter migration into the intrathecal space when an epidural infusion has been implemented (McCaffery and Pasero, 1999; Rathmell et al, 2005). Evaluation of the pump must also be conducted to ensure it is functioning properly. The use of an electronic infusion device with anti–free-flow protections should be utilized. Additionally, the patient should

be assessed for responses to therapy at regular intervals (INS, 2006). In patients who have used systemic opioids, the risk of respiratory depression is small (McCaffery and Pasero, 1999; Mercadante, 1999; Rathmell et al, 2005).

Urinary retention

Urinary retention is common with the intraspinal administration of opiates. It may be due to the opioid's inhibition of the parasympathetic nervous system on the bladder, which leads to detrusor muscle relaxation and an increase in bladder capacity (Kuipers et al, 2004; Rathmell et al, 2005). The decrease in bladder function is directly related to the medication, and is dose-dependent with effects on bladder function occurring as early as 1 hour after medication administration. Patients receiving morphine versus sufentanil require longer recovery time (Kuipers et al, 2004). Important nursing actions may include palpating the bladder for distention, monitoring intake and output, and providing catheterization as appropriate. Also, simple nursing measures may need to be provided, such as allowing the patient privacy or running the water in the sink (Slowikowski and Flaherty, 2000).

Hypotension

Hypotension has been identified to occur more frequently in epidural analgesia administration than in systemic analgesia (Choi et al, 2003). Hypotension may be due to numerous factors including hypovolemia, decreased venous return, adjuvant medications, or overdoses of opioids. Careful patient assessment is warranted as is the implementation of patient safety strategies. These strategies might include elevating the lower extremities to promote venous return, monitoring intake and output, administering oxygen or fluid boluses, and assisting in cautious ambulation (Slowikowski and Flaherty, 2000).

Constipation

Constipation is known to occur with the administration of opiates regardless of the route of administration. It is the only side effect to which patients do not develop tolerance (McCaffery and Pasero, 1999). It is commonly treated with laxatives such as stimulants, stool softeners, and enemas. Prevention is the key to management of this side effect; therefore management should be preemptive. It also appears that this complication is more prevalent in epidural and intrathecal administration than in intraventricular administration (Ballantyne and Carwood, 2005).

Sedation and confusion

Sedation and confusion may be more prevalent in intraventricular methods of administration; however, this has not been verified.

COMPLICATIONS OF CATHETERS/PUMPS
Infection

Although infections are rare, they do occur. Estimates vary depending on the population studied, type of access device utilized (e.g., epidural versus intrathecal), and study design, but range from 2% to 5%. Infection may be related to the length of time of infusion, the type of catheter used (e.g., if a short-term catheter is used for long-term infusions), the patients' condition and age, if the dressing at the insertion site was compromised, and if anticoagulants were used (Byerly et al, 1998; Simpson et al, 2000; Yentur et al, 2003; Bubeck et al, 2004; DuPen, 2005; Holmfred et al, 2006; Ruppen et al, 2006). Infections may be divided into those that occur at the catheter insertion site or those involving the pump pocket. Additionally, infections may be systemic such as in the case of meningitis. Signs and symptoms of infection may include inflammation, warmth, drainage at the catheter site or pump pocket site, tenderness at the site of insertion, and/or complaints of back pain by the patient. Two local signs of inflammation are strong predictors of local and epidural catheter infections (Darchy et al, 1996; Mercadante, 1999; Folett et al, 2004). If pump pocket infections are not treated aggressively and infection spreads, removal of the entire system may be warranted (Mercadante, 1999). Bacterial colonization of the insertion site, catheter, or catheter tip has been identified as a possible source of infection; however, this does not correlate with infection. Therefore careful patient assessment on a continuous basis is warranted. Aseptic technique during insertion and while providing routine care is important in preventing infections (Folett et al, 2004; Holmfred et al, 2006; INS, 2006).

Abscess

Abscess formation is a true medical emergency and early identification and intervention is of paramount importance to prevent long-term neurological damage. With the formation of an epidural abscess, the patient is usually febrile and complains of pain. Pain may begin with local back pain and some percussion tenderness; however, the pain is often severe and may radiate in a nerve root distribution. Compression of the cord leads to weakness, which progresses to paralysis over hours to days. Prompt decompression is required, as well as the commencement of antibiotics appropriate for the offending agent. The incidence of epidural abscess formation is less than 0.1% (Wang et al, 1999). Delays in identification of 24 hours or more can lead to paralysis (Wang et al, 1999; Murdoch, 2005). Epidural abscess formation may be more prevalent in patients with longer catheterization times; however, the level of catheter insertion has not been identified to play a part in the formation of abscesses (Wang et al, 1999). Any signs of infection merit notifying the provider and monitoring the patient for fever, signs of systemic infection, and meningitis (headache, nuchal rigidity, irritability). An aseptic sample of CSF and skin swabs may be obtained and sent for analysis. Care must be taken to avoid catheter puncture.

Hematoma

Hematoma formation is considered to be a rare complication. In obstetric patients, studies have identified incidence in obstetrics to be 6 per 1 million (Ruppen et al, 2006). The incidence of spinal hematoma in other populations is not known but is estimated to be 1 in 150,000 (Wheatley et al, 2001). Despite its low incidence, hematoma formation can have devastating consequences. The formation of a spinal hematoma is a true medical emergency that merits early detection and intervention. The hematoma is a collection of blood within the epidural spaces that ultimately leads to spinal cord compression. Presentation is similar to that of an abscess and may begin with local back pain and percussion tenderness. The pain is often severe and may radiate in a nerve root distribution. Compression

of the cord leads to weakness and then progresses to paralysis, usually within minutes to several hours. Prompt decompression and medical intervention are warranted (Mahlmeister, 2003; Murdoch, 2005). An increasing level of motor blockade may be indicative of hematoma formation. Neurological signs and symptoms will occur at the level of cord compression. Any continued complaints of paresthesia in lower extremities or continued motor block over 1 hour after discontinuation of epidural analgesia may signal hematoma formation (Mahlmeister, 2003). Risk for development of hematoma formation is increased in those using anticoagulants or those with thrombocytopenia.

Guidelines regarding the concomitant use of anticoagulants and intraspinal infusions have been established. Low–molecular-weight heparins (LMWHs) should be held 12 hours before initiation of the intraspinal infusion and not resumed for 2 hours after removal of devices. The use of other anticoagulants such as warfarin merits more intensive care. Most typically, unless the International Normalized Ratio (INR) is equal to or less than 1.4, intraspinal analgesia should not be initiated (Wheatley et al, 2001). Patients may often be "bridged" with a LMWH during intraspinal infusions, which allows less risk for clot formation. In the case of implanted devices, the LMWH should be discontinued 24 hours before implantation and resumed 12 hours postoperatively. Heparin infusions, with discontinuation 4 to 6 hours before implantation or insertion of an inferior vena cava filter, may also be options for those at highest risk (Stearns et al, 2005). The use of antiplatelet medications appears to be safe (Wheatley et al, 2001).

Fibrosis

Fibrosis formation is typically seen in long-term infusions of intraspinal opiates. The use of a silicone or polyurethane catheter and use of morphine without additives are thought to prevent the formation of catheter fibrosis. The catheter tip may need to be repositioned or epidural steroids may need to be administered for treatment (Mercadante, 1999). Current recommendations are that all patients who receive long-term intrathecal infusion for analgesia are screened periodically to assess for mass formation (McMillan et al, 2003). Additionally, any decrease in medication effectiveness should merit further investigation for the possibility of mass or fibrosis (Murphy et al, 2006).

Catheter migration

Migration of the catheter may occur either into or out of the intended delivery site. Signs of catheter migration may include decrease in effective pain control in a patient who previously had adequate pain relief (intrathecal to epidural migration), or the patient may experience an increase in medication side effects if migration is from the epidural to the intrathecal space (McCaffery and Pasero, 1999). Catheters should be assessed routinely for changes in external catheter length. Application of a dressing for securing the catheter, which allows the insertion site to be inspected and maintains sterility, is the ideal for temporary catheters. Some studies have advocated the use of dual fixation of the catheter to prevent migration (Burns et al, 2001). In the cases of implanted pumps, migration may also lead to pump failure and necessitate internal pump replacement (Pasquier et al, 2003). Treatment may include reimplantation of the pump (Ross et al, 2005).

Puncture of the dura mater during epidural insertion

Puncture of the dura mater may occur with the insertion of an epidural catheter, leading to leakage of CSF, which may cause headache (Morley-Forster et al, 2006; Weetman and Allison, 2006). The most common indication of puncture of the dura mater is headache. Patients may complain of headache that is worse with sitting or standing and improves with lying in the supine position. Patients may indicate the headache is throbbing, diffuse, or localized. There may be some indication of photosensitivity. Careful evaluation of the patient every shift or with each visit will allow the nurse to investigate the leaking of CSF (Weetman and Allison, 2006). The most effective remedy for spinal headache is a blood patch. This is performed by drawing approximately 10 mL of blood from the patient's arm and injecting the blood epidurally near the level of the original insertion site of the intrathecal needle (Weetman and Allison, 2006). The administration of a prophylactic epidural blood patch in the obstetric population after inadvertent dural puncture has been identified to shorten the length of time the patients experienced symptoms related to the headache (Scavone et al, 2004). Additionally, the types of needles used to initiate epidural analgesia are being evaluated in an effort to decrease the incidence of post–dural-puncture headaches (Morley-Forster et al, 2006). Patients who experience a new onset of headache after a period of catheterization with no headache merit further evaluation to rule out other potentially life-threatening conditions that may mimic the post–dural-puncture headache (meningitis, intracranial hemorrhage, intracranial metastasis, tumor, cerebrovascular accident [CVA], or cerebral venous thrombosis). The use of epidural blood patches in those who have implanted ports is very difficult and may require removal of the system (Stearns et al, 2005).

 ## NURSING CONSIDERATIONS

PREINSERTION

The nurse should perform a preinsertion assessment of the patient, notifying the provider of any relative or absolute contraindications to the use of intraspinal catheters and access devices. The nurse should also provide education to the patient and/or significant others about the insertion procedure and ensure informed consent is obtained. The clinician inserting the access device is expected to provide the patient with informed consent and written verification of the same.

All intraspinal infusions are accessed using aseptic technique. The initial implementation may occur in the operating room or at the bedside of the patient, such as in the obstetrical patient for epidural and intrathecal infusions. Insertion of an Ommaya reservoir is completed while the patient is sedated with a local or general anesthetic. All supplies should be maintained sterile. Sterile technique, including mask and gloves, should be used when accessing and maintaining an intraspinal access device as well as when providing patient care (Burke et al, 2001). Ensure all necessary supplies and equipment are available. Effective pain management should be ensured with a trial catheter before insertion of intrapinal analgesia. In addition, bridging patients from oral analgesia to intraspinal analgesia may be a challenge. It is important to prevent withdrawal in patients who are opioid tolerant. Suggestions include a 50% reduction in the oral opioid dose, substituted with an intrathecal equivalent during

the first day of the trial, and administering orally the remaining 50%. Subsequent adjustments may include a decrease in the oral dose by 20% daily while simultaneously increasing the intrathecal dose by 20% (Krames, 2002).

CLEANSING OF SKIN

Adequate skin disinfection before catheter placement is of paramount importance for prevention of colonization of the skin and to stave off catheter-associated infections. The debate regarding the most effective disinfectant continues. Studies have compared povidine-iodine solution and iodophor-in-isopropyl alcohol solutions; nevertheless, the skin must be prepped and cleaned before the initiation of intraspinal infusions (Kinirons et al, 2001). Alcohol, disinfectants containing alcohol, and acetone should never be used for site preparation or for cleaning the catheter hub because of the potential deleterious neurotoxic effects to the spinal cord. Spray disinfection has been identified to be equally efficacious in comparison with conventional swab disinfection (Debreceni et al, 2007). Birnbach et al (2003) found that DuraPrep™ solution provided a greater decrease in the number of positive skin cultures immediately after disinfection as well as in colonization of the epidural catheter. Studies documenting bacterial colonization in intraspinal access devices are summarized in the Focus on Evidence box.

PATIENT POSITIONING

Three primary methods of patient positioning exist for intraspinal catheter placement including lateral decubitus, sitting, and prone. The position used will depend on the provider's choice for best access based on the patient's age, level of alertness for cooperation, and body habits (e.g., an obese patient may have a difficult time maintaining adequate positioning, or a patient may be uncooperative because of lack of understanding). Positioning for children most often occurs in the lateral decubitus position because it allows for ease of maintenance of a patent airway and identification of appropriate landmarks. In the prone position, a pillow may be used to improve access to the appropriate insertion site. The nurse can assist with the procedure by placing the patient in the most comfortable position (Miller, 2000). Current practice has dictated that patients remain awake during the insertion of epidural catheters to ensure no significant neurological sequelae develop. Recent studies are challenging this practice and have studied the placement of catheters after the induction of anesthesia and tracheal intubation or after the completion of the surgical procedure (Horlocker et al, 2002).

POSTINSERTION

Patient assessment should be conducted following insertion to evaluate neurological status, including level of anesthesia and return of motor function as applicable. Vital signs should be monitored per organizational protocol. Evaluation should include monitoring the catheter, port, and pump pocket for edema, leaking of fluid (particularly CSF), and/or bleeding. Findings should be documented and communicated to the provider as appropriate. Ensuring that all ports and catheters are labeled clearly to avoid inadvertent administration of neurotoxic agents is of utmost importance (Kingsley, 2001). Most major complications of spinal infusion occur during or shortly after the initial administration of agents and during rebolusing procedures (Mahlmeister, 2003).

FOCUS ON EVIDENCE

Bacterial Colonization in Intraspinal Access Devices

- A convenience sample of 100 pediatric patients were randomly assigned to receive either 0.5% chlorhexidine gluconate or 10% povidone-iodine for cutaneous cleansing before epidural catheter insertion by computer. Data were analyzed for 96 catheters: 44 in the povidone-iodine group and 52 in the chlorhexidine group. No patients developed an epidural space infection, but the study demonstrated that in the pediatric population, a solution of 0.5% chlorhexidine gluconate was more effective than the 10% povidone-iodine in preventing catheter colonization in children (Kinirons et al, 2001).

- In a convenience sample of 60 women in active labor and requesting epidural analgesia, assignment was made to randomly receive either povidone-iodine solution or DuraPrep™ (iodophor-in-isopropyl alcohol) for skin cleansing before epidural insertion. Disinfection with either substance decreased the number of bacteria detected; however, those in the DuraPrep™ group had negative cultures immediately after skin disinfection more often than those in the povodine-iodine group. Additionally, DuraPrep™ was also more effective at limiting regrowth of the skin flora than povodine-iodine. DuraPrep™ solution may also inhibit bacterial regrowth (Birnbach et al, 2003).

- In a prospective study of 205 patients with epidural analgesia for postoperative pain, the infusate, the inside of the catheter injection port or hub, the skin surrounding the insertion site, the catheter tip, and the subcutaneous section of the catheter were cultured upon catheter removal. The positive culture rates for the subcutaneous and tip segments of the catheter were 10.5% and 12.2%, respectively. The authors suggest that bacterial migration along the epidural catheter track is the most common route of epidural catheter colonization and that maintaining sterile skin around the catheter insertion site would reduce colonization of the epidural catheter tip (Yuan et al, 2008).

- A retrospective review of records for 1810 patients who had received epidural analgesia over a 4-year period was completed. Culture results of epidural catheter tips were available for 1443 patients. A total of 1027 of the tips were sterile, with 416 being positive for at least 1 microorganism. No epidural catheter site infections were identified. Positive microorganisms were usually normal skin flora; however, other contaminants such as *Escherichia coli* were found. The authors concluded that routinely obtaining cultures of epidural catheter tips is clinically irrelevant in the vast majority of cases and the identification of a positive catheter tip is not a good predictor of the presence of epidural space infection (Simpson et al, 2000).

The optimal time interval for changing dressings is dependent on the dressing material, age and condition of the patient, infection rate reported by the organization, environmental conditions, and manufacturer's labeled use(s) and directions for product use (INS, 2006). One study found a reduction in bacterial colonization of epidural short-term catheter exit sites with the use of chlorhexidine-impregnated dressings (Mann et al, 2001). Nurses are responsible for inspecting the catheter site every shift in the acute care setting, or more often if patient status dictates. In the outpatient setting, each visit with the patient should merit evaluation of the catheter and pump pocket sites. Placement should always be confirmed before use of the intraspinal device. During the initial 24 hours of use, the patient must have an intravenous access in place for the initial administration of reversal agents if needed (Otto, 1998; Mercadante, 1999). Postinsertion monitoring includes assessing the patient for any signs of hypotension, neurological changes, speech difficulties, cognitive changes, and signs and symptoms of infection.

Access of the intraspinal catheter or device should be with aseptic technique using sterile gloves, masks, and gown. A procedure outlining the steps in accessing an epidural or intrathecal port can be found in Box 27-1. Maintenance of sterile skin around the catheter insertion site will reduce colonization of the epidural catheter tip, which may decrease the incidence of infection (Yuan et al, 2008). Studies have all focused on insertion site preparation, with conflicting recommendations for the use of povidone-iodine and chlorhexidine (Kinirons et al, 2001; Kasuda et al, 2002). Regardless, all antibacterial agents have the potential to be neurotoxic, and should be allowed to air-dry according to the manufacturers' instructions. Any excess fluid should be removed with sterile gauze. All medications and diluents must be preservative-free and labeled for intraspinal infusion. Once the intraspinal infusion is initiated, patients should be assessed for paresthesias, which may result from contact of

Box 27-1   ACCESSING EPIDURAL/INTRATHECAL PORTS

1. Assess patient (neurological status, vital signs). Obtain informed consent. Explain procedure.
2. Assemble appropriate equipment: sterile gloves (two pairs), antibacterial cleansing agent; sterile gauze, noncoring needle, syringe; preservative-free 0.9% sodium chloride; appropriate intraspinal medication.
3. Perform hand hygiene; don sterile gloves using aseptic technique.
4. Cleanse port site using antibacterial cleansing agent; allow site to air-dry per manufacturer's instructions; remove any moist agent with sterile gauze.
5. Access port with noncoring needle; gently aspirate 1 mL. If blood or more than 0.5 mL of clear fluid is aspirated, medication is NOT administered and provider is notified. Aspirate is discarded along with syringe.
6. Proceed with medication administration if aspirate was appropriate. Administer slowly and steadily.
7. Flush catheter with 2 to 3 mL of preservative-free 0.9% sodium chloride.
8. Evaluate patient response, catheter, and insertion site as appropriate.
9. Discard materials appropriately; perform hand hygiene.
10. Document findings, nursing actions, and patient response.

the catheter with neural tissue, neurotoxic drug administration, or spinal cord compression (Mercadante, 1999). Routine dressing changes of short-term epidural and intrathecal infusions are not recommended because this practice will help avoid introduction of bacteria and prevent dislodgement of catheters

(Weetman and Allison, 2006). After the insertion of the Ommaya reservoir, a pressure dressing is placed and remains for 24 hours; then the site may be left open to air (Otto, 1998). Patients are monitored for side effects of medications and managed per organizational protocol. For intraspinal infusions, a 0.2-micron filter that is surfactant-free, particulate-retentive, and air-eliminating is used (INS, 2006).

REMOVAL OF CATHETERS

Catheter removal is to be completed using aseptic technique. Only nurses with specialized training should remove intrathecal catheters. Epidural catheters should not be removed if there is resistance or difficulty in removing, as there could be kinking of the catheter or breakage with a retained catheter tip. Additionally, before removal, evaluation of the use of anticoagulants in patients must be completed to decrease the chance of hematoma formation. After intraspinal access device removal, an occlusive sterile dressing should be applied. The access site should be assessed every 24 hours until the site is epithelialized. The condition and length of the intraspinal access device should be ascertained upon removal. Nursing actions and observation should be documented in the patient's permanent medical record (McCaffery and Pasero, 1999; Stearns et al, 2005; INS, 2006).

PATIENT EDUCATION

Patient education must include explanation of the technique of medication injection and catheter care instructions. Additionally, patient education must also include information regarding dressing changes, as applicable, infection precautions, and signs and symptoms to report to the physician. Patient education must be documented in the patient's permanent medical record. Written information provided for the patient and/or caregiver to reference may also be helpful.

 ## SUMMARY

Nurses who provide direct patient care at the bedside, in the office exam room, or in the patient's home are able to effectively assist in identifying appropriate patients for intraspinal medication infusions. Nurses should understand spinal neuroanatomy and the properties and uses of intraspinal medications, and be aware of potential complications that can accompany the intraspinal route of administration. Should complications arise from intraspinal infusions, the competent nurse will be able to troubleshoot them, ensuring patient safety and positive patient outcomes.

 ## REFERENCES

Albright AL, Awaad Y, Muhonen M et al: Performance and complications associated with the Synchromed 10-ml infusion pump for intrathecal baclofen administration in children, *J Neurosurg* 101(1 Suppl):S64-S68, 2004.

American Pain Society: *Principles of analgesic use in the treatment of acute pain and cancer pain*, ed 5, Glenview, Ill, 2003.

Ballantyne JC, Carwood CM: Comparative efficacy of epidural, subarachnoid, and intracerebroventricular opioids in patients with pain due to cancer, *Cochrane Database Syst Rev* 2(CD005178):1-25, 2005.

Birnbach DJ, Meadows W, Stein DJ et al: Comparison of povidone iodine and DuraPrep™, and iodophor-in-isopropyl alcohol solutions, for skin disinfection prior to epidural catheter insertion in parturients, *Anesthesiology* 98(1):164-169, 2003.

Brant JM: The use of access devices in cancer pain control, *Semin Oncol Nurs* 11(3):203-212, 1995.

Brogan SE: Intrathecal therapy for the management of cancer pain, *Curr Pain Headache Rep* 10(4):254-259, 2006.

Bubeck J, Boos K, Krause H et al: Subcutaneous tunneling of caudal catheters reduces the rate of bacterial colonization to that of lumbar epidural catheters, *Anesth Analg* 99(3):689-693, 2004.

Burke MB, Wilkes GM, Ingwerson K: *Cancer chemotherapy: a nursing process approach* ed 3, Sudbury, Mass, 2001, Jones and Bartlett.

Burns SM, Cowan CM, Barclay PM et al: Intrapartum epidural catheter migration: a comparative study of three dressing applications, *Br J Anaesth* 86(4):565-567, 2001.

Byerly SK, Tobin JR, Greenburg RS et al: Bacterial colonization and infection rate of continuous epidural catheters in children, *Anesth Analg* 86(4):712-716, 1998.

Choi JH, Lee J, Choi JH et al: Epidural naloxone reduces pruritus and nausea without affecting analgesia by epidural morphine in bupivacaine, *Can J Anaesth* 47(1):33-37, 2000.

Choi PT, Bhandari M, Scott J et al: Epidural analgesia for pain relief following hip or knee replacement, *Cochrane Database Syst Rev* (3):CD003071, 2003.

Cohen SP, Dragovich A: Intrathecal analgesia, *Med Clin North Am* 91(2):251-270, 2007.

Darchy B, Forcevill X, Bavoux E et al: Clinical and bacteriologic survey of epidural analgesia in patients in the intensive care unit, *Anesthesiology* 85(5):988-998, 1996.

Debreceni G, Meggyesi R, Mestyán G: Efficacy of spray disinfection with a 2-propanol and benzalkonium chloride containing solution before epidural catheter insertion—a prospective, randomized, clinical trial, *Br J Anaesth* 98(1):131-135, 2007.

Dolin SJ, Cashman JN: Tolerability of acute postoperative pain management: nausea, vomiting, sedation, pruritus, and urinary retention. Evidence from published data, *Br J Anaesth* 95(5):584-591, 2005.

DuPen A: Care and management of intrathecal and epidural catheters, *J Infus Nurs* 28(6):377-381, 2005.

Farrow-Gillespie A, Kaplan KM: Intrathecal analgesic drug therapy, *Curr Pain Headache Rep* 10(1):26-33, 2006.

Folett K, Boorts-Marx RL, Drake JM et al: Prevention and management of intrathecal drug delivery and spinal cord stimulation system infections, *Anesthesiology* 100(6):1582-1594, 2004.

Ghafoor VL, Epshteyn M, Carlson GH et al: Intrathecal drug therapy for long-term pain management, *Am J Health Syst Pharm* 64(23):2447-2461, 2007.

Golembiewski J, Torrecer S, Katke J: The use of opioids in the postoperative setting: focus on morphine, hydromorphone, and fentanyl, *J Perianesth Nurs* 20(2):141-143, 2005.

Gooch JL, Oberg WA, Grams B et al: Complications of intrathecal baclofen pumps in children, *Pediatr Neurosurg* 39(1):1-6, 2003.

Heitz JW, Viscusi ER: The evolving role of spinal agents in acute pain, *Curr Pain Headache Rep* 9(1):17-23, 2005.

Holmfred A, Vikerfors T, Berggren L et al: Intrathecal catheters with subcutaneous port systems in patients with severe cancer-related pain managed out of hospital: the risk of infection, *J Pain Symptom Manag* 31(6):568-572, 2006.

Horlocker TT, Abel MD, Messick JM et al: Small risk of serious neurologic complications related to lumbar epidural catheter placement in anesthetized patients, *Anesth Analg* 96(6):1547-1552, 2002.

Infusion Nurses Society: Infusion nursing standards of practice, *J Infus Nurs* 29(1 Suppl), S1-S92, 2006.

Kasuda H, Fukuda H, Togashi H et al: Skin disinfection before epidural catheterization: a comparative study of povidone-iodine versus chlorhexidine ethanol, *Dermatology* 204(S1):42-46, 2002.

Kedlaya D, Reynolds L, Waldman S: Epidural and intrathecal analgesia for cancer pain, *Best Pract Res Clin Anaesthesiol* 16(4):651-665, 2002.

Kim MK, Nam SB, Cho MJ et al: Epidural naloxone reduces postoperative nausea and vomiting in patients receiving epidural sufentanil for postoperative analgesia, *Br J Anaesth* 99(2):270-275, 2007.

Kingsley C: Epidural analgesia: your role, *RN* 64(3):53-57, 2001.

Kinirons B, Mimoz O, Lafendi L et al: Chlorhexidine versus povidone iodine in preventing colonization of continuous epidural catheters in children: a randomized, controlled trial, *Anesthesiology* 94(2):239-244, 2001.

Krames E: Implantable devices for pain control: spinal cord stimulation and intrathecal therapies *Best Pract Res Clin Anaesthesiol* 16(4):619-649, 2002.

Kuipers PW, Kamphuis ET, vanVenrooij GE et al: Intrathecal opioids and lower urinary tract function: a urodynamic evaluation, *Anesthesiology* 100(6):1497-1503, 2004.

Maher AB, Salmond SW, Pellino TA: *Orthopaedic nursing,* ed 3, Philadelphia, 2002, Saunders.

Mahlmeister L: Nursing responsibilities in preventing, preparing for, and managing epidural emergencies, *J Perinat Neonatal Nurs* 17(1):19-32, 2003.

Mann TJ, Orlikowski CE, Gurrin LC et al: The effect of the BIOPATCH, a chlorhexidine impregnated dressing, on bacterial colonization of epidural catheter exit sites, *Anaesth Intensive Care* 29(6):600-603, 2001.

McCaffery M, Pasero C: *Pain: clinical manual,* ed 2, St Louis, 1999, Mosby.

McMillan MR, Doud T, Nugent W: Catheter-associated masses in patients receiving intrathecal analgesic therapy, *Anesth Analg* 96(1):186-190, 2003.

Mercadante S: Problems of long-term spinal opioid treatment in advanced cancer patients *Pain* 79:1-13, 1999.

Miller RD: *Anesthesia,* ed 5, Philadelphia, 2000, Churchill Livingstone.

Morley-Forster PK, Singh S, Angle P et al: The effect of epidural needle type on postdural puncture headache: a randomized trial, *Can J Anaesth* 53(6):572-578, 2006.

Murdoch J: Ensuring prompt diagnosis and treatment of epidural abscess, *Nurs Times* 101(20):17-23, 2005.

Murphy PM, Skouvaklis DE, Amadeo RJ et al: Intrathecal catheter granuloma associated with isolated baclofen infusion, *Anesth Analg* 102(3):848-852, 2006.

Otto SE: *Oncology nursing,* ed 4, St Louis, 1998, Mosby.

Pasero C: Epidural analgesia for postoperative pain, *Am J Nurs* 103(10):62-64, 2003.

Pasquier Y, Cahana A, Schnider A: Subdural catheter migration may lead to baclofen pump dysfunction, *Spinal Cord* 41(12):700-702, 2003.

Potter P, Perry AG: *Fundamentals of nursing: concepts, process, and practice,* ed 6, St Louis, 2007, Mosby.

Prager JP: Neuraxial medication delivery: the development and maturity of a concept for treating chronic pain of spinal origin, *Spine* 27(22):2593-2605, 2002.

Rathmell JP, Lair TR, Nauman B: The role of intrathecal drugs in the treatment of acute pain, *Anesth Analg* 101(5 Suppl):S30-S43, 2005.

Rauck RL, Wallace MS, Leong MS et al: A randomized, double-blind, placebo-controlled study of intrathecal ziconotide in adults with severe chronic pain, *Pain Sympt Manag* 31(5):393-406, 2006.

Ruppen W, Derry S, McQuay H et al: Incidence of epidural hematoma, infection, and neurologic injury in obstetric patients with epidural analgesia/anesthesia, *Anesthesiology* 105(2):394-399, 2006.

Saladin KS, Porth CM: *Anatomy & physiology: the unity of form and function* ed 1, Boston, 1998, McGraw-Hill.

Scavone BM, Wong CA, Sullivan JT et al: Efficacy of a prophylactic epidural blood patch in preventing post dural puncture headache in parturients after inadvertent dural puncture, *Anesthesiology* 101(6):1422-1427, 2004.

Simpson RS, Macintyre PE, Shaw D et al: Epidural catheter tip cultures: results of a 4-year audit and implications for clinical practice, *Reg Anesth Pain Med* 24(4):360-367, 2000.

Skyryabina EA, Dunn TS: Disposable infusion pumps, *Am J Health-Syst Pharm* 63(13):1260-1268, 2006.

Sloan PA: Neuraxial pain relief for intractable cancer pain, *Curr Pain Headache Rep* 11(4):283-289, 2007.

Slowikowski RD, Flaherty SA: Epidural analgesia for postoperative orthopaedic pain, *Orthop Nurs* 19(1):23-31, 2000.

Staats PS, Yearwood T, Charapata SG et al: Intrathecal ziconotide in the treatment of refractory pain in patients with cancer or AIDS: a randomized controlled trial, *JAMA* 291(1):63-70, 2004.

Stearns L, Boortz-Marx R, DuPen S et al: Intrathecal drug delivery management of cancer pain; a multidisciplinary consensus of best clinical practices, *J Supportive Oncol* 3(6):399-408, 2005.

Wang LP, Hauerberg J, Schmidt JS: Incidence of spinal epidural abscess after epidural analgesia, *Anesthesiology* 91(6):1928-1936, 1999.

Weetman C, Allison W: Use of epidural analgesia in post-operative pain management, *Nurs Stand* 20(44):54-64, 2006.

Wheatley RG, Schug SA, Watson D: Safety and efficacy of postoperative epidural analgesia, *Br J Anaesth* 87(1):47-61, 2001.

Yarbro CH, Frogge MH, Goodman M et al: *Cancer nursing principles and practice,* ed 5, Sudbury, Mass, 2000, Jones and Bartlett.

Yentur EA, Luleci N, Topcu I et al: Is skin disinfection with 10% povidone iodine sufficient to prevent epidural needle and catheter contamination, *Reg Anesth Pain Med* 28(5):389-393, 2003.

Yuan HB, Zuo Z, Yu KW et al: Bacterial colonization of epidural catheters used for short-term postoperative analgesia: microbiological examination and risk factor analysis, *Anesthesiology* 108(1):130-137, 2008.

Zahavi A, Geertzen JH, Middel B et al: Long term effect (more than 5 years) of intrathecal baclofen on impairment, disability, and quality of life in patients with severe spasticity of spinal origin: *J Neurol Neurosurg Psychiatry* 75(11):1553-1557, 2004.

28 DOCUMENTATION

Brenda Dugger, MSHA, RN, CRNI®, CNA-BC

HISTORICAL OVERVIEW

Documentation of the nursing process has always been viewed as a necessary but time-consuming chore. Over the past 20 years, nursing documentation has become more important and has changed to respond to the requirements of state and federal regulatory agencies, changes in nursing practice, determination of reimbursement fees, and legal ramifications.

Until around 3000 BC, when a system of writing was developed in Egypt, no formal records were kept by attendants to the sick. With the advent of Christianity, patient care records of nursing became organized and continuous. No one person contributed more to nursing than Florence Nightingale (1986). Documentation in 1820 to 1910 was used primarily to communicate the implementation of physicians' orders. Nursing notes were not viewed as an important part of the patient's medical record and were often discarded when the patient was discharged from the hospital.

In the 1930s a written plan of care was developed. In 1951 nursing standards became formalized, and the Joint Commission on Accreditation of Healthcare Organizations (now The Joint Commission) was formed. In the mid-1960s documentation in nurses' notes evolved as an essential method of evaluating nursing care that met the requirements of regulatory agencies, provided evidence in litigation, and delineated professional responsibility. When diagnosis-related groups (DRGs) were implemented in the early 1980s, documentation in the medical record served as a mechanism for determining reimbursement guidelines. In the 1990s the emphasis was on quality improvement, with a focus on evaluating organizational and clinical performance outcomes. In the 2000s documentation emphasizes outcomes. It is important to emphasize activities that improve clinical performance and facilitate the continuous collection and evaluation of statistical data to improve care. Quality and outcomes will be tied to reimbursement. Publicly reported data will be available and health care providers and consumers will expect cost-effective positive outcomes. Documentation plays a key role in providing the information necessary to track and evaluate quality and patient care outcomes.

Electronic documentation offers many benefits to health care providers for data retrieval, avoidance of duplicate documentation, and analysis of care, interventions, and outcomes. Documentation systems should be designed in consultation with the nursing staff and their concerns should be addressed before the system is implemented. Entry and retrieval processes should be user friendly and help nurses think more critically to improve patient outcomes. This information would include the nursing-sensitive indicators such as patient falls, pressure ulcers, staff mix, nursing hours per patient day, job satisfaction, and nurse education (Monarch, 2007).

The Institute of Medicine (IOM) made additional recommendations in 2003 that all clinicians gain competency in delivering patient-centered care, working in interdisciplinary teams, practicing evidence-based medicine, focusing on quality improvement, and in using information technology (Chiverton and Witzel, 2008). They cited the need to expand use of bedside clinical testing technologies, electronic medical records, personal health records, and telehealth programs for which improved skills of documentation are imperative.

PURPOSE AND SCOPE

Documentation in the medical record is the best evidence that appropriate care was done and that the care was reasonable under the circumstances. Standards of care are based on the skill, care, and judgment used by an average health care provider under similar situations (Ferrell, 2007). Standards of care are determined by practice acts, state and federal regulatory agencies, The Joint Commission, organizational policies, and specialty organizations. Documentation validates that these standards are followed and assists with continuity of care among the health care team.

The *Infusion Nursing Standards of Practice*, published by the Infusion Nurses Society (2006), states that nursing documentation shall contain complete information regarding infusion therapy and vascular access in the patient's permanent medical record. Specific documentation is required by state statutes and regulatory agencies and must include the documentation of invasive procedures such as infusion therapy. The underlying reason for these regulations is to protect the health care consumer by delineating professional responsibility and accountability. Nurses are responsible for assessment of the patient, development of the nursing plan of care to reach established goals, and evaluation of the effectiveness of the care given. This process along with determination of best practices to achieve quality outcomes constitutes evidence-based practice.

Nurses are responsible for data collection and for the documentation process. A coherent record of the patient care event or encounter should be evident through the medical record. Objective assessments use the nurses' senses of sight, touch, hearing, and smell (Austin, 2006). Documentation provides the pathway to continuity of care. Each specialty or point of service reveals a part of the patient's clinical picture or story. Documentation should clearly include the following:

- Diagnosis
- Assessment of the patient's condition
- Care given to the patient
- Any unusual circumstances or complications
- Interventions performed to correct the situation
- Interactions with the physician, supervisor, or other health care professionals
- Evaluation of all interventions
- Outcomes

The necessity of effective documentation is an integral part of prudent patient care. The medical record is proof of the nursing process and the steps used to reach the resulting outcomes. Studies have shown that nurses often spend up to 30% of their time in the documentation process (Ferrell, 2007). As nursing responsibilities expand, professional roles and accountability increase. With this expanded role, critical thinking becomes essential to improve positive patient outcomes (INS, 2006). Hospital nurses often work by protocol to treat certain symptoms. For example, a protocol may direct the nurse to titrate a medication to obtain a certain effect. Home health nurses may work according to specific physicians' orders, such as medication dosage ranges. While working alone in the community, home health nurses must make independent decisions about the patient's condition and determine when a change in condition merits physician notification. Infusion nurses are called on to lead other health care professionals in recommending catheter selection or improving catheter function. These activities are orchestrated by good communication and should be evidenced throughout the documentation.

No longer are episodes of illness viewed as separate. A focus on wellness chooses to look at the life of the individual in its entirety and all of the influences that affect the health of the individual. Comprehensive documentation of care in all settings provides invaluable information to guide future treatment.

▮ DOCUMENTATION GUIDELINES

Documentation should contain only factual information pertaining to the patient's condition, diagnosis, and treatment. Speculation, conjecture, or demeaning comments are inappropriate and may be damaging to the patient, nurse, and the organization. Charting should never cover up an incident or document care that was not given. Inappropriate bias should be avoided, such as describing a patient as obnoxious, belligerent,

hostile, or rude. Personal opinions should not be referenced. The medical record is confidential and is protected by the Health Insurance Portability and Accountability Act of 1996 (HIPAA). Access to this documentation should be monitored and controlled according to organizational policy.

WRITTEN DOCUMENTATION

Written documentation in the medical record should be legible and concise. Illegible writing may become the focal point for a plaintiff's attorney, even if a mistake or error was not made. Scribbling, writing over another word or statement, and erasing an incorrect entry are unacceptable practices that can lead to disciplinary action in some organizations. In addition, writing over another word or statement or erasing an incorrect entry admits fault and can lead to serious consequences if the case is litigated. Errors should be corrected by drawing a line through the incorrect word or words and writing "error" or "mistaken entry" (Austin, 2006). The entry should be accompanied by the initials of the individual making the entry.

Common terminology, approved by the organization and written into policy, defines the accepted terms and clarifies misconceptions about meanings or interpretations. Abbreviations should be used only if accepted as the standard for the organization. The Joint Commission (2007c) has a *Do Not Use* list of abbreviations that should never be used because of their potential for confusion or misinterpretation (Table 28-1).

All observations should be recorded accurately. The date and the organization's accepted method of keeping time (military or regular) should be used for every entry. Liability cases have used the documented time of treatment to determine the appropriateness of nurse response time and judgment relative to patient care.

The propensity for accurate documentation often arises from fear of litigation. Charting should always be written with potential legal review in mind. Investigation, deposition, and testimony often occur months or several years after the questionable event. Failure to appropriately document nursing assessment, interventions, or outcomes may cast doubt on the nurse's actions. Comprehensive documentation often shows that the nurse is competent and cognizant of good nursing practice.

Documentation may be the difference in accusation of negligence or malpractice. The Joint Commission (2007d) defines negligence as "failure to use such care as a reasonably prudent and careful person would use under similar circumstances," and malpractice as "improper or unethical conduct to unreasonable lack of skill by a holder of a professional or official position" (Box 28-1).

TABLE 28-1 **Examples of "Do Not Use List"**

Write out	Avoid
Unit, International Unit	Using U or IU
Daily, every other day	Q.D., QD, qd, Q.O.D., QOD, q.o.d., qod
Write X mg or 0.X mg	X.0 mg, .X mg
Morphine sulfate, magnesium sulfate	MS, MSO$_4$, MgSO$_4$

Data from The Joint Commission: *Do not use list*, 2007c. Accessed 11/13/07 at www.jointcommission.org/patientsafety/donotuselist.

Box 28-1 DOCUMENTATION ISSUES THAT RISK PROFESSIONAL NEGLIGENCE CLAIMS

- Lack of informed consent, treatment, patient teaching, or discharge instructions
- Delays, substandard or inappropriate treatment
- Charting inconsistencies, late entries, improper alterations of the record
- Reference to an unusual occurrence report, conflicting documentation
- Missing records or destruction of records

Box 28-2 BENEFITS OF AN ELECTRONIC MEDICAL RECORD (EMR)

- Instant access to patient data
- Secure information
- Multiple end users
- Smooth flow inside and outside of hospital
- Data retrieval through report writing
- Reduction of medical errors
- Reduction of paperwork

From Doyle M: Promoting standardized nursing language using an electronic medical record system, *AORN* 83(6):1336, 2006; Wolf DM et al: Community hospital successfully implements eRecord and CPOE, *Comput Inform Nurs* 24(6):307-316, 2006.

A signature is mandatory after every entry. Chart reviews are difficult when entry ownership is not established or difficult to read. Initials are acceptable if the complete signature is on the bottom of the page or at the end of the documentation segment.

Flow sheets are often used for IV therapy records. They offer a concise list of IV fluids and medications given and the dates and time of IV catheter insertion and site checks. The flow sheet should include the type, length, gauge, removal, replacement, or rotation of the vascular access device. Degrees of phlebitis should be documented within the medical record each time a device is removed because of phlebitis. The degree of infiltration should also be documented in the medical record each time a device is removed when an infiltration has occurred. Considering the potency and venous irritability of many medications, charting observations about a discontinued device may help identify a postinfusion phlebitis.

COMPUTERIZED DOCUMENTATION

Most organizations are moving to electronic systems because of legibility and the ease of storage and retrieval of information. Along with enormous initial investment costs, concerns about moving to computerized documentation systems include fears that rapidly changing technology will make the system obsolete after only a few years. These systems are continually improved for easier user access, such as touch screens, handwriting interpretation, bar coding, and voice recognition.

Other considerations include the extensive hours required to build the screens and dictionaries, the variability of employee computer expertise, the reluctance of staff and physicians to learn the system, the amount of education and training needed for staff, and the maintenance of the system to meet changing regulatory requirements, new medications, or terminology changes. The availability of information is improved and easily attainable from episode to episode, whether inpatient or outpatient, to improve care through the continuum. When the patient's entire clinical history is available, treatment can be more effective. Past illnesses may show trends and help reveal patterns of positive or negative outcomes from different courses of treatment. Online nursing documentation potentially improves overall documentation requirements because of the ability to halt screen progression until missing mandatory information is included (Langowski, 2005). Point of care technology keeps documentation data near the patient yet accessible by multiple parties in different locations at the same time. Opportunity for errors can be reduced and reduction of data entry can be accomplished (Box 28-2). Ease of implementation and the success of a computerized system are dependent upon the acceptance by the physicians and clinicians. It is essential that they understand the benefits for them, their organization, and their patients (Geibert, 2006).

The nurse's signature is attached to the record by an individual password that the nurse uses to gain access to the system. The password should never be shared or used by anyone other than the person to whom it is assigned. Passwords should be changed often to prevent misuse and protect the system. Confidentiality must be emphasized so that the information is not used in an illegal or inappropriate manner. Entrance to the medical record can usually be tracked and an unauthorized chart entry may result in disciplinary action.

Using a computer is usually a simple process to document the selection of the insertion site and catheter gauge, purpose of therapy, degree of phlebitis or infiltration, and time of device removal (Figure 28-1). Such documentation can usually be accomplished by selecting the appropriate key words or phrases already programmed on the screen or by typing them onto the screen (Figure 28-2). The system should always allow options to add narrative notes to further explain or describe abnormal or unusual events or situations. Home care nurses may use handheld, tabletop, or laptop computers to document in the home setting. Although computerized records are more legible than handwriting, the format is not always clearly delineated, especially when the record is not printed in color. Computerized systems take time to master, but wil l be faster to use and accessed more quickly after several weeks of practice.

Some infusion pumps are computer-driven and have downloading capabilities that record information directly into the patient's electronic health record. These systems have drug libraries that match the patient's name, patient's medical record number, physician's order, drug name, drug dose, and nurse's name to ensure verification of the right patient, the right drug, and the right dose.

Bar coding offers a computer driven process by which the nurse, the patient's identification band, and the drug label are verified for accuracy and safety. Challenges have slowed faster adoption of these systems as a result of nonstandardized manufacturer's drug labeling and bar coding. Charting and charging for the medication can also be accomplished by utilizing a bar coding system.

DOCUMENTATION SYSTEMS

Critical, or clinical, pathways should be developed using evidence-based best practices. Care is outlined, or "mapped," for a predictable length of stay and progression of recovery. Using

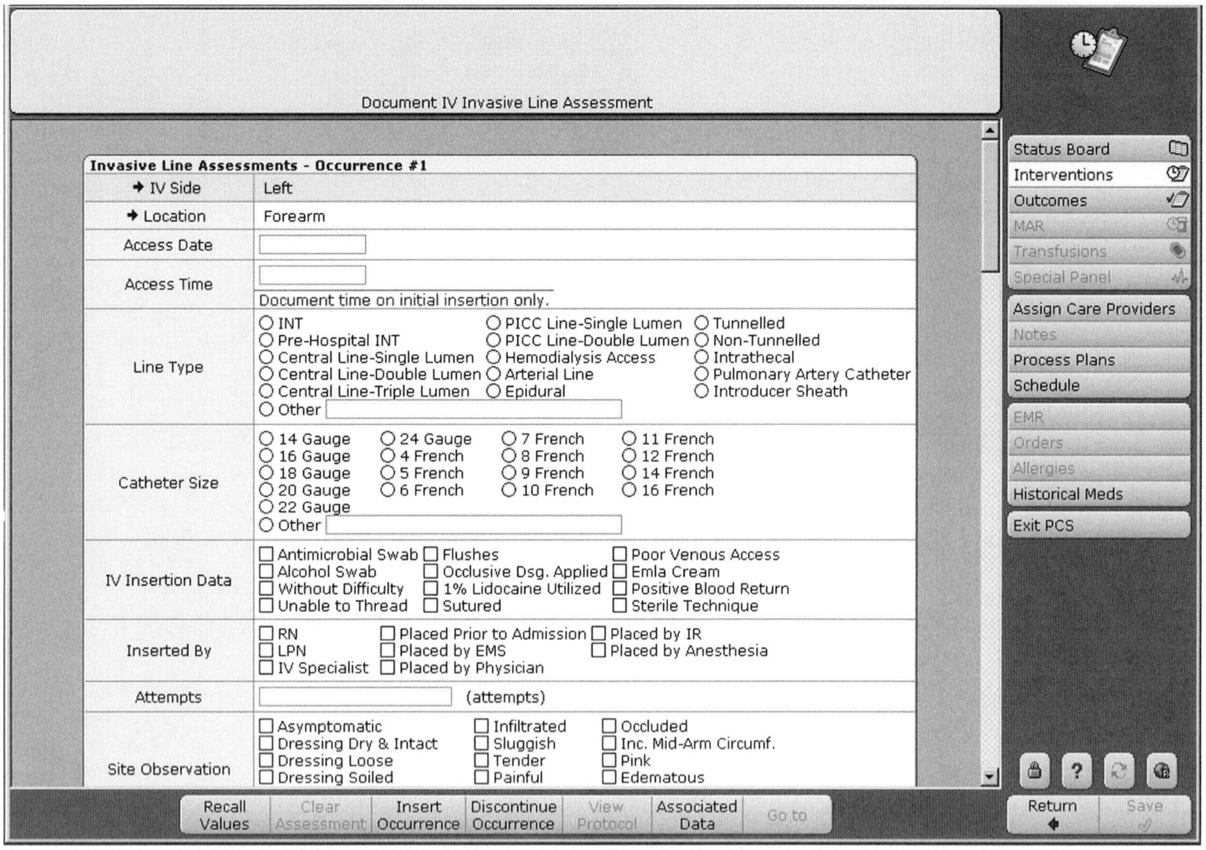

FIGURE 28-1 Computerized charting IV invasive line assessment screen. (From Meditech PCS documentation system, St. Mary's Health Care System, Athens, Ga.)

critical pathways requires increased interdisciplinary collaboration and efficiency facilitated by streamlined documentation procedures. The care plan is developed for a disease-specific episode of illness or surgical procedure. It should always be individualized to the patient's condition and changed according to the physician orders as necessary. It provides data to track variances based on expected outcomes or failure to meet certain criteria. Monitoring progress along the pathway may indicate variances in the plan of care; this information can be used to improve recovery time or identify opportunities to adjust patient care interventions.

Commonly used critical pathways provide an outline of care for acute care procedures with predictable outcomes and treatments, such as total knee replacement, hip replacement, or percutaneous transluminal coronary angioplasty. In home health care, pathways are used for conditions with predictable courses of care such as heart failure and home IV antibiotic therapy.

Critical pathways often reflect the most frequently seen, highest risk, or most costly conditions within an organization. However, some organizations have critical pathways for almost every diagnosis and procedure. Pathways provide a plan of care for the patient on the stated day, and plans are provided for subsequent days until the patient is discharged (examples of subsequent days are not provided in this chapter because of space limitations). Vascular access options should be addressed in the plan of care during the acute phase of care and after discharge.

Critical pathways are usually documented with the *charting by exception* method, which records only abnormal findings and condenses normal findings. Normal findings are assumed unless otherwise indicated. Detailed descriptions of acceptable normal findings should be clearly defined in organizational standards of care (TJC, 2007a).

Documentation by exception, better known as charting by exception, was created in an effort to reduce documentation time and to make trends in the patient's status more obvious. Documentation by exception records only those events that do not reflect the normal. This form of documentation, reflected in Figure 28-3, requires an understanding of what is normal so that the abnormal (exception) is recognized. It is necessary that there be clear delineation of what is defined as normal findings for comprehensive and abbreviated assessments.

Education about concise, accurate documentation is paramount. Statements should be specific and descriptive. Some indication in the record should refer to observations within normal limits, even if only a check mark or a symbol is used.

Charting by exception does not negate the need for effective documentation of assessments performed and unusual symptoms noted. Negative outcomes of infusion therapy, such as gross infiltration or severe phlebitis, often suggest that observations were *not normal*. In the absence of adequate documentation, such negative outcomes can imply insufficient observation by the nurse.

ACUTE CARE DOCUMENTATION

The Joint Commission (2007a) states that the goal for information management is to support decision-making to improve patient outcomes, patient safety, health care documentation,

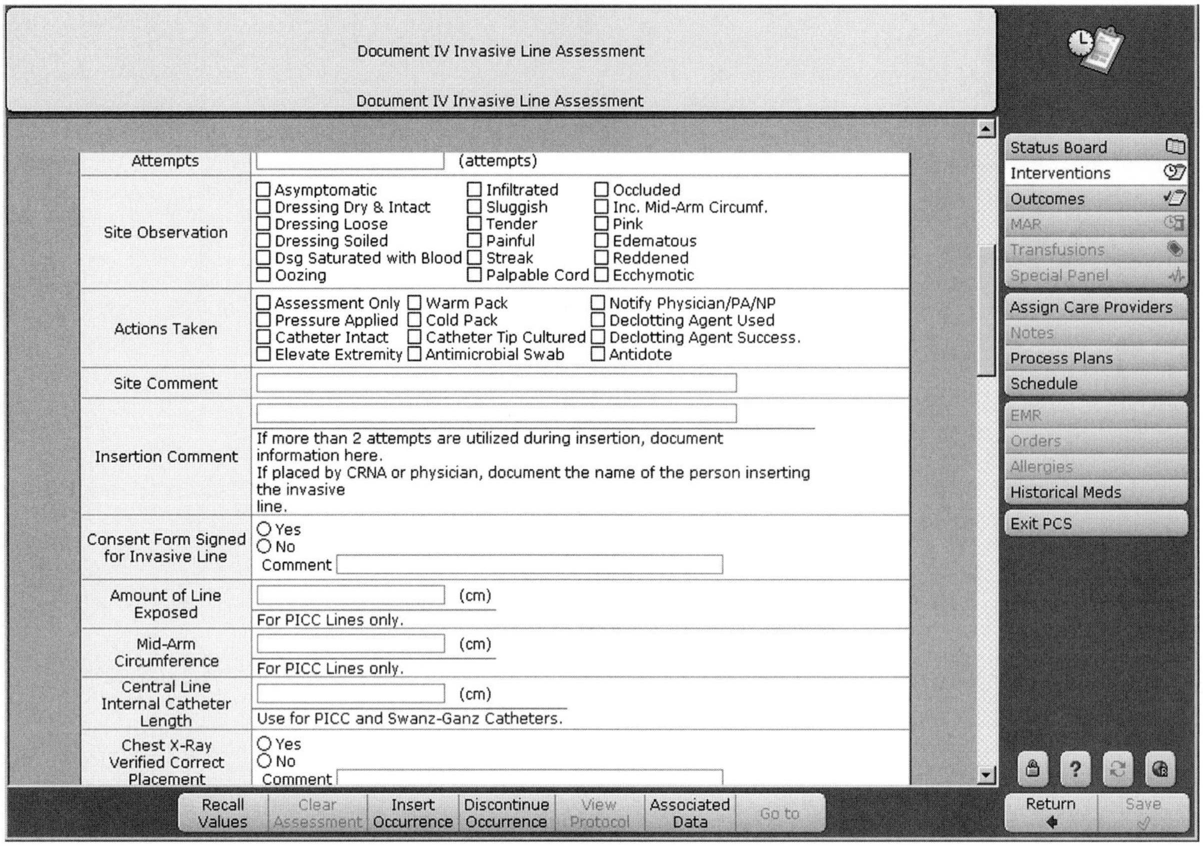

FIGURE 28-2 Computerized charting IV invasive line assessment screen. (From Meditech PCS documentation system, St. Mary's Health Care System, Athens, Ga.)

performance in patient care, treatment, services, governance, management, and support processes. Patient assessment activities are defined in writing so that scope, responsibility, and accountability are clearly delineated. The initial assessment must be accomplished and documented by the registered nurse within the first 24 hours of admission. Because most hospitalized patients have some form of infusion therapy, the assessment should also include an access device assessment and evaluation of current infusion treatment regimens, and include consideration in discharge planning for future or continuing infusion needs. The Joint Commission also requires reassessment at regular intervals or in response to significant changes in the patient's condition or diagnosis (for example, when a malignancy is discovered and long-term venous access for chemotherapy is needed, or if the patient's condition worsens to cardiac arrest and an emergency central line is established during the code). The infusion needs to be changed in both of the preceding situations, necessitating not only a change in the type of venous access but also a change in the plan of care for different infusion therapy modalities. Care decisions should be based on identified patient needs and care priorities (Geibert, 2006).

The initial assessment documentation should include the patient's psychological and social concerns as well as physiological status. The level of family and caregiver support available for the patient in the home may determine the type of infusion therapy used and the type of catheter inserted. An implantable access device may be indicated if the patient needs intermittent therapy or daily flushing of an infusion device, or if routine care is unavailable. Cultural influences, financial concerns, gender, age, and the availability of health care resources

should be considered. Documentation records should reflect external and internal restraints and provide justification for payment or future treatment decisions. Younger patients may be embarrassed about an exposed peripherally inserted central catheter (PICC), or a woman of ethnic origin may have cultural restrictions for catheter placement. Documentation of these concerns facilitates the decision-making process in developing the plan of care.

Successful continuity of care requires careful assessment and discharge planning. Infusion access must be appropriate to the level of care required and accessible to the patient. Managed care groups, insurance companies, governmental agencies, and other payers require precise, appropriate documentation, and the transfer needs must be justified to smoothly transition the patient from one unit to another within the acute care setting, the home, or another facility.

HOME CARE DOCUMENTATION

Requirements for clinical documentation are generally the same for acute care and home care settings except for environmental issues. In addition, documentation of home care services must include information that justifies the need for home care visits. Home care documentation should be interdisciplinary and require communication and documentation between disciplines. The record must reflect total patient care, including the assessment, care plan, implementation of care, evaluations, and outcomes. Reimbursement under Medicare for

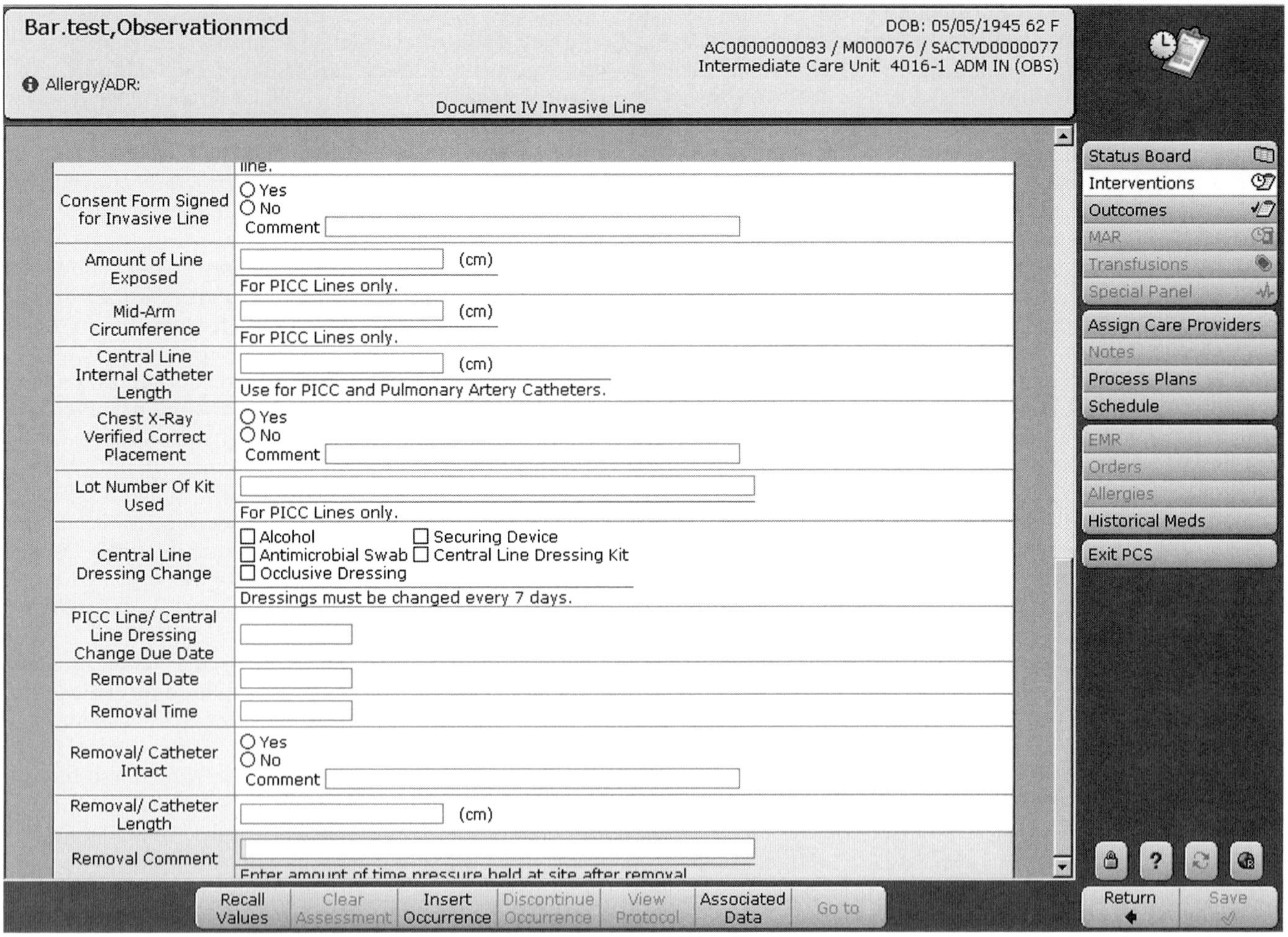

FIGURE 28-3 Charting by exception: comprehensive and modified assessments. (From Meditech PCS documentation system, St. Mary's Health Care System, Atlanta, Ga.)

home heath is complex and is based upon a combination of the patient's primary diagnosis, the first five secondary diagnoses, and the patient's level of acuity based upon completion of selected OASIS (Outcome Assessment Information Set) questions. OASIS is a standardized patient data collection and assessment tool (CMS). There is an OASIS question that asks about the need for infusion therapies at home, including parenteral and enteral nutrition.

PATIENT ASSESSMENT

The Joint Commission (2006-2007) standards for home care (TJC, 2007b) require an agency or organization to document the use of clinical practice guidelines, critical pathways, and standards of practice in the decision-making process. The documentation should include observations about safety of the environment, medications, storage and handling of supplies, use of medical gases, and instructions concerning handling and disposal of hazardous or infectious materials.

Written assessments should also include the following:
- Medical history
- Pertinent physical findings
- Age- and gender-specific findings
- Laboratory results
- History of chemical dependency

- Psychological and nutritional status
- Use of herbal and over-the-counter medications
- Condition of the home and surroundings
- Patient and family educational needs, abilities, and readiness to learn

There should be documentation about the environment indicating that it is safe and has water, electricity, and refrigeration.

The patients' learning needs—such as knowledge of their disease, prognosis, medication administration and schedules, procedure and treatments, personal access, emergency plans, infection control, and safety—should be documented. Assessments should also include reporting victims of abuse or neglect. Discharge needs (termination of therapy) should be assessed and a follow-up plan of care should be established to provide the patient with ongoing health care.

INFUSION THERAPY

In addition to general nursing documentation, vascular access details and assessment and other information are required for infusion therapy patients. Documentation must demonstrate that the risks and benefits of the prescribed therapy or access device have been explained. Appropriate consents must be signed. The physicians' orders must include the medication name, dose, route, rate and volume, and frequency of administration as well as the duration of the infusion therapy. The *Infusion Nursing Standards of Practice* (2006) includes specific information about the insertion and care of vascular access devices and administration practices that should be included in documentation, and the *Standards* should always be the ultimate authority. Documentation should include the type, brand, length, and size of the vascular access device; the number of attempts, anatomical location, and patient's response to the infusion procedure; and the use of visualization or guidance technologies during the infusion procedure (INS, 2006). Flush solution and frequency of flushing should be documented. Anaphylactic orders, if indicated, should also be included with the physicians' orders or outlined in organizational policy and procedure guidelines. Organizational policy should be specific as to the acceptability of administering medications that have not been approved by the U.S. Food and Drug Administration.

The patient or caregiver should receive written instructions about the infusion therapy. Interventions or treatments should be described. Documentation should include a description of written or verbal instructions with results of return demonstration for technical procedures.

Subsequent documentation should include the following (TJC, 2007b):

- Changes in the initial assessment
- Procedure performed
- Local anesthetics, if used
- Description of device (gauge and length)
- Location of insertion site and number of attempts
- External length of catheter left outside the skin
- Location of catheter tip, if necessary (e.g., central venous catheter)
- Equipment used
- Infusate or medication and volume infused
- Patient's response and compliance
- Supply disposal procedures
- Unusual or unexpected sequelae

Documentation of catheter removal should include the integrity and length of the catheter, any complications incurred, and the dressing applied to the insertion site. Symptoms, interventions for complications encountered, and physician communications should be described and recorded, including the time. If extravasation has occurred, documentation should include insertion site appearance, amount of medication infused, amount and method of administering the antidote, and the patient's response to the interventions.

Documentation of periodic evaluations of therapy should include the patient's clinical status, complications and sequelae encountered, potential problems, the patient's or caregiver's response and compliance to the therapy and care administered, telephone conversations that may support or reinforce education to the patient, and verbal communications between other members of the health care team.

INSURANCE REQUIREMENTS

Insurance companies generally authorize the number of home care visits required to provide needed care. The goal, in most cases, is to teach the patient or a caregiver how to administer infusions at home. Ongoing need for home care is justified by specific descriptions of the patient's condition and the patient's severity of illness. Communication between the insurance case manager and the home care nurse is essential. Home care nursing documentation must indicate progress towards expected outcomes, barriers interfering with safe progress (such as cognitive or functional limitations), and need for further home visits. Because the insurance case manager or reviewer may not have the complete chart, concise and pertinent documentation on the assessment form is imperative. Factual descriptions should be used, including details such as "redness extends 3 cm around insertion site in the left antecubital area." Documentation of patient teaching should be specific, such as, "taught patient how to use aseptic technique when attaching IV tubing to the catheter injection port," or "the patient will demonstrate how to clean and maintain PICC dressing." The documentation of patient education should reflect, for example, that the patient knows the name, correct dose, and times the medication is administered. If reteaching is necessary, the reason for repeating instructions must be documented. Descriptions of patient progress should be specific, such as "the patient experiences nausea within 30 minutes from the start of the infusion." Documentation must describe a chronic or acute problem. Payment may be denied based on the assumption that the care is custodial or maintenance in nature.

Evidence, including clinical diagnosis and significant clinical findings, must be given to justify the need for skilled care. A description of services should include the assessment, procedures needed, teaching activities, and the services needed to meet these requirements. Documentation should also include the patient's response, measurable outcomes, and progress as a result of the therapy or services delivered. The nurse should note appropriate and timely interventions related to identified nursing diagnoses, changes in condition, notification and communication with the physician, interventions made, patient response and progress, and evidence of coordination of other services.

 ## NON–ACUTE NURSING CARE FACILITIES

Infusion therapy is often delivered in skilled nursing, rehabilitation, long term care facilities or hospice units. Documentation requirements are like those for home care if rehabilitation is needed, and similar to acute care documentation if infusion therapy is temporary and short term.

 ## INFUSION THERAPY DOCUMENTATION

ASSESSMENT

The rationale for infusion therapy should be recorded to ensure the appropriateness of device selection and the purpose of the intended treatment. An accurate initial infusion therapy assessment documents the patient's general condition, the condition of the patient's skin, and the reason for therapy. A PICC may be inserted for long-term antibiotics, or a large-gauge catheter may be placed for open-heart surgery. General information about the patient is helpful in determining the type of therapy that is most beneficial. The patient's cognitive mental condition, whether confused, combative, or restless, may affect placement preference.

MONITORING

It is imperative that infusion sites be monitored and that monitoring assessments be documented at frequent intervals, according to organizational policy. A site assessment should be specific and describe the site using the degree or grade of phlebitis, such as "0+ phlebitis," which indicates no clinical symptoms of phlebitis or swelling (INS, 2006). Any unusual symptoms noted, such as pain, tenderness, swelling, or poor function, should be addressed and followed throughout the documentation process. Skin condition should be assessed to document potential difficulties in placing, positioning, or securing the infusion device. Documentation for patients who have diabetes, have been taking steroids or anticoagulants, or are undergoing chemotherapy should be specific because these patients may experience changes in skin fragility and thickness.

Many cases of legal liability hinge on the adequacy and timeliness of corrective action. Clearly, inadequate monitoring of an infusion site or incomplete documentation of monitoring activities can put the nurse and organization at a disadvantage in court. When vesicants (such as dopamine) or highly acidic or irritating medications (such as chlorpromazine) are administered, site monitoring and documentation should be more frequent.

TREATMENT

Documentation of infusion therapy should include the type of access device, catheter gauge and length, location and condition of the insertion site, and date and time of insertion. There are many designs and materials used for catheters. Allergies to the catheter material may develop. If an agency or organization uses only one brand of catheter, documentation of brand is not as crucial as in facilities where many types are available. However, catheter care and use may be specific for a certain catheter type, or the patient may be transferred to another facility. In these instances, documentation of catheter type would help the nurse provide appropriate care. The catheter size and length provide important functional information; for example, blood products, surgery, chemotherapy, vesicants, or other special therapies require different catheter gauges. Documentation also needs to include details about administration when medications require dilution or extended administration time.

Patient response to an infusion procedure should be documented. Excessive anxiety, patient movement, or an untoward response should be reported to others on the health care team. This information may forewarn subsequent infusion care providers that device dwell time may be adversely affected or that the next venipuncture may be difficult.

Documentation of the exact insertion site is essential in tracking appropriateness of site selection, presence of phlebitis, and dates for catheter rotation. If therapy was established in the upper arm or feet, additional documentation is needed to support limited or unavailable IV access in the hands, forearms, or antecubital fossa.

Infection control data and performance improvement activities require that all bloodstream infections and local peripheral infections be researched to determine, if possible, the cause of the infection. An accurate description of the insertion date and the condition of the insertion site not only will help determine when the site should be rotated, but also will help track possible causes of any complications.

OBSERVATIONS AND INTERVENTIONS

Observation of the patient and delivery of infusion therapy provide the necessary information for documentation. Infusion sites should be observed and palpated, if possible. Documentation of infusion site observations should include the following:

- Tenderness
- Temperature at and around the site
- Discoloration
- Swelling
- Drainage

Organizational policy should quantify the frequency of required nursing observation and documentation. Home care policies should provide thorough education of the patient or designated caregiver in the importance of observing and caring for the infusion site and of documenting observations and care.

Documentation of infusion device removal is crucial. Documentation of a peripheral device removal should include the site condition, date, time, and initials of the person removing the device. Documentation of a central venous catheter removal should include a description of how the device was removed, the length of time pressure was held on the insertion site after removal, the character and type of dressing applied, any ointment applied, the patient's response to the procedure, any patient restrictions after removal, and the initials of the nurse or name of the health care provider removing the device. For both peripheral and central device removal, the integrity of the catheter must be assessed by comparing the length to the original insertion length to ensure that the entire device is removed intact.

COMPLICATIONS

Complications associated with infusion therapy (such as pain, phlebitis, infiltration, extravasation, infection, and drainage) and any unusual symptom or event should be recorded. For central devices, the lack of blood return or poor blood return, positional problems, catheter dysfunction (e.g., malposition), shortness of breath, or air embolism should be reported and documented. When interventions are necessary, the following should be documented:

- Date and time symptoms occurred that required an intervention
- Assessment of the patient's condition
- Notification of physician
- Communication with patient and family, if necessary
- Treatment interventions taken
- Ongoing monitoring and further interventions
- Patient response until the problem is resolved

Particular care should be given to documentation when unusual or unanticipated occurrences happen. Organizational policies need to be followed for identification and reporting of unusual occurrences or sentinel events.

PATIENT QUALITY OUTCOMES

Ongoing and reliable information is necessary so that key clinical decisions can be made to improve nursing care. Positive and negative outcomes of infusion therapy should be addressed in the patient's record. Outcomes, or results of therapy, complete the procedure and indicate whether therapy was successful. Positive outcomes may be simple, such as "termination of therapy," or slightly more complex, such as "termination of therapy without complications." Negative outcomes should be described in detail, including interventions and sequelae. For example, extravasation documentation should include the following:

- Assessment of the site (e.g., degree of extravasation, discoloration)
- Estimation of the amount of drug infused into the tissue
- Notification of the physician
- Medications injected to reverse or minimize damage to surrounding tissue
- Device removal (how and by whom)
- Any other necessary interventions, such as application of heat or cold
- Patient response to the procedure

After an extravasation the nurse should observe the site often and document each observation until the site has healed or the patient is discharged.

 COMMUNICATION

Documentation is the best way for health care professionals to communicate with one another. A medical record reveals the history, treatment, and outcomes for a given period. Documentation should include pertinent information about communication between patients, families, physicians, and other members of the health care team. Information about physician notification orders and directives should be noted. Communication to supervisors or others in authority should be noted if their response seems important to the patient's outcome.

 PATIENT TEACHING AND UNDERSTANDING

Documentation should include the responses of the patient, family, and caregiver to teaching. All infusion therapy modalities should be explained to all those involved in patient care. The explanation should include the following:

- Purpose of the procedure
- Use of and care for the infusion device
- Observation of the therapy and site
- Sign and symptoms of infection
- Recognition of other potential complications
- Interventions for problems and complications
- Any restrictions necessary while receiving therapy

Written information regarding infusion therapy is often given to the patient before the procedure. The information should be individualized and reflect the patient's specific needs. Receipt and understanding of the information by the patient, family, and caregiver should be recorded. Written instructions at discharge are necessary, especially for the patient receiving continuing therapy at home.

 NURSING RESPONSIBILITIES

ACCOUNTABILITY

Infusion nurses are accountable for their practices, including the elements of the nursing process: assessment, planning, implementation, and evaluation. Documentation needs to reflect

these steps. Even if the infusion nurse's primary responsibility is working on an infusion team or in home infusion therapy, basic nursing skills and assessments are no less important.

COMPETENCY

Regulatory agencies require that staff competencies be evaluated and maintained. Written policies and standards are determined by the organization as to the frequency and depth of the validation process. Competency in infusion therapy should be assessed and documented. This may be accomplished by testing and return demonstration. Standards define acceptable practice guidelines for performance. Organizations should have written standards that establish the expectation for positive patient outcomes and should provide guidelines to accomplish those outcomes. Staff education and IV validation records should be kept in personnel files.

PATIENT OUTCOMES

Expected outcomes with documentation include:
- The patient will have an accurate medical record.
- The patient will be able to retrieve his or her medical and medication records.

The Infusion Nurses Certification Corporation established a credentialing program for infusion therapy in 1983. Through testing designed to document the knowledge of practitioners of infusion nursing, an individual is awarded the trademarked credential Certified Registered Nurse Infusion (CRNI®). The CRNI designation provides national recognition and documentation of knowledge, skills, and experience of the infusion nurse. Courts of law recognize the *Infusion Nursing Standards of Practice* as the basis for optimal infusion care. The signature of the registered nurse along with the CRNI designation indicate the acquisition of additional education and knowledge in infusion nursing.

PERFORMANCE IMPROVEMENT

Performance improvement activities are an integral part of the delivery of infusion therapy. Complications are not always avoidable; they should be investigated and issues should be evaluated to help prevent an unfavorable outcome. Efforts toward and results of performance improvement are part of the documentation of infusion therapy.

Documenting data and trends allows specific patient events to be retrieved and future developments to be predicted. The Joint Commission requires that all sentinel events (that is, near misses, events that are life-threatening or have a life-limiting potential) be investigated for root and cause. When outcomes are unexpected or need to be improved, previous documentation provides important information and clues to help understand why the outcome occurred. An analysis of the root causes provides the basis for creating an action plan for improvement. Corrective efforts to improve infusion therapy outcomes may include education; change of policies and procedures, such as for dressing care or frequency of peripheral rotation; and product changes. The *Infusion Nursing Standards of Practice* provides clearly stated standards and practice criteria information related to the practice of infusion therapy.

Any agency or organization delivering infusion therapy should maintain records concerning the infusion devices inserted (volume and type) and the rates of phlebitis, infiltration, and infection. These data are necessary to measure the effectiveness and monitor outcomes of infusion therapy.

 REIMBURSEMENT

Inadequate or inappropriate documentation affects patient safety and care, and may decrease or negate payment. Pay for performance practices penalize organizations for hospital-acquired infections not present when the patient was admitted, poor outcomes, or hospital-incurred injury such as a fractured hip after a fall. Therefore it is important to comply with payers' rules and guidelines. Careful complete assessment, appropriate diagnosis, treatment, intervention, and expected outcomes are reported to describe and justify payment. Thorough knowledge and close monitoring are necessary to ensure proper coding to allow payment. Incomplete documentation may lead to full or partial denial of payment or possible fraud charges. For example, if a blood transfusion was ordered and a charge was generated but there is no record the patient received the blood and the record is not corrected before billing, it appears that the hospital may be billing for services not delivered (Childers, 2005).

 SUMMARY

Documentation offers a permanent record of events, behaviors, and responses to infusion therapy. It is the most important vehicle for validating the care performed by the infusion nurse. It provides the details necessary to understand the care given and the patient's response to that care. Documentation provides the information necessary for concurrent and retrospective reviews and information that allows the total performance of the infusion department to be evaluated and benchmarked against other organizations and national standards. Periodic concurrent and retrospective reviews of infusion practices provide medical information that can determine future treatment. Quality of patient care is improved through redesign, restructure, and innovation in nursing care (Johnson et al, 2006). The accuracy and completeness of infusion care documentation can help improve patient outcomes by adding pertinent information to the analysis of the patient's clinical picture. Documentation in the medical record is recognized in legal settings as

proof of infusion care administered. Although it takes time, a commodity often in short supply, care must be taken to document all infusion care concisely, precisely, and accurately to create a valid, reliable medical record.

 REFERENCES

Austin S: Ladies and gentlemen of the jury, I present…the nursing documentation, *Nurs* 36(1):56-63, 2006.

Centers for Medicare & Medicaid Services: *Home health prospective PPS overview.* Accessed 5/18/08 at http://www.cms.hhs.gov/HomeHealthPPS/01_overview.asp#TopOfPage.

Childers K: Paying a price for poor documentation, *Nurs* 35(11):32-33, 2005.

Chiverton P, Witzel P: What CNO's really want, *Nurs Manag* 39(1):33, 2008.

Doyle M: Promoting standardized nursing language using an electronic medical record system, *AORN* 83(6):1336, 2006.

Ferrell K: Documentation, part 2: the best evidence of care, *AJN* 107(7):61-64, 2007.

Geibert RC: Using diffusion of innovation concepts to enhance implementation of an electronic health record to support evidence-based practice, *Nurs Adm Q* 30(3):203-210, 2006.

Health Insurance Portability and Accountability Act of 1996. Accessed 11/13/07 at http://aspe.hhs.gov/amnsimp/p1104191.htm.

Infusion Nurses Society: Infusion nursing standards of practice, *J Infus Nurs* 29(1):S3-S43, S53, S59, 2006.

Johnson K, Hallary D, Meridith R et al: A nurse-driven system for improving patient quality outcomes, *J Nurs Care Qual* 21(2):6168-6175, 2006.

Langowski C: The times they are a changing: effects of online nursing documentation systems, *Qual Manag Health Care* 14(2):121-125, 2005.

Monarch K: Documentation, part I: principles for self-protection, *AJN* 107(7):58-60, 2007.

Nightingale F: *Notes on nursing: what it is, and what it is not,* New York, NY, 1986, Dover.

The Joint Commission: *Comprehensive accreditation manual for hospitals: the official hand book, CAMH Refreshed Core,* Oakbrook Terrace, Ill, 2007a, Author.

The Joint Commission: *2006-2007 Comprehensive accreditation manual for homecare: the official hand book, CAMH Refreshed Core,* Oakbrook Terrace, Ill, 2007b, Author.

The Joint Commission: *Do not use list,* 2007c. Accessed 11/13/07 at www.joint commission.org/patient safety/donotuselist.

The Joint Commission: *Sentinel event glossary of terms,* 2007d. Accessed 11/13/07 at http://www.jointcommission.org/sentinelevents/se-glossary.htm.

Wolf DM, Greenhouse PK, Diamond JN et al: Community hospital successfully implements eRecord and CPOE, *Comput Inform Nurs* 24(6):307-316, 2006.

CHAPTER

29   INFUSION THERAPY IN CHILDREN

Anne Marie Frey, BSN, CRNI® and Janet Pettit, MSN, NNP-BC, CNS

Administering intravenous infusions to neonates and children poses unique challenges to the clinicians responsible for their care. Not only are children very different from adults, but they also display variations among their different age groups, including physical, physiological, developmental, cognitive, and emotional variables. The nurse performing infusion techniques in children should be knowledgeable of the child's developmental stage and highly skilled in the basic principles of safe administration of infusion solutions and medications. This skill set includes the ability to calculate small doses and low infusion rates, select appropriate venipuncture sites and equipment, and develop creative measures to distract curious little minds and hands. This chapter focuses on the needs of children as they relate to infusion therapy and on the unique aspects of caring for children and their families.

ANATOMICAL AND PHYSIOLOGICAL DIFFERENCES IN CHILDREN

PHYSIOLOGY
Thermoregulation

The large surface area in relation to volume, the thin layer of subcutaneous fat, and unique methods for producing heat predispose the neonate to excessive heat loss. Premature and sick infants are predisposed to cold, stress, and hypoglycemia, demonstrating an increased metabolism, which results in higher oxygen and caloric requirements and ultimately acidosis (Hockenberry and Wilson, 2007).

Measures must be taken to protect the neonate from hypothermia during all aspects of care, including obtaining vascular access and performing site care. A neutral thermal environment (one that permits the infant to maintain a normal core temperature with minimum oxygen consumption and calorie expenditure) must be provided during all caregiving functions, including venipuncture. Use of radiant warming beds, incubators, warming lamps, warm blankets, and head coverings are all measures that may be employed to protect the infant from heat loss.

Vessel size

Venous and arterial vessels in the infant and child are smaller than those in the adult. Although the vessels are anatomically positioned in the same locations throughout life, the small size and presence of subcutaneous fat may contribute to difficulty locating suitable veins. Vasodilation, caused by application of heat to the extremity, before performing venipuncture may facilitate venous identification and catheter insertion. Other vein location measures include transillumination (Goren et al, 2001) and use of infrared and near-infrared technologies.

Renal function

The newborn has an anatomically complete renal system; however, in the infant younger than 6 weeks of age, glomerular filtration and the ability to concentrate urine function less precisely than in the mature child. Mature kidney function is complete by approximately 2½ to 3 years of age. The young infant's renal system has difficulty coping with changes in fluid and electrolyte status. Dehydration, conditions of hyperosmolality, and sometimes overhydration are problems for the infant. Not only are infants more prone to develop these conditions, but also the effects progress more rapidly. Infants have a greater urine volume per kilogram of body weight. Expected urine output with adequate intake should be 0.5 to 1.0 mL/kg/hour for the newborn and 1.0 to 2.0 mL/kg/hour for the infant (Hockenberry and Wilson, 2007).

Hepatic function

Throughout the first year of life, the liver remains immature and this resultant decrease in hepatic function affects the ability to metabolize drugs, form plasma proteins and ketones, store glycogen and vitamins, and break down amino acids. Digestive

TABLE 29-1 Circulating Blood Volumes in Children

Age	mL/kg of body weight
Neonate	85-90
Infant	75-80
Child	70-75
Adolescent	65-70

From Hazinski MF: *Nursing care of the critically ill child*, ed 2, St Louis, 1992, Mosby.

and metabolic processes are usually completely developed by the beginning of toddlerhood.

Endocrine function

The endocrine system in the newborn is intact anatomically; however, it functions at an immature level. The entire endocrine system interrelates and affects body homeostasis. Decreased functioning of this system affects the ability of the infant to cope with stress. For example, endocrine-secreted hormones that affect fluid and electrolyte equilibrium and metabolism include adrenocorticotropic hormone, antidiuretic hormone, and vasopressin. The immature endocrine system, in concert with other immature body systems, predisposes the infant to such conditions as dehydration and unstable blood glucose levels.

BODY COMPOSITION
Subcutaneous fat

The percentage of body fat gradually increases over the first 6 months of life with the highest percentages of body fat seen in the toddler and prepubescent years. Additional adipose tissue may add to the difficulty of locating veins for IV access. In addition, the percentage of body fat can affect therapeutic requirements of lipid-soluble IV medications such as the benzodiazepines (e.g., diazepam [Valium], lorazepam [Ativan], and midazolam [Versed]).

Circulating blood volume

In children, the circulating blood volume is much greater per unit of body weight than in the adult, but the absolute blood volume is small (Table 29-1). In a small infant, hypovolemia can occur from only a small amount of blood loss. The following equations compare the relative impact of an absolute-volume loss on a 7-kg infant and a 70-kg adult:

25-mL blood loss from 7 - kg infant
= 5% of total circulating blood volume (500 mL)

25-mL blood loss from 70 - kg adult
=< 0.6% of total circulating blood volume (4150 mL)

When blood samples are obtained for laboratory examination, the smallest amount of blood required for accurate results should be removed. Blood replacement should be considered when blood loss is greater than 10% of the total circulating volume (Cahill-Alsip and McDermott, 2001). Some hospitals with acutely ill infants record the blood sample amount in the output section of the intake and output record. In neonates, other physiological criterion is used to measure if blood replacement is needed.

Fluid and electrolyte metabolism

The ratio of fluid to body mass is greater in the newborn than at any other time of life; this ratio decreases steadily with age. The newborn has the largest proportion of free water in the extracellular spaces. This results in higher levels of total body sodium and chloride and lower levels of potassium, magnesium, and phosphate than in the adult. At a rate of exchange seven times greater than that of the adult, the infant exchanges approximately half of its total extracellular fluid daily. The basal metabolism rate is also twice as great in relation to body weight in the infant than it is in the adult. Insensible water losses are greater in infants because of their larger body surface/body weight ratio. These factors, in addition to the inability of the kidneys to concentrate urine in infants, can cause dehydration, acidosis, and overhydration (Fann, 1998).

The daily fluid requirement (per kilogram of body weight) for an infant is three times greater than that of an adult and increases under stress. The normal daily caloric requirements are also greater than those of the adult because of the child's increased basal metabolism rate and rapid growth rate. Children who are ill, especially those with fever or who have had major surgery, require more calories than are required for regular maintenance (see Table 17-7).

PEDIATRIC DEVELOPMENTAL AND ASSESSMENT CONSIDERATIONS

Successful pediatric infusion therapy relies on more than technical skill and knowledge of the physiological differences between children and adults. An understanding of the psychological aspects of the child's growth and development and the application of appropriate interventions is essential when interacting with children. Table 29-2 outlines the various developmental stages of childhood and suggests nursing actions for IV placement for each stage.

HISTORY

Although in most cases the assigned nurse or nurse practitioner will obtain a nursing history, the infusion nurse can contribute to this ongoing database by assessing criteria related to infusion therapy. This includes information such as IV history, current plan of treatment, expectations of the child and family, and special considerations that might affect IV access, such as hand dominance or thumb sucking if peripheral IV access in the upper extremities is considered. Reviewing maternal prenatal and delivery records, as well as an assessment of maternal health in the immediate postpartum period, contributes to the history of the newborn. Additionally, events in the immediate newborn transition period may be critical.

PHYSICAL ASSESSMENT

Before and during the course of infusion therapy, the clinical assessment of the child should include weight; height; vital signs; condition of skin, mucous membranes, and fontanels; urine volume; and neurological status. Some elements of the

TABLE 29-2 Developmental Stages of Childhood and Nursing Implications for Venous Access Device Insertion

Age group	Developmental stage and characteristics	Nursing implications
Infant (birth to 1 yr)	Basic Trust vs. Mistrust Develops trust as basic needs are met. Separation anxiety and fear of strangers with infant >6 months. Communicates by crying.	Keep infant warm. Use a pacifier. Avoid feeding immediately before procedure (risk of vomiting and aspiration). Use assistants other than family to restrain infant. Encourage parental tactile contact and soothing verbal stimuli immediately after procedure and throughout duration of therapy. Protect site from infant's reach.
Toddler (1-3 yr)	Autonomy vs. Shame Has little understanding of cause and effect. Communicates by crying, pointing, using basic words. May calm with security items. May regress in developmental milestones.	Prepare immediately before procedure. Use simple and honest explanations; tell child of impending IV insertion right before procedure. Use positioning for comfort techniques to restrain. Transitional objects provide comfort (blanket, toy). Likes rewards (e.g., stickers). NOTE: Secure anchoring of IV site is essential for this age group.
Preschool (4-6 yr)	Initiative vs. Guilt Follows directions but has short attention span. Needs support with invasive procedures and may perceive pain as punishment. Involve in decisions when possible.	Prepare just before procedure. Use equipment to teach (with dolls and stuffed animals). Use short simple words (e.g., "small straw" for "catheter"). Explain that holding still is a big help and that it is OK to cry. Curious about IV but able to keep from touching with frequent reminders. Never bribe or threaten. ("If you don't drink, you'll get an IV.") Praise cooperation.
School age (6-12 yr)	Sense of Industry Understands directions and likes to see cause and effect. Magical thinking exists. May try to delay procedure, likes sense of control, participation. Can conceptualize the element of time.	Prepare several hours in advance. Provide privacy. Provide distraction during procedure. Parents present at child's choice. Allow child to help and give tasks, such as ripping tape, holding still, slow breathing. Explain each step. Offer choices as much as possible. Reassure that crying is OK.
Adolescence (13-19 yr)	Sense of Identity Vacillates between dependence and independence. Questions authority figures. Exaggerated response to pain; minor illness magnified. Fears altered body image.	Preparation several hours to days in advance is vital. Show equipment, and explain function and allow time for questions. Offer choices such as site location, if peers or family can be present. Explain therapy as to an adult patient. Provide privacy. Teach adolescent to report observations about IV.

Adapted from Doellman D: Pediatric PICC insertions: easing the fears in infants and children, *JAVA* 9(2):68-71, 2004; and Hockenberry MJ, Wilson D, editors: *Wong's nursing care of infants and children* (pp 1158-1177), St Louis, 2007, Mosby.

clinical assessment may be performed simultaneously with the nursing history interview. When possible, the young child should be allowed to sit in the parent's lap or the parent should be allowed to be in proximity to the child. This helps the child feel more secure and enhances the child's ability to cooperate. The physician or nurse practitioner, along with the assigned staff nurse, obtain and document physical assessment data.

Height and weight

Height and weight measures are essential for accurate calculations to be made in fluid and medication administration. The comparison of prior weight with current weight is an accurate indicator of fluid-volume deficit or fluid-volume excess. Children younger than 2 years of age are more susceptible to weight changes resulting from fluid balance than from a change in body mass. In this age group, the proportion of body fluid to total body weight is greater and most of this fluid is in the extracellular space.

Changes in weight must be monitored closely. Approximately 1 g of body weight is equal to 1 mL of body fluid. Thus weight loss or gain of 1 kg (2.2 pounds) within 24 hours represents 1 L of fluid loss or gain. Weight changes in a 24-hour period of plus or minus 50 g in an infant, 200 g in a child, or 500 g in an adolescent may be significant, and the physician should be notified. For consistency, infants should be weighed without clothing and on the same scale each time. With small infants, the infusion equipment should be weighed or the weight approximated before venipuncture, and that amount should be subtracted from the total weight obtained. Calculations for fluid replacement are based on the percentage of weight lost; the amount of fluid restriction is based on the amount of weight gained (Mott, James, and Sperac, 1990; Cahill-Alsip and McDermott, 2001).

Vital signs

A listing of normal pediatric vital signs is provided in Table 29-3.

Body temperature may initially be elevated during dehydration but becomes subnormal as dehydration progresses. With each degree of rise or fall in body temperature, the basal metabolic rate increases. This increase in basal metabolic rate results in additional fluid and caloric maintenance requirements of 10% to 12% above maintenance requirements. In many health care settings, the traditional method of using the rectal route has been replaced by safer methods of body temperature recording, such as axillary, which is the primary route in infants, children up to 4 to 6 years of age, or any child who is uncooperative, unconscious, seizure-prone, or has had recent oral surgery. The oral route can be used in children older than 2 years of age who are cognitively able. Rectal temperature assessment has the risk of perforating the wall of the rectum, and is contraindicated in conditions such as thrombocytopenia, neutropenia, and imperforate anus, or after rectal surgery (Wilshaw et al, 1999). More recently, devices that measure tympanic temperature have been used; these devices provide quick measurements and are comfortable, but are accurate only if the probe fits well in the ear canal (usually in children older than 1 year of age).

TABLE 29-3 Pediatric Vital Signs (Normal Values)

Age	Temperature* Fahrenheit	Temperature* Celsius	Pulse rate (Beats/min)	Respiratory rate (Breaths/min)	Blood pressure (mmHg)†
Newborn	96.8-99 (axillary)	36-37.2 (axillary)	120-160	30-60	Systolic: 60-99 (Doppler) Diastolic: 30-62
4 years	97.5-98.6 (axillary)	36.4-37 (axillary)	80-125	20-30	Girls Systolic: 91-104 Diastolic: 52-66 Boys Systolic: 93-107 Diastolic: 50-65
10 years	97.5-98.6 (oral)	36.4-37 (oral)	70-110‡	16-22	Girls Systolic: 102-115 Diastolic: 60-74 Boys Systolic: 102-115 Diastolic: 61-75
16 years	97.5-98.6 (oral)	36.4-37 (oral)	55-90	15-20	Girls Systolic: 111-124 Diastolic: 66-80 Boys Systolic: 116-130 Diastolic: 65-80

*The normal range of the child's temperature will depend on the measuring method used. Temperatures exhibit circadian rhythms at all ages.
†From the National Heart, Lung, and Blood Institute: *The fourth report on the diagnosis, evaluation, and treatment of high blood pressure in children and adolescents* (pp 10-11), Bethesda, Md, 2005, Author. Retrieved 6/11/08 from www. nhlbi.nih.gov.
‡After age 12 years, a boy's pulse rate is 5 beats/min slower than that of a girl in this age group.
From McKinney ES et al: *Maternal-child nursing,* ed 3, St Louis, 2009, Saunders.

The apical pulse is the best site for auscultation of the heart rate in an infant and child. As the child grows older, the heart rate decreases to adult values. An apical rate in a resting infant of 80 to 100 beats per minute is considered *bradycardia,* and an apical rate greater than 160 to 180 beats per minute is considered *tachycardia.* Changes in rate and rhythm may indicate changes in circulating blood volume or electrolyte imbalances.

The normal range of respiration in the infant is 30 to 60 breaths per minute, and diminishes slowly during the toddler stage to near adult levels. An infant with a respiratory rate greater than 60 breaths per minute is generally considered *tachypneic.* *Apnea* is defined as a 20-second or longer period without respiration. The infant's respiratory rate may be increased in either fluid depletion or fluid overload. Alterations in respiratory rate may represent inadequate oxygenation or an attempt to compensate for metabolic acid-base imbalances (i.e., respiratory rate is increased in acidosis and is decreased in alkalosis). The child who is hyperventilating either from anxiety or from a disease process may develop respiratory alkalosis. Breath sounds and rate should be noted when respirations are assessed. Moist breath sounds (rales) may be an indication of fluid overload.

Blood pressure (BP) readings in children normally are much lower than adult levels and vary upward with age. To obtain an accurate blood pressure, the appropriate sized cuff should be used. The width of the BP cuff should be sufficient to cover 75% of the upper arm between the top of the shoulder and the olecranon. The length of the cuff must completely surround the circumference of the limb with or without overlapping. Sites other than the brachial artery that can be used to obtain a BP measurement include the radial, popliteal, dorsalis pedis, and posterior tibial arteries (Mott et al, 1990). If an electronic BP monitor is used, the manufacturer's instructions and guidelines for correct cuff size should be followed. Even with an oscillometric device, movement interferes with the accuracy of measurement. The child should be quiet and the extremity stabilized during the procedure. Changes in BP may indicate a change in circulating blood volume. In fluid-volume deficit, the BP is usually decreased. When a fluid-volume overload exists, the BP is generally elevated. In infants and children, however, the BP should *not* initially be relied on as an accurate measurement of shock. Normal BP may be maintained as the circulatory system compensates with vasoconstriction, tachycardia, and increased cardiac contractility. The other assessment signs discussed, including skin color, temperature, fluid volume, quality of peripheral pulses, mental status, heart rate, and urinary output, are the best status indicators to determine shock (International Consensus on Science, 2000).

Skin

Skin color, turgor (elasticity), temperature, moisture, and texture all relate to the child's state of hydration and nutrition. With fluid-volume deficit, the skin tends to be cool and dry and exhibits poor color return when pressure is gently applied to skin. Cyanosis and mottling usually occur in more advanced stages of fluid deficit. If fever is also present, the skin may be warm and moist. Skin turgor is generally a good indicator of fluid-volume status. Skin turgor is assessed by gently grasping the skin on the abdomen or inner thigh between the thumb and index finger and then quickly releasing. Good hydration is exhibited by an immediate return of the skin to its normal position. Fluid deficit may be present when the skin remains suspended (called *tenting*) for a brief period after being released (Barkin, 1990).

Edema is a sign of fluid-volume overload or fluid shift from the intravascular space to the interstitial space. In infants, edema is most noticeable in the periorbital and scrotal/perineal areas, especially after the infant has been lying flat for a period. The presence and severity of edema can be assessed by indenting the skin with a finger and then releasing to determine if pitting occurs.

Circulation, or end-organ perfusion, is assessed via the skin, brain, and kidneys. Decreased perfusion in the skin is an early sign of shock. As cardiac output decreases, the extremities become cool and blanched and capillary refill is delayed (more than 2 to 3 seconds in neonates and greater than 3 seconds with infants). Mottling, pallor, cyanosis, and peripheral cyanosis, except in newborns who normally have acrocyanosis, are additional signs of poor perfusion (International Consensus on Science, 2000).

Mucous membranes

Moistness of the mucous membranes provides information regarding the hydration status of a child. Dryness of the mucous membranes occurs early in dehydration. The area of the mouth where the gums and cheek meet is often the best place to assess moistness because it remains moist, even during mouth breathing. The lack of tears and the presence of dark circles around sunken eyes are signs of dehydration that occur later in the progression of the condition (Barkin, 1990; Mott et al, 1990).

Fontanels

The anterior fontanel remains open until the child is approximately 2 years of age. This characteristic provides an additional tool to assess hydration status. The anterior fontanel is either completely flat or slightly sunken in a normal state, depressed in states of fluid deficit, and bulging with increased pressure caused by cerebral edema, hemorrhage, or fluid-volume excess.

Urine

An accurate record of urinary output is an important element in the management of fluid balance. A specific gravity value between 1.002 and 1.030 is usually an indication of fluid balance. Fluid restriction or deficit is reflected by a high specific gravity, whereas a low measurement reflects fluid retention or overload or the poor concentrating ability of the premature kidney. In young infants, however, the immature renal system is less able to concentrate urine, causing the results of the measurement to be less accurate (Mott et al, 1990).

When hourly output records are necessary, the child in intensive care may require a urinary catheter for assessment of accurate output; otherwise, the usual practice is to weigh the diapers. The weight of the dry diaper is subtracted from that of the wet diaper, allowing the nurse to determine urinary output. The weight in grams equals the volume voided in milliliters.

Neurological status

In young children, neurological status is more difficult to assess than in adults. Developmentally, young children are unable to respond verbally to questions regarding orientation to surroundings. Changes in behavior or mood, such as hyperirritability when touched or refusal to drink fluids, may indicate a change in the child's neurological status. A child older than 2 months of age should be able to normally focus on his or her parent's face and be attracted by bright objects. Failure to recognize parents may be an early sign of hypoperfusion to the brain. The family is usually the first to detect this but may only be able to interpret this change as "something wrong." A usual sign of neurological involvement in the infant is a high-pitched cry. Changes in the level of consciousness may be an indication of fluid-volume or electrolyte imbalance. Infants are more sensitive to hypo- and hypernatremia and abruptly demonstrate signs of lethargy, somnolence, and hypersensitivity to noise and touch. Twitching, tremors, or convulsions may be noted in more advanced cases. Cerebral edema caused by fluid retention can be displayed by vomiting, restlessness, irritability, and even convulsions, as well as complaints of headache in older children (Barkin, 1990; Mott et al, 1990).

FLUID THERAPY

MAINTENANCE FLUID REQUIREMENTS

Maintenance fluid requirements for a 24-hour period are based on the child's age and change in weight. The standard regimen for normal maintenance fluids is based on water and electrolyte output through insensible fluid losses (particularly transcutaneous and respiratory in the neonate), gastrointestinal fluids, and urine. Because the metabolic rate in infants and children is higher than that in adults, fluid losses are also greater than in adults, and maintenance requirements are increased. The amount of fluid lost before treatment is determined by comparison of preillness and current weights and by clinical signs of deficit. Maintenance fluid requirements for children are usually calculated according to the guidelines in Table 17-7 (Barkin, 1990; Mott et al, 1990; Fann, 1998).

Example: Fluid maintenance for a 14-kg infant would be 1200 mL/24 hours:

$$\frac{1000 \text{ mL(for first 10kg)}}{+ 200 \text{ mL(50mL} \times 4 \text{ kg)}}$$
$$1200 \text{ mL/24 hr}$$

Once the 24-hour maintenance fluid requirement has been calculated, the need for additional fluids must be evaluated. Conditions in which fluid requirements are increased include fluid loss before treatment (e.g., gastroenteritis), increased metabolism (e.g., fever, hyperthyroidism), concurrent losses (e.g., wound drainage, nasogastric suction), or the need to dilute urine (e.g., before chemotherapy). Very-low–birth weight infants (those less than 1500 grams) possess thinner skin layers, allowing significant evaporative water loss through the skin.

REPLACEMENT (DEFICIT) THERAPY

Replacement therapy is divided into phases. The first phase is initial management or rapid delivery of fluid therapy; the second phase, repletion and maintenance therapy; and the third phase, early recovery.

TABLE 29-4 Replacement and Maintenance Requirements

Amount of deficit	Formula for calculating amount of replacement fluid
Mild (5%)	Maintenance + (maintenance × 0.5)
Moderate (10%)	Maintenance + (maintenance × 1.0)
Severe (15%)	Maintenance + (maintenance × 1.5)

Phase I: initial management

In children with fluid-volume deficit, replacement of vascular volume is essential. These children require immediate infusion of fluids (20 mL/kg 0.9% sodium chloride or lactated Ringer's) infused rapidly over 20 to 60 minutes, especially if there is evidence of poor tissue perfusion or changes in vital signs and neurological status. If the child has a documented normal blood glucose level or is known to have diabetes, dextrose solutions should be omitted to prevent hyperglycemia, which may induce an osmotic diuresis. The child's condition is then reassessed. If the response to the therapy is poor, an additional bolus of the initial solution is given. The child continues to be evaluated for the need of additional boluses, invasive monitoring, or the implementation of repletion (maintenance) therapy (Barkin, 1990; Fann, 1998).

Phase II: repletion and maintenance therapy

During this second phase (2 to 24 hours after onset of the deficit), replacement is combined with maintenance requirements. Acid-base and electrolyte disturbances are partially corrected. The simple formulas in Table 29-4 incorporate replacement and maintenance requirements for mild, moderate, and severe volume deficit.

Example: A 10-kg infant has a maintenance fluid requirement of 1000 mL/24 hours. The replacement amounts for 24 hours are shown in the following equations:

Mild (5%)	Maintenance + ½ maintenance 1000 + (1000 × 0.5) = 1500 mL/24 hr
Moderate (10%)	Maintenance + full maintenance 1000 + (1000 × 1.0) = 2000 mL/24 hr
Severe (15%)	Maintenance + 1½ maintenance 1000 + (1000 × 1.5) = 2500 mL/24 hr

Note: The bolus of fluid infused during the initial phase of replacement should be subtracted from the 24-hour volume, and any ongoing losses sustained should be added to these amounts.

Phase III: early recovery

Early recovery, which can last from 24 to 96 hours, is aimed at correcting the remaining deficits occurring in hypertonic dehydration. These electrolyte deficits need to be corrected slowly so as not to impair neurological status. By this time, the child usually is well enough to ingest some fluids orally.

FLUID-VOLUME DEFICIT

Any abnormal fluid loss or reduction in fluid intake can lead to depletion of fluid in the extracellular and intracellular compartments. The most common cause of fluid loss in children is gastroenteritis with diarrhea accompanied by nausea or vomiting. Oral fluid intake is reduced in response to the symptoms, and therefore the amount of fluid lost through the stools or vomiting cannot be balanced. A fluid-volume deficit results, and physiological changes occur that progress as the condition worsens. The infusion of IV solutions into infants and children with fluid-volume deficit requires an understanding of the various types of deficit and the specific therapies required. In addition to being characterized by degree of fluid loss, fluid-volume deficit (dehydration) is also categorized by type—isotonic, hypotonic, or hypertonic, depending on the changes in the child's serum sodium level (Table 29-5).

Hypovolemic shock is a common problem in children who are in need of emergency care. Trauma and burns are obvious causes, but hypovolemic shock can also occur with gastroenteritis and diabetic ketoacidosis. Sepsis in a child can develop into septic shock, which is not classified as hypovolemic but equally requires fluid resuscitation. The initial therapies for hypovolemic and septic shock are similar, and both require immediate vascular access. In traumatic shock, large volumes of blood and fluid are required; therefore IV access sites should be adequate to meet these needs. In emergency situations in which large volumes of fluids are needed, two peripheral catheters, in 24-, 22-, or 20-gauge size, or a short-term emergency central access device, such as a nontunneled femoral line or an intraosseous needle, can provide adequate vascular access in a child (International Consensus on Science, 2000; Hockenberry and Wilson, 2007; Lavelle and Costarino, 2007). The clinical assessment and laboratory data determine the urgency and the type of therapy required. The degree of fluid loss is categorized according to the percentage of total body weight lost: mild (less than 5%), moderate (5% to 10%), and severe (more than 10%).

OTHER INFUSION THERAPIES

In addition to the administration of solutions, venous access devices in children are also used for therapies such as medication administration, parenteral nutrition (PN), and transfusion of blood products. An overview of these therapies as they relate to children is provided in this section. See Chapters 14 and 17 for additional information on blood component therapy and parenteral nutrition, respectively.

MEDICATION ADMINISTRATION

The most commonly used calculations for medication administration in pediatrics are those based on body weight and body surface area (calculated by using a nomogram). Dosing of pediatric medications is usually ordered as milligrams (mg) per kilogram (mg/kg), or in the case of chemotherapeutic agents, milligrams per meter squared (mg/m^2).

Techniques

All methods of IV medication administration, such as IV bolus or push and intermittent and continuous infusions, are used in the pediatric patient. In children, however, the dose and

TABLE 29-5 Clinical Assessment and Infusion Treatment for Types of Fluid-Volume Deficit (Dehydration)

Description	Isotonic	Hypotonic	Hypertonic
Type of Loss			
	Solute and water loss proportional	Greater solute loss than water	Greater water loss than solute
ICF and ECF fluid shift	None	From ECF to ICF	From ICF to ECF
Plasma volume	Decreased	Decreased	Maintained
Serum sodium level (mEq/L)	125-150	<125	>150
Cause	GI fluid loss	GI fluid loss with hypotonic oral intake (glucose in water, ginger ale)	GI fluid loss with hypertonic oral intake (boiled skim milk)
	Urine loss		Diabetes insipidus
	Decreased oral intake		Fever
			Hyperventilation
Clinical Signs			
Skin	Poor turgor, cold, dry, dusky	Very poor turgor, cold, clammy, dusky	Fair turgor; cold, thick, and "doughy" skin
Eyes	Sunken	Sunken	Sunken
Mucous membranes	Dry	Slightly dry	Parched
Fontanels	Depressed	Depressed	Depressed
Pulse rate	Rapid	Rapid	Moderately rapid
Blood pressure	Low	Very low	Moderately low
Neurological status	Irritable or lethargic	Lethargic, coma, seizure	Hyperirritable, high-pitched cry, seizure
Infusion	Half of deficit replaced in first 8 hr, remaining over next 16 hr	Half of deficit replaced in first 8 hr, remaining over next 16 hr	Slow and gradual over 48 hr
Sodium level	2-3 mEq/kg/24 hr	2-3 mEq/kg/24 hr plus replacement; sodium should only be increased ≤2 mEq/L/hr up to serum level of 120 mEq/L	Sodium should not be reduced >2 mEq/L/hr
Potassium level	2-3 mEq/kg/24 hr	2-3 mEq/kg/24 hr	2-3 mEq/kg/24 hr

ECF, extracellular fluid; *GI,* gastrointestinal; *ICF,* intracellular fluid.

volume can be different from those used in adults, depending on the age and the size of the child. In neonates and infants, medications are commonly calculated to the tenths of a milligram or milliliter. Continuous infusions are used primarily to administer drugs that require maintenance of a constant blood level, and potent drugs that must be precisely titrated to individual needs.

Infusion of intermittent medications can be administered by several different methods. The in-line calibrated chamber is commonly used in general pediatric settings for continuous and intermittent infusions in small children. The medication is injected into the in-line calibrated chamber, diluted to a recommended concentration with a compatible IV solution, and infused at a prescribed rate. At the completion of the infusion, the usual practice is to flush the chamber with a volume of a compatible IV solution. The advantages of this method include eliminating the risk of fluid overload and providing accuracy in fluid delivery. A disadvantage of this method is that it is not practical for small infants who are fluid and volume restricted. Also, the drug must be compatible with the primary solution or a second IV administration set-up is required. Recent evidence shows that at least two times the flush volume of the administration set is necessary to clear medication from the line and ensure complete dosage delivery to the patient (Ford et al, 2003).

Administering medications via a syringe pump is commonly used for neonates and children and provides an accurate method of IV medication administration. The syringe pump can be connected via an extension set directly onto an intermittent venous access device or in a piggyback fashion into the primary administration set closest to the insertion site to ensure timely administration. A syringe containing the properly diluted medication is attached to a microbore tubing and pump set to infuse at a prescribed rate.

The retrograde method of medication infusion is less commonly used in the neonatal intensive care unit. A specific low-volume (less than 1 mL) retrograde administration set, with an access port at each end, is attached and primed along with the primary administration set. To administer medications via the system, a medication-filled syringe is attached to the port most proximal to the patient, an empty syringe is connected to the port most distal from the patient, the clamp between the port and the child is closed, and the medication is injected distally up the tubing (away from the child). The solution in the retrograde tubing is displaced upward in the tubing into the empty syringe. Both syringes are removed, the lower clamp is opened, and the medication is then infused into the patient at the prescribed rate. The medication volume is then automatically incorporated into the regulated amount of fluid to be infused. This method is often used in infants who cannot tolerate a rapid infusion rate or additional fluid volume; in this method, the medication infuses at the same rate set for the IV infusion.

PARENTERAL NUTRITION

Parenteral nutrition (PN) is administered when patients cannot or will not fully use their gastrointestinal tract for nutrition or when they require supplemental calories for growth or healing. The goal of parenteral nutrition is to meet anabolic needs and allow normal growth and development. Conditions requiring PN include prematurity, children with congenital or acquired anomalies of the digestive tract (e.g., inflammatory bowel disease, Hirschsprung's disease, short-bowel syndrome, pancreatitis, necrotizing enterocolitis, omphalocele, gastroschisis), surgical conditions, or disease states that may increase the risk of starvation (e.g., cancer, cystic fibrosis, acquired immunodeficiency syndrome [AIDS]). Candidates for parenteral nutrition therapy are identified by medical diagnosis, physical examination, and nutritional evaluation, including such measurements as weight loss, below normal percentiles for height and weight on the growth chart, and abnormal laboratory values such as albumin level (Bilodeau, Poon, and Mascarenhas, 1998).

The parenteral nutrition solution is made up of several components, depending on the status of the child; these solutions can be individualized to fit calorie and nutrient needs (Heird, 1993; ASPEN 2002). The basic components of PN are protein, carbohydrates, fat, electrolytes, vitamins, trace elements, and minerals. Protein, for growth, is administered in the form of crystalline amino acids; infants younger than 6 months require a special amino acid mixture that mimics that of breast milk (ASPEN 2002). Dextrose is used as the carbohydrate source, providing energy so that the body does not break down protein or fat to meet metabolic needs. Fat emulsions or lipids provide a high calorie content per volume, making them ideal sources of calories for children (ASPEN 2002). Fat emulsions also buffer the irritating effects that glucose tends to exert on the vein. Lipids should be infused cautiously in patients with infections, compromised renal function, or hyperbilirubinemia. Compromised liver function and an increased risk of fungal infections have been associated with lipid infusions (Weiss et al, 1991). Fat emulsions may be infused over a 24-hour period, or given over several hours with a break in therapy to allow clearance before proceeding to the next daily infusion. In VLBW preterm and small gestational age infants, lipids are cleared more slowly and patients are at a greater risk of developing hyperlipidemia.

When treating children, it is often difficult to balance fluid needs with calorie needs. A large volume may be necessary to infuse through a peripheral vein to meet a child's caloric needs. Therefore PN is often concentrated in a smaller volume and administered via a central vein. Dextrose 10% may be administered peripherally; central access should be considered when the dextrose percentage exceeds 10%. Fluids containing greater than 10% dextrose concentration can be very irritating to the vein intima and cause local injury.

For children receiving long-term PN, continued growth can change the nutritional requirements, so careful monitoring is essential. PN can be administered in the home or hospital. Home PN is often administered via the central route and cycled over 12 to 18 hours, usually at night, so that the child may function normally during the day. Usually, home PN is initiated in the hospital. When the child is stable and the infusion process for home PN has been mastered by the caregiver(s) with appropriate participation of the child (depending on his or her level of development), home PN may be instituted.

Continuous monitoring is required to ensure safe, efficacious infusion of PN that meets the changing needs of the child. This includes monitoring the following on a scheduled basis:

- Parenteral nutrition base solution or formula
- Electrolytes, vitamins, and trace elements
- Fat emulsion
- Infusion rate
- Laboratory results
- Nutritional measurements

A multidisciplinary team approach can result in the successful clinical application and monitoring of PN while preventing complications.

TRANSFUSION THERAPY

Children are unique with regard to maturation of their hematopoietic system and need special consideration when transfusing blood products because of their smaller vein size and the volume of blood to be infused. During the last few weeks of intrauterine life, maternal gamma-immunoglobulin crosses the placenta into the fetus; therefore the mother's serum is used for compatibility testing during the first few days of life. The fetus does not produce its own antibodies until exposed to foreign substances after birth. After about 1 week of life, or sooner if the newborn underwent transfusion during the first week, serum from the baby may be used for compatibility testing (Nathan et al, 2003). Differences between children and adults include blood volume (see Table 29-1), red cell life span, and hemoglobin level. The red blood cell of the premature newborn has a life span of 35 to 50 days, and the red blood cell of a full-term baby survives 60 to 70 days, compared with 100 to 120 days in an adult (Nathan et al, 2003).

General indications for pediatric transfusion therapy include acute hemorrhage, anemia, abnormal component function (either congenital or acquired), and the presence of toxic substances. The most commonly used products for transfusion in children are packed red blood cells and platelets. The fluid volume in a "unit" of packed red cells is 220 mL. Replacement of red blood cells and platelets is indicated when the hemoglobin level is decreased from chemotherapy and with hematological disorders such as anemia.

In infants and children, hemorrhage can be defined as an acute reduction of blood volume (30% to 40%) or a 20% blood volume loss with chance for recurrence (Nathan et al, 2003). Hemoglobin and hematocrit values are considered less reliable indicators of blood loss. Children can compensate and have normal activity functions despite low hemoglobin and hematocrit levels. Activity level and cardiopulmonary status should be assessed before transfusion therapy is initiated in a child, because an unstressed child can tolerate hemoglobin levels of 3 to 6 g/dL without signs of heart failure or tissue hypoxia. Children usually undergo transfusion if hemoglobin levels fall below 6 g/dL.

Young children, particularly neonates, may become anemic because of repeated blood withdrawals for laboratory testing. Blood withdrawal volumes, especially for neonates, should be recorded in the output section of the nursing flow sheet and monitored daily. Thrombocytopenia can result from maternally induced causes (e.g., aspirin ingestion during pregnancy), pregnancy-induced hypertension, acquired disorders (e.g., idiopathic thrombocytopenia purpura), chemotherapy, or congenital dysfunction of platelets.

Platelet transfusions are indicated when bleeding time is longer than 15 minutes or the platelet count is less than 20,000/mm³ with active bleeding, less than 5000/mm³ with or without active bleeding, or less than 50,000/mm³ before surgery (Landier, Barrell, and Styffe, 1987; NIH, USDHHS, 1990). Rarely is 1 whole unit used for a pediatric transfusion. The average fluid volume for a unit of whole blood is 440 mL. Children and infants require the transfusion of whole blood for volume replacement in the presence of trauma or gastrointestinal bleeding. Blood products are usually administered in increments of milliliters per kilogram based on body weight and estimated blood loss. A packed red blood cell dose is 10 to 15 mL/kg; platelet dose is 1 unit (50 to 70 mL) per 7 to 10 kg of body weight (Landier et al, 1987; NIH, USDHHS, 1990).

The basic principles of blood component therapy for adults (refer to Chapter 14) also apply to children. Transfusion equipment is similar to that for an adult; differences for children include use of smaller gauge needles for transfusion (25- or 23-gauge winged-steel needles or 22- or 24-gauge catheters). Studies show that 27-gauge needles can be used to give packed red blood cells at a rate of up to 50 mL/hr without significant hemolysis (Keller, 1995). Because of volume restrictions in many children, packed red blood cells are not usually diluted with 0.9% sodium chloride; rather, a 0.9% sodium chloride flush is given through the IV administration set to prevent mixing red cells with incompatible solutions that may cause hemolysis. In-line blood filters are used, which may be specially designed, low-volume filters for children. In some cases, small aliquot bags or syringes of blood are transfused; these products are usually prefiltered by blood bank personnel during transfer to the smaller container, eliminating the need to add a filter when administering the blood product. For accuracy, blood products are usually infused using an electronic infusion device approved for use with blood and blood products. The rate of infusion for packed red cells is initially 5% to 10% of the total transfusion volume, given over 15 minutes (Landier et al, 1987; NIH, USDHHS, 1990).

If no adverse reaction is noted, the rate is then increased to 2 to 5 mL/kg/hour or as tolerated. Platelets are given by IV bolus or IV infusion over 30 minutes to 4 hours (NIH, USDHHS, 1990). Because of the absence of foreign antibodies and antigens, titration of the transfusion in the initial stages is not performed in neonates. During transfusion, vital signs and monitoring guidelines are similar to those recommended for adults. In addition, all neonates should be monitored for cold, stress, hypoglycemia, and hypocalcemia. These reactions can occur because of the temperature of the blood product or the presence of a preservative in the blood, which can affect calcium and glucose levels. Another consideration in young infants and immunosuppressed patients is cytomegalovirus; it is important that the blood products be free of this virus. Although adults may also contract cytomegalovirus, infants who contract it suffer much greater consequences that can lead to death (Yeager et al, 1981).

Immunosuppressed pediatric patients—such as premature infants and children with malignancies, end-stage renal disease, or AIDS; infants undergoing an exchange transfusion; or those receiving directed donation of blood from a parent—are at risk of developing graft-versus-host disease (GVHD) if they receive transfusions of blood products that contain lymphocytes. GVHD can be prevented by giving these children transfusions with blood products that are rendered leukocyte poor, either by irradiating the product or by filtering or washing the cells before transfusion. Other transfusion reactions and complications are described in Chapter 14. Documenting transfusions in children is similar to requirements used with the adult patient.

When transfusing a child, the child's and family's view of the transfusion, prior experience, and cultural and religious practices must be examined. Preparation should be age appropriate, as outlined earlier in this chapter. With proper preparation and consent of the caregiver, close monitoring, and follow-up, infusion nurses can ensure safe, efficacious transfusion therapy delivery.

EXCHANGE TRANSFUSION

A therapeutic transfusion modality performed infrequently and almost exclusively in neonates and infants is exchange transfusion, which replaces the infant's blood with donor blood. The most common indication is severe unconjugated hyperbilirubinemia carrying the risk of bilirubin encephalopathy and kernicterus if untreated. This is most often the result of maternal-fetal blood type or group incompatibility leading to maternal antibodies crossing the placenta and causing hemolysis of the fetal and newborn's red blood cells. Performing an exchange transfusion will lower serum bilirubin levels, correct anemia, and remove sensitized erythrocytes. Additional indications for exchange transfusion may include severe anemia, polycythemia, removal of toxins or overdose of medication, disseminated intravascular coagulation, and sepsis (MacDonald and Ramasethu, 2007).

The procedure requires one to two vascular catheters, most commonly umbilical catheters, but other central or peripheral devices are acceptable, allowing for both the withdrawal and the infusion of blood. Monitoring for complications during the procedure is imperative, with the most common being respiratory and cardiac instability, metabolic disorders (hypocalcemia, hypo- or hyperglycemia, and hyperkalemia), hematological disorders, and catheter-associated complications (MacDonald and Ramasethu, 2007).

 ## PERIPHERAL ACCESS

SITE SELECTION

Whether the prescribed therapy is infused via the central or peripheral route, the main goal of therapy is to provide the treatment with the maximum amount of safety and efficiency, while meeting the infant's and child's emotional needs and considering the developmental level.

Characteristics of the therapy that must be considered include type of therapy, expected duration and location for delivery of the therapy (e.g., hospital, home), and rate of infusion. Physical considerations of the child include age, degree of prematurity, ability to tolerate the procedure, size and condition of the veins, reason for the therapy, general patient condition, and mobility of the child. Just as important are the child's developmental considerations: level of activity (e.g., turns, crawls, walks); gross and fine-motor skills (e.g., sucks fingers, plays with own hands, holds bottle, draws, colors); sense of body

TABLE 29-6 Intravenous Sites in Children

Site	Patient age	Veins used	Advantages	Disadvantages
Scalp	Infant, toddler	Superficial temporal, frontal, occipital, posterior auricular, supraorbital	Easily observed, readily dilates, no valves, hands kept free, head easily stabilized, allows accessibility to extremities	Hair must be shaved, arteries hidden, infiltrates easily, disfigurement with infiltration, difficult to secure device, greater family anxiety
Foot	Infant, toddler	Saphenous, median marginal, dorsal arch	Readily dilates, hands kept free, less rolling, more visible in chubby infants, easy to splint	Decreases mobility with walking, limited to smaller gauge sizes, more difficult to advance catheter, near arteries, increased risk of phlebitis in older patients
Fingers	Toddler through adolescent	Digital	Useful if unable to access other sites, easily stabilized on tongue blade in older child	Infiltrates easily, limited to smaller gauge sizes, dependent edema masks infiltration, difficult to stabilize in small infant
Hand	All ages	Metacarpal, dorsal venous arch, tributaries of cephalic and basilic	Easily accessible, readily visible, large enough for larger size catheter, distal location, bones act as natural splints	Increased nerve endings means increased pain, difficult to anchor catheter on infant, interferes with child's activity
Forearm	All ages	Cephalic, basilic, median antebrachial	Same as for hand, keeps hands free	Difficult to observe in chubby toddlers
Antecubital	All ages	Cephalic, basilic, median	Large veins visible and palpable, preferred site in infants	Elbow joint must be maintained in extended position, limits activity, limits sites for phlebotomy, limits sites for possible peripherally inserted central catheter placement

image; fear of mutilation; and cognitive ability (i.e., understands and can follow directions).

The infant and younger child have the advantage of additional optional site locations, including the scalp, foot, and leg. Although the anatomical locations of the vessels are similar in both children and adults, the child's smaller body and vessel size may make it more difficult to successfully achieve access. Along with the individual preference of the clinician, each site has its own characteristics and its own advantages and disadvantages as described in Table 29-6.

PERIPHERAL VENOUS ACCESS SITES
Upper extremity

As with adults, upper extremity sites are readily chosen for venous access in children. Similarly, the veins in the most distal part of the extremity are used first for access, choosing sites from hand to forearm, antecubital, and upper extremity veins (INS, 2006). The dorsal metacarpal veins are smaller but sometimes may be the only vessels visible in the hand. Other veins of the hand, including the dorsal venous arch and tributaries of the cephalic and basilic veins, are generally easier to locate. The cephalic, median basilic, and median antebrachial veins in the forearm may be difficult to locate in children, especially chubby babies and toddlers. Antecubital veins, although more easily located in children needing emergent IV access, should be preserved for phlebotomy or peripherally inserted central catheter (PICC) placement (Figure 29-1).

Foot

The foot is commonly used in neonates, infants, and young children but generally avoided in the child who has mastered walking. Foot vein sites are also used in children older than walking age for special circumstances, such as short-term

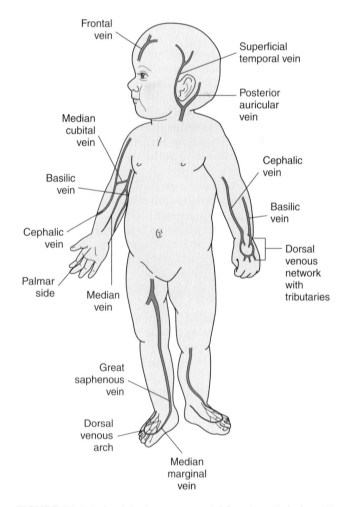

FIGURE 29-1 Preferred sites for venous access in infants. (From Hockenberry MJ, Wilson D: *Wong's nursing care of infants and children,* ed 8, St Louis, 2007, Mosby.)

emergency (24- to 48-hour use) or intensive care situations, where other access sites may be unavailable. Several veins are highly visible and easily accessible. The curve of the foot, especially around the ankle, may make venous entry and catheter advancement difficult. Because the dorsum of the foot has little subcutaneous tissue, it is prone to extravasation injuries and should be avoided unless absolutely necessary (Brown, Hoelzer, and Piercy, 1979).

Infants have great strength in their legs and kick their feet vigorously, so the site should be securely taped to a padded limb board, carefully maintaining normal joint configuration and site visibility. After the age of approximately 10 years, children start to experience phlebitis at rates approaching that of adults, and care should be taken to avoid using lower extremities for IV insertion unless the special circumstances identified previously are documented; other access choices should be used as soon as possible (Nelson and Garland, 1987).

Scalp

The scalp veins are readily visible and easily accessed, and allow free movement of the extremities, but the catheter can be more difficult to secure because of the shape of the head and the presence of hair. Scalp veins can be used in children as old as approximately 18 months, when hair follicles mature and the epidermis toughens. The superficial temporal, frontal, occipital, and posterior auricular veins of the scalp are most commonly used for IV access. The temporal artery is located near the temporal vein and can be easily palpated. Scalp veins do not contain valves, which allows for bidirectional blood flow. Instead of a tourniquet, a rubber band with a piece of tape attached may be used as a tourniquet, or digital pressure may be applied proximal to the insertion site to distend the vein. The needle or catheter should be aimed downward, toward the heart, so that the flow of the infusion can follow the same direction as the venous blood returning to the heart.

Using the scalp for an IV catheter is often most traumatic for the parents. It is important to fully explain the procedure to the parents and to give the removed hair to them as a keepsake. Their lack of understanding can lead to additional anxiety and fear, and they may believe that the IV catheter is directly infusing into the child's brain.

PERIPHERAL ACCESS DEVICES

The guidelines for choosing the appropriate gauge catheter are the same for children as for adults. Peripheral catheters used in children range from 26 to 20 gauge. Peripheral access devices are available in various types and styles. Although personal preference for a certain type of device is a consideration, other factors, such as safety, patient comfort, type and length of therapy, and site of insertion, are also important.

Winged-steel needle set

The winged-steel needle set, also known as a scalp vein needle, is available in odd-number sizes from 27 to 19 gauge, with the 25 gauge being the most common size used in neonates and the 23 gauge being the most common size used in children. Because these devices can easily become dislodged,

the risk of infiltration is increased, and the dwell time of the device is shortened, they are best used for obtaining blood samples or for performing a one-time infusion of short duration. More contemporary types of peripheral venous access catheters have replaced this once popular and sole therapeutic option.

Over-the-needle catheter

These devices consist of a flexible catheter made of Teflon or polyurethane over an internal stylet. They are commonly used in infants and children for peripheral short-term or intermediate-term therapy. The selected size depends on the child's age, vein size, and the therapy prescribed. Gauge sizes range from 26 to 14; the size most commonly used for neonates is 24 gauge, and for children, 24 and 22 gauge, in lengths of 2 inches or shorter. Over-the-needle catheters are available with built-in wings and extension sets. Safety-engineered catheters lessen the risk of needlestick injury and have become the standard of practice.

The flexibility of over-the-needle catheters may add to the dwell time of the device. According to the CDC Guidelines (2002) and the *Infusion Nursing Standards of Practice* (INS, 2006), peripheral IV sites are not routinely rotated in neonates or pediatric patients.

Midline catheter

The midline catheter, composed of polyurethane or silicone, is longer than a peripheral IV catheter and is intended for use in neonates and children who require therapy of intermediate duration. The catheter is inserted into a peripheral vein in the antecubital area and is advanced into the upper arm veins, but not past the axilla. Other sites for midline insertion include the leg (with the tip away from areas of flexion and below the groin) and in the scalp (with the tip located in the neck and above the thorax) (Pettit and Wyckoff, 2007). Because the tip is still located in a peripheral vein, infusate limitations mimic those safe for peripheral infusions. The average dwell time of a midline catheter in the neonate is 6 to 10 days, making it a less desirable option in this pediatric population (Leick-Rude and Haney, 2006). Additionally, approximately 50% of neonatal midline catheters are removed as a result of complications related to catheter migration and infiltration. More published studies, depicting outcomes related to midline catheter use in children, are needed.

VENIPUNCTURE

The actual method of venipuncture is the same for children as for adults. However, certain techniques facilitate successful venipuncture in a small infant or child.

Techniques for neonates and infants

Unlike adults, children fail to understand the need for venipuncture, and evidence shows that neonates and children experience a high degree of fear, pain, and trauma from needlesticks.

One should not attempt a venipuncture on an infant or a young child without extra assistance and use of pharmacological and/or nonpharmacological techniques for pain reduction (Box 29-1).

Box 29-1   TECHNIQUES FOR PAIN REDUCTION DURING VENIPUNCTURE

NONPHARMACOLOGICAL

Imagery
- Distraction (e.g., TV, videotapes, personal music players, comfort boxes)
- Auditory/music

Positioning for comfort

Touch/massage
- Non-nutritive/nutritive sucking
- Rocking/holding
- Reduce lighting/noise
- Visual/mobiles/toys
- Swaddling/nesting
- Sucrose pacifier
- Ice/heat
- Security object/blanket or toy

PHARMACOLOGICAL

Topical local anesthetic creams

Vapocoolant spray

Subcutaneous or intradermal injection:
- 0.9% sodium chloride with preservative
- Lidocaine

Iontophoresis

Oral analgesics

Oral nonsteroidal medications

Oral opioids

Oral benzodiazepines

IV sedation

General anesthesia

From Koh et al, 1999, 2004; Eichenfield et al, 2002; Fetzer, 2002; Kleiber et al, 2002; Priestley et al, 2003; Zempsky and Cravero, 2004; Zempsky et al, 2004, 2008; Sethna et al, 2005; Barclay and Murata, 2006; Jimenez et al, 2006.

Preferably, someone other than a family member should help hold and position the child. Child life therapists can assist with positioning-for-comfort techniques and help distract the child during the procedure. The American Academy of Pediatrics (AAP) and the American Pain Society issued joint guidelines recommending the use of local anesthetics and strategies to soothe and minimize distress associated with all procedures, including venipuncture (AAP and American Pain Society, 2001). Methods to manage pain in neonates are defined by the National Association of Neonatal Nurses (Walden and Gibbins, 2008). The Infusion Nurses Society also calls for the implementation of protocols for the use of local anesthetics based on the nurse's assessment of patient needs (INS, 2006). A comprehensive/interactive website dedicated to decreasing discomfort of peripheral venous access has multiple resources: www.manageIVpain.com.

The child's room needs to remain a "safe space." When possible, all attempts to insert a venous access device should occur in the treatment room or in an area separate from the child's room. The need to explain the procedure and completely prepare the child and family was discussed earlier in this chapter.

Limited venous access sites in infants and children necessitate every effort be made to decrease the number of venipunctures. To reduce the number of additional punctures, blood samples for laboratory tests may be collected at the time of venipuncture when inserting an IV catheter. Once the blood sample has been collected, the catheter is flushed with 0.9% sodium chloride and connected to the prescribed therapy to maintain patency. Maintaining the IV catheter securely in place in an infant or child can be more difficult than the initial insertion. Studies in adult patients have demonstrated extended catheter life span and decreased risk of complications when using manufactured catheter stabilization devices with peripheral IV catheters (Frey and Schears, 2001). Unfortunately, these devices are not available for all IV catheters currently used. As an alternative, application of a sterile transparent dressing and tape can be used to effectively secure an IV catheter in place (Figure 29-2). The tape should be transparent and not obscure the area above the insertion site so that visual assessments can be performed (Figure 29-3).

Clear, plastic site protectors placed over the site help prevent accidental dislodgment or vein damage. Roller bandages should not be used to cover or secure the catheter site; the catheter site should remain readily visible for inspection.

Although some IV complications (e.g., dislodgment, infiltration) are expected to occur in infants and children, careful securement of the venous access device and frequent observation of the site can minimize these complications. Placing the catheterized extremity on a specially designed limb board is necessary for devices placed near a joint. Caution should be taken to maintain normal body alignment and prevent pressure points when taping the extremity to the board. Fingers should be allowed to extend beyond the end of the board rather than being taped down. Limb boards are not considered a restraint (JCAHO, 2005; INS, 2006). In all cases, site assessment should be completed and documented hourly for infusing IVs and at least once every 8 hours for devices that are locked (Brown, Hoelzer, and Piercy; Pettit, 2003).

Heparin locks versus saline locks

In adults, 0.9% sodium chloride has replaced heparinized saline solution for maintaining patency of intermittently used peripheral venous access devices (VADs). In the early 1990s published studies indicated that saline alone can be used to maintain patency of 22-gauge or larger catheters in children (Danek and Noris, 1992; McMullen et al, 1993; Hanrahan, Kleiber and Fagan, 1994).

However, these results cannot be applied to all subgroups (e.g., neonates) or all gauges of catheters. Today, heparin and 0.9% sodium chloride are both being used in management of peripheral VADs, and there are anecdotal reports of success in maintaining patency with 0.9% sodium chloride in neonates and conflicting reports in pediatrics (Gyr et al, 1995; Krueger-Paisely, Brown, and Ganong, 1997; Heilskov et al, 1998; Mok, Kwong, and Chan, 2007). To prevent respiratory depression, solution without benzyl alcohol should be used in neonates. Small catheter size, a hypercoagulable state, an increased incidence of catheter occlusion, and difficulty in achieving and maintaining access in neonates and children are concerns to be addressed when maintaining patency of venous access devices. Solutions used to clear catheters may vary based on the technique used to lock the device. Flushing technique will vary depending on the device and needleless cap that are used. Effective heparin/0.9% sodium chloride ratios for maintaining the patency of venous access devices in neonates and children are outlined in Table 29-7.

FOCUS ON EVIDENCE

Pain Related to Venipuncture—Pediatrics

- A descriptive study examined the prevalence and sources of pain in a pediatric hospital. The study period was 3 weekdays during which inpatient interviews were conducted with 102 parents of children <5 years and with 98 children >5 years. Subjects reported source of pain, and used ratings of worst, usual, and current to rank intensity within the last 24 hours. Causes of pain were variable and included disease, surgery, and intravenous (IV) lines. Children ranked IV insertion as the most frequent procedure associated with the worst pain. Pain intensity was not significantly related to age, gender, patient type (medical, surgical), or diagnostic category. Children were given significantly less medication than was prescribed, regardless of their reported pain level. Medications and nonpharmacological methods were reported as helpful in managing pain. The authors concluded that many children endure unacceptable levels of pain during hospitalization (Cummings et al, 1996).

- A descriptive study examined stress levels experienced by children undergoing routine venipunctures. Trained observers evaluated 223 different children: toddlers, described as 2½ to 6 years (N = 70); preadolescents, described as 7 to 12 years (N = 55); and adolescents, described as 12 years and older (N = 98). Level of distress was rated using a scale of 1 to 5 where 1 = calm, 2 = timid/nervous, 3 = serious distress, but still under control, 4 = serious distress with loss of control, and 5 = panic. The authors determined that 83% of the toddler group, 51% of the preadolescent group, and 28% of the adolescent group experienced high distress levels during venipuncture. The authors concluded that age, not gender, correlates with venipuncture distress, high levels of distress are common, and interventions to relieve distress should be provided especially for those in the toddler and preadolescent groups (ages 2½ to 12 years) (Humphrey et al, 1992).

- In this clinical trial, 31 children were randomized to 1 of 2 arms before venipuncture: (1) no preparation; or (2) preparation that included local anesthesia of the skin, sensory and procedural information, and parental involvement. Raters who were blinded to the randomization viewed videotapes of children and rated distress levels. The authors concluded that children prepped for venipuncture with a local anesthetic, teaching, and support exhibited less distress (Kolk, van Hoof, and Fiedeldij Dop, 2000).

- In this double-blind randomized controlled trial, children aged 1 month to 17 years were randomized to receive either topical liposomal lidocaine 4% (N = 69) or placebo (N = 73) before venous cannulation. The purpose was to determine the success rate of cannulation, analgesic effectiveness, procedure duration, and rate of adverse skin reactions. Cannulation on the first attempt occurred in 74% of children who received a local anesthetic, but only 55% of children who received placebo. Children who received topical analgesia exhibited lower mean pain scores and shorter procedure duration. Transient dermal changes were reported as 23% in both groups. The authors concluded that use of liposomal lidocaine was associated with a higher intravenous cannulation success rate, less pain, shorter total procedure time, and minor dermal changes among children undergoing cannulation. Routine use of topical analgesia for painful cutaneous procedures should be considered whenever feasible (Taddio et al, 2005).

- A descriptive survey of 51 effective dose (ED) programs with fellowships was conducted to determine the one most commonly used pain or sedation management option for five clinical scenarios: facial laceration repair, cranial computed tomography in a toddler, closed fracture reduction, neonatal lumbar puncture, and intravenous catheter insertion. Thirty-eight responses (75%) to the survey were received. Only 38% of those responding reported use of pharmacological pain management for intravenous catheter insertion. The authors concluded that pain and sedation management methods for pediatric procedures continue to evolve. Despite guideline recommendations and literature supporting the benefits of topical local anesthetics, venous access pain in children remains undermanaged (Bhargava and Young, 2007; MacLean Obispo, and Young, 2007).

- The American Academy of Pediatrics (AAP) and the American Pain Society issued joint guidelines recommending the use of local anesthetics and strategies to soothe and minimize distress associated with all procedures, including venipuncture (AAP and American Pain Society, 2001). The Infusion Nurses Society in its *Infusion Nursing Standards of Practice* calls for the implementation for the use of local anesthetics based on the nurse's assessment of patient needs (INS, 2006).

COMPLICATIONS

Complications related to peripheral IV therapy are discussed in detail in Chapter 23. However, some complications occur more often or can be more serious in the neonatal and pediatric population, such as catheter occlusion and infiltration. Small-sized veins, use of smaller-gauge IV catheters, and the slow rates of infusion contribute to an increased risk of catheter occlusion.

Vessel fragility and high activity levels in young children can increase the chance of infiltration. Infiltration is the most commonly identified complication of peripheral infusion therapy, with a reported incidence of 23% to 78% (Figure 29-4) (Pettit, 2003). When an irritant or vesicant solution infiltrates, an extravasation injury, with swelling, blistering, and skin necrosis, may occur (Figure 29-5).

These injuries can be devastating in children, causing loss of tissue and function of the affected area (Brown et al, 1979). Standardized management of extravasation is hampered by

limited research. Treatment may consist of administration of an antidote (hyaluronidase, phentolamine, nitroglycerin ointment) or 0.9% sodium chloride into the extravasation, elevation of the injection site, application of warm or cool compresses (based on substance extravasated), and care for the resultant wound (Clifton-Koeppel, 2006; Thigpen, 2007). An early landmark study of extravasation injuries demonstrated that sites located where there is little subcutaneous tissue, such as the dorsum of the foot, use of pumps with high pressures, infusion of parenteral nutrition solutions, inability to visualize the site, and treatment with hot compresses postinfiltration increased extravasation injury risk and extent (Brown et al, 1979).

Phlebitis is seen less often in children than adults until after the age of 10, when the incidence of phlebitis begins to approach adult rates (Nelson and Garland, 1987). In addition, as discussed earlier, fluid-volume overload can be a serious complication in an infant or small child.

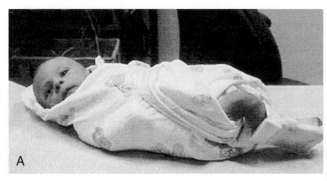

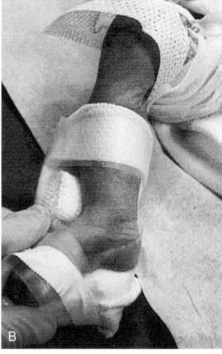

FIGURE 29-2   A, Baby wrapped in blanket "mummy" restraint before placing foot IV. **B,** Foot taped to padded board before IV placement, maintaining normal joint configuration and site visibility. (Courtesy Anne Marie Frey.)

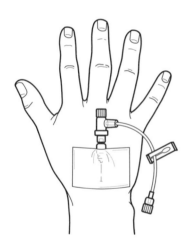
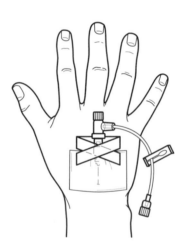
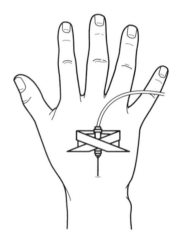

FIGURE 29-3   Securing an IV.

CENTRAL ACCESS

CENTRAL VENOUS ACCESS DEVICES

A central venous access device (CVAD) is a catheter whose tip is located in a central vein, defined as the superior vena cava for catheters inserted via the arms, scalp, or neck and as the thoracic aspect of the inferior vena cava for catheters inserted via veins of the lower extremities (INS, 2006). Many catheter types and protocols for care of central venous access devices exist. Catheter type should be based on the age and size of the child, his or her cognitive and compliance ability, the type and duration of the therapy, infusate characteristics, vein quality and ability to access, body image considerations, and home care needs. Central venous access devices are recommended for therapies to be administered in a subacute or home care setting, for a duration that ranges from several days to weeks or longer, and for the administration of solutions or medications that are hyperosmolar (>600 mOsm/L), have a pH less than 5 or greater than 9, or are considered vesicants (INS, 2006). Care of CVADs is based on the type of catheter, tip location, and manufacturer recommendations (refer to flushing protocols in Table 29-7).

Care of central venous catheters varies by device, but includes site assessment, flushing protocols or infusion systems

TABLE 29-7 Recommended Flush Volumes/Solutions for Various Vaenous Access Devices in Neonates and Children

Venous access device and approximate priming volume (APV)	Locked device: Volume, frequency, and solution All 0.9% NaCl should be preservative free	Medications: Before and after administration Administration systems/ methods: Large-volume pump, gravity set, syringe pump method, and IV push	Blood product administration and sampling Withdrawal volume for blood sampling accuracy
APV: 0.05- 0.07 mL	NICU patients: 1 mL 0.9% NaCl every 6 hr Pediatrics: 1-3 mL 0.9% NaCl every 8 hr	2 times administration tubing and add-on set volume	Before and after blood administration: 1-3 mL 0.9% NaCl N/A for routine sampling; for short-term studies follow locked device protocol; discard 1.5 mL for short-term studies from PIV dedicated to sampling
APV: 0.05- 0.07 mL	N/A	N/A for medication administration	Administration: N/A Withdrawal volume for sampling: Stopcock method: 1.6 mL (Davies and Molloy, 2006) Closed blood sampling system: refer to manufacturer recommendations Post sampling: up to 1 mL 0.9% NaCl or heparinized 0.9% NaCl solution in 24-gauge catheters and until clear for all other catheters
APV: Each lumen, 0.15-0.32 mL	Umbilical venous catheter (UVC):1 mL 0.9% NaCl + 10 units/mL heparin every 6 hr if locked Umbilical arterial catheter (UAC): typically not locked	1 mL 0.9% NaCl solution or heparinized 0.9% NaCl solution with ≤1 unit/mL heparin, or 2 times administration tubing and add-on set volume	Before and after blood administration or sampling: 1 mL 0.9% NaCl or 1 mL 0.9% NaCl + ≤1 unit/mL heparin and until clear Withdrawal volume for sampling when using a stopcock on catheter hub: 1.6 mL (Davies and Molloy, 2006) Closed blood-sampling system: refer to manufacturer's recommendations
Midline APVs (mL): 3F: 0.16 4F: 0.19 5F: 0.22	2F: 1 mL 0.9% NaCl + 10 units/mL heparin every 6 hr 2.6F and larger: 2-3 mL 0.9% NaCl + 10 units/mL heparin every 12 hr	2 times administration tubing and add-on set volume	Before and after blood administration: 1-3 mL 0.9% NaCl followed by locking solution or resume infusion N/A for routine sampling: For short-term studies follow locked device protocol; discard 1.5 mL for short-term studies from midline dedicated to sampling
PICC APVs (mL): 1.9F: 0.06 3-3.5F: 0.2-0.5 4F: 0.6 5F: 0.4-0.8 6F: 0.5-0.6	2F: 1 mL 0.9% NaCl + 10 units/mL heparin every 6 hr 2.6F and larger: 2-3 mL 0.9% NaCl + 10 units/mL heparin every 12 hr	2 times administration tubing and add-on set volume	2F sampling and before and after blood administration: 1 mL to clear line and then flush with 1 mL 0.9% NaCl or saline solution with ≤1 unit/mL heparin and until clear 2.6F and larger: Sampling and before and after blood administration: 1-3 mL 0.9% NaCl followed by locking solution or resume infusion Withdrawal volume: 3 times administration tubing and add-on set volume (Frey, 2003)
Tunneled and nontunneled APVs (mL): 2-3F: 0.12- 0.15 4F: 0.3 5F: 0.5 6F: 0.6-0.8 7F: 0.6-0.9 9F: 0.6-1.3	_NICU patients:_ 1-3 mL 0.9% NaCl + 10 units/mL heparin every 12-24 hr _Pediatrics:_ 2 mL 0.9% NaCl + 10 units/mL heparin every 24 hr	2 times administration tubing and add-on set volume	Before and after blood administration: 1 mL 0.9% NaCl for NICU patients and 3 mL 0.9% NaCl for all others followed by locking solution or resume infusion Withdrawal volume for sampling: 3 times administration tubing and add-on set volume Variation in size makes it difficult to recommend one volume for all patients
Ports APVs (mL): 0.8-mm ID: 0.8 1.0-mm ID: 1.1-1.2 1.1-mm ID: 1.2 1.4-mm ID: 1.7 1.6-mm ID: 2	If used for more than 1 medication daily: 3-5 mL 0.9% NaCl + 10 units/mL heparin Monthly maintenance flush: 3-5 mL 0.9% NaCl + 100 units/mL heparin	2 times administration tubing and add-on set volume	Before and after blood administration: 3-5 mL 0.9% NaCl followed by locking solution or resume infusion Withdrawal volume for sampling: 3 times administration tubing and add-on set volume Variation in size makes it difficult to recommend one volume for all patients

_ID,_ Inner diameter.

* Adapted from Finishing Protocols.

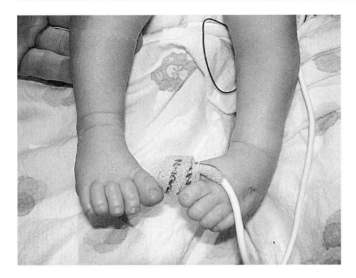

FIGURE 29-4 Infiltration of IV fluid in left leg of infant. (Courtesy Anne Marie Frey.)

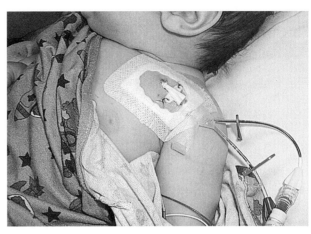

FIGURE 29-6 Subclavian nontunneled catheter in infant. (Courtesy Anne Marie Frey.)

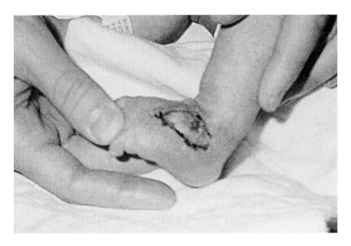

FIGURE 29-5 Intravenous infiltration in an infant's foot. (From Hockenberry MJ, Wilson D: *Wong's nursing care of infants and children,* ed 8, St Louis, 2007, Mosby.)

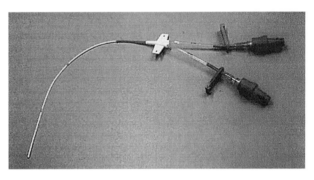

FIGURE 29-7 Pediatric-sized peripherally inserted central catheter.

to maintain patency, and periodic dressing changes, depending on the type of catheter dressing and securement device (Frey and Schears, 2001). No conclusive evidence is available on which to evaluate the effectiveness of flushing and locking with heparin to prolong PICC, umbilical, and other central venous catheter life in the neonatal population. CVADs should continue to be locked with heparin in the neonatal and pediatric population until conclusive evidence is presented.

Central venous site assessments can be every hour, every shift, or daily depending on the patient's age and condition and the infusate. The most common complications of central venous catheters in children include occlusion, migration, and infection, which may lead to premature catheter removal. Essential components of assessment include noting the securement of the catheter, any change in the external catheter

length if applicable, integrity of the dressing, and absence of visible complications at the exit/insertion site.

Nontunneled percutaneous central venous access devices

Percutaneously placed CVADs are available in single- or multiple-lumen configurations and are generally made of polyurethane. These catheters are placed directly into the superior vena cava by way of the right or left subclavian vein, the internal or external jugular veins, or the inferior vena cava via the femoral veins at the groin. Nontunneled catheters are usually placed by physicians and are used for short-term emergency access in critical care patients. Site preferences in children—in order of preference, safety, and accessibility—are the femoral vein, internal jugular veins, and subclavian vein (Figure 29-7) (Lavelle and Costarino, 2008).

Peripherally inserted central catheters

The peripherally inserted central catheter is a thin, single- or double-lumen catheter inserted through a breakaway or peel-away introducer, or using a modified Seldinger technique by specially trained nurses, nurse practitioners, and physicians. The device is beneficial for patients needing several days, weeks, or months of therapy. Available sizes for infants and children include 1.1 to 5 French (F) (Figure 29-7).

PICCs are inserted into a peripheral vein and threaded in the vena cava. Sites used include the arm in all ages and the leg, foot, or scalp/neck in infants (Pettit and Wyckoff, 2007). The addition of heparin to the infusate has been shown to decrease catheter occlusion and lengthen dwell of PICCs in neonates (Shah et al, 2007).

Tunneled catheters

Surgically placed tunneled catheters are single-lumen or multi-lumen silicone catheters with one or two Dacron polyester cuffs to anchor the catheter in the subcutaneous tissue. An example of this type of catheter is the Broviac catheter. These catheters are surgically tunneled under the skin of the chest into the superior vena cava. An alternative site is the inferior vena cava, with the catheter tunneled to the abdomen, thigh, or back. Indications for use of tunneled catheters are long-term parenteral nutrition or cancer treatment (Figure 29-8).

Implanted port

An implanted port is a surgically placed central venous access device that is made up of a totally implanted metal or plastic dome containing a self-sealing injection port. An implanted port may be sutured to the chest wall under the skin with the catheter tip located in the superior or inferior vena cava. Another type of port can be implanted and positioned near the antecubital fossa in the arm. With the "arm" port, the catheter is threaded via the basilic vein to the superior vena cava. Ports are also indicated for long-term intravascular access, particularly when intermittent infusion therapy is needed, such as in children with cancer or cystic fibrosis (Figure 29-9).

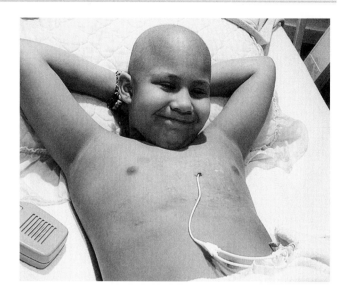

FIGURE 29-8 Child with tunneled cuffed central venous catheter. (From Hockenberry MJ, Wilson D: *Wong's nursing care of infants and children*, ed 8, St Louis, 2007, Mosby.)

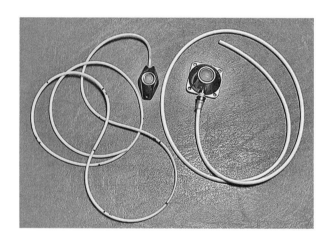

FIGURE 29-9 Pediatric-sized implanted ports. (Courtesy Anne Marie Frey.)

OTHER INTRAVASCULAR ROUTES

UMBILICAL VEIN AND ARTERY

The umbilical cord of the neonate provides a route for vascular access and can be readily accessed during the first few days of life. Three vessels are present in the umbilical cord: one vein (thin walled with a large-diameter lumen) and two arteries (thick walled with a small-diameter lumen). Catheter sizes range from 2.8F to 8F; they are made of silicone or polyurethane, and can have single-, dual-, or triple-lumen configurations.

The umbilical vein is the preferred vessel for emergency infusion of medications and volume in the neonate and is commonly used for infusions lasting several days to 2 weeks (Bradshaw and Furdon, 2006; Wortham, and Rais-Bahrami, 2007). Catheters placed in the vein are also used for solution and medication administration, central venous pressure measurement, venous blood sampling, and exchange transfusion. The catheter tip in the inferior vena cava is located at approximately the eighth to ninth rib (Wortham and Rais-Bahrami, 2007).

Umbilical artery cannulation is indicated for conducting hemodynamic monitoring, performing frequent arterial blood gas measurements, and obtaining laboratory specimens. Infusion of many solutions and medications or exchange transfusions may also be accomplished through this route. The catheter tip is kept in the aorta either at T7-9 (considered a high-lying line) or at L3-4 (considered a low-lying line) and is generally removed within 2 weeks. Low-lying lines are associated with a greater incidence of vascular symptoms noted in the lower extremities. The addition of heparin to the infusate of the umbilical arterial catheter (UAC) prevents catheter occlusion (Rajani et al, 1979; Horgan et al, 1987; Barrington, 1998a,b). Heparinization of flushes used with the UAC without heparinizing the infusate is ineffective in decreasing catheter occlusion.

Complications of umbilical catheterization include catheter malposition and subsequent vascular or organ injury, vascular compromise, hemorrhage, air embolism, infection, thrombosis, and vascular perforation (Wortham, Gaitatzes, and Rais-Bahrami, 2007). The nursing assessment for evaluating catheter function and identifying potential complications is usually performed hourly. Essential components include noting the security of the catheter, length of the indwelling catheter, quality of the hemodynamic waveform, and signs of surrounding erythema and drainage from the umbilicus. Symptoms of pericardial effusion and tamponade should be noted for infants having an umbilical venous catheter (UVC). Additional considerations for an indwelling UAC include assessment of distal pulses, perfusion, and any discoloration (cyanosis or blanching) of the buttocks or lower extremities that may signal the presence of thromboemboli or vascular spasm (Wortham et al, 2007b).

Catheter removal is accomplished by stopping the infusion, removing the suture and securement device, and placing an umbilical tie around the umbilical stump, if able, followed by slow, controlled withdrawal. The umbilical artery catheter is removed slowly until 5 cm remains, and then pulled at a rate of 1 cm/minute until it is completely removed; this minimizes spasm of the artery and prevents significant bleeding (Wortham et al, 2007). Compressing the umbilical stump or remaining cord may be required to avoid tamponade bleeding.

INTRAOSSEOUS ROUTE

The intraosseous (into the bone) route is an important adjunct to emergency measures used in infant and child resuscitation. For this technique, see Chapter 26.

 ## ADMINISTRATION EQUIPMENT

FLUID CONTAINERS

A plastic rather than glass solution container should be used whenever possible to avoid breakage if the container falls off the pole. To prevent the risk of fluid-volume overload, the volume of the fluid container should be based on the age and size of the child and the 24-hour volume needs (INS, 2006). In premature infants and neonates, smaller fluid containers should be considered.

ADMINISTRATION SETS

The fluid delivery system for infants and children is different from that of adults in that the flow rate requirements are minimal, necessitating the proper choice of administration set. Precise infusion rates are required to prevent the possibility of medication overdose or fluid-volume overload.

Microdrip tubing (60 drops/minute) and microbore administration sets are used for infants and children. IV administration sets with an in-line, calibrated, volume-control chamber (50-, 100-, and 150-mL sizes are available) should be used on all children whose prescribed fluid rate is less than 100 mL/hour, unless another volume-control method, such as an electronic infusion pump, is used. The use of an in-line chamber can provide an increased measure of volume control for gravity infusions and also provides a mechanism for diluting and administering medication.

Because acutely ill patients often need multiple therapies, microbore extension sets with multiple limbs are often used. The use of stopcocks capped with a dead-end cap or removable syringe is not recommended because of the increased risk of contamination (Casey et al, 2007). If stopcocks are used, capping with a needleless connector, that needs to be swabbed with an antimicrobial agent before entry, is recommended (Bouza et al, 2003).

ELECTRONIC MONITORING DEVICES

Electronic infusion devices or pumps that regulate fluid delivery are used in neonates, infants, and children and should demonstrate ±5% accuracy, guard against free flow, and have occlusion alarm ratings that fall within safety limits. Infusion pumps are necessary in infants and children who require arterial lines and highly accurate infusions, such as PN, chemotherapy, and vasoactive and other rate-dependent medications that must be delivered accurately to achieve desired effect. Infusion pumps are available commercially in various styles and delivery options. Pumps exert varying degrees of pressure when they meet resistance during infusion. Considerations for evaluating a pump for pediatric use should include its ability to set variable pressure limits, have low alarm limits, program as low as tenths of milliliters per hour, and have tamper-proof features. Also recommended for use is smart pump technology with medication libraries that afford an additional level of safety (TJC, 2007).

A popular volumetric pump often used for children is the syringe pump. This portable pump incorporates a syringe as the volume chamber to deliver the infusate. The syringe pump is indicated in children for infusion of intermittent doses of medications, such as antibiotics, low-volume therapy, and medications that need to infuse at very low flow rates.

Mechanical controllers, such as dial mechanisms on tubing, may help regulate flow rate; however, in the infant and child with flow rates of only several milliliters per hour, their accuracy cannot be guaranteed. In addition, these mechanisms are often accurate only when used in conjunction with larger gauge IV devices or correct position of the patient. Complete manufacturer's information should be examined before these devices are used.

Electronic infusion devices for use at home should be portable, require minimal programming, be easy for the caregiver and possibly child to operate, and be able to tolerate activity of a mobile child. Such systems include syringe pumps and positive-pressure devices. One such device is an elastomeric infusion device that incorporates a fillable balloon inside a plastic housing. This system eliminates gravity flow concerns and delivers antibiotic and chemotherapy infusions at a constant rate. Elastomeric infusion devices are available in different sizes (i.e., volumes) and delivery rates. Advantages to the child and family are that these devices come prefilled by the pharmacy, the set-up time is minimal, and the devices are small and lightweight, a characteristic that promotes ambulation. For school-aged children or adolescents, such devices can be hidden in their clothes or be carried in a user-friendly pouch.

 ## ALTERNATIVE-SITE INFUSION THERAPY

SUBACUTE CARE

Recovery from a long-term illness or injury may be accomplished in a subacute care facility. These facilities provide a step between hospital and home, and in addition to nursing services provide such services as physical, occupational, and respiratory therapy, and developmental and feeding teams. Children in subacute care may need short-term infusion therapy intermittently, or continue on long-term therapies such as parenteral nutrition via a tunneled catheter. In any case, nurses and other providers need to be educated in care of the devices and safe administration of the infusions when providing rehabilitative therapies.

HOME INFUSION THERAPY

Home infusion therapy for the child is viewed as a positive alternative to hospitalization, but it certainly has its challenges for the child and family, as well as for the health care team responsible for the family's care. After discharge criteria have been met, the caregivers and the child (if appropriate) begin educational preparation for maintaining the prescribed infusion treatment at home. Such therapies as antibiotics, antifungals, chemotherapy, parenteral nutrition, blood and blood components, and solutions and medications can be delivered in the home. These therapies, delivered using a team approach by a company dedicated to pediatrics or with an experienced pediatric division along with a strong nursing component, have been shown to be critical to optimal patient outcomes (Johnson et al, 2008). The psychosocial and developmental needs of the child and family are an issue, more frequently at home than in the acute care setting. The child may be returning to school and will need assistance on how to deal with issues such as body image and remarks from peers. Returning to a sport or other activity may be important to the child and will require support. If siblings are in the home, they may feel neglected because of their parents' attention to the child receiving therapy. At home, parents do not have the security of having reliable health care providers always available. Alternative caregivers should be identified early in the process so that the parents can have respite periods.

SUMMARY

Infusion therapy in infants and children is highly specialized, requiring sophisticated technology and diligence in care delivery and monitoring. Individual policies and procedures in the hospital, outpatient department, subacute facilities, and the home should be developed using established standards of practice, available published evidence and guidelines, and practitioners' experience, keeping in mind the unique developmental needs of the child.

REFERENCES

American Academy of Pediatrics and American Pain Society: The assessment and management of acute pain in infants, children, and adolescents, *Pediatrics* 108(3):793-797, 2001.

ASPEN Board of Directors and the Clinical Guidelines Task Force: ASPEN guidelines for the use of parenteral and enteral nutrition in adult and pediatric patients, *JPEN* 26(1 Suppl):1-138SA, 2002.

Barclay L, Murata P: TV viewing has analgesic effect during venipuncture in children, *Medscape Medical News*, 2006. Accessed 12/5/2006 at http://www.medscape.com/view article 548718.

Barkin RM: Treatment of the dehydrated child, *Pediatr Ann* 19(10):597, 1990.

Barrington KJ: Umbilical artery catheters in the newborn: effects of position of the catheter tip, *Cochrane Database Syst Rev*, 1998a. Accessed at http://www.nichd.nig.gov/cochrane/Barring1/Barrington.htm.

Barrington KJ: Umbilical artery catheters: heparin usage. *Cochrane Database Syst Rev*, 1998b. Accessed at http://ww.nichd.nih.gov/cochranebarring3/barring3.htm.

Bhargava R, Young K: Procedural pain management patterns in academic pediatric emergency departments, *Acad Emerg Med* 14(5):479-482, 2007.

Bilodeau JA, Poon C, Mascarenhas MR: Parenteral nutrition and care of central venous lines. In Altschuler SM, Liacouras CA, editors: *Clinical pediatric gastroenterology*, Philadelphia, 1998, Churchill Livingstone.

Bouza E, Munoz P, Lopex-Rodriguez J et al: A needleless closed system device (CLAVE) protects from intravascular catheter tip and hub colonization: a prospective randomized study, *J Hosp Infect* 54:279-287, 2003.

Bradshaw WT, Furdon SA: A nurse's guide to early detection of umbilical venous catheter complications in infants, *Adv Neonatal Care* 6:127-138, 2006.

Brown AS, Hoelzer D, Piercy SA: Skin necrosis from extravasation of intravenous fluids in children, *Plast Reconstr Surg* 64:145, 1979.

Cahill-Alsip C, McDermott B: Hematologic critical care problems. In Curley MQ, Smith JB, Moloney-Harmon P, editors: *Critical care nursing of infants and children*, Philadelphia, 2001, Saunders.

Casey AL, Burnell S, Whinn H et al: A prospective clinical trial to evaluate the microbial barrier of a needleless connector, *J Hosp Infect* 65:212-218, 2007.

Centers for Disease Control and Prevention: Guidelines for the prevention of intravascular catheter-related infections, *MMWR Recommend Rep* 51(RR10):1-29, 2002.

Clifton-Koeppel R: Wound care after peripheral intravenous extravasation: what is the evidence? *Newborn Infant Nurs Rev* 6:202-211, 2006.

Cummings EA, Reid GJ, Finley GA et al: Prevalence and source of pain in pediatric inpatients, *Pain* 68:25-31, 1996.

Danek GD, Noris EM: Pediatric IV catheters: efficacy of saline flush, *Pediatr Nurs* 18:111, 1992.

Davies EH, Molloy A: Comparison of ethyl chloride spray with topical anaesthetic in children experiencing venipuncture, *Paediatr Nurs* 8(3):39-43, 2006.

Doellman D: Pediatric PICC insertions: easing the fears in infants and children, *JAVA* 9(2):68-71, 2004.

Eichenfield LF, Funk A, Fallon-Friedlander S et al: A clinical study to evaluate the efficacy of ELA-Max (4% liposomal lidocaine) as compared with eutectic mixture of local anesthetics cream for pain reduction of venipuncture in children, *Pediatrics* 109(6):1093-1099, 2002.

Fann BD: Fluid and electrolyte balance in the pediatric patient, *J Intrav Nurs* 21(3):153, 1998.

Fetzer SJ: Reducing venipuncture and intravenous insertion pain with eutectic mixture of local anesthetic: a meta-analysis, *Nurs Res* 51(2):119-124, 2002.

Ford NA, Drott HR, Cieplinski-Robertson JA: Administration of IV medications via soluset, *Pediatr Nurs* 29(4):283-286, 319, 2003.

Frey AM: Drawing blood samples from vascular access devices: evidence-based practice, *J Infus Nurs* 26(5):285-293, 2003.

Frey AM, Schears G: Evidenced based practice: dislodgment rates and impact of securement methods for peripherally inserted central catheters (PICCs) in children, *Pediatric Nurs* 27(2).

Goren A, Laufer J, Yativ N et al: Transillumination of the palm for venipuncture in infants, *Pediatr Emerg Care* 17(2):130-131, 2001.

Gyr P, Burroughs T, Smith K et al: Double blind comparison of heparin and saline flush solutions in maintenance of peripheral infusion devices, *Pediatr Nurs* 21(4):383, 1995.

Hanrahan KS, Kleiber C, Fagan CL: Evaluation of saline for IV locks in children, *Pediatr Nurs* 20:549, 1994.

Hazinski MF: *Nursing care of the critically ill child,* ed 2, St Louis, 1992, Mosby.

Heilskov J, Kleiber C, Johnson K et al: A randomized trial of heparin and saline for maintaining intravenous locks in neonates, *JSPN* 3(3):111, 1998.

Heird WC: Parenteral support of the hospitalized child In Suskind RM, Lewinter-Suskind L, editors: *Textbook of pediatric nutrition,* ed 2 , New York, 1993, Raven.

Hockenberry MJ, Wilson D, editors: *Wong's nursing care of infants and children* (pp 1158-1177), St Louis, 2007, Mosby.

Horgan MJ, Bartoleti A, Polansky S et al: Effect of heparin infusates in umbilical arterial catheters on frequency of thrombotic complications, *J Pediatr* 111:774, 1987.

Humphrey GB, Boon CM, van Linden van den Heuvell GF et al: The occurrence of high levels of acute behavioral distress in children and adolescents undergoing routine venipunctures, *Pediatrics* 90(1 pt 1):87-91, 1992.

Infusion Nurses Society: Infusion nursing standards of practice, *J Infus Nurs* 29(1 Suppl), S1-S92, 2006.

International Consensus on Science: Guidelines 2000 for cardiopulmonary resuscitation and emergency cardiovascular care, *Circulation* 102(suppl 1):I-291-342, 2000.

Jimenez N, Bradford H, Seidel KD et al: A comparison of a needle-free injection system for local anesthesia versus EMLA for intravenous catheter insertion in the pediatric patient, *Anesth Analg* 102(2):411-414, 2006.

Johnson et al: Multidisciplinary approach to improving pediatric home infusion, *Am J Health Syst Pharm* 56:473-474, 2008.

Joint Commission, 2005. Accessed Oct 2008 from http://www. jointcommission.org/AccreditationPrograms/BehavioralHealthCare/ Standards/FAQs/Provision+of+Care+Treatment+and+Services/ Restraint+and+Seclusion/Restraint_Seclusion.htm.

Keller S: Small gauge needles promote safe blood transfusions, *Oncol Nurs Forum* 22(4):718, 1995.

Kleiber C, Sorenson M, Whiteside K et al: Topical anesthetics for intravenous insertion in children: a randomized equivalency study, *Pediatrics* 110(4):758-761, 2002.

Koh JL, Fanurik D, Stoner PD et al: Efficacy of parenteral application of eutectic mixture of local anesthetics for intravenous insertion, *Pediatrics* 103(6):79, 1999.

Koh JL, Harrison D, Myers R et al: A randomized, double-blind comparison study of EMLA and ELA-Max for topical anesthesia in children undergoing intravenous insertion, *Paediatr Anaesth* 14(12):977-982, 2004.

Kolk AM, van Hoof R, Fiedeldij Dop MJ: Preparing children for venepuncture. The effect of an integrated intervention on distress before and during venepuncture, *Child Care Health Dev* 26(3):251-260, 2000.

Krueger-Paisely M, Brown N, Ganong LH: The use of heparin and normal saline flushes in neonatal intravenous catheters, *Pediatr Nurs* 23(5):521, 1997.

Landier WC, Barrell ML, Styffe DJ: How to administer blood components to children, *Am J Matern Child Nurs* 12:178, 1987.

Lavelle J, Costarino A: Central venous access and central venous pressure monitoring In Henretig FM, King C, editors: *Textbook of pediatric emergency procedures,* Philadelphia, 2007, Lippincott Williams and Wilkins.

Leick-Rude MK, Haney B: Midline catheter use in the intensive care nursery, *Neonatal Network* 25:189-199, 2006.

MacDonald MG, Ramasethu J, editors: *Atlas of procedures in neonatology,* Philadelphia, 2007, Lippincott Williams and Wilkins.

MacLean S, Obispo J, Young KD: The gap between pediatric emergency department procedural pain management treatments available and actual practice, *Pediatr Emerg Care* 23(2):87-93, 2007.

McKinney ES et al: *Maternal-child nursing,* ed 3, St Louis, 2009, Saunders.

McMullen A et al: Heparinized saline or normal saline as a flush solution in intermittent intravenous lines in infants and children, *Matern Child Nurs J* 18:78, 1993.

Mok E, Kwong TY, Chan MF: A randomized controlled trial for maintaining peripheral intravenous lock in children, *Int J Nurs Pract* 13:33-45, 2007.

Mott SR, James SR, Sperac AM: *Nursing care of children and families,* ed 2, Redwood City, Calif, 1990, Addison-Wesley.

Nathan DG, Orkin SH, Look AT et al: *Nathan and Oski's hematology of infancy and childhood,* ed 6, Philadelphia, 2003, Saunders.

National Blood Resource Program: *Transfusion therapy guidelines for nurses,* Bethesda, Md, 1990, U.S. Department of Health and Human Services.

National Heart, Lung, and Blood Institute: *The fourth report on the diagnosis, evaluation, and treatment of high blood pressure in children and adolescents* (pp 10-11), Bethesda, Md, 2005, Author. Retrieved 6/11/08 from www. nhlbi.nih.gov.

Nelson DB, Garland JS: The natural history of catheter associated phlebitis in children, *Am J Dis Child* 141:1090, 1987.

Pettit J: Assessment of an infant with a peripheral intravenous device, *Adv Neonatal Care* 3(5):230-240, 2003.

Pettit J, Wyckoff MM: *Peripherally inserted central catheters: guidelines for practice,* ed 2, Glenview, Ill, 2007, National Association of Neonatal Nurses.

Priestley S, Kelly AM, Chow L et al: Application of topical local anesthetic at triage reduces treatment time for children with lacerations: a randomized controlled trial, *Ann Emerg Med* 42(1):34-40, 2003.

Rajani K, Goetman BW, Wennberg RP et al: Effects of heparinization of fluids infused through an umbilical artery catheter on catheter patency and frequency of complications, *Pediatrics* 63:552, 1979.

Sethna NF, Verghese ST, Hannallah RS et al: A randomized controlled trial to evaluate S-Caine patch for reducing pain associated with vascular access in children, *Anesthesiology* 102(2):403-408, 2005.

Shah PS, Kalyn A, Satodia P, et al: A randomized, controlled trial of heparin versus placebo infusion to prolong the usability of peripherally placed percutaneous central venous catheter (PCVCs) in neonates: The HIP (Heparin Infusion for PCVC) study, *Pediatrics* 119:e284-291, 2007. Retrieved 3/19/07 from www.pediatrics.org/ cgi/content/full/119/1/e284.

Taddio A, Soin HK, Schuh S et al: Liposomal lidocaine to improve procedural success rates and reduce procedural pain among children: a randomized controlled trial, *CMAJ* 172(13):1691-1695, 2005.

The Joint Commission (TJC): *2007 National patient safety goals: FAQs.* Accessed 5/18/08 from www.jointcommission.org/NR/rdonlyres/ B423198E-8EB1-468C-B01E-JDBB0324B5C60/0/07_NPSG_FAQs_3.pdf.

Thigpen JL: Peripheral intravenous extravasation: nursing protocol for initial treatment, *Neonatal Network* 26:379-384, 2007.

Transfusion therapy guidelines for nurses, Bethesda, Md, 1990, National Blood Resource Education Program, Public Health Service, National Institutes of Health, U.S. Department of Health and Human Services.

Walden M, Gibbins S: *Pain assessment and management: guidelines for practice,* ed 2, Glenview, Ill, 2008, National Association of Neonatal Nurses.

Weiss SJ, Schoch PE, Burke AC: Malassezia furfur fungemia associated with central venous catheter lipid emulsion infusion, *Heart Lung* 20:87-90, 1991.

Wilshaw R, Beckstrand R, Waid D et al: A comparison of the use of tympanic, axillary, and rectal thermometers in infants, *J Pediatr Nurs* 14(2):88, 1999.

Wortham BM, Gaitatzes CG, Rais-Bahrami K: Umbilical artery catheterization. In MacDonald MG, Ramasethu J, editors: *Atlas of procedures in neonatology,* ed 4 , Philadelphia, 2007, Lippincott Williams and Wilkins.

Wortham BM, Rais-Bahrami K: Umbilical vein catheterization. In MacDonald MG, Ramasethu J, editors: *Atlas of procedures in neonatology,* ed 4, Philadelphia, 2007, Lippincott Williams and Wilkins.

Yeager AS et al: Prevention of transfusion acquired cytomegalovirus infections in newborn infants, *J Pediatr* 98:281, 1981.

Zempsky WT, Bean-Lijewski J, Kauffman RE et al: Needlefree powder lidocaine delivery system provides rapid and effective analgesia for venipuncture or cannulation pain in children: the COMFORT-003 trial, *Pediatrics* 121(5):979-987, 2008.

Zempsky WT, Cravero J, Committee on Pediatric Emergency Medicine and Section on Anesthesiology and Pain Medicine: Relief of pain and anxiety in pediatric patients in emergency medical systems *Pediatrics* 114:1348-1356, 2004.

Zempsky WT, Sullivan J, Paulson DM et al: Evaluation of a low-dose lidocaine iontophoresis system for topical anesthesia in adults and children: a randomized, controlled trial, *Clin Ther* 26(7):1110-1119, 2004.

30 Infusion Therapy in the Older Adult

Beth Fabian, BA, RN, CRNI®*

THE AGING POPULATION

With medical advances, infusion nursing faces the challenges of an ever-expanding aging population; the mean age of adults has increased to an unprecedented level. The older adult presents a unique set of concerns for which health care professionals do not yet have a complete solution. Ironically, gerontology, the study of the aged, is one of the newest specialties in the medical world. Primary goals of infusion nursing with the older adult include selecting the correct venous access device, type of therapy, and medication. To achieve these goals, the infusion nurse needs to have a broad understanding of geriatric assessment and the impact the aging and infusion processes will have on the older adult patient.

Gerontology has become a specialty in its own right. The development of gerontological *Scope and Standards of Gerontology Nursing Practice* (Congdon et al, 2001), in collaboration with the National Gerontological Nursing Association, the National Association of Nursing Administrators of Long Term Care, the National Conference of Gerontological Nurse Practitioners, and the American Nurses Association, set a standard of care for the older adult. The standards directed a holistic approach be incorporated throughout the continuum of care with the elderly patient to achieve the most positive outcome. The role of the infusion nurse is expanding to different health care delivery settings. Chronic diseases such as cardiovascular dysfunction, diabetes, and cancer continue to have a major impact on the world population. The elderly patient can present with all three diseases, thereby significantly increasing the challenges of infusion nursing. Accurate assessment of the older patient by health care professionals ensures timely and less costly interventions.

STATISTICS AND PROJECTED GROWTH

According to the United Nations Department of Economic and Social Affairs Population Division, the world's population will increase by 2.5 billion people from 2007 to 2050. Today's 6.7 billion people will grow to an estimated 9.2 billion in 2050.

The *2007 Revision* of their *World Urbanization Prospects* indicates that by 2008 the world population living in urban areas will exceed that of the rural areas. Urban population growth will continue moving beyond the 3.3 billion in 2007 to more than 6.4 billion in 2050 (United Nations, 2008).

The urbanization growth of the population allows for more convenient access to health care. Combined with a sharp reduction in mortality as a result of increasing medical and pharmacological advances, a declining birth rate, and increased longevity, the growing population is also an aging population (United Nations, 2008). The United Nations *World Population Prospects: The 2006 Revision* estimates that from 2005 to 2050, the growth in the population aged 60 or older will account for half of the total worldwide population. In 2005 the number of persons aged 60 or older was estimated at 673 million. By the year 2050 that number will exceed 2 billion. The most dramatic increases will be in the developing countries, where the older population is expected to grow from 171 million in 1998 to 1594 million in 2050. This reflects a shift of the over 60 population—comprising 64% of the population in 2005 to nearly 84% in 2050 (United Nations, 2007). Within the aging population, the 80 or older category is projected to increase from 88 million in 2005 to 402 million in 2050.

These numbers demonstrate the impact this population will have on the health care delivery system. It will tremendously affect the way that health care is delivered and the types of services that are offered. Infusion therapy will advance with various types of medical devices and will be a significant factor in maintaining the expanding (and aging) population. With the dramatic increases in life expectancy and the gradual decline in fertility rates, the proportion of older adults has now exceeded that of younger children for the first time in history. This phenomenon has been termed *population aging* and has required a shift in health care, focusing on the elderly. Understanding the global implications of population aging will empower the health care professional to provide the best possible care for older adults.

AGING THEORIES

Many theories exist regarding the population and the process of aging. No one theory can fully describe the inevitable aging that the body endures. Eliopoulos (2005) describes the many

*The author and editors wish to acknowledge the contributions made by Kathleen Walther in the second edition of *Infusion Theraphy in Clinical Practice*.

theories of aging and categorizes them into two areas: biological theories and psychosocial theories. The common denominator in the theories is that currently, no single factor is responsible for the aging process.

Aging is unique for each individual, beginning at conception. Aging depends on nutritional, environmental, educational, genetic, societal, physiological, and spiritual factors. Aging uses the life experiences and shapes the future needs of the older adult. Because of the complexities of the aging process, it is much more difficult to assess the older adult than the younger adult. When assessment is made even more difficult by acute or chronic cognitive deficits in the patient, the role of the infusion nurse becomes extremely difficult.

Older people are classified into the following three major groups:

1. Young old: 65 to 74 years
2. Middle old: 75 to 84 years
3. Old old: 85 years and older

The population experiencing the most change is the old-old age group. Advances in medicine and education provide the practitioner a wealth of knowledge about this group (Congdon et al, 2001; Eliopoulos, 2005).

 ## LEGAL AND ETHICAL CONSIDERATIONS

ADVANCE DIRECTIVES

To understand the requests of the older adult in the delivery of health care, there must be a clear understanding of advance directives. The desires of the elderly are often ignored, especially when a metabolic imbalance has rendered the older adult cognitively deficient. Chronic illnesses, medications, and fluid and electrolyte imbalances can impair the patient's ability to make clear-cut decisions about infusion therapy. The health care professional must advocate for the wishes of the patient. When an elderly person is treated, the entire family is affected. Many complex emotional and ethical issues arise regarding the treatment of the older adult. These issues need to be discussed in a controlled setting, before the onset of an acute illness that requires infusion therapy. The patient may have a variety of documents or persons designated responsible for the plan of care. These may include advance directives, which are legally binding documents set forth by the patient in anticipation of future health care needs. These documents are reviewed before providing any treatment. In the case of infusion therapy, a review is particularly important if the practitioner is not familiar with the patient and has been called as the specialist to perform an invasive procedure.

The living will, a part of the advance directives, is a comprehensive document specifying the holistic aspects of the patient's care. Another document often used confers a durable power of attorney for health care to a friend, family member, advisor, or guardian. This person is appointed to make decisions when the patient is considered legally incompetent or incapable of making decisions regarding health care (Congdon et al, 2001; Loengard and Boal, 2004).

DO-NOT-RESUSCITATE ORDERS

As with advance directives, do-not-resuscitate (DNR) orders are reviewed with the patient and family before the order is written. A DNR order must be written on the physician's order sheet and progress notes. A DNR order may be written in the absence of or in conjunction with a living will (Phillips, 2005). The patient or legal guardian must participate in the decision-making process. If the patient resides in a long-term care setting, cardiopulmonary resuscitation (CPR) must be available to the patient if the patient does not have a DNR order. If the facility is unable to perform CPR, the patient must be informed. This is of particular importance to the health care professional consulting on an emergent basis to perform a venipuncture.

INFORMED CONSENT

The initiation of infusion therapy without consent is construed as assault and battery (Phillips, 2005; Weinstein, 2007). The older adult does not give up the right to refuse treatment. Health care professionals must recognize that the elderly person needs to feel a sense of independence and control over his or her environment. In the acute care setting, much of a patient's care and environment is out of his or her control. This circumstance must be met with reasoning and discussion, not force.

The patient who is confused does not relinquish his or her rights to refuse treatment. The determination of what is best for the care and safety of the patient must be weighed against a careful evaluation of the patient's mental and emotional ability to make rational decisions. The patient's life and safety are always the first priority to the health care provider. If a patient cannot make these judgments, the patient, the family, or the hospital representative can ask the court to appoint a patient advocate to oversee the best interests of the patient. The determination of who will speak for the patient must be made early in the course of care so that proper therapy can be continued with the appropriate consent. See Box 30-1 for additional factors that should be considered when obtaining informed consent from the older adult.

Box 30-1   CONSIDERATIONS FOR THE OLDER ADULT: INFORMED CONSENT

Before informed consent can be obtained, it is necessary to assess the older adult's mental status. Mental status can be impaired for many reasons. If impaired memory or confusion is due to a reversible condition, it is important to address the underlying condition. If pain is affecting the older adult's ability to think clearly, appropriate management strategies must be in place before obtaining informed consent.

The nurse should assess any sensory deficits, such as vision or hearing, provide written consent forms that are printed in an easy-to-read font, and adapt spoken information for any hearing deficits. The use of unfamiliar language should be avoided, and written material should be provided at the patient's reading level. Pausing periodically allows the patient time to process the information given, and can enhance comprehension. The nurse may have to adapt the signed consent process if the older adult has developed upper extremity problems, such as fine tremors or eye-hand coordination or range-of-motion limitations.

The nurse must be knowledgeable about advance directives and existing health care proxies.

From Infusion Nurses Society: *Policies and procedures for infusion nursing for the older adult,* Norwood, Mass, 2004, Author.

GERONTOLOGICAL ASSESSMENT

HOLISTIC APPROACH TO CARE

The older population is a very diverse group. Everyone ages differently, taking into consideration climate, geographic locations, family size, life skills, and experiences. Individual variations in biological characteristics tend to be greater in the older population than in the younger population. This diversity makes it difficult to categorize older people. The health care professional needs to do a complete, holistic assessment of the older adult before initiating therapy. All aspects of life need to be respected when an older person requires infusion therapy. It is important to take into account that this particular generation has survived many global changes and medical advances. This generation has seen the advances in antibiotic therapy and has witnessed the virtual eradication of diseases such as polio and whooping cough. Decisions regarding infusion therapy are very important to the process of completing therapy with the fewest complications and the most positive outcomes for the older adult (Hogstel, 2001).

ACTIVITIES OF DAILY LIVING

Activities of daily living are a common criterion used by health care professionals to determine the care that an elderly person will require in the event of an illness. Determining a patient's optimal level of functioning is a key component when addressing this issue.

In the holistic plan for care, bathing, dressing, housekeeping, mobility, and cognitive function are factors in determining overall wellness. When infusion therapy is considered, other factors need to be identified before initiating therapy (Box 30-2).

If there is a question about the patient's cognitive level, many quick and easy assessments can be performed to determine whether the patient understands the impending therapy. It is important to have an understanding of the patient's entire 24-hour day. Issues such as insomnia, depression, or sundowner's syndrome are some common examples that may complicate care (Fetter, 2003).

THE AGING PROCESS

CARDIOVASCULAR FUNCTION

Changes occurring in the cardiovascular system of the older adult are one of the most important systemic changes that should be assessed by the health care professional. With advancing age, the left atrium enlarges to enhance ventricular

---

Box 30-2   FACTORS TO CONSIDER BEFORE INITIATING THERAPY

- What were the locations of prior IV cannulations? Determine degrees of phlebitis, if known.
- Will the patient be receiving occupational or physical therapy? If so, the catheter should not be placed in the affected arm because of increased risk of manipulation of the catheter.
- Can the patient or caregiver be taught to take care of the infusion site, dressings, and medication administration?

---

filling. In most healthy older adults, a fourth audible heart sound can occur from the enlargement. The overall size of the heart increases in mass; the increase is estimated at 1 gram per year in men and 1.5 grams per year in women after the age of 30 (Phillips, 2005; Weinstein, 2007). In both genders, the intraventricular septal thickness increases with age, creating a stiffness in the ventricular walls. This impedes the heart's ability to contract and relax. The heart valves may also become thicker and less flexible from lipid accumulation, collagen degeneration, and fibrosis. Decreased efficiency of the heart muscle reduces the cardiac output by approximately 1% per year in adulthood (Hogstel, 2001). The vessels have greater peripheral resistance because of calcium deposits, crosslinking of collagen, and a reduction in elastin content. The capillary walls are thicker, which may impede the effective exchange of nutrients. In older adults, the venous elasticity also slowly declines, making the veins more difficult for venipuncture. The body's ability to store blood volume is reduced, and the peripheral valve efficiency is decreased. In areas of high venous pressure, the adult is at risk for varicosities. The older adult's lack of mobility may also impair venous return.

RESPIRATORY FUNCTION

Assessment of the respiratory system is paramount to providing the best possible care for the geriatric patient. The respiratory system changes begin with an overall decrease in vital capacity resulting from the loss of elastic recoil and decreased respiratory mass. There is an increase in dead space along with a decrease in the amount and effectiveness of the cilia along the tracheobronchial tree (Hogstel, 2001; Eliopoulos, 2005). Because of the loss of elasticity and decreased effectiveness of the alveoli, the older adult is at increased risk for respiratory tract infections and dyspnea.

The older adult compensates for the flattening diaphragm and decrease in the capacity of respiratory muscles by using abdominal accessory muscles for respirations. These muscles make breathing increasingly difficult for the patient. Surgeries with anesthesia can make the older patient more prone to aspiration. The blood oxygen level decreases by 10% to 15% (Eliopoulos, 2005). Oxygen perfusion decreases and the elderly are more prone to hypoxemia. Care and consideration should be given to the amount of medication, number of infections, and co-morbidity when determining respiratory function. Hypoxemia can result in cognitive impairment, which can be misconstrued in the older adult. Swallowing deficits can result in right lower lobe and right middle lobe pneumonia that is often undiagnosed and undertreated because of inadequate assessment skills.

ENDOCRINE FUNCTION

The body's immune system changes with the normal aging process. The immune system becomes hyporesponsive to foreign antigens and hyperresponsive to self (Phillips, 2005). These changes can result in decreased resistance to infection, increased incidence of cancers, and increased autoimmunity. Infusion nurses must consider that older adults may be more susceptible to infection and may not show the same signs and symptoms of infection they did when they were younger (Hogstel, 2001; Eliopoulos, 2005). Because of this change, the use of aseptic technique and appropriate use of antimicrobial agents with all infusion-related procedures are essential.

The pituitary gland loses weight and vascularity with age, and there are changes in the thyroid gland. Hypothyroidism is a common diagnosis in the elderly that is often misdiagnosed because of its vague symptomatology, such as mild depression, weight gain, chest pain, atrial fibrillation, and cold intolerance.

Acquired immunodeficiency syndrome (AIDS) also affects older adults. Human immunodeficiency virus (HIV) may be misdiagnosed or missed entirely in the elderly because the early symptoms of fatigue, anorexia, and weight loss can be misinterpreted. Cognitive impairment, for example, is often diagnosed as Alzheimer's disease or dementia rather than a symptom of HIV. About 10% of adults over the age of 50 are diagnosed with HIV/AIDS. This percentage is thought to be low as a result of misdiagnosis (Hogstel, 2001; Eliopoulos, 2005).

Because the risk of pregnancy is eliminated, older adults need education on barrier protection. Also, the introduction of sildenafil citrate (Viagra) has led to a significant increase in sexual activity among older adults (Hogstel, 2001). Care and consideration should be given to the older adult's sexual history when the early symptoms of HIV occur. The health care professional cannot be lax in using standard precautions, such as wearing gloves, during a venipuncture on the older adult (INS, 2006).

GASTROINTESTINAL FUNCTION

The gastrointestinal function of the older adult can be complex and requires a comprehensive assessment. The life experiences and nutritional status of the older adult define and shape his or her future health and welfare. Co-morbidities, such as a cardiovascular accident or hypertension, can lead to inadequate flow to the gastrointestinal tract or dysphagia.

The dentition of the elderly does not change with age (Hogstel, 2001; Eliopoulos, 2005). However, studies have shown that by the age of 65, many elders are edentulous. Poor dental hygiene in younger years leads to loss of teeth, which impairs proper chewing of food. The salivary glands secrete less ptyalin and amylase as age advances and the saliva becomes more alkaline. The taste buds also atrophy with a decrease in discrimination between salt and sweet flavors.

By the age of 60, gastric secretions decrease by 20% to 30% (Hogstel, 2001; Eliopoulos, 2005). A decrease in pepsin secretion may hinder protein digestion, and decreased hydrochloric acid and intrinsic factor levels can lead to malabsorption of iron, vitamin B_{12}, calcium, and folic acid. Pernicious anemia is also a concern for the older adult.

Constipation or diarrhea is not attributable to the aging process as was once commonly believed (Eliopoulos, 2005). A slight decrease in intestinal motility comes with aging but does not lead to chronic changes in bowel patterns. The health care practitioner should pay attention to the medications that the patient is taking. Polypharmacy, the taking of multiple medications, in the elderly is a common problem; this practice can produce an array of side effects, including the loss of fluids and electrolytes.

INTEGUMENTARY FUNCTION

The integumentary system is the largest and most complex organ in the body. The skin can divulge a wealth of information to the health care professional during assessment. Accurate skin assessment can help determine hydration status, potential for infection, amount of sun exposure, and attention to personal appearance. The skin plays a key role in influencing self-esteem and appearance in the older adult.

The skin is the first body system affected by venipuncture. Changes in the skin, texture, depth, and integrity result from the natural aging process and from the onset of certain disease states. The changes affect all layers of the skin, including the epidermis, the dermis, and the superficial fascia (Eliopoulos, 2005).

The *epidermis,* the outermost layer of the integumentary system, has four cellular layers. The *stratum corneum* consists of dead squamous cells that form a protective barrier for the body. The *stratum granulosum* helps organize the keratin layer. The *stratum spinosum* produces the fibrous portion of the keratin layer. The *basal cell* layer is responsible for pigmentation. These layers play a role in thermal regulation of the body. With aging, the epidermis becomes thinner, thereby resulting in decreased healing rates and barrier protection. The cell replacement rate of the stratum corneum declines by 50% in the older adult (Eliopoulos, 2005).

The *dermis* is the middle layer of the skin consisting of protein structures, blood vessels, nerve endings, and appendages such as hair follicles and nails. As the body ages, the dermis decreases in thickness by 20% (Eliopoulos, 2005). The number of sweat glands and nerve endings also decreases. In regard to nerve endings, this is of particular importance in relation to pain perception and tactile sensation. The infusion nurse should consider the lack of sensation when performing a venipuncture and minimize catheter manipulation. This will help decrease the risk of a serious infiltration caused by the patient being unable to feel the pain or pressure caused by fluid leaking into the tissue. Because of the decreased thickness, the skin is at great risk for tears, which can lead to ulceration. Caution should be taken during insertion and removal of a venous access device and removal of the tape securing the device.

The subcutaneous layer of fat in the skin helps provide insulation from cold and serves as a shock absorber from blunt trauma. As the body ages, this layer becomes thinner and redistributes to the abdomen and thighs. With the thinning of this layer, the older patient is more at risk for hypothermia and skin tears.

SENSORY FUNCTION

Sensory functional changes occurring in the elderly can have a dramatic impact on quality of life. These changes, both normal and those associated with a disease process, can be misdiagnosed as a cognitive functional loss. Care and consideration should be given to accurate assessment of all functions when initiating infusion therapy (Hogstel, 2001; Eliopoulos, 2005).

If the patient's visual acuity is impaired, the patient may appear withdrawn and unable to participate in the plan of care. Cataracts and glaucoma are easily treated with medications and surgery if detected in a timely manner.

Hearing deficits are also thought to be a part of the normal aging process. The deficits are usually part of the high-frequency range (Hogstel, 2001; Eliopoulos, 2005). One of the most common reasons for hearing loss is increased cerumen in the ear canal. This can lead to gait disturbances and more commonly a withdrawal from daily activities. The ear canal curves as the person ages, and proper visualization is important in cleaning the ear canal.

Olfactory deficits can be another area for assessment in the elderly population. Some studies have shown an olfactory deficit in response to smells such as smoke. This is of importance to the patient at home, where the risk of fire is greater for the elderly population.

Tactile sensation is decreased and the skin is more susceptible to injury with aging. Infiltration may go unnoticed because of the skin's decreased integrity and loose skin folds. A large amount of fluid may infuse subcutaneously before the patient experiences pain. Phlebitis may develop without pain but with significant vein inflammation resulting from the decreased sensitivity of the skin's nerve endings (Hogstel, 2001; Eliopoulos, 2005). Close monitoring of infusions, especially with potentially irritating medications, must be performed often because severe tissue necrosis, infection, or compartment syndrome can be the catastrophic result (Weinstein, 2007).

The elderly person with a peripheral catheter may not be able to alert the nursing staff of pain at the insertion site resulting from chemical or mechanical phlebitis. Caution should be exercised in the selection of the appropriate venous access device.

The elderly may experience multiple sensory losses. The practitioner needs to be aware of any deficits when caring for the patient. Sensory deficits or disorders can also affect how the patient reacts and responds to the infusion nurse and the delivery of infusion therapies. Sensory deficits can dramatically affect older patients' understanding of procedures, their independence, and their ability to cooperate with prescribed therapies. Therefore these changes must be kept in mind so that a personal connection is established with the patient and successful infusion therapies are administered (INS, 2004; INS, 2006).

MUSCULOSKELETAL FUNCTION

Changes in the musculoskeletal function occur with age. Muscle mass gradually decreases with the muscle being replaced by fibrous connective tissue. The decreased elasticity in the ligaments, tendons, and cartilage can lead to a general overall stiffness in the older adult (Hogstel, 2001; Eliopoulos, 2005).

Decreased density in bone structure may lead to osteoporosis and place the patient at risk for falls. Falls are a significant concern in the elderly population. Assessment of the patient's environment, medications, and history of disease is crucial in preventing potentially life-threatening falls.

Changes related to arthritis can have a particular impact on placement of an IV catheter. Areas of flexion should not be cannulated because of the impact of restricted movement on arthritic joints. Arm boards should be avoided when possible for the same reason.

FLUID AND ELECTROLYTE BALANCE

Fluid changes in the elderly can lead to a significant imbalance because of the decrease in fluid ratios overall. As the body ages, changes occur in fluid to body mass ratios. Over the age of 65, overall body fluid gradually decreases to 33% in females and approximately 45% in males. As a result, the elderly can exhibit significant signs of fluid and electrolyte loss within a 4-hour period. An accurate assessment is essential to promote well-being and prevent fluid and electrolyte imbalances (Hogstel, 2001; Eliopoulos, 2005).

A fluid and electrolyte deficit can result in behavioral changes. The elderly become inflexible to change, especially in the presence of cognitive impairment. If the patient with Alzheimer's disease paces the floor continuously and then appears lethargic and sits in a chair, this can easily be interpreted as tiredness or lack of interest. A quick fluid assessment should be performed to determine whether rehydrating the elderly patient instead of waiting for significant electrolyte changes will make a difference in the patient's condition (Figure 30-1).

COGNITIVE FUNCTION

Psychological factors in the older adult can affect how the patient responds to infusion therapy. The cognitively impaired patient may have problems determining recent versus remote memory. For instance, the patient may understand the procedure while the IV catheter is inserted but an hour later may pull it out. Difficulties with short-term memory may also dramatically affect the older adult who is receiving instruction for home infusion therapies (Hogstel, 2001; Eliopoulos, 2005). Depression may affect the older adult's attitude toward the venous access device and decisions regarding the alternatives in the care and treatment of the illness. Causes for such behavior can be mental deterioration, effects of medications, thyroid disorders, Alzheimer's disease, stroke, or electrolyte imbalances.

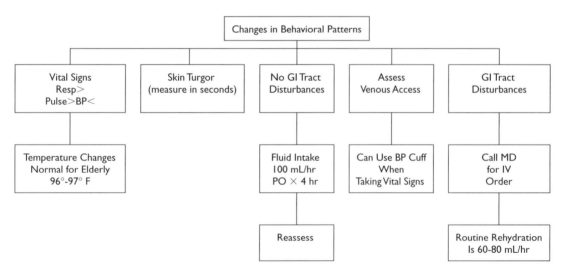

FIGURE 30-1 Fluid deficit assessment.

CONSIDERATIONS IN INFUSION NURSING

VEIN SELECTION

Selecting the appropriate vein for IV access in the older adult can provide the infusion nurse with a great clinical challenge. The infusion nurse must possess clinical and anatomical knowledge specific to the older adult and must have the physical dexterity and high level of expertise needed to place a venous access device into an appropriate vein.

Primary principles of IV site selection in the younger adult are applicable to the older adult. For instance, initial venipuncture should be in the most distal portion of the extremity, allowing for subsequent venipuncture to move progressively upward (Phillips, 2005; Weinstein, 2007). This method provides new IV access away from the previous site or area of complication. However, certain factors for site selection are specific to the older adult. For instance, the veins of the hands may not be the best choice for the initial distal site because of the loss of subcutaneous fat and the thinning of the skin. A venous access device inserted into such a site could quickly lead to mechanical inflammation of the vein and infiltration (Phillips, 2005; Weinstein, 2007). In addition to this factor, one must take into account the number of venipunctures performed and the outcomes. Therapies that produce a high degree of phlebitis, such as medications with a high or low pH along with increased osmolarity, are factors to consider in determining vein selection.

Vein selection begins by evaluating the patient's peripheral access for potential sites that can accommodate the duration of the infusion therapy. The entire surface of both arms should be inspected for potential sites. When possible, an insertion site that will not hamper the performance of activities of daily living should be selected. Physiological changes in the skin and veins should also be considered when a venipuncture site is selected. For instance, stabilization of a venous access catheter may be affected by decreased skin turgor; therefore areas where sufficient tissue and skeletal support exist should be selected if possible. The condition of the vein should be evaluated by careful palpation. The nurse should be aware of the more fragile nature of the vein and should begin at distal sites to preserve future access sites. The nurse should avoid previously used, bruised areas and articulating surfaces. In choosing a site, the nurse should also consider the need for future venipuncture sites and promote vein conservation as indicated (Box 30-3) (Phillips, 2005; Weinstein, 2007). In patients who have limited venous access, hypodermoclysis may be used to administer a prescribed therapy. More information on this method of infusion delivery is described in Chapter 26.

To help locate a vein, adequate lighting should be used. Bright examination lights located directly overhead may tend to obscure veins. The use of side lighting may highlight the skin's color and texture and allow visualization of the vein shadow below the skin (Phillips, 2005).

The use of a tourniquet may be helpful in distending and locating an appropriate vein. However, important considerations regarding the use of tourniquets for older adults should be kept in mind. The tourniquet should be applied in a flat fashion, snugly but not too tightly. Venous distention may take a few moments longer in the older adult because of the slower venous return in this population. Excessive distention of the vein must be avoided because it might cause vein damage when the vein is punctured, resulting in a hematoma. In addition,

---

Box 30-3   CONSIDERATIONS FOR THE OLDER ADULT: SITE SELECTION

Because of loss of subcutaneous fat and thinning of the skin in the older adult, placement of a VAD can be challenging. Lack of supporting tissues may make catheter insertion and securement more difficult, while increasing the potential risk for bruising, phlebitis, and infiltration. The nurse should select areas with more subcutaneous tissue and skeletal support for better device stabilization, keeping in mind the need to conserve peripheral access for future therapy.

Length and type of treatment must be taken into consideration when selecting potential sites. If the older adult is independent, it is important for him or her to continue these activities. A VAD site that allows for use of the hands and does not restrict range of motion is ideal.

Patient handedness is an important consideration. It is acceptable for the older adult to have input as to where the catheter will be placed, for example, in the nondominant arm. Many older adults have had previous experience with infusion therapy and can indicate what has and has not worked for them in the past. If the older adult must use an ambulatory aid to maintain independence, determine the side on which the aid will be used. It is important to avoid VAD placement in the hands and areas of flexion if possible. For the less mobile patient, consider using the extremity that most easily allows access to the bathroom or commode to minimize inadvertent catheter dislodgment or entanglement in the administration set.

From Infusion Nurses Society: *Policies and procedures for infusion nursing for the older adult,* Norwood, Mass, 2004, Author.

---

the tourniquet itself may create bruising. Because of these factors, it may be preferable to eliminate the use of a tourniquet in the older adult, especially if the vein to be used is visible and already somewhat distended without the use of a tourniquet (Phillips, 2005).

During venous distention, the veins should be palpated to determine their condition. Adequate time should be taken to carefully evaluate all potential venipuncture sites. Palpation is the key to determining which veins have soft, bouncy vein walls. Resilient veins feel very different from those that are sclerosed and hard. Veins that feel ribbed or rippled may distend readily when a tourniquet is applied. However, these corded veins are enlarged as a result of thickening of the vein wall, which may be so thick that the lumen may be extremely narrow or occluded (Phillips, 2005; Weinstein, 2007). These sites are almost impossible to access, causing pain for the patient and frustration for the infusion nurse.

The thickening that occurs in the vein wall also affects the function of the valves, which become stiff and less effective. In many elderly patients, these valves can be seen and palpated because of vessel sclerosis. The valves appear as small bumps along the vein path. The infusion nurse must be aware of the potential problems associated with attempting vein access close to or through a valve area. For instance, venous circulation may be sluggish, resulting in slow venous return and distention, venous stasis, and dependent edema. These factors may inhibit the nurse's ability to thread a catheter into the vein. Inflexible valves can make catheter threading difficult or impossible. In these situations, it may be necessary to reduce catheter size by several gauges to thread a catheter through an inflexible valve. Sclerosed valves impede venous circulation and may result in

FOCUS ON EVIDENCE

Subcutaneous Infusion of Hydration Fluids in the Older Adult Patient

- Patients on hospital geriatric units with a diagnosis of mild to moderate dehydration were randomly assigned to receive either a subcutaneous (Sub-Q) (n = 48) or an IV infusion (n = 48) of 0.45% sodium chloride. Patients received median solution volumes of 750 mL (Sub-Q) and 1000 mL per day (IV). There were few systemic adverse reactions but they included acute cardiac failure and hyponatremia with no significant difference between the groups. There also were no significant differences in the incidence of local side effects between the groups. In 13 patients, therapy was switched from Sub-Q to IV because of addition of IV drugs or poor absorption, and in 17 patients therapy was switched from IV to Sub-Q because of peripheral IV problems. The researchers concluded that rehydration using Sub-Q infusion was feasible and well-accepted by the patients and is an easier administration method for patients with difficult venous access and in those who were confused (Slesak et al, 2003).

- A review of 57 long-term care patients who received Sub-Q infusion of hydration solutions for dehydration was conducted. The mean duration of infusions was 15.9 days and the mean volume of the daily infusion was 1161 mL. Clinical improvement was shown in 77% of the patients, by evidence of improvement in cognitive status, general condition, and oral intake; there was no evidence of fluid overload. The researchers concluded that Sub-Q infusion was a safe and effective alternative to IV rehydration (Arinzon et al, 2004).

- Through a systematic literature review researchers aimed to evaluate the safety of Sub-Q hydration compared to IV hydration with 5% dextrose solutions. Four studies—including two randomized controlled trials, one systematic literature review, and one cohort study—met the inclusion criteria. Five percent dextrose solutions were found to be effective in the treatment of dehydration with similar rates of adverse reactions to IV infusions. However, the researchers acknowledge that the research is limited and recommend larger randomized clinical trials to validate the findings (Turner and Cassano, 2004).

- In a review of the literature examining the safety and efficacy of Sub-Q administration of fluids to treat mild to moderate dehydration, eight studies were reviewed—two randomized controlled trials and six cohort studies. The mean ages of patients in the studies were between 71 years and 85 years. The authors concluded that based on the studies, Sub-Q administration of hydration solutions was as effective as IV administration and may potentially reduce the need for hospitalization for patients in long-term care facilities, and also reduce the cost of care. While absorption of Sub-Q fluids is slower than IV absorption, it is still important to monitor the patient for fluid overload (Remington and Hultman, 2007).

- The use of recombinant human hyaluronidase to facilitate absorption of Sub-Q hydration and drug infusion was reported in a hospice setting. There were 32 patients treated over a 6-month period; 26 received Sub-Q hydration solutions for either dehydration or to control delirium symptoms. Flow rates of up to 500 mL per hour were achieved; there was induration at the infusion site in one patient. The authors state interest in expanding the use of hyaluronidase based on its initial success (Pirrello et al, 2007).

---

slow or sluggish flashback, causing the nurse to advance the catheter too far, resulting in intima damage or vessel rupture (Phillips, 2005; Weinstein, 2007).

Small, surface peripheral veins appear as thin, tortuous veins with many bifurcations. Only a few short, straight branches may sustain an IV catheter. Appropriate catheter gauge and length selections are critical to achieve successful venous access device (VAD) placement in these veins.

VENOUS ACCESS DEVICE SELECTION

When a patient's venous access device needs are evaluated, a judicious analysis of many factors is necessary, particularly the type and duration of infusion therapy. For instance, are hydration solutions, chemotherapy, antibiotics, parenteral nutrition, or supplemental infusions such as potassium chloride solutions to be administered? The nurse must recognize potentially irritating agents and consider decreasing the concentration or infusing into a larger vessel to promote hemodilution (INS, 2006). For example, continuous infusion of vesicant chemotherapy must be administered through a central venous access catheter to avoid the potential complication of peripheral extravasation. In addition, solutions with glucose concentrations greater than 10%, such as parenteral nutrition solutions, must be administered through central venous access devices to prevent peripheral vein damage. The duration of therapy is also a factor in determining whether a patient's needs are best met by a central or peripheral VAD. If therapy is required for several weeks, central venous access may be the most cost-effective method for delivery, and it conserves the patient's peripheral access. Another indication for a central venous access catheter is the patient who has no peripheral access available. The selection of the type of central venous access device (CVAD) should be based on the evaluation of potential access sites and the anticipated duration of therapy (INS, 2006).

In catheter selection, the skin and vein changes that occur with the older adult should be considered to enhance successful catheter placement and initiation of infusion therapies. In particular, consideration should be given to catheter design and gauge size. Catheters can be made of silicone, various polyurethane formulations, or polytetrafluoroethylene (Teflon®). Softer, more flexible materials may allow increased dwell time and reduce complications. In addition, the needle-bevel tip design of a peripheral catheter should be considered when selecting an infusion access device to provide the least traumatic insertion. The smallest possible gauge size appropriate for therapy and a vein that will provide adequate hemodilution around the catheter should be selected (INS, 2006). The use of 22- and 24-gauge catheters is appropriate for delivery of many infusion therapies. These sizes are recommended when possible for the older adult to reduce insertion-related trauma and provide greater hemodilution, by reducing irritation of the intima of the vein resulting from catheter insertion trauma or from medication administration (INS, 2004).

When a midline or a peripherally inserted central catheter (PICC) is placed in an elderly patient, prehydration is often necessary. With the significant loss of fluid or the introduction of medications that have the potential for irritation or extravasation, this is important. On day 1 of therapy, assessment for intravascular depletion is performed with diagnostic tests such as blood urea nitrogen level and accurate intake and output. If a 22- or 24-gauge catheter is inserted and slow rehydration occurs, the insertion of the larger venous access device, such as a midline or PICC, will be easier.

When a central venous access device is necessary, the need for a long-term versus a short-term device should be evaluated, as should the older adult's ability to care for the device. Percutaneously placed central venous catheters designed for short-term use may be appropriate for several weeks of therapy. A PICC may provide an excellent alternative for intermediate access and may reduce the complications associated with subclavian and jugular insertions. Tunneled catheters may be appropriate when long-term, frequent access is required; however, associated catheter care needs should be considered carefully. The patient and/or caregiver may have difficulty maintaining and coping with dressing changes and flushing procedures. In this instance, an implantable vascular access port may be a better alternative because of its limited catheter care requirements (INS, 2004; Phillips, 2005; INS, 2006).

ADMINISTRATION EQUIPMENT SELECTION

Because of the dangers associated with overadministration or underadministration of infusion therapies, the type of equipment selected should provide safe, consistent delivery of required medications or solutions. To prevent fluid overload, the use of microdrip administration sets, if appropriate for the delivery rate required, should be considered. When rapid flow rates or more exact delivery is required, volume-controlled administration sets and electronic monitoring devices may be needed (Phillips, 2005).

Advanced technology in stationary and ambulatory electronic monitoring devices, such as pumps, of all types and sizes are used to administer solutions and medications. Because of the fragile nature of the veins of the older adult, the nurse must recognize the potential complications associated with pressures generated by mechanical infusion devices. In addition, because of the dangers associated with overadministration or underadministration of prescribed therapies, monitoring devices must have safety features to protect the patient and still ensure delivery of the required medication or solutions.

An internal diagnostic system should evaluate the pump's basic programming to maintain a standard volume and rate of delivery. Variations from the settings should trigger alarms and stop the infusion until the problem can be corrected. Pump infusion pressures should be monitored carefully to ensure the appropriate delivery of fluids and medications. Pump line pressure can be calibrated in millimeters of mercury (mm Hg) or pounds per square inch (psi).

Technical pump information may refer to pressure limits in terms of pounds per square inch. A pump with a fixed pressure alarm of 4 psi will sound an alarm when the peripheral venous pressure reaches 200 mm Hg (1 psi = 50 mm Hg) (Weinstein, 2007). This setting can result in a significant infiltration before any pump alarm sounds. Dramatic infiltrations can occur when pumps simply continue to pump or when gravity infusion is used because the loose peripheral skin of the older adult does not offer any peripheral tissue resistance to stop a subcutaneous infusion (Phillips, 2005).

An electronic flow control device is reliable only if it is used correctly. The device must not be so cumbersome that it inhibits the patient's movement. The older adult needs to maintain mobility to keep a sense of independence. If applicable to the type of pump and infusion, the pump should have a lock-out feature to prevent tampering with the programming once it has been set. This feature can be of significant importance with medications whose dosing can be critical. The older adult may feel overwhelmed by the prospect of home infusion therapy, and one of the most intimidating components may be the high-technology electronic monitoring device (see Chapter 20).

SPECIAL CONSIDERATIONS FOR THE OLDER ADULT
Skin preparation

The first step in venipuncture is careful preparation of the proposed venipuncture site. The technique used to apply the cleansing agent can be as important as the antimicrobial effect of the agent. Adequate friction is necessary to cleanse the skin. However, older skin is more delicate, and too vigorous an action may damage surface skin tissue.

Appropriate cleansing agents for skin preparation include alcohol, 2% tincture of iodine, 10% povidone-iodine, and chlorhexidine gluconate—as single agents or in combination (INS, 2006). Although practices vary, generally, preparatory cleansing with a combination skin antiseptic that is allowed to dry for 30 to 60 seconds is best for germicidal effect. The site can be cleansed with alcohol pads until the pads no longer show soil after cleansing. Because older skin has lost some of its natural moisture as a result of aging, excessive use of alcohol may add to skin dryness and cracking (INS, 2004).

Excessive amounts of hair over the infusion site can be removed by clipping. Care must be taken to prevent nicking the skin. Shaving is not recommended to remove hair from potential venipuncture sites because it may cause microabrasions (INS, 2006). In the older adult, shaving could easily cause multiple cuts and nicks because of the fragile thinner skin layers; these cuts could provide an open pathway for bacteria to invade the tissue in and around the venipuncture site (INS, 2004).

Technique

A key factor for successful venipuncture in the older adult is stabilization of the vein. In the older adult, the vessels may lack stability as a result of loss of tissue mass, and veins may tend to roll. Attempting to access such veins can result in the needle's tip nicking the vein or pushing the vein continually away. Skin tension is established by first determining the direction or axis of the vessel. Initial traction is accomplished by placing the thumb directly along the vein axis approximately 2 to 3 inches below the intended venipuncture site. The palm and fingers of the traction hand serve to hold and stabilize the extremity. The index finger of the traction hand can be used to further stretch the skin alongside the intended venipuncture site. Once traction has been initiated, it should be maintained throughout the venipuncture and catheter advancing procedure (Phillips, 2005).

The directional line of the vein should be observed. (Each vessel follows its own route.) By palpation, the infusion nurse locates the vein and its route. When skin tension is established, palpating the vessel may be difficult or impossible. If the vein is a small, thin surface vessel, the venous distention may not be sufficient for extensive palpation. In these cases, the nurse should attempt to imagine the vein's track along the skin surface. This perceived path assists in aligning the catheter for insertion along the vein route after skin traction has been established.

As stated in *Infusion Nursing Standards of Practice* (2006), 0.9% sodium chloride or lidocaine should not be routinely injected subcutaneously at the insertion site to anesthetize the area. These preparations are most commonly used in anesthesiology before large-bore, 14- or 16-gauge catheters are inserted. In the elderly population, any additional needle puncture in the area for IV access may make successful venous access more difficult or impossible as a result of subcutaneous tissue swelling, vessel injury, or hemorrhage.

An IV catheter with a sharp, atraumatic bevel tip should be selected. The contour cuts on the bevel tip are designed for sharpness and ease of skin penetration. With the vessel held securely and the vein track visualized, the catheter should be aligned parallel to the vein track. The catheter should be brought close to the skin directly above the potential insertion site. The angle of insertion should be lowered to 20 to 30 degrees to reduce vein trauma on insertion (Weinstein, 2007).

The insertion technique can be either direct or indirect. When a direct technique is used, once skin traction is established, the vein is directly accessed at a 20- to 30-degree angle in a single motion, thereby penetrating the skin and the vein simultaneously. This method can be routinely used for patients with good vein access or those whose veins are easily stabilized. For patients with small, delicate veins or whose vessels are difficult to secure, an indirect or two-step insertion technique may be necessary (Phillips, 2005). With this technique, the skin is penetrated close to the vein by using the same firm motion as that used for a direct access method. If a stabbing or thrusting motion is used with the catheter, there is a danger of going too deep or accidentally damaging the vein. Once the surface of the skin has been penetrated, the insertion angle of the catheter should be lowered to 10 to 15 degrees, the access vein should be restabilized, and the IV catheter bevel tip should be realigned to penetrate the vein wall. With a steady motion, the bevel tip should be advanced gently through the vein wall and into the lumen. The nurse should then check for backflow of blood into the flashback chamber of the catheter. As soon as the bevel and part of the catheter tip have advanced into the vein, the nurse should push the catheter forward off the stylet into the vein while stabilizing the stylet. During catheter-stylet separation, the nurse should observe the flashback chamber to ensure a continuing backflow of blood (Weinstein, 2007). The stylet should not be pulled out of the catheter; rather, the catheter should always be pushed forward off the stylet into the vein. This method ensures that the bevel and part of the catheter are well into the vein before the stylet is removed.

If the veins are extremely fragile, it may be necessary to release the tourniquet as soon as a blood return occurs and catheter separation is achieved. This may prevent vein wall damage from high-pressure backflow of blood from the point where the catheter enters the vein (Weinstein, 2007).

A "hooded" technique can be effectively used to advance the catheter into the vein. In this technique, the catheter is advanced forward over the bevel tip into the vein. This measure retracts the stylet tip inside the catheter. Then, the nurse threads the catheter into the vein by grasping the hub of the catheter and advancing the catheter-stylet as one unit up the vein, with the blunt catheter tip leading the way up the vessel. This process reduces the possibility of an accidental penetration of the

vein wall during the threading. Vein stabilization and skin tension must be maintained from the time of insertion throughout the threading of the catheter. Only after the catheter has been advanced as far as possible can the tension from stabilization be eased slowly. The hooding technique can be essential to successfully threading the catheter without damaging or rupturing the fragile vessels of the older patient. If the skin tension is released before the catheter is threaded, the rebound of the skin and vein being released may cause the catheter to rupture the vein (Phillips, 2005; Weinstein, 2007).

IV access in the older adult may test all of the skill and knowledge of the infusion nurse. However, the use of special techniques may enhance the success of venipuncture in these patients.

Device maintenance

Adequate stabilization of a venous access device is essential to reduce the degree of mechanical irritation that results when the catheter shifts inside the vein. The key to maintaining a venipuncture site in an older adult is to anticipate potential problems and to apply preventive measures before problems occur. Protective devices can be used to secure the catheter.

Site care begins with VAD stabilization and application of a dressing. The catheter is more unstable because of the decrease in subcutaneous fat and tissue in the elderly. The use of soft-winged catheters and securement devices also enhances the nurse's ability to stabilize and secure the catheter. These catheters offer another advantage; the extension tubing is a part of the catheter, thereby greatly reducing mechanical manipulation at the insertion site. IV devices that have stiff wings or flanges must be used with caution on the delicate skin of the elderly. Hard, stiff edges can cause skin irritation, soreness, or even ulceration. To prevent irritation when this type of device is used, any portion of the device that may cause skin irritation may need to be protected with a small gauze pad.

Securing the catheter to prevent accidental dislodgment is necessary; however, the amount of tape applied to the skin should be minimized in patients with delicate skin. Consideration should also be given to the kind of tape used on delicate skin. Some tapes may easily tear the fragile, thin skin of the older adult. Therefore the patient should be assessed for any reaction to the tape product used. The patient should also be questioned about previous experiences with tape products before the tape is applied. Adaptations to the taping technique or product used should be implemented as necessary. To help reduce irritation or damage to the skin of the older adult, the additional protection provided by a skin polymer solution should be considered. This added skin barrier protects the skin from the effects of adhesives and from the drying nature of cleansing agents that occurs with repeated tape removal and dressing changes. While stabilizing the catheter, the nurse should apply the polymer solution in a circular motion around the site, starting ½ to ¾ inch out from the insertion point. The nurse should then allow the solution to air-dry before applying the dressing. A gauze or transparent semipermeable membrane (TSM) dressing can be placed over the site (Box 30-4).

The infusion nurse must anticipate potential hazards that could affect the successful delivery of the infusion therapy. The older adult is not always as aware of his or her surroundings as other patients and is slower to adapt to environmental changes. These factors may result in accidents that might disturb or interrupt the patency of an IV catheter. For example, the older

Box 30-4   CONSIDERATIONS FOR THE OLDER ADULT: DRESSING CHANGE

Because of age-related changes, especially in the immune system, the older adult will be more susceptible to infectious processes. Remote infections may predispose the older adult to catheter-associated bloodstream infections. Changes in sensorium and cognition may predispose the older adult to accidental manipulations of the infusion catheter and dressing materials, disrupting protective care and maintenance practices (such as dressing maintenance) and contaminating the catheter-skin junction and administration system. Urinary incontinence and accidental separation or dislodgement of enteral feeding systems may also affect catheter dressing integrity. Extra securement measures such as additional taping and wraps that obscure the venipuncture site as protective measures will hinder daily site observations and implementation of appropriate interventions.

In the older adult, skin care is of utmost importance. Nonocclusive or compromised dressing materials must be changed as soon as possible. Antimicrobial cleansing agents are often very drying or irritating to the skin. The skin must be inspected with each dressing change for any adverse reaction to antiseptic solutions or adhesives, for changes in any pressure areas (from catheter hubs or administration sets and add-on devices), or for the macerating effects of leakage of infusates or bodily fluids from the catheter-skin junction. These are a medium for bacterial growth and their presence may necessitate more frequent dressing changes or VAD replacement.

From Infusion Nurses Society: *Policies and procedures for infusion nursing for the older adult,* Norwood, Mass, 2004, Author.

adult may not remember that an IV catheter is in place or may not have a good view of the set-up and may become tangled in the tubing, resulting in an accidental disconnection. Excessive lengths of tubing can become a physical hazard to the elderly patient who is trying to ambulate or to perform his or her own activities of daily living. The IV administration set should be long enough to give adequate range of motion, but not to dangle on the floor or get caught under an IV pole or pump wheels. A segment of the administration set should be looped to the patient's arm so that inadvertent tugging pulls on the loop and not directly on the venipuncture site. Another important consideration is the type of administration sets connected to the catheter. A Luer-Lok™ connector provides a more secure connection and greater protection against accidental disconnection than do male-female connectors, which can easily pull apart.

Occasionally, the catheter site may need to be covered to prevent the patient from inadvertently removing the catheter. An alternative method used to stabilize the catheter is to stretch properly sized site-protection material over the venipuncture site. This measure provides coverage and stability for the site and protects the catheter from snagging on bed clothes, pumps, or other encumbrances. The site-protection material allows unimpeded peripheral circulation for the infusion site while stabilizing the catheter and dressing. This material can also be used to help stabilize the device and minimize the need for tape. However, roller-type gauze or any covering that is not easily removed should not be used because it decreases the ability to observe the site.

Another approach to covering a venipuncture site is to place the patient in a long-sleeved gown or pajamas. If the

venipuncture site is covered from the patient's view, the patient may not disturb it.

Arm boards should be used with care to stabilize VADs over areas of flexion. These boards must be padded and support the hand or arm in a functional position. The fingers should be allowed some motion to encourage circulation and to decrease the potential for dependent edema. The tape used to secure the board should be prebacked with gauze or tape so that the adhesive does not contact the patient's skin, thereby permitting good control of the extremity without circulatory impediment. The venipuncture site and the vein path above the site should still be visible for frequent evaluation. When any extremity is immobilized, increased peripheral edema may occur as a result of slowed venous return in the restricted extremity. This problem can be critical in the older adult with peripheral vascular changes or limited mobility. Any decrease in activity to an extremity increases venous stasis and the resultant dependent edema; therefore these venipuncture sites must be monitored often and the observations documented regularly.

Occasionally, some kind of immobilization device must be used to prevent the patient from dislodging the venous access device. A physician's order is required for use of such a device. Immobilization policies vary between institutions, but regular monitoring and documentation are always required. Soft wrist immobilizers can be placed below an infusion site but should never be placed directly over the site. If the venipuncture site is in the wrist or hand, the immobilizer should be placed around an arm board, and then the extremity should be secured on the arm board. The extremity with the VAD is secured by the board while the board takes the pulling stress of the immobilizer.

Site monitoring

The venipuncture site should be observed regularly (as set by organizational policy) to ensure patency. Nursing practice policy may recommend observing the area every 1 to 2 hours to verify site patency, condition, and flow rate and then documenting the observation in the patient medical record. With the older adult, a small infiltrate could easily lead to a severe complication.

Site rotation is recommended every 72 hours, according to the *Infusion Nursing Standards of Practice* (INS, 2006). Variations from this standard may be acceptable if they are justified through documented and statistically substantiated clinical practice. If a routine site change is not performed because of limited access or patient condition, a full description of the site evaluation, dressing change, and reasons for the inability to rotate the site should be well documented in the patient's medical record (INS, 2006).

PATIENT EDUCATION
Family involvement

The patient education process begins with the physician's or authorized prescriber's order for infusion therapy. It is important for the patient's self-esteem that all procedures be explained fully before they are performed. Such communication gives the patient a sense of participation in the process.

The nurse should speak slowly, clearly, and directly to the older adult. The patient should be addressed by name, and anyone who is involved in performing the procedure should be introduced by name and identification (Hogstel, 2001;

Eliopoulos, 2005). Steps in any procedure, such as catheter insertion, should be described as they are performed. The patient will be more cooperative if he or she can anticipate the elements of his or her care and if trust is established.

Important ongoing infusion therapy–related considerations should be clearly and simply explained to the patient and family. For instance, while cleansing and dressing a venipuncture site, the nurse should provide instructions of basic care that protect the venipuncture site from infection or dislodgment. In this way, the patient and family can become partners in the maintenance of the venous access device. If a pump or monitoring device is used, the nurse should explain potential alarms and how to prevent possible problems. The nurse should not use unfamiliar terminology, but instead should use clear, concise phrases that leave no doubt as to the meaning (Hogstel, 2001; Eliopoulos, 2005).

ACUTE CARE CONSIDERATIONS

Infusion therapy in the acute care setting can be a challenging experience for both the practitioner and the patient. The rules of assessment for the younger adult are not appropriate for the elderly. The elderly are at an increased risk of misdiagnosis of a cognitive deficit resulting from acute illness, change in environment, or medications. Rapid decision-making around the elderly can make them uncomfortable and withdrawn. The health care practitioner must not forget to include the elderly patient in his or her own plan of care. The practice of placing large-gauge catheters also needs to be carefully evaluated. If the elderly patient is not to receive blood or a large volume of solution, a 22- or even 24-gauge catheter is a much better choice. Pathways and decision-making tools can address these issues with the least amount of conflict.

HOME CARE CONSIDERATIONS

The infusion nurse must balance many elements when planning the delivery of infusion therapies in the home setting. The infusion nurse's role includes evaluating the type and duration of therapy, and the venous access device and infusion equipment required. These factors are all crucial to determining the appropriateness of home infusion therapy. Careful evaluation of the home physical environment, family members in the home, designated home health provider and other care providers, cost of the therapy, and insurance coverage must be performed. If these physical needs cannot be met, the environment for the patient and family may be too stressful for learning and retention (Loengard and Boal, 2004).

Educating older adults in the administration of home infusion therapy presents certain challenges. As people age, they may less readily adapt to environmental changes, especially those they cannot easily control or that affect their independence. Therefore the infusion nurse must have a high degree of motivation and patience when instructing the older adult. Teaching the older adult complex drug admixtures, tubing connections, maintenance, pump programming, and accessing and deaccessing various venous access devices is a step-by-step, individualized process. A progressively organized training program should include a written teaching manual or a program module using large print and, more importantly, direct demonstrations of specific procedures with return demonstration evaluated by the potential home care provider (Fetter, 2003; Loengard and Boal, 2004).

The medical knowledge and nursing care required of an older patient or family in a short time can be particularly overwhelming. The infusion nurse must evaluate the older adult for the ability to perform and the willingness to comply with the required skills. With the older patient or designated primary care provider, time must be spent evaluating the emotional stability, intellectual capacity, and physical ability to perform the required skills. For instance, is the patient emotionally able to cope with care at home by a family member or a home health worker? The family members or significant others must be able to provide support for the patient and each other. In addition, can the learner understand the necessary health care concepts? A gap in comprehension may result from the aging process and language or cultural differences. The nurse should consider whether interpreters could be used to enhance learning. The use of pictorial step-by-step manuals can dramatically facilitate learning for those with a reading, language, or hearing deficit. Sign language interpreters and lip reading can help the hearing impaired. In addition, videotapes of procedures can permit the patient and family to refresh skills at home (Hogstel, 2001; Eliopoulos, 2005).

With patient education, the content must be taught in exactly the same way to each caregiver. Tasks can become easily confusing to the lay caregiver if different methods are used for procedures. Precise training examples should be used and repeated exactly the same way each time. This consistency and repetition will reduce the potential for errors or patient complications in the home.

The patient and family should have an understanding of what complications or problems could occur and the appropriate interventions for these problems. This information should be included in the patient teaching module and should be reviewed several times before discharge or independent administration. The information should include care of the venipuncture site and the venous access device, the proper use of the pumps (intermittent, continuous, patient-controlled analgesia, ambulatory, stationary), knowledge of the medications and their side effects, administration procedures for delivery of parenteral nutrition (cyclic or continuous), emergency procedures, emergency access to health care personnel, record keeping, storage of medical supplies, and proper disposal of medical wastes.

The impact of sensory changes that occur with aging, particularly changes in visual acuity, hearing, and manual dexterity, should also be considered. The importance of visual acuity is seen when administering small medication dosages for IV admixtures, adjusting pump rates, accessing VADs, and making tubing connections. The primary care provider must be able to see and read the directions for medication administration and for the care and maintenance of the venous access devices. Changes in hearing may affect the patient's ability to hear and respond to pump alarms in a timely manner. Manual dexterity is another important requirement for many home infusion procedures. The older adult may have significant problems handling the necessary equipment because of illness-related changes resulting from arthritis, cardiovascular accidents, partial or full paralysis, amputation, or other physical impairments. For instance, the older adult may have difficulty attaching administration sets and handling the small caps attached to these sets. The older adult should be carefully observed working with the various devices and alternatives should be used as are deemed appropriate.

The infusion nurse providing care in the home is a partner in the development of a safe, home-based, infusion delivery system. The concerns of the home care provider include the following:

- A clean, dry space for supplies
- A clean work preparation area
- Special refrigeration needs
- Pets
- Parasites and infestations in the home
- Necessary electrical outlets
- Batteries and sufficient supplies
- Telephone
- Names of people to call in an emergency

The hospital and home care provider must evaluate all of these factors to determine whether the home is a safe place for the administration of infusion therapy.

LONG-TERM CARE CONSIDERATIONS

The long-term care setting provides a unique set of conditions for the patient receiving infusion therapy. Prospective payment systems, managed care, and the drive for patients to be discharged from the acute care environment have placed patients with much higher acuity in settings that traditionally were not equipped to handle such patients. The lack of laboratory, x-ray, and on-call physician services once posed a barrier to acceptance of these patients in long-term care settings. However, long-term care is now seeing the influx of all types of therapies. Hydration and antibiotic therapy have been common in long-term care for many years. Recently, therapies such as inotropic medications and chemotherapy have made their way into the long-term care environment. These therapies require strict monitoring and staff members who have the validated competencies required to effectively manage patients requiring infusion therapy.

Educational requirements for the nursing staff and nursing assistants need to be defined. PICCs and midlines can be placed in this environment by qualified nursing staff. Currently, the model most commonly used is the pharmacy or outside agency contracting with nurses to place these VADs. Because they are not considered emergency devices and the elderly often require prehydration before insertion, it may be 24 to 48 hours before the nurse is available to place the device, which will depend on the patient's condition and geographic location of the facility (Hogstel, 2001; Eliopoulos, 2005).

 SUMMARY

Infusion therapy in the older adult is one of the most challenging responsibilities of the infusion nurse. However, it can be one of the most rewarding. The ability to accurately assess

and care for the older adult requires a very clear understanding of the aging process. Listening and learning from the older adult enable the infusion nurse to be the best possible patient advocate. The ability to communicate with other members of the health care team along the continuum of care regarding the patient's needs will ensure the successful completion of therapy and minimize complications. Society is aging—it is essential that health care professionals be prepared to deal with the specific issues of older adults.

 REFERENCES

Arinzon Z, Feldman J, Fidelman Z et al: Hypodermoclysis (subcutaneous infusion) effective mode of treatment of dehydration in long-term care patients, *Arch Gerontol Geriatr* 38(2):167-173, 2004.

Congdon JG et al: *Scope and standards of gerontological nursing practice,* Silver Spring, Md, 2001, ANA.

Eliopoulos C: *Gerontologic nursing,* ed 6 , Philadelphia, 2005, Lippincott, Williams & Wilkins.

Fetter MS: Geriatric assessment and management protocols, *J Infus Nurs* 26(3), 153-160, 2003.

Hogstel MO: *Gerontology: nursing care of the older adult, United States,* Albany, NY, 2001, Delmar Thompson Learning.

Infusion Nurses Society: *Policies and procedures for infusion nursing for the older adult,* Norwood, Mass, 2004, Author.

Infusion Nurses Society: Infusion nursing standards of practice, *J Infus Nurs* 29(1 suppl), S1-S92, 2006.

Loengard AU, Boal J: Home care of the frail elderly, *Clinical geriatric medicine,* St Louis, 2004, Elsevier.

Phillips LD: *Manual of I.V. therapeutics,* ed 4, Philadelphia, 2005, FA Davis.

Pirrello RD, Ting CC, Thomas SH: Initial experiences with subcutaneous recombinant human hyaluronidase, *J Palliat Med* 10(4):861-864, 2007.

Remington R, Hultman T: Hypdermoclysis to treat dehydration: a review of the evidence, *J Am Geriatr Soc* 55:2051-2055, 2007.

Slesak G, Schnurle JW, Kinzel E et al: Comparison of subcutaneous and intravenous rehydration in geriatric patients: a randomized trial, *J Am Geriatr Soc* 51:155-160, 2003.

Turner T, Cassano AM: Subcutaneous dextrose for rehydration of elderly patients—an evidence-based review, *BMC Geriatr* 4(2), 2004. Accessed 12/5/08 from http://www.biomedcentral.com/1471-2318/4/2.

United Nations Department of Economic & Social Affairs: Population Division: *World population prospects: the 2006 revision,* United Nations, NY, 2007.

United Nations Department of Economic & Social Affairs: Population Division: *World urbanization prospects: the 2007 revision, executive summary,* United Nations, New York, Feb 26, 2008.

Weinstein S: *Plumer's principles and practices of intravenous therapy,* ed 8, Philadelphia, 2007, Lippincott, Williams & Wilkins.

INDEX

Note: Page numbers followed by *b, f* and *t* indicate boxes, figures and tables, respectively.